Therapeutic Immunology
Second Edition

Therapeutic Immunology
Second Edition

Edited by

K. Frank Austen, MD

Theodore Bevier Bayles Professor of Medicine
Harvard Medical School
Director, Inflammation & Allergic Diseases Research Section
Division of Rheumatology, Immunology, and Allergy
Department of Medicine
Brigham and Women's Hospital
Boston, Massachusetts

Steven J. Burakoff, MD

Laura and Issac Perlmutter Professor of Pathology
Professor of Medicine and Pediatrics
New York University School of Medicine
Director of the New York University Kaplan Comprehensive Cancer Center
Director of the Skirball Institute for Biomolecular Medicine
New York, New York

Fred S. Rosen, MD

James L. Gamble Professor of Pediatrics
Harvard Medical School
President
The Center for Blood Research
Boston, Massachusetts

Terry B. Strom, MD

Professor of Medicine
Harvard Medical School
Director of Immunology
Beth Israel Deaconess Medical Center
Boston, Massachusetts

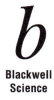

**Blackwell
Science**

Editorial Offices:
Commerce Place, 350 Main Street, Malden, Massachusetts 02148, USA
Osney Mead, Oxford OX2 0EL, England
25 John Street, London WC1N 2BL, England
23 Ainslie Place, Edinburgh EH3 6AJ, Scotland
54 University Street, Carlton, Victoria 3053, Australia
Other Editorial Offices:
Blackwell Wissenschafts-Verlag GmbH, Kurfürstendamm 57, 10707 Berlin, Germany
Blackwell Science KK, MG Kodenmacho Building, 7-10 Kodenmacho Nihombashi, Chuo-ku, Tokyo 104, Japan

Acquisitions: Chris Davis
Development: Julia Casson
Production: Andover Publishing Services
Manufacturing: Lisa Flanagan
Marketing Manager: Anne Stone
Director of Marketing: Lisa Larsen
Cover design by Electronic Illustrators Group
Typeset by Best-set Typesetter Ltd., Hong Kong
Printed and bound by Edwards Brothers/Ann Arbor

Printed in the United States of America
00 01 02 03 5 4 3 2 1

Distributors:
USA
  Blackwell Science, Inc.
  Commerce Place
  350 Main Street
  Malden, Massachusetts 02148
  (Telephone orders: 800-215-1000 or 781-388-8250;
  fax orders: 781-388-8270)

Canada
  Login Brothers Book Company
  324 Saulteaux Crescent
  Winnipeg, Manitoba, R3J 3T2
  (Telephone orders: 204-837-2987)

Australia
  Blackwell Science Pty, Ltd.
  54 University Street
  Carlton, Victoria 3053
  (Telephone orders: 03-9347-0300;
  fax orders: 03-9349-3016)

Outside North America and Australia
  Blackwell Science, Ltd.
  c/o Marston Book Services, Ltd.
  P.O. Box 269
  Abingdon
  Oxon OX14 4YN
  England
  (Telephone orders: 44-01235-465500;
  fax orders: 44-01235-465555)

Library of Congress Cataloging-in-Publication Data

Therapeutic immunology / by K. Frank Austen . . . [et al.].—2nd ed.
    p.; cm.
  Includes bibliographical references and index.
  ISBN 0-632-04359-8
  1. Immunotherapy.   I. Austen, K. Frank (Karl Frank)
  [DNLM: 1. Immunotherapy. 2. Immune System—drug effects.
  QW 940 T398 2001]
  RM275 .T44 2001
  615¢37—dc21
                                                    00-044408

Contents

Contributors

Abul K. Abbas, MD
Professor and Chair
Department of Pathology
University of California, San Francisco
San Francisco, California

John P. Atkinson, MD
Professor of Medicine and Molecular Microbiology
Washington University School of Medicine
Department of Medicine
Barnes Jewish Hospital
St. Louis, Missouri

Shairaz Baksh, PhD
Department of Pediatric Oncology
Dana-Farber Cancer Institute
Boston, Massachusetts

Barbara E. Bierer, MD
Professor of Pediatrics
Department of Pediatric Oncology
Dana-Farber Cancer Institute
Boston, Massachusetts
Senior Investigator and Chief
Laboratory of Lymphocyte Biology
National Heart, Lung, and Blood Institute
National Institutes of Health
Bethesda, Maryland

R. Michael Blaese, MD
Chief Scientific Officer and President, Pharmaceutical
   Division
Valigen, Inc.
Newtown, Pennsylvania

Francisco A. Bonilla, MD, PhD
Children's Hospital
Division of Immunology
Department of Pediatrics
Harvard Medical School
Boston, Massachusetts

Myles Brown
Department of Adult Oncology
Dana-Farber Cancer Institute
Boston, Massachusetts

Steven J. Burakoff, MD
Laura and Issac Perlmutter Professor of Pathology
Professor of Medicine and Pediatrics
New York University School of Medicine
Director of the New York University Kaplan
   Comprehensive Cancer Center
Director of the Skirball Institute for Biomolecular
   Medicine
New York, New York

Fabio Candotti, MD
Head, Disorders of Immunity Section
Clinical Gene Therapy Branch
NHGRI, National Institutes of Health
Bethesda, Maryland

Lucienne Chatenoud, MD, Dsc
Director of Research
Necker Hospital
Paris, France

Leonard Chess, MD
Professor of Medicine and Pathology
Columbia University College of Physicians and Surgeons
New York, New York

David K.C. Cooper, MD, PhD, FRCS
Associate Professor of Surgery
Harvard Medical School
Immunologist, Transplantation Biology Research Center
Massachusetts General Hospital
Harvard Medical School
Boston, Massachusetts

Nicola Cooper, BSc
Senior Group Leader, Biology
Celltech Chiroscience
Cambridge, England

David L. DeWitt, PhD
Associate Professor
Department of Biochemistry
Michigan State University
East Lansing, Michigan

John P. Doweiko
Assistant Professor of Medicine
Harvard Medical School
Division of Infectious Disease and Division of
    Hematology and Oncology
Beth Israel Deaconess Medical Center
Boston, Massachusetts

Glenn Dranoff, MD
Assistant Professor of Medicine
Harvard Medical School
Department of Adult Oncology
Dana-Farber Cancer Institute
Boston, Massachusetts

Jeffrey M. Drazen, MD
Partners Asthma Center
Pulmonary and Critical Care Division
Department of Medicine
Brigham and Women's Hospital
Harvard Medical School
Boston, Massachusetts

Ronald W. Ellis, PhD
Senior Vice President, Vaccine R&D, and General
    Manager
BioChem Pharma, Inc.
Northborough, Massachusetts

Douglas T. Fearon, MD
Wellcome Trust Immunology Unit
University of Cambridge School of Medicine
Cambridge, England

James L.M. Ferrara, MD
Professor of Medicine and Pediatrics
Director, Combined BMT Program
University of Michigan Cancer Center
Ann Arbor, Michigan

Jeff Friedman, MD, PhD
Department of Pediatric Oncology
Dana-Farber Cancer Institute
Boston, Massachusetts

Leslie Garrison, MD, MPH
Vice President, Clinical Development
Immunex Corporation
Seattle, Washington

Roberto Gedaly, MD
Clinical Fellow, Liver and GI Transplantation
Jackson Memorial Hospital
University of Miami School of Medicine
Miami, Florida

Raif S. Geha, MD
Children's Hospital
Division of Immunology
Department of Pediatrics
Harvard Medical School
Boston, Massachusetts

Philip D. Greenberg, MD
Fred Hutchinson Cancer Research Center
Departments of Medicine and Immunology
University of Washington
Seattle, Washington

Siân V. Griffin, PhD, MRCP
Registrar
Cambridge University Department of Medicine
Addenbrooke's Hospital,
Cambridge, England

Robert Gristwood, PhD
Research and Development Director
Arachnova Ltd
Cambridge, United Kingdom

Jerome E. Groopman, MD
Professor of Medicine
Harvard Medical School
Chief of Hematology/Oncology
New England Deaconess Hospital
Boston, Massachusetts

Hilde-Kari Guttormsen, MD, PhD
Instructor in Medicine
Harvard Medical School
Associate Physician in Medicine
Brigham and Women's Hospital
Boston, Massachusetts

Stephen T. Holgate, MD, DSc, FRCP
MRC Clinical Professor of Immunopharmacology
Medical Specialties (RCMB Division)
University of Southampton
Honorary Consultant Physician
Southampton General Hospital
Southampton, Hampshire, United Kingdom

Luca Inverardi, MD
Associate Professor of Medicine, Microbiology, and
    Immunology
Co-Director, Cell Transplant Center
Diabetes Research Institute
University of Miami School of Medicine
Miama, Florida

Roger L. Jenkins, MD, FACS
Section Head of Hepatobiliary Surgery
Institute for Transplantation
Lahey Clinic Medical Center
Burlington, Massachusetts

Carl H. June, MD
Professor of Molecular and Cellular Engineering
University of Pennsylvania School of Medicine
Philadelphia, Pennsylvania

Dennis L. Kasper, MD
William Ellery Channing Professor of Medicine
Professor of Microbiology and Molecular Genetics
Harvard Medical School
Director, Channing Laboratory
Brigham and Women's Hospital
Boston, Massachusetts

Arthur F. Kavanaugh, MD
Associate Professor of Medicine
Director, Center for Innovative Therapy
University of California, San Diego
San Diego, California

A.B. Kay, FRCP, FRCPath, Dsc, PhD, FRSE
Professor and Head
Department of Allergy and Clinical Immunology
National Heart and Lung Institute
Imperial College School of Medicine
London, England

Abdallah G. Kfoury, MD
Assistant Professor of Medicine
Associate Medical Director
Utah Cardiac Transplant Program
University of Utah Health Sciences Center
Salt Lake City, Utah

Lloyd B. Klickstein, MD, PhD
Assistant Professor of Medicine
Harvard Medical School
Division of Rheumatology, Immunology
    and Allergy
Department of Medicine
Brigham and Women's Hospital
Boston, Massachusetts

Mamidipudi Thirumala Krishna, PhD, MRCP (UK), DNB
Specialist Registrar in Allergy and Clinical
Immunology and Honorary Clinical Lecturer
Southampton General Hospital and University of
    Southampton
Southampton, United Kingdom

M. Larché, PhD
National Asthma Campaign Senior Research Fellow
Lecturer, Department of Allergy and Clinical Immunology
National Heart and Lung Institute
Imperial College School of Medicine
London, England

Jeffrey A. Ledbetter, PhD
Pacific Northwest Research Foundation
Seattle, Washington

Peter E. Lipsky, MD
Scientific Director
National Institute of Arthritis and Musculoskeletal and
    Skin Diseases
National Institutes of Health
Bethesda, Maryland

C. Martin Lockwood, FRCP, FRCPath
Reader in Therapeutic Immunology
Cambridge University Department of Medicine
Addenbrooke's Hospital
Cambridge, England

Richard P. MacDermott, MD
Chief, Division of Gastroenterology
The Albert M. Yunich MD Professor of Medicine
The Albany Medical College
Albany, New York

Donald MacGlashan, Jr., MD, PhD
Professor of Medicine
Johns Hopkins University School of Medicine
Johns Hopkins Asthma and Allergy Center
Baltimore, Maryland

Steven J. Mentzer, MD
Lung Transplant Program
Division of Thoracic Surgery
Brigham and Women's Hospital
Harvard Medical School
Boston, Massachusetts

Jeffrey N. Miner
Department of Endocrine Research
Ligand Pharmaceuticals
San Diego, California

Richard N. Mitchell, MD, PhD
Associate Professor
Immunology Research Division
Department of Pathology
Brigham and Women's Hospital and Harvard Medical
    School
Boston, Massachusetts

Kendall M. Mohler, PhD
Senior Director, Immunobiology
Immunex Corporation
Seattle, Washington

Francis D. Moore, Jr., MD
Associate Professor of Surgery
Harvard Medical School
Department of Surgery
Brigham and Women's Hospital
Boston, Massachusetts

James J. Pomposelli, MD, PhD
Assistant Professor of Surgery
Tufts Medical School
Institute for Transplantation
Lahey Clinic Medical Center
Burlington, Massachusetts

Alberto Pugliese
Research Associate Professor of Medicine, Microbiology,
    and Immunology
Diabetes Research Institute
Unversity of Miami School of Medicine
Miami, Florida

Charles D. Pusey, MSc, FRCP, FRCPath
Professor of Renal Medicine
Imperial College School of Medicine
Hammersmith Hospital
London, England

Voravit Ratanatharathorn, MD
Associate Professor of Internal Medicine
University of Michigan Cancer Center
Ann Arbor, Michigan

Dale G. Renlund, MD
Professor of Medicine
University of Utah School of Medicine
Director, Heart Failure Prevention and Treatment
    Program
Intermountain Healthcare, Inc.
Salt Lake City, Utah

Camillo Ricordi, MD
Stacy Joy Goodman Professor of Surgery and Medicine
Chief, Division of Cellular Transplantation
Scientific Director and Chief Academic Officer
Diabetes Research Institute
University of Miami School of Medicine
Miami, Florida

Stanley R. Riddell, MD
Fred Hutchinson Cancer Research Center
Department of Medicine
University of Washington
Seattle, Washington

Harriet L. Robinson, PhD
Chief, Division of Microbiology and Immunology
Yerkes Regional Primate Research Center
Asa Griggs Candler Professor
Department of Microbiology and Immunology
School of Medicine
Emory University
Atlanta, Georgia

Fred S. Rosen, MD
James L. Gamble Professor of Pediatrics
Harvard Medical School
President
The Center for Blood Research
Boston, Massachusetts

Robert H. Rubin, MD, FACTP, FCCP
Chief of Surgical and Transplant Infectious Disease
Massachusetts General Hospital
Director of the Center for Experimental Pharmacology
    and Therapeutics
Harvard-M.I.T. Division of Health Sciences and
    Technology
Gordon and Marjorie Osborne Professor of Health
    Sciences and Technology and Professor of Medicine
Harvard Medical School
Boston, Massachusetts

Tomasz Sablinski, MD, PhD
Global Head, Transplantation and Organ Engineering
Clinical Research and Development
Novartis Pharmaceuticals Corporation
East Hanover, New Jersey

David H. Sachs, MD
Associate Professor of Surgery (Immunology)
Harvard Medical School
Director, Transplantation Biology Research Center
Massachusetts General Hospital
Boston, Massachusetts

Robert D. Schreiber, PhD
Alumni Endowed Professor of Pathology
Department of Pathology and Immunology and Center for
    Immunology
Washington University School of Medicine
St. Louis, Missouri

Vijay Shankaran
Graduate Research Assistant,
Department of Pathology
Washington University School of Medicine
St. Louis, Missouri

Michael E. Shapiro, MD
Chief of Transplantation
Department of Surgery
Hackensack University Medical Center
New Jersey Medical School/UMDNJ
Hackensack, New Jersey

Colin A. Sieff, MB, BCh
Department of Pediatric Oncology
Dana-Farber Cancer Institute
Division of Hematology
Children's Hospital
Department of Pediatrics
Harvard Medical School
Boston, Massachusetts

F. Estelle R. Simons, MD, FRCPC
Bruce Chown Professor and Head
Section of Allergy and Clinical Immunology
Department of Pediatrics and Child Health
University of Manitoba
Winnipeg, Manitoba, Canada

Kendall Smith, MD
Professor of Medicine
Division of Immunology
Department of Medicine
Weill Medical College
Cornell University
New York, New York

William L. Smith, PhD
Professor and Chair
Department of Biochemistry
Michigan State University
East Lansing, Michigan

Alfred D. Steinberg, MD
Senior Fellow
Mitretek Systems
McLean, Virginia

Terry Strom, MD
Professor of Medicine
Harvard Medical School
Director of Immunology
Beth Israel Deaconess Medical Center
Boston, Massachusetts

Manikkam Suthanthiran, MD
Stanton Griffis Distinguished Professor of Medicine
Weill Medical College of Cornell University
Chief, Department of Transplantation Medicine and
    Extracorporeal Therapy
New York-Presbyterian Hospital
New York, New York

Scott J. Swanson
Lung Transplant Program
Division of Thoracic Surgery
Brigham and Women's Hospital
Harvard Medical School
Boston, Massachusetts

David O. Taylor, MD
Associate Professor of Medicine
Medical Director
Utah Cardiac Transplant Program
University of Utah School of Medicine
Salt Lake City, Utah

Nina E. Tolkoff-Rubin, MD, FACP
Director of the Hemodialysis and CAPD Units
Massachusetts General Hospital
Associate Professor of Medicine
Harvard Medical School
Boston, Massachusetts

Emil R. Unanue, MD
Department of Pathology and Immunology
Washington University School of Medicine
St. Louis, Missouri

Martin D. Valentine, MD
Maryland Asthma and Allergy Center
Professor of Medicine
Johns Hopkins University School of Medicine
Clinical Professor of Medicine
University of Maryland School of Medicine
Baltimore, Maryland

Andrew F. Walls, PhD
Immunopharmacology Group
University of Southampton
Southampton General Hospital
Southampton, England

A. Thomas Waytes, MD, PhD
Clinical Assistant Professor of Internal Medicine
Wayne State University School of Medicine
Vice President of Medical Affairs
Community Bio-Resources, Inc.
Medical Director, Medical Affairs & Clinical
    Development
Hyland Immuno Division, Baxter Healthcare
Medical Staff
Department of Medicine
Veterans Administration Medical Center
Detroit, Michigan

Michael E. Weinblatt, MD
Professor of Medicine
Harvard Medical School
Director of Rheumatology
Brigham and Women's Hospital
Boston, Massachusetts

Michael B. Widmer, PhD
Vice-President, Director of Biological Sciences
Immunex Corporation
Seattle, Washington

Preface

In the preface to the first edition, we highlighted the rationale for initiating a volume to address the particular area of therapeutic maneuvers in the management of human diseases of immunologic origin. We emphasized that while other volumes would be directed principally to basic immunology, disease-oriented clinical immunology, and "organ-directed immunopathology," *Therapeutic Immunology* would be directed to intervention, with clinical issues serving as the framework and background for such intervention. At that time, we presumed that the immediate future would be highlighted by the clinical deployment of therapeutic strategies with a conceptual design for efficacy based on the therapeutic target.

That projection has, indeed, been supported by the advances in the biotherapeutic management of human disease. The reasons for the progress in biotherapeutic intervention are several-fold. They include the humanization technologies and other molecular approaches to increase binding affinities for monoclonal antibodies. In addition to these technical advances, there has been an important conceptual recognition that monoclonal antibodies or soluble receptors can be used to define subgroups of responders within a clinical entity and to highlight a direction for small-molecule intervention at a future point in time. The biotherapeutics do not have the unexpected "side effects" of small molecules; for the most part, they exhibit side effects that are predictable and target-related.

Immunology, as a rapidly maturing discipline in the basic sciences, continues to provide insights into the development of novel therapeutic strategies. As a field, immunology is particularly well positioned to bridge the divide between laboratory science and clinical application, an area termed translational research. We anticipate that the continued development of the fields of genomics and bioinformatics will have a significant impact on the field of immunology. This impact will lead to exciting and unexpected therapies that will affect the outcome of diseases. Thus, we envision *Therapeutic Immunology* as a continuing work-in-progress, and we expect the next edition to be vastly different from the one we present to you today.

The task of organizing and editing a text with multiple authors in order to address the range of therapeutic interventions for diseases suitable for immunologic intervention is complex and multi-system. We deeply appreciate the support that we each received from the staff of our individual offices. We thank Joanne Miccile, Darlene Chase, and Fran Pechenick, and also Julia Casson of Blackwell Science, for their attention to the volume and execution of the needed tasks. We are most appreciative of Ms. Arlene Stolper Simon for the countless hours she spent editing various chapters as well as the index, and in reviewing the proofs. Finally, and certainly most of all, the editors are appreciative of the integrative thinking and knowledge that the authors brought to each chapter, and we thank them for sharing their wisdom and their knowledge of unresolved issues with our readers.

KFA
SJB
FSR
TBS

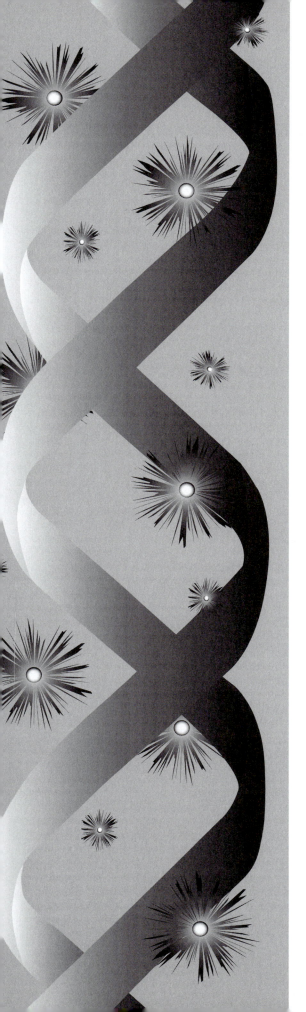

I

Introduction

Chapter 1

Adaptive Immunity

Emil R. Unanue

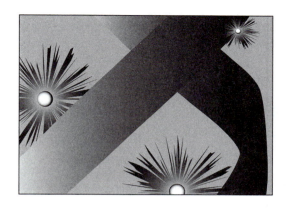

This chapter is an overview of the immune system. It discusses some of the major events taking place in the response to antigen and places them in a historical perspective. (Citations of the literature are limited, and place particular emphasis on key reports and on review papers.) The immune system operates physiologically to curb microbial infection and therefore has a major survival value for the species. It operates through the coordinated interaction of various cell lines, one of which, the lymphocyte lineage, endows the system with an incredible degree of specificity in molecular recognition. Cells of the mononuclear phagocyte system, including the dendritic cells (DCs) and the macrophages, natural killer (NK) cells, granulocytes, and mast cells, represent lineages that interact rapidly with pathogens—they can recognize the pathogen and respond by inducing inflammation, in great part mediated by cytokines. These sets of cells—the old term "reticuloendothelial system" (RES) was most appropriate and is used herein—intimately participate with the lymphocyte ("Innate immunity" is a useful term, much in vogue now, that encompasses the early cellular reaction to microbes by nonlymphocytic cells.) We have used the term "symbiosis" to define this very intimate collaboration among both sets of cells (1). Each cellular lineage influences the others in profound ways.

To simplify in order to start this discussion, the innate system interacts first with pathogens and responds in one of two major ways. First, it releases the mediators that change the environment of the tissue and also influence the responses of the surrounding cells: blood vessels are dilated and blood flow increases, and a variety of cells are attracted into the site and are activated. Second, the innate system presents antigen to the T cells, which respond specifically to the antigens from the pathogen and become activated. Antigen presentation plus the presence of cytokines released by the RES constitute the two major stimuli necessary for the lymphocyte to respond. Lymphocyte activation means an increase in proliferation and the functional differentiation of the various lymphocyte lineages. Clones of lymphocytes proliferate, antibody molecules are released as B cells differentiate, CD4 and CD8 T cells are activated and a whole gamut of new cytokines are released that influence the inflammatory response, and infected cells are killed in a variety of ways, but particularly by CD8 T cells. Following this first stage, the innate system then responds more exuberantly in response to the stimuli from the lymphocytes, hence the use of the term "symbiosis" to characterize these dual interactions between lymphocytes and the RES. The end result is the elimination of the phlogogen. Subsequently, inflammation subsides, many of the cells die, and homeostasis sets in. An important consequence is the development of immunological memory—that is to say, the lymphocyte system can now recognize the antigens in a very effective way in the event of a new encounter. This is the principle behind vaccination, one of the most successful therapies in medicine. Indeed, it is through vaccination that immunology began as a discipline—in 1796, when Jenner discovered cowpox vaccination (2). But the immune system can be involved in diseases. Diseases can result from a genetic or acquired impairment of a cellular response; from the abnormal response to self-proteins—i.e., the autoimmunities; or from the normal response to an abnormal challenge with antigen.

The Specificity and Diversity of the Immune Response

A major distinguishing feature of the immune response is the high degree of specificity in the recognition of different chemical species. The immune system can discriminate among chemical entities that differ in subtle ways, such as—in a single amino acid side chain, for example—a tyrosine in a peptide from a phenyl alanine, the position of a group in a ring structure, or the number of monosaccharides in a polysaccharide (3,4). The fine specificity of recognition is the property of the antigen receptors in B and T cells.

Lymphocytes recognize molecules by way of specific surface-bound receptors, an issue first brought forward in 1900 when Ehrlich postulated the side-chain theory: cells should have side chains as extensions of their "protoplasm" that would capture toxins and would lead to cell stimulation (5). "The antitoxins represent nothing more than the side chains reproduced in excess during regeneration, and therefore pushed off from the protoplasm and so coming to exist in a free state." This was remarkable forward thinking in what turned out to be correct in its general features. The identification of the actual receptors was difficult and did not take place until the two major cellular systems were clearly identified in the 1960s (6–8). Highly influential in guiding much of the research in this area was the development of the selective theories that superseded the template theories. The selective theories, starting with Niels Jerne in 1955 (9), stated that antibody molecules, found prior to antigenic stimulation, served to select antigen and to start the process of cellular response. The clonal-selection theories that followed, through MacFarland Burnett (10) and David Talmage (11), correctly placed the selection on lymphocytes through unique and specific antigen-receptor molecules present on their plasma membranes.

Lymphocytes express only one set of mature receptors prior to antigenic stimulation. The immune system functions as a system in which antigen selects those lymphocytes that bear their complementary receptors. In such a Darwinian system, those lymphocytes with the best-fitting receptors for antigen are the ones that will be preferentially activated (12). The antigen receptor of the B cell is an antibody molecule that is surface bound. The T-cell receptor (TCR) is a unique molecule different from the antibody molecule but bearing important structural features in common. On productive activation of the lymphocytes, there is expansion by proliferation, with the development of clones all bearing the same recognition unit as that of their progenitor cell. This expansion and the maintenance of the specific clones constitute, of course, a major component of immunological memory. The size of the clonal expansion is the result of many factors, including the strength of the stimulus and the balance between those lymphocytes that survive and those that die.

Surface-bound immunoglobulin (Ig) of the B cells was the first antigen receptor identified both cytologically and chemically (13–15). The B cells express the antibody molecule in two ways: as a receptor for the binding and selection of antigen in close cellular interactions with CD4 T cells; and as a secreted protein that in blood and extracellular tissue complexes to antigen molecules and mediates their elimination. Thus, the antibody molecule displays two functions: the specific one of binding antigen, and a non-antigen-specific one that varies among the various Ig classes or isotypes.

The B cells display about 100,000 copies of a membrane form of IgM and IgD, both of which contain a transmembrane segment that serves to bind them to the plasma membrane. On successful engagement of this B-cell receptor (BCR), the B cell undergoes activation. With activation there are changes in the physiology of the cell. The B cell can evolve into a rich antibody-secreting cell— the plasma cell; these were the first cells shown to contain Ig, based on their high content of Ig in the endoplasmic reticulum. The fundamental change in the B cell following successful activation is the change in the molecular display of Ig from a BCR to a secreted protein. The specificity of the secreted Ig molecules is the same as that exhibited by the BCR. However, as the immune response matures, two other important biochemical changes take place: isotype or class switch, and affinity maturation. In class switch, the isotype-specific domains are expressed as the response develops. So, from an IgM and IgD expressed only as a membrane molecule, the secreted Ig is predominantly IgG. With affinity maturation, the quality of the antibody improves markedly (16).

The biology and chemistry of the antibody molecule were the focus of immunology research for several decades, since von

Behring and Kitasato first identified antitoxins (17). It is a molecule made of two identical half-molecules, each with one heavy and one light chain (18), well constructed to carry out its two main functions: antigen binding, and mediation of effector reactions (19). These latter properties are associated with distinct regions of the molecule. At the amino terminal ends of the two component chains, there are the variable Ig domains in which the interaction with parts of the antigen molecule takes place. The Ig domain (20,21) is a particular fold of the polypeptide that contains two series of antiparallel beta strands; the Ig-like domain is common to many proteins of the immune system and is thought to represent the ancestral structure that was involved in modulating cell-to-cell interactions and that diversified during evolution. The remaining portions of the heavy chain and the light chain are also made of Ig-like constant domains that mediate distinct effector functions depending on each immunoglobulin isotype (22). To highlight two of the most important immunoglobulin isotypes, antibody molecules of the IgG isotype are used to eliminate extracellular pathogens or toxins by various ways, including opsonization, neutralization of their sites of attachment to the pathogen, and production of inflammation, having neutrophils as a conspicuous component. Some of these effects are mediated through interactions with the complement system. Antibody molecules of the IgA isotype are involved in mucosal immunity.

Because of its very high specificity for antigen, the secreted antibody molecule has been used extensively, either as a reagent for laboratory testing or in clinical medicine, an issue that is well analyzed in later chapters. Preparations of Ig are used in the treatment of B-cell deficiencies. Antibodies to Rh blood groups are used in the control of Rh incompatibility, in the prevention of hemolytic disease of the newborn (23). Revolutionary was the finding of Kohler and Milstein (24) that a single B cell could be selected and immortalized in culture by fusing it to a myeloma cell. These B-cell hybridomas not only have served to study the biology of B cells but also have opened a new era of "serotherapy." Monoclonal antibodies, because of their homogeneity and relative ease of production, are finding more applications in a number of clinical situations, including their use for the neutralization of cytokines, in cases of septic shock, in combinations with toxins, for killing tumor cells, and for the inhibition of costimulator molecules to control T-cell reactions in graft rejection.

The identification of the T-cell receptor (TCR) for antigen followed later in time, after the findings of the BCR in B cells. The identification of the BCR was possible in part because of the available information and reagents derived from the study of serum antibodies. This was not the case with the TCR, which is only a membrane protein. On activation, the T cells release instead a series of modulatory proteins, the cytokines, that have no antigen specificity. The identification and analysis of the TCR was solved at the laboratories of Mark Davis and Tak Mak by application of modern gene cloning approaches (25–27). The TCR of most T cells is made of a pair of transmembrane chains, the alpha and beta chains. (A small set of T cells contains two other distinct chains, the gamma/delta TCR.) The binding site of the TCR in common with Ig is made of an Ig-like variable

Table 1-1. Comparison of the Responses to Carbohydrates and Proteins

	Pure Polysaccharide	**Globular Protein**
Recognition by BCR	Yes	Yes
Recognition by TCR	No	Yes, after processing
Binding to MHC	No	Only after processing by APC
Involvement of CD4 T cells	No	Yes
Memory	Poor	Strong
Affinity maturation	Poor	Strong

domain. In contrast to the BCR, the TCR does not engage proteins directly, but only recognizes peptides or unfolded proteins complexed to histocompatibility molecules (see below).

There is, of course, much diversity in the recognition properties of the receptors. Presumably, the number of entities that the receptors can recognize reaches 10^{10}. This ensures that most chemical conformations can eventually be identified by the lymphocyte and that most pathogens can be recognized. The molecular explanation for diversity was first solved at the laboratory of Susumu Tonegawa when various DNA segments were found to encode for the mature light chain of the BCR (28). The same findings were later made regarding the TCR. The gene that encodes the mature receptor is generated by recombining distinct gene segments found in the germ line (28–31). This selection of DNA segments from a finite number of V (for variable), J, and, for some chains, D gene segments plus addition or deletion of nucleotides at their coding ends (N-region diversity) is responsible for the generation of the very diverse library of B- and T-cell receptors. (For the Ig genes, the heavy chain is encoded by V, D, and J genes, while the light chain is encoded by V and J genes. The mature T-cell receptor alpha chain is encoded by recombination of V and J, while the beta chain encodes for V, D, and J gene segments. The VDJ exon is then spliced to genes encoding the constant segments of the heavy or light chain of Ig, or the TCR chains.) During their differentiation, the immature B and T cells express genes encoding two enzymes involved in the recombination process (these are the recombination-activating genes, RAG-1 and RAG-2) (32). These proteins are responsible for DNA scission and their joining (together with other proteins such as DNA ligase, Ku70, and Ku80). The RAG proteins are expressed at particular stages in the differentiation of B and T cells, a point that we discuss later.

Does the specificity of the antigen receptors change during an immune response? In the B cell, the quality of antigen recognition improves markedly as the response "matures." Affinity maturation was discovered by studying the response to haptens and finding by equilibrium dialysis that the affinity increased by several fold (33). At the molecular level, the change in affinity is explained by the presence of somatic mutations. During the B-cell response in germinal centers, the rate of mutation of the genes encoding the BCR increases markedly. This hypermutation was first indicated by Weigert, Cohn, and associates (34) when

studying lambda light chains in the mouse. It results in point mutations in the variable genes, while the genes encoding the constant region are not affected. Somatic mutation takes place in the germinal centers of the follicles and is accompanied by extensive proliferation. It requires interaction of the B cells with CD4 T cells. Indeed, the response to pure polysaccharides that trigger B cells to a limited amount and do not stimulate T cells shows limited if any affinity changes. (For a comparison of the responses to proteins and polysaccharides, see Table 1-1.) Many of the growing B cells die, while those having the highest-affinity receptors survive and become the predominant clones. Thus, as a combination of somatic mutation and selection, the B-cell response improves for the best. These changes in affinity are not found in the T-cell response.

Antigen Presentation

The modes of interaction with antigen of the two major lineages of cells are different. B cells can directly recognize antigen molecules through their BCR: they can recognize pure carbohydrate as well as proteins in their native or tertiary configuration (Table 1-1). It is apparent that this direct recognition was the case when the specificity of serum antibodies was studied: antibodies raised against globular proteins bind only to the native molecule and not to the denatured proteins (reviewed in 1). Thus, most B-cell clones have been selected by protein antigens prior to their extensive catabolism by the host. This is not the case for T cells, where an antigen-presenting cell (APC) has to come into operation in order to promote the recognition. T cells recognize a linear sequence of amino acids, either segments of an unfolded protein or peptides of a few amino acids. Indeed, the TCR will not interact directly with protein antigens unless they are part of a complex with the major histocompatibility complex (MHC) molecules. Thus, protein antigens need to be processed and presented by the APC as peptides or unfolded molecules bound to MHC proteins (35). Pure polysaccharides do not bind to MHC proteins and do not stimulate T cells (Table 1-1).

The differences in antigen recognition between T and B cells was a major puzzle for many years. The early literature had indicated two sets of reactions to proteins. As mentioned above,

Table 1-2. Comparison of Class I and II MHC Molecules

	MHC-I	**MHC-II**
Expression	Most cells	Primarily in APC and in some specialized epithelial cells
Structure	A heavy transmembrane chain (~44 Kd) together with β2 microglobulin (12 Kd)	Two transmembrane chains α and β of ~30 Kd
Peptide binding	Usually 8–10 residues in length	Normally large, >5 residues
Peptide loading	In endoplasmic reticulum	In vesicles
Site of catabolism of the protein	Cytosol: proteasome	Vesicles
Chaperonins	Tapasin, calreticulin	Invariant chain, AL-A DM
Biology	Antiviral and antitumor immunity	Immunity to intracellular pathogenesis and foreign proteins
	Interacts with CD8 T cells	Interacts with CD4 T cells

serum antibodies reacted with conformational-dependent epitopes of a globular protein. The same results applied to immunopathologic reactions, such as the Arthus reaction or the acute anaphylactic reactions, both of which needed to be elicited with the native proteins. In contrast were the reactions now known to be elicited by T cells, such as the delayed sensitivity reactions. These reactions were identified when Koch first reported the reaction to tuberculin, and were later shown, by the classical experiments of Chase and Landsteiner, to be transferred by lymphocytes (36,37). These reactions did not discriminate between denatured and native proteins and showed marked dependency on the "carrier," in the examples of hapten-carrier protein conjugates. (The antibody-mediated reactions were infiltrated by neutrophils, while the delayed reactions were rich in activated macrophages, an indication of the different patterns of inflammation, which involved complement and cytokines, respectively.)

The seminal molecules responsible for the APC–T cell interaction are those encoded in the major histocompatibility gene complex (MHC) of the species. The APC informs the T cell of the molecular status of its environment by displaying peptides bound to either their class I or class II MHC molecules (Table 1-2). MHC molecules are peptide-binding proteins that rescue peptides from intracellular digestion (38). The peptide-MHC complex constitutes the epitope that the TCR recognizes. The TCR contacts both the peptide as well as residues of the MHC molecule, an issue that has now been settled by x-ray crystallographic analysis of TCR complexed to their specific peptide-MHC complex (39–41). This double interaction creates a situation whereby the T cell that is selected in the thymus must have two specificities, one for peptides and the other for its own MHC. This interaction results in the phenomenon of MHC

restriction—that is to say that T cells recognize foreign elements, but always in the framework of also recognizing a self-MHC protein (42–45).

The MHC molecules were discovered in the context of transplantation reactions (46,47). Indeed, it is the strong reaction to allogeneic MHC proteins that is responsible for graft rejection, creating the difficulties in transplanting tissues within members of the species. These proteins were found to be part of a complex genetic system with a high degree of allelism. It is the most polymorphic gene system of the species.

The human leukocyte antigen (HLA) system was discovered when sera from mutiparous women or highly transfused individuals were found to contain leukoagglutinins—i.e., anti-HLA antibodies, which is the basis of tissue typing for transplantation reactions (48,49). However, it was through mouse genetics and the development of inbred strains of mice that the major advances in this field were made (50). These lines were developed through the laborious work of many, including CC Little and George Snell at the Jackson Laboratory. These strains provided a homogeneous genetic population that enabled the fine genetic dissection of the mouse MHC (the H-2) and cell transfers and organ grafts to be carried out (51). The basic laws of transplantations were developed through the use of inbred strains of mice. The physiological role of MHC was discovered in part through serendipity, but by very astute researchers who followed the leads and pinpointed the essential role of the MHC in T-cell recognition. Indeed, the realization that some strains of mice and guinea pigs were either high or low responders to peptides and that this response was linked genetically to the MHC laid the groundwork for such discoveries (52–55). Finally, considering this topic of inbred mice, the next major advance of the past decade has been the production of mice bearing transgenes or having mutations or ablations of a given gene. The advances with the use of trans-genes or gene knockout mice has been revolutionary, dramatically changing biology and immunology (56).

There are two sets of MHC molecules encoded in the MHC gene complex, the class I and class II molecules (57–60) (Table 1–2). Each MHC gene complex may contain more than one gene encoding class I or II molecules. In the human HLA there are three major class I proteins, HLA A, B, and C, and three major class II proteins, HLA DR, DQ, and DP. Each has multiple allelic variants. The class I molecules are made up of a heavy chain and a small polypeptide beta-2 microglobulin (61). The heavy chain is a transmembrane protein that contains three external domains; the two most distal to the membrane assemble to form the combining site while the one closest to the membrane is made of an Ig-like fold. The class II molecules are composed of two transmembrane chains, each having an external domain that contributes to the formation of the peptide combining site (62). The peptide combining site of both sets of molecules has a similar basic structure, made up of a platform of seven beta pleated sheet strands, bordered by two walls made of alpha helices, with the peptide sitting at about the center between the helices. The amino acids responsible for the allelic polymorphisms are all located in the helices and platform, in contact with the peptide. Thus, the driving force in evolution for diversification of the MHC is at the level of peptide binding.

MHC molecules do not discriminate between self-peptides and foreign peptides—both bind or do not bind (63). Indeed, these molecules are normally occupied by autologous peptides that bind with varying degrees of affinity (64–66). It is estimated that for each APC, about 2000 peptides are contained in each set of MHC molecules. The importance of these self-peptides is threefold. First, it allows for the elimination in the thymus of T cells that are autoreactive. This is the important process of "negative selection" or central tolerance, which is discussed below. Second, binding of such peptides gives stability and structure to the MHC molecule, which otherwise would not be correctly expressed: depending on the binding affinity, the MHC molecule will be able to exchange some of these self-peptides with other peptides, including those from foreign molecules. But third, and very importantly, the self-peptides bound to the MHC molecule are the basis for T-cell recognition in autoimmunities. There is a relationship between a particular autoimmunity and an MHC allele such as occurs in type I or insulin-dependent diabetes (67). At this point in time, the number of autologous peptides identified as responsible for an autoimmune process is very limited, but the approaches and technologies are now available, and information should be forthcoming.

Class I molecules interact with peptides of 8–10 residues in length, but of much larger length in the case of class II molecules (61,65,68,69). Peptides bind through two major sets of interactions. One set of interactions is at the level of amino acid side chains with sites (or pockets) in the combining site that are allele specific: in a class I molecule, there are two major sites located at each end. Four sites are involved in peptide binding to class II, although usually one becomes the dominant site of interaction. A second set of interactions involves a complex hydrogen

bonding network between conserved residues of the MHC and the peptide backbone (for examples, see 70 and 71).

Peptides vary in their strength of binding to MHC, depending on their amino acid composition as well as on the particular MHC alleles (72). In general, binding is in the low nM to μM affinity range. Each allele binds to many peptides. So there is specificity, but at the same time the binding is broad. This binding repertoire allows an individual to recognize multiple peptides. This was well stated by Benacerraf: "The evolutionary significance of the commitment of T cells to MHC antigens should be assessed from several vantage points. From the point of view of the individual concerned, the existence of such a broadly polymorphic system to determine specific responsiveness and suppression will inescapably result in individuals with different immunological potential to a given challenge. Some will clearly be at risk, whereas others will be better prepared to resist certain infectious agents, and it is not surprising that immunological diseases are linked to the MHC. As far as the species is concerned, this polymorphic defense system results in a very significant survival advantage to unforeseen challenges and a better possibility for the immune system to adapt to evolutionary pressures" (55).

The probable reason for the development of two sets of MHC molecules is because each samples a distinct cellular compartment. Thus, the class I MHC proteins sample the peptides from the cytosol (73, reviewed in 74). These peptides result from proteasomal digestion, passing into the endoplasmic reticulum (ER) by way of peptide transporters of the ABC type (which also happen to be encoded in the HLA gene complex). In the ER, the complex assembles with nascent class I MHC molecules and is then transported to the plasma membrane (75). Several chaperonin-like molecules such as tapasin and calreticulin are involved, allowing for the proper folding of the heavy chain, the peptide, and beta-2 microglobulin. It follows that the MHC class I system is the one that evolved to deal with viral infections, since it is in the cytosol that viral proteins are assembled and processed. Of the two major subsets of T cells, the CD8 T cells recognize the peptide-MHC class I complex. The CD8 molecule has affinity for the class I MHC molecule and contributes to the cellular interaction. CD8 T cells protect against viral infections by killing infected cells and also by releasing interferon-gamma (reviewed in 76 and 77).

In contrast, the class II MHC system is best suited to handle peptides from proteins that have been taken into the APC by endocytosis (69). The internalized protein, either free or as part of a microbial structure, is processed in organelles of low pH and the protein is unfolded and subjected to partial proteolysis—the peptide or unfolded protein binds to nascent class II molecules in a complex series of steps that involve a number of auxiliary or chaperoning proteins (invariant chain, HLA-Dm). So it follows that the class II system is primarily involved in the reactions to exogenous proteins or to microbes that reside in phagolysosomes. Infections with intracellular bacteria depend on the action of the CD4 T-cell subset interacting with the microbial peptides selected by the class II MHC molecules. The CD4 molecule, as in the case of the CD8 molecule, contributes to the interaction while at the same time serving to mark this subset. CD4 T cells are involved in activating macrophages by releasing interferon-gamma, promoting growth via IL-2, and regulating B-cell differentiation by way of IL-4 release (reviewed in 78).

The three cells involved in antigen presentation are the dendritic cell, which derives from monocytes, expresses a high level of MHC molecules, and is specially endowed for very effective close contact with lymphocytes (79,80); the monocyte/macrophage, which modulates its expression of MHC molecules and responds to interferon gamma by increasing the number of them; and the B cell, which expresses MHC molecules constitutively. These three cells are denoted as antigen-presenting cells, or APCs. Antigen presentation in a lymph node takes place in two main contexts. First is the activation of the CD4 T-cell clones when antigen enters the node and is captured by the dense network of dendritic cells in the deep cortex. The dendritic cells are powerful APC with a high density of MHC molecules and a large surface made by cytoplasmic extensions that favor close cellular interactions (79). The second context is that of B cell interacting with the activated CD4 T cell (81). The B cell captures the native antigen by way of surface Ig and then internalizes it and processes it, placing peptides bound to its class II MHC molecules. The interaction with the T cell then takes place. Anatomically it is thought that it arises in the deep cortex next to the follicle. The APC/T cell interaction leads to reciprocal effects. These double effects are particularly pointed in the case of B cell/T cell interaction. The B cell is activated and differentiates while the T cell likewise continues on its activation pathway. The result is the dual recognition and specificity: a B cell that makes antibody reactive to the native protein antigen and the T cell that reacts with the peptides derived from intracellular processing.

Following these first interactions, the cellular interactions move to the follicles (81). There the follicular dendritic cell (FDC) traps the soluble antigen molecules as an antigen-antibody-complement complex. In the follicle, the B cells undergo extensive proliferation with differentiation. It is at this site where class switch and affinity maturation take place. Presumably the B cells are interacting with the FDC-bound complex in the context also of receiving signals from the activated T cells.

The Discrimination Between Self and Nonself by the Immune System

The molecular mechanisms that generate a diverse BCR and TCR library do not discriminate between receptors to foreign antigens or to self-proteins. Autoreactive cells do develop and have the potential to produce the autoimmune diseases. This is the price that we pay for having a vast repertoire of receptors. Actually, autoimmunity was first mentioned by Ehrlich using the term "horror autotoxicus" to describe what he foresaw as a disastrous event for the individual. After much debate, it is now well established that these conditions do take place and constitute a serious cause, or at least a component, of many diseases. Indeed,

many if not all organs can be the spontaneous targets of autoimmunity in humans or can be induced targets in experimental animals strongly immunized with autologous antigens. The spontaneous human diseases with an autoimmune component include hemolytic anemias and thrombocytopenias, type I or insulin-dependent diabetes mellitus, lupus erythematosus, rheumatoid arthritis, some forms of thyroiditis, myasthenia gravis, and multiple sclerosis. But these are disease states because the normal immune system has developed mechanisms to control either the development or the activation of the autoreactive clones.

Several points stand out for explaining the control of self-reactivity, a subject of much research at present. As initially theorized by Joshua Lederberg (82), in the development of lymphocytes, the immature cells pass through a stage in which they become highly sensitive to the engagement of their receptors by antigen and die if this engagement takes place (Fig. 1-1). Thus, many autoreactive cells are deleted by a process called clonal anergy that involves the death of the cells by apoptosis. Much attention has now been given to how the differentiation of the early T and B cells takes place and how the selection of the cells reactive to foreign antigen (called positive selection) and those reactive to autologous antigen (called negative selection) takes place (83–87). In the former case, the cells live to form part of the peripheral lymphocyte pool that permits the species to confront the environment. In the latter case, the cells die and autoreactivity to some antigens is avoided. The differentiation of T cells and B cells has common and also distinct features that we now address in the context of analyzing self-reactivity.

The thymus gland is the primary lymphoid organ in which stem cells differentiate to thymocytes. This differentiation takes place most vigorously during fetal life and in early postnatal development. The essential role of the thymus was first noted by Jacques Miller: he thymectomized mice immediately after birth and before there was an opportunity for seeding of the secondary lymphoid organs (88,89). While thymectomy of the adult did not result in impairment of immune response, the mice thymectomized at birth were T-cell and immune deficient. [Birds also have a defined organ for B-cell development, the bursa of Fabricius (90); in mammals, however, B cells develop mostly in bone marrow. It follows that birds show with great distinction the pathways of B- and T-cell differentiation: bursectomy results in selective loss of B cells but with a healthy T-cell system, while in contrast thymectomy impairs selectively the T-cell development (91).]

The early T cell goes through defined stages as it moves in very close contact through the gland by means of a network of epithelial cells and dendritic cells that express class II MHC molecules. The differentiation can be tracked by following the expression of the CD4 and CD8 coreceptors. From the "double negative" stage the cells develop both coreceptors (the "double positive" stage) and then differentiate to either CD4 or CD8 T cells, some of which emigrate to constitute the peripheral population. At the double negative stage, the cells express the RAG enzymes and undergo recombination of their V, D, and J genes that encode the TCR beta chain, through an order rearrangement, first of the D and J gene segments and then with a V gene.

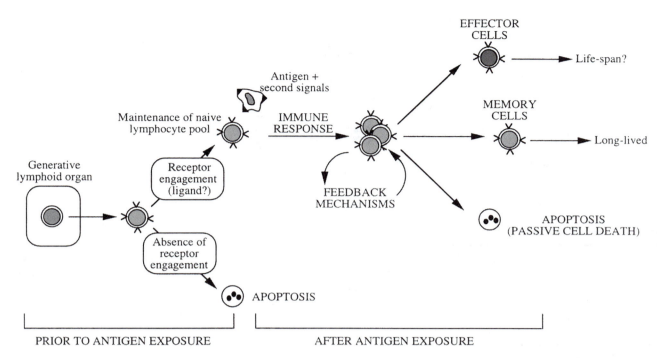

Figure 1-1. The different fates of early lymphocytes and their response once there is antigenic stimulation. (Reproduced by permission from Abbas AK, van Parijs L. Maintaining homeostasis in the immune system: turning lymphocytes off. Science 1998;280:243–251.)

Subsequently, the beta chain pairs with a surrogate alpha T-cell receptor gene called the pre-T alpha. At this point, the cells segregate into "double positives" and the alpha chain undergoes recombination and eventual pairing with the beta chain, to form the mature TCR. Single positives, with either CD4 or CD8 T cells, now develop and are committed to react to either class II or class I MHC molecules, respectively.

The specificity of the TCR is skewed to react with MHC molecules (92,93). Three events are believed to be taking place in the differentiation of thymocytes (reviewed in 94 and 95) as the various TCRs are expressed. The first event is the strong engagement of the TCR by self-molecules displayed by APC of the thymus that process their own proteins as well as blood proteins. The result is death by apoptosis; this negative selection process, to be significant, needs to be highly sensitive, and indeed can take place when the APC displays as few as two to three MHC-peptide complexes per APC. The second event is weak interactions of the TCR to self-MHC that does not display the correct peptide; here the T cell matures and leaves the thymus gland to form part of the recirculating pool of lymphocytes. The third event is no interaction because the TCR of the developing thymocyte does not match the MHC; here the cells die by "neglect," also by apoptosis. About 90% of thymocytes die in the gland. The deletion of the double positive to single positive stage has been masterfully explored by using transgenic mice that bear a single

TCR for antigen and introducing the antigen into the thymus in different ways. Harold von Boehmer and his associates, who first reported this result, used a CD8 T cell with specificity against an antigen encoded by the Y chromosome: in transgenic mice expressing the TCR, the TCR-bearing thymocytes were deleted in the males (which presented the peptide encoded by the Y chromosome) but not in the females. In the females, the TCR-bearing T cells appeared in the secondary lymphoid organs (85) (Table 1-3).

The end result of these events is the survival of T cells that are restricted to react with foreign peptides, but always presented by their own MHC molecules. As a result, the repertoire of T cells reactive to blood proteins and antigens of the APC is effectively deleted. However, many self-proteins are confined to their organs and do not have a blood stage. Therefore, these proteins are not expected to reach the thymus gland to induce negative selection. Thus, many autoreactive cells with specificity to these hidden antigens will peripheralize. This happens, for example, with proteins of the central nervous system or of the beta cells of the islets of Langerhans. Knowing these events, we can understand well and reinterpret the pioneering studies from Peter Medawar's laboratory, where "acquired immunological tolerance" was first described (96). Indeed, the introduction of cells (in this case, allogeneic cells) or of foreign proteins into the thymus resulted in the lack of immune reactivity to them. [Medawar based some of his

Table 1-3. Positive and Negative Thymic Selection

Thymus	Positive Selection	Negative Selection	Neglect	Peripheral T Cells
K^b male	−	+	−	Poor
K^b female	+	−	−	Abundant
K^d female	−	−	+	Poor

This table is a summary adapted from the experiment in reference 85. TCR transgenic mice contain CD8 T cells that react with a peptide encoded in the Y chromosome presented by the class I MHC molecule K^b. Indicated are the various outcomes depending on the genotype and sex of the mouse (under "Thymus").

experiments on the work of Ray Owen, who had examined cattle twins in which there was mixing of the placental circulation. The resulting twins were chimeric; the cells of each recirculated and were not eliminated (97).]

A comparable series of events takes place in the B cell, but a distinct primary lymphoid organ, such as the thymus, is not present. Primarily in the bone marrow, the B cells develop through a series of well-defined stages, regulated by the activity of transcription factors that influence the expression of various genes and their encoded proteins. The first defined cell in the lineage, called the pre-B cell, expresses the RAG-1 and RAG-2 genes, allowing recombination of the heavy chain to take place. On successful recombination and assembly of the heavy chain gene from one chromosome, no further activation of the second chromosome takes place (allelic exclusion) and the pre-B cell stage is identified; here the mu heavy chain pairs with a surrogate light chain (lambda 5 or VpreB). At this checkpoint, the expression of the RAG genes is stopped and the cells divide, stimulated by interaction with stromal cells and by the cytokine IL-7. In the next stage, the RAG genes are expressed again, and light chain gene rearrangement proceeds, leading to the immature B cell that expresses the mu chain. At this point, the B cell is highly sensitive to interaction of its BCR with antigen. If the specificity of the BCR is toward a self-antigen, three possible events may transpire: the B cell may die by apoptosis (the clonal deletion process akin to what transpired in the thymocyte); the B cell may survive but become hyporesponsive (clonal anergy) (86,87); or, lastly and very interestingly, the cell may replace the transcribed light chain and express a new rearranged one, a process termed "receptor editing" (98,99). The interaction of the immature B cell may also take place in secondary lymphoid tissue. Subsequently, the B cells express IgD together with IgM, the mature B cell.

In summary, there are developmental stages in which the differentiating T and B cells that express autoreactive receptors can be eliminated. This sensitive stage purges the system of many autoreactive clones. How about the autoreactive cells that escaped clonal deletion to form part of the peripheral lymphoid pool? This is a subject that will require more research, since at this time we do not fully understand how autoimmunity develops. Nevertheless, several factors have been identified that keep the autoreactive cells in a dormant state. For T cells, we know that many epithelial and connective cells in the various organs do not express the class II MHC molecules, and therefore are not capable of presenting their own antigens. Second, the threshold of activation of the immature T cells is now relatively high; compared with thymocytes, about 100 times more MHC-peptide complexes are required. Such levels are not easy to reach with most autoantigens (100). Finally, cells in most organs do not express molecules that are important for stimulating T cells, such as the costimulatory molecules. In the case of B cells, an encounter of the mature B cell with an autoantigen in the absence of T-cell interaction is nonproductive and may lead to the anergy state, to be described below.

The Life of a Lymphocyte before Contact with Antigen: Recirculation, Migration, and Survival

In a quiet situation where no antigen is in the system, the lymphocytes are in a state of continuous circulation from blood into lymph and back to blood (101,102). This recirculation of lymphocytes is a most important process, since it ensures that the various clones can sample their environment in their search for the complementary antigen molecules. Lymphocytes enter a lymph node, attaching first to the specialized endothelium of the postcapillary venules and then crossing into the parenchyma of the node, into the deep cortex. The deep cortex is made primarily of T cells, while the superficial cortex contains the follicles, the site of B-cell accumulation. Thus, in a quiescent state the two major sets of lymphocytes are segregated from each other. Neither the attachment nor the migration is a random event: first, the attachment of lymphocytes involves cell adhesion molecules in a tight cell-to-cell contact; second, their migration is a response to chemoattractants.

The attachment of the lymphocytes to the postcapillary endothelium, or to any other vascular bed, takes place by ligand-receptor interactions involving molecules on the lymphocytes with their respective acceptors on the endothelium (reviewed in 103 and 104). Having this information, therapeutic strategies can be devised to block one of the members of the pair and therefore stop unwanted inflammation such as in graft rejection.

The molecules involved in the physiological crossing from blood to lymph nodes are the selectins—particularly L-selectin, which is normally expressed in lymphocytes (other members of the selectin family include P- and E-selectin) (103,105). The acceptor molecules of selectins are cell surface carbohydrates on glycoproteins of the endothelia. The other major set of adhesion molecules are the integrins (106). Integrins constitute a very large family of molecules involved in a range of cell-to-cell interactions both in and outside the immune system. Characterized by two chains, these molecules are grouped by families, depending on the particular kind of alpha or beta chain. In the immune system, the integrins that are of particular importance are the beta-2 integrins. These include three distinct molecules, each bearing a distinct alpha chain associated with a common beta-2 chain: the LFA-1, Mac-1, and p150/95 molecules (107). The coreceptors for the beta-2 integrins are the intercellular adhesion molecules (ICAMs) expressed on a variety of cells, including the APC. Under conditions of inflammation, the lymphocytes as well as the monocytes and granulocytes can bind to inflamed vessels, which acquire sets of adhesion molecules. Both integrins and selectins are involved in these interactions (104). The studies of selectins and integrins using gene knockout mice have indicated the important role that cell adhesion molecules play in regulating traffic from blood to various lymphoid tissues, and also within the lymphoid tissue and extravascular sites.

The distribution and migration of lymphocytes in the lymph nodes, and also at sites of inflammation, are programmed and regulated by low-molecular-weight proteins, now termed collectively as chemokines (reviewed in 108). Chemotaxis was first studied in cultures of neutrophils, in response to small peptides derived from activation of some complement proteins (such as C5a) or bacterial peptides or arachidonate derivatives. Their biological role had been suspected but not fully established. Discovery of the presence and importance of a large family of small proteins with some specificity in their cellular target is a recent development. Chemokines belong primarily to two distinct families (distinguished by the presence of cysteines at conserved positions, the CC and CXC chemokines). Chemokine receptors are specific to sets of chemokines and are members of a family of seven transmembrane G coupled receptors (for example, 109–111). Chemokines are expressed by lymphocytes, dendritic cells, stromal cells, and endothelia. The release of the various chemokines and the expression of their receptors are complex and depend on the state of maturation and activation of the cells. Evidence has now been brought forth that the migration of T cells, after crossing into the node, is dictated by one set of chemokines (SLC acting on the CCR7 receptor), while the migration of the B cell to the follicle involves a second distinct molecule (BLC acting on CXCR5) (109–111).

Lymphocytes maintain a relatively constant number in blood, under normal homeostatic conditions (112). This number is the result of many factors, including survival, normal rate of proliferation, the fraction that die, and the contribution of recent emigrants to the peripheral pool. Under conditions of lymphopenia, the transfusion of normal lymphocytes in small numbers restores the level to (but not beyond) normal in the absence of antigenic stimulation.

The survival of both T and B cells depends on the continuous "basal" engagement of their receptors. Indeed, B cells that lack surface Ig have a short life, leading to the thinking that perhaps a low-affinity interaction with BCR promotes their survival (113). The same happens with T cells: the number of T cells in blood depends very much on the presence of MHC class I and II molecules: mice deficient in these molecules exhibit a loss of peripheral T cells. As with the B cell, this survival appears to depend on a level of low-affinity interaction between the TCR and MHC molecules (114).

The Lymphocyte Response to Antigen

The introduction of antigen into an individual can result in a variety of responses and the breakdown of the homeostasis described above. There are various outcomes, depending on the amounts and forms of antigen. The intrinsic immunogenic strength of the antigen depends on the chemical complexity of the molecules and the degree to which they differ from host proteins (all this results in having more potential clones capable of being selected by the antigen). Furthermore, the form of the antigen and its initial fate with the RES is of utmost importance. Antigens that form part of the structure of viruses or bacteria are the strongest antigens. In stark contrast is the response to soluble proteins, which may not trigger much of a response. For example, foreign serum proteins can circulate for periods of time without causing a response. However, if the same protein is administered in adjuvants (water in oil emulsions containing dead tubercle bacilli, or in alum, or, more recently, as naked DNA encoding for the protein), a brisk response is elicited.

These two opposite patterns of lymphocyte responses have been explained on the basis of whether or not the APC system is activated: the APC becomes the central regulator deciding the outcome of the lymphocyte response. Thus, the interactions of APC with microbes or antigens in adjuvants induce in them the expression of sets of molecules important in fostering the cell-to-cell interaction and the activation of the T cell. The first set is the adhesion molecules, represented by the ICAM molecules (104). These molecules interact with the LFA-1 molecule, a beta-2 integrin, to promote strong adhesion between the two cells. A second set of molecules consists of the costimulators, molecules that are required to promote the activation of the T cell following the recognition of the peptide-MHC complex of the APC. Normally in limited amounts from resting APC, costimulators include three groups of proteins: the B7 molecules (B7-1 and B7-2) that match with the CD28 molecule of the T cell (115,116); the CD58 molecule that binds to the CD2 molecule (117); and finally, the CD40 on APC including B cells and the CD40 Ligand on the T cell (118,119). A final set of molecules are soluble instead of membrane bound and are represented by cytokines that regulate the type of response of the T cell (see below).

The stimulus for the identification of costimulators came from the observation that interactions of T cells with APC (120), or of B cells with antigen molecules (121), do not result in their activation despite the engagement of their antigen receptors. In fact, such interactions are not productive and may leave the T cell or the B cell in a state of unresponsiveness. These observations led to the "two-signal hypothesis," meaning that at least two events were needed to take the resting cell to an activated state (121). As was referred to above, this lack of response, which has been termed anergy, is believed to be the other mechanism for controlling autoreactive lymphocytes that have not been negatively selected during their primary differentiation. Thus, in the circumstance that autoreactive T cells of the recirculating pool encounter a peptide-MHC complex in an otherwise resting APC, such an encounter generates a T cell that will not be productively triggered by a subsequent encounter with a fully two-signal-competent APC (for examples, see 122,123). A similar event takes place in B cells, where an encounter with a self-antigen in the absence of T-cell "help" results in a negative event in which the cell dies or becomes unresponsive (87).

For the T cell, engagement of CD28 brings about the transcription of various cytokine genes including IL-2, a major cytokine responsible for clonal growth (115,116,124). The T cells also express an antiapoptotic intracellular molecule, bcl-xL, that promotes their survival. In the case of the B cell, the second signal is brought about by close interaction with the activated T cell. The T cell delivers its second signal by engagement of its CD40 ligand with the B cell's CD40, an event that results in expression of B7 molecules that interact with the CD28 molecules (119). It follows that interruption of the molecules involved in the second signaling—i.e., the costimulators—should be an effective way to modulate the response; this manipulation has been tried experimentally in blocking the CD40 ligand. Likewise, expression of costimulators in cells that lack them should improve the response, a point made experimentally by stimulation of antitumor immunity using tumor cells expressing B7.

If there is a productive event, the immune system is activated. The activation of the lymphocyte involves clonal expansion and the change from a resting cell to a cell that is in DNA synthesis. The first interaction is that of the CD4 and/or CD8 T cells with the activated APC. In a lymph node, it takes place in the deep cortex among a network of dendritic cells that trap and present the antigen. Clonal expansion of specific lymphocytes can now be determined by testing with soluble MHC-peptide complexes, a recent approach taken by Mark Davis and his associates. Because of the polyvalent nature of the complex (it is made with streptavidin binding four biotinylated peptide-MHC complexes, hence the popular name "tetramer MHC"), the binding to the T cell is of sufficient avidity to be detected (125). With viruses and bacteria, the expansion of CD8-specific T cells can be detected with this new approach and shown to be quite notable, up to about a 100-fold increase in clone size, during the initial days after infection (126,127). Much work is now in progress evaluating this response both in experimental animals and in humans.

Following clonal expansion, there is differentiation of the T and B cells with transcription of new genes and the consequent expression of new proteins (128). CD4 T cells, on interactions with cytokines produced by APC, and other T cells will differentiate into two general sets of cells with unique patterns of cytokine production (129). Early in their interaction with APC, the T cells produce IL-2, a cytokine that promotes their growth in an autocatalytic fashion, since the T cells express the receptor for it. Then T cells differentiate into more mature patterns of cytokine expression, much depending on the cytokines that the cell first encounters (130). The Th1 cells release IL-2, and also interferon-gamma, the cytokine that distinguishes this set. This is caused by the release of IL-12 by the APC (131). In fact, many microbes are strong stimulants for IL-12 release. In contrast, the Th2 pattern involves the production of IL-4 and other cytokines that influence B-cell differentiation, such as IL-5 and IL-6. This pattern of differentiation is highly influenced by the amounts of IL-4 in the environment of the T cell (132). (Cytokines such as IL-1 and IL-18 also modulate these outcomes.) Although these two patterns of response were first reported in T-cell clones, by Coffman and Mosman (129), they were later shown to apply to in vivo situations (133). Particular attention is now being paid to the control of this differentiation. For example, a skewed differentiation to a Th2 pattern does not favor the response to infections with intracellular pathogens because of poor macrophage activation. This situation has been well documented in the response to leishmania among strains of mice (133). In humans, the two extremes are best found in leprosy characterized by T cells showing the Th1/Th2 patterns: the former is seen in the tuberculoid form with the activated macrophage that contains bacillary load; in contrast is the lepromatous form associated with the Th2 pattern and with a lack of control of the bacteria by activated macrophages (134).

At this point, a comment on the cytokines is pertinent (Table 1-4). A large number of cytokines are released during the development of the response, and these cytokines are responsible for the magnitudes and the various patterns of responses by lymphocytes and by cells in tissues, including blood vessels. A description of these cytokines is beyond the scope of this review, but suffice it to say that cytokines represent the major vehicle by which the immune system informs surrounding cells and modulates an extensive range of responses. One can broadly identify cytokines, depending on the stage in which they appear and their scope of action. Early in the process, the RES releases important cytokines that influence and poise the lymphocyte response. These include IL-1, and, as already stated, IL-12 and IL-18, among several. Also of note is the TNF family of molecules that have extensive effects from promoting macrophage activation to activating the vascular endothelium, thus promoting cell migration (for a recent review, see 135). Later, as the response develops, the lymphocytes themselves release a large spectrum of cytokines. Important examples are IL-2, which regulates growth; IL-4 and IL-5, which modulate B-cell differentiation; and interferon-gamma, which leads to macrophage activation. Finally, cytokines are also responsible for the demise of the

Table 1-4. Cytokines

Cytokines released by the RES, early in the response

IL-1	Two proteins, IL-1 α and β, made as precursor proteins in macrophages and dendritic cells. Made also by some epithelial cells. Involved in the early inflammatory response. Induces fever.
TNFα	Involved in activation of many cells, including endothelial cells and macrophages. Can induce apoptosis of many cells, including tumors. Can induce vascular shock.
Interferon-α and -β	Type I interferons. Produced in many cells in response to viral infection. Antiviral effect. Enhance expression of class I MHC molecules.
IL-18	Produced by macrophages. Potentiates the response of NK cells and T cells to produce interferon-γ.
IL-12	Released by macrophages and dendritic cells in response to microbial challenge. Required for NK cells to produce IFN-γ and for T cells to differentiate to Th1 cells.
IL-6	Made by monocytes. Promotes B-cell differentiation and IgG production. Induces acute phase reactants from liver cells.
TGB-β	Made by macrophages, epithelial cells, and connective tissue cells. Inhibits proliferation of lymphocytes and macrophage activation.

Modulating cytokines primarily made by T cells

IL-2	Produced by T cells. A T-cell growth factor that promotes the replication of T cells.
IL-4	Produced by T cells. Promotes growth of T and B cells. Favors class switch in B cells, to IgE. Favors Th2 differentiation.
IL-5	Released by T cells. Promotes B-cell growth and IgA production. Enhances eosinophil differentiation.
IL-7	Produced by bone marrow stromal cells. Stimulates growth of early immature B and T cells.
IL-10	Made by macrophages and Th2 T cells. Inhibits macrophage activation; reduces IFN-γ, IL-1, and IL-6 production.
Interferon-γ	Made by T cells and NK cells. Constitutes the major cytokine that activates macrophages. Induces class II molecules in many cells. Promotes B-cell differentiation.
Colony stimulating factor (CSF)	Three distinct proteins: GE-CSF, which stimulates production of granulocytes and macrophages from stem cells; G-CSF, which stimulates granulocyte differentiation; and M-CSF, which stimulates monocyte differentiation.

This table considers a number of selected cytokines and is intended to illustrate the wide spectrum of action of this family of molecules.

---

response; the most prominent ones appear to be IL-10 and TGF beta (Table 1-4).

Following the phase of cellular growth and activation, the response to antigen subsides. It is vital to terminate the response and to control cellular activation: cytokines, cytocidal molecules, and activated macrophages and T cells are all highly inflammatory and can lead to pathology in the tissues, if not restricted both in their intensity and in time. Several components bring about the cooling of the response. First, there is the elimination of the stimulus for the response to continue, which is the antigen itself. For example, this happens, depending on the antigen in question, as macrophages get activated and become cytocidal for intracellular pathogens, or as neutrophils infiltrate and take up opsonized antigen, or as CD8 T cells kill the virally infected cells. The end result is that antigen is no longer found and antigen presentation ceases. At the same time, many of the expanded clones of lymphocytes die, and the response is markedly constricted (136). The death of these lymphocytes may be caused by several mechanisms. One involves the loss of any further stimulants, as growth factors and antigen become limiting (136). [Here the balance of intracellular proapoptotic and antiapoptotic molecules of the bcl-2 family becomes critical. The role of bcl-2 was actually discovered through the finding that overexpression in certain lymphomas led to B-cell growth and neoplasia (137,138).] However, a prominent cause of the demise of the lymphocyte is through activation-induced cell death, which decreases the number of lymphocytes to a nearly normal level (136,139). The actual mechanisms in vivo are not entirely elucidated at this point. One well-studied process involves the protein fas-ligand on T cells, expressed after TCR engagement (140). Interaction with fas also expressed on lymphocytes brings about the intracellular death program. The discovery of the fas pathway was brought about by the finding by Ed Murphy of the Jackson Laboratories with strains of mice in which the proteins were defective or absent (reviewed in 140). Such mice developed massive lymphadenopathy, as the cell death program was no longer operative (141). In association with the lymphocyte proliferation, autoantibodies developed. The fas pathway may be operative in eliminating cells that react to autoantigens. However, its role in reducing the normal response to antigen has not been established.

Two other factors bring about the control of the response by dampening cellular activation. Indeed, during cellular activation the T cell produces, in addition to CD28 as costimulator, a contrasting molecule, CTLA-4, that also binds to B7 (142). The result is the inhibition of the T cell. Thus, there is a balance between a positive and a negative regulatory protein, both reacting with the same ligand. Since CTLA-4 appears late in the activation of T cells, it serves then as a control mechanism, stopping activation. Genetic mutation of this molecule is also characterized by increased lymphocyte proliferation. Finally, the cytokines IL-10 and TGF beta participate in inhibiting macrophage activation.

B and T cells responsible for the memory or secondary response develop after the primary immunization. There has been much discussion on whether or not persistence of antigen is a requisite for maintenance of the memory response, the essence of prophylactic immunization (139,143,144). Recent studies tend to suggest that memory B and T cells do not need continuous stimulation by the original antigen. Memory cells do cycle, apparently spontaneously, and their numbers under physiological conditions—when antigen is not available—are controlled differently from that of naive T cells (112,139). Aside from the presence of lymphocytes with the memory property, plasma cells may survive for long periods, maintaining a titer of antibody for some time (145). Memory cells show markers of activation that are maintained (146).

Conclusion

We have considered general features of the adaptive response. Since the late 1960s, the field has been dominated by the analysis of the cellular response. (This followed a long period in which the analysis of the "humoral" or antibody response had become central.) Since the 1960s, we have seen notable advances in cellular biology, genetics, and molecular biology, including the manipulations of genes in mice. Immunology has now entered a new stage of research in which the emphasis is on the analysis of cellular and molecular mechanisms. How each cell responds and the signaling pathways that control the spectrum of cell responses will be major focuses of research for the immediate future. Signaling involves complex, apparently chaotic pathways of which the main components will need to be placed in the proper framework. The events following the engagement of TCR and BCR, and the cytokine receptors, the mechanisms of regulation of lymphocyte response in tissues, the nature of the death programs and of the activation, deletion, death, and anergy are the issues that will have to be sorted out in the future.

References

1. Unanue ER. The regulatory role of macrophages in antigenic stimulation. Part Two: Symbiotic relationship between lymphocytes and macrophages. Adv Immunol 1981;31:1–48.
2. Jenner E. An inquiry into the causes and effects of the variolae vaccinae, a disease discovered in some of the western countries of England, particularly Gloucestershire, and known by the name of the cow pox. Soho, London: Sampson Low, 1798.
3. Landsteiner K. The specificity of serological reactions. Rev. ed. Boston: Harvard University Press, 1945.
4. Sela M. Antigenicity: some molecular aspects. Science 1969;166:1365–1371.
5. Ehrlich P. The Croonian lecture: on immunity with special reference to cell life. Proc Roy Soc London (Biol) 1900;66:424–435.
6. Claman HN, Chaperon EA, Triplett RF. Thymus-marrow cell combinations. Synergism in antibody production. Proc Soc Exp Biol Med 1966;122:1167–1175.
7. Davies AJS, Leuchars E, Wallis V, et al. The failure of thymus-derived cells to produce antibody. Transplantation 1976;5:222–231.
8. Mitchell GM, Miller JFAP. Immunological activity of thymus and thoracic duct lymphocytes. Proc Natl Acad Sci USA 1968;59:296–302.
9. Jerne NK. The natural-selection theory of antibody formation. Proc Natl Acad Sci USA 1955;41:849–855.
10. Burnett FM. Modification of Jerne's theory of antibody production using the concept of clonal selection. Aust J Sci 1957;20:67–73.
11. Talmage DW. A century of progress: beyond molecular immunology. J Immunol 1988;141:S5–S16.
12. Siskind GW, Benacerraf B. Cell selection by antigen in the immune response. Adv Immunol 1969;10:1–14.
13. Pernis B, Forni L, Amante L. Immunoglobulin spots on the surface of rabbit lymphocytes. J Exp Med 1970;132:1001–1012.
14. Raff MC, Sternberg M, Taylor RB. Immunoglobulin determinants on the surface of mouse lymphoid cells. Nature 1970;225:553–559.
15. Vitetta ES, Baur S, Uhr JW. Cell surface immunoglobulin. II. Isolation and characterization of immunoglobulin from mouse splenic lymphocytes. J Exp Med 1971;134:242–250.
16. Rajewsky K. Clonal selection and learning in the antibody system. Nature 1996;381:751–758.
17. Behring E von, Kitasato S. Über das zustandekommen der diphtherie-immunität und der tetanus-immunität bei thieren. Dtsch Med Wochenschr 1890;16:1113–1133.
18. Edelman GM. Dissociation of γ-globulin. J Am Chem Soc 1959;81:3155–3166.
19. Porter RR. The hydrolysis of rabbit γ-globulin and antibodies with crystalline papain. Biochem J 1959;73:119–129.
20. Williams AF. A year in the life of the immunoglobulin superfamily. Immunol Today 1987;8:298–303.
21. Barclay AN. Ig-like domains: evolution from simple interaction molecules to sophisticated antigen recognition. Proc Natl Acad Sci USA 1999;96:14672–14674.
22. Frazer K, Capra JD. Immunoglobulins structure and function. In: Paul WE, ed. Fundamental immunology. 4th ed. New York: Raven Press, 1998.

23. Levine P. The protective action of ABO incompatibility on Rh isoimmunization and Rh hemolytic disease—theoretical and clinical implications. Am J Hum Genet 1959;11:418–429.
24. Kohler G, Milstein C. Continuous culture of fused cells secreting antibody of predefined specificity. Nature 1975; 256:495–501.
25. Hedrick SM, Nielsen EA, Kavaler J, et al. Sequence relationships between putative T-cell receptor polypeptides and immunoglobulins. Nature 1984;308:153–158.
26. Chien Y, Becker DM, Lindsten T, et al. A third type of murine T-cell receptor gene. Nature 1984;312:31–34.
27. Saito H, Kranz D, Takagai Y, et al. A third rearranged and expressed gene in a clone of cytotoxic T lymphocytes. Nature 1984;312:36–40.
28. Bernard O, Hozumi N, Tonegawa S. Sequences of mouse immunoglobulin light chain genes before and after somatic changes. Cell 1978;15:1133–1144.
29. Early P, Huang H, Davis M, et al. An immunoglobulin heavy chain variable region gene is generated from three segments of DNA: VH, D and JH. Cell 1980;19:981–990.
30. Seigman JG, Leder A, Nau M, et al. The structure of cloned immunoglobulin genes suggests a mechanism for generating new sequences. Science 1978;202:11–14.
31. Alt FW, Oltz EM, Young F, et al. VDJ recombination. Immunol Today 1992;13:306–314.
32. Schatz DG, Oettinger MA, Baltimore D. The V(D)J recombination activating gene (RAG-1). Cell 1989;59:1035–1048.
33. Eisen HN, Siskind GW. Variations in affinities of antibodies during the immune response. Biochem 1964;3:996–1006.
34. Weigert MG, Cesari IM, Yonkovich SJ, Cohn M. Variability in the lambda light chain sequences of mouse antibodies. Nature 1970;228:1045–1052.
35. Ziegler K, Unanue ER. Decrease in macrophage antigen catabolism by ammonia and chloroquine is associated with inhibition of antigen presentation to T cells. Proc Natl Acad Sci USA 1982;78:175–182.
36. Chase MW. The cellular transfer of cutaneous hypersensitivity to tuberculin. Proc Soc Exp Biol Med 1945;59:134–145.
37. Landsteiner K, Chase MW. Experiments on transfer of cutaneous sensitivity to simple compounds. Proc Soc Exp Biol Med 1942;49:688–675.
38. Babbitt BP, Allen PM, Matsueda G, et al. Binding of immunogenic peptides to Ia histocompatibility molecules. Nature 1985;317:359–364.
39. Garcia KC, Dagano M, Stanfield RL, et al. An αβ T cell receptor structure at 2.5A and its orientation in the TCR-MHC complex. Science 1996;274:209–219.
40. Garcia KC, Teyton L, Wilson IA. Structural basis of T cell recognition. Ann Rev Immunol 1999;17:369–397.
41. Reinherz EL, Tan K, Tang L, et al. The crystal structure of a T cell receptor in complex with peptide and MHC class II. Science 1999;286:1913–1921.
42. Katz DH, Hamaoka T, Dorf ME, et al. Cell interactions between histoincompatible T and B lymphocytes. IV. Involvement of immune response (Ir) gene control of lymphocyte interaction controlled by the gene. J Exp Med 1973;138:734–745.
43. Zinkernagel RM, Doherty PC. Activity of sensitized thymus-derived lymphocytes in lymphocytic choriomeningitis reflects immunological surveillance against altered self components. Nature 1974;251:547–552.
44. Zinkernagel RM, Doherty PC. Restriction of in vitro T cell-mediated cytotoxicity in lymphocytic choriomeningitis within a syngeneic or semiallogeneic system. Nature 1974; 248:701–706.
45. Rosenthal AS, Shevach EM. Function of macrophages in antigen recognition by guinea pig T lymphocytes. I. Requirement for histocompatibility macrophages and lymphocytes. J Exp Med 1973;138:1194–1201.
46. Klein J, Takahata N. The major histocompatibility complex and the quest for origins. Immunol Rev 1990; 113:5–14.
47. Klein J, Satta Y, O'hUigin C. The molecular descent of the major histocompatibility complex. Ann Rev Immunol 1993; 11:269–283.
48. Dausset J. Leuco-agglutinins. Vox Sang 1954;6:190–210.
49. Rood JJ van, Eernisse JG, van Leeuwen A. Leukocyte antibodies in sera from pregnant women. Nature 1958;181: 1735–1741.
50. Gorer PA. The detection of antigenic differences in mouse erythrocytes by the employment of immune sera. Br J Exp Pathol 1936:17:42–55.
51. Snell GD. Methods for the study of histocompatibility genes. J Genet 1948:49:87–98.
52. Benacerraf B, McDevitt HO. Histocompatibility-linked immune response genes. Science 1972;175:273–285.
53. McDevitt HO, Sela M. Genetic control of the antibody response. I. Demonstration of determinant-specific differences in response to synthetic polypeptide antigens in two strains of inbred mice. J Exp Med 1965;122:517–529.
54. McDevitt HO, Chinitz A. Genetic control of the antibody response: relationship between immune response and histocompatibility (H-2) type. Science 1969;163:1207–1215.
55. Benacerraf B. Role of MHC gene products in immune regulation. Science 1981;212:1229–1237.
56. Allen PM, Murphy KM, Schreiber RD, Unanue ER. Immunology at 2000. Immunity 1999;11:649–651.
57. Campbell RD, Trowsdale J. A map of the major histocompatibility complex. Immunol Today 1997;18:43–58.
58. Parham P. Virtual reality in the MHC. Immunol Rev 1999; 167:5–15.
59. Beck S, Trowsdale J. Sequence organization of the class II region of the human MHC. Immunol Rev 1999;167:201–210.
60. MHC Sequencing Consortium. Complete sequence and gene map of the human major histocompatibility complex. Nature 1999;401:921–923.
61. Bjorkman PJ, Saper B, Samraoui B, et al. The foreign antigen binding site and T cell recognition regions of class I histocompatibility regions. Nature 1987;329:512–520.
62. Stern L, Brown G, Jardetsky T, et al. Crystal structure of the human class II MHC protein HLA-DR1 complexed with an antigenic peptide from influenza virus. Nature 1994;368: 215–222.
63. Babbitt BP, Matsueda G, Haber E, et al. Antigenic competition at the level of peptide-Ia binding. Proc Natl Acad Sci USA 1986;83:4509–4513.
64. Falk K, Rötzschke O, Rammensee H-G. Cellular peptide composition governed by major histocompatibility complex class I molecules. Nature 1990;348:248–251.
65. Chicz RM, Urban RG, Lane WS, et al. Predominant naturally processed peptides bound to HLA-DR1 are derived

from MHC-related molecules and are heterogeneous in size. Nature 1992;358:764–768.

66. Hunt DF, Henderson RA, Shabanowitz J, et al. Characterization of peptides bound to the class I MHC molecule HLA-A2.1 by mass spectrometry. Science 1992;255:1261–1263.

67. Todd JA, Bell JI, McDevitt HO. HLA-DQ β gene contributes to susceptibility and resistance to insulin-dependent diabetes mellitus. Nature 1987;329:599–604.

68. Matsumura M, Fremont DH, Peterson DA, Wilson IA. Emerging principles for the recognition of peptide antigens by MHC class I molecules. Science 1992;257:927–934.

69. Unanue ER. Chemical features of peptide selection by the class II histocompatibility molecules. Am J Path 1999;154:651–664.

70. Fremont DH, Hendrickson WA, Marrack P, Kappler JW. Structures of an MHC class II molecule with covalently bound single peptides. Science 1996;272:1001–1004.

71. Dessen A, Lawrence CM, Cupo S, et al. X-ray crystal structure of HLA-DR4 (DRA*0101, DRB1*0401) complexed with a peptide from human collagen II. Immunity 1997;7:473–481.

72. Rötzschke O, Falk K. Origin, structure and motifs of naturally processed MHC class II ligands. Curr Opin Immunol 1994;6:45–51.

73. Townsend ARM, Rothbard J, Gotch FM, et al. The epitopes of influenza nucleoprotein recognized by cytotoxic T lymphocytes can be defined with short synthetic peptides. Cell 1986;44:959–968.

74. Pamer E, Cresswell P. Mechanisms of MHC class I-restricted antigen processing. Ann Rev Immunol 1998;16:323–358.

75. Sadasivan B, Lehner P, Ortman B, et al. Roles for calreticulin and a novel glycoprotein, tapasin, in the interaction of MHC class I molecules with TAP. Immunity 1996;5:103–114.

76. Klenerman P, Zinkernagel R. What can we learn about human immunodeficiency virus infection from a study of lymphocytic choriomeningitis virus? Immunol Rev 1997;159:5–17.

77. Parham P, ed. Anti viral immunity. Immunol Rev 1997;159:5–178.

78. Parham P, ed. Pathways of antigen processing and presentation. Immunol Rev 1999;172:5–336.

79. Banchereau J, Steinman RM. Dendritic cells and the control of immunity. Nature 1998;392:245–252.

80. Inaba K, Steinman RM, Van Voorhis WC, Muramatsu S. Dendritic cells are crucial accessory cells for thymus-dependent antibody responses in mouse and man. Proc Natl Acad Sci USA 1983;80:6041–6045.

81. MacLennan ICM, Gulbrandson-Judge A, Toellner KM, et al. The changing preference of T and B cells for partners as T-dependent antibody responses develop. Immunol Rev 1997;156:53–66.

82. Lederberg J. Genes and antibodies. Science 1959;129:1649–1653.

83. Hengartner H, Odermatt B, Schneider R, et al. Deletion of self-reactive T cells before entry into the thymus medulla. Nature 1988;336:388–395.

84. Kappler JW, Roehm N, Marrack P. T cell tolerance by clonal elimination in the thymus. Cell 1987;49:273–381.

85. Kisielow P, Bluthman H, Staerz UD, et al. Tolerance in T cell receptor transgenic mice involves deletion of nonmature CD4⁺8⁺ thymocytes. Nature 1988;333:742–749.

86. Nemazee D, Burki K. Clonal deletion of B lymphocytes in a transgenic mouse bearing anti-MHC class I antibody genes. Nature 1989;337:562–571.

87. Goodnow CG, Crosbie J, Jorgensen H, et al. Induction of self-tolerance in mature peripheral B lymphocytes. Nature 1989;342:385–392.

88. Miller JFAP. Immunological function of the thymus. Lancet 1961;2:748–760.

89. Miller JFAP. Effect of thymectomy on the immunological responsiveness of the mouse. Proc Roy Soc London Ser B 1962;156:415–422.

90. Glick B, Chang TS, Jaap RG. The bursa of Fabricius and antibody production. Poultry Sci 1956;35:224–234.

91. Warner NL, Szenberg A, Burnet FM. The immunological role of different lymphoid organs in the chicken. I. Dissociation of immunological responsiveness. Aust J Exp Biol Med Sci 1962;40:373–388.

92. Zerratin J, Held W, Raulet DH. The MHC reactivity of the T cell repertoire prior to positive and negative selection. Cell 1997;88:627–636.

93. Merkenschlager M, Graf D, Lovatt M, et al. How many thymocytes audition for selection? J Exp Med 1997;186:1149–1158.

94. Jamieson SC, Bevan M. T cell selection. Curr Opin Immunol 1998;10:214–219.

95. Bevan MJ. In thymic selection, peptide diversity gives and takes away. Immunity 1997;7:175–178.

96. Billingham RE, Brent L, Medawar PB. Actively acquired tolerance of foreign cells. Nature 1953;172:603–608.

97. Owen RD. Immunogenetic consequences of vascular anastomoses between bovine twins. Science 1945;102:400–409.

98. Chen C, Prak EL, Weigert M. Editing disease-associated autoantibodies. Immunity 1997;6:97–105.

99. Melamed D, Nemazee D. Self-antigen does not accelerate immature B cell apoptosis, but stimulates receptor editing as a consequence of development arrest. Proc Natl Acad Sci USA 1997;94:9267–9272.

100. Peterson DA, DiPaolo RJ, Kanagawa O, Unanue ER. Negative selection of immature thymocytes by a few peptide-MHC complexes: differential sensitivity of immature and mature T cells. J Immunol 1999;162:3117–3120.

101. Gowans JL, Knight EJ. The route of recirculation of lymphocytes in the rat. Proc Roy Soc Series B 1964;159:257–270.

102. Gowans JL. The recirculation of lymphocytes from blood to lymph in the rat. J Physiol 1959;14:654–662.

103. Butcher EC. Leukocyte-endothelial cell recognition: three (or more) steps to specificity and diversity. Cell 1991;67:1033–1037.

104. Springer TA. Traffic signals for lymphocyte recirculation and leukocyte emigration: the multistep paradigm. Cell 1994;76:301–314.

105. Siegelman MH, van de Rijn M, Weissman IL. Mouse lymph node homing receptor cDNA clone encodes a glycoprotein revealing tandem interaction domains. Science 1989;243:1165–1172.

106. Hynes RO. Integrins: versatility, modulation and signaling in cell adhesion. Cell 1992;69:11–25.

107. Kurzinger K, Springer TA. Purification and structural characterization of LFA-1, a lymphocyte function-associated

antigen, and Mac-1, a related macrophage differentiation antigen associated with the type three complement receptor. J Biol Chem 1982;257:12412–12418.

108. Baggiolini M. Chemokines and leukocyte traffic. Nature 1998;392:565–568.
109. Gunn MD, Tangemann K, Tam C, et al. A chemokine expressed in lymphoid high endothelial venules promotes the adhesion and chemotaxis of naive T lymphocytes. Proc Natl Acad Sci USA 1995;95:258–263.
110. Gunn MD, Ngo VN, Ansel KM, et al. A B cell-homing chemokine made in lymphoid follicles activates Burkitt's lymphoma receptor-1. Nature 1998;391:799–803.
111. Ngo VN, Tang HL, Cyster JG. Epstein-Barr virus-induced molecule 1 ligand chemokine is expressed by dendritic cells and strongly attracts naive T cells and activated B cells. J Exp Med 1998;188:181–191.
112. Freitas AA, Rocha B. Peripheral T cell survival. Curr Opin Immunol 1999;11:152–156.
113. Kitamura D, Roes J, Kuhn R, Rajewsky K. A B cell deficient mouse by targeted disruption of the membrane exon of the immunoglobulin mu chain gene. Nature 1991;350:423–426.
114. Tanchot C, Lemonnier FA, Perarnau B, et al. Differential requirements for survival and proliferation of CD8 naive or memory T cells. Science 1997;276:2057–2062.
115. Bluestone JA. New perspectives of CD28-B7-mediated T cell costimulation. Immunity 1995;2:739–745.
116. Lenshow DJ, Walunas TL, Bluestone JA. CD28/B7 system of T cell costimulation. Ann Rev Immunol 1996;14:233–258.
117. Merwe PA van der. A subtle role for CD2 in T cell antigen recognition. J Exp Med 1999;190:1371–1374.
118. Ramesh N, Fuleihan R, Geha R. Molecular pathology of x-linked immunoglobulin deficiency with normal or elevated IgM. Immunol Rev 1994;138:87–104.
119. Grewal IS, Flavell RA. CD40 and CD154 in cell-mediated immunity. Ann Rev Immunol 1998;16:111–136.
120. Jenkins MK, Schwartz RH. Antigen presentation by chemically modified splenocytes induces antigen-specific T cell unresponsiveness *in vitro* and *in vivo*. J Exp Med 1997;165:302–319.
121. Bretscher P, Cohn M. A theory of self-nonself discrimination: paralysis and induction involve the recognition of one and two determinants on an antigen, respectively. Science 1970;169:1042–1049.
122. Burkly LC, Lo D, Kanagawa O, et al. T cell tolerance by clonal anergy in transgenic mice with nonlymphoid expression of MHC class II I-E. Nature 1989;342:564–566.
123. Morahan G, Allison J, Miller JF. Tolerance of class I histocompatibility antigen expressed extrathymically. Nature 1989;339:622–624.
124. Harding FA, McArthur JG, Gross JA, et al. CD28-mediated signalling co-stimulates murine T cell and prevents induction of anergy in T cell clones. Nature 1992;356:607–609.
125. Altman JD, Moss PAH, Goulder PJR, et al. Phenotypic analysis of antigen specific T lymphocytes. Science 1996;274:94–96.
126. Murali-Krishna K, Altman JD, Suresh M, et al. Counting antigen specific CD8 T cells: a reevaluation of bystander activation during viral infection. Immunity 1998;8:177–187.

127. Butz EA, Bevan MJ. Massive expansion of antigen-specific CD8+ T cells during an acute virus infection. Immunity 1988;8:167–175.
128. Leevwen JEM van, Samelson LE. T cell antigen receptor signal transduction. Curr Opin Immunol 1999;11:242–248.
129. Mosman TR, Cherwinski H, Bond M, et al. Two types of murine helper T cell clones. 1. Definition according to profiles of lymphokine activities and secreted proteins. J Immunol 1986;136:2348–2359.
130. Abbas AK, Murphy KM. Functional diversity of helper T lymphocytes. Nature 1996;383:787–793.
131. Hsieh CS, Macatonia SE, Tripp CS, et al. Development of TH1 CD4+ T cells through IL-12 produced by *Listeria*-induced macrophages. Science 1993;260:547–549.
132. Swain SL, Weinberg AD, English M, Huston G. IL-4 directs the development of Th2-like helper effectors. J Immunol 1990;145:3796–3806.
133. Locksley R, Heinzel F, Holaday B, et al. Induction of Th1 and Th2 CD4 subsets during murine L. major infection. Res Immunol 1991;142:2832–2875.
134. Yamamura M, Uyemura K, Deans RJ, et al. Defining protective responses to pathogens—cytokine profiles in leprosy lesions. Science 1992;254:277–285.
135. Wallach D, Varfolomeev EE, Malinin NL, et al. Tumor necrosis factor receptor and fas signaling mechanism. Ann Rev Immunol 1999;17:331–367.
136. Abbas AK, van Parijs L. Maintaining homeostasis in the immune system: turning lymphocytes off. Science 1998;280:243–251.
137. Vaux DL, Cory S, Adams JM. Bcl-2 gene promotes hemopoietic cell survival and cooperates with c-myc to immortalize pre-B cells. Nature 1988;335:440–445.
138. Nunez G, London L, Hockenbery D, et al. Deregulated bcl-2 gene expression selectively prolongs survival of growth factor-deprived hemopoietic cell lines. J Immunol 1990;144:3602–3611.
139. Goodrath AW, Bevan MJ. Selecting and maintaining a diverse T cell repertoire. Nature 1999;402:255–262.
140. Cohen PL, Eisenberg RA. Lpr and gld: single gene models of systemic autoimmunity and lymphoproliferative disease. Ann Rev Immunol 1991;9:243–269.
141. Watanabe-Fukunaga R, Brannan CI, Copeland NG, et al. Lymphoproliferation disorder in mice explained by defects in fas antigen that mediates apoptosis. Nature 1992;356:314–319.
142. Thompson CB, Allison JP. The emerging role of CTLA-4 as an immune attenuator. Immunity 1997;7:445–460.
143. Lau LL, Jamieson BD, Somasundaran T, Ahmed R. Cytotoxic T-cell memory without antigen. Nature 1994;369:648–652.
144. Mullbacher A. The long term maintenance of cytotoxic T-cell memory without antigen. J Exp Med 1994;179:317–321.
145. Slitka MK, Ahmed R. Long-lived plasma cells: a mechanism for maintaining persistent antibody production. Curr Opin Immunol 1998;10:252–258.
146. Budd RC, Cerottini J-C, Horvath C, et al. Distinction of virgin and memory T lymphocytes. J Immunol 1987;138:3120–3129.

Chapter 2

Innate Immunity and Instruction of the Adaptive Immune Response

Douglas T. Fearon

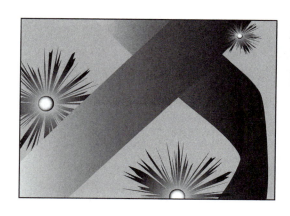

Innate immunity is an immense topic. It includes all the cellular and humoral elements of recognition and killing of microorganisms that are available to invertebrate and vertebrate species and that are not mediated by B and T lymphocytes. Rather than presenting all of these systems, this chapter will focus on that aspect of innate immunity unique to vertebrates: the capacity of innate immune systems for instructing the adaptive immune response. Until the past 3 to 4 years immunologists had not considered an integrated immune response because their principal interests were usually directed toward either innate or adaptive immunity but not both. With the conceptual integration of these two systems has come a better understanding of how the adaptive immune response can be regulated by phylogenetically ancient systems (1–4). This new understanding offers potential for therapeutic approaches to modifying responses to microbial antigens in infectious diseases. Readers who are interested in other antimicrobial functions of innate immune systems that are unrelated to its instructive role in the adaptive immune response are referred to several excellent reviews (5–7).

Definition and Background

Two general systems of immunity to infections have developed during the evolution of multicellular organisms: innate (natural) and adaptive (acquired). The phylogenetically older system, innate immunity, is that form of resistance to infection that does not require prior exposure to the infectious organism for an antimicrobial response. Adaptive immunity, which did not appear until approximately 400 million years ago with the evolution of cartilaginous fish, is found only in vertebrates. The essential difference between the two systems is that the receptors of innate immunity (Table 2-1) are encoded in the germ line, whereas those of adaptive immunity, the antigen receptors of B and T lymphocytes, are encoded by somatically rearranging genes. This distinction indicates that only the receptors of innate immune systems can reflect evolutionary selection for an ability to recognize microbial determinants. The determinants that have been selected for recognition are usually carbohydrate or a complex of carbohydrate and lipid. Presumably, these determinants have been chosen for recognition by innate immune receptors because they must be conserved to maintain viability or infectivity of the microorganism. In essence, recognition of microbial determinants

by innate immune systems is based on the biologic association of infectivity with these determinants.

The shortcoming of this strategy of innate immunity is that relatively few microbial structures can be recognized because insufficient space exists in the genome to encode all possible receptors. Even if there were genetic space, many microbial structures can mutate without deleterious functional consequences and alter recognition by host receptors. Mutants would be selected at a rate that exceeded compensatory mutation and selection of new receptors encoded in the host germ line, leading to microbial escape. It is precisely this limitation of innate immunity that has been overcome by adaptive immunity. As reviewed in Chapter 1, receptor genes are assembled through a process of somatic rearrangement and recombination of two or three separate genetic segments—the V, (D), and J segments of the antibody and T-cell receptor genes. The presence of multiple copies of each of these segments, each copy with a unique sequence, and the imprecise nature of the joining process itself, which allows the addition and subtraction of nucleotides, ensure an almost limitless variety of potential antigen receptors. Each lymphocyte clone expresses its own unique receptor, and the immune response then involves the growth and activation of those clones possessing receptors that bind microbial antigens. When viewed in this perspective, adaptive immunity can be seen to be a form of evolutionary selection on the "fast track," occurring in a few days rather than in thousands of years.

In adopting this clever strategy, however, adaptive immunity sacrificed its connection to the germ line and, therefore, to any inherited ability to recognize microbial determinants. Possible exceptions to this loss of evolutionary linkage may be those V regions of antibody and T-cell receptors that carry microbial recognition functions in complementarity-determining regions (CDRs) 1 and 2. As these regions are in the germ line, in contrast to CDR-3, they may have been selected to enable some lymphocyte clones to recognize preferentially microbial determinants. Examples of such lymphocytes may be the B-1 cells that produce most of the serum IgM, and natural killer (NK) 1.1$^+$ αβ T cells that express an invariant α chain and secrete large amounts of cytokines. Nevertheless, other than a few examples such as these, antigen receptors of a naïve, unprimed, adaptive immune system have no ability to distinguish nonmicrobial antigens from other nonself structures. They have a remarkable ability to recognize many structures, but they have achieved this capability at the cost of biologic recognition.

Table 2-1. The Major Recognition Proteins of the Innate Immune System as Extracellular and Cellular Receptors

Molecule	Structure	Location	Ligands	Function
		Humoral Receptors		
C-reactive protein	Pentraxin; Ca²⁺-dependent lectin	Primary synthesis in liver; part of acute-phase response	Microbial polysaccharides	Activates complement; enhances phagocytosis
Serum amyloid protein	Pentraxin; Ca²⁺-dependent lectin	Primary synthesis in liver, acute-phase response	Extracellular matrix proteins; microbial cell-wall carbohydrates	Enhances phagocytosis; stabilizes extracellular matrix proteins
Mannan-binding protein	Collectin, contains 18 CRDs per molecule on helical collagenous domains	Primary synthesis in liver; normal levels vary with allelic variants; up to 10µg/mL	Microbial cell-wall saccharides	Binds collectin (C1q) receptor; activates complement; promotes phagocytosis; modulates CD14-induced cytokine production
LPS-binding protein	Lipid transferase	Primary synthesis in liver; normal Levels <0.5µg/mL, increase to 50 µg/mL with acute-phase response	Catalytically transferred LPS to CD 14 and from CD14 to serum lipoproteins	Enhances sensitivity to LPS; system for inactivating LPS
C3	Disulfide-linked dimer	Primary synthesis in liver; normal levels 1 mg/mL; induced by acute-phase response	Forms ester linkage to OH- groups on carbohydrates and proteins	Attachment of ligand for receptors such as CD21 and CD35
Mannose receptors:				
Macrophage mannose receptor	8 CRDs	Tissue macrophages; hepatic endothelial cells; dendritic cells; thymic epithelium	Multiple carbohydrates	Potentially targets antigens to class II–loading compartment
DEC-205	Mannose-type receptor; 10 CRDs	Dendritic cells; thymic epithelium	Multiple carbohydrates	Potentially targets class II–loading compartment
Scavenger receptors:				
Type I	Type II trimeric transmembrane protein with helical collagenous stalk domain and terminal SRCR domain	Tissue macrophages: hepatic endothelial cells; high endothelial venules	Bacterial and yeast cell walls	Clearance of LPS and microbes; adhesion
Type II	Alternatively spliced form missing the terminal SRCR domain			
MARCO	Extended form resembling type I	Marginal zone of spleen; medullary lymph node; macrophages	Bacterial cell walls	Bacterial clearance
CD14	Lipid-anchored glycoprotein; leucine-rich protein	Monocyte-macrophages; PMNs	LPS; numerous microbial cell-wall components	LPS sensitivity; clearance of microbes; proinflammatory cytokine induction
Toll-like receptors	Drosophila Toll homolog	Monocyte-macrophages		Macrophage activation
CD35 (CR1)	30 SCRs	Monocyte-macrophages; PMNs; lymphocytes	LPS-CD14 complexes? C3b; C4b	Enhances C3b and C4b cleavage
CD21 (CR2)	15 SCRs	B lymphocytes; follicular dendritic cells	IC3d; C3dg; C3d	Augments B-cell activation
CD11b, CD18(CR3)	Integrin	Monocyte-macrophages; PMNs; NK cells	IC3b; LPS fibrinogen	Adhesion; LPS clearance

Abbreviations: CRD, Ca2+-dependent carbohydrate recognition domain; LPS, lipopolysaccharide; PMN, polymorphonuclear leukocyte; SRCR, scavenger receptor cysteine-rich; SCR, short consensus repeat; NK, natural killer

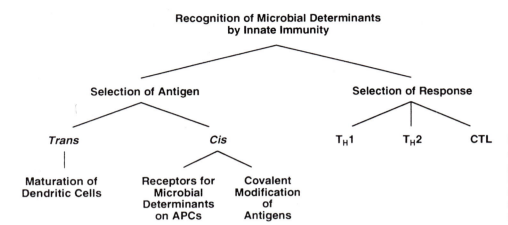

Figure 2-1. Recognition of microbial determinants by innate immunity guides the adaptive immune response, influencing the selection of antigen and the nature of the adaptive response. APC, antigen-presenting cell; CTL, cytotoxic T lymphocyte.

Vertebrates, therefore, possess two immune systems with different but complementary attributes. Innate immunity can recognize a relatively limited number of structures that have the biologic association of "infectious" organisms, and adaptive immunity can distinguish an almost unlimited number of structures, but without any preference for those that may be associated with infectious organisms. In an ideal immune response, these two systems would be integrated. Indeed, we now recognize that molecular pathways exist that transmit information from innate to adaptive immunity to allow the biologic recognition of microbial determinants by the former to guide the responses of the latter. Guidance refers to the selection of both the antigen and the type of adaptive immune response (Fig. 2-1). This function of innate immunity is critical during the first interaction of the naïve host with microbial antigens. Thereafter, the establishment of "immunologic memory" through the clonal expansion of lymphocytes that are specific for microbial antigens lessens the need for this function of innate immunity. Analysis of the collaborative interaction that occurs between innate and adaptive immune systems during primary immune responses is the focus of this chapter.

Receptors of Innate Immunity: Targeting and Signaling

Receptors of innate immune systems have two general functions with respect to modifying the adaptive immune response: targeting antigens to cells with immunologic functions and triggering the immunologic functions of these cells. Accordingly, receptors that mediate endocytosis such as mannose receptors, the various types of scavenger receptors, and some of the complement receptors (see Table 2-1) may have evolved in invertebrates for the purpose of clearing microbial products. However, in vertebrates these receptors have the additional function of capturing antigens for presentation to T cells. For example, the mannose receptor on macrophages mediates the uptake of mycobacterial lipoglycan lipoarabinomannan for delivery to the compartment for MHC

class II antigen loading onto CD1b molecules and subsequent presentation to T cells (8). This selection by innate immunity of those antigens with microbial determinants gives an "infectious" bias to the repertoire of antigens that are presented to the adaptive immune system.

The capacity of innate immune receptors to announce the presence of an infectious process by inducing signals in cells with immunologic functions has been inferred from the potent biologic effects of certain microbial products such as bacterial lipopolysaccharide (LPS). To the clinician, LPS represents a potential cause of mortality and morbidity because it induces gram-negative bacteremic shock, but this function is an exaggeration of an immunologically important host response to this microbial determinant. LPS induces the secretion by macrophages of cytokines such as interleukin (IL)-1, IL-12, tumor necrosis factor (TNF), and lymphotoxin that, when locally produced at the site of infection rather than systemically as in endotoxic shock, enhance the functions of macrophages and NK cells and promote the development of T_H1 cells (see below). These and other cellular responses to LPS have indicated the existence of a receptor-mediated signaling system that promotes communication between innate and adaptive systems of immunity, the molecular identification of which has remained elusive until recently.

The importance of gram-negative bacteria as pathogens has caused the evolution of a complex system for the recognition of LPS that involves at least three components: a soluble, LPS-binding protein; CD14, a membrane protein of macrophages that has an extracellular domain comprised of leucine-rich repeats, a characteristic of many receptors of innate immunity, and a glycophosphatidylinositol (GPI) tail for anchoring the protein to the plasma membrane; and one or more members of the recently identified family of Toll-like receptors (TLRs) (9–13). LPS-binding protein is a plasma protein lipid transferase that binds LPS and transfers it to CD14 on cells of the myelomonocytic lineage. However, CD14 does not activate the cells, presumably because its GPI-anchor cannot transduce signals. Rather, signaling is dependent on a third component, which genetic and biochemical studies have recently identified as one or more members of the TLR family.

The background to this important discovery begins with Drosophila in which Toll is a receptor that mediates both development and host resistance. Toll signals through a transduction pathway similar to that involved in plant resistance to infection and in IL-1 receptor (IL-1R) signaling, indicating a remarkable level of conservation of this pathway. A human homolog of Toll was then discovered that, when expressed in macrophages, induced the secretion of inflammatory cytokines and the upregulation of the membrane proteins B7.1 (CD80) and B7.2 (CD86), that engage CD28, the coreceptor of T cells (10). This seminal finding has been amplified by subsequent discoveries of a family of mammalian TLRs (TLR1-5) (11) and their role in responses to LPS (12,13).

Analysis of the C3H/Hej mouse strain that is resistant to bacterial endotoxin uncovered a missense mutation in the *Tlr4* gene that causes a substitution of histidine for proline at position 712 in the cytoplasmic domain. Macrophages from a separate mouse strain, C57BL/10ScCr, that also is unresponsive to LPS was found not to have mRNA for TLR4, further supporting a role for TLR4 in mediating responses to LPS in the mouse. However, biochemical studies examining the ability of recombinant TLRs to mediate cellular responses to LPS in vitro have suggested that TLR2, but not TLR4, has this function. Furthermore, TLR2 required CD14 for its functions, apparently because the receptor interacts weakly, if at all, with LPS. Thus, it is envisioned that CD14 captures LPS from the LPS-binding protein–LPS complex and then interacts with TLR2 to induce transmembrane signaling. Signaling by TLR2 requires a region in the cytoplasmic domain that is homologous to the IL-1 receptor (IL-1R) and is involved with the activation of the IL-1R–associated kinase. Consistent with this observation is the finding that a human TLR also uses MyD88, a cytosolic adaptor protein involved in IL-1R signaling, to induce nuclear translocation of nuclear factor κB (NFκB) (14). Thus, TLR2 and TLR4 confer some, and possibly all, innate immune responses to LPS. The apparently discordant conclusions of the relative roles of these two receptors must indicate that additional components of these systems remain to be identified. One anticipates that other members of the TLR family may have roles in responses to other microbial determinants. It is relevant to note that the transcription factor, NFκB, and its homologs are activated by IL-1R/Toll-type receptors in plants, Drosophila, and mammals, indicating that this mechanism for regulating the expression of genes involved inflammation and immunity has been conserved through evolution (15).

The Maturation of Dendritic Cells by Innate Immunity: *Trans* Regulation of Antigen Selection

There are two general means by which innate immune recognition of microbial antigens can target these antigens for an adaptive immune response, *trans* and *cis* (see Fig. 2-1). These terms refer to innate immune recognition affecting the immunogenicity of only those antigens carrying a determinant, a *cis* effect, or

altering the adaptive immune response to other, non–physically associated antigens that happen to be in the same microenvironment of a microbial product, which would indicate a *trans* mechanism. Dendritic cells represent the most striking example of the *trans* effect of innate immunity.

The activation of unprimed T cells requires that antigen be presented by dendritic cells. These cells of hematopoietic origin have two major phases in their development: first, the immature phase, characterized by the uptake of potential antigens, and second, the mature phase, characterized by the presentation of antigen to T cells (Fig. 2-2) (16). Immature dendritic cells reside in nonlymphoid tissues, primarily epithelial, where they may be known by other names such as the Langerhans cells of the skin. In these locations they are endocytically active, both by macropinocytosis and adsorptive, receptor-mediated endocytosis, and they continuously sample their microenvironment for potential antigens. However, as long as the dendritic cells remain

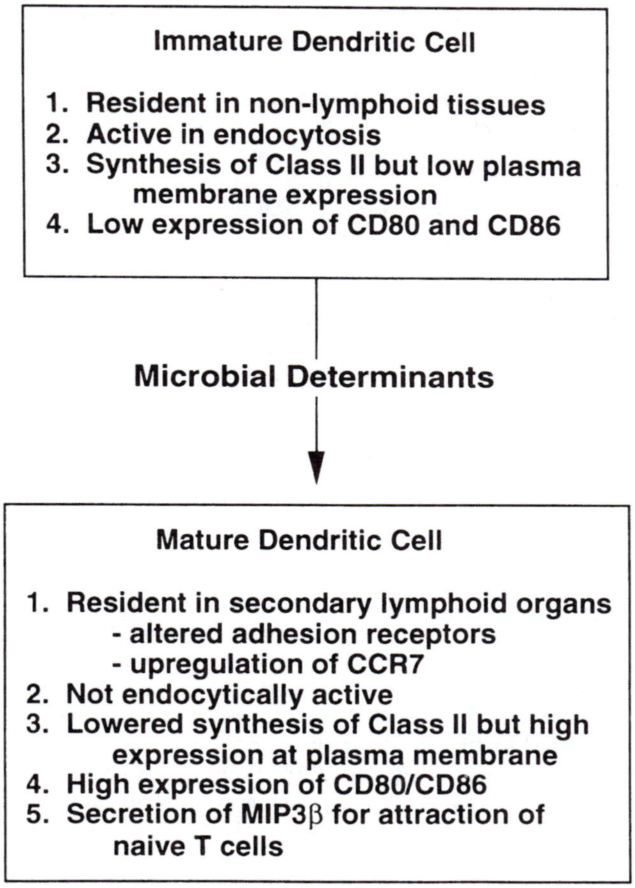

Immature Dendritic Cell

1. **Resident in non-lymphoid tissues**
2. **Active in endocytosis**
3. **Synthesis of Class II but low plasma membrane expression**
4. **Low expression of CD80 and CD86**

↓ **Microbial Determinants**

Mature Dendritic Cell

1. **Resident in secondary lymphoid organs**
   - **altered adhesion receptors**
   - **upregulation of CCR7**
2. **Not endocytically active**
3. **Lowered synthesis of Class II but high expression at plasma membrane**
4. **High expression of CD80/CD86**
5. **Secretion of MIP3β for attraction of naive T cells**

Figure 2-2. Microbial determinants induce the maturation of dendritic cells, changing their function from that of antigen uptake in peripheral tissues to antigen presentation in secondary lymphoid organs. CCR7, Epstein-Barr virus–induced molecule 1; MIP-3β, macrophage inflammatory protein-3β.

immature, such sampling is biologically meaningless because at this stage of development they do not make antigens available for presentation to T cells. Their newly synthesized MHC class II complexes do not traffic to the intracellular sites where the internalized proteins are degraded to peptides, and they are restricted from moving to the plasma membrane (17). Dendritic cells also express low levels of the costimulatory proteins, CD80 and CD86, and they remain in peripheral sites away from naïve T lymphocytes.

Dendritic cells mature and acquire antigen-presenting function when they interact with microbial products such as LPS or unmethylated CpG dinucleotides of bacterial origin, or with the cytokines, TNF-α and IL-1, that are made in response to microbial products. The molecular correlates of this maturational process are many. Newly synthesized class II complexes now intersect with a post-Golgi, vesicular site into which are delivered peptides that have been generated by the breakdown of proteins present in endosomal compartments, including those inhabited by certain intracellular parasites and mycobacteria. Following HLA-DM–mediated dissociation of the CLIP peptide of the invariant chain, the class II complexes take up these peptides. The fully assembled class II-peptide complexes then move to the plasma membrane where they can stimulate T cells. Mature dendritic cells also increase their biosynthesis and expression of CD80 and CD86 to ligate CD28 and provide the necessary costimulatory signals, and they down-regulate their expression of adhesion proteins such as E-cadherin (18) on Langerhans cells, to enable them to leave the periphery. In this coordinated response, the maturing dendritic cells also augment their complement of chemokine receptors, inducing the expression of CCR7 (Epstein-Barr virus–induced molecule 1), so that they can respond to the chemokine, macrophage inflammatory protein-3β (MIP-3β), that is produced in secondary lymphoid organs (19–22). Mature dendritic cells in the lymph node also express MIP-3β to mediate the attraction of naïve T lymphocytes. Finally, terminally differentiated dendritic cells turn off their endocytic activity and MHC class II synthesis so that they can reflect the antigenic repertoire of the peripheral antigenic microenvironment from which they migrated.

This maturational process of dendritic cells biases the pool of antigens that is presented to T lymphocytes toward a microbial origin because it is triggered directly or indirectly by microbial products. A microenvironment containing LPS, for example, is likely also to contain other microbial antigens suitable for processing and presentation to T lymphocytes. The process is not perfectly discriminating, however, since host antigens that are in the microenvironment of the immature dendritic cell at the time of microbial stimulation also will be taken up by dendritic cells and offered to T cells. Therefore, the *trans* effect of this mechanism of innate immunity for selecting antigens may contribute to autoimmunity. Examples of autoimmunity resulting from microbial determinants inducing responses to self-antigens by activation of dendritic cells may be diseases in which there is a link between infection and autoimmunity, such as reactive arthritis, and those in which complete Freund's adjuvant promotes vigorous immune responses to coadministered self-antigens.

Cis Regulation of Antigen Selection by Innate Immunity

Receptors for Microbial Determinants on Cells with Antigen-Presenting Function

Innate immunity has a more discriminating means by which it can select antigens for adaptive immune responses that are termed *cis*. The *cis* regulatory mechanisms are accomplished in two ways: 1) by receptors that are specific for certain microbial determinants and mediate the binding and uptake of their microbial ligands, and 2) by reactions that covalently modify antigens to "tag" them for adaptive immune recognition (see Fig. 2-2). The first mechanism involves both soluble and cell-associated carbohydrate binding proteins such as C-reactive protein, serum amyloid protein, mannose-binding protein, and mannose receptors (23) (see Table 2-1). Scavenger receptors, which have multiple specificities, including apoptotic cells that may harbor viruses, also can localize microbial antigens to cells with specialized presenting function. For example, mice in which the macrophage type I scavenger receptor is deleted have an impaired immune response to *Listeria monocytogenes* and herpes simplex virus type-1 (24). The phenomenon of "cross-priming," which is important for the induction of antiviral cytotoxic T lymphocytes in the absence of direct viral infection of dendritic cells, may be based on the phagocytosis of virally infected cells through scavenger receptors specific for apoptotic cells (25). The common characteristic of these receptors is that they "hard-wire" the recognition of structures for which an adaptive immune response would be biologically appropriate.

Covalent "Tagging" of Antigens by Innate Immunity: Complement and Glycolaldehyde

Innate immunity also has an ability to "tag" covalently any antigens to enhance their recognition by adaptive immunity. Although this process may have initially evolved to label microorganisms for recognition by phagocytic cells in invertebrates, receptors have evolved that link tagged antigens to the stimulation of lymphocytes. The process extends the range of structures that can be made more immunogenic to include proteins that lack microbial determinants but does so in a discrete manner; only those proteins with the modification demonstrate increased immunogenicity. An example of the covalent modification of antigen is provided by the complement system.

Complement is a complex system of humoral innate immunity in invertebrates and vertebrates that is comprised of more than 20 components. Complement can be activated on the first exposure of the host to microbial determinants by several mechanisms: the alternative pathway; the pathway involving the mannan-binding protein and the mannan-binding protein–associated serine proteases, MASP-1 and MASP-2 (26); and the classical pathway when triggered by collectins (27). Each of these pathways converges on C3 by the formation of C3 convertases, which are highly specific proteases that cleave C3. A reactive thiol ester results that participates in a transesterification reaction to mediate the covalent attachment of C3 to nearby proteins and carbohydrates. The short half-life of the thiol ester, which is hydrolyzed by H_2O in a competing reaction, limits the physical extent to which the C3 can diffuse away from its site of activation and still covalently bind, thereby biasing its attachment to the microbial surfaces that initiated the complement activation process. Once an initial C3b has bound to a target, it can catalyze the covalent attachment of additional molecules through an amplification pathway in which the C3b participates in the formation of additional C3 convertases.

The bound C3b and its proteolytic fragments that remain covalently attached to the activator, iC3b and C3dg (C3d), serve as tags for both innate and adaptive cellular immune recognition by interacting with three types of C3 receptors: CR1 (CD35), CR2 (CD21), and CR3 (CD11b/CD18). CR1 binds the C3b fragment and is expressed by myelomonocytic cells and B lymphocytes. Its most important biologic function may be the blocking of further complement activation and the redistribution of complement-activating substances to the other C3 receptors. CR1 accomplishes this function by serving as a cofactor for the factor I–mediated cleavage of C3b to the iC3b and C3dg fragments. CR3 on myelomonocytic cells binds the iC3b fragment to promote the phagocytosis of complement-activating complexes and therefore has a role in the innate immune clearance of microorganisms. However, it is CR2, which binds C3dg and its tryptic cleavage fragment, C3d, that is most relevant to the focus of this chapter, as it is expressed by B lymphocytes and follicular dendritic cells, two cellular elements of the humoral adaptive immune response. C3d and CR2 constitute the bridge that links complement to adaptive immunity.

The first evidence that complement could alter adaptive immunity was provided more than 25 years ago when mice depleted of C3 were found to have a diminished IgG response to a T-dependent antigen (28). Understanding the basis for this function of complement required advances in both complement and lymphocyte research. C3b, and its terminally processed fragment, C3d, were shown subsequently to bind covalently to targets of complement activation, indicating that highly stable, "tagged" forms of antigen complexes could be formed. CR2 was then discovered on B cells and follicular dendritic cells (FDCs), directing attention to this receptor and its ligand, C3d. CR2 on FDCs was assumed to concentrate C3d-tagged antigen in the germinal center, but the role of CR2 on B cells awaited a fuller understanding of signaling by membrane Ig. Thus, CR2 was found to costimulate B-cell activation when coligated with membrane Ig, but not when ligated alone, indicating that the receptor functioned in concert with membrane Ig, a circumstance that is consistent with the unique ability of a C3d-antigen complex to cross-link CR2 and membrane Ig (Fig. 2-3). Altered immunogenicity of the C3d-tagged antigen was formally demonstrated by finding that recombinant fusion proteins containing antigen linked to two or three copies of C3d were 10^3-fold to 10^4-fold more immunogenic in vivo than was unmodified antigen (29).

An essential role in vivo for CR2 has been established by studies of mice in which the *Cr2* gene has been interrupted through

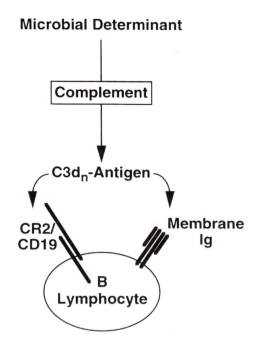

Figure 2-3. Microbial determinants cause the complement system to "tag" antigens with C3d for recognition by the costimulatory complex of CR2 and CD19 on B lymphocytes. Ig, immunoglobulin.

homologous recombination (30–32). Through adoptive transfer experiments, expression of CR2 on both FDCs and B lymphocytes was found to be required. The aspect of the humoral response that is most impaired appears to be the germinal center reaction. In this reaction somatic mutation of Ig genes occurs, leading to high affinity Ig, the development of memory B cells, and the production of long-lived plasma cells. Therefore, innate immunity, through the tagging of antigen with C3d and the presence of CR2 on FDCs and B cells, can regulate the most critical step in the humoral immune response. Interestingly, in $Cr2^{-/-}$ mice there is also a decrease in the number of peritoneal B-1 cells, which are self-renewing and may produce polyreactive IgM that binds many multimeric microbial determinants in the nonimmunized host.

A full presentation of the cell biology that is related to the costimulatory function of CR2 on B cells is beyond the scope of this chapter. However, the finding that it forms a molecular complex with CD19 is relevant because the CR2-CD19 complex represents a molecular junction of innate and adaptive immunity (33,34). Mice in which the *Cd19* gene has been interrupted share with $Cr2^{-/-}$ mice an absence of germinal centers after immunization with T-dependent antigens, markedly impaired antibody responses with low titer and no affinity maturation, and an absence of long-lived plasma cells (35,36). Although these abnormalities can be overcome to some extent in $Cr2^{-/-}$ mice by the administration of antigen with a potent microbial adjuvant, the response in $Cd19^{-/-}$ mice cannot be rendered normal by this means. The role of CD19 in the costimulation of signaling by membrane Ig has been clarified by several in vitro biochemical findings. Coligating CD19 to membrane Ig lowers the threshold at which membrane Ig activates the B cell by two to three orders of magnitude and amplifies the activation of intracellular signaling pathways such as the Ca^{2+} response and the activation of MAP kinases (37). Therefore, CD19 is absolutely required for a normal humoral immune response, and the evolution of a means by which the complement system can ligate this essential coreceptor is an excellent example of *cis* regulation of the adaptive immune response by innate immunity.

Glycolaldehyde [$CH_2(OH)CHO$] can be produced at sites of inflammation when extracellular serine is hydrolyzed by hypochlorous acid (HOCl) (38). HOCl is generated during acute inflammatory reactions in the presence of Cl when H_2O_2 that has been formed by the activated oxidase of neutrophils and monocytes reacts with a peroxidase, which may be myeloperoxidase of these cells or other, possibly extracellular, peroxidase. Glycolaldehyde shares with other aldehydes a capacity for forming Schiff-base adducts with protein -NH_2 groups, but it differs in that the presence of the hydroxyl allows the Schiff base to undergo Amadori rearrangement to create an aldoamine. The aldoamine is then available for formation of an intramolecular or intermolecular Schiff base. These reactions of glycolaldehyde have been shown recently to enable it to be a mediator of innate immunity that tags antigens for adaptive immune recognition.

Treatment in vitro of model protein antigens such as ovalbumin and pigeon cytochrome C with glycolaldehyde generates 1 to 2 aldoamines/mole of protein. Antigens that have been modified in this manner are up to 100-fold more immunogenic when administered to mice in the absence of adjuvant than are unmodified antigens. The enhancement of immunogenicity is sufficient to render immunogenic a self-antigen and a relatively nonimmunogenic recombinant antigen being developed as a vaccine. The enhanced immunogenicity is not a consequence merely of modifying lysines, which might conceivably alter proteolytic processing and presentation of peptides, because the presence of $NaCNBH_3$ during the reaction of glycolaldehyde with antigen, which reduces the initial Schiff base and prevents Amadori rearrangement, prevents the enhancement in immunogenicity. Rather, augmented immunogenicity induced by the covalent tagging of antigen with glycolaldehyde requires the formation of the aldoamine adduct, suggesting that the formation of intermolecular Schiff bases between the antigen and other proteins is the basis for this biologic response. The means by which this recently discovered mechanism tags antigens for adaptive immune recognition is not known.

Innate Immunity and the Development of T Helper Cells

The targeting of microbial antigens by innate immunity for recognition by adaptive immunity is not sufficient to generate an immune response that is optimally suited to a particular microbial infection. Innate immunity must also dictate the type of adaptive immune response, that is, whether it promotes the killing of virally infected cells, the intracellular killing of microorganisms by macrophages, or a mucosal immune response. These three types of responses are dependent on different types of T cells, class I–restricted cytotoxic T lymphocytes, and class II–restricted T_H1 and T_H2 cells. For the purpose of this overview, the ability of innate immunity to regulate the development of class II–restricted αβ T_H1 and T_H2 cells will be examined, although innate immunity has roles in cytotoxic T lymphocyte responses.

T_H1 cells promote the microbicidal activity of macrophages by secreting cytokines such as interferon (IFN)-γ and TNF-α. They induce the expression of nitric oxide synthase (type II, iNOS), which, together with reactive oxygen species produced by these cells, accounts for almost all of their bactericidal activity (39). IFN-γ also augments the expression of class II complexes to enable macrophages that have ingested microorganisms to recruit additional T-cell help for the killing of intracellular organisms. Another, indirect effect of IFN-γ on intracellular killing by macrophages is the induction of isotype switching in the B cell to IgG1 (IgG2a in the mouse). This isotype mediates the phagocytosis of target organisms through interacting with Fc receptors and activation of complement. For these and other reasons, in the absence of T_H1 cells the immunologic recognition of pathogens does not provide an effective host defense against most microorganisms.

Innate immunity has an essential role in the development of T_H1 cells by directing the production of three cytokines that are required for this process: IL-12 (40–42), IL-18 (43), and IFN-γ. Activation of macrophages by LPS or unmethylated CpG–containing microbial oligonucleotides causes the secretion of both IL-12 and IL-18. An initial source of IFN-γ, before its secretion by T_H1 cells, is the NK cell responding to IL-12. Thus, a feedback reaction is initiated by the macrophage that, in response to pathogens for which intracellular killing is required, secretes cytokines that select the genetic program of T_H1 cells for the production of IFN-γ. This interleukin both activates the microbicidal activities of the macrophage and reinforces T_H1-cell development (Fig. 2-4).

Another potential source of early IFN-γ is found in an unusual subset of T cells in which the distinction between innate and adaptive immunity is blurred; these cells express a restricted set of V(D)J genes, sharing with innate immunity the characteristic of having a "hard-wired" form of recognition. These T cells, which have rearranged the Vγ2Vδ2 genes, are activated in a non–MHC-dependent manner by antigens containing prenyl pyrophosphate to secrete IFN-γ and TNF-α (44,45). Therefore, V(D)J rearrangements may occur in subsets of T cells that are selected for the production of IFN-γ, perhaps to promote a T_H1-cell response required for the elimination of certain microorganisms.

The alternative type of adaptive immune response is mediated by T_H2 cells and is characterized by the secretion of IL-4, IL-5, IL-6, IL-10, and IL-13. These cytokines promote the growth and activation of mast cells and eosinophils, direct the Ig class switching in B cells to IgG4 (IgG1 in the mouse) and IgE, suppress the activation of macrophages, and impair the IL-12 respon-

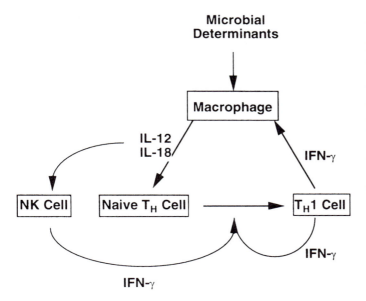

Microbial
Determinants

Macrophage

IL-12
IL-18

IFN-γ

NK Cell   Naive T$_H$ Cell   T$_H$1 Cell

IFN-γ

IFN-γ

Figure 2-4. Microbial determinants can induce T$_H$1-cell responses by establishing a macrophage-dependent, cytokine feedback loop involving interleukin (IL)-12, IL-18, and interferon γ (IFN-γ). NK, natural killer.

currently be used in humans is alum, which serves only to provide a depot of antigen and does not recruit any components of innate immunity. In the past, crude antigen preparations for vaccines may have been relatively immunogenic because they were contaminated with a biologically significant amount of microbial products. Such contaminants probably enhanced the adaptive response by inducing the maturation of dendritic cells. With the development of highly purified recombinant subunit antigens for vaccination, the immune response of humans to vaccines has diminished. The inclusion in such vaccines of defined microbial determinants of limited toxicity, for example, unmethylated CpG–containing oligonucleotides (52), or of interleukins or cytokines may overcome this problem. However, these determinants act in *trans* and may have unwanted side effects. The development of DNA vaccines (53), carrying not only sequences encoding the relevant antigens but also the microbial CpG sequences (54), may elicit both the desired antigen-specific and T$_H$-cell–specific response. Other approaches may be the covalent modification of antigens by attachment of C3d or aldehydes or the chemical alteration of the microenvironment of the antigen with Schiff base–forming agents. With the enormous problem that infectious diseases pose for Third World countries and the increasing antibiotic resistance of pathogens, which do not respect international boundaries, a breakthrough leading to an improved efficacy of vaccines would have extraordinary benefits for humankind.

siveness of T$_H$ cells. These responses are adapted to the elimination of mucosal pathogens, especially parasites, and also have suppressive, regulatory roles in dampening T$_H$1-cell responses to control damage to host tissues.

The development of T$_H$2 cells requires IL-4 and IL-13 during the priming of naïve T$_H$ cells (46,47), but the sources in innate immune systems for these interleukins are not clear. There are suggestions that mast cells, eosinophils, and NK cells can provide these interleukins and that infectious agents regulate this process, presumably through innate immune receptors. For example, *Schistosoma mansoni* eggs induce early IL-4 in a reaction that requires IL-5 and eosinophils (48). NK cells, in addition to being non–T-cell sources of IFN-γ, also can secrete IL-5, although the physiologic circumstances in which this function occurs are not defined (49). A subpopulation of T cells that expresses NK cell markers and is either CD4$^+$ or CD4$^-$CD8$^-$ has a relatively invariant T-cell receptor comprised of Vα24JαQ (Vα14Jα281 in the mouse). In mice, these natural T cells rapidly produce large amounts of IL-4 on binding the nonclassical MHC antigen, CD1 (the homolog of CD1d in humans) (50). However, because the elimination of these cells does not impair the development of T$_H$2-cell responses under some circumstances (51), their biologic role remains to be determined.

Therapeutic Potential of Innate Immunity

A clinical area that will benefit from this newly recognized role of innate immunity is that of vaccination. The only adjuvant that can

References

1. Janeway CA Jr. Approaching the asymptote? Evolution and revolution in immunology. Cold Spring Harb Symp Quant Biol 1989;54:1–13.
2. Matzinger P. Tolerance, danger, and the extended family. Annu Rev Immunol 1994;12:991–1045.
3. Fearon DT, Locksley RM. The instructive role of innate immunity in the acquired immune response. Science 1996; 272:50–53.
4. Medzhitov R, Janeway CA Jr. Innate immunity: the virtues of a nonclonal system of recognition. Cell 1997;91:295–298.
5. Ganz T. Biosynthesis of defensins and other antimicrobial peptides. Ciba Found Symp 1994;186:62–71.
6. Boman HG. Peptide antibiotics and their role in innate immunity. Annu Rev Immunol 1995;13:61–92.
7. Hoffmann JA, Reichhart JM, Hetru C. Innate immunity in higher insects. Curr Opin Immunol 1996;8:8–13.
8. Prigozy TI, Sieling PA, Clemens D, et al. The mannose receptor delivers lipoglycan antigens to endosomes for presentation to T cells by CD1b molecules. Immunity 1997;6:187–197.
9. Ulevitch RJ, Tobias PS. Receptor-dependent mechanisms of cell stimulation by bacterial endotoxin. Annu Rev Immunol 1995;13:437–457.
10. Medzhitov R, Preston-Hurlburt P, Janeway CA Jr. A human homologue of the Drosophila Toll protein signals activation of adaptive immunity. Nature 1997;388:394–397.
11. Rock FL, Hardiman G, Timans JC, et al. A family of human receptors structurally related to Drosophila Toll. Proc Natl Acad Sci USA 1998;95:588–593.
12. Kirschning CJ, Wesche H, Ayres TM, Rothe M. Human Toll-like receptor 2 confers responsiveness to bacterial lipopolysaccharide. J Exp Med 1998;188:2091–2097.

13. Poltorak A, He X, Smirnova I, et al. Defective LPS signaling in C3H/Hej and C57BL/10ScCr mice: mutations in *Tlr4*. Science 1998;282:2085–2088.
14. Medzhitov R, Preston-Hurlburt P, Kopp E, et al. MyD88 is an adaptor protein in the hToll/IL-1 receptor family signaling pathways. Mol Cell 1998;2:253–258.
15. Baeuerle PA, Baltimore D. NK-κ B: ten years after. Cell 1996;87:13–20.
16. Cella M, Sallusto F, Lanzavecchia A. Origin, maturation and antigen-presenting function of dendritic cells. Curr Opin Immunol 1997;9:10–16.
17. Pierre P, Mellman I. Developmental regulation of invariant chain proteolysis controls MHC class II trafficking in mouse dendritic cells. Cell 1998;93:1135–1145.
18. Jakob T, Walker PS, Krieg AM, et al. Activation of cutaneous dendritic cells by CpG-containing oligodeoxynucleotides: a role for dendritic cells in the augmentation of Th1 responses by immunostimulatory DNA. J Immunol 1998;161:3042–3049.
19. Dieu MC, Vanbervliet B, Vicari A, et al. Selective recruitment of immature and mature dendritic cells by distinct chemokines expressed in different anatomic sites. J Exp Med 1998; 188:373–386.
20. Ngo VN, Tang HL, Cyster JG. Epstein-Barr virus–induced molecule 1 ligand chemokine is expressed by dendritic cells in lymphoid tissues and strongly attracts naive T cells and activated B cells. J Exp Med 1998;188:181–191.
21. Sozzani S, Allavena P, D'Amico G, et al. Differential regulation of chemokine receptors during dendritic cell maturation: a model for their trafficking properties. J Immunol 1998;161:1083–1086.
22. Yanagihara S, Komura E, Nagafune J, et al. EBI1/CCR7 is a new member of dendritic cell chemokine receptor that is upregulated upon maturation. J Immunol 1998;161:3096–3102.
23. Stahl PD, Ezekowitz RA. The mannose receptor is a pattern recognition receptor involved in host defense. Curr Opin Immunol 1998;10:50–55.
24. Suzuki H, Kurihara Y, Takeya M, et al. A role for macrophage scavenger receptors in atherosclerosis and susceptibility to infection. Nature 1997;386:292–296.
25. Albert ML, Pearce SF, Francisco LM, et al. Immature dendritic cells phagocytose apoptotic cells via alphavbeta5 and CD36, and cross-present antigens to cytotoxic T lymphocytes. J Exp Med 1998;188:1359–1368.
26. Matsushita M, Endo Y, Nonaka M, Fujita T. Complement-related serine proteases in tunicates and vertebrates. Curr Opin Immunol 1998;10:29–35.
27. Reid KB, Colomb MG, Loos M. Complement component C1 and the collectins: parallels between routes of acquired and innate immunity. Immunol Today 1998;19:56–59.
28. Pepys MB. Role of complement in induction of antibody production in vivo. Effect of cobra factor and other C3-reactive agents on thymus-dependent and thymus-independent antibody responses. J Exp Med 1974;140:126–145.
29. Dempsey PW, Allison ME, Akkaraju S, et al. C3d of complement as a molecular adjuvant: bridging innate and acquired immunity. Science 1996;271:348–350.
30. Ahearn JM, Fischer MB, Croix D, et al. Disruption of the Cr2 locus results in a reduction in B-1a cells and in an impaired B-cell response to T-dependent antigen. Immunity 1996;4: 251–262.
31. Molina H, Holers VM, Li B, et al. Markedly impaired humoral immune response in mice deficient in complement receptors 1 and 2. Proc Natl Acad Sci USA 1996;93:3357–3361.
32. Croix DA, Ahearn JM, Rosengard AM, et al. Antibody response to a T-dependent antigen requires B-cell expression of complement receptors. J Exp Med 1996;183:1857–1864.
33. Matsumoto AK, Kopicky-Burd J, Carter RH, et al. Intersection of the complement and immune systems: a signal transduction complex of the B lymphocyte–containing complement receptor type 2 and CD19. J Exp Med 1991;173: 55–64.
34. Tedder TF, Inaoki M, Sato S. The CD19-CD21 complex regulates signal transduction thresholds governing humoral immunity and autoimmunity. Immunity 1997;6:107–118.
35. Engel P, Zhou LJ, Ord DC, et al. Abnormal B-lymphocyte development, activation, and differentiation in mice that lack or overexpress the CD19 signal transduction molecule. Immunity 1995;3:39–50.
36. Rickert RC, Rajewsky K, Roes J. Impairment of T-cell–dependent B-cell responses and B-1-cell development in CD19-deficient mice. Nature 1995;376:352–355.
37. Tooze RM, Doody GM, Fearon DT. Counterregulation by the coreceptors CD19 and CD22 of MAP kinase activation by membrane immunoglobulin. Immunity 1997;7:59–67.
38. Anderson MM, Hazen SL, Hsu FF, Heinecke JW. Human neutrophils employ the myeloperoxidase-hydrogen peroxide-chloride system to convert hydroxy-amino acids into glycolaldehyde, 2-hydroxypropanal, and acrolein. A mechanism for the generation of highly reactive alpha-hydroxy and alpha, beta-unsaturated aldehydes by phagocytes at sites of inflammation. J Clin Invest 1997;99:424–432.
39. Shiloh MU, MacMicking JD, Nicholson S, et al. Phenotype of mice and macrophages deficient in both phagocyte oxidase and inducible nitric oxide synthase. Immunity 1999;10:29–38.
40. Trinchieri G. Interleukin-12: a proinflammatory cytokine with immunoregulatory functions that bridge innate resistance and antigen-specific adaptive immunity. Annu Rev Immunol. 1995;13:251–276.
41. Hsieh CS, Macatonia SE, Tripp CS, et al. Development of TH1 CD4+ T cells through IL-12 produced by Listeria-induced macrophages. Science 1993;260:547–549.
42. Gately MK, Renzetti LM, Magram J, et al. The interleukin-12/interleukin-12-receptor system: role in normal and pathologic immune responses. Annu Rev Immunol 1998;16: 495–521.
43. Takeda K, Tsutsui H, Yoshimoto T, et al. Defective NK cell activity and Th1 response in IL-18–deficient mice. Immunity 1998;8:383–390.
44. Constant P, Davodeau F, Peyrat MA, et al. Stimulation of human γ δ T cells by nonpeptidic mycobacterial ligands. Science 1994;264:267–270.
45. Morita CT, Beckman EM, Bukowski JF, et al. Direct presentation of nonpeptide prenyl pyrophosphate antigens to human γ δ T cells. Immunity 1995;3:495–507.
46. Constant SL, Bottomly K. Induction of Th1 and Th2 CD4+ T-cell responses: the alternative approaches. Annu Rev Immunol 1997;15:297–322.
47. McKenzie GJ, Emson CL, Bell SE, et al. Impaired development of Th2 cells in IL-13–deficient mice. Immunity 1998;9: 423–432.

48. Sabin EA, Kopf MA, Pearce EJ. Schistosoma mansoni egg–induced early IL-4 production is dependent upon IL-5 and eosinophils. J Exp Med 1996;184:1871–1878.

49. Warren HS, Kinnear BF, Phillips JH, Lanier LL. Production of IL-5 by human NK cells and regulation of IL-5 secretion by IL-4, IL-10, and IL-12. J Immunol 1995;154:5144–5152.

50. Bendelac A, Lantz O, Quimby ME, et al. CD1 recognition by mouse NK1+ T lymphocytes. Science 1995;268:863–865.

51. Smiley ST, Kaplan MH, Grusby MJ. Immunoglobulin E production in the absence of interleukin-4–secreting CD1-dependent cells. Science 1997;275:977–979.

52. Krieg AM, Yi AK, Matson S, et al. CpG motifs in bacterial DNA trigger direct B-cell activation. Nature 1995;374:546–549.

53. Ulmer JB, Donnelly JJ, Parker SE, et al. Heterologous protection against influenza by injection of DNA encoding a viral protein. Science 1993;259:1745–1749.

54. Davis HL. Plasmid DNA expression systems for the purpose of immunization. Curr Opin Biotechnol 1997;8:635–646.

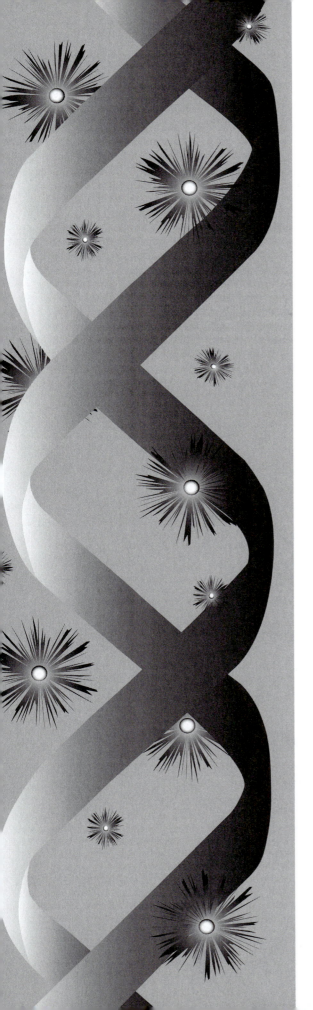

II
Drugs

Antimetabolites and Radiomimetics

Corticosteroids

Anti-Inflammatory Agents

Chapter 3

Cyclophosphamide

Alfred D. Steinberg

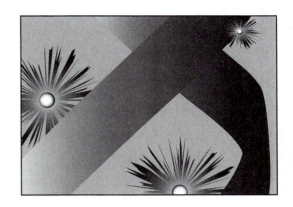

Cyclophosphamide (Cytoxan) is a cytotoxic alkylating agent originally developed as a nitrogen mustard analog and introduced for the treatment of malignancies more than 40 years ago (1). It has been used widely in the therapy of immune-mediated disorders, in cancer chemotherapy, and in the preparation for hematopoietic stem-cell reconstitution. The drug is capable of killing cells throughout the cell cycle, but is especially toxic to proliferating cells. Cyclophosphamide is administered orally or intravenously. It can be given as a single agent or as one agent in a combined chemotherapy program. Cyclophosphamide may be administered daily in low doses or intermittently in larger doses. Because of substantial side effects, the drug is reserved for serious illness.

Structure and Metabolism

Cyclophosphamide, *N,N*-bis (2-chlorethyl)-*N',O*-propylene phosphoric acid ester diamine monohydrate, is a cyclic phosphamide mustard (Fig. 3-1). As such, it falls into the family of alkylating agents of which nitrogen mustard is the prototype. However, there are two fundamental differences between cyclophosphamide and nitrogen mustard: 1) unlike nitrogen mustard, which is active in its native state, cyclophosphamide is largely inactive until the bis-(2-chloroethyl) alkylating sites are freed to ionize by cleavage of the phosphamide ring; and 2) although both drugs alkylate, unlike nitrogen mustard, cyclophosphamide is also able to phosphorylate.

The drug is readily soluble in body fluids and therefore is widely distributed. Cyclophosphamide binds minimally to plasma proteins; however, several of its metabolites are protein bound (2). The parent compound and the active metabolites are eliminated primarily by the kidney. Because metabolites accumulate in patients with severe renal insufficiency, the dose of drug should be reduced in such individuals (2–5).

Cyclophosphamide is primarily metabolized in the liver by the mixed-function oxidase, cytochrome P-450 system, to 4-hydroxy-cyclophosphamide (6–8) as shown in Figure 3-1. The 4-hydroxy compound enters the plasma and circulates throughout the body; it is able to cross cell membranes and enter cells. It spontaneously tautomerizes to aldophosphamide with breakage of the phosphamide ring structure at the N-C bond (see Fig. 3-1). Aldophosphamide is unstable; it breaks down spontaneously

(by beta elimination) to form the highly reactive phosphoramide mustard (with the chloroethyl side chains) and acrolein (see Fig. 3-1).

The major active principle of cyclophosphamide is the metabolite phosphoramide mustard (9). Acrolein is the principal cause of bladder toxicity, but it also is able to interact with and alter DNA (10). Other metabolites are capable of alkylating cellular macromolecules. Phosphoramidases convert phosphoramide mustard to nor-nitrogen mustard, which is believed to be important in the alkylating effects of cyclophosphamide. In addition to its major metabolism in the liver, cyclophosphamide may be converted to its active metabolites in other organs, especially lung and kidney (11–16). Four-hydroxy-cyclophosphamide can be metabolized to the less-reactive 4-ketophosphamide or to the nontoxic alcophosphamide (by alcohol dehydrogenase) and to carboxyphosphamide (by aldehyde oxidase/aldehyde dehydrogenase). Measurable amounts of aldehyde oxidase and aldehyde dehydrogenase are absent in the lung (13); this circumstance conceivably could predispose to lung toxicity because aldophosphamide would not be as readily broken down to nontoxic metabolites.

Drugs that activate the hepatic mixed-oxidase, cytochrome P-450 system such as corticosteroids, phenobarbital, and phenytoin may lead to more complete metabolism of the drug and, thereby, a greater drug effect. Cyclophosphamide itself may increase its own metabolism by this mechanism (5,17).

Cyclophosphamide is very well absorbed from the gastrointestinal tract. As a result, the oral dose approximates the intravenous dose. The average half-life of cyclophosphamide in humans is approximately 5 hours (range, 3 to 11 hours). The half-life is shorter in children and longer in patients with renal insufficiency. The half-life of 4-hydroxycyclophosphamide is approximately 1.5 to 6 hours, depending on the rate of formation from cyclophosphamide in the liver (18). There is a longer half-life of phosphoramide mustard adducts of DNA than nitrogen mustard adducts (8.5 hours versus 1.6 hours).

Mechanisms of Action

The metabolites of cyclophosphamide, especially phosphoramide mustard, alkylate and cross-link cellular macromolecules, including DNA, RNA, and proteins, in a manner similar to that of other

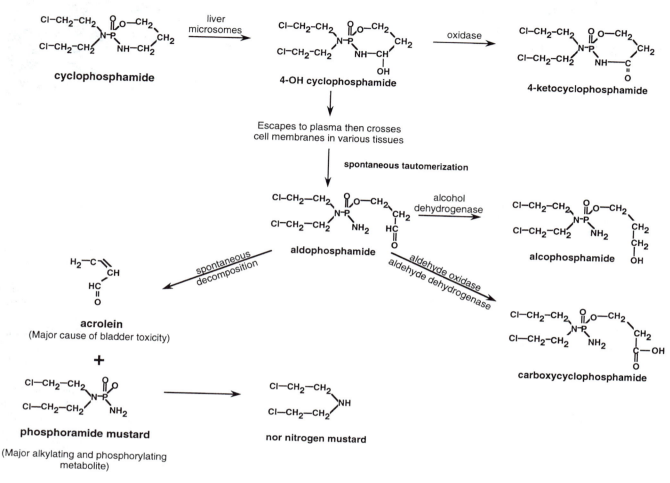

Figure 3-1. Schematic diagram of the major metabolic steps in the in vivo metabolism of cyclophosphamide. The drug is first metabolized in the liver by the mixed-oxidase cytochrome P-450 system to yield 4-hydroxycyclophosphamide. This metabolite escapes to the blood and travels throughout the body, ultimately crossing the cell membranes of various tissues. Within these cells, there is a spontaneous tautomerization to aldophosphamide and then decomposition to phosphoramide mustard (the major alkylating and phosphorylating metabolite) plus acrolein (the major cause of bladder toxicity). Aldophosphamide is also converted to less active metabolites by tissue enzymes.

bifunctional alkylating agents. The 7-nitrogen of guanosine is the major site of DNA alkylation. Intrastrand and interstrand DNA cross-links result in dysfunction of the DNA template and cell death (19). Unlike alkylating agents such as nitrogen mustard and chlorambucil, cyclophosphamide phosphorylates as well as alkylates. The intracellular biochemical reactions of cyclophosphamide metabolites lead to cell death. Therefore, cyclophosphamide is a cytotoxic drug. Studies have suggested that many cytotoxic drugs bring about their effects through apoptosis (programmed cell death).

Cyclophosphamide can damage cells throughout their cell cycle—when they are resting or during the various phases of division. However, its greatest action is during the S phase of the cell cycle, when cells are undergoing DNA synthesis. Thus, cyclophosphamide has its greatest effects on cells that are rapidly dividing.

As a result, cyclophosphamide acts as an immunosuppressive drug by killing activated lymphocytes, but it also causes bone marrow depression. Because cyclophosphamide damages DNA, it can predispose to malignancies, especially leukemia and lymphoma (20–22).

Immune Effects

Cyclophosphamide administered daily to patients with a variety of immune-mediated diseases induces a progressive reduction in the number of circulating lymphocytes (23–26). The lymphopenia is out of proportion to the granulocytopenia. Indeed, at low doses of drug, the reduction in lymphocyte counts can occur with minimal changes in granulocyte counts. At higher drug dosages, granulocytes as well as lymphocytes are reduced in number.

Chronic, low-dose therapy appears to affect cell-mediated responses more than intermittent bolus therapy, which primarily impairs antibody production (27). Monthly boluses of intravenous cyclophosphamide lead to a reduction in the numbers of B cells and T cells (both CD 4 and CD 8) (28). B cells return more rapidly than T cells (28), but the effects on lymphocyte subsets are dose dependent. The lowest doses of bolus cyclophosphamide ($<600\,mg/m^2$) reduce the numbers of B cells to a greater extent than T cells and CD8$^+$ T cells to a greater extent than CD4$^+$ T cells. Cyclophosphamide doses $>600\,mg/m^2$ reduce the numbers of CD4$^+$ and CD8$^+$ T cells almost equivalently (29). Thus, a dose of $1000\,mg/m^2$ leads to a 30% to 40% reduction on day 7 of the numbers of B cells, CD8$^+$ T cells, and CD4$^+$ T cells (30).

Recovery from the effects of cyclophosphamide after the cessation of therapy may vary. In patients with multiple sclerosis, B-cell and CD4$^+$ and CD8$^+$ T-cell lymphopenia was observed with 1 year of monthly cyclophosphamide therapy. After therapy was stopped, CD8$^+$ T-cell numbers returned first, B-cell numbers second, and CD4$^+$ T-cell numbers last (>4 months) (31).

Cyclophosphamide interferes with both B-cell and T-cell function in patients and experimental animals (32–35). As a result, the drug has been effective in preventing allograft rejection, antibody production, and both B-cell– and T-cell–mediated diseases. Like other drugs that kill rapidly dividing cells, cyclophosphamide is more effective than cytostatic drugs in inducing tolerance to an antigen given within a day or two of drug (36). In experimental animals, cyclophosphamide has been remarkably effective therapy for antibody-mediated murine lupus (37,38) and also cell-mediated experimental allergic encephalomyelitis (39). In rheumatoid vasculitis, cyclophosphamide causes a reduction in IgG rheumatoid factor titers and in immune complex levels, as well as in elevated levels of circulating activated T cells (40).

In animals, low doses of cyclophosphamide may paradoxically potentiate immune activity (34,35,41–44) or allow immune responses that otherwise would not be expressed (45). These potentiation effects have been attributed to a selective inhibition of suppressor T-cell function. Indeed, suppressor T-cell function is more susceptible to the effects of cyclophosphamide than is helper T-cell function (44). This phenomenon has been observed in humans as well. Whereas standard therapeutic doses of cyclophosphamide (at least $500\,mg/m^2$ monthly or at least $1\,mg/kg/day$) cause a reduction in the numbers of CD3$^+$ T cells, CD4$^+$ T cells, CD8$^+$ T cells, CD19$^+$ T cells, CD4$^+$CD45$^+$ T cells, and CD4$^+$CDw29$^+$ T cells, lower doses cause a reduction only in the number of CD4$^+$CD45$^+$ T cells, which are thought to include suppressor-inducer cells (28,30,46). It is not at all clear what, if any, clinical relevance might be attributable to the effects of low-dose cyclophosphamide. In one clinical study of patients with rheumatoid arthritis (47), the control group of patients was given a low dose of cyclophosphamide, and it is not clear that this therapy had a deleterious effect.

In cancer chemotherapy, multiple immunosuppressive drugs may be used together in an attempt to kill tumor cells. It is possible that the use of several immunosuppressive drugs in immune-mediated diseases could lead to additive or even synergistic effects (48). The potential synergy in immunosuppression of cyclophosphamide with other drugs (e.g., azathioprine, methylprednisolone, methotrexate) has not been well evaluated in humans, and only a few well-performed studies have been conducted in animals.

In one well-performed animal study of synergy, methylprednisolone and methotrexate each acted synergistically with a nontolerogenic dose of cyclophosphamide to induce tolerance to a nucleic acid antigen (36). Three drugs together, azathioprine, methylprednisolone, and cyclophosphamide, acted synergistically in the induction of tolerance (36). Tolerance was induced with antigen plus cyclophosphamide or methotrexate, the two agents that preferentially damage actively proliferating cells. Synergy was not observed between methotrexate and cyclophosphamide, the two study drugs that preferentially incapacitate rapidly dividing cells.

Cyclophosphamide also acts synergistically with other drugs in the treatment of lupus-prone New Zealand mice. Low doses of cyclophosphamide, methylprednisolone, and azathioprine together were more effective than higher doses of each individual agent (37). This form of therapy has been used to treat patients with lupus nephritis (49).

Use in Nonmalignant Diseases

General Considerations

Cyclophosphamide was not originally developed for the treatment of nonmalignant diseases; such use occurs through the adaptation of an agent designed for cancer chemotherapy (1). Like many other anticancer drugs, cyclophosphamide was found to be effective as an immunosuppressive agent. It was a short step to try it in the treatment of immune-mediated, nonmalignant diseases; however, such use assumes that the disease process being treated is mediated by the immune system and that immunosuppression will be beneficial.

In cancer chemotherapy, it may not be possible to give a single drug such as cyclophosphamide in high enough doses to bring about the desired cytoreductive effect. Therefore, cyclophosphamide often is given with other agents in a combined chemotherapy program. Analogously, the therapeutic window for cyclophosphamide in certain nonmalignant disorders is rather narrow. The therapeutic window is defined as the dosage range that provides adequate benefit in most patients with side effects in very few (Fig. 3-2).

Figure 3-2 implies that there is individual variation in responsiveness to cyclophosphamide. This observation undoubtedly has many bases, including such factors as the severity of the illness, the responsiveness of the cells mediating the illness, the amount of drug that can be reasonably given without toxicity, the rate and other details of the metabolism of the drug, the rate

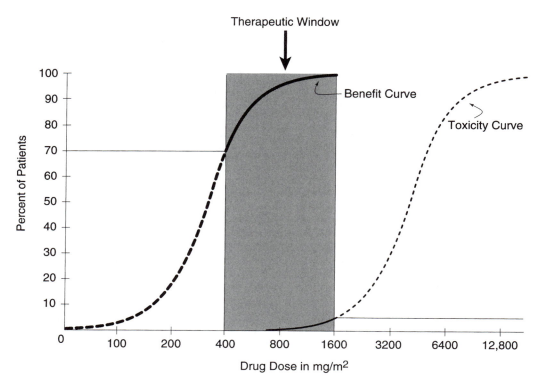

Figure 3-2. An idealized diagram of the therapeutic window. The therapeutic window is the dosage range of a drug in which the majority of patients benefit and few have untoward effects. In this example, the therapeutic window has been defined arbitrarily as the dosage of drug providing benefit to 70% of patients with toxicity in less than 5%. It is shown by the gray area as well as the solid lines on the benefit curve and the toxicity curve.

and magnitude of lymphocyte generation, and the degree of recall immune responses already generated. The differences in the dose at which toxicity occurs must include the resiliency of the bone marrow and metabolic factors. These differences might not be very important if there were a 100-fold difference between the therapeutic dose and the toxic dose, but for many human disorders the therapeutic dose of cyclophosphamide is a toxic dose (Fig. 3-3). Therefore, although many patients reach the therapeutic dose before the toxic dose, others reach a toxic dose before a therapeutic one.

Although cyclophosphamide currently is being used to treat several nonmalignant disorders, support for that use through randomized clinical trials may be lacking. In some of these situations, the results of cyclophosphamide therapy for a disease have been compared with the courses of different patients observed in earlier eras (historic controls). The problem with such comparisons is that the disease itself may evolve or that adjunctive therapy (antibiotics, antihypertensives) or diagnostic procedures (MRI, CT scans) may allow better care and therefore a better outcome unrelated to the immunosuppressive agent. Under such circumstances, any new therapy that was not deleterious might be seen as an improvement over previous therapies.

Another issue is the specific drug regimen. A cyclophosphamide dose of 50 mg/day may provide no significant benefit to patients with a given disease, whereas 100 mg/day would. To patients with another disorder, a dose of 75 mg/day may provide benefit, but monthly boluses of 0.75 g/m² may not. Thus, a study that does or does not show benefit of cyclophosphamide to patients with a specific disorder may be applicable to other patients only in the context of the exact dosage regimen followed. Similarly, the demonstration of benefit with one cyclophosphamide regimen does not imply benefit with another cyclophosphamide regimen (an assumption too often made in clinical practice). For example, patients with polymyositis or rheumatoid arthritis may respond to daily cyclophosphamide therapy but not monthly bolus therapy. Indeed, adult patients with those disorders may respond to 100 to 125 mg/day but not to 50 to 75 mg/day.

Choosing between daily and bolus therapy may be difficult and is a cause of considerable uncertainty. Because daily therapy is superior at suppressing cell-mediated immunity, that method would be used when suppression of cell-mediated immunity is important. In contrast, for treatment of antibody-mediated diseases, bolus therapy might be chosen to minimize toxicity. In bolus therapy, the patient is exposed to the drug and its toxic effects only intermittently (and the total drug dose often is less than with daily therapy). Indeed, with bolus therapy, there has been less infection, bladder irritation, and malignancy (49–51).

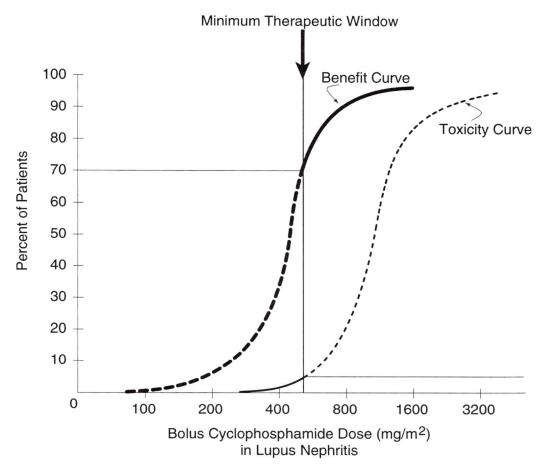

Figure 3-3. An idealized diagram of the therapeutic window for bolus cyclophosphamide in patients with lupus nephritis. The window is defined as in Figure 3.2. Seventy percent of patients should receive benefit, whereas fewer than 5% experience toxicity. Unfortunately, there is no therapeutic window because there is already toxicity in 5% of patients at a dosage at which 70% of patients benefit. Indeed, in actual practice, the benefit and toxicity curves may be much closer, giving an even greater percentage of patients experiencing toxicity at 70% benefit.

Nevertheless, if bolus therapy is not of sufficient benefit in most patients with a given disorder, the administration of the drug in that manner in an attempt to reduce its toxicity may not be appropriate.

Often, a relatively toxic therapy such as cyclophosphamide treatment is reserved until all efforts with less toxic but less effective agents have failed. Although reserving more toxic therapy for serious problems is appropriate, there are two general problems with this approach. First, by delaying therapy with the more toxic but more effective medication, one may have passed the period in which that medication may have been able to do the most good. This approach is especially problematic when a major organ is involved. If one has reversible CNS disease, reversible renal disease, or reversible myocardial disease and there is a delay in therapy, it may be more difficult at the later time for the medication to bring about a remission. A corollary is that there already may have been irreversible damage by the time the more

toxic therapy is instituted. To avoid these dilemmas, it may be necessary to make an early decision that the disease is serious enough to warrant the more toxic medication and institute it early (38,52). For example, it is easier to bring about an adequate resolution of lupus nephritis in both mice and humans when cyclophosphamide therapy is begun early in the disorder and more difficult later in the disorder (37,38).

Second, by delaying therapy with a drug such as cyclophosphamide, one may end up treating a mixture of reversible and irreversible lesions or largely irreversible problems. Cyclophosphamide cannot bring back glomeruli or myocardial cells or neurones from scar tissue. Such a delay may even result in increased toxic side effects 1) because the drug is pushed when results are not rapidly forthcoming or 2) because the treatment is continued in the hope of ultimate effect, even though there is less possibility of benefit than might have been the case had the drug been started earlier in the course of the disease. This practice shifts the therapeutic-toxic ratio substantially from that of studies that justified the use of drug initially.

Drug Dosage and Route of Administration

Cyclophosphamide may be given in many different dosage regimens. Typical regimens in patients with inflammatory diseases are 1) a modest daily oral dosage or 2) intermittent administration of larger amounts of drug. The amount of the daily oral dose is typically constrained by the peripheral white count, which usually falls over time in patients receiving daily cyclophosphamide at doses of 2 mg/kg/day or greater. It is often possible to maintain daily therapy for several years by tapering the dose before a major chronic reduction in leukocyte counts. The intermittent regimen (which can be given intravenously or orally) is typically 500 mg/m² to 1500 mg/m² every 3 to 4 weeks. The dosage is again constrained by acute reduc-

tions in the white cell counts, which occur between days 8 and 14 and are dose dependent (Fig. 3-4). Greater amounts of drug or more frequent boluses have been given to patients with multiple sclerosis and other diseases. In general, repeated boluses spaced at least 24 days apart provide rather similar degrees of reduction of white cell counts (Fig. 3-5) provided there have not been any major changes such as in the corticosteroid dose. More frequent administration (more often than every 3 weeks) of full-dose cyclophosphamide boluses may kill bone marrow cells just as they are recovering from the previous dose, and dangerous marrow suppression may occur.

Daily or intermittent cyclophosphamide therapy may be administered orally or intravenously. A typical daily dosage in adults is approximately 1.5 to 3 mg/kg/day, given as a combination of 50-mg and 25-mg tablets. Unlike azathioprine, cyclophosphamide does not carry the threat of idiosyncratic

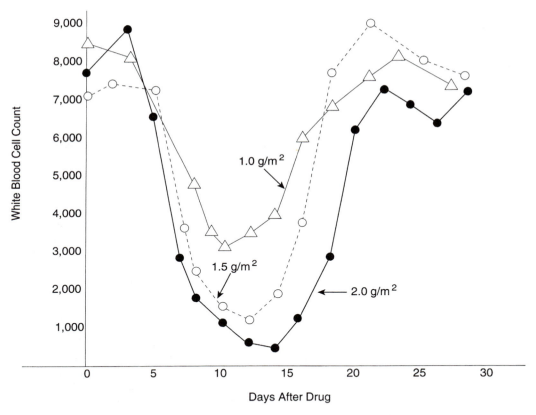

Figure 3-4. Diagram of the dose- and time-dependent reduction in peripheral white cell count in patients receiving different doses of cyclophosphamide. In this example, a dose of 1.0 g/m² caused a white blood cell count reduction from 8500/μL to 3050/μL, with a nadir on day 10. Increasing doses led to greater degrees of leukopenia as well as a nadir on progressively later days. In all cases, there was a return to a normal white blood cell count by day 21. Sometimes there is a white blood cell count overshoot on approximately day 20. This illustration should not be taken as a guide to dose selection because patients vary markedly in their susceptibility to cyclophosphamide-induced leukopenia; some have marked leukopenia with as little as 0.5 to 0.75 g/m². Indeed, patients with systemic lupus erythematosus appear to be more susceptible to cyclophosphamide-induced leukopenia than those with other disorders. Therefore, it is often necessary to determine the maximum tolerated dose for a given individual. If boluses are given more frequently than every 4 weeks, greater leukopenia may occur in later courses than was experienced after the first dose.

agranulocytosis in the first week of therapy. However, the white blood cell count must be monitored regularly over time because it tends to fall after weeks to months of therapy, and the drug dosage may need to be adjusted downward to avoid dangerous leukopenia. Because cyclophosphamide and its major metabolites are cleared by the kidney, drug doses must be reduced in renal failure to prevent profound bone marrow suppression (53); nevertheless, the drug may be given, in reduced dosage, to patients on dialysis (54).

Therapy with 1 to 2 mg/kg/day of cyclophosphamide does not usually cause nausea sufficient to require antinausea medication. However, the metabolites of daily low doses of cyclophosphamide, especially acrolein, frequently cause bladder irritation. Therefore, a high urine volume must be maintained throughout the entire course of cyclophosphamide. This is a problem in both genders during hot weather. Some individuals, especially women, have learned to limit their intake of fluids to avoid the need to urinate at socially difficult times. This cultural effect damages the

bladder when such people take daily cyclophosphamide. They must be re-educated to both drink more and to urinate more frequently. In addition, cyclophosphamide can be given with a reducing agent to minimize the bladder toxicity.

Low-dose daily cyclophosphamide causes alopecia in some individuals. Patients with lupus who have a predisposition to telogen effluvium may be especially susceptible to alopecia. Nevertheless, the hair typically regrows, often while the drug is continued. A wig may be desired by an occasional patient.

Herpes zoster may occur during a course of cyclophosphamide therapy (55). Some physicians stop the drug and add an antiviral agent (e.g., acyclovir), even for dermatomally confined herpes zoster. Many patients without dissemination have not received antiviral therapy, and some of these patients have continued cyclophosphamide therapy despite the dermatomally confined zoster. Disseminated zoster is a more serious condition requiring a different approach, typically hospitalization, discontinuation of cyclophosphamide, and full antiviral therapy.

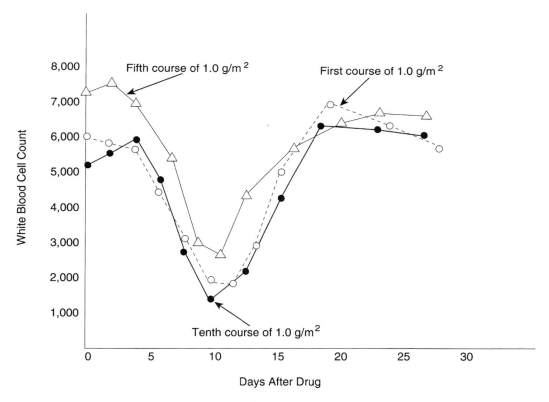

Figure 3-5. Diagram of the time-dependent reduction in peripheral white blood cell count in a single patient given repeated monthly boluses of cyclophosphamide, all at a dose of 1.0 g/m² body surface area. Provided there are no major changes in the dosage of corticosteroids (or other drugs with major effects on cyclophosphamide-induced leukopenia), there is a remarkable consistency in the time course and nadir of the leukopenia induced by repeated courses of the drug at a given dosage. However, if repeated boluses are given during major corticosteroid tapering, there may be progressively greater degrees of leukopenia. (This may be less of a problem if dexamethasone is given to reduce ondansetron dosage.) It should be noted that the patient on whom this diagram is based experienced greater leukopenia at 1.0 g/m² than the patient on whom Figure 3-4 is based. Indeed, some individuals cannot be given more than 0.5 g/m² monthly without experiencing worrisome leukopenia.

Protection against pregnancy is urged for both males and females receiving cyclophosphamide to avoid potential deleterious effects on offspring (or grandchildren). Some males store sperm before therapy for use afterwards. Although the drug reduces fertility in women, many have had successful pregnancies after their courses of cyclophosphamide ended (and others have become pregnant and given birth to normal children during a course of cyclophosphamide against the advice of their physicians).

The administration of bolus cyclophosphamide at the time of menstruation may help to reduce the risk of ovarian failure (56); however, for convenience, many physicians prefer to see patients at times other than menstruation to obtain an uncontaminated urine specimen. The therapy and the urinalysis clearly do not have to occur on the same day.

Bolus therapy, typically $500 \, \text{mg/m}^2$ to $1500 \, \text{mg/m}^2$ of cyclophosphamide every 3 to 4 weeks (eventually spread out to every 3 months), has somewhat different requirements for monitoring and adjunctive therapy than does daily low-dose cyclophosphamide. Bolus therapy may be given orally or intravenously. Antinausea medication is necessary for most patients. Indeed, patients have recall of prior nausea and may become nauseated on entering the treatment room—before any new therapy. Experiences with ondansetron (Zofran), a serotonin antagonist, have been most favorable (57,58). This drug blocks both peripheral and central serotonin type 3 receptors involved in the pathophysiology of acute, chemotherapy-induced emesis without affecting other types of receptors. Other type 3 serotonin receptor antagonists may also provide benefit.

Typically, a patient receives an initial dose of ondansetron orally (4 to 8 mg) or intravenously (10 mg) 4 hours after the infusion of cyclophosphamide is begun. The same dose is given every 4 hours for three additional doses. The risk period for emesis usually passes in <24 hours. The concomitant administration of dexamethasone (10 to 20 mg) allows the ondansetron to be effective at a lower dosage than without the dexamethasone. Although ondansetron has provided excellent protection from emesis for patients with systemic lupus erythematosus who are receiving up to $1000 \, \text{mg/m}^2$ boluses of cyclophosphamide, as well as for other patients, different antiemetics, even in combination, may be suitable for some individuals (59).

Careful monitoring of hematologic parameters is always appropriate for patients receiving cyclophosphamide. Figures 3-4 and 3-5 provide an example of changes in peripheral white blood cell counts after bolus cyclophosphamide; however, there is substantial individual variation among patients receiving either bolus or daily therapy. Patients with some diseases, for example, systemic lupus erythematosus, may be more sensitive to the leukopenic effects of cyclophosphamide than patients with other diseases. Typically, an attempt is made to keep the nadir of the white blood cell count above $1500/\mu\text{L}$ after bolus therapy and above $3000/\mu\text{L}$ during daily therapy.

The bladder must be protected from the adverse effects of acrolein to avoid hemorrhagic cystitis, bladder fibrosis, and possible bladder malignancy. During bolus therapy and for the next 24 hours, the patient is hydrated with $2.5 \, \text{L/m}^2$ of fluid if tolerated.

The fluid should contain solute (e.g., normal saline or normal saline containing 5% dextrose) to avoid hyponatremia from the inappropriate antidiuretic hormone (ADH) syndrome induced by bolus cyclophosphamide (60,61). Frequent voiding is encouraged. If urine output does not keep up with fluid input, furosemide may be given; this drug also counteracts the potential for hyponatremia (62). If the patient is oliguric, an irrigation catheter (e.g., three-way Foley) may be placed in the bladder for the postcyclophosphamide period and the bladder irrigated appropriately.

Reducing agents such as *N*-acetylcysteine or, in the past decade, MESNA (2-mercaptoethane sodium sulfonate) have markedly diminished the risk of bladder irritation (63–65). With very high doses of cyclophosphamide, it was found that a dose of 60% weight of MESNA/weight of cyclophosphamide was sufficient to protect the bladders of children, whereas adults required a higher dose of 120% to 160% weight of MESNA/weight cyclophosphamide (66). Many physicians believe that for patients with nonmalignant diseases, a single episode of hemorrhagic cystitis is a contraindication to continued cyclophosphamide use.

There may be questions regarding the concomitant administration of other immunosuppressive drugs with cyclophosphamide. Other alkylating agents (nitrogen mustard, chlorambucil) or drugs that also preferentially kill rapidly dividing cells (e.g., methotrexate) typically are not given with full doses of cyclophosphamide to patients with nonmalignant disorders. In contrast, cytostatic drugs (e.g., azathioprine, 6-mercaptopurine, 6-thioguanine) may be given with cyclophosphamide. Indeed, there is substantial experience with the combination of cyclophosphamide plus azathioprine in lupus nephritis (49). Of course, with any combination, special care must be exercized in monitoring hematologic parameters.

Corticosteroids may be given with cyclophosphamide in any dosage that would be used without cyclophosphamide. There may be an additive or even synergistic effect of administering the agents together. The peripheral leukocyte count is better maintained after cyclophosphamide therapy when corticosteroids are also administered. Nevertheless, a frequent goal of cyclophosphamide therapy is the reduction in corticosteroid requirements, and the combination of prolonged high doses of corticosteroids and cyclophosphamide markedly predisposes to infection. This predisposition is not seen with low doses of corticosteroids and cyclophosphamide.

Agents that alter the activity of the hepatic mixed-oxidase, cytochrome P-450 system such as phenobarbital and phenytoin may alter the metabolism of cyclophosphamide. This phenomenon is often of greater interest to pharmacologists than physicians. In practice, a dose-finding effort is carried out for each patient. The amount of drug tolerated is based on many individual factors, only one of which is concomitant medication. Nevertheless, a change in other medications may alter the effects of a given, previously well-tolerated, cyclophosphamide dose, especially if corticosteroid tapering leads to a dangerous reduction in the peripheral leukocyte count of a patient on a fixed dose of cyclophosphamide.

Bone Marrow Stimulants for Patients Receiving Cyclophosphamide

Recombinant DNA technology has led to the development of human factors able to stimulate marrow production and release formed elements of the blood. Some of these factors are used in patients receiving various types of chemotherapy, but they are not routinely used in the management of patients with nonmalignant diseases who are being treated with cyclophosphamide as a single agent.

Recombinant Human Erythropoietin (rHuEPO)

Erythropoietin stimulates committed erythroid precursors both to survive and to differentiate terminally into nucleated erythroid elements. Normally, local hypoxia (induced by anemia) is a critical signal for the release of erythropoietin. However, inflammatory cytokines produced by patients are able to inhibit the erythropoietin response to hypoxia (67). Moreover, alkylating agents, including cyclophosphamide, inhibit renal erythropoietin production (68). Although recombinant human erythropoietin is not recommended as standard therapy in patients treated chronically with cyclophosphamide, it has been effective in the treatment of the anemia of chronic renal failure (69) and of rheumatoid arthritis (70), as well as of the chemotherapy-induced anemia of patients with malignancies (71). Thus, it might be helpful in selected patients. There is a delay of about 2 weeks between the start of therapy with recombinant human erythropoietin and clinical effects. A typical dose is 150 units/kg subcutaneously three times per week.

Factors That Stimulate Granulocyte Production

Human granulocyte colony-stimulating factor (G-CSF) is a glycoprotein that stimulates selective stimulation of neutrophil production from committed precursors (72). It stimulates neutrophil progenitor production, neutrophil differentiation, and neutrophil function (72,73). A commercial recombinant human G-CSF (Neupogen) has been used in drug-induced neutropenic states, especially in patients who have received high-dose chemotherapy for malignancy (74–76). The producer's recommended dose is 5 µg/kg/day, and the recommended course is until postnadir neutrophil counts reach 10,000/µL. This recommendation is usually not a problem for patients with malignancies, because excessive white blood cell counts are uncommon. (Indeed, leukocyte counts of 40,000 to 100,000/µL are not rare after such a company-recommended course of Neupogen.) In contrast, an excessive leukocyte count may be less well tolerated by patients with inflammatory nonmalignant diseases for which the cyclophosphamide is given. Although it is a largely theoretic point that the excess leukocytes may exacerbate the underlying inflammatory process, the author is aware of patients with immune-mediated, inflammatory, nonmalignant diseases whose condition worsened after bolus cyclophosphamide therapy and who had an excessive leukocyte response to Neupogen. Thus, if a patient with a serious inflammatory disease is given cyclophosphamide, develops a leukocyte count that is dangerously low, and is given Neupogen,

it may be desirable to give fewer doses of the drug and only until the patient is beyond the risk of infection rather than until the leukocyte count reaches 10,000/µL. Moreover, in selected situations, it may be possible that a patient could benefit from the combination of higher doses of cyclophosphamide and be "rescued" with Neupogen from the more severe neutropenia that results; this approach has been used in patients with cancer. The author is aware of at least one individual with lupus and dose-limiting neutropenia who so benefitted. Nevertheless, this maneuver is life-threatening, and extreme caution should be used on both sides of the Neupogen issue for patients with nonmalignant disorders until solid information becomes available.

Another issue is the potential for compromising hematopoietic precursors by giving cyclophosphamide after marrow stimulation with colony-stimulating factors. If a cytotoxic drug is given after stimulation of marrow precursors, excess destruction of the precursors may occur (77,78).

Finally, some investigators have expressed concern that pulmonary toxicity may be increased by the combination of chemotherapy and G-CSF (79).

Toxicity

Although alkylating agents often are grouped together and do share some toxicities, there also are differences. For example, cyclophosphamide does not cause local irritation if it infiltrates (as is the case with nitrogen mustard), and cyclophosphamide rarely causes the thrombocytopenia more commonly noted with chlorambucil. In contrast, cyclophosphamide does have bladder toxicity not observed with nitrogen mustard or chlorambucil. Although there are short-term toxicities of cyclophosphamide, of concern are the long-term complications (80). Like other alkylating agents, cyclophosphamide has been linked with the development of lymphoma and leukemia, especially with prolonged therapy, a risk that has been estimated to be between 0.1% and 1% (20).

Bladder

Bladder toxicity is caused by the direct action of cyclophosphamide metabolites, especially acrolein, on transitional epithelium (81–88). The risks of bladder toxicity are substantial even for patients with nonmalignant diseases who are receiving low daily doses of the drug.

Very high dose cyclophosphamide given for marrow transplantation increases the risk of hemorrhagic cystitis from 2% (related to thrombocytopenia) to ten times that (89,90). In some of these patients, viral infection may contribute to cystitis (91).

After treatment with cyclophosphamide, symptoms of cystitis may occur, including suprapubic discomfort, frequency, urgency, dysuria, and nocturia. Severe involvement may give rise to incontinence and gross hematuria. In the milder cases, laboratory findings may disclose microscopic hematuria or only excess sloughing of transitional epithelial or bladder cells. Repeated insults with the metabolites of cyclophosphamide can lead to fibrosis and telangiectasia of the bladder (85–87,92); these conditions may lead, in turn, to life-threatening hemorrhage and/or a dysfunctional, noncompliant bladder. Bladder symptoms may occur shortly after cyclophosphamide administration or up to many years after cessation of therapy. Although bladder fibrosis and malignancy may follow hemorrhagic cystitis, they may also occur in the absence of clinically overt cystitis. Malignant transformation to transitional cell carcinoma has been reported to occur in 2% to 5% of patients receiving oral cyclophosphamide for nonmalignant disease (83,84,93,94).

Cystitis may occur after a single oral dose of cyclophosphamide. Generally, however, the greater the dose of drug and the longer the duration of therapy, the greater is the probability of bladder toxicity. Thus, cumulative damage to transitional epithelium occurs with repeated insults by the metabolites of cyclophosphamide. A high urine flow tends to reduce the risk by both diluting the metabolites and reducing bladder contact as a result of more frequent bladder emptying. Intermittent bolus cyclophosphamide therapy puts the patient at risk for this and other toxicities only periodically. Careful attention to the bladder during those times can greatly decrease bladder toxicity. Reducing agents such as *N*-acetylcysteine or MESNA have markedly diminished the risk of bladder irritation (63–66).

Nausea

Nausea is a common complication of high-dose cyclophosphamide therapy. After bolus treatment, there may be protracted vomiting. On subsequent administration, recall of the prior therapy and its attendant nausea may cause worse vomiting or even severe nausea on arrival at the scene of treatment and before the drug is even given. This complication can be ameliorated with anti-nausea medications. One very effective drug is ondansetron (Zofran), which blocks the peripheral and central serotonin type 3 receptors involved in the pathophysiology of acute chemotherapy-induced emesis.

Alopecia

Hair loss is a common complication of high-dose cyclophosphamide treatment. Although this side effect tends to be dose dependent, some patients lose substantial amounts of hair at doses below those at which other individuals suffer little hair loss. The alopecia is typically diffuse and reversible. Indeed, many patients experience regrowth even while continuing to take the drug.

Allergic Reaction

Immediate hypersensitivity reactions varying from urticaria to acute anaphylaxis have occurred in several patients after a dose of intravenous cyclophosphamide (28,95,98). In many of these patients, subsequent skin testing with either cyclophosphamide or one of its metabolites such as 4-hydroperoxycyclophosphamide was positive (95–98). IgE antibodies to cyclophosphamide also

have been found (96). However, not all allergic responses that occur after cyclophosphamide are necessarily caused by an allergic reaction to the drug. Cyclophosphamide appears to be capable of inactivating cells that ordinarily serve to suppress allergic responses (34,41–44). As a result, cyclophosphamide therapy may release allergic responses to other antigens (45,99).

Gonadal Failure

Cyclophosphamide, like other alkylating agents, is capable of damaging germ cells in both males and females. In general, the effect is dose dependent, although boluses of cyclophosphamide may have less toxicity on the gonads (as has been long recognized for the bladder) than daily doses (100). Premature menopause may occur after courses of drug in adult women. In general, the older the patient, the greater the likelihood (56,101). In females of all ages, cyclophosphamide therapy may lead to ovarian failure with ovarian atrophy and loss of follicles and ova (101,102).

Male sterility with testicular atrophy may occur after cyclophosphamide therapy (103). The frequent use of cyclophosphamide in minimal change renal disease of children has led to studies of the effect on their gonads. The deleterious action of cyclophosphamide on male gonads appears to have a threshold of about 300 mg/kg total dose (104–106). Cyclophosphamide is much less toxic in this regard than chlorambucil with a threshold of 8 to 10 mg/kg (107,108).

Teratogenicity

Conception during the course of cyclophosphamide therapy is associated with a risk of fetal malformations in both experimental animals and humans, although normal offspring may result (109–114). In experimental animals, a number of specific types of defects have been described. The malformations appear to arise from the excess death of cells undergoing rapid cell division without an effect on cells undergoing physiologic death (113).

In addition to therapy during embryogenesis, prior cyclophosphamide treatment of animals has led to an increase in postimplantation loss, decreased fetal weight, and an increase in malformed fetuses. Moreover, grandchildren of cyclophosphamide-treated animals have had similar abnormalities. This finding is true even of grandchildren of males treated with cyclophosphamide (110,114). Indeed, defective grandchildren may be born to phenotypically normal parents whose own parents had been treated with the drug. It appears that cyclophosphamide can cause sufficient damage to induce intrauterine death, or less damage that leads to a malformation or alterations in DNA of a recessive nature.

Carcinogenicity

Cyclophosphamide therapy has been associated with an increased risk of malignancy (20–22,93,94,115). Presumably the DNA damage caused by the drug contributes importantly to leukemia and lymphomas; there is an increased frequency of hypoxanthine-guanine phosphoribosyl transferase mutants (116), and there is increased sister-chromatid exchange in peripheral blood mononuclear cells from patients treated with the drug (117).

Baltus et al (115) found that fifteen of eighty-one patients treated with cyclophosphamide developed malignancies, mainly lymphoid and hematologic. This was a 14-fold risk compared with disease controls. Indeed, it has been suggested that the threat of malignancies limits effective, cyclophosphamide-containing treatments for rheumatoid arthritis (118).

The cause of bladder cancer is very different. Chronic irritation by the cyclophosphamide metabolite, acrolein, (and perhaps other metabolites) is the major cause of bladder cancer, which occurred in 2% to 5% of patients receiving oral cyclophosphamide for nonmalignant disease (83,84,93,94). This cancer is largely preventable with proper bladder care (e.g., hydration, MESNA).

Foods containing carotenoids and various other reducing agents may limit in vitro clastogenicity after cyclophosphamide administration or the in vitro effect of its metabolites. Whether such reducing agents interfere in vivo with either the beneficial actions of cyclophosphamide or its malignant potential remains to be determined.

Infection

There have been long-standing fears that patients with nonmalignant diseases receiving moderate doses of cyclophosphamide might develop infectious complications, including serious infections. There is no question that patients made severely leukopenic are subject to infection. This condition may occur if a bolus therapy drives the white count too low (see Fig. 3-4) or if the marrow cannot continue to tolerate a previously tolerated daily dose. Moreover, patients with serious immune-mediated disorders who are given the drug also may be predisposed to infection by the underlying disease or by recent or concomitant therapy, especially with corticosteroids (119). The latter situation is especially important because many patients who are given cyclophosphamide are already receiving corticosteroids, often in high dosage. Corticosteroids, especially in high daily doses, markedly predispose patients to infections, promote dissemination of infections, and mask the early signs of infections, often resulting in a delay in treatment.

When a patient fails to respond adequately to high doses of corticosteroids and cyclophosphamide is added, the physicians often fail to taper the corticosteroids until there is a clinical effect of the cyclophosphamide therapy. This practice subjects the patient to a much greater risk of infection than if the steroids had been reduced to a low dose. Moreover, maintaining the high steroid dose is usually inappropriate because the risk-benefit ratio is far in favor of risk. Thus, when cyclophosphamide is added to a corticosteroid regimen, in most cases it is necessary to taper the steroids before a response is obtained from the cyclophosphamide to prevent infectious complications. Indeed, both the National Institutes of Health (NIH) lupus protocol (49,120) and the NIH Wegener's granulomatosis protocol (121,122) call for steroid tapering. The lupus protocol calls for a lower initial dose of prednisone (30 mg/day or 0.5 mg/kg/day) and is associated with fewer infections.

Many patients have developed serious infections during cyclophosphamide therapy. It appears that most of the serious infections have occurred in patients who also have received prolonged daily therapy with prednisone at dosages of at least 30 mg/day and often in the range of 60 mg/day (122–125). The infections are those also seen in patients treated with high doses of corticosteroids alone (e.g., *S. aureus* and other bacterial infections, herpes viruses, fungi, and *Pneumocystis carinii*). Patients receiving, at most, low doses of corticosteroids do not experience an increase in infections (with the exception of herpes zoster) (47,49).

Cardiac

High doses of bolus cyclophosphamide, especially those used to prepare patients for hematopoietic stem-cell reconstitution, have been associated with acute hemorrhagic myocarditis and congestive heart failure, which have led to death (126,127).

One recent study suggested that cardiac toxicity was especially a problem at doses greater than $1.55\,g/m^2$ (128). Another found that people who maximally metabolize the drug are at special risk for cardiac toxicity (129).

Most patients who receive 120 to 240 mg/kg of cyclophosphamide over a few days have electrocardiograms with reduced voltage in the QRS complex and decreased systolic function. In these cases congestive heart failure may be induced by the large amounts of fluid often given to patients receiving the drug to prevent bladder complications. Arrhythmias may result from direct toxic effects of drug on the cardiac conducting system or may be secondary to toxic effects on the myocardium. Sinus tachycardia may indicate early myocardial damage.

Pulmonary

High doses of cyclophosphamide may cause histologic findings in the lung similar to those that occur with other cytotoxic agents such as endothelial swelling, intra-alveolar exudation, interstitial inflammation, fibroblast proliferation, and fibrosis. Pulmonary fibrosis developed after cyclophosphamide in experimental animals and in approximately 1% of patients (8,130–132). Genetic factors appear to play a role in that mouse strains show substantial differences in susceptibility (8). Pulmonary toxicity can appear from weeks to many years after cyclophosphamide administration. The major symptom is dyspnea. Typically, nonproductive cough, dyspnea, fatigue, and malaise may be present. Bibasilar end-inspiratory ("velcro") rales may occur, but the physical examination may be normal. There may be a fever. Hemoptysis is not common and should suggest another diagnosis. Chest x-rays show a bibasilar or diffuse reticular pattern. There may be a diffuse pulmonary edema pattern, especially early in the disorder. In some cases of biopsy-proven fibrosis, the x-ray may be nondiagnostic. Pleural effusion is not a feature of this toxicity. High-resolution CT scans, gallium scans, and MRI may be more sensitive than the plain chest x-ray in detecting the abnormalities of cyclophosphamide-induced pulmonary fibrosis. Sputum containing bizarre pneumocytes is suggestive. A definitive diagnosis is made by open lung biopsy. Treatment is withdrawal of drug. Corticosteroids often have been given, but do not appear to modify the effect on mortality, which may be as high as 35% in severe cases.

It has been suggested that the pulmonary-damaging effects of cyclophosphamide are related to co-oxidation by way of the prostaglandin H synthetase system because high levels of the prostaglandin H synthetase are found in the lung (132). The pulmonary toxicity of cyclophosphamide is worsened by simultaneous or even subsequent oxygen therapy because of loss of antioxidant defense mechanisms through complex reactions involving the formation of oxygen free radicals, lipid peroxidation, and membrane damage (13).

Although the bulk of the initial metabolism of cyclophosphamide occurs in the liver, the drug may be converted to its active metabolites in other organs, especially the lung and kidney (11,13–16,19). Ordinarily, the 4-hydroxy-cyclophosphamide produced can be metabolized to the less reactive 4-ketophosphamide or to the nontoxic alcophosphamide (by alcohol dehydrogenase) and to carboxyphosphamide (by aldehyde oxidase/aldehyde dehydrogenase). The absence in the lung of measurable amounts of aldehyde oxidase and aldehyde dehydrogenase may contribute to lung toxicity; in other tissues these enzymes metabolize aldophosphamide to nontoxic metabolites (see Fig. 3-1) (13). Acrolein also may contribute to the pulmonary damage (13).

Liver

It is not completely clear whether liver disease is a rare complication of cyclophosphamide therapy. It has been suggested that cyclophosphamide itself might induce hepatotoxicity (133) on the basis of a few patients who experienced liver toxicity after cyclophosphamide therapy. However, other possible reasons must be considered for the appearance of liver disease after cyclophosphamide therapy such as reactivation of a viral liver disorder or even an exacerbation of azathioprine-induced hepatitis (134).

Inappropriate Secretion of Antidiuretic Hormone

The ADH secreted after cyclophosphamide therapy may have direct adverse effects on renal tubules, leading to severe hyponatremia, seizures, and sudden death in patients hydrated with salt-free fluids. Therefore, the drug should not be administered with 5% dextrose in water (60–62).

Effects in Specific Nonmalignant Diseases

Rheumatoid Arthritis

When cyclophosphamide became available for experimental use in nonmalignant disorders, it was tried in the treatment of patients with rheumatoid arthritis. In an early uncontrolled study, cyclophosphamide was given to 38 patients for 6 to 40 months; improvement occurred in 75% (135). A 32-week randomized trial was reported by a committee of the Arthritis Foundation (47). There were two cyclophosphamide regimens: 1) high dose, up to 150 mg/day, regarded as the potentially effective dose; and 2) low dose, up to 15 mg/day, regarded as the negative control dose. The high-dose group had clinical improvement, decline in immunoglobulin levels, reduced rheumatoid factor titers, and slowing of radiographic changes.

Several additional controlled trials have affirmed the ability of cyclophosphamide to inhibit the disease process in patients with rheumatoid arthritis (118,136–139), including erosions (136,139). In a subsequent, 32-week, double-blind study comparing two doses of cyclophosphamide (150 mg/day versus 75 mg/day) in 88 patients with rheumatoid arthritis, improvement occurred in patients in both groups, but greater improvement occurred in patients receiving the higher dose (140). The side effects were similar in the two groups, suggesting that if a patient is going to be put at risk of side effects, there ought to be maximal chance of benefit.

In another early study, cyclophosphamide was found to reduce the requirement for corticosteroids (141). All of these early studies in patients with rheumatoid arthritis involved daily cyclophosphamide therapy, generally in the range of 50 mg/day to 150 mg/day. Such therapy was occasionally associated with hemorrhagic cystitis, clearly a result of the cyclophosphamide therapy, and later with malignancy, which initially was not clearly attributed to drug. Since then, however, it has become clear that daily oral cyclophosphamide poses an unacceptable risk of malignancy in patients with rheumatoid arthritis (115,118,142). In an attempt to retain efficacy but reduce potential toxicity, intravenous cyclophosphamide has been tried in patients with rheumatoid arthritis, but it generally has not been effective (143–144).

Daily cyclophosphamide suppresses both cell-mediated immunity and antibody production; bolus cyclophosphamide suppresses antibody production well, but is less effective at suppressing cell-mediated immune function. As a result, it would be expected that a cell-mediated disorder such as rheumatoid synovitis would respond better to daily therapy. In contrast, if rheumatoid vasculitis includes a pathogenetic component of antibody-mediated disease, bolus, as well as daily, cyclophosphamide might be expected to be effective. Indeed, both daily and bolus cyclophosphamide have been given to patients with necrotizing rheumatoid vasculitis (145). Bolus therapy is now preferred, although this use is not supported by randomized trials. Patients may have a good response to intravenous cyclophosphamide with regard to the vasculitis and yet develop new or worsening arthritis (50), consistent with the view that bolus therapy is effective for the antibody-mediated disorder but not the cell-mediated disease.

Wegener's Granulomatosis

The usefulness of cyclophosphamide in patients with Wegener's granulomatosis was documented by Novack and Pearson in 1971

(146) and confirmed by several reports (121,147–149). Before immunosuppressive drugs were used in the therapy of this disorder, the outlook for patients with serious forms of the disease was bleak. With cyclophosphamide, the outlook was improved substantially. For many years, the NIH group used cyclophosphamide in patients with Wegener's granulomatosis without ever performing a randomized trial. They reported that a daily dose of cyclophosphamide (2 to 4 mg/kg body weight) plus prednisone (1 mg/kg body weight) resulted in remission in almost 90% of patients (121). The 5-year survival rate was 80% compared with a 1-year survival rate of less than 20% in historic controls who were treated with corticosteroids alone. However, as milder forms of Wegener's granulomatosis were diagnosed and toxicity from long-term cyclophosphamide therapy became a difficulty, the lack of comparative studies with other agents (e.g., azathioprine, methotrexate) became apparent. Such studies might have pointed to adequate therapy of milder disease with a less toxic drug.

The NIH daily cyclophosphamide regimen led to hemorrhagic cystitis in 43% of 158 patients and a 2.4-fold increase in malignancies, especially bladder cancer (122). Almost half of the patients had serious infections, and 3% of the 158 patients died of the infections.

In an attempt to provide the benefits of cyclophosphamide with less toxicity, one group administered pulse cyclophosphamide to patients with Wegener's granulomatosis in the manner used to treat patients with systemic lupus erythematosus: IV boluses monthly for 6 months in a dose of 350 to 909 mg/m^2 to keep the white blood cell count at about 3000/μL; a bolus of 100 mg prednisone also was given (150). They confirmed that pulse cyclophosphamide was relatively safe: serious side effects occurred in only one patient. However, only 42% of patients showed complete or partial remission lasting 6 months (150). Pulse cyclophosphamide was effective in those patients with mild-to-moderate disease activity and low titers of antibodies reactive with neutrophil cytoplasmic antigens. The regimen was of little benefit in patients with more severe Wegener's granulomatosis (150). The authors suggested that pulse cyclophosphamide not be used as first-line therapy in severe Wegener's granulomatosis. Because the dose of cyclophosphamide was rather modest, averaging 667 mg/m^2, it is possible that this test of bolus therapy was not adequate and that larger doses of bolus cyclophosphamide, perhaps given a little more frequently, might have yielded a different result. This idea is supported by a recent report of the benefit of bolus cyclophosphamide in patients with Wegener's granulomatosis (151).

The attention to drug dosage is particularly important in view of the narrow therapeutic window of cyclophosphamide in most nonmalignant diseases (see Fig. 3-2). Indeed, in cancer chemotherapy, small differences in the amount of bolus chemotherapy can lead to significant increases in patients' survival (152). Nonetheless, the modest therapeutic benefits in Wegener's granulomatosis are consistent with the idea that bolus cyclophosphamide therapy is more useful for antibody-mediated than cell-mediated or granulomatous disease.

Three groups (51,153,154) found that bolus cyclophosphamide was especially effective in patients with Wegener's granulomatosis and renal disease. It may be that cyclophosphamide is especially effective in patients with renal disease; however, Reinhold-Keller et al (150) claim that the patients really did not have Wegener's granulomatosis. A higher cyclophosphamide dose used to treat the patients who showed benefit may have been as relevant to the favorable response as the organs involved.

Systemic Lupus Erythematosus

The mainstays of treatment in systemic lupus erythematosus are nonsteroidal anti-inflammatory drugs, hydroxychloroquine, and low doses of corticosteroids. For patients with serious disease, especially those with vasculitis, nonthrombotic CNS involvement, and glomerulonephritis, cyclophosphamide therapy can be lifesaving and/or organ preserving. Patients with lupus nephritis have been treated successfully with daily cyclophosphamide (1 to 2.5 mg/kg/day) or with intermittent bolus therapy (500 to 1000 mg/m^2 every 4 weeks to every 3 months), a therapy based on randomized clinical trials (49,120,155). Typically, therapy is continued for 18 to 24 months after the clearing of renal inflammation as determined by urinalyses. The decision to begin or to withhold cyclophosphamide therapy in a patient with lupus nephritis may be clear cut in cases of severe or minimal nephritis, respectively, but may be difficult in marginal cases (52,156).

In addition, substantial anecdotal evidence supports the use of cyclophosphamide to treat CNS lupus syndromes not related to infection, bleeding, or thrombosis (including those with antiphospholipid antibodies), but including some serious psychiatric syndromes in addition to vasculitic problems. Some patients have responded to a few boluses of 500 to 1000 mg/m^2 every 3 to 4 weeks. Others have required somewhat more prolonged therapy. Occasionally, patients with systemic lupus erythematosus have other disease manifestations that do not respond to corticosteroid therapy. Many such patients, including those with myocarditis and thrombocytopenia (157), respond to the addition of cyclophosphamide. Rare patients with suppression of bone marrow products (e.g., autoimmune neutropenia) have responded to cyclophosphamide therapy.

In recent years, there has been a move to induce a remission of disease with one form of therapy and to maintain that remission with another (potentially less toxic) therapy. For example, treatment with several courses of bolus cyclophosphamide would be followed by treatment with azathioprine (49). Large clinical trials are needed to support this approach, which has some theoretic merit.

Polymyositis

In the standard treatment of polymyositis, high doses of corticosteroids are given initially. If that therapy is inadequate or if the corticosteroids cannot be tapered reasonably, methotrexate is added. Some individuals with polymyositis have benefitted from other immunosuppressive drugs. Uncontrolled studies have suggested that daily cyclophosphamide benefits patients with polymyositis and dermatomyositis (158); however, monthly bolus therapy was not effective (159). It appears that dermatomyositis is especially responsive. There are few guidelines to determine when or whether daily cyclophosphamide should be given to patients with either polymyositis or dermatomyositis. Patients with poorly responsive polymyositis may have inclusion body disease, which responds very slowly to all therapies. In addition, therapy can only help the immune and inflammatory component of the disease; it should not be expected to correct weakness resulting from permanent loss of muscle fibers.

Idiopathic Nephrotic Syndrome

One of the early clinical uses of cyclophosphamide was to treat children with idiopathic nephrotic syndrome and minimal-change disease (160,161). Short courses of cyclophosphamide (2 mg/kg/day) have been advocated in children with minimal-change disease who have relapsed after receiving intensive corticosteroid therapy. Typically, an 8-week course of cyclophosphamide is given to those who have relapsed and who are not corticosteroid dependent. A 12-week course is given to those who have relapsed and are steroid dependent (107,108). Cyclophosphamide also has been given to avoid toxicity from corticosteroids, especially in patients who relapse frequently.

Adults with minimal-change disease also respond to cyclophosphamide administration, but somewhat more slowly and less completely than children. Nevertheless, approximately 60% of adults respond to prolonged cyclophosphamide therapy with remission of their proteinuria (162–164). Cyclophosphamide also has been used successfully to treat patients with membranous disease (165).

As a general principle, the nephrotic syndrome itself may be associated with a risk of atherogenesis. Similarly, corticosteroid therapy may be associated with such a risk. Therefore, the combination may be especially deleterious. Compared with corticosteroids, cyclophosphamide is an excellent drug for the treatment of nephrotic syndrome because it does not predispose to atherogenesis and it eliminates the nephrotic syndrome more rapidly than do corticosteroids.

Polyarteritis Nodosa and Other Vasculitides

Uncontrolled reports indicate that cyclophosphamide treatment is effective for patients with polyarteritis nodosa and other necrotizing vasculitides with or without the concomitant use of corticosteroids. Indeed, the response and survival rates of patients with systemic necrotizing vasculitis have risen from less than 20% to greater than 80% with cyclophosphamide therapy, 2 mg/kg/day (166). In practice, cyclophosphamide has been added to corticosteroid therapy in patients with inadequate responses, or both cyclophosphamide and corticosteroids are initiated simultaneously, especially in patients with rapidly progressive vasculitic syndromes (167). If daily therapy is chosen, the dose of drug that can be given is usually limited by the leukopenia that develops after 6 to 12 months of therapy. In general, treatment is continued for 12 to 18 months after a clinical remission is obtained. Sepsis has been

reported as a complication of therapy (123). Patients with "microscopic polyarteritis" do not respond as well to cyclophosphamide as other patients with polyarteritis (168).

Multiple Sclerosis

Cyclophosphamide has been evaluated in uncontrolled and controlled trials in patients with multiple sclerosis, primarily of the chronic progressive type. Several studies used very intensive therapy (larger boluses than given to patients with lupus were given more frequently early in the therapeutic course). Daily cyclophosphamide proved to be of no significant benefit in some studies (169,170) and of benefit in others (171). Several studies showed benefit with intensive therapy. Among those, the overall results show that relatively short-term benefits are not maintained unless therapy is continued for long periods (162–175). Patients younger than 40 years of age appear to benefit the most (175). Even when treatment was stopped and the patient has relapsed, reinstitution of cyclophosphamide may provide therapeutic benefit.

In those who respond, the mechanism of action has been difficult to elucidate. Recent studies have pointed to an immune modulatory effect rather than just a cytotoxic or immunosuppressive action (176). In these studies, Th-1 type T-lymphocyte effects predominated in patients with multiple sclerosis and correlated with disease activity. Cyclophosphamide therapy led to a normalization of Th-1/Th-2 effects, with an increase in Th-2 effects and a decrease in Th-1 effects. A post-cyclophosphamide increase in Th-2 effects was also found by another group (177). Such an immune mechanism in multiple sclerosis may be the mirror image of systemic lupus erythematosus in which Th-2 effects may dominate and where therapy is aimed at a relative reduction in such Th-2 effects (178,179).

Other Diseases

In addition to the disorders just discussed, patients with many other immune-mediated diseases have been treated successfully with cyclophosphamide, usually in uncontrolled situations. These diseases include hematologic disorders such as autoimmune hemolytic anemia and autoimmune thrombocytopenia; renal diseases such as Goodpasture's syndrome and antiglomerular basement membrane disease (the drug has been used in conjunction with plasma exchange); neurologic disorders such as chronic inflammatory polyneuropathy; and Behçet's syndrome (both the ocular and extraocular manifestations have been controlled) (180–182). Controlled trials comparing different regimens would help physicians evaluate their relative merits. Cyclophosphamide has been effective in treating patients with inflammatory cardiac disease associated with immune-mediated rheumatic diseases (e.g., systemic lupus erythematosus and dermatomyositis) but only occasional patients with chronic idiopathic myocarditis. Indeed, in animals with experimental myocarditis, cyclophosphamide is of no benefit (183).

There are some suggestions that cyclophosphamide may be more effective than its relative, chlorambucil, for patients with certain diseases; however, there are too few comparative studies to draw a firm conclusion (184,185).

Cyclophosphamide As an Inducer of Hematopoietic Stem Cells

In recent years, the use of hematopoietic stem-cell reconstitution has increased dramatically. One reason has been the relative ease of obtaining stem cells from blood through the use of various conditioning regimens, many of which use cyclophosphamide (along with marrow stimulants such as granulocyte colony-stimulating factor). Moreover, engraftment may be accelerated when peripheral stem cells are used rather than marrow cells to reconstitute individuals after they have been treated with high doses of chemotherapeutic agents. The exact composition of peripheral stem cells (and their function) may vary depending on the induction regimen (186).

Drugs Related to Cyclophosphamide

Ifosphamide is a drug similar to cyclophosphamide in which one of the two 2-chloroethyl groups is shifted to the nitrogen atom of the oxazaphosphorine ring. It is activated by the hepatic P-450 mixed-function oxidase (187). It causes less myelosuppression than cyclophosphamide and more bladder and central nervous system toxicity. Cerebellar dysfunction, seizures, and altered mental status occur in more than 25% of patients receiving high doses of drug. Neurotoxicity correlates with hepatic dysfunction. More chloroacetaldehyde is produced, which gives greater levels of urologic and neurologic toxicity (188). As a result, the drug must be given with MESNA or a comparable agent.

Another related drug, 4-hydroxycyclophosphamide, can be directly activated by tumor cells. It has been used in conjunction with high-dose chemotherapy programs in association with autologous bone marrow rescue (189). Marrow is removed and then the patient undergoes high-dose chemotherapy to eliminate leukemic cells. Patients are rescued by the marrow that had been removed prior to chemotherapy. The autologous marrow is treated in vitro with the 4-hydroxycyclophosphamide to remove leukemic cells before reinfusion (189). This method may be modified when peripheral stem cells are used.

Since cyclophosphamide and ifosphamide must be activated (and only a limited number of organs are capable of doing so), investigators have sought a related drug that might be used for regional therapy. Recently, mafosfamide, which does not require liver metabolism for activity, has been used intrathecally (190).

Concluding Comments

Cyclophosphamide has been a mainstay of several cancer chemotherapy regimens and is an important drug for inducing marrow suppression prior to transplantation. Several once-fatal non-malignant diseases, including severe Wegener's granulo-matosis, severe systemic lupus erythematosus, and necrotizing rheumatoid vasculitis (as well as other vasculitides), have responded dramatically to cyclophosphamide therapy. Proper use of the drug can provide efficacy while minimizing toxicity. Still, potential toxicities are worrisome. New methods should be sought for maintaining efficacy while further reducing toxicity and for developing less toxic but equally effective agents.

With advances in molecular genetics, cyclophosphamide has been swept into the revolution with the identification of genes that cause drug resistance in tumors and constructs that may be used to deliver genes to increase cells' susceptibility to the drug. A discussion of such issues is beyond the scope of this chapter.

References

1. Arnold H, Bourseaux F, Brock N. Chemotherapeutic action of a cyclic nitrogen mustard phosphamide ester (B518-ASTA) in experimental tumours of the rat. Nature 1958; 181:931.
2. Bagley CM Jr, Bostick FW, Devita VT. Clinical pharmacology of cyclophosphamide. Cancer Res 1973;33:226–233.
3. Cohen JL, Jao JY, Jusko WJ. Pharmacokinetics of cyclophosphamide in man. Br J Pharmacol 1970;43:677–680.
4. Mouridsen HT, Jacobsen E. Pharmacokinetics of cyclophosphamide in renal failure. Acta Pharmacol Toxicol 1975; 36:409–414.
5. Ren S, Kalhorn TF, McDonald GB, et al. Pharmacokinetics of cyclophosphamide and its metabolites in bone marrow transplantation patients. Clin Pharmacol Ther 1998;64:289–301.
6. Brock N, Hohorst HJ. Metabolism of cyclophosphamide. Cancer 1967;20:900–904.
7. Torkelson AR, LaBudde JA, Weikel JH Jr. Metabolic fate of cyclophosphamide. Drug Metab Rev 1974;3:131–165.
8. Kanekal S, Fraiser L, Kehrer JP. Pharmacokinetics, metabolic activation, and lung toxicity of cyclophosphamide in C57/B16 and ICR mice. Toxicol Appl Pharmacol 1992;114:1–8.
9. Fischer DS. Alkylating agents. In: Fischer DS, Marsh JC, eds. Cancer therapy. Boston: GK Hall, 1982.
10. McDiarmid MA, Itpe PT, Kolodner K, et al. Evidence for acrolein-modified DNA in peripheral blood leukocytes of cancer patients treated with cyclophosphamide. Mutat Res 1991;248:93–99.
11. Dormeyer BE, Sladek NE. Kinetics of cyclophosphamide biotransformation in vivo. Cancer Res 1980;40:174–180.
12. Friedman OM, Myles A, Colvin M. Cyclophosphamide and related phosphoramide mustards: current status and future prospects. Adv Cancer Chemother 1979;1:143–204.
13. Patel JM. Metabolism and pulmonary toxicity of cyclophosphamide. Pharmacol Ther 1990;47:137–146.
14. Acosta D, Mitchell DB. Metabolic activation and cytotoxicity of cyclophosphamide in primary cultures of postnatal hepatocytes. Biochem Pharmacol 1981;30:3225–3230.
15. Hipkens JH, Struck RF, Gurtao HL. Role of aldehyde dehydrogenase in the metabolism-dependent biological activity of cyclophosphamide. Cancer Res 1981;41:3571–3583.
16. Colvin M, Hilton J. Pharmacology of cyclophosphamide and metabolites. Cancer Treat Rep 1981;65:89–95.
17. Joqueviel C, Martino R, Gilard V, et al. Urinary excretion of

cyclophosphamide in humans. Drug Metab Dispos 1998;26: 418–428.

18. Sladek NE, Powers JF, Grage GM. Half-life of oxazaphosphorines in biological fluids. Drug Metab Dispos 1984;12: 553–559.

19. Brookes P, Lawley PD. The action of alkylating agents on deoxyribonucleic acid in relation to biological effects of the alkylating agents. Exp Cell Res 1963;9:512–520.

20. Kahn MF, Arlet J, Bloch-Michel H. Leucemies aigues apres traitment par agents cytotoxiues en rheumatologie-19 observations chez 2006 patients. Nouv Presse Med 1979;8: 1393–1397.

21. Krause JR. Chronic idiopathic thrombocytopenic purpura (ITP): development of acute non-lymphocytic leukemia subsequent to treatment with cyclophosphamide. Med Pediatr Oncol 1982;10:61–65.

22. Puri HC, Cambell RA. Cyclophosphamide and malignancy. Lancet 1977;1:1306.

23. Brinkman CJJ, Nillesen WM, Hommes OR. The effect of cyclophosphamide on T lymphocytes and T lymphocyte subsets in patients with chronic progressive multiple sclerosis. Acta Neurol Scand 1984;69:90–96.

24. Clements RJ, Yu DTY, Levy J. Effects of cyclophosphamide on B- and T-lymphocytes in rheumatoid arthritis. Arthritis Rheum 1974;17:347–353.

25. Hurd ER, Giuliano VJ. The effect of cyclophosphamide on B and T lymphocytes in patients with connective tissue diseases. Arthritis Rheum 1975;18:67–75.

26. Moody DJ, Fahey JL, Grable E, et al. Administration of monthly pulses of cyclophosphamide in multiple sclerosis patients: delayed recovery of several immune parameters following discontinuation of long-term cyclophosphamide treatment. J Neuroimmunol 1987;14:175–182.

27. Hersh EM, Wong VG, Freireich EJ. Inhibition of the local inflammatory response in man by antimetabolites. Blood 1966;27:38–48.

28. McCune WJ, Golbus J, Zeldes W, et al. Clinical and immunologic effects of monthly administration of intravenous cyclophosphamide in severe systemic lupus erythematosus. N Engl J Med 1988;318:1423–1431.

29. Bast RC Jr, Reinherz EL, Maver C, et al. Contrasting effects of cyclophosphamide and prednisolone on the phenotype of human peripheral blood lymphocytes. Clin Immunol Immunopathol 1983;28:101–114.

30. Berd D, Mastrangelo MJ. Effect of low dose cyclophosphamide on the immune system of cancer patients: depletion of CD4+, w2H4+ suppressor-inducer T-cells. Cancer Res 1988;48:1671–1675.

31. Moody DJ, Kagan J, Liao D, et al. Administration of monthly pulses of cyclophosphamide in multiple sclerosis patients: effects of long-term treatment on immunologic parameters. J Neuroimmunol 1987;14L:161–173.

32. Cupps TR, Edgar LC, Fauci AS. Suppression of human B lymphocyte function by cyclophosphamide. J Immunol 1982;128:2453–2457.

33. Zhu L-P, Cupps TR, Whalen G. Selective effects of cyclophosphamide therapy of activation, proliferation, and differentiation of human B cells. J Clin Invest 1987;79:1082–1090.

34. Turk JL, Parker D. The effect of cyclophosphamide on the immune response. J Immunopharmacol 1979;1:127–137.

35. Turk JL, Parker D. Effect of cyclophosphamide on immunological control mechanisms. Immunol Rev 1982;65:99–113.

36. Hyman LR, Kovacs K, Steinberg AD. Durg-induced tolerance: selective induction with immunosuppressive drugs and their synergistic interaction. Int Arch Allergy Appl Immunol 1975;48:248–260.

37. Steinberg AD, Gelfand MC, Hardin JA, Lowenthal DT. Therapeutic studies in NZB/W mice. III: relationship between renal status and efficacy of immunosuppressive drug therapy. Arthritis Rheum 1975;18:9–14.

38. Steinberg AD, Krieg AM, Takashi T, Gourley MF. Timing of immunosuppression in the natural history of autoimmune diseases. J Autoimmun 1992;5(suppl A):197–203.

39. Paterson PY. Cyclophosphamide treatment of experimental allergic encephalomyelitis in Lewis rats. J Immunol 1971; 106:1473–1479.

40. Scott DG, Bacon PA, Allen C, et al. IgG rheumatoid factor, complement and immune complexes in rheumatoid synovitis and vasculitis: comparative and serial studies during cytotoxic therapy. Clin Exp Immunol 1981;43:54–63.

41. Chiorazzi N, Fox DA, Katz DH. Hapten specific IgE antibody responses in mice. VI. Selective enhancement of IgE antibody production by low doses of x-irradiation and by cyclophosphamide. J Immunol 1976;117:1629–1637.

42. Chiorazzi N, Fox DA, Katz DH. Hapten specific IgE antibody responses in mice. VII: conversion of IgE non-responder strains to IgE responders by elimination of suppressor T cell activity. J Immunol 1977;118:48–54.

43. Drossler K, Klima F, Ambrosius H. Influence of cyclophosphamide and 6-mercaptopurine on the IgG1 and IgG2 immune response in guinea pigs. Immunol 1981;44:61–66.

44. Askanese PW, Hayden BJ, Gershon RK. Augmentation of delayed-type hypersensitivity by doses cyclophosphamide which do not affect antibody responses. J Exp Med 1975;141:697–705.

45. Debre P, Waltenbaugh C, Dorf ME, Benacerraf B. Genetic control of specific immune suppression. IV: responsiveness to the random copolymer L-glutamic acid^{50}-L-tyrosine^{50} induced in Balb/c mice by cyclophosphamide. J Exp Med 1976;144:277–281.

46. Uitdehaag BMJ, Nillesen WM, Hommes OR. Long-lasting effects of cyclophosphamide on lymphocytes in peripheral blood and spinal fluid. Acta Neurol Scand 1989;79:12–17.

47. Cooperating Clinics Committee of the American Rheumatism Association. A controlled trial of cyclophosphamide in rheumatoid arthritis. N Engl J Med 1970;283:883–889.

48. Steinberg AD. Principles in the use of immunosuppressive agents. In: Schumacher HR, ed. Primer on the rheumatic diseases. 9th ed. Atlanta, GA: The Arthritis Foundation, 1988: 288–294.

49. Steinberg AD, Steinberg SC. Long-term preservation of renal function in patients with lupus nephritis randomized to receive cyclophosphamide-containing regimens as compared with prednisone only. Arthritis Rheum 1991;34:945–950.

50. Bacon PA. Vasculitis—clinical aspects and therapy. Acta Med Scand Suppl 1987;715:157–163.

51. Hoffman GS, Leavitt RY, Fleisher TA, et al. Treatment of Wegener's granulomatosis with intermittent high-dose intravenous cyclophosphamide. Am J Med 1990;89:403–410.

52. Steinberg AD. The treatment of lupus nephritis. Kidney Int 1986;30:769–787.
53. Juma FD. Effect of liver failure on the pharmacokinetics of cyclophosphamide. Eur J Clin Pharmacol 1984;26:591–593.
54. Galletti PM, Pasqualino A, Geering RG. Haemodialysis in cancer chemotherapy. Trans Am Soc Artif Org 1966;12: 20–25.
55. Moutsopoulos HM, Gallagher JD, Decker JL, Steinberg AD. Herpes zoster in patients with systemic lupus erythematosus. Arthritis Rheum 1978;21:798–802.
56. Boumpas DT, Austin HA III, Vaughan EM, et al. Risk for sustained amenorrhea in patients with systemic lupus erythematosus receiving intermittent pulse cyclophosphamide therapy. Ann Intern Med 1993;119:366–369.
57. Clavel M, Soukop M, Greenstreet YL. Improved control of emesis and quality of life with ondansetron in breast cancer. Oncology 1993;50:180–195.
58. Beck TM, Ciociola AA, Jones ES, et al. Efficacy of oral ondansetron in the prevention of emesis in outpatients receiving cyclophosphamide-based chemotherapy. Ann Intern Med 1993;118:407–413.
59. Grunberg SM, Hesketh PJ. Control of chemotherapy-induced emesis. N Engl J Med 1993;329:1790–1796.
60. DeFronzo RA, Braine H, Colvin OM, Davis PJ. Water intoxication in man after cyclophosphamide therapy: time course and relation to drug activation. Ann Intern Med 1973;78: 861–869.
61. Bressler RB, Huston DP. Water intoxication following moderate-dose intravenous cyclophosphamide. Arch Intern Med 1985;145:548–551.
62. Green TP, Mirken BL. Prevention of cyclophosphamide-induced antidiuresis by furosemide infusion. Clin Pharmacol Ther 1981;29:634.
63. Brock N, Phol J. Prevention of urotoxic side effects by regional detoxification with increased selectivity of oxazophosphorine cytostatics. IARC Sci Publ 1986;78:269.
64. Droller MJ, Saral R, Santos G. Prevention of cyclophosphamide-induced hermorrhagic cystitis. Urology 1982;20:256.
65. Andrioli GL, et al. The efficacy of MESNA (2-mercaptoethane sodium sulfonate) as a uroprotectant in patients with hemorrhagic cystitis receiving further oxazaphosphorine chemotherapy. J Clin Oncol 1987;5:799–805.
66. Blacklock H, Ball L, Knight C, et al. Experience with mesna in patients receiving allogeneic bone marrow transplants for poor prognosis leukaemia. Cancer Treat Rev 1983;10:45–52.
67. Faquin WC, Schneider TJ, Goldberg MA. Effect of inflammatory cytokines on hypoxia-induced erythropoietin production. Blood 1992;79:1987–1994.
68. Fischer JW, Roh BL. Influence of alkylating agents on kidney erythropoietin production. Cancer Res 1964;24:983–988.
69. Eschbach JW, Kelly MR, Haley NR, et al. Treatment of the anemia of progressive renal failure with recombinant human erythropoietin. N Engl J Med 1989;321:158–161.
70. Pincus T, Olsen NJ, Russell IJ, et al. Multicenter study of recombinant human erythropoietin in correction of anemia in rheumatoid arthritis. Am J Med 1990;89:161–168.
71. Miller CB, Plantanias LC, Ratain MJ, et al. A phase I/II trial of erythropoietin in the treatment of chemotherapy-induced anemia in patients with cancer. J Natl Cancer Inst 1992;84:98–103.
72. Duhrsen U, Villefal JL, Boyd J, et al. Effects of recombinant human granulocyte colony-stimulating factor on hematopoietic progenitor cells in cancer patients. Blood 1988;72:2074–2081.
73. Souza LM, Boone TC, Gabrilove K, et al. Recombinant human granulocyte colony-stimulating factor: effects on normal and leukemic myeloid cells. Science 1986;232:61–65.
74. Morstyn G, Souza L, Keech J, et al. Effect of granulocyte colony-stimulating factor on neutropenia induced by cytotoxic chemotherapy. Lancet 1988;1:667–672.
75. Gabrilove JL, Jakubowski A, Scher H, et al. Effect of granulocyte colony-stimulating factor on neutropenia and associated morbidity due to chemotherapy for transitional cell carcinoma of the uroepithelium. N Engl J Med 1988;318: 1414–1422.
76. Bronchud MH, Howell A, Crowther D, et al. The use of granulocyte colony-stimulating factor to increase the intensity of treatment with doxorubicin in patients with advanced breast and ovarian cancer. Br J Cancer 1989;60:121–128.
77. Tjan-Heijnen VC, Biesma B, Feszten J, et al. Enhanced myelotoxicity due to granulocyte colony-stimulating factor administration. J Clin Oncol 1998;16:2708–2714.
78. van Os R, Robinson S, Sheridan T, et al. Granulocyte colony-stimulating factor enhances bone marrow stem cell damage caused by repeated administration of cytotoxic agents. Blood 1998;92:1950–1956.
79. Yokose N, Ogata K, Tamura H, et al. Pulmonary toxicity after granulocyte colony-stimulating factor-combined chemotherapy. Br J Cancer 1998;77:2286–2290.
80. Schein PS, Winokur ST. Immunosuppressive and cytotoxic chemotherapy: long term complications. Ann Intern Med 1975;82:84–95.
81. Brock N, Stekar J, Pohl J, et al. Acrolein: the causative factor of urotoxic side-effects of cyclophosphamide, ifosfamide, trofostamide and sufosafamide. Arzneimittel-Forsch 1979; 29:659–661.
82. Cox PJ. Cyclophosphamide cystitis—identification of acrolein as the causative agent. Biochem Pharmacol 1979; 28:2045–2049.
83. Fairchild WV, Spence CR, Solomon HD, Gangai MP. The incidence of bladder cancer after cyclophosphamide therapy. J Urol 1979;122:163–164.
84. Stillwell TJ, Benson RC Jr, DeRemee RA, et al. Cyclophosphamide-induced bladder toxicity in Wegener's granulomatosis. Arthritis Rheum 1988;31:465–470.
85. Ansell ID, Castro JE. Carcinoma of the bladder complicating cyclophosphamide therapy. Br J Urol 1975;47:413–418.
86. Johnson WW, Meadows DC. Urinary bladder fibrosis and telangiectasia associated with long term cyclophosphamide therapy. N Engl J Med 1971;284:290–294.
87. Plotz PH, Klippel JH, Decker JL, et al. Bladder complications in patients receiving cyclophosphamide for systemic lupus erythematosus or rheumatoid arthritis. Ann Intern Med 1979;91:221–223.
88. Lawrence HJ, Simone A, Aur RJ. Cyclophosphamide-induced hemorrhagic cystitis in children with leukemia. Cancer 1975;36:1572–1576.
89. Brugieres L, Hartmann O, Travagli JP, et al. Hemorrhagic cystitis following high-dose chemotherapy and bone

marrow transplantation in children with malignancies: incidence, clinical course, and outcome. J Clin Oncol 1989;7: 194–199.

90. Thomas AE, Patterson J, Prentice HG, et al. Hemorrhagic cystitis in bone marrow transplantation patients: possible increased risk associated with prior busulfan therapy. Bone Marrow Transplant 1987;1:347–355.

91. Arthur RR, Shah VK, Baust SJ, et al. Association of BK viruria with hemorrhagic cystitis in recipients of bone marrow transplants. N Engl J Med 1986;315:230–234.

92. Manohoran A. Carcinoma of the urinary bladder in patients receiving cyclophosphamide. Aust N Z J Med 1984;14: 507–512.

93. Baker GL, Kahl LE, Zee BC, et al. Malignancy following treatment of rheumatoid arthritis with cyclophosphamide: long term case controlled follow up study. Am J Med 1987;83:1–9.

94. Kinlen LJ. Incidence of cancer in rheumatoid arthritis and other disorders after immunosuppressive treatment. Am J Med 1985;78(suppl 1):A44–A49.

95. Knysak DJ, McLean JA, Solomon WR, et al. Immediate hypersensitivity reaction to cyclophosphamide. Arthritis Rheum 1994;37:1101–1104.

96. Lakin JD, Cahill RA. Generalized urticaria to cyclophosphamide: type I hypersensitivity to an immunosuppressive agent. J Allergy Clin Immunol 1976;58:160–171.

97. Cromar BW, Colvin M, Casale TB. Validity of skin tests to cyclophosphamide and metabolites. J Allergy Clin Immunol 1991;88:965–967.

98. Weiss RB, Bruno S. Hypersensitivity reactions to cancer chemotherapeutic agents. Ann Intern Med 1981;94:66–72.

99. Yasunami R, Bach J-F. Anti-suppressor effect of cyclophosphamide on the development of spontaneous diabetes in NOD mice. Eur J Immunol 1988;18:481–484.

100. Haubitz M, Ehlerding C, Kamino K, et al. Reduced gonadal toxicity after i.v. cyclophosphamide administration in patients with non-malignant diseases. Clin Nephrol 1998;49: 19–23.

101. Warne GL, Fairley KF, Hobbs JB, Martin FIR. Cyclophosphamide-induced ovarian failure. N Engl J Med 1973;289:1159–1162.

102. Miller JJ III, Williams GF, Lessing JC. Multiple late complications of therapy with cyclophosphamide including ovarian destruction. Am J Med 1971;50:530–535.

103. Fairley KF, Barrie JG, Johnson W. Sterility and testicular atrophy related to cyclophosphamide therapy. Lancet 1972;1:568–569.

104. Etteldorf JN, West CD, Pitcock JA, Williams DL. Gonadal function, testicular histology, and meiosis following cyclophosphamide therapy in patients with nephrotic syndrome. J Pediatr 1976;88:206.

105. Watson AR, Rance CP, Bain J. Long-term effects of cyclophosphamide on testicular function. Br Med J 1985; 291:1457.

106. Trompeter RS, Evans PR, Barratt TM. Gonadal function in boys with steroid-responsive nephrotic syndrome treated with cyclophosphamide for short periods. Lancet 1981;1: 1177–1179.

107. APN (Arbeitsgemeinschaft fur Padiatrische Nephrologie). Effect of cytotoxic drugs in frequently relapsing nephrotic syndrome with and without steroid dependence. N Engl J Med 1982;306:451–457.

108. APN (Arbeitsgemeinschaft fur Padiatrische Nephrologie). Cyclophosphamide treatment of steroid-dependent nephrotic syndrome: comparison of eight weeks with twelve weeks course. Arch Dis Child 1987;62:1102–1119.

109. Kirshon B, Wasserstrum N, Willis R, et al. Teratogenic effects of first-trimester cyclophosphamide therapy. Obstet Gynecol 1988;72:462–464.

110. Auroux M, Dulioust E, Selva J, Rince P. Cyclophosphamide in the F_0 male rat: physical and behavioral changes in three successive adult generations. Mutat Res 1990;229:189–200.

111. Gibson JE, Becker BA. The teratogenicity of cyclophosphamide in mice. Cancer Res 1968;28:475–480.

112. Porter AJ, Singh S. Teratogenesis and mutagenesis in mouse fetuses treated with cyclophosphamide. Teratogenesis Carcinog Mutagen 1988;8:191–203.

113. Singh S, Sanyal AK. Eye anomalies induced by cyclophosphamide in rat fetuses. Acta Anat (Basel) 1976;94:490–496.

114. Hales BF, Crossman K, Robaire B. Increased postimplantation loss and malformations among the F_2 progeny of male rats chronically treated with cyclophosphamide. Teratology 1992;45:671–678.

115. Baltus JAM, Boersma JW, Hartman AP, Vandenbrouke JP. The occurrence of malignancies in patients with rheumatoid arthritis treated with cyclophosphamide: a controlled retrospective follow-up. Ann Rheum Dis 1983;42:368–373.

116. Palmer RG, Smith-Burchnell CA, Pelton BK, et al. Use of T cell cloning to detect in vivo mutations induced by cyclophosphamide. Arthritis Rheum 1988;31:757–761.

117. Palmer RG, Dore S, Denman AM. Cyclophosphamide induces more chromosome damage than chlorambucil in patients with connective tissue diseases. Q J Med 1986; 59:395–400.

118. Csuka M, Carrera GF, McCarty DJ. Treatment of intractable rheumatoid arthritis with combined cyclophosphamide, azathioprine, and hydroxychloroquine: a follow-up study. JAMA 1986;255:2315–2319.

119. Dale DC. Defects in host defense mechanisms in compromised patients. In: Rubin RH, Young LS, eds. Clinical approach to infections in the compromised host. New York: Plenum, 1981:35–74.

120. Steinberg AD, Kaltreider HB, Staples PJ, et al. Cyclophosphamide in lupus nephritis: a controlled trial. Ann Intern Med 1971;75:165–171.

121. Fauci AS, Haynes BF, Katz P, Wolff SM. Wegener's granulomatosis: prospective clinical and therapeutic experience with 85 patients for 21 years. Ann Intern Med 1983;98:76–85.

122. Hoffman GS, Kerr GS, Leavitt RY, et al. Wegener's granulomatosis: an analysis of 158 patients. Ann Intern Med 1992;116:488–498.

123. Bradley JD, Brandt KD, Katz BP. Infectious complications of cyclophosphamide treatment for vasculitis. Arthritis Rheum 1989;32:45–53.

124. Morgan MC, Matteson E, Dunne R, et al. Complications of intravenous cyclophosphamide: association of infection with high daily doses of prednisone in lupus patients. Arthritis Rheum 1995;33(suppl 5):R27.

125. Kattwinkel N, Cook L, Agnello V. Overwhelming infection in a young woman after intravenous cyclophosphamide therapy for lupus nephritis. J Rheum 1991;18:79–81.

126. Gottdeiner JS, Appelbaum FR, Ferrans VJ, et al. Cardiotoxicity associated with high-dose cyclophosphamide therapy. Arch Intern Med 1981;141:758.

127. Cazin B, Gorin NC, Laporte JP, et al. Cardiac complications after bone marrow transplantation: a report on a series of 63 consecutive transplantations. Cancer 1986;57:2061.
128. Braverman AC, Antin JH, Plappert MT, et al. Cyclophosphamide cardiotoxicity in bone marrow transplantation: a prospective evaluation of new dosing regimens. J Clin Oncol 1991;9:1215–1223.
129. Ayash LJ, Wright JE, Trettakov O, et al. Cyclophosphamide pharmacokinetics: correlation with cardiac toxicity and tumor response. J Clin Oncol 1992;10:995–1000.
130. Cooper JAD Jr, White DA, Matthay RA. Drug-induced pulmonary disease. Am Rev Respir Dis 1986;133:321–340.
131. Fraiser LH, Kanekal S, Kehrer J. Cyclophosphamide toxicity: characterizing and avoiding the problem. Drugs 1992; 42:781–795.
132. Smith DR, Kehrer JP. Cooxidation of cyclophosphamide as an alternative pathway for its bioactivation and lung toxicity. Cancer Res 1991;51:542–548.
133. Goldberg JW, Lidsky MD. Cyclophosphamide-associated hepatotoxicity. South Med J 1985;78:222–223.
134. Shaunak S, Munro JM, Weinbren K, et al. Cyclophosphamide-induced liver necrosis: a possible interaction with azathioprine. Q J Med 1988;67:309–317.
135. Fosdick WM, Parsons JL, Hill DF. Long term cyclophosphamide therapy in rheumatoid arthritis. Arthritis Rheum 1968;11:151–161.
136. Currey HL, Harris J, Mason RM, et al. Comparison of azathioprine, cyclophosphamide, and gold in treatment of rheumatoid arthritis. Br Med J 1974;3:763–766.
137. Felson DT, Anderson JJ, Meenan RF. The comparative efficacy and toxicity of second-line drugs in rheumatoid arthritis: results of two meta-analyses. Arthritis Rheum 1990;33: 1449–1461.
138. Hawley DJ, Wolfe F. Are the results of controlled clinical trials and observational studies of second line therapy in rheumatoid arthritis valid and generalizable as measures of rheumatoid arthritis outcome: analysis of 122 studies. J Rheumatol 1991;18:1008–1014.
139. Davis JD, Muss HB, Turger RA. Cytotoxic agents in the treatment of rheumatoid arthritis. South Med J 1978;71: 58–64.
140. Williams HJ, Reading JC, Ward JR, O'Brien WM. Comparison of high and low dose cyclophosphamide therapy in rheumatoid arthritis. Arthritis Rheum 1980;23:521–527.
141. Urowitz MB. Immunosuppressive therapy in rheumatoid arthritis. J Rheumatol 1974;1:364–373.
142. Keysser G, Keysser C, Keysser M. Treatment of refractory rheumatoid arthritis with low-dose cyclophosphamide. Long-term follow-up of 108 patients. Z Rheumatol 1998;57: 101–107.
143. Hall ND, Bird HA, Ring EFJ, Bacon PA. A combined clinical and immunological assessment of four cyclophosphamide regimens in rheumatoid arthritis. Agents Actions 1979;9:97–102.
144. Walters MT, Cawley MID. Combined suppressive drug treatment in severe refractory rheumatoid disease: an analysis of the relative effects of parenteral methylprednisolone and cyclophosphamide. Ann Rheum Dis 1988;47: 924–929.
145. Scott DG, Bacon PA. Intravenous cyclophosphamide plus methylprednisolone in treatment of systemic rheumatoid vasculitis. Am J Med 1984;76:377–384.
146. Novack SN, Pearson CM. Cyclophosphamide therapy in Wegener's granulomatosis. N Engl J Med 1971;284:938–942.
147. Wolff SM, Fauci AS, Horn RG, Dale DC. Wegener's granulomatosis. Ann Intern Med 1974;81:513–525.
148. Reza MJ, Dornfield L, Goldberg LS, et al. Wegener's granulomatosis: long-term follow-up of patients treated with cyclophosphamide. Arthritis Rheum 1975;18:501–506.
149. Israel HL, Patchefsky AS, Saldana MI. Wegener's granulomatosis, lymphomatoid granulomatosis, and benign lymphocyte angiitis and granulomatosis of lung: recognition and treatment. Ann Intern Med 1977;87:691–699.
150. Reinhold-Keller E, Kekow J, Schnabel A, et al. Influence of disease manifestation and anti-neutrophil cytoplasmic antibody titer on the response to pulse cyclophosphamide therapy in patients with Wegener's granulomatosis. Arthritis Rheum 1994;37:919–924.
151. Koldingsnes W, Gran JT, Omdal R, Husby G. Wegener's granulomatosis: long-term follow-up of patients treated with pulse cyclophosphamide. Br J Rheumatol 1998;37:659–664.
152. Arriagada R, LeChevalier T, Pignon J-P, et al. Initial chemotherapeutic doses and survival in patients with limited small-cell lung cancer. N Engl J Med 1993;329: 1848–1852.
153. Falk RJ, Hogan S, Carey TS, Jennette C. Clinical course of anti-neutrophil cytoplasmic autoantibody-associated glomerulonephritis and systemic vasculitis. Ann Intern Med 1990;113:656–663.
154. Steppat D, Gross WL. Stage adapted treatment of Wegener's granulomatosis: first results of a prospective study. Klinische Wochenschrift 1989;67:666–671.
155. Boumpas DT, Austin HA III, Vaughan EM, et al. Severe lupus nephritis: controlled trial of pulse methylprednisolone versus two different regimens of pulse cyclophosphamide. Lancet 1992;340:741–745.
156. Steinberg AD. Reply: a critique of the NIH lupus nephritis survey. Arthritis Rheum 1992;35:605–607.
157. Roach BA, Hutchinson GJ. Treatment of refractory systemic lupus-associated thrombocytopenia with intermittent low-dose intravenous cyclophosphamide. Arthritis Rheum 1993;36:682–684.
158. Cairo-Glasgow Study Group. Dermatomyositis: observations on the use of immunosuppressive therapy and review of literature. Postgrad Med 1978;54:516–527.
159. Cronin ME, Miller FW, Hicks JE, et al. The failure of intravenous cyclophosphamide therapy in refractory idiopathic inflammatory myopathy. J Rheumatol 1989;16:1225–1228.
160. International Study of Kidney Disease in Children. Prospective controlled trial of cyclophosphamide therapy in children with the nephrotic syndrome. Lancet 1974;2:423–427.
161. Chiu J, Drummond KN. Long-term follow-up of cyclophosphamide therapy in frequent-relapsing minimal-lesion nephrotic syndrome. J Pediatr 1974;84:825.
162. Cameron JS, Chantler C, Ogg CS, White RPR. Long-term stability of remission in nephrotic syndrome after treatment with cyclophosphamide. Br Med J 1974;274:7–11.
163. Al-Kader AA, Lien JWK, Aber GM. Cyclophosphamide alone in the treatment of adult patients with minimal-change glomerulonephritis. Clin Nephrol 1979;11:26–30.
164. Nolasco F, Cameron JS, Heywood EF, et al. Adult-onset minimal-change nephrotic syndrome: a long-term follow-up. Kidney Int 1986;29:1215–1223.

165. West ML, Jindal KK, Bear RA, Goldstein MB. A controlled trial of cyclophosphamide in patients with membranous glomerulonephritis. Kidney Int 1987;31:579–584.

166. Fauci AS, Katz P, Haynes BF, Wolff SM. Cyclophosphamide therapy of severe systemic necrotizing vasculitis. N Engl J Med 1979;301:234–238.

167. Fauci AS, Haynes BF, Katz P. The spectrum of vasculitis: clinical, pathologic, immunologic and therapeutic considerations. Ann Intern Med 1978;89:660–676.

168. Adu D, Howie AJ, Scott DI, et al. Polyarteritis and the kidney. Q J Med 1987;62:221–237.

169. The Canadian Cooperative Multiple Sclerosis Study Group. The Canadian cooperative trial of cyclophosphamide and plasma exchange in progressive multiple sclerosis. Lancet 1991;337:441–446.

170. Likosky WH, Fireman B, Elmore R, et al. Intense immunosuppression in chronic progressive multiple sclerosis: the Kaiser study. J Neurol Neurosurg Psychiatry 1991;54: 1055–1060.

171. Mauch E, Kornhuber HH, Pfrommer U, et al. Effective treatment of chronically progressive multiple sclerosis with low-dose cyclophosphamide with minor side-effects. Eur Arch Psychiatry Neurol Sci 1989;238:115–117.

172. Wajgt A, Szyrocka-Szwed K, Gadomska B, Szczechowski L. Evaluation of the results of treating progressive multiple sclerosis with cyclophosphamide. Neurol Neurochir Pol 1988;22:518–523.

173. Carter JL, Hafler DA, Dawson DM, et al. Immunosuppression with high-dose i.v. cyclophosphamide and ACTH in progressive multiple sclerosis: cumulative 6-year experience in 164 patients. Neurology 1988;38:9–14.

174. Trouillas P, Neuschwander P, Nighoghossian N, et al. Intensive immunosuppression in progressive multiple sclerosis: an open study comparing 3 groups: cyclophosphamide, cyclophosphamide-plasmapheresis and control subjects: results after 3 years. Rev Neurol (Paris) 1989;145:369–377.

175. Weiner HL, Mackin GA, Orav EJ, et al. Intermittent cyclophosphamide pulse therapy in progressive multiple sclerosis: final report of the Northeast Cooperative Multiple Sclerosis Treatment Group. Neurology 1993;43:910–918.

176. Comabella M, Balashov K, Issazadeh S, et al. Elevated interleukin-12 in progressive multiple sclerosis correlates with disease activity and is normalized by pulse cyclophosphamide therapy. J Clin Invest 1998;102:671–678.

177. Takashima H, Smith DR, Fukara H, et al. Pulse cyclophosphamide plus methylprednisolone induced specific IL-4-secreting T cells in multiple sclerosis patients. Clin Immunol Immunopathol 1998;88:28–34.

178. Steinberg AD, Klinman DM. Studies on the immunological basis of systemic lupus. Immunol Rev 1995;144:157–193.

179. Steinberg AD. Systemic lupus erythematosus. In: Kaplan AP, ed. Allergy. Orlando: WB Saunders, 1997.

180. Urgancioglu M, Saylan T, Akarcay K, Sezen T. Immunosuppressive therapy in Behçet's disease. In: Dilsen N, Konice M, Ovul C, eds. Behçet's disease. Amsterdam: Excerpta Medica, 1979.

181. Firat IK. Immunosuppressive treatment in Behçet's disease (report of 100 cases). In: Dilsen N, Konice M, Ovul C. eds. Behçet's disease. Amsterdam: Excerpta Medica, 1979.

182. Hijikata K, Ezawa Y, Masuda K, Ohara K. An evaluation of immunosuppressant therapy in Behçet's disease. In: Dilsen N, Konice M, Ovul C, eds. Behçet's disease. Amsterdam: Excerpta Medica, 1979.

183. Lange LG, Schreiner GF. Mechanisms of disease: immune mechanisms of cardiac disease. N Engl J Med 1994;330: 1129–1135.

184. Branten AJ, Reichert LJ, Koene RA, Wetzels JF. Oral cyclophosphamide versus chlorambucil in the treatment of patients with membranous nephropathy and renal insufficiency. QJM 1998;91:359–366.

185. Ivanova MM, Nasanova VA, Solovyov SK, et al. Controlled trial of cyclophosphamide, azathioprine, and chlorambucil in lupus nephritis. A double-blind trial. Rheumatisma 1981;2:11–18.

186. Sammarelli G, Caramatti C, Tabilio A, et al. CD34+ cells mobilized by cyclophosphamide and granulocyte colony-stimulating factor are functionally different from CD34+ cells mobilized by G-CSF. Bone Marrow Transplant 1998;21:561–568.

187. Brock N, Hilgard P, Peukert M, et al. Basis and new developments in the field of oxazaphosphorines. Cancer Invest 1988;6:513–532.

188. Goren MP, Wright RK, Pratt CB, et al. Dechloroethylation of isofosfamide and neurotoxicity. Lancet 1986;2:1219–1220.

189. Yeager AM, Kaizer H, Santos GW, et al. Autologous bone marrow transplantation in patients with acute non-lymphocytic leukemia using ex vivo marrow treatment with 4-hydroperoxycyclophosphamide. N Engl J Med 1986;315: 141–147.

190. Slavc I, Schuller E, Czech T, et al. Intrathecal mafosfamide therapy. J Neurooncol 1998;38:213–218.

Chapter 4

The Purine Antagonists: Azathioprine and Mycophenolate Mofetil

Nina E. Tolkoff-Rubin
Robert H. Rubin

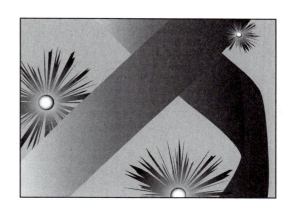

The potential clinical applications of immunosuppressive therapy are many, ranging from the control and prevention of transplant rejection to the treatment of an ever-increasing array of diseases in which self-directed inflammatory processes result in tissue injury and/or systemic symptoms. Such "autoimmune" or "autoinflammatory" processes include the collagen vascular diseases, inflammatory bowel disease, certain forms of hepatitis, a variety of skin conditions such as pemphigus and discoid lupus, such neurologic diseases as myasthenia gravis and multiple sclerosis, sarcoidosis and other idiopathic inflammatory conditions of the lung, a variety of renal diseases, and type I diabetes mellitus. All these conditions have several characteristics in common: Tissue injuring inflammation and immune injury are central to the pathogenesis of the clinical disease; the clinical course of these conditions tends to be chronic, progressive, and/or relapsing; and there is at least suggestive evidence that corticosteroids, if administered in high enough doses for sufficiently long periods, can attenuate the extent of tissue injury and alleviate many of the patients' symptoms.

As immunosuppressive therapy has emerged to become the cornerstone of patient management for a number of conditions, certain basic principles have emerged: The consequences of sustained corticosteroid therapy are many, ranging from the metabolic to the skeletal, with perhaps the most important being their broad-based inhibitory effect on virtually all elements of host defense. Thus, it is now clearly recognized that there is a limit to the amount of corticosteroid therapy that can be administered to an individual on a continuous basis and still achieve a balance between therapeutic benefit and an acceptable rate of side effects. As a result, considerable effort has been expended over the past 3 decades in developing so-called "steroid-sparing" immunosuppressive regimens. Such regimens have been based on the concept that the addition of moderate doses of more specific immunosuppressive agents to the therapeutic program will permit the use of lower doses of steroids, thus achieving the desired therapeutic effect but with fewer side effects. The drug that established the validity of this concept is azathioprine, which is still an important part of immunosuppressive therapy today, more than 30 years after its first use therapeutically as an immunosuppressive agent in humans (1). The purpose of this chapter is to review the pharmacology, mechanism of action, toxicities, and clinical applications of this drug, as well as those of a new drug, mycophenolate mofetil, which has been developed to play a role similar to that of azathioprine but with the pos-

sibility of increased efficacy without a significant increment in toxicity.

Azathioprine

History

The development of azathioprine was a direct outgrowth of an effort led by Gertrude Elion and George Hitchings to synthesize antimetabolites of the nucleic acid bases as cancer chemotherapeutic agents. Within 2 years of the synthesis of 6-mercaptopurine in 1951, Joseph Burchenal had shown that this drug could produce remissions in childhood leukemia. The next step was the obervation that 6-mercaptopurine, when administered to cancer patients, had both cytotoxic and immunosuppressive effects (2,3). Very quickly thereafter, experimental studies showed that 6-mercaptopurine prolonged the survival of skin allografts in rodent models (4), as well as the survival of kidney allografts in dogs (5). Azathioprine, an N-methyl-nitroimidazole thiopurine (Fig. 4-1), had been synthesized previously with the intent of developing a slow-release prodrug of 6-mercaptopurine. Although this was not the case, it became apparent that azathioprine had similar immunosuppressive effects to 6-mercaptopurine and, at least in the canine model, was less toxic. By 1963 a protocol in which azathioprine and corticosteroids were combined in renal transplantation had been successful (6), and the modern era of organ transplantation and immunosuppressive therapy had begun. With success in transplantation and with the increasing recognition of the importance of autoimmunity in a number of diseases and its resemblance pathogenetically to allograft rejection, similar regimens were tested in many of the previously listed diseases (3,7,8). Azathioprine emerged as an important immunosuppressive agent itself, as well as a model for the development of other steroid-sparing immunosuppressive agents.

Pharmacology and Mechanism of Action

Azathioprine interacts with sulfhydryl-containing compounds in the intestinal wall, liver, and red blood cells to release 6-mercaptopurine. 6-Mercaptopurine is then converted to a series of intracellularly active metabolites, most notably thioinosinic acid and

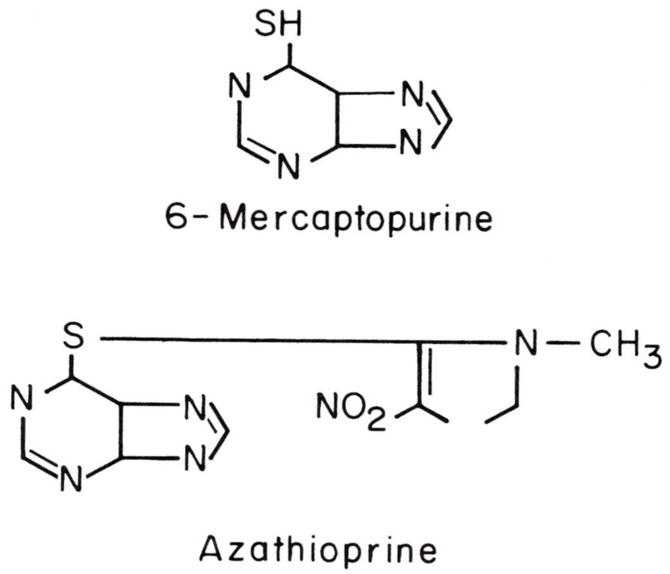

Figure 4-1. Structural formulas of 6-mercaptopurine and azathioprine.

6-thioguanine nucleotides. Thioinosinic acid inhibits phosphoribosylpyrophosphate amidotransferase, which catalyzes an early step of de novo purine synthesis (Fig. 4-2*A*). In addition, thioinosinic acid inhibits a number of enzymes involved in the purine salvage pathway (Fig. 4-2*B*). The net effect is depletion of cellular purine stores, thus suppressing DNA and RNA synthesis. This effect is most notable during the S phase (DNA synthesis) of the cell cycle; that is, actively dividing lymphocytes responding to antigenic stimulation are particularly susceptible to this effect. In contrast, there is little impact on mature elements of antigenic memory or end-stage lymphocyte function. Not surprisingly, azathioprine exerts its maximal immunosuppressive effect when administered immediately following antigenic challenge (3,7,8).

Although the relatively selective toxicity of azathioprine for replicating, antigen-responsive cells probably accounts for most of its immunosuppressive action, additional immunomodulatory effects may also be of importance. For example, 6-thioguanosine triphosphate, when incorporated into cellular DNA, may give rise to delayed cytotoxicity by causing chromosomal breaks and nucleic acid malformations. These events contribute to immunosuppression, myelotoxicity, and perhaps an increased risk for malignancy. In addition, azathioprine itself may block antigen recognition by alkylating thiol groups on T-cell surface membranes; and a 6-mercaptopurine metabolite (6-methylmercaptopurine ribonucleotide) may also inhibit purine synthesis. However, the quantitative importance of these last two effects in determining the immunosuppressive impact of azathioprine is unclear (7,8).

Both azathioprine and 6-mercaptopurine disappear rapidly from the plasma, with half-lives of 50 and 74 minutes, respectively. In contrast, the active metabolites thioinosinic acid and 6-

thioguanine persist over many hours, particularly intracellularly, making possible once-a-day therapy. Renal dysfunction does not have a significant effect on the pharmacokinetics or immunosuppressive effects of azathioprine or 6-mercaptopurine.

There are two major pathways of azathioprine and 6-mercaptopurine degradation: The first involves S-methylation of these compounds, which inactivates them. A cytoplasmic enzyme, thiopurine methyltransferase (TPMT), catalyzes this process. There is considerable genetic polymorphism is this enzyme, such that intermediate TPMT activity is found in approximately 10% of individuals (patients who are heterozygous for an altered TPMT) and low activity is found in about 1 in 300 (patients who are homozygous for the recessive trait of an altered TPMT). These individuals, when given standard doses of azathioprine either to prevent allograft rejection or to treat rheumatic disease, are at high risk for the development of azathioprine toxicity, both myelosuppression and gastrointestinal intolerance. The major inactivating mutations at the human TPMT locus have been identified, and both genotypic (by polymerase chain reaction) and phenotypic (by enzymatic assay) assays are available. It is now apparent that most instances of myelosuppression are caused by this mechanism and are potentially avoidable through measurement of TPMT function and subsequent dosage adjustment (9–13).

The second pathway of metabolic degradation is direct oxidation by xanthine oxidase to 8-hydroxy-6-mercaptopurine and then to 6-thiouric acid. An important aspect of the xanthine oxidase pathway is that allopurinol (a xanthine oxidase inhibitor commonly used in the treatment of gout and hyperuricemia) can block this pathway, thereby potentiating both the immunosuppressive and myelotoxic effects of azathioprine. Thus, a decrease in the dose of azathioprine by 60% to 80% is necessary, with close monitoring of bone marrow function if allopurinol therapy is instituted (14,15).

Clinical Usefulness

Transplantation

The use of azathioprine and prednisone in combination, first reported in 1963, remained the basis for management of clinical transplantation for the next 2 decades, transforming renal transplantation from an interesting experiment in human immunobiology to a practical means of rehabilitating patients with end-stage renal disease. A typical immunosuppressive regimen during this era was as follows: azathioprine, 5 mg/kg/day for 5 days and tapering to 2 to 2.5 mg/kg/day by the tenth day; prednisone, 2 mg/kg/day at 1 week and tapering to 40 mg/day at 30 days and 25 mg/day at 60 days. In addition, antilymphocyte antibody preparations were used either as induction therapy or as antirejection therapy, with pulse doses of intravenous methylprednisolone (500 to 1000 mg) also being used to treat rejection. With programs such as these, 1-year allograft survival rates of 70% for living-related donor kidneys and 50% for cadaver donor kidneys were achieved (7,8,16).

The advent of cyclosporine-based immunosuppressive regimens increased the success of organ transplantation (in fact,

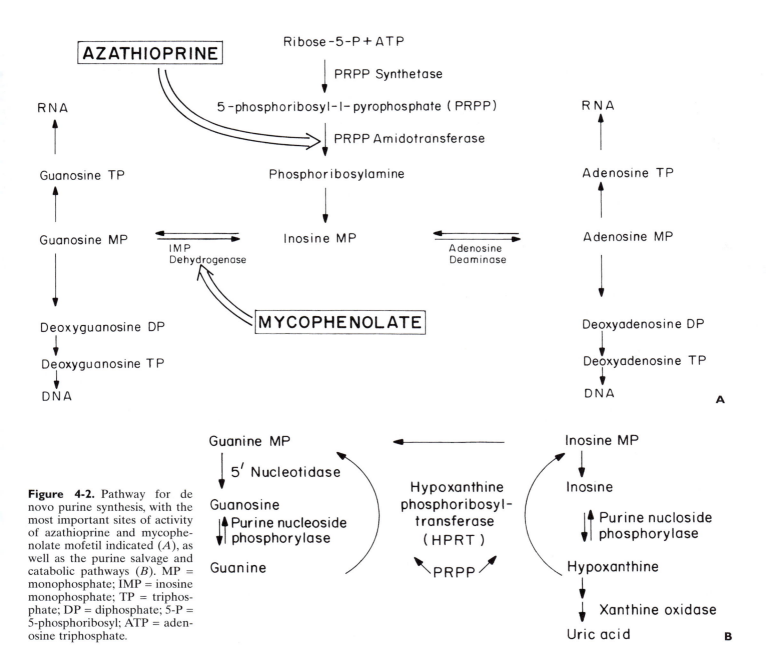

Figure 4-2. Pathway for de novo purine synthesis, with the most important sites of activity of azathioprine and mycophenolate mofetil indicated (*A*), as well as the purine salvage and catabolic pathways (*B*). MP = monophosphate; IMP = inosine monophosphate; TP = triphosphate; DP = diphosphate; 5-P = 5-phosphoribosyl; ATP = adenosine triphosphate.

cyclosporine was a major factor in the development of heart, liver, and lung transplantation, in addition to improving the success of renal transplantation). One-year allograft survival rates for cadaver donor organs rose to greater than 80%. In addition, the role of azathioprine was changed from that of a major component of the immunosuppressive regimen to that of a useful, ancillary agent that is deployed in one of the following ways.

First, the addition of azathioprine, usually at a dose of 1.5 to 2.0 mg/kg/day, to the basic regimen of cyclosporine and pred-

nisone (with or without an initial 5 to 7-day induction course of antilymphocyte antibody) permits the use of a lower dose of cyclosporine (with a corresponding reduction in cyclosporine nephrotoxicity), without decreasing the excellent allograft-survival results achieved with the higher-dose cyclosporine regimens. In a variant of this strategy, higher doses of azathioprine (initial dose of 5 mg/kg/day) are used, and then the dose is titrated on the basis of measured levels of red cell 6-thioguanine, with an aim to achieve a level of 100 to 200 pmol/8×10^8 red cells. This form of triple therapy has been associated with a significantly lower rate of rejection activity than that occurring with standard triple therapy (17). Such triple-drug regimens (or quadruple if induction antilymphocyte antibody programs are used as well) represent the modern extension of the concept of "steroid-sparing" immunosuppression: the desired net state of immunosuppression is most safely achieved when multiple drugs with different mechanisms of action are combined in a regimen that uses submaximal doses of these agents, thus minimizing the specific toxicities of the individual agents. The analogy to modern cancer chemotherapy is clear. These multiple-drug regimens that include azathioprine have become increasingly common in the management of heart, liver, and lung transplants, as well as cadaver kidney transplants, particularly if the patient had previously rejected an allograft or had a high level of presensitization to HLA antigens (8,18,19).

Second, azathioprine may be used as part of a sequential therapy regimen to minimize acute cyclosporine nephrotoxicity after cadaver kidney transplantation. Delayed graft function is associated with prolonged hospitalization and may be associated with decreased long-term allograft function. When cyclosporine is used immediately, particularly if the allograft has been harvested in less than optimal circumstances, the incidence of delayed graft function may be greater than 50%. Hence, to avoid superimposing cyclosporine nephrotoxicity on acute ischemia-reperfusion injury engendered in the harvesting process, while still avoiding rejection, sequential therapy was devised. In this program, azathioprine, prednisone, and an antilymphocyte antibody are used initially, and cyclosporine is substituted for the antilymphocyte antibody and azathioprine once the serum creatinine level falls to less than 2.5 mg/dL. With this approach 2-year allograft survival rates of 85% and 72% for primary and secondary cadaver renal allografts, respectively, have been reported, with the incidence of delayed graft function falling to 7.6% and that of primary nonfunction falling to 1.9%. In a variation of this approach azathioprine is continued as part of a three-drug regimen after the initiation of cyclosporine. More recent studies have suggested that this sequential approach is not required for every cadaver renal allograft recipient; rather, it should be reserved for those who are oliguric in the first few days after transplantation and would thus benefit from a cessation of cyclosporine therapy while recovering from peritransplant ischemia. This approach represents a positive example in which antirejection therapy is individualized to fit the particular clinical circumstances, rather than the treatment of every patient according to a rigid immunosuppressive protocol (20,21).

Third, although most centers use triple (or quadruple) regimens that include cyclosporine or tacrolimus for the first 3 to 6 months after transplantation, many of them attempt to pare down these regimens after that period. Because of the nephrotoxicity that can occur with either cyclosporine or tacrolimus, a number of centers slowly taper the doses of these drugs in selected patients while seeking to maintain the patients on azathioprine/prednisone regimens for the long term. When this approach is successful, improvement can occur in both renal function and blood pressure control. However, great care in patient selection for such a conversion is mandatory (e.g., first transplant, no pre-

sensitization, no acute rejection episodes for less than 6 months, and no severe episodes at any time) to avoid postconversion rejection activity (22–25). Similarly, some groups eliminate steroids from the treatment regimen of the same kind of stable patient and manage patients long term with cyclosporine or tacrolimus plus azathioprine (26–29). This option is particularly attractive for use in children, in patients with derangements in carbohydrate or lipid metabolism, in patients with posttransplant obesity or osteoporosis, and in patients with other major side effects resulting from the chronic use of corticosteroids.

Although its primary use in transplantation has been after organ transplantation, azathioprine has also been used as adjunctive therapy in the management of chronic graft-versus-host disease. Administered in conjunction with prednisone, azathioprine is effective in ameliorating graft-versus-host disease, although measurable clinical improvement may take several months. Again, an important aspect of the usefulness of azathioprine in this clinical situation is that it provides a practical approach for lowering steroid doses while still maintaining control of the graft-versus-host disease.

Rheumatoid Arthritis

Azathioprine has been approved by the Food and Drug Administration (FDA) for the treatment of severe, active, and erosive rheumatoid arthritis that has been refractory to such standard therapies as salicylates, nonsteroidal anti-inflammatory drugs, chloroquine, gold, and D-penicillamine. In such patients, azathioprine has produced response rates of 30% to 82%, with a therapeutic response usually occurring within 6 to 12 weeks of initiating therapy. In these studies, azathioprine has been used in doses ranging from 50 to 200 mg/day and in a variety of ways: short-term daily administration for 6 months, high-dose pulse therapy three times per week, and long-term therapy on a daily basis for years. In general, daily treatment programs used dosage regimens comparable to those used in organ transplantation (50 to 150 mg/day), and higher doses are used in the nondaily regimens (30).

There are multiple expected benefits of azathioprine for patients with severe, refractory rheumatoid arthritis. Significant improvement can take place in such indices of rheumatoid activity as articular index, joint count, grip strength, and synovial effusions, as well as in such subjective measures as morning stiffness, pain, and general well-being. In patients requiring corticosteroids for control of their disease, the addition of azathioprine to the therapeutic regimen can have a significant steroid-sparing effect while still maintaining control of disease manifestations. This effect is particularly beneficial in children with juvenile rheumatoid arthritis (31). Finally, some evidence suggests that azathioprine administered over a prolonged period can delay the radiologic progression of joint destruction. Azathioprine appears to be more effective in maintaining disease remission rather than in inducing a remission. As such, it has been used effectively in combination with such other drugs as gold, methotrexate, and the combination of cyclophosphamide and hydroxychloroquine; the azathioprine is maintained once disease control has been achieved (32–34).

Azathioprine therapy cannot be relied on to normalize such laboratory markers of rheumatoid arthritis as the erythrocyte sedimentation rate, latex titer, or levels of immunoglobulins in the serum. When azathioprine therapy is stopped in patients who responded to treatment, the remission is not sustained. Recrudescence of disease when azathioprine therapy is withdrawn is to be expected in this group of patients with the severe, refractory disease for which azathioprine is approved therapy, unless some other maintenance program is substituted. In patients whose disease flares when the drugs are discontinued, the resumption of therapy can once again provide control, usually within 3 months of reintroduction (35). Comparative studies would suggest that azathioprine is less effective than methotrexate in the treatment of refractory rheumatoid arthritis. However, it is clear that early institution of disease-modifying, antirheumatic drug–based treatment strategies, whether they be methotrexate, azathioprine, antimalarials, or gold therapy, will decrease long-term disability in patients with rheumatoid arthritis. The task of the clinician is to find such a program for the individual patient (32,36–38).

Systemic Lupus Erythematosus

Although not approved by the FDA for this purpose, azathioprine is used not uncommonly in the treatment of systemic lupus erythematosus, particularly in those with lupus nephritis. The combination of azathioprine and prednisone is more effective than prednisone alone in controlling disease activity and preventing the progression to end-stage renal disease. Although well-controlled studies comparing the two are not available, there is a general belief that weekly intravenous cyclophosphamide therapy is somewhat more effective in inducing remission than daily azathioprine. As a result, most patients are now being treated with intravenous cyclophosphamide and prednisone until remission is induced; and then they are maintained with azathioprine and prednisone, often with eventual tapering of the prednisone (39–44).

Azathioprine therapy may also be of use in the management of other manifestations of systemic lupus erythematosus that are resistant to more conventional therapies. For example, patients with generalized discoid skin lesions and cutaneous leukocytoclastic vasculitis who are unresponsive to therapies other than high-dose systemic steroids have been reported to respond to azathioprine (45,46). Similarly, in such other collagen diseases as Reiter's syndrome (47), there is anecdotal experience suggesting possible clinical benefit from azathioprine therapy.

Inflammatory Bowel Disease

Although not approved by the FDA for these conditions, azathioprine has been extensively studied in the treatment of both ulcerative colitis and Crohn's Disease. Azathioprine appears to be of little benefit in the management of acute flares of ulcerative colitis. In contrast, the addition of azathioprine to the therapeutic regimen of patients with chronic disease can permit the doses of corticosteroids required to be decreased and, in some cases, even stopped. It also appears to have efficacy against steroid-resistant disease, particularly in combination with cyclosporine; long-term maintenance therapy with azathioprine alone becomes possible in many instances. Maintenance therapy with azathioprine appears to decrease the relapse rate in patients with chronic ulcerative colitis in whom remission has been induced with other regimens, particularly corticosteroids (48–52). As has been the experience in transplant patients receiving azathioprine, successful outcomes of pregnancy have occurred in patients with inflammatory bowel disease who were receiving azathioprine (53–55).

Less information is available on the treatment of Crohn's disease with azathioprine, although the published experience suggests that the effects are similar to those obtained in the treatment of ulcerative colitis. Particular indications for azathioprine use include the following: pediatric Crohn's disease (especially for the steroid-sparing effect to maximize growth), refractory Crohn's disease, fistulizing Crohn's disease, recurrent disease after ileoanal anastamosis, and extraintestinal complications of Crohn's disease (56–60).

Neurologic Disease

Azathioprine has been studied in the treatment of both myasthenia gravis and multiple sclerosis, although it is not approved by the FDA in the treatment of either condition. In myasthenia gravis, both azathioprine and cyclosporine have been reported to cause significant improvement in clinical performance scores and pyridostigmine consumption. The beneficial effects of azathioprine in the treatment of myasthenia gravis are gradual in onset and may be delayed, with peak benefits not observed for 18 to 24 months. In general, however, it appears that azathioprine therapy has a beneficial effect in the management of myasthenia gravis, again primarily for chronic rather than acute disease. When azathioprine is stopped after remission has been obtained, clinical disease may recur. Although azathioprine may be used alone or in combination with corticosteroids, it appears to be most useful in combination. In many patients the disease may be effectively managed with the combination of azathioprine and alternate-day steroids (61–63).

Azathioprine has modest beneficial effects in multiple sclerosis, restricted primarily to the most severe cases, namely, those with relapsing or relentlessly progressive disease. In these individuals, azathioprine, perhaps best given in combination with other modalities, appears to have some effect in decreasing the lesion load as demonstrated by magnetic resonance imaging. These modest effects need to be carefully weighed in view of the potential toxicities of azathioprine therapy (see below) (64–66).

Other Conditions

Azathioprine therapy has been attempted in a wide variety of disease states in which autoimmune phenomena are believed to play a significant role. However, in none of these conditions have sufficient data been submitted to win FDA approval for these therapeutic indications. In the field of dermatology, azathioprine, often at least initially and in combination with corticosteroids, has been reported to be efficacious in the treatment of chronic eczematous dermatitides, a variety of bullous diseases, pemphigus vulgaris, severe polymorphous light eruption, actinic reticuloid, chronic actinic dermatitis, and pyoderma gangrenosa (67–70).

In children with the recent onset of type I diabetes mellitus, azathioprine, particularly in combination with prednisone, can have some beneficial effects in improving glucose control and in some instances in inducing a temporary remission. However, the lack of sustained benefit, coupled with the potential for toxicity, argues against this approach to diabetes (71,72). In contrast, azathioprine, especially as a steroid-sparing therapy, has shown promise in the treatment of Behçet's syndrome (73–75), sarcoidosis (76), idiopathic pulmonary fibrosis (77), chronic idiopathic thrombocytopenic purpura (78), nephrotic syndrome caused by minimal-change disease (79), autoimmune hepatitis (80), refractory myositis (81), and even asthma (82). In all these instances, further study is needed to define the relative value of azathioprine therapy as opposed to other treatment regimens, as well as the details of optimal management. As a first approximation, if azathioprine is to be used, initial therapy should be at a dose of 1.5 to 2.5 mg/kg/day.

Adverse Effects

The potential adverse effects of azathioprine can be grouped into the categories of myelotoxicity, hepatic and gastrointestinal toxicity, hypersensitivity, and participation in the pathogenesis of certain infections and malignancies. The most complete information available on adverse effects comes from the study of renal transplant recipients and those with rheumatoid arthritis. The most common side effects are nausea, vomiting, and leukopenia, with at least a temporary cessation of therapy being necessary in as many as 30% of individuals being treated with azathioprine for rheumatoid arthritis and neuromuscular disease. In patients with rheumatoid arthritis, methotrexate appears to have a similar rate of gastrointestinal side effects, raising the possibility that the underlying disease may be of importance in determining the rate of side effects. The incidence of side effects requiring interruption of azathioprine therapy is markedly less in transplant patients (and is primarily the result of dose-related myelotoxicity), perhaps related to the concomitant therapies being administered (83–85).

At doses of greater than 2 mg/kg/day, azathioprine can cause dose-related hepatotoxicity, with progression to chronic active hepatitis. At lower doses, however, particularly in organ transplant recipients, azathioprine-induced, chronic, active hepatitis and/or cirrhosis is very rare. The substitution of cyclophosphamide for azathioprine in patients with hepatic dysfunction only occasionally results in clinical or laboratory improvement. Clinical hepatitis induced by azathioprine is uncommon, although the combination of this condition with chronic hepatitis B or C infection can be problematic (86). Other forms of hepatic abnormality resulting from the chronic administration of this drug are seen but very infrequently. These include hepatic veno-occlusive disease, peliosis hepatis, perisinusoidal (Disse's space) fibrosis, and nodular regenerative hyperplasia. It has been proposed that azathioprine can damage the endothelial cells lining the hepatic sinusoids and the terminal hepatic venules, thereby producing this array of uncommon entities. This form of hepatic injury does resolve with cessation of azathioprine (87–91).

An azathioprine hypersensitivity syndrome characterized by fever, myalgias, arthralgias, malaise, and variable amounts of nausea, vomiting, and diarrhea has been described. Leukocytosis and even eosinophilia may be present. In patients with severe gastrointestinal symptoms, duodenal biopsy has revealed an eosinophilic infiltrate. Pancreatitis can occur. Rarely, the hypersensitivity reaction may be so severe that hypotension occurs. Also, as a rare consequence of azathioprine therapy, a multiorgan system condition suggesting vasculitis has occurred. Not surprisingly, such hypersensitivity reactions are most common in nontransplant patients who are not receiving other concomitant immunosuppressive therapies (92–96).

There is little doubt that azathioprine is an effective immunosuppressive agent that contributes significantly to the patient's net state of immunosuppression. As such, the major life-threatening complications associated with azathioprine use are infection and certain malignancies. In assessing the importance of these risks, several observations are appropriate. First, potent immunosuppressive regimens, including those using azathioprine, should be prescribed only for clinically important disease.

Second, when the consequences of immunosuppressive therapy are considered, the total regimen, rather than the effects of one or another component, should be assessed. In general, if bone marrow function is adequately monitored and appropriate adjustments in drug dose are made for the marrow abnormalities that are produced, the risks of azathioprine therapy (at doses of 1.0 to 1.5 mg/kg/day) are outweighed by the benefits that occur in terms of control of the disease process and the ability to lower the doses of such other drugs as prednisone and cyclosporine.

Third, azathioprine-induced leukopenia is associated with an increased risk of bacterial and candidal infection. If leukopenia is not present, then the major classes of infection that are of concern are the herpes group viruses (particularly cytomegalovirus and Epstein-Barr virus), *Mycobacteria tuberculosis*, and the opportunistic fungal agents. The risk of these infections is determined primarily by the interaction of two factors, the patient's net state of immunosuppression (to which azathioprine contributes) and the epidemiologic exposures encountered.

Fourth, azathioprine-based immunosuppressive programs will decrease the host's response to influenza, hepatitis B, and pneumococcal vaccines. More potent vaccines such as tetanus and diphtheria remain effective in these patients (97).

Fifth, the most important malignancies associated with immunosuppressive therapy (including azathioprine) are those associated with viruses: posttransplant lymphoproliferative disease (associated with Epstein-Barr virus), Kaposi's sarcoma (associated with human herpesvirus–8), warts and squamous cell carcinoma (associated with papillomavirus), and hepatocellular carcinoma (associated with hepatitis B and C virus). The key host defense associated with the control of these viruses is that mediated by virus-specific, cytotoxic T cells (i.e., the limb of host defense being most inhibited by immunosuppressive programs, including those using azathioprine). In addition, the chronic bone marrow effects of azathioprine can be associated with the development of myeloid malignancies that range from a myeloid dysplastic syndrome to frank leukemia. Rarely, soft-tissue sarcomas have been associated with chronic azathioprine administration (98–106).

Mycophenolate Mofetil

History

If the 1970s were the years in which the potential usefulness of immunosuppressive therapy in clinical medicine was firmly established, the years since have been spent seeking new compounds that could accomplish this task more effectively. Mycophenolate mofetil has come from efforts to find and develop a new immunosuppressive agent that functions by way of reversible antiproliferative effects specific for lymphocytes and that is free of the hematopoietic, hepatic, renal, and neurologic toxicity associated with currently available immunosuppressive agents (107). This effort was founded on important observations on children with devastating genetic defects in purine metabolism. Children with inherited adenosine deaminase deficiency, which affects a key step in de novo purine synthesis (Fig. 4-2*A*), were shown to have a major defect in the function and number of T and B lymphocytes but normal numbers of neutrophils, erythrocytes, and platelets, as well as normal brain function (108). In contrast, children with the Lesch-Nyhan syndrome, which is caused by the absence of hypoxanthine-guanine phosphoribosyltransferase, a key enzyme in the purine salvage pathway (Fig. 4-2*B*), have normal T and B lymphocyte numbers and function but devastating neurologic dysfunction (mental deficiency and compulsive self-mutilation) (109,110). Subsequently, it was confirmed that adequate levels of guanosine and deoxyguanosine nucleotides are required to allow lymphocytes to proliferate in response to antigenic stimulation. On the basis of these observations, it was hypothesized that an agent that reversibly inhibited the final stages of purine synthesis, thus depleting the supply of guanosine and deoxyguanosine nucleotides (Fig. 4-2), could provide effective immunosuppression and yet have the potential for a more favorable side-effect profile than the immunosuppressive drugs currently available. Mycophenolate mofetil was developed to fulfill these requirements (107).

Pharmacology and Mechanism of Action

Mycophenolic acid is a potent, noncompetitive, reversible inhibitor of inosine monophosphate dehydrogenase, the enzyme that catalyzes the final step in the synthesis of guanosine (Fig. 4-2*A*). Unlike nucleoside analogs, including azathioprine, mycophenolic acid does not inhibit DNA repair enzymes or produce chromosomal breaks, a property that is at least theoretically appealing in terms of teratogenicity and oncogenesis (107). Mycophenolate mofetil, the morpholinoethyl ester of mycophe-

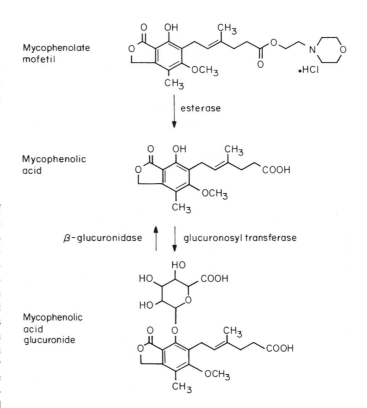

Figure 4-3. Structural formulas of mycophenolate mofetil, its active form (mycophenolic acid), its major glucuronide metabolite, and the interconversions among them.

nolic acid, was synthesized as a prodrug with increased bioavailability on oral administration (111). This drug is rapidly hydrolyzed in vivo to the active agent, mycophenolic acid, which is converted by the liver into its principal metabolite, mycophenolic acid glucuronide (Fig. 4-3). Mycophenolic acid glucuronide is biologically inactive and is primarily excreted in the urine. An enterohepatic recirculation of the drug probably occurs, although its quantitative importance in humans is currently unknown. The mycophenolate area under the curve (AUC) measurement is predictive of rejection activity: the higher the AUC, the less the amount of rejection. Tacrolimus, but not cyclosporine, appears to increase the mycophenolate AUC, possibly by affecting glucuronidation. Neither renal failure nor hemodialysis significantly affects the concentration of active drug present, although peritoneal dialysis does lower the AUC by a factor of approximately 35% (107,112–117).

Mycophenolate mofetil inhibits the proliferative response of human peripheral blood mononuclear cells to both T- and B-lymphocyte mitogens, as well as mixed lymphocyte reactions at concentrations of drug that have no effects on most other cell types (118). However, clinically attainable concentrations of the drug both inhibit the proliferation of human smooth muscle cells and block ongoing mixed lymphocyte reactions; these properties are of potentially great importance in the treatment of chronic vascular rejection of allografts, particularly cardiac allografts (107). In particular, mycophenolate mofetil blocks neointimal thickening and intimal hyperplasia in rat aortic allograft models (119–121). The ability of mycophenolate mofetil to block antibody formation is illustrated by studies in which mycophenolate mofetil, but not cyclosporine, was able to block the secondary responses of human spleen cells to tetanus toxoid (122). Mycophenolate mofetil blocks the glycosylation of adhesion molecules that mediate the attachment of leukocytes to endothelial cells and target cells, which could decrease the recruitment of lymphocytes and monocytes into sites of chronic inflammation and rejection. Mycophenolate mofetil has no effect on neutrophil chemotaxis, superoxide production, and microbiocidal capacity (107).

Although the clinical significance is unclear, mycophenolate mofetil appears to have some antimicrobial effects. In animal models, it blocks the development of *Pneumocystis carinii* pneumonia. Both in vitro and in animal models, mycophenolate mofetil potentiates the antiherpes group virus activity of a variety of antiviral drugs (including acyclovir, ganciclovir, penciclovir, and certain experimental agents) (123–126).

In experimental animals mycophenolate mofetil has been shown to inhibit the generation of cytotoxic T cells and the rejection of allogeneic cells; to block the formation of antibodies in a dose-dependent fashion; and to be effective in preventing and treating allograft rejection in both rodent and large animal models of organ transplantation, particularly when combined with cyclosporine (107,127–132). Mycophenolate mofetil decreases renal damage and prolongs life in mouse lupus autoimmune disease (133,134). In addition, it appears to attenuate renal injury in the rat remnant kidney; this nonimmunologic effect is of potential interest in kidney transplantation (135).

In humans, a twice-a-day dosage of 1 to 1.5 grams appears to be well tolerated and produces effects similar to those observed in the experimental studies (107).

Clinical Usefulness

Transplantation

Mycophenolate mofetil has been used increasingly in place of azathioprine, particularly in combination with cyclosporine and prednisone in a triple-therapy regimen. Currently available data suggest that the use of such regimens results in less frequent rejection episodes than occur with azathioprine-containing regimens. In addition, mycophenolate mofetil has been reported to permit lower cyclosporine dosages (especially appealing in patients with delayed graft function), to be useful in the treatment of refractory rejection, to be effective in combination with plasma exchange and tacrolimus in the management of humoral rejection, to suppress circulating panel reactive antibodies (that mediate positive cross matches), and to inhibit the development of antimouse antibodies induced by the administration of OKT3. African-American kidney allograft recipients appear to receive less clinical benefit from mycophenolate mofetil than Caucasians. Mycophenolate mofetil appears not be be useful in reversing chronic rejection of the renal allograft (136–148).

Although there is significantly less information available on the efficacy of mycophenolate mofetil in other forms of organ transplantation, the available data are quite promising. The outcome of pancreas-kidney transplantation is improved by the substitution of mycophenolate mofetil for azathioprine. In liver, cardiac, and lung transplant recipients, there appear to be similar benefits (107,149–158).

In addition to its efficacy as part of a three-drug prophylactic regimen, emerging data suggest that mycophenolate mofetil will be useful in several specific ways: in the development of strategies that will permit sparing of both corticosteroids and cyclosporine without an undue risk of rejection; as "rescue therapy" in patients with refractory acute and chronic rejection; and as maintenance therapy, particularly in such high-risk patients as those who have rejected previous transplants or who have a high level of pretransplant sensitization (107,159–163).

Rheumatoid Arthritis

Initial studies with mycophenolate mofetil have been quite promising: objective improvements were noted in more than 50% of patients with severe, refractory disease, including those who had previously not responded to cyclooxygenase inhibitors, methotrexate, and other treatments. Of particular interest, mycophenolate mofetil, unlike azathioprine, causes a fall in rheumatoid factor titers, immunoglobulin levels, and the total number of circulating T-lymphocytes in the peripheral blood (164–167).

Other Conditions

Preliminary data suggest that mycophenolate mofetil might be useful in the management of psoriasis, lupus nephritis and other forms of immunologic renal injury, graft-versus-host disease in bone marrow transplant recipients, and inflammatory bowel disease (168–173).

Adverse Effects

The dose-limiting and the most frequently observed adverse effect of mycophenolate mofetil is gastrointestinal toxicity: nausea, vomiting, abdominal pain, and diarrhea. In most instances this toxicity requires only a decrease in dose or temporary cessation of therapy; it is unusual for a patient to require permanent discontinuation of this drug. Bone marrow toxicity appears to be less common than with azathioprine, and significant nephrotoxicity and hepatotoxicity caused by this drug have not been issues. Not yet determined are what the long-term effects of this agent will be on the occurrence of infections and certain malignancies (107,136–158).

With respect to infection, the apparent decreased incidence of neutropenia is an important benefit. However, it is likely that mycophenolate mofetil will attenuate the benefits of vaccine administration, as well as amplify the effects of those infections against which a cytotoxic T-cell response is the critical host defense. Thus, herpes group virus infection, particularly that caused by cytomegalovirus and Epstein-Barr virus, and opportunistic fungal infection probably would be exacerbated by therapy with this agent. The previously described antimicrobial effects of mycophenolate mofetil may be of some benefit in this instance. In addition, as previously discussed for azathioprine, this adverse effect should be manageable by one or more of the following strategies: inclusion of mycophenolate mofetil in immunosuppressive regimens that achieve the desired net immunosuppressive effect, while the dosage required of such other agents as cyclosporine and prednisone is decreased; use of effective antimicrobial strategies whose intensity is linked to the immunosuppressive therapy being employed; and implementation of appropriate caution in protecting patients from excessive environmental exposures to opportunistic infectious agents. In the studies carried out thus far with mycophenolate mofetil, no effort has been made to optimize antimicrobial strategies, so that the incidence of infection (which appears to be slightly greater than with azathioprine) is probably greater than if appropriate antimicrobial strategies had been implemented. Even then, this risk in the first 12 to 24 months of therapy does not appear to be excessive (136–158).

Similarly, it would be expected that immunosuppressive programs that include mycophenolate mofetil would be associated with somewhat higher incidence of malignancies in which viral infection plays a significant role in the oncogenic process; that is, Epstein-Barr virus–associated lymphoproliferative disease, hepatocellular carcinoma associated with hepatitis B, and perhaps squamous cell carcinoma associated with papillomavirus infection. Thus far, the magnitude of this increased risk appears to be small; and it is hoped that some of the antimicrobial strategies that are emerging will diminish the risk further (136–158).

References

1. Rubin RH, Ikonen T, Gummert JF, Morris RE. The therapeutic prescription for the organ transplant recipient: the linkage of immunosuppression and antimicrobial strategies. Transplant Infect Dis 1999;1:29–39.
2. Elion GB, Callahan S, Bieber S, et al. A summary of investigations with 6-(1-methyl-2-nitro-5-imidazole) thiopurine. Cancer Chemother Reports 1961;14:93–98.
3. Elion GB. The George Hitchings and Gertrude Elion Lecture: The pharmacology of azathioprine. Ann NY Acad Sci 1993;685:400–407.
4. Schwartz R, Dameshek W. The effects of 6-mercaptopurine on homograft reactions. J Clin Invest 1960;39:952–958.
5. Calne RY, Alexandre GPJ, Murray JE. A study of the effects of drugs in prolonging survival of homologous renal transplants in dogs. Ann NY Acad Sci 1962;99:743–761.
6. Starzl TE, Marchioro TL, Waddell WR. The reversal of rejection in human renal homografts with subsequent development of homograft tolerance. Surg Gynecol Obstet 1963;117:385–395.
7. Spina CA. Azathioprine as an immune modulating drug: clinical applications. Clin Immunol Allergy 1984;4:415–446.
8. Chan GLC, Canafax DM, Johnson CA. The therapeutic use of azathioprine in renal transplantation. Pharmacotherapy 1987;7:165–177.
9. Yates CR, Krynetski EY, Loennechen T, et al. Molecular diagnosis of thiopurine S-methyltransferase deficiency: genetic basis for azathioprine and mercaptopurine intolerance. Ann Intern Med 1997;126:608–614.
10. Leipold G, Schutz E, Hass JP, Oellerich M. Azathioprine-induced severe pancytopenia due to a homozygous two-point mutation of the thiopurine methyltransferase gene in a patient with juvenile HLA-B27-associated spondylarthritis. Arthritis Rheum 1997;40:1896–1898.
11. Stolk JN, Boerbooms AM, de Abreu RA, et al. Reduced thiopurine methyltransferase activity and development of side effects of azathioprine treatment in patients with rheumatoid arthritis. Arthritis Rheum 1998;41:1858–1866.
12. Black AJ, McLeod HL, Capell HA, et al. Thiopurine methyltransferase genotype predicts therapy-limiting severe toxicity from azathioprine. Ann Intern Med 1998;129:716–718.
13. Escousse A, Guedon F, Mounie J, et al. 6-Mercaptopurine pharmacokinetics after use of azathioprine in renal transplant recipients with intermediate or high thiopurine methyl transferase activity phenotype. J Pharm Pharmacol 1998; 50:1261–1266.
14. Cummins D, Sekar M, Halil O, Banner N. Myelosuppression associated with azathioprine-allopurinol interaction after heart and lung transplantation. Transplantation 1996;61: 1661–1662.
15. Kennedy DT, Hayney MS, Lake KD. Azathioprine and allopurinol: the price of an avoidable drug interaction. Ann Pharmacother 1996;30:951–954.
16. Starzl TE, Rosenthal JT, Hakala TR, et al. Steps in immunosuppression for renal transplantation, Kidney Int 1983;23 (suppl 14):60–65.
17. Bergan S, Rugstad HE, Bentdal O, et al. Monitored high-dose azathioprine treatment reduces acute rejection episodes after renal transplantation. Transplantation 1998; 66:334–339.
18. Rubin RH, Cosimi AB. Therapy, both immunosuppressive and antimicrobial, for the transplant patient in the 1990s. In: Brent L, Sells RA, eds. Organ transplantation: current clinical and imunological concepts. London: Bailliere Tindall, 1989:71–89.
19. Amenabar JJ, Gomez-Ullate P, Garcia-Lopez FJ, et al. A randomized trial comparing cyclosporine and steroids with cyclosporine, azathioprine, and steroids in cadaveric renal transplantation. Transplantation 1988;65:653–661.
20. Sommer BG, Henry M, Ferguson RM. Sequential antilymphoblast globulin and cyclosporine for renal transplantation. Transplantation 1987;43:85–90.
21. Deierhoi MH, Sollinger HW, Kalayoglu M, Belzer FO. Quadruple therapy for cadaver renal transplantation. Transplant Proc 1987;19:1917–1919.
22. Aichberger C, Eberl T, Riedmann B, et al. Long-term outcome after switch from cyclosporine-based triple-drug immunosuppression to double therapy at three months. Clin Transplant 1996;10:209–212.
23. Hilbrands LB, Hoitsma AG, Wetzels JF, Koene RA. Detailed study of changes in renal function after conversion from cyclosporine to azathioprine. Clin Nephrol 1996;45:230–235.
24. Hilbrands LB, Hoitsma AJ, Koene RA. Randomized, prospective trial of cyclosporine monotherapy versus azathioprine-prednisone from three months after renal transplantation. Transplant 1996;61:1038–1046.
25. MacPhee IA, Bradley JA, Briggs JD, et al. Long-term outcome of a prospective randomized trial of conversion

from cyclosporine to azathioprine treatment one year after renal transplantation. Transpl 1998;66:1186–1192.

26. Ratcliffe PJ, Dudley CR, Higgins RM, et al. Randomized controlled trial of steroid withdrawal in renal transplant recipients receiving triple immunosuppression. Lancet 1996;348:643–648.

27. Fraser GM, Grammoustianos K, Reddy J, et al. Long-term immunosuppression without corticosteroids after orthotopic liver transplantation: a positive therapeutic aim. Liver Transpl Surg 1996;2:411–417.

28. Van den Dorpel MA, Ghanem H, Rischen-Vos J, et al. Conversion from cyclosporine A to azathioprine treatment improves LDL oxidation in kidney transplant recipients. Kidney Int 1997;51:1608–1612.

29. Sanfey H, Haussman G, Isaacs I, et al. Steroid withdrawal in kidney transplant recipients: is it a safe option? Clin Transplant 1997;11:500–504.

30. Cseuz R, Zimmerman J, Panayi GS. Daily and alternate-day azathioprine treatment in rheumatoid arthritis: a twelve-week controlled clinical trial. Br J Rheumatol 1992;31:501–504.

31. Savolainen HA, Kautiainen H, Isomaki H, et al. Azathioprine in patients with juvenile chronic arthritis: a long-term follow-up study. J Rheumatol 1997;24:2444–2450.

32. Willkens RF, Urowitz MB, Stablein DM, et al. Comparison of azathioprine, methotrexate, and the combination of both in the treatment of rheumatoid arthritis. Arthritis Rheum 1992;35:849–856.

33. Paulus HE, Williams HJ, Ward JR, et al. Azathioprine versus D-penicillamine in rheumatoid arthritis patients who have been treated unsuccessfully with gold. Arthritis Rheum 1984;27:721–727.

34. Csuka ME, Carrera GF, McCarty DJ. Treatment of intractable rheumatoid arthritis with combined cyclophosphamide, azathioprine, and hydroxychloroquine. A follow-up study. JAMA 1986;255:2315–2319.

35. Ten wolde S, Hermans J, Breedveld FC, Dijkmans BA. Effect of resumption of second line drugs in patients with rheumatoid arthritis that flared up after treatment discontinuation. Ann Rheum Dis 1997; 56:235–239.

36. Fries JF, Williams CA, Morfeld D, et al. Reduction in long-term disability in patients with rheumatoid arthritis by disease-modifying antirheumatic drug-based treatment strategies. Arthritis Rheum 1996;39:616–622.

37. Jeurissen MEC, Boerbooms AMT, van de Putte LBA, et al. Methotrexate versus azathioprine in the treatment of rheumatoid arthritis: a forty-eight-week randomized, double-blind trial. Arthritis Rheum 1991;34:961–972.

38. Jeurissen MEC, Boerbooms AMT, van de Putte LBA, et al. Influence of methotrexate and azathioprine on radiologic progression in rheumatoid arthritis: a randomized, double-blind study. Ann Intern Med 1991;114:999–1004.

39. Sambrook PN, Champion GD, Browne CD, et al. Comparison of methotrexate with azathioprine or 6-mercaptopurine in refractory rheumatoid arthritis: a life-table analysis. Br J Rheumatol 1990;29:120–125.

40. Felson DT, Anderson J. Evidence for the superiority of immunosuppressive drugs and prednisone over prednisone alone in lupus nephritis; results of a pooled analysis. N Engl J Med 1984;311:1528–1533.

41. Rahman P, Humphrey-Murto S, Glladman DD, Urowitz MG. Cytotoxic therapy in systemic lupus erythematosus.

Experience from a single center. Medicine 1997;76:432–437.

42. D'Cruz D, Cuadrado MJ, Mujic F, et al. Immunosuppressive therapy in lupus nephritis. Clin Exp Rheumatol 1997;15:275–282.

43. Bansal VK, Beto JA. Treatment of lupus nephritis: a meta-analysis of clinical trials. Am J Kidney Dis 1997;29:193–199.

44. Dooley MA, Falk RJ. Immunosuppressive therapy of lupus nephritis. Lupus 1998;7:630–634.

45. Tsokos GC, Caughman SW, Klippel JH. Successful treatment of generalized discoid skin lesions with azathioprine. Its use in a patient with systemic lupus erythematosus. Arch Dermatol 1985;121:1323–1325.

46. Callen JP, Spencer LV, Burruss JB, Holtman J. Azathioprine. An effective, corticosteroid-sparing therapy for patients with recalcitrant cutaneous lupus erythematosus or with recalcitrant cutaneous leukocytoclastic vasculitis. Arch Dermatol 1991;127:515–522.

47. Calin A. A placebo controlled, crossover study of azathioprine in Reiter's syndrome. Ann Rheum Dis 1986;45:653-655.

48. Fernandez-Banares F, Bertran X, Esteve-Comas M, et al. Azathioprine is useful in maintaining long-term remission induced by intravenous cyclosporine in steroid-refractory severe ulcerative colitis. Am J Gastroenterol 1996;91:2498–2499.

49. Ramakrishna J, Langhans N, Calenda K, et al. Combined use of cyclosporine and azathioprine or 6-mercaptopurine in pediatric inflammatory bowel disease. J Pediatr Gastroenterol Nutr 1996;22:296–302.

50. Kader HA, Mascarenhas MR, Piccoli DA, et al. Experiences with 6-mercaptopurine and azathioprine therapy in pediatric patients with severe ulcerative colitis. J Pediatr Gastroenterol Nutr 1999;28:54–58.

51. Ardizzone S, Molteni P, Imbesi V, et al. Azathioprine in steroid-resistant and steroid-dependent ulcerative colitis. J Clin Gastroenterol 1997;25:330–333.

52. Kashimura H, Hassan M, Shibahara K, et al. Steroid-refractory severe ulcerative colitis responding to cyclosporine and long-term follow-up. J Gastroenterol 1998;33:566–570.

53. Ramsey-Goldman R, Schilling E. Immunosuppressive drug use during pregnancy. Rheum Dis Clin North Am 1997;223:149–167.

54. Armenti VT, Moritz MJ, Davison JM. Drug safety issues in pregnancy following transplantation and immunosuppression: effects and outcomes. Drug Saf 1998;19:219–232.

55. Ostensen M, Ramsey-Goldman R. Treatment of inflammatory rheumatic disorders in pregnancy: what are the safest treatment options? Drug Saf 1998;19:389–410.

56. Ewe K, Press AG, Singe CC, et al. Azathioprine combined with prednisolone or monotherapy with prednisolone in active Crohn's disease. Gastroenterology 1993;105:367–372.

57. Berrebi W, Chaussade S, Bruhl AL, et al. Treatment of Crohn's disease recurrence after ileoanal anastomosis by azathioprine. Dig Dis Sci 1993;38:1558–1560.

58. D'Haens G, Geboes K, Ponette E, et al. Healing of severe recurrent ileitis with azathioprine therapy in patients with Crohn's disease. Gastroenterology 1997;112:1475–1481.

59. Sandborn WJ. Azathioprine: state of the art in inflammatory bowel disease. Scand J Gastroenterol Suppl 1998;225:92–99.

60. Kirschner BS. Safety of azathioprine and 6-mercaptopurine in pediatric patients with inflammatory bowel disease. Gastroenterology 1998;115:813–821.
61. Cosi V, Lombardi M, Erbetta A, Piccolo G. Azathioprine as a single immunosuppressive drug in the treatment of myasthenia gravis. Acta Neurol 1993;15:123–131.
62. Kuks JB, Djojoatmodjo S, Oosterhuis HJ. Azathioprine in myasthenia gravis: observations in 41 patients and a review of literature. Neuromuscul Disord 1991;1:423–431.
63. Palace J, Newsom-Davis J, Lecky B. Myasthenia Gravis Study Group. A randomized double-blind trial of prednisolone alone or with azathioprine in myasthenia gravis. Neurology 1998;50:1778–1783.
64. Goodkin DE, Bailly RC, Teetzen ML, et al. The efficacy of azathioprine in relapsing-remitting multiple sclerosis. Neurology 1991;41:20–25.
65. Yudkin PL, Ellison GW, Ghezzi A, et al. Overview of azathioprine treatment in multiple sclerosis. Lancet 1991;388:1051–1055.
66. Cavazzuti M, Merelli E, Tassone G, Mavilla L. Lesion load quantification in serial MR of early relapsing multiple sclerosis patients in azathioprine treatment. A retrospective study. Eur Neurol 1997;38:284–290.
67. Aberer W, Wolff-Schreiner EC, Stingl G, Wolff K. Azathioprine in the treatment of pemphigus vulgaris. A long-term follow-up. J Am Acad Dermatol 1987;16:527–533.
68. Guillaume JC, Vaillant L, Bernard P, et al. Controlled trial of azathioprine and plasma exchange in addition to prednisolone in the treatment of bullous pemphigoid. Arch Dermatol 1993;129:49–53.
69. Adam DJ, Nawroz I, Petrie PW. Pyoderma gangrenosum severely affecting both hands. J Hand Surg [Br] 1996;21:792–794.
70. Dutz JP, Ho VC. Immunosuppressive agents in dermatology. An update. Dermatol Clin 1998;16:235–251.
71. Silverstein J, Maclaren N, Riley W, et al. Immunosuppression with azathioprine and prednisone in recent-onset insulin-dependent diabetes mellitus. N Engl J Med 1988;319:599–604.
72. Cook JJ, Hudson I, Harrison LC, et al. Double-blind controlled trial of azathioprine in children with newly diagnosed type I diabetes. Diabetes 1989;38:779–783.
73. Yazici H, Pazarli H, Barnes CG, et al. A controlled trial of azathioprine in Behcet's syndrome. N Engl J Med 1990;322:281–285.
74. Kotter I, Durk H, Saal J, et al. Therapy of Behcet's disease. Ger J Ophthalmol 1996;5:92–97.
75. Hamuryudan V, Ozyazgan Y, Hizli N, et al. Azathioprine in Behcet's syndrome: effects on long-term prognosis. Arthritis Rheum 1997;40:769–774.
76. Pacheco Y, Marechal C, Marechal F, et al. Azathioprine treatment of chronic pulmonary sarcoidosis. Sarcoidosis 1985;2:107–113.
77. Raghu G, Depaso WJ, Cain K, et al. Azathioprine combined with prednisone in the treatment of idiopathic pulmonary fibrosis: a prospective double-blind, randomized, placebo-controlled clinical trial. Am Rev Respir Dis 1991;144;291–296.
78. Quiquandon I, Fenaux P, Caulier MT, et al. Re-evaluation of the role of azathioprine in the treatment of adult chronic idiopathic thrombocytopenic purpura: a report on 53 cases. Br J Haematol 1990;74:223–228.
79. Cade R, Mars D, Privette M, et al. Effect of long-term azathioprine administration in adults with minimal-change glomerulonephritis and nephrotic syndrome resistant to corticosteroids. Arch Intern Med 1986;146:737–741.
80. Stellon AJ, Keating JJ, Johnson PJ, et al. Maintenance of remission in autoimmune chronic active hepatitis with azathioprine after corticosteroid withdrawal. Hepatology 1988;8:781–784.
81. Villalba L, Hicks JE, Adams EM, et al. Treatment of refractory myositis: a randomized crossover study of two new cytotoxic regimens. Arthritis Rheum 1998;41:392–399.
82. Saadeh C, Urban RS. Azathioprine in the treatment of chronic refractory steroid-dependent asthma. South Med J 1993;86:94–95.
83. Singh G, Fries JF, Spitz P, Williams CA. Toxic effects of azathioprine in rheumatoid arthritis. A national post-marketing perspective. Arthritis Rheum 1989;32:837–843.
84. McKendry RJ, Cyr M. Toxicity of methotrexate compared with azathioprine in the treatment of rheumatoid arthritis. A case-control study of 131 patients. Arch Intern Med 1989;149:685–689.
85. Kissel JT, Levy RJ, Mendell JR, Griggs RC. Azathioprine toxicity in neuromuscular disease. Neurology 1986;36:35–39.
86. Pol S, Cavalcanti R, Carnot F, et al. Azathioprine hepatitis in kidney transplant recipients. A predisposing role of chronic viral hepatitis. Transplantation 1996;61:1774–1776.
87. Haboubi NY, Ali HH, Whitwell HL, et al. Role of endothelial cell injury in the spectrum of azathioprine-induced liver disease after renal transplant: light microscopy and ultrastructural observations. Am J Gastroenterol 1988;83:256–260.
88. Lemley DE, DeLacey LM, Seeff LB, et al. Azathioprine induced hepatic veno-occlusive disease in rheumatoid arthritis. Ann Rheum Dis 1989;48:342–346.
89. Read AE, Wiesner RH, LaBrecque DR, et al. Hepatic veno-occlusive disease associated with renal transplantation and azathioprine therapy. Ann Intern Med 1986;104:651–655.
90. Katska DA, Saul SH, Jorkasky D, et al. Azathioprine and hepatic venocclusive disease in renal transplant patients. Gastroenterology 1986;90:446–454.
91. Azoulay D, Castaing D, Lemoine A, et al. Successful treatment of severe azathioprine-induced hepatic veno-occlusive disease in a kidney-transplanted patient with transjugular intrahepatic portosystemic shunt. Clin Nephrol 1998;50:118–122.
92. Jeurissen ME, Boerbooms AM, van de Putte LB, et al. Azathioprine induced fever, chills, rash, and hepatotoxicity in rheumatoid arthritis. Ann Rheum Dis 1990;49:25–27.
93. Blanco R, Martinez-Taboada VM, Gonzalez-Gay MA, et al. Acute febrile toxic reaction in patients with refractory rheumatoid arthritis who are receiving combined therapy with methotrexate and azathioprine. Arthritis Rheum 1996;39:1016–1020.
94. Wilmink T, Frick TW. Drug-induced pancreatitis. Drug Saf 1996;14:406–423.
95. Beckett CG, Hill P, Hine KR. Leucocytoclastic vasculitis in a patient with azathioprine hypersensitivity. Postgrad Med J 1996;72:437–438.
96. Brown G, Boldt C, Webb JG, Halperin L. Azathioprine-induced multisystem organ failure and cardiogenic shock. Pharmacotherapy 1997;17:815–818.

97. Enke BU, Bokenkamp A, Offner G, et al. Response to diphtheria and tetanus booster vaccination in pediatric renal transplant recipients. Transplantation 1997;64:237–241.

98. Rubin RH. Infection in organ transplant recipients. In: Rubin RH, Young LS, eds. Clinical approach to infection in the compromised host. 4th ed. New York: Plenum Press, in press.

99. Confavreux C, Saddier P, Grimaud J, et al. Risk of cancer from azathioprine therapy in multiple sclerosis: a case-control study. Neurology 1996;46:1607–1612.

100. Jones M, Symmons D, Finn J, Wolfe F. Does exposure to immunosuppressive therapy increase the 10 year malignancy and mortality risks in rheumatoid arthritis? A matched cohort study. Br J Rheumatol 1996;35:738–745.

101. Bouwes Bavinck JN, Hardie DR, Green A, et al. The risk of skin cancer in renal transplant recipients in Queensland, Australia. A follow-up study. Transplantation 1996;61:715–721.

102. Vandercam B, Lachapelle JM, Janssens P, et al. Kaposi's sarcoma during immunosuppressive therapy for atopic dermatitis. Dermatology 1997;194:180–182.

103. Lesnoni La Parola I, Masini C, Nanni G, et al. Kaposi's sarcoma in renal-transplant recipients: experience at the Catholic University in Rome, 1988–1996. Dermatology 1997;194:229–233.

104. Kwong YL, Au WY, Liang RH. Acute myeloid leukemia after azathioprine treatment for autoimmune diseases: association with −7/7q−. Cancer Genet Cytogenet 1998;104:94–97.

105. Renneboog B, Hansen V, Heimann P, et al. Spontaneous remission in a patient with therapy-related myelodysplastic syndrome (t-MDS) with monosomy 7. Br J Haematol 1996;92:696–698.

106. Csuka ME, Hanson GA. Resolution of a soft-tissue sarcoma in a patient with rheumatoid arthritis after discontinuation of azathioprine therapy. Arch Intern Med 1996;156:1573–1576.

107. Allison AC, Eugui EM. Mycophenolate mofetil, a rationally designed immunosuppressive drug. Clin Transplantation 1993;7:96–112.

108. Giblett ER, Anderson JE, Cohen F, Meuwissen HJ. Adenosine deaminase deficiency in two patients with severely impaired cellular immunity. Lancet 1972;2:1067–1069.

109. Allison AC, Hovi T, Watts RWE, Webster ADB. Immunological observations on patients with the Lesch Nyhan syndrome, and on the role of *de novo* purine synthesis in lymphocyte transformation. Lancet 1975;2:1179–1183.

110. Allison AC, Hovi T, Watts RWE, Webster ADB. The role of *de novo* purine synthesis in lymphocyte transformation. Ciba Foundation Symp Purine Pyrimidine Metabol 1977;48:207–223.

111. Lee WA, Gu L, Miksztal AR, et al. Bioavailability improvement of mycophenolic acid through amino ester derivitization. Pharm Res 1990;7:161–166.

112. Langman LJ, LeGatt DF, Halloran PF, Yatscoff RW. Pharmacodynamic assessment of mycophenolic acid-induced immunosuppression in renal transplant recipients. Transplantation 1996;62:666–672.

113. Zucker K, Rosen A, Tsaroucha A, et al. Unexpected augmentation of mycophenolic acid pharmacokinetics in renal transplant patients receiving tacrolimus and mycophenolate

114. Hale MD, Nicholls AJ, Bullingham RE, et al. The pharmacokinetic-pharmacodynamic relationship for mycophenolate mofetil in renal transplantation. Clin Pharmacol Ther 1998;64:672–683.

115. Morgera S, Neumayer HH, Fritsche L, et al. Pharmacokinetics of mycophenolate mofetil in renal transplant recipients on peritoneal dialysis. Int J Clin Pharmacol Ther 1998;36:159–163.

116. Johnson HJ, Swan SK, Heim-Duthoy KL, et al. The pharmacokinetics of a single oral dose of mycophenolate mofetil in patients with varying degrees of renal function. Clin Pharmacol Ther 1998;63:512–518.

117. Bullingham RE, Nicholls AJ, Kamm BR. Clinical pharmacokinetics of mycophenolate mofetil. Clin Pharmacokinet 1998;34:429–455.

118. Eugui EM, Almquist S, Muller CD, Allison AC. Lymphocyte-selective cytostatic and immunosuppressive effects of mycophenolic acid *in vitro*: role of deoxyguanosine nucleotide depletion. Scand J Immunol 1991;33:161–173.

119. Fraser-Smith EB, Rosete JD, Schatzman RC. Suppression by mycophenolate mofetil of the neointimal thickening caused by vascular injury in a rat arterial stenosis model. J Pharmacol Exp Ther 1995;275:1204–1208.

120. Raisanen-Sokolowski A, Vuoristo P, Myliarniemi M, et al. Mycophenolate mofetil (MMF, RS-61443) inhibits inflammation and smooth muscle cell proliferation in rat aortic allografts. Transplant Immunol 1995;3:342–351.

121. Hullett DA, Geraghty JG, Stoltenberg RL, Sollinger HW. The impact of acute rejection on the development of intimal hyperplasia associated with chronic rejection. Transplant 1996;62:1842–1846.

122. Grailer A, Nichols J, Hullett D, et al. Inhibition of human B cell responses *in vitro* by RS-61443, cyclosporine A and FK506. Transplant Proc 1991;23:314–315.

123. Oz HS, Hughes WT. Novel anti-Pneumocystis carinii effects of the immunosuppressant mycophenolate mofetil in contrast to provocative effects of tacrolimus, sirolimus, and dexamethasone. J Infect Dis 1997;175:901–904.

124. Neyts J, Andrei G, De Clercq E. The novel immunosuppressive agent mycophenolate mofetil markedly potentiates the antiherpesvirus activities of acyclovir, ganciclovir, and penciclovir in vitro and in vivo. Antimicrob Agents Chemother 1998;42:216–222.

125. Neyts J, De clercq E. Mycophenolate mofetil strongly potentiates the antiherpesvirus activity of acyclovir. Antiviral Res 1998;40:53–56.

126. Neyts J, Andrei G, De clercq E. The antiherpesvirus activity of H2G [(R)-9-[r-hydroxy-2-(hydroxymethyl)butyl] guanine] is markedly enhanced by the novel immunosuppressive agent mycophenolate mofetil. Antimicrob Agents Chemother 1998;42:3285–3289.

127. Eugui EM, Mirkovich A, Allison AC. Lymphocyte-selective antiproliferative and immunosuppressive effects of mycophenolic acid in mice. Scand J Immunol 1991;33:175–183.

128. Hao L, Lafferty KJ, Allison AC, Eugui E. RS-61443 allows islet allografting and specific tolerance induction in adult mice. Transplant Proc 1990;22:1659–1662.

129. Morris RE, Hoyt EG, Murphy MP, et al. Mycophenolic acid morpholinoethylester (RS-61443) is a new immunosuppressant that prevents and halts heart allograft rejection by selective inhibition of T and B cell purine synthesis. Transplant Proc 1990;22:1659–1662.

130. Morris RE, Wang J, Blum JR, et al. Immunosuppressive effects of the morpholinoethyl ester of mycophenolic acid (RS-61443) in rat and nonhuman primate recipients of heart allografts. Transplant Proc 1991;23(suppl 2):19–25.

131. Platz KP, Sollinger HW, Hullett DA, et al. RS-61443, a new, potent immunosuppressive agent. Transplantation 1990;51:27–31.

132. Platz KP, Eckhoff D, Bechstein WO, et al. RS-61443 for reversal of acute rejection in canine renal allografts. Surgery 1991;110:736–741.

133. McMurray RW, Elbourne KB, Lagoo A, Lal S. Mycophenolate mofetil suppresses autoimmunity and mortality in the female NZB X NZW F1 mouse model of systemic lupus erythematosus. J Rheumatol 1998;25:2364–2370.

134. Corna D, Morigi M, Facchinetti D, et al. Mycophenolate mofetil limits renal damage and prolongs life in murine lupus autoimmune disease. Kidney Int 1997;51:1583–1589.

135. Fujihara CK, Malheiros DM, Zatz R, Noronha ID. Mycophenolate mofetil attenuates renal injury in the rat remnant kidney. Kidney Int 1998;54:1510–1519.

136. Sollinger HW. U.S. Renal Transplant Mycophenolate Mofetil Study Group. Mycophenolate mofetil for the prevention of acute rejection in primary cadaveric renal allograft recipients. Transplantation 1995;60:225–232.

137. European Mycophenolate Mofetil Cooperative Study Group. Placebo-controlled study of mycophenolate mofetil combined with cyclosporin and corticosteroids for prevention of acute rejection. Lancet 1995;345:1321–1325.

138. The Tricontinental Mycophenolate Mofetil Renal Transplantation Study Group. A blinded, randomized clinical trial of mycophenolate mofetil for the prevention of acute rejection in cadaveric renal transplantation. Transplantation 1996;61:1029–1037.

139. Halloran P, Mathew T, Tomlanovich S, et al. The International Mycophenolate Mofetil Renal Transplant Study Groups. Mycophenolate mofetil in renal allograft recipients: a pooled efficacy analysis of three randomized, double-blind, clinical studies in prevention of rejection. Transplantation 1997;63:39–47.

140. The Mycophenolate Mofetil Renal Refractory Rejection Study Group. Mycophenolate mofetil for the treatment of refractory, acute, cellular renal transplant rejection. Transplantation 1996;61:722–729.

141. Neylan JF. U.S. Renal Transplant Mycophenolate Mofetil Study Group. Immunosuppressive therapy in high-risk transplant patients: dose-dependent efficacy of mycophenolate mofetil in African-American renal allograft recipients. Transplantation 1997;64:1277–1282.

142. Schweitzer EJ, Yoon S, Fink J, et al. Mycophenolate mofetil reduces the risk of acute rejection less in African-American than in Caucasian kidney recipients. Transplantation 1998;65:242–248.

143. Ducloux D, Fournier V, Bresson-Vautrin C, et al. Mycophenolate mofetil in renal transplant recipients with cyclosporine-associated nephrotoxicity: a preliminary report. Transplantation 1998;65:1504–1506.

144. Mathew TH. Tricontinental Mycophenolate Mofetil Renal Transplantation Study Group. A blinded, long-term, randomized multicenter study of mycophenolate mofetil in cadaveric renal transplantation: results at three years. Transplantation 1998;65:1450–1454.

145. Pascual M, Saidman S, Tolkoff-Rubin N, et al. Plasma exchange and tacrolimus-mycophenolate rescue for acute humoral rejection in kidney transplantation. Transplantation 1998;66:1460–1464.

146. Hueso M, Bover J, Seron D, et al. Low-dose cyclosporine and mycophenolate mofetil in renal allograft recipients with suboptimal renal function. Transplantation 1998;66:1727–1731.

147. Broeders N, Wissing KM, Crusiaux A, et al. Mycophenolate mofetil, together with cyclosporin A, prevents anti-OKT3 antibody response in kidney transplant recipients. J Am Soc Nephrol 1998;9:1521–1525.

148. Glicklich D, Gupta B, Schurter-Frey G, et al. Chronic renal allograft rejection: no response to mycophenolate mofetil. Transplantation 1998;66:398–399.

149. Stegall MD, Simon M, Wachs ME, et al. Mycophenolate mofetil decreases rejection in simultaneous pancreas-kidney transplantation when combined with tacrolimus or cyclosporine. Transplantation 1997;64:1695–1700.

150. Odorico JS, Pirsch JD, Knechtle SJ, et al. A study comparing mycophenolate mofetil to azathioprine in simultaneous pancreas-kidney transplantation. Transplantation 1998;66:1751–1759.

151. Sollinger HW, Odorico JS, Knechtle SJ, et al. Experience with 500 simultaneous pancreas-kidney transplants. Ann Surg 1998;228:284–296.

152. Eckhoff DE, McGuire BM, Renette LR, et al. Tacrolimus (FK506) and mycophenolate mofetil combination therapy versus tacrolimus in adult liver transplantation. Transplantation 1998;65:180–187.

153. Fisher RA, Ham JM, Marcos A, et al. A prospective randomized trial of mycophenolate mofetil with neoral or tacrolimus after orthotopic liver transplantation. Transplantation 1998;66:1616–1621.

154. Jain AB, Hamad I, Rakela J, et al. A prospective randomized trial of tacrolimus and prednisone versus tacrolimus, prednisone, and mycophenolate mofetil in primary adult liver transplant recipients: an interim report. Transplantation 1998;66:1395–1398.

155. Ross DJ, Waters PF, Levine M, et al. Mycophenolate mofetil versus azathioprine immunosuppressive regimens after lung transplantation: preliminary experience. J Heart Lung Transplant 1998;17:768–774.

156. O'Hair DP, Cantu E, McGregor C, et al. Preliminary experience with mycophenolate mofetil used after lung transplantation. J Heart Lung Transplant 1998;17:864–868.

157. Kobashigawa J, Miller L, Renlund D, et al. Mycophenolate Mofetil Investigators. A randomized active-controlled trial of mycophenolate mofetil in heart transplant recipients. Transplantation 1998;66:507–515.

158. Kobashigawa JA. Mycophenolate mofetil in cardiac transplantation. Curr Opin Cardiol 1998;13:117–121.

159. Van Gelder T, Klaassen RJ, van Riemsdijk-van Overbeeke I, et al. Mycophenolate mofetil and prednisone as maintenance treatment after kidney transplantation. Transplantation 1997;63:1530–1531.

160. Stegall MD, Wachs ME, Everson G, et al. Prednisone withdrawal 14 days after liver transplantation with mycophenolate: a prospective trial of cyclosporine and tacrolimus. Transplantation 1997;64:1755–1760.

161. Grinyo JM, Gil-Vernet S, Seron D, et al. Steroid withdrawal in mycophenolate mofetil-treated renal allograft recipients. Transplantation 1997;63:1688–1690.

162. Birkeland SA. Steroid-free immunosuppression after kidney transplantation with antithymocyte globulin induction and cyclosporine and mycophenolate mofetil maintenance therapy. Transplantation 1998;66:1207–1210.

163. Zanker B, Schneeberger H, Rothenpieler U, et al. Mycophenolate mofetil-based, cyclosporine-free induction and maintenance immunosuppression: first three months analysis of efficacy and safety in two cohorts of renal allograft recipients. Transplantation 1998;66:44–49.

164. Goldblum R, McHugh D, Schiff M, et al. 2-Morpholino-ethyl mycophenolic acid (ME-MPA) inhibits lymphocyte mitogen responses in rheumatoid arthritis. Clin Pharmacol Ther 1990;47:193–197.

165. Allison AC, Eugui EM. Immunosuppressive and long-acting anti-inflammatory activity of mycophenolic acid and derivatives. Br J Rheumatol 1991;30(suppl 2):57–61.

166. Schiff MH, Goldblum R, Rees MMC. 2-Morpholino-ethyl mycophenolic acid (ME-MPA) in the treatment of refractory rheumatoid arthritis (RA). Arthritis Rheum 1990;33 (suppl 9):S155.

167. Goldbum R. Therapy of rheumatoid arthritis with mycophenolate mofetil. Clin Exp Rheumatol 1993;11(suppl 8):S117–S119.

168. Gomez EC, Menendez L, Frost P. Efficacy of mycophenolic acid for the treatment of psoriasis. J Am Acad Dermatol 1979;1:531–537.

169. Haufs MG, Beissert S, Grabbe S, et al. Psoriasis vulgaris treated successfully with mycophenolate mofetil. Br J Dermatol 1998;138:179–181.

170. Glicklich D, Acharya A. Mycophenolate mofetil therapy for lupus nephritis refractory to intravenous cyclophosphamide. Am J Kidney Dis 1998;32:318–322.

171. Briggs WA, Choi MY, Scheel Pj Jr. Successful mycophenolate mofetil treatment of glomerular disease. Am J Kidney Dis 1998;31:213–217.

172. Fickert P, Hinterleitner TA, Wenzl HH, et al. Mycophenolate mofetil in patients with Crohn's disease. Am J Gastroenterol 1998;93:2529–2532.

173. Basara N, Blau WI, Romer E, et al. Mycophenolate mofetil for the treatment of acute and chronic GVHD in bone marrow transplant patients. Bone Marrow Transplant 1998;22:61–65.

Chapter 5

Methotrexate

Michael E. Weinblatt

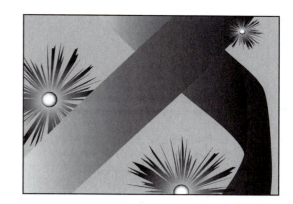

Methotrexate, a folate acid antagonist, has been used in clinical practice for more than 4 decades. It was initially developed as an anticancer drug; it is now used at lower doses for a variety of diseases, including psoriasis and rheumatoid arthritis. In 1948 Farber and colleagues (1) reported their classic study of aminopterin, the parent compound of methotrexate, in the treatment of childhood leukemia. This study established the role of folic acid antagonists in the treatment of malignancy. In 1951 Gubner and colleagues (2) reported the first open study of aminopterin in patients with nonmalignant disorders, including psoriasis, rheumatoid arthritis, and psoriatic arthritis. Further refinement of the aminopterin compound led to the synthesis of methotrexate. Dermatologists extensively studied methotrexate in the treatment of psoriasis in the 1950s and 1960s. There was a natural progression from the use of methotrexate in psoriasis to its successful use in psoriatic arthritis. Despite the observation by Gubner et al in 1951 (2) of the beneficial effects of aminopterin in the treatment of rheumatoid arthritis, it took another 20 years for there to be additional reports on the effects of methotrexate in the treatment of rheumatoid arthritis. In 1972 Hoffmeister (3) reported that low-dose methotrexate had beneficial effects in patients with rheumatoid arthritis. Open studies in the late 1970s and randomized controlled studies in the early 1980s confirmed the efficacy of low-dose, weekly methotrexate in the treatment of active rheumatoid arthritis. In 1988 the U.S. Food and Drug Administration approved low-dose, weekly methotrexate as a therapy for rheumatoid arthritis. Methotrexate has now become the most widely prescribed second-line therapy in the United States for rheumatoid arthritis. As such, it is used both alone and in combination with gold salts, sulfasalazine, hydroxychloroquine, and cyclosporine. It is also being studied in combination with leflunomide, a pyrimidine inhibitor, and a variety of biologic response modifiers such as the interleukin (IL) 1 receptor antagonist, IL-10, and inhibitors of tumor necrosis factor α (TNFα) (including monoclonal antibodies and etanercept, the p75 TNF receptor). It has become the standard comparator drug in trials of investigational therapies for rheumatoid arthritis.

Chemical Structure

Methotrexate (4-amino-N^{10}-methylpteroylglutamic acid, amethopterin) is a structural analog of folic acid (Fig. 5-1). Folic acid (pteroylglutamic acid) consists of three elements: a multiring pteridine group linked to para-aminobenzoic acid, which is connected to a terminal glutamic acid residue. Structurally, methotrexate differs from folic acid only in that an amino acid group substitutes for a hydroxyl group in position 4 of the pteridine portion of the molecule and a methyl group is added in position 10 of the 4-amino-benzoic acid structure. Methotrexate differs from its parent compound aminopterin in that aminopterin is devoid of the methyl group at the N^{10} position. The pteridine ring in methotrexate serves as the active site for the molecule.

Mechanisms of Action

Dietary folic acid is reduced enzymatically to dihydrofolate, tetrahydrofolate, and other reduced folates. These reduced folates participate in multiple biochemical reactions, including the conversion of homocysteine to methionine, the metabolism of histidine, the synthesis of purines, and the synthesis of thymidylate, which is essential for DNA synthesis. The primary enzyme responsible for the reduction of folic acid to these metabolically active reduced folates is dihydrofolate reductase (DHFR). Methotrexate inhibits the activity of this enzyme. The binding of DHFR by methotrexate is reversible. This inhibition of DHFR results in cessation of the biosynthesis of thymidilic acid, inosinic acid, and other purine metabolites. Methotrexate also affects protein biosynthesis by interrupting or preventing amino acid interconversions. Two important interconversions necessary for protein synthesis are the conversion of glycine to serine and homocysteine to methionine; both are blocked by methotrexate. Methotrexate inhibits DNA synthesis to a greater extent than RNA or protein synthesis. The complete inhibition of DHFR is not essential for the efficacy of the drug in rheumatoid arthritis. The inhibition of other folate-dependent enzymes may be as important in the actions of methotrexate in rheumatoid arthritis (4,5).

Most circulating folates in the blood have a single-terminal, glutamic structure (monoglutamated), whereas intracellular folates are converted from a monoglutamated to a polyglutamated compound. Folate polyglutamates have a longer cellular retention and are more efficient cofactors than the monoglutamated compounds. Similar to folate cofactors, methotrexate is also metabolized from a monoglutamated to a polyglutamated compound. This

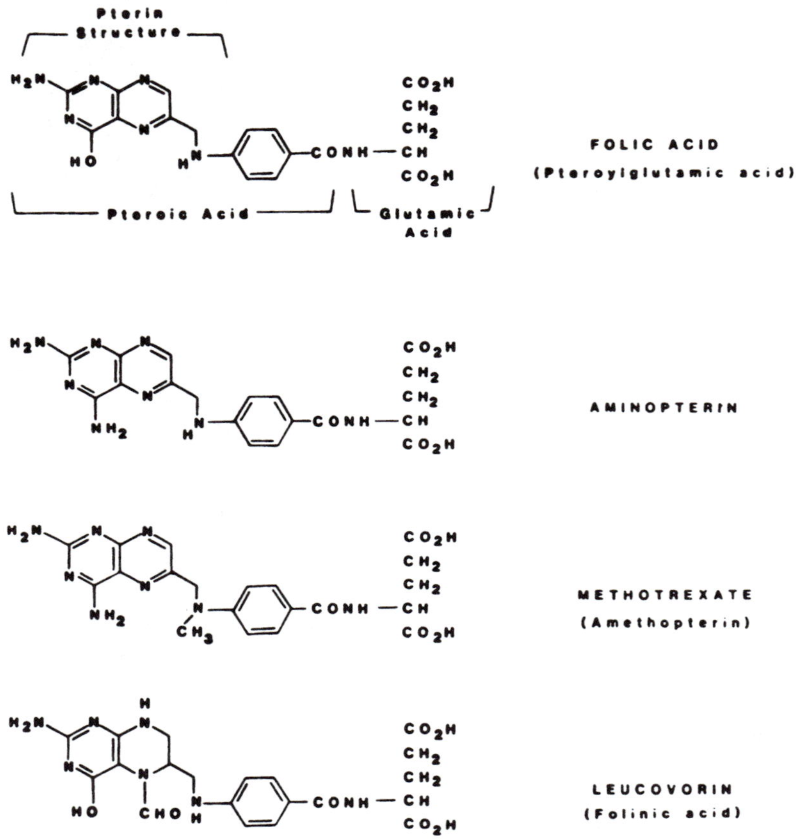

Figure 5-1. Structure of folic Acid, aminopterin, methotrexate, and leucovorin.

process of polyglutamation is essentially complete in 24 hours. Methotrexate polyglutamates have a stronger cellular retention, are more potent inhibitors of DHFR, and remain in the cell in the absence of extravascular drug (6). The synthesis of the methotrexate polyglutamates increases with chronic therapy. Methotrexate polyglutamates inhibit other folate-dependent enzymes that are not directly inhibited by methotrexate. Methotrexate polyglutamates are also more potent direct inhibitors of both thymidylate synthetase and 5-aminoimidazole-4-carboxamide ribonucleotide (AICAR) transformylase than the parent compound. Thymidylate synthetase and AICAR transformylase are required for de novo purine synthesis. The partial inhibition of these enzymes could lead to inhibition of both thymidylate and purine biosynthesis. It has been suggested that inhibition of AICAR transformylase may be one of the primary mechanisms of action of methotrexate in rheumatoid arthritis.

Methotrexate polyglutamates predominate in hepatic tissue (7). Whether polyglutamated methotrexate is more toxic to the liver than the monoglutamated compound is unknown. There is a decrease in the hepatic methotrexate polyglutamate concentration after folinic acid therapy (7).

Folinic acid (leucovorin) restores thymidylate, purine, and methionine biosynthesis in the presence of methotrexate. Folinic acid is a fully reduced, metabolically active folate coenzyme. It functions without the need for reduction by the enzyme DHFR. The fact that normal cells are more permeable to folinic acid and are more likely to possess the necessary enzymes for activation than are aberrant malignant cells has been the basis for the use of folinic acid as a rescue agent in cancer chemotherapy. Folinic acid is also used as a therapy for acute methotrexate overdose and to reduce side effects of low-dose, weekly methotrexate.

The antineoplastic effects of methotrexate are postulated to be the result of inhibition of DHFR leading to folate depletion and inhibition of purine and pyrimidine synthesis. In neoplastic disease methotrexate exerts its maximum inhibitory effect on cells actively undergoing DNA synthesis, particularly those cells in the S-phase of the cell cycle. Cells undergoing rapid turnover such as cells of the skin and gastrointestinal tract are the most susceptible to the cytotoxic effect of the drug. Folate depletion may not, however, account for all the therapeutic effects of methotrexate in an inflammatory disease such as rheumatoid arthritis.

Mechanisms of Action in Rheumatoid Arthritis

The effects of low-dose methotrexate on a variety of immune and inflammatory parameters have been extensively studied.

Methotrexate works on multiple levels of the disease process in rheumatoid arthritis.

Low-dose methotrexate has a variable effect on humoral immunity. A significant decrease in serum levels of immunoglobulin G (IgG), IgM, and IgA has been reported with methotrexate therapy (8). A suppression of both in vivo IgA and IgM rheumatoid factor titers and in vitro synthesis of IgM rheumatoid factor has been observed (9).

Several studies have investigated the effects of methotrexate on cytokine levels, production, and activity. IL-1, TNFα, IL-2, and IL-6 have all been postulated to be important in the pathogenesis of rheumatoid arthritis. Methotrexate has a variable effect on these cytokines. There was no inhibition of IL-1 synthesis or secretion in either rheumatoid arthritis patients or mice treated with methotrexate (10). Methotrexate had no cytotoxic effect on IL-1-producing cells and no inhibitory effect on IL-1 secretion by peripheral blood mononuclear cells from patients with rheumatoid arthritis. However, methotrexate inhibited IL-1 activity in vitro. These studies suggested that methotrexate inhibits IL-1 activity without affecting IL-1 production or secretion. The fact that this inhibition of IL-1 activity in vitro was abrogated by the addition of folinic acid but not folic acid (11) suggests that some of the effects of methotrexate on IL-1 activity are folate dependent. There was no consistent effect on IL-1 levels or on stimulated IL-1 production from peripheral blood mononuclear cells from patients with rheumatoid arthritis treated with methotrexate. After 6 weeks of therapy there was, however, a decrease in IL-1 synthesis. A decrease in both serum (12) and synovial fluid IL-1 β levels (13) has been noted with low-dose methotrexate.

Soluble IL-2 receptor levels are decreased (14) and the production of IL-2 ex vivo is increased from baseline in patients with rheumatoid arthritis who are treated with chronic methotrexate (15). This enhanced IL-2 production after methotrexate therapy was also reported in the streptococcal cell-wall–induced arthritis model in rats (16).

Methotrexate also strongly inhibited in vitro IL-6 activity; this inhibition was blocked by folinic acid (11). In contrast, TNF activity was not affected by methotrexate. A reduction in soluble TNF receptor levels but not TNFα levels occurred in patients who experienced clinical improvement during treatment with methotrexate (14). A reduction in IL-6 levels (14,15) and IL-8 levels (15) has also been observed in patients being treated with methotrexate.

In one study methotrexate increased both IL-10 and IL-4 gene expression in vitro, whereas IL-2 and interferon gamma gene expression were decreased (17). This increase in the Th-2 cytokines with a decrease in Th-1 cytokines could account for some of the beneficial effects of methotrexate.

Low-dose methotrexate, unlike high-dose therapy, does not have a significant effect on cellular immunity. In two short-term, randomized, placebo-controlled trials, no changes were detected in lymphocyte subsets after methotrexate therapy (8,18). After 2 years of therapy, the percentages of CD3+ and CD4+ cells increased significantly (19), but this change may have been caused by the reduction in prednisone dose and overall improvement in disease activity rather than to a selective effect of the drug. Over-

all, no consistent change in either lymphocyte or monocyte populations has been observed with low-dose methotrexate (19). Methotrexate in vitro induces apoptosis of activated T cells and clonal deletion of activated T cells (20). Adenosine release accounted for only a small portion of this effect. The process was blocked by the addition of folinic acid. There must be some effect on cellular immunity as evidenced by reports of opportunistic infections occurring in patients receiving low-dose methotrexate for treatment of rheumatoid arthritis.

Methotrexate exerts an antiproliferative effect on peripheral blood mononuclear cells in vitro. In a rabbit corneal model low-dose methotrexate inhibited neovascularization (21), suggesting an antiangiogenic effect that could contribute to the drug's mechanism of action by suppressing proliferation of small blood vessels in the rheumatoid synovium. Methotrexate inhibits in vitro the formation of S-adenosyl-methionine (SAMS), a methyl donor required for protein and lipid methylation and synthesis of polyamines (22). Because polyamines play a role in the disease process, inhibition of polyamines by methotrexate would be another mechanism for the efficacy of this drug in rheumatoid arthritis.

Many of the effects of methotrexate are mediated through inhibition of the enzyme DHFR or other folate-dependent enzymes. Methotrexate may also interfere with de novo purine biosynthesis by inhibition of the enzyme AICAR transformylase (23). Inhibition of AICAR transformylase increases the intracellular concentration of its substrate AICAR, which stimulates the release of adenosine (Fig. 5-2). Adenosine is a potent inhibitor of stimulated neutrophil function and thus has antiinflammatory properties. In the mouse air-sac model of inflammation methotrexate increased the intracellular accumulation of AICAR, which in turn increased adenosine concentrations in the exudates and inhibited leukocyte accumulation in the inflamed air pouch (4). This reduction in leukocyte accumulation was partially reversed by the injection of adenosine deaminase into the air pouch and was completely reversed by the injection of a specific adenosine A_2 receptor antagonist. An A_1 receptor antagonist had no effect. Adenosine also inhibited the production of several inflammatory cytokines that might be critical in rheumatoid arthritis, including TNFα, IL-6, and Il-8.

The facts that methotrexate has a rapid onset of action and the disease flares when the drug is discontinued suggest that methotrexate has an anti-inflammatory effect. Within days of a single injection of methotrexate, both the C-reactive protein level and the erythrocyte sedimentation rate are reduced (24). In the air-sac model of inflammation pretreatment of mice with low-dose methotrexate inhibited neutrophil migration induced by leukotriene B_4 (LTB$_4$) (25). In patients with psoriasis, in vivo chemotaxis of neutrophils induced by LTB$_4$ and C5a was blocked with methotrexate (26,27). Total generation of LTB$_4$ in neutrophils stimulated ex vivo was suppressed a mean of 53% compared with predose levels in patients receiving chronic methotrexate therapy (28). Patients with rheumatoid arthritis beginning therapy with methotrexate had a 27% reduction of LTB$_4$ from neutrophils stimulated ex vivo after the first 7.5-mg dose of methotrexate (29). A mean reduction of 43% in the

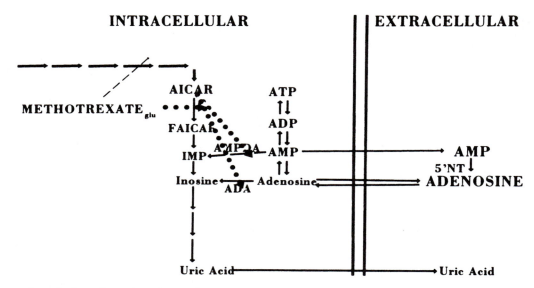

Figure 5-2. Promotion of adenosine release by methotrexate. ATP = adenosine triphosphate; ADP = adenosine diphosphate; AMP = adenosine monophosphate; AICAR = 5-aminoimidazole-4-carboxamide ribonucleotide; FAICAR = 5-formamidoimidazole-4-carboxamide ribonucleotide; IMP = inosine monophosphate (inosinic acid); AMPDA = AMP deaminase; ADA = adenosine deaminase; 5'NT = ecto-5'-nucleotidase. (Reproduced by permission from Cronstein B. Molecular therapeutics: methotrexate and its mechanisms of action. Arthritis Rheum 1996;39:1951.)

generation of LTB$_4$ in neutrophils stimulated ex vivo was observed after 6 to 8 weeks of methotrexate therapy as compared with predose levels. Another group observed a 32% decrease in ex vivo LTB$_4$ generation 24 hours after the first dose of intramuscular methotrexate in patients with rheumatoid arthritis (30). Another effect of methotrexate on inflammatory mediators is the reduction of superoxide production as demonstrated ex vivo from stimulated cells of patients with rheumatoid arthritis treated with methotrexate (31). In vitro studies also report an inhibitory effect on prostaglandin PGE$_2$ release without affecting cyclooxygenase mRNA expression (32).

Neutral metallocollagenolytic enzyme levels in synovial tissue from patients with rheumatoid arthritis were significantly lower in those patients being treated with methotrexate than in those receiving other treatment modalities, including nonsteroidal anti-inflammatory drugs or corticosteroids (33). Methotrexate was the only drug that consistently decreased neutral protease levels in joint tissue. In another study of patients with rheumatoid arthritis (34), synovial biopsies were obtained before treatment and after 5 months of treatment with either a nonsteroidal anti-inflammatory drug alone or methotrexate plus a nonsteroidal anti-inflammatory drug. The numbers of CD3+ and CD4+ cells in the synovium were decreased in the group receiving methotrexate, but no changes were observed in the group receiving only the nonsteroidal anti-inflammatory drug. In a third study, patients with rheumatoid arthritis underwent closed synovial biopsies before treatment and after 3 to 4 months of methotrexate therapy (35). Clinical improvement and a slight decrease in the synovial inflammatory score were noted. In situ hybridization studies showed a significant decrease in collagenase

gene expression but no effect on tissue inhibitor of metalloproteinase 1 or stromelysin mRNA levels.

Pharmacology

At the low doses used to treat rheumatoid arthritis, methotrexate can be administered either orally or parenterally. Methotrexate is actively transported across the proximal small intestine through pathways shared with folic acid. The absorption of oral methotrexate is variable. At a dose of 10 mg/m^2 (the dose used in rheumatoid arthritis) a mean bioavailability of 70% (range 40% to 100%) was achieved (36). The mean absorption time was 1.2 hours, and the terminal half-life was approximately 6 hours. Absorption was not affected by the presence of food (37,38). Synovial fluid concentrations were equal to serum concentrations 4 hours after methotrexate administration. Methotrexate diffused into synovial fluid at concentrations equal to serum levels (36). The pharmacokinetics of low-dose methotrexate were similar after both intramuscular and subcutaneous injections (39). Rapid absorption occurred with both methods of parenteral administration, and a maximum serum concentration was obtained within 2 hours (39). Because the absorption of oral methotrexate is variable, a trial of parenteral methotrexate is recommended for patients not responding to oral therapy. In pharmacokinetic studies, the tablet form and the parenteral solution administered orally yielded similar bioavailability (38). The parenteral solution administered orally offers potential cost savings over the tablet (40).

Methotrexate is approximately 50% bound to plasma protein. Methotrexate is distributed from plasma in a triphasic manner. The first phase of less than 1 hour corresponds to the distribution of methotrexate into body fluids, while the second and third stages, lasting 2 to 3 hours and 8 to 9 hours, respectively, reflect renal clearance and the combined effect of the drug being released from peripheral compartments, enterohepatic recirculation, and tubular reabsorption. Methotrexate is distributed throughout the body, with higher concentrations found in intestinal epithelium and hepatic cells. Methotrexate may undergo limited hepatic metabolism by the enzyme aldehyde oxidase to the 7-hydroxymethotrexate metabolite. The intracellular conversion of methotrexate from the monoglutamated to the polyglutamated derivative produces potent inhibitors of DHFR, which are retained intracellularly in preference to the monoglutamated parent compound.

Methotrexate accumulates in third-space fluid collections such as large pleural effusions. Such accumulations can lead to toxic levels of drug when reabsorption of the fluid and drug occurs.

Methotrexate is excreted primarily by glomerular filtration and active tubular transport. Organic acids such as probenecid competitively inhibit tubular secretion and thereby delay methotrexate clearance. The plasma half-life of methotrexate is less than 10 hours, but increases in the setting of renal insufficiency.

Because methotrexate is only 50% bound to plasma protein, an increase can occur in free methotrexate as a result of its displacement from albumin by more highly protein-bound drugs such as nonsteroidal anti-inflammatory drugs and sulfonamides. This displacement appears to have limited clinical significance with low-dose methotrexate because the increase in free methotrexate is generally modest. In several pharmacokinetic studies, no significant interaction was detected between low-dose methotrexate and a variety of nonsteroidal anti-inflammatory drugs, including sulindac, diclofenac, indomethacin, and naproxen (41–43). Two other studies reported a change in the kinetics of low-dose methotrexate with aspirin and ibuprofen (44,45). A reduction in the renal clearance of methotrexate was reported when methotrexate at higher doses (mean 16 mg/wk) was coadministered with nonsteroidal anti-inflammatory drugs (46). With higher doses of methotrexate, as used in cancer chemotherapy, the coadministration of nonsteroidal anti-inflammatory drugs or aspirin may be toxic and even fatal. Non-steroidal anti-inflammatory drugs must be avoided with high-dose methotrexate as used in cancer chemotherapy. Drugs that inhibit tubular secretion such as probenecid must also be avoided.

Trimethoprim/sulfamethoxazole should be used with great caution with methotrexate; several case reports revealed hematologic toxicity with this combination (47,48). Possible mechanisms for this synergistic toxicity include an additive antifolate effect from trimethoprim, decreased methotrexate clearance resulting from inhibition of tubular secretion by sulfamethoxazole, and altered methotrexate plasma protein binding.

Therapeutic indications

Low-dose, weekly methotrexate is approved by the Food and Drug Administration for the treatment of psoriasis and rheuma-toid arthritis. It is also being used to treat a variety of other rheumatologic, inflammatory, and autoimmune diseases. At higher doses the drug has established efficacy in neoplastic diseases but this use is not reviewed in this chapter.

Rheumatoid Arthritis

Extensive experience with methotrexate in psoriasis led to formalized studies of the drug in the treatment of psoriatic arthritis and then rheumatoid arthritis. Open studies in patients with rheumatoid arthritis, primarily performed by community-based rheumatologists, reported efficacy with an acceptable tolerability profile (49–53). On the basis of the positive results from these uncontrolled studies, four placebo-controlled trials were initiated in patients who had not responded to traditional second-line therapies, including gold salts and d-penicillamine. In a 35-patient, 24-week double-blind, placebo-controlled, crossover study, the standard rheumatoid arthritis disease activity parameters improved in the methotrexate-treated group (18). This improvement in clinical disease activity began within 3 weeks of the start of methotrexate therapy. Individual patient response criteria, defined as greater than a 50% improvement in the joint pain or joint swelling index, occurred in 54% and 34% of the methotrexate-treated patients, respectively. In this crossover study, disease activity increased within 3 weeks after methotrexate was discontinued. The doses of methotrexate used in this study were 7.5 mg/wk initially and 15.0 mg/wk maximum. In an 18-week, double-blind, placebo-controlled trial of 189 patients, methotrexate was again found to be superior to placebo (54). The dose of oral methotrexate was again 7.5 mg/wk initially and 15.0 mg/wk maximum. Significant improvement in all variables occurred in the methotrexate-treated group. These two studies served as the pivotal studies for the review by the U.S. Food and Drug Administration of methotrexate as a therapy for rheumatoid arthritis. Two other randomized, placebo-controlled trials, including a 6-week parallel study (55) and a 24-week, placebo-controlled, crossover study (8), noted similar improvements with methotrexate therapy.

A meta-analysis of these four randomized trials confirmed the significant clinical response that had been observed in each of the individual studies (56). In this meta-analysis, patient benefit was defined as the percentage of improvement from baseline achieved in the methotrexate-treated group over and above that attributable to the placebo response. There was a 46% improvement in the duration of morning stiffness, a 27% improvement in the number of painful joints, and a 26% improvement in the number of swollen joints in the methotrexate-treated group. The four placebo-controlled trials and the meta-analysis demonstrated the efficacy of methotrexate as compared with placebo in patients with active rheumatoid arthritis.

Several studies have compared methotrexate to other standard therapies in rheumatoid arthritis. In a 48-week, multicenter study of 64 patients, methotrexate was found to be superior to azathioprine in both clinical response and tolerability (57). Methotrexate was also found to be superior to oral gold (auranofin) in both efficacy and tolerability in a 9-month, 282-patient,

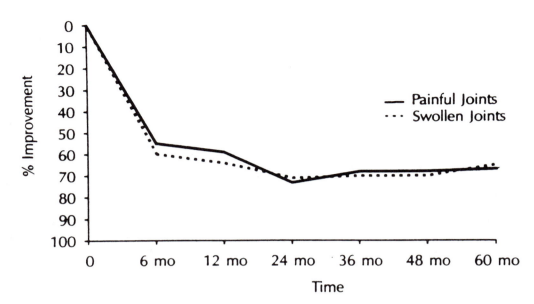

Figure 5-3. Long-term response to methotrexate. Shown is the mean percent change from baseline in the number of painful joints and the number of swollen joints, in patients with rheumatoid arthritis treated with methotrexate. The number of patients at each visit was as follows: 120 patients at 12 months, 109 patients at 24 months, 98 patients at 36 months, 88 patients at 48 months, and 70 patients at 60 months. (Reproduced by permission from Weinblatt ME, Kaplan H, Germain BF, et al. Methotrexate in rheumatoid arthritis: a 5-year prospective multicenter trial. Arthritis Rheum 1994;37:1492–1498.)

multicenter trial (58). Using the American College of Rheumatology Criteria for response (59), 68% of patients in the methotrexate-treated group achieved a positive response as compared with 30% in the auranofin-treated group. Methotrexate was also superior to cyclosporine in a large multicenter study (60). Smaller studies comparing methotrexate to parenteral gold reported a similar clinical response, to both agents, but gold salts were more toxic (61–63). A meta-analysis of all second-line therapies reported that methotrexate was the most effective second-line therapy in the treatment of rheumatoid arthritis (64).

There have been several, long-term, prospective studies of methotrexate in rheumatoid arthritis. In one, 26 patients who had successfully completed a 24-week, placebo-controlled, crossover study of methotrexate (18) entered into a long-term prospective study lasting 130 months (65,66). At the completion of the study, 10 (38%) patients still remained in therapy, and they continued to note a sustained beneficial effect with methotrexate. The maximum beneficial effects were achieved by 6 months. Fifty percent of the patients were also able to discontinue background prednisone therapy.

A second study reported a sustained clinical response after a mean of 13.3 years of therapy (67). The clinical response plateaued after the initial 6 months of treatment. Ten of 29 patients completed this long-term study, and a sustained clinical effect was again observed.

In a third, long-term, prospective study, 123 patients who had successfully completed a 9-month randomized trial comparing methotrexate with auranofin (58) enrolled in a 5-year open study of methotrexate (68) (Fig. 5-3). Patients could not have received prior intramuscular gold or *d*-penicillamine, thereby making this population different from the patient populations in all the other prospective studies. This study included patients with less refractory and untreated disease. At 5 years 64% remained on drug therapy. A significant improvement was observed in all parameters, including a reduction in the erythrocyte sedimentation rate.

In another long-term study, 271 patients were treated with methotrexate for up to 108 months (69). At five years 60% of patients remained on drug therapy. A sustained improvement in disease activity was noted.

Other investigators have confirmed the high retention rate in these studies of patients being treated with methotrexate. In a study of 152 patients with rheumatoid arthritis, 71% remained on methotrexate at 1 year (70). It was projected that at 6 years 49% of the patients would remain on methotrexate. In this study the major reason for withdrawal was drug toxicity. Studies from community-based rheumatologists further support the concept of longer therapy durations with methotrexate compared with those with other second-line therapies (71). The rate of methotrexate continuation was approximately double that seen with the other second-line treatments.

Discontinuation of methotrexate is generally associated with a return in disease activity. Two short-term, placebo-controlled, crossover studies (8,18) and two longer studies (72,73) reported a flare of arthritis activity when methotrexate was discontinued.

Methotrexate effects on radiographic progression are variable. Erosions healed within the first 29 months of methotrexate therapy in a limited number of patients (74). However, after a mean of 54 months of therapy new erosions were observed (75). In another long-term study, erosion healing with a marked loss of joint space was observed in a small number of patients after 28 months of therapy (19). In a study comparing patients treated with methotrexate to those treated with azathioprine, the rate of radiographic progression was less with methotrexate than with azathioprine (76). The rate of radiographic progression, as defined by joint erosions and joint space narrowing, was decreased in patients treated with methotrexate compared with those treated with auranofin (77).

To summarize, the efficacy profile of methotrexate in rheumatoid arthritis has been established by open studies; short-term, randomized, placebo-controlled trials; randomized comparative studies with other second-line therapies; and long-term retrospective and prospective studies. It is currently the most effective second-line therapy for rheumatoid arthritis as defined by both the beneficial clinical response and its duration.

Other Rheumatic Diseases

Methotrexate at doses of 30 to 50 mg per week by parenteral administration has been used to treat corticosteroid-resistant polymyositis and dermatomyositis (78). Several open studies reported an improvement in patients with Felty's syndrome who were treated with low-dose, weekly methotrexate (79–81). The leukocyte count improved within 3 to 12 weeks after starting methotrexate, but the leukopenia returned promptly when the drug was discontinued. Methotrexate has also been used to treat patients with Reiter's syndrome (82). The doses of methotrexate required for improving the skin and joint disease range from 10 to 50 mg per week. A small randomized study reported a beneficial response to methotrexate in patients with scleroderma (83). Open studies in patients with giant cell arteritis (84), cutaneous vasculitis (85), multicentric reticulohistiocytosis (86,87), systemic lupus (arthritis and dermatitis) (88,89), Takayasu's arteritis (90), and Wegener's granulomatosis (91,92) all suggest a role for methotrexate in the treatment of these conditions. Studies in patients with polymyalgia rheumatica have yielded conflicting results, and the use of methotrexate to treat this disease requires further study (93,94).

In juvenile rheumatoid arthritis, methotrexate has become the standard therapy for children with resistant polyarthritis. The efficacy of low-dose methotrexate as compared with placebo in children with resistant juvenile rheumatoid arthritis was established in an international multicenter trial (95). Efficacy was achieved with a dose of methotrexate of $10 \, mg/m^2$; a lower dose ($5 \, mg/m^2$) was no better than placebo. In children with juvenile rheumatoid arthritis higher mean doses of methotrexate based on body weight are used as compared with doses used in adults with rheumatoid arthritis.

Open (96) and short-term randomized studies (97,98) reported efficacy of methotrexate in the treatment of patients with corticosteroid-dependent asthma. However, other randomized, short-term, placebo-controlled trials reported no difference in pulmonary function, corticosteroid reduction, or airway reactivity with methotrexate compared with placebo (99,100). There is less enthusiasm for the use of methotrexate in the treatment of asthma because studies to confirm its efficacy are lacking.

Methotrexate has been used to treat a variety of other inflammatory and autoimmune diseases, including primary biliary cirrhosis (101,102), inflammatory bowel disease (103), sclerosing cholangitis (104,105), granulomatous hepatitis (106), and sarcoidosis (107). Most of these studies have been either short-term, open studies or small, randomized trials. In a large, multicenter, double-blind, placebo-controlled study of patients with Crohn's disease, methotrexate was found to be superior to placebo in controlling the disease and in reducing background dose requirements for prednisone (108). Methotrexate is also being used in the treatment of inflammatory eye disease, primarily to reduce doses of steroids and cyclosporine.

Dose and Drug Administration

Methotrexate can be administered either orally or by parenteral injection. It should be given only on a weekly basis; more frequent administration is associated with a greater incidence of acute and chronic toxicity. For the treatment of rheumatoid arthritis, the initial methotrexate dose is generally 7.5 mg per week. The optimal dose is unknown, but doses of 7.5 to 20 mg per week have been used in most studies. If a positive response has not occurred in 4 to 6 weeks and there has been no toxicity, the dose is increased. In one study, a dose response effect was seen with placebo, $5 \, mg/m^2$ methotrexate, and $10 \, mg/m^2$ methotrexate, with a greater response with the $10 \, mg/m^2$ dose (109). Some patients may require higher doses over time to maintain the clinical response. Doses above 20 mg per week are generally administered parenterally because of decreased oral bioavailability at higher doses. Once a satisfactory response is achieved, the dose of methotrexate may be slowly reduced. Frequent dose titrations (up and down) may be required to maintain response and reduce toxicity. In one study, patients, whose disease was stable at a particular dose of methotrexate were tapered to an every-other-week dose regimen without a flare of disease activity (110). In patients who have a beneficial response to therapy, but develop gastrointestinal toxicity or fatigue, increasing the interval to every 10 to 14 days may be worthwhile. Higher doses of methotrexate have been used to treat patients with refractory disease. In a pilot study an initial intravenous dose of $40 \, mg/m^2$ induced a beneficial clinical response in patients who had not responded to oral therapy (111). After 12 weeks the mean dose was $26 \, mg/m^2$. In another pilot study, patients with refractory rheumatoid arthritis being treated with high-dose intravenous methotrexate ($500 \, mg/m^2$ with folinic acid therapy) appeared to have a beneficial clinical response over the 8-week trial period (112). A randomized trial based on these preliminary results was terminated prematurely because of issues related to efficacy and toxicity (113).

Toxicity

Adverse events occur throughout methotrexate treatment, but are most frequent during the first 6 months (Fig. 5-4). The most common side effects associated with low-dose, weekly methotrexate are gastrointestinal, including anorexia, nausea, vomiting, diarrhea, and stomatitis. Many of these toxicities improve with dose reduction or a change from oral to parenteral administration. Both folic acid (114) and folinic acid (115) may reduce the gastrointestinal toxicity. Newer antiemetics such as ondanestron may also be of value in treating nausea (116). In most patients these toxicities occur shortly after the drug is administered, are mild, and usually resolve within several days. Of 587 patients who received low-dose methotrexate for rheumatoid arthritis, 10% experienced gastrointestinal toxicity; 2.5% of the patients had a moderate to severe event, which led to drug withdrawal (117).

Hematologic toxicity occurs with low-dose methotrexate; it has been reported in approximately 5% of patients being treated with the drug for rheumatoid arthritis (117). In almost all cases an identifiable risk factor for this toxicity was present such as unrecognized renal insufficiency; concomitant folic acid deficiency; use of the drug during acute infection, including viral illnesses; use in patients undergoing dialysis; and the concomitant use of probenecid or trimethoprim/sulfamethoxazole (47,48,118–120). Pancytopenia has also been reported in the setting of acute parvovirus infection (121). An elevation in the mean corpuscular volume (MCV) may serve as a predictor of potential hematologic toxicity (122). Folic acid or folinic acid is recommended for patients receiving methotrexate. In patients with a sustained elevation of the MCV, vitamin B-12 and red blood cell folate levels should be measured. Folinic acid should be administered immediately to patients who develop hematologic toxicity. Folinic acid is generally most effective when administered within 24 to 48 hours of the methotrexate dose. Methotrexate is poorly cleared by either hemodialysis or peritoneal dialysis.

Renal toxicity with low-dose methotrexate is rare. Renal insufficiency from any cause can lead to sustained and toxic levels of methotrexate. Regular monitoring of renal function in patients being treated with methotrexate is essential.

Cutaneous reactions to methotrexate include urticaria, reactivation of ultraviolet light–induced erythema, and alopecia. An increase in the number and size of rheumatoid nodules despite an improvement in the articular disease has been observed in patients with rheumatoid arthritis receiving methotrexate (19,123). Nodules have also been reported in patients with psoriasis (124) and juvenile rheumatoid arthritis receiving methotrexate (125). The mechanism for this accelerated nodulosis is unknown. Nodulosis might be related to the promotion of multinucleated giant cell formation by the adenosine A_1 receptor (126). The therapy for the nodulosis is unknown, but attempts to control it have included discontinuation of methotrexate or reduction of the dose, the injection or systemic administration of corticosteroids, the addition of another second-line therapy, or colchicine therapy. There have been no formal studies to assess these approaches.

Methotrexate is a definite teratogenic agent. It should not be administered to women of childbearing age unless adequate birth control measures are used. Women should discontinue methotrexate for at least one ovulatory cycle before attempting conception. The parent compound of methotrexate, aminopterin,

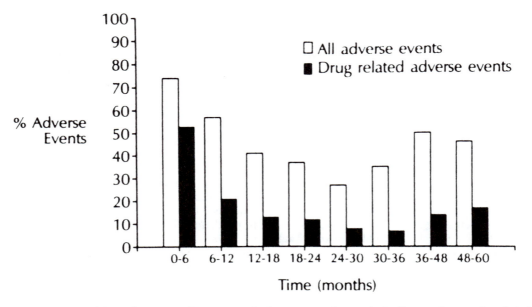

Figure 5-4. Toxicity frequency with methotrexate. Frequency of adverse experiences, including methotrexate-related and non-drug-related experiences, over the course of the study. (Reproduced by permission from Weinblatt ME, Kaplan H, Germain BF, et al. Methotrexate in rheumatoid arthritis: a 5-year prospective multicenter trial. Arthritis Rheum 1994;37:1492–1498.)

was associated with specific fetal abnormalities described as the "aminopterin syndrome" (127). It was also used as an abortifacient. Methotrexate is again being used as a medical therapy to terminate pregnancy (128). Congenital abnormalities similar to those produced by aminopterin have been reported with low-dose methotrexate (129).

Ovarian dysfunction has not been reported with the drug. Transient but reversible oligospermia has been reported in males receiving high-dose methotrexate for cancer chemotherapy (130). Reversible oligospermia has been reported in patients being treated with low-dose methotrexate for psoriasis (131). It is suggested that males discontinue methotrexate 90 days before attempting conception.

Methotrexate has not been identified as a carcinogenic agent in humans, and no carcinogenic effect has been detected in animal studies (132). Patients receiving high doses of methotrexate for the treatment of choriocarcinoma exhibited no increase in the appearance of second malignancy (133). In several large studies in patients with psoriasis, a carcinogenic effect was also not observed (134,135). There are, however, reports of patients who developed non-Hodgkin's lymphoma while taking low-dose methotrexate for treatment of rheumatoid arthritis or polymyositis (136–142). In many cases this lymphoma was extranodal in location, including skin, soft tissue, lung, and salivary gland; Epstein-Barr virus (EBV) was detected in many of the tumor cells. In these cases the non-Hodgkin's lymphoma frequently resolved when methotrexate was discontinued. Resolution of the lymphoma suggests a cause-and-effect relationship with methotrexate. The reversible nature of the lymphoproliferative disorder in these cases is similar to that reported with immunosuppressive therapy associated with organ transplant, that is, the posttransplant lymphoproliferative disease that occurs with cyclosporine and azathioprine therapy. The role of EBV in the modulation of this lymphoproliferative disorder is still under study. In patients receiving methotrexate, azathioprine, or cyclosporine who develop a lymphoma, the tumor should be examined for the presence of EBV, and these drugs should be withdrawn. Spontaneous regression of the lymphoma (if it occurs) will begin 4 to 6 weeks after the drug is discontinued. Except for EBV-associated lymphoma, there are no data that methotrexate therapy is associated with an increased risk for lymphoma or solid tumors. Of 16,263 patients seen during 16 years at the Mayo Clinic, 39 patients who had been treated with a second-line therapy for rheumatoid arthritis subsequently developed a hematologic malignancy (143). In this study there was no relationship between these malignancies and methotrexate therapy or any other second-line therapy.

Central nervous system toxicity, including headache, fatigue, mood alteration, depression, and dizziness has been observed (144). An increased adenosine concentration in the cerebral spinal fluid has been suggested as a cause of the neurotoxicity seen with methotrexate in the treatment of leukemia (145). This toxicity was reversed with the administration of aminophylline, an adenosine receptor antagonist.

Fatigue, fever, and polyarthralgias are unusual effects seen after methotrexate administration. Opportunistic infections such as Pneumocystis carinii, localized and disseminated herpes zoster, and fungal infections have been reported in patients with rheumatoid arthritis receiving low-dose methotrexate therapy (146–149).

Localized osteoporosis presenting as severe bone pain and nontraumatic fractures occurred in children receiving high doses of methotrexate for the treatment of acute leukemia and resolved when the drug was discontinued (150–152). In animals, short-term administration of high-dose methotrexate was associated with a reduction in the volume of trabecular bone and the rate of bone formation (153). Osteopenia with suppression of osteoblast activity and stimulation of osteoclast recruitment occurred in rats receiving methotrexate at doses similar to those used to treat rheumatoid arthritis (154,155). The cells were unable to synthesize and calcify bone matrix. Methotrexate had no effects on bone density in adults with rheumatoid arthritis (156).

Acute and chronic pulmonary toxicity occurs with methotrexate therapy (157–160). The clinical syndrome includes fever, cough, dyspnea, hypoxemia, and the development of interstitial pulmonary infiltrates. In a study of 29 patients who met the criteria for methotrexate lung disease, the predominant symptom was dyspnea, which was present for 3 weeks before the diagnosis; cough and fever were reported in greater than 50% of the patients (161). This toxicity generally occurred earlier in the course of methotrexate therapy (mean 66 weeks) and at any dose. Pathologic examination classically shows alveolar and interstitial infiltrates consisting of mononuclear cells, giant cells with granuloma formation, bronchiolitis, and fibrosis. The lung pathology may be indistinguishable from that of rheumatoid lung disease. In a case-control study of 29 rheumatoid arthritis patients with methotrexate-induced lung disease and 82 patients without methotrexate-induced lung disease, increased age, rheumatoid pleuropulmonary disease, and diabetes were the risk factors for this toxicity (162). Underlying pulmonary disease, particularly interstitial fibrosis, has also been suggested as a risk factor (163). The chest radiograph may initially be normal, but generally progresses to show interstitial and occasionally alveolar infiltrates. Treatment includes discontinuation of methotrexate, respiratory support, exclusion of opportunistic infections, and the administration of systemic corticosteroids. The outcome is variable, but most patients have recovered. In a review of the literature 17% of patients with methotrexate-induced lung disease died from complications associated with this toxicity. Rechallenge was associated with reoccurrence of lung disease in one-third of the patients (161). Occasionally, the fibrosis progresses and leads to chronic interstitial lung disease and even death (164–166). In a patient with underlying lung disease, a baseline chest radiograph is suggested before starting methotrexate. Surveillance pulmonary function testing is of limited value in identifying patients at risk for this toxicity.

The development of serious liver disease in patients with rheumatoid arthritis receiving methotrexate is uncommon. This finding is in contradistinction to the experience in patients with psoriasis; in one study more than 20% of patients with psoriasis developed cirrhosis after 5 years of methotrexate treatment (167). In patients with psoriasis, the increase in serious liver disease may be caused by a number of factors, including greater alcohol consumption, preexisting histologic abnormalities independent of drug exposure, and higher weekly doses. The natural history of methotrexate-associated liver disease in psoriasis is unknown, but it has been suggested that the liver disease does not progress once the drug is discontinued. In psoriasis the risk factors for methotrexate-associated hepatic toxicity include insulin-dependent diabetes, morbid obesity, alcohol consumption, and total cumulative dose of the drug (168). The characteristic pathology associated with methotrexate is fibrosis and cirrhosis. Dermatologists have developed a series of guidelines for patients receiving the drug for psoriasis, which include liver biopsies after 1500 mg of therapy and repetitive liver biopsies thereafter (168). Liver biopsies in patients with psoriasis before treatment have also been recommended, but this recommendation is controversial. These recommendations for patients with psoriasis need to be reexamined because the patients on whom the recommendations were based were not advised to abstain from alcohol and their liver blood tests were not performed on a regular basis.

The data for patients with rheumatoid arthritis receiving methotrexate are much more encouraging and complete. Of 714 patients who underwent liver biopsy after receiving approximately 1.5 grams of methotrexate, mild fibrosis was observed in 8% and moderate fibrosis was noted in 0.5% (4 patients) (169). One case of cirrhosis was present on a pretreatment biopsy. In 23 patients with rheumatoid arthritis who received methotrexate for more than 10 years, there were no cases of cirrhosis (170). There

have been isolated reports of both cirrhosis (171,172) and acute decompensated liver disease (173,174). In a case-control study, which included a survey of members of the American College of Rheumatology, 24 cases of serious liver disease were identified (175). The estimated risk of developing serious liver disease after 5 years of treatment was projected at less than 1 per 1000. Elevations in serum transaminase levels and a decrease in serum albumin were observed more frequently in the population who developed serious liver disease than in the control population. Two independent risk factors for liver toxicity, age and duration of therapy, have been noted. A committee organized by the American College of Rheumatology published guidelines for monitoring patients with rheumatoid arthritis receiving methotrexate (176) (Table 5-1). The committee defined an abnormality in the serum transaminase level as a test result above the upper range of the laboratory normal. It is important to note that clinically serious liver disease has been found in only one patient with normal liver blood tests; this patient was an insulin-dependent diabetic receiving methotrexate for rheumatoid arthritis whose values for albumin and serum transaminases were consistently normal during regular monitoring (177). The Committee recommended that serum transaminase and albumin levels be monitored every 4 to 8 weeks. A biopsy should be performed if the serum alanine or aspartate aminotransferase level is elevated into the abnormal range in 5 of 9 yearly determinations or if the serum albumin level falls below the lower limit of

Table 5-1. Recommendations for Monitoring for Hepatic Safety in Patients with Rheumatoid Arthritis Receiving Methotrexate

A. Baseline
  1. Tests for all patients
    a. Liver blood tests (aspartate aminotransferase [AST], alanine aminotransferase [ALT], alkaline phosphatase, albumin, bilirubin), hepatitis B and C serologic studies
    b. Other standard tests, including complete blood cell count and serum creatinine
  2. Pretreatment liver biopsy (Menghini suction-type needle) only for patients with:
    a. Prior excessive alcohol consumption
    b. Persistently abnormal baseline AST values
    c. Chronic hepatitis B or C infection
B. Monitor AST, ALT, albumin at 4–8-week intervals
C. Perform liver biopsy if:
  1. Five of 9 determinations of AST within a given 12-month interval (6 of 12 if tests are performed monthly) are abnormal (defined as an elevation above the upper limit of normal)
  2. There is a decrease in serum albumin below the normal range (in the setting of well-controlled rheumatoid arthritis)
D. If results of liver biopsy are:
  1. Roenigk grade I, II, or IIIA, resume methotrexate and monitor as in B, C1, and C2 above
  2. Roenigk grade IIIB or IV discontinue methotrexate
E. Discontinue methotrexate in patients with persistent liver test abnormalities, as defined in C1 and C2 above, who refuse liver biopsy

From Kremer JM, Alarcón GS, Lightfoot RW Jr, et al. Methotrexate for rheumatoid arthritis: suggested guidelines for monitoring liver toxicity. Arthritis Rheum 1994;37:316–328.

normal in the setting of well-controlled rheumatoid arthritis. Two studies of the guidelines have determined that they are clinically useful and cost effective, with 80% sensitivity and 82% specificity (177,178).

Folic acid is now routinely used to reduce many of the side effects associated with methotrexate therapy. In a randomized, 24-week, placebo-controlled trial, folic acid (1 mg/day) did not abrogate the beneficial effects of methotrexate, but did reduce the number and severity of side effects (114). In a follow-up study, folic acid doses of both 5 mg per week and 27.5 mg per week were superior to placebo in reducing the side effects of methotrexate without blocking efficacy (179). The higher dose of folic acid had no advantage in this study. Clinical experience suggests that folic acid might reduce some of the gastrointestinal toxicity associated with methotrexate. Folic acid also maintains red blood cell folate levels, thereby reducing the risk of hematologic toxicity. Folinic acid has also been reported to reduce side effects associated with low-dose methotrexate therapy. In a 52-week, placebo-controlled study, patients who received weekly folinic acid had fewer side effects and a lower rate of withdrawal from the study than those who received placebo (115). Folinic acid was administered 24 hours after methotrexate at a dose that ranged from 2.5 to 5.0 mg per week. In this study folinic acid did not interfere with the efficacy of methotrexate. However, another study determined that higher dose folinic acid administered within the half-life of methotrexate and for 2 additional days eliminated existing toxicity, but attenuated the efficacy of methotrexate (180). A randomized, placebo-controlled study reported that low-dose folinic acid (1 mg) administered simultaneously with methotrexate did not block the efficacy of methotrexate (181). These studies suggest that the effects of folinic acid on efficacy might be related to the dose and time of administration. A trial comparing folic acid to folinic acid has not yet been performed in patients with rheumatoid arthritis. A meta-analysis confirms that folic acid and folinic acid reduce gastrointestinal and oral toxicity (182). Because the cost of folinic acid is greater than that of folic acid, it is reasonable to use folic acid initially either for prevention of or as therapy for mild side effects associated with methotrexate. In patients receiving folic acid who continue to experience gastrointestinal toxicity, stomatitis, folate depletion, fatigue, or central nervous system toxicity, a trial of folinic acid is recommended. Folinic acid is also recommended for methotrexate overdose or hematologic toxicity. There are no data to show that either folic acid or folinic acid is useful as prophylaxis or as therapy for pulmonary toxicity.

Indications and Monitoring

Methotrexate is used in patients with active rheumatoid arthritis. Women of childbearing potential who do not use adequate birth control and patients with renal insufficiency, untreated folate deficiency, active liver disease, chronic hepatitis B or C infection, excessive alcohol consumption, or serious concomitant medical illnesses should not receive methotrexate therapy. Baseline laboratory parameters include a complete blood count, serum creatinine, liver blood tests, hepatitis B and C serologies, and in selected cases a chest radiograph. After the initiation of therapy, complete blood counts should be obtained monthly, and every 4 to 8 weeks the levels of serum alanine and aspartate transferase, albumin, and serum creatinine should be measured. Methotrexate should be temporarily discontinued during acute infections and during the immediate preoperative and postoperative periods for major surgical procedures. Supplemental daily folic acid (1 mg) reduces some of the adverse experiences associated with methotrexate. Detailed discussion must be held with the patient about the side-effect profile and the rationale for monitoring, including the potential need for liver biopsies.

Methotrexate has become the major therapy for rheumatoid arthritis. It is regarded as one of the most significant advances during the past decade for the treatment of rheumatoid arthritis (183).

References

1. Farber S, Diamond LK, Mercer RD, et al. Temporary remissions in acute leukemia in children produced by folic acid antagonist, 4-aminopteroyl-glutamic acid (aminopterin). N Engl J Med 1948;238:787–793.
2. Gubner R, August S, Ginsberg V. Therapeutic suppression of tissue reactivity. II. Effect of aminopterin in rheumatoid arthritis and psoriasis. Am J Med Sci 1951;22:176–182.
3. Hoffmeister RT. Methotrexate in rheumatoid arthritis. Arthritis Rheum 1972;15:114. Abstract.
4. Cronstein BN, Naime D, Ostad E. The antiinflammatory mechanism of methotrexate. Increased adenosine release at inflamed sites diminishes leukocyte accumulation in an in vivo model of inflammation. J Clin Invest 1993;92:2675–2682.
5. Baggott JE, Morgan SL, Alarcón GS, Krumdieck CL. Antifolates in rheumatoid arthritis: a hypothetical mechanism of action. Clin Exp Rheumatol 1993;11(suppl 8):S101–S105.
6. Jolivet J, Cowan KH, Curt GA, et al. The pharmacology and clinical use of methotrexate. N Engl J Med 1983;309:1094–1104.
7. Kremer JM, Galivan J, Streckfuss A, Kamen B. Methotrexate metabolism analysis in blood and liver of rheumatoid arthritis patients. Association with hepatic folate deficiency and formation of polyglutamates. Arthritis Rheum 1986;29:832–835.
8. Andersen PA, West SG, O'Dell JR, et al. Weekly pulse methotrexate in rheumatoid arthritis. Clinical and immunologic effects in a randomized, double-blind study. Ann Intern Med 1985;103:489–496.
9. Olsen NJ, Callahan LF, Pincus T. Immunologic studies of rheumatoid arthritis patients treated with methotrexate. Arthritis Rheum 1987;30:481–488.
10. Segal R, Mozes E, Yaron M, Tartakovsky B. The effects of methotrexate on the production and activity of interleukin-1. Arthritis Rheum 1989;32:370–377.
11. Segal R, Yaron M, Tartakovsky B. Rescue of interleukin-1 activity by leucovorin following inhibition by methotrexate in a murine in vitro system. Arthritis Rheum 1990;33:1745–1748.

12. Kremer JM, Lawrence DA. Correlation of immune parameters with clinical and laboratory effects in prospective cohort of patients with rheumatoid arthritis receiving methotrexate. Arthritis Rheum 1992;35:S144. Abstract.

13. Thomas R, Carroll GJ. Reduction of leukocyte and interleukin-1β concentrations in the synovial fluid of rheumatoid arthritis patients treated with methotrexate. Arthritis Rheum 1993;36:1244–1252.

14. Barrera P, Boerbooms AMT, Janssen EM, et al. Circulating soluble tumor necrosis factor receptors, interleukin-2 receptors, tumor necrosis factor α, and interleukin-6 levels in rheumatoid arthritis: longitudinal evaluation during methotrexate and azathioprine therapy. Arthritis Rheum 1993;36:1070–1079.

15. Kremer JM, Petrillo GF, Lawrence DA. Methotrexate induces significant changes in IL-1, IL-2, IL-6, and IL-8 but not lymphocyte markers in patients with rheumatoid arthritis. Arthritis Rheum 1993;36:S77. Abstract.

16. Kerwar SS, Oronsky AL. Methotrexate in rheumatoid arthritis: studies with animal models. Adv Enzyme Regul 1989;29:247–265.

17. Constantin A, Loubet-Lescoulié P, Lambert N, et al. Antiinflammatory and immunoregulatory action of methotrexate in the treatment of rheumatoid arthritis—evidence of increased interleukin-4 and interleukin-10 gene expression demonstrated in vitro by competitive reverse transcriptase polymerase chain reaction. Arthritis Rheum 1998;41:48–57.

18. Weinblatt ME, Coblyn JS, Fox DA, et al. Efficacy of low-dose methotrexate in rheumatoid arthritis. N Engl J Med 1985;312:818–822.

19. Weinblatt ME, Trentham DE, Fraser PA, et al. Long-term prospective trial of low-dose methotrexate in rheumatoid arthritis. Arthritis Rheum 1988;31:167–175.

20. Genestier L, Paillot R, Fournel S, et al. Immunosuppressive properties of methotrexate: apoptosis and clonal deletion of activated peripheral T cells. J Clin Invest 1998;102:322–328.

21. Hirata S, Matsubara T, Saura R, et al. Inhibition of in vitro vascular endothelial cell proliferation and in vivo neovascularization by low-dose methotrexate. Arthritis Rheum 1989;32:1065–1075.

22. Nesher G, Moore TL. The in vitro effects of methotrexate on peripheral blood mononuclear cells: modulation by methyl donors and spermidine. Arthritis Rheum 1990;33: 954–959.

23. Cronstein BN, Eberle MA, Gruber HE, Levin RI. Methotrexate inhibits neutrophil function by stimulating adenosine release from connective tissue cells. Proc Natl Acad Sci USA 1991;88:2441–2445.

24. Segal R, Caspi D, Tishler M, et al. Short term effects of low dose methotrexate on the acute phase reaction in patients with rheumatoid arthritis. J Rheumatol 1989;16:914–917.

25. Suarez CR, Pickett WC, Bell DH, et al. Effect of low dose methotrexate on neutrophil chemotaxis induced by leukotriene B₄ and complement C5a. J Rheumatol 1987;14:9–11.

26. van de Kerkhof PC, Bauer FW, Maassen-de Grood RM. Methotrexate inhibits the leukotriene B₄ included intraepidermal accumulation of polymorphonuclear leukocytes. Br J Dermatol 1985;113:251a–255a.

27. Ternowitz T, Bjerring P, Andersen PH, et al. Methotrexate inhibits the human C5a-induced skin response in patients with psoriasis. J Invest Dermatol 1987;89:192–196.

28. Sperling RI, Coblyn JS, Larkin JK, et al. Inhibition of leukotriene B₄ synthesis in neutrophils from patients with rheumatoid arthritis by a single oral dose of methotrexate. Arthritis Rheum 1990;33:1149–1155.

29. Sperling RI, Benincaso AI, Anderson RJ, et al. Acute and chronic suppression of leukotriene B₄ synthesis ex vivo in neutrophils from patients with rheumatoid arthritis beginning treatment with methotrexate. Arthritis Rheum 1992;35:376–384.

30. Leroux JL, Damon M, Chavis C, et al. Effects of a single dose of methotrexate on 5- and 12-lipoxygenase products in patients with rheumatoid arthritis. J Rheumatol 1992;19: 863–866.

31. Laurindo IMM, Mello SBV, Cossermelli W. Influence of low doses of methotrexate on superoxide anion production by polymorphonuclear leukocytes from patients with rheumatoid arthritis. J Rheumatol 1995;22:633–638.

32. Vergne P, Liagre B, Bertin P, et al. Methotrexate and cyclooxygenase metabolism in cultured human rheumatoid synoviocytes. J Rheumatol 1998;25:433–440.

33. Martel-Pelletier J, Cloutier J-M, Pelletier J-P. *In vivo* effects of antirheumatic drugs on neutral collagenolytic proteases in human rheumatoid arthritis cartilage and synovium. J Rheumatol 1988;15:1198–1204.

34. Balsa A, Gamallo C, Martín-Mola E, Gijón-Baños J. Histologic changes in rheumatoid synovitis induced by naproxen and methotrexate. J Rheumatol 1993;20:1472–1477.

35. Firestein GS, Paine MM, Boyle DL. Mechanisms of methotrexate action in rheumatoid arthritis: selective decrease in synovial collagenase gene expression. Arthritis Rheum 1994;37:193–200.

36. Herman RA, Veng-Pedersen P, Hoffman J, et al. Pharmacokinetics of low-dose methotrexate in rheumatoid arthritis patients. J Pharm Sci 1989;78:165–171.

37. Oguey D, Kölliker F, Gerber NJ, Reichen J. Effect of food on the bioavailability of low-dose methotrexate in patients with rheumatoid arthritis. Arthritis Rheum 1992;35:611–614.

38. Jundt JW, Browne BA, Fiocco GP, et al. A comparison of low dose methotrexate bioavailability: oral solution, oral tablet, subcutaneous and intramuscular dosing. J Rheumatol 1993;20:1845–1849.

39. Brooks PJ, Spruill WJ, Parish RC, Birchmore DA. Pharmacokinetics of methotrexate administered by intramuscular and subcutaneous injections in patients with rheumatoid arthritis. Arthritis Rheum 1990;33:91–94.

40. Marshall PS, Gertner E. Oral administration of an easily prepared solution of injectable methotrexate diluted in water: a comparison of serum concentrations vs. methotrexate tablets and clinical utility. J Rheumatol 1996;23:455–458.

41. Skeith KJ, Russell AS, Jamali F, et al. Lack of significant interaction between low dose methotrexate and ibuprofen or flurbiprofen in patients with arthritis. J Rheumatol 1990;17:1008–1010.

42. Stewart CF, Fleming RA, Arkin CR, Evans WE. Coadministration of naproxen and low-dose methotrexate in patients with rheumatoid arthritis. Clin Pharmacol Ther 1990;47: 540–546.

43. Ahern M, Booth J, Loxton A, et al. Methotrexate kinetics in rheumatoid arthritis: is there an interaction with nonsteroidal antiinflammatory drugs? J Rheumatol 1988;15: 1356–1360.

44. Seleznick MJ, Vasey FB, Evans WE, et al. Effect of aspirin (ASA) on the disposition of methotrexate (MTX) in

patients with rheumatoid arthritis (RA). Arthritis Rheum 1990;33:S39. Abstract.

45. Krohn K, Bradley J, Tracy T, et al. Effect of NSAIDs on methotrexate disposition in rheumatoid arthritis. Arthritis Rheum 1990;33:S39. Abstract.

46. Kremer JM, Hamilton RA. The effects of nonsteroidal anti-inflammatory drugs on methotrexate (MTX) pharmacokinetics: impairment of renal clearance of MTX at weekly maintenance doses but not at 7.5 mg. J Rheumatol 1995;22:2072–2077.

47. Thomas MH, Gutterman LA. Methotrexate toxicity in a patient receiving trimethoprim-sulfamethoxazole. J Rheumatol 1986;13:440–441.

48. Maricic M, Davis M, Gall EP. Megaloblastic pancytopenia in a patient receiving concurrent methotrexate and trimethoprim-sulfamethoxazole treatment. Arthritis Rheum 1986;29:133–135.

49. Willkens RF, Watson MA. Methotrexate: a perspective of its use in the treatment of rheumatic diseases. J Lab Clin Med 1982;100:314–321.

50. Steinsson K, Weinstein A, Korn J, Abeles M. Low dose methotrexate in rheumatoid arthritis. J Rheumatol 1982;9:860–866.

51. Hoffmeister RT. Methotrexate therapy in rheumatoid arthritis: 15 years experience. Am J Med 1983;75:69–73.

52. Weinstein A, Marlowe S, Korn J, Farouhar F. Low-dose methotrexate treatment of rheumatoid arthritis. Long-term observations. Am J Med 1985;79:331–337.

53. Michaels RM, Nashel DJ, Leonard A, et al. Weekly intravenous methotrexate in the treatment of rheumatoid arthritis. Arthritis Rheum 1982;25:339–341.

54. Williams HJ, Willkens RF, Samuelson CO Jr, et al. Comparison of low-dose oral pulse methotrexate and placebo in the treatment of rheumatoid arthritis. A controlled clinical trial. Arthritis Rheum 1985;28:721–730.

55. Thompson RN, Watts C, Edelman J, et al. A controlled two-centre trial of parenteral methotrexate therapy for refractory rheumatoid arthritis. J Rheumatol 1984;11:760–763.

56. Tugwell P, Bennett K, Gent M. Methotrexate in rheumatoid arthritis. Indications, contraindications, efficacy, and safety. Ann Intern Med 1987;107:358–366.

57. Jeurissen MEC, Boerbooms AMT, van de Putte LBA, et al. Methotrexate versus azathioprine in the treatment of rheumatoid arthritis: a forty-eight-week randomized, double-blind trial. Arthritis Rheum 1991;34:961–972.

58. Weinblatt ME, Kaplan H, Germain BF, et al. Low-dose methotrexate compared with auranofin in adult rheumatoid arthritis. A thirty-six-week, double-blind trial. Arthritis Rheum 1990;33:330–338.

59. Felson DT, Anderson JJ, Boers M, et al. American College of Rheumatology preliminary definition of improvement in rheumatoid arthritis. Arthritis Rheum 1995;38:727–735.

60. Cohen S, Rutstein J, Luggen M, et al. Comparison of the safety and efficacy of cyclosporin A and methotrexate in refractory rheumatoid arthritis: a randomized, multicentered placebo-controlled trial. Arthritis Rheum 1993;36:S56. Abstract.

61. Morassut P, Goldstein R, Cyr M, et al. Gold sodium thiomalate compared to low dose methotrexate in the treatment of rheumatoid arthritis—a randomized, double blind 26-week trial. J Rheumatol 1989;16:302–306.

62. Suarez-Almazor ME, Fitzgerald A, Grace M, Russell AS. A randomized controlled trial of parenteral methotrexate compared with sodium aurothiomalate (Myochrysine) in the treatment of rheumatoid arthritis. J Rheumatol 1988;15:753–756.

63. Rau R, Herborn G, Menninger H, Blechschmidt J. Comparison of intramuscular methotrexate and gold sodium thiomalate in the treatment of early erosive rheumatoid arthritis: 12 month data of a double-blind parallel study of 174 patients. Br J Rheumatol 1997;36:345–352.

64. Felson DT, Anderson JJ, Meenan RF. The comparative efficacy and toxicity of second-line drugs in rheumatoid arthritis: results of two metaanalyses. Arthritis Rheum 1990;33:1449–1461.

65. Weinblatt ME, Maier AL, Fraser PA, Coblyn JS. Longterm prospective study of methotrexate in rheumatoid arthritis: conclusion after 132 months of therapy. J Rheumatol 1998;25:238–242.

66. Weinblatt ME, Weissman BN, Holdsworth DE, et al. Long-term prospective study of methotrexate in the treatment of rheumatoid arthritis: eighty-four-month update. Arthritis Rheum 1992;35:129–137.

67. Kremer JM. Safety, efficacy, and mortality in a long-term cohort of patients with rheumatoid arthritis taking methotrexate: follow-up after a mean of 13.3 years. Arthritis Rheum 1997;40:984–985.

68. Weinblatt ME, Kaplan H, Germain BF, et al. Methotrexate in rheumatoid arthritis: a five-year prospective multicenter trial. Arthritis Rheum 1994;37:1492–1498.

69. Rau R, Schleusser B, Herborn G, Karger T. Longterm treatment of destructive rheumatoid arthritis with methotrexate. J Rheumatol 1997;24:1881–1889.

70. Alarcón GS, Tracy IC, Blackburn WD Jr. Methotrexate in rheumatoid arthritis. Toxic effects as the major factor in limiting long-term treatment. Arthritis Rheum 1989;32:671–676.

71. Pincus T, Marcum SB, Callahan LF. Longterm drug therapy for rheumatoid arthritis in seven rheumatology private practices. II. Second line drugs and prednisone. J Rheumatol 1992;19:1885–1894.

72. Kremer JM, Rynes RI, Bartholomew LE. Severe flare of rheumatoid arthritis after discontinuation of long-term methotrexate therapy. Double-blind study. Am J Med 1987;82:781–786.

73. Szanto E. Low-dose methotrexate in rheumatoid arthritis: effect and tolerance. An open trial and a double-blind randomized study. Scand J Rheumatol 1986;15:97–102.

74. Kremer JM, Lee JK. The safety and efficacy of the use of methotrexate in long-term therapy for rheumatoid arthritis. Arthritis Rheum 1986;29:822–831.

75. Kremer JM, Lee JK. A long-term prospective study of the use of methotrexate in rheumatoid arthritis. Update after a mean of fifty-three months. Arthritis Rheum 1988;31:577–584.

76. Jeurissen MEC, Boerbooms AMT, van de Putte LBA, et al. Influence of methotrexate and azathioprine on radiologic progression in rheumatoid arthritis. A randomized, double-blind study. Ann Intern Med 1991;114:999–1004.

77. Weinblatt ME, Polisson R, Blotner SD, et al. The effects of drug therapy on radiographic progression of rheumatoid arthritis: results of a 36-week randomized trial comparing

methotrexate and auranofin. Arthritis Rheum 1993;36: 613–619.

78. Arnett FC, Whelton JC, Zizic TM, Stevens MB. Methotrexate therapy in polymyositis. Ann Rheum Dis 1973;32:536–546.

79. Isasi C, Lopez-Martin JA, Angeles Trujillo M, et al. Felty's syndrome: response to low dose oral methotrexate. J Rheumatol 1989;16:983–985.

80. Fiechtner JJ, Miller DR, Starkebaum G. Reversal of neutropenia with methotrexate treatment in patients with Felty's syndrome. Correlation of response with neutrophil-reactive IgG. Arthritis Rheum 1989;32:194–201.

81. Allen LS, Groff G. Treatment of Felty's syndrome with low-dose oral methotrexate. Arthritis Rheum 1986;29:902–905.

82. Lally EV, Ho G Jr. A review of methotrexate therapy in Reiter syndrome. Semin Arthritis Rheum 1985;15:139–145.

83. Van den Hoogen FHJ, Boerbooms AMT, Swaak AJG, et al. Comparison of methotrexate with placebo in the treatment of systemic sclerosis: a 24 week randomized double-blind trial, followed by a 24 week observational trial. Br J Rheumatol 1997;35:364–372.

84. Krall PL, Mazanec DJ, Wilke WS. Methotrexate for corticosteroid-resistant polymyalgia rheumatica and giant cell arteritis. Cleve Clin J Med 1989;56:253–257.

85. Espinoza LR, Espinoza CG, Vasey FB, Germain BF. Oral methotrexate therapy for chronic rheumatoid arthritis ulcerations. J Am Acad Dermatol 1986;15:508–512.

86. Gourmelen O, Le Loët X, Fortier-Beaulieu M, et al. Methotrexate treatment of multicentric reticulohistiocytosis. J Rheumatol 1991;18:627–628.

87. Cash JM, Tyree J, Recht M. Severe multicentric reticulohistiocytosis: disease stabilization achieved with methotrexate and hydroxychloroquine. J Rheumatol 1997; 24:2250–2253.

88. Rahman P, Humphrey-Murto S, Gladman DD, Urowitz MB. Efficacy and tolerability of methotrexate in antimalarial resistant lupus arthritis. J Rheumatol 1998;25:243–246.

89. Wise CM, Vuyyuru S, Roberts WN. Methotrexate in nonrenal lupus and undifferentiated connective tissue disease—a review of 36 patients. J Rheumatol 1996;23:1005–1010.

90. Hoffman GS, Leavitt RY, Kerr GS, et al. Treatment of glucocorticoid-resistant or relapsing Takayasu arteritis with methotrexate. Arthritis Rheum 1994;37:578–582.

91. Hoffman GS, Leavitt RY, Kerr GS, Fauci AS. The treatment of Wegener's granulomatosis with glucocorticoids and methotrexate. Arthritis Rheum 1992;35:1322–1329.

92. Sneller MC, Hoffman GS, Talar-Williams C, et al. An analysis of forty-two Wegener's granulomatosis patients treated with methotrexate and prednisone. Arthritis Rheum 1995;38:608–613.

93. Ferraccioli G, Salaffi F, De Vita S, et al. Methotrexate in polymyalgia rheumatica: preliminary results of an open, randomized study. J Rheumatol 1996;23:624–628.

94. Feinberg HL, Sherman JD, Schrepferman CG, et al. The use of methotrexate in polymyalgia rheumatica. J Rheumatol 1996;23:1550–1552.

95. Giannini EH, Brewer EJ, Kuzmina N, et al. Methotrexate in resistant juvenile rheumatoid arthritis—results of the U.S.A.-U.S.S.R. double-blind, placebo-controlled trial. N Engl J Med 1992;326:1043–1049.

96. Mullarkey MF, Webb DR, Pardee NE. Methotrexate in the treatment of steroid-dependent asthma. Ann Allergy 1986; 56:347–350.

97. Mullarkey MF, Lammert JK, Blumenstein BA. Long-term methotrexate treatment in corticosteroid-dependent asthma. Ann Intern Med 1990;112:577–581.

98. Shiner RJ, Nunn AJ, Chung KF, Geddes DM. Randomised, double-blind, placebo-controlled trial of methotrexate in steroid-dependent asthma. Lancet 1990;336:137–140.

99. Erzurum SC, Leff JA, Cochran JE, et al. Lack of benefit of methotrexate in severe, steroid-dependent asthma. A double-blind, placebo-controlled study. Ann Intern Med 1991;114;353–360.

100. Coffey MJ, Sanders G, Eschenbacher WL, et al. The role of methotrexate in the management of steroid-dependent asthma. Chest 1994;105:117–121.

101. Kaplan MM, Knox TA. Treatment of primary biliary cirrhosis with low-dose weekly methotrexate. Gastroenterology 1991;101:1332–1338.

102. Kaplan MM, DeLellis RA, Wolfe HJ. Sustained biochemical and histologic remission of primary biliary cirrhosis in response to medical treatment. Ann Intern Med 1997;126: 682–688.

103. Baron TH, Truss CD, Elson CO. Low-dose oral methotrexate in refractory inflammatory bowel disease. Dig Dis Sci 1993;38:1851–1856.

104. Knox TA, Kaplan MM. Treatment of primary sclerosing cholangitis with oral methotrexate. Am J Gastroenterol 1991;86:546–552.

105. Knox TA, Kaplan MM. A double-blind controlled trial of oral-pulse methotrexate therapy in the treatment of primary sclerosing cholangitis. Gastroenterology 1994;106: 494–499.

106. Knox TA, Kaplan MM, Gelfand JA, Wolff SM. Methotrexate treatment of idiopathic granulomatous hepatitis. Ann Intern Med 1995;122:592–595.

107. Lower EE, Baughman RP. The use of low dose methotrexate in refractory sarcoidosis. Am J Med Sci 1990;299: 153–157.

108. Feagan BG, Rochon J, Fedorak RN, et al. Methotrexate for the treatment of Crohn's disease. N Engl J Med 1995;332: 292–297.

109. Furst DE, Koehnke R, Burmeister LF, et al. Increasing methotrexate effect with increasing dose in the treatment of resistant rheumatoid arthritis. J Rheumatol 1989;16:313–320.

110. Kremer JM, Davies JMS, Rynes RI, et al. Every-other-week methotrexate in patients with rheumatoid arthritis: a double-blind, placebo-controlled prospective study. Arthritis Rheum 1995;38:601–607.

111. Gabriel S, Creagan E, O'Fallon WM, et al. Treatment of rheumatoid arthritis with higher dose intravenous methotrexate. J Rheumatol 1990;17:460–465.

112. Shiroky J, Allegra C, Inghirami G, et al. High dose intravenous methotrexate with leucovorin rescue in rheumatoid arthritis. J Rheumatol 1988;15:251–255.

113. Shiroky JB, Neville C, Skelton JD. High dose intravenous methotrexate for refractory rheumatoid arthritis. J Rheumatol 1992;19:247–251.

114. Morgan SL, Baggott JE, Vaughn WH, et al. The effect of folic acid supplementation on the toxicity of low-dose

methotrexate in patients with rheumatoid arthritis. Arthritis Rheum 1990;33:9–18.

115. Shiroky JB, Neville C, Esdaile JM, et al. Low-dose methotrexate with leucovorin (folinic acid) in the management of rheumatoid arthritis: results of a multicenter randomized, double-blind, placebo-controlled trial. Arthritis Rheum 1993;36:795–803.

116. Blanco R, González-Gay MA, García-Porrúa C, et al. Ondansetron prevents refractory and severe methotrexate-induced nausea in rheumatoid arthritis. Br J Rheumatol 1998;37:590–592.

117. Weinblatt ME. Toxicity of low dose methotrexate in rheumatoid arthritis. J Rheumatol 1985;12(suppl)12:35–39.

118. MacKinnon SK, Starkebaum G, Willkens RF. Pancytopenia associated with low dose pulse methotrexate in the treatment of rheumatoid arthritis. Semin Arthritis Rheum 1985;15:119–126.

119. Gutierrez-Ureña S, Molina JF, García CO, Cuéllar ML, Espinoza LR. Pancytopenia secondary to methotrexate therapy in rheumatoid arthritis. Arthritis Rheum 1996;39:272–276.

120. Ellman MH, Hou S, Ginsberg D. Low-dose methotrexate and severe neutropenia in patients undergoing renal dialysis. Arthritis Rheum 1990;33:1060–1061.

121. Naides SJ. Acute parvovirus B19-induced pancytopenia in the setting of methotrexate therapy for rheumatoid arthritis. Arthritis Rheum 1995;38:1023–1024.

122. Weinblatt ME, Fraser P. Elevated mean corpuscular volume as a predictor of hematologic toxicity due to methotrexate therapy. Arthritis Rheum 1989;32:1592–1596.

123. Segal R, Caspi D, Tishler M, et al. Accelerated nodulosis and vasculitis during methotrexate therapy for rheumatoid arthritis. Arthritis Rheum 1988;31:1182–1185.

124. Berris B, Houpt JB, Tenenbaum J. Accelerated nodulosis in a patient with psoriasis and arthritis during treatment with methotrexate. J Rheumatol 1995;22:2359–2360.

125. Falcini F, Taccetti G, Ermini M, et al. Methotrexate-associated appearance and rapid progression of rheumatoid nodules in systemic-onset juvenile rheumatoid arthritis. Arthritis Rheum 1997;40:175–178.

126. Merrill JT, Shen C, Schreibman D, et al. Adenosine A₁ receptor promotion of multinucleated giant cell formation by human monocytes—a mechanism for methotrexate-induced nodulosis in rheumatoid arthritis. Arthritis Rheum 1997;40:1308–1315.

127. Warkany J. Aminopterin and methotrexate: folic acid deficiency. Teratology 1978;17:353–357.

128. Hausknecht RU. Methotrexate and misoprostol to terminate early pregnancy. N Engl J Med 1995;333:537–540.

129. Buckley LM, Bullaboy CA, Leichtman L, Marquez M. Multiple congenital anomalies associated with weekly low-dose methotrexate treatment of the mother. Arthritis Rheum 1997;40:971–973.

130. Shamberger RC, Rosenberg SA, Seipp CA, Sherins RJ. Effects of high-dose methotrexate and vincristine on ovarian and testicular functions in patients undergoing postoperative adjuvant treatment of osteosarcoma. Cancer Treat Rep 1981;65:739–746.

131. Sussman A, Leonard JM. Psoriasis, methotrexate, and oligospermia. Arch Dermatol 1980;116:215–217.

132. Rustia M, Shubik P. Life-span carcinogenicity tests with 4-amino-N10-methylpteroylglutamic acid (methotrexate) in Swiss mice and Syrian golden hamsters. Toxicol Appl Pharmacol 1973;26:329–338.

133. Rustin GJ, Rustin F, Dent J, et al. No increase in second tumors after cytotoxic chemotherapy for gestational trophoblastic tumors. N Engl J Med 1983;308:473–476.

134. Bailin PL, Tindall JP, Roenigk HH Jr, Hogan MD. Is methotrexate therapy for psoriasis carcinogenic? A modified retrospective-prospective analysis. JAMA 1975;232:359–362.

135. Stern RS, Zierler S, Parrish JA. Methotrexate used for psoriasis and the risk of noncutaneous or cutaneous malignancy. Cancer 1982;50:869–872.

136. Kamel OW, Van de Rijn M, Weiss LM, et al. Reversible lymphomas associated with Epstein-Barr virus occurring during methotrexate therapy for rheumatoid arthritis and dermatomyositis. N Engl J Med 1993;328:1317–1321.

137. Shiroky JB, Frost A, Skelton JD, et al. Complications of immunosuppression associated with weekly low dose methotrexate. J Rheumatol 1991;18:1172–1175.

138. Salloum E, Cooper DL, Howe G, et al. Spontaneous regression of lymphoproliferative disorders in patients treated with methotrexate for rheumatoid arthritis and other rheumatic diseases. J Clin Oncol 1996;14:1943–1949.

139. Kamel OW, Van de Rijn M, LeBrun DP, et al. Lymphoid neoplasms in patients with rheumatoid arthritis and dermatomyositis: frequency of Epstein-Barr virus and other features associated with immunosuppression. Human Pathol 1994;25:638–643.

140. Bachman TR, Sawitzke AD, Perkins SL, et al. Methotrexate-associated lymphoma in patients with rheumatoid arthritis—report of two cases. Arthritis Rheum 1996;39:325–329.

141. Lioté F, Pertuiset É, Cochand-Priollet B, et al. Methotrexate related B lymphoproliferative disease in a patient with rheumatoid arthritis. Role of Epstein-Barr virus infection. J Rheumatol 1995;22:1174–1178.

142. Ferraccioli GF, Casatta L, Bartoli E, et al. Epstein-Barr virus-associated Hodgkin's lymphoma in a rheumatoid arthritis patient treated with methotrexate and cyclosporin A. Arthritis Rheum 1995;38:867–868.

143. Moder KG, Tefferi A, Cohen MD, et al. Hematologic malignancies and the use of methotrexate in rheumatoid arthritis: a retrospective study. Am J Med 1995;99:276–281.

144. Wernick R, Smith DL. Central nervous system toxicity associated with weekly low-dose methotrexate treatment. Arthritis Rheum 1989;32:770–775.

145. Bernini JC, Fort DW, Griener JC, et al. Aminophylline for methotrexate-induced neurotoxicity. Lancet 1995;345:544–547.

146. Perruquet JL, Harrington TM, Davis DE. Pneumocystis carinii pneumonia following methotrexate therapy for rheumatoid arthritis. Arthritis Rheum 1983;26:1291–1292. Letter.

147. Keegan JM, Byrd JW. Nocardiosis associated with low dose methotrexate for rheumatoid arthritis. J Rheumatol 1988;15:1585–1586. Letter.

148. Altz-Smith M, Kendall LG Jr, Stamm AM. Cryptococcosis associated with low-dose methotrexate for arthritis. Am J Med 1987;83:179–181.

149. Leff RL, Case JP. Rheumatoid arthritis, methotrexate therapy, and Pneumocystis pneumonia. Ann Intern Med 1990;112:716. Letter.

150. O'Regan S, Melhorn DK, Newman AJ. Methotrexate-induced bone pain in childhood leukemia. Am J Dis Child 1973;126:489–490.

151. Ragab AH, Frech RS, Vietti TJ. Osteoporotic fractures secondary to methotrexate therapy of acute leukemia in remission. Cancer 1970;25:580–585.

152. Stanisavljevic S, Babcock AL. Fractures in children treated with methotrexate for leukemia. Clin Orthop 1977;139–144.

153. Friedlaender GE, Tross RB, Doganis AC, et al. Effects of chemotherapeutic agents on bone. I. Short-term methotrexate and doxorubicin (adriamycin) treatment in a rat model. J Bone Joint Surg [Am] 1984;66:602–607.

154. May KP, West SG, McDermott MT, Huffer WE. The effect of low-dose methotrexate on bone metabolism and histomorphometry in rats. Arthritis Rheum 1994;37:201–206.

155. May KP, Mercill D, McDermott MT, West SG. The effect of methotrexate on mouse bone cells in culture. Arthritis Rheum 1996;39:489–494.

156. Buckley LM, Leib ES, Cartularo KS, et al. Effects of low dose methotrexate on the bone mineral density of patients with rheumatoid arthritis. J Rheumatol 1997;24:1489–1494.

157. Engelbrecht JA, Calhoon SL, Scherrer JJ. Methotrexate pneumonitis after low-dose therapy for rheumatoid arthritis. Arthritis Rheum 1983;26:1275–1278.

158. Cannon GW, Ward JR, Clegg DO, et al. Acute lung disease associated with low-dose pulse methotrexate therapy in patients with rheumatoid arthritis. Arthritis Rheum 1983;26:1269–1274.

159. St Clair EW, Rice JR, Snyderman R. Pneumonitis complicating low-dose methotrexate therapy in rheumatoid arthritis. Arch Intern Med 1985;145:2035–2038.

160. Carson CW, Cannon GW, Egger MJ, et al. Pulmonary disease during the treatment of rheumatoid arthritis with low dose pulse methotrexate. Semin Arthritis Rheum 1987;16:186–195.

161. Kremer JM, Alarcón GS, Weinblatt ME, et al. Clinical, laboratory, radiographic, and histopathologic features of methotrexate-associated lung injury in patients with rheumatoid arthritis—a multicenter study with literature review. Arthritis Rheum 1997;40:1829–1837.

162. Alarcón GS, Kremer JM, Macaluso M, et al. Risk factors for methotrexate-induced lung injury in patients with rheumatoid arthritis—a multicenter, case-control study. Ann Intern Med 1997;127:356–364.

163. Searles G, McKendry RJ. Methotrexate pneumonitis in rheumatoid arthritis: potential risk factors. Four case reports and a review of the literature J Rheumatol 1987;14:1164–1171.

164. Bedrossian CW, Miller WC, Luna MA. Methotrexate-induced diffuse interstitial pulmonary fibrosis. South Med J 1979;72:313–318.

165. Kaplan RL, Waite DH. Progressive interstitial lung disease from prolonged methotrexate therapy. Arch Dermatol 1978;114:1800–1802.

166. Van der Veen MJ, Dekker JJ, Dinant HJ, et al. Fatal pulmonary fibrosis complicating low dose methotrexate therapy for rheumatoid arthritis. J Rheumatol 1995;22:1766–1768.

167. Nyfors A. Liver biopsies from psoriatics related to methotrexate therapy. III Findings in post-methotrexate liver biopsies from 160 psoriatics. Acta Pathol Microbiol Scand [A] 1977;85:511–518.

168. Roenigk HH Jr, Auerbach R, Maibach HI, Weinstein GD. Methotrexate in psoriasis: revised guidelines. J Am Acad Dermatol 1988;19:145–156.

169. Weinblatt ME, Kremer JM. Methotrexate in rheumatoid arthritis. J Am Acad Dermatol 1988;19:126–128.

170. Aponte J, Petrelli M. Histopathologic findings in the liver of rheumatoid arthritis patients treated with long-term bolus methotrexate. Arthritis Rheum 1988;31:1457–1464.

171. Phillips CA, Cera PJ, Mangan TF, Newman ED. Clinical liver disease in patients with rheumatoid arthritis taking methotrexate. J Rheumatol 1992;19:229–233.

172. Augur NA, Anderson LC, Cogen L, et al. Prospective study of hepatotoxicity in patients receiving methotrexate for rheumatoid arthritis. Arthritis Rheum 1990;33:S60. Abstract.

173. Clegg DO, Furst DE, Tolman KG, Pogue R. Acute, reversible hepatic failure associated with methotrexate treatment of rheumatoid arthritis. J Rheumatol 1989;16:1123–1126.

174. Kujala GA, Shamma'a JM, Chang WL, Brick JE. Hepatitis with bridging fibrosis and reversible hepatic insufficiency in a woman with rheumatoid arthritis taking methotrexate. Arthritis Rheum 1990;33:1037–1041.

175. Walker AM, Funch D, Dreyer NA, et al. Determinants of serious liver disease among patients receiving low-dose methotrexate for rheumatoid arthritis. Arthritis Rheum 1993;36:329–335.

176. Kremer JM, Alarcón GS, Lightfoot RW Jr, et al. Methotrexate for rheumatoid arthritis: suggested guidelines for monitoring liver toxicity. Arthritis Rheum 1994;37:316–328.

177. Erickson AR, Reddy V, Vogelgesang SA, West SG. Usefulness of the American College of Rheumatology recommendations for liver biopsy in methotrexate-treated rheumatoid arthritis patients. Arthritis Rheum 1995;38:1115–1119.

178. Bergquist SR, Felson DT, Prashker MJ, Freedberg KA. The cost-effectiveness of liver biopsy in rheumatoid arthritis patients treated with methotrexate. Arthritis Rheum 1995;38:326–333.

179. Morgan SL, Baggott JE, Vaughn WH, et al. Supplementation with folic acid during methotrexate therapy for rheumatoid arthritis. A double-blind, placebo-controlled trial. Ann Intern Med 1994;121:833–841.

180. Tishler M, Caspi D, Fishel B, Yaron M. The effects of leucovorin (folinic acid) on methotrexate therapy in rheumatoid arthritis patients. Arthritis Rheum 1988;31:906–908.

181. Weinblatt ME, Maier AL, Coblyn JS. Low dose leucovorin does not interfere with the efficacy of methotrexate in rheumatoid arthritis: an 8-week randomized placebo-controlled trial. J Rheumatol 1993;20:950–952.

182. Ortiz Z, Shea B, Suarez-Almazor ME, et al. The efficacy of folic acid and folinic acid in reducing methotrexate gastrointestinal toxicity in rheumatoid arthritis. A metaanalysis of randomized controlled trials. J Rheumatol 1998;25:36–43.

183. Fries JF. Advances in management of rheumatic disease 1965 to 1985. Arch Intern Med 1989;149:1002–1011.

Chapter 6

Immunosuppressants and Immunophilin Binding Agents: Current Research and Clinical Applications

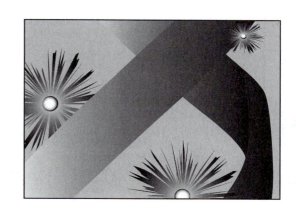

Shairaz Baksh

Jeff Friedman

Steven J. Burakoff

Barbara E. Bierer

Antigen-specific immunity is dependent on the timely and specific activation of B and T lymphocytes; the inappropriate or unwanted activation of these cells underlies the pathophysiology of many clinical disorders. T lymphocytes are the primary effector cells mediating allograft rejection and graft-versus-host disease (GVHD) as well as many manifestations of autoimmune disease. B-lymphocyte activation, largely dependent on T-cell cytokine production, is necessary for maintaining humoral immunity. Autoimmune diseases may result from the activation of host T lymphocytes to endogenous antigens, while T-cell unresponsiveness or anergy may result in infections or permit the development of malignant clones. In each of these situations, lymphocyte function depends on the transmission of signals from the cell surface to the nucleus, where gene expression (and thus cell function) is regulated. In recent years, several immunosuppressive compounds have been identified that are able to regulate immune responsiveness. These compounds have been used as probes to identify novel molecules involved in lymphocyte signal transduction, and have helped to delineate signaling pathways. In turn, many of the components of lymphocyte signaling pathways are of fundamental importance in cell biology, having highly analogous counterparts in a wide variety of cell types.

Immunosuppressive agents are commonly used in the treatment of both transplant rejection and autoimmune disorders. Over the last two decades, the number of agents available for use has increased rapidly, as has our understanding of the molecular pathways these drugs affect. In the mid-1970s, cyclosporine, also termed cyclosporin A (CsA), was isolated from cultures of the soil fungus *Tolypocladium inflatum Gams* by its ability to inhibit the proliferation of alloreactive T lymphocytes (1). Cyclosporine, an 11 amino acid cyclic polypeptide (Fig. 6-1), is now commonly used in the prevention and treatment of graft rejection and has improved the outcome of allograft and stem cell transplantation dramatically (2,3). Tacrolimus (FK506, Prograf), another immunosuppressive agent, was isolated from cultures of soil microorganisms in the 1980s, again by its ability to inhibit the activation of alloreactive T cells (see Fig. 6-1) (2–4). It has been approved by the U.S. Food and Drug Administration (FDA) for

use in the prevention (and treatment) of organ rejection in patients receiving allogeneic liver or kidney transplants (5) and is now widely used in solid organ and stem cell transplantation, and in a variety of other disorders. Cyclosporine and tacrolimus were shown to share qualitatively identical effects in various lymphocyte activation assays (2,3), a finding that led to speculation that they might have a common target. In T lymphocytes, these actions result in inhibition of transcriptional activation of lymphokine and other genes essential for T-cell proliferation and function (2,3,6) (reviewed later).

The discovery of tacrolimus and cyclosporine (CsA) led to the isolation and analysis of their intracellular binding proteins, collectively termed the immunophilins. Tacrolimus binds to a number of endogenous binding ligands, the FK506-binding proteins (or FKBPs) (7), while CsA binds to a family of proteins termed the cyclophilins (8). Several mammalian FKBPs and cyclophilins have been isolated, and members of both protein families are found in all tissue types, some expressed at very high levels. In the absence of drugs, the immunophilins (Tables 6-1 and 6-2) are involved in numerous cellular processes that include protein folding, control of calcium channel function, and intracellular receptor signaling.

Immunophilins are petidyl-prolyl isomerases (rotamases) that are able to catalyze the *cis-trans* isomerization of petidyl-prolyl bonds, suggesting that they may be involved in the regulation of protein folding and trafficking (9). Rotamase activity is potently inhibited by the binding of either tacrolimus to FKBPs or CsA to cyclophilins (10). However, in addition to inhibition of rotamase activity, drug binding to immunophilins unmasks a novel property of the drug/receptor complex that is now recognized as the biologically relevant action leading to immunosuppression. Both tacrolimus binding to FKBPs and CsA binding to cyclophilins inhibit the activity of calcineurin, a calcium- and calmodulin-activated serine/threonine phosphatase (11–13). Calcineurin controls the activity and subcellular localization of several intracellular enzymes and transcription factors—most notably the nuclear factor of activated T cells (NFAT) (reviewed in 14). While tacrolimus is a more potent inhibitor of calcineurin

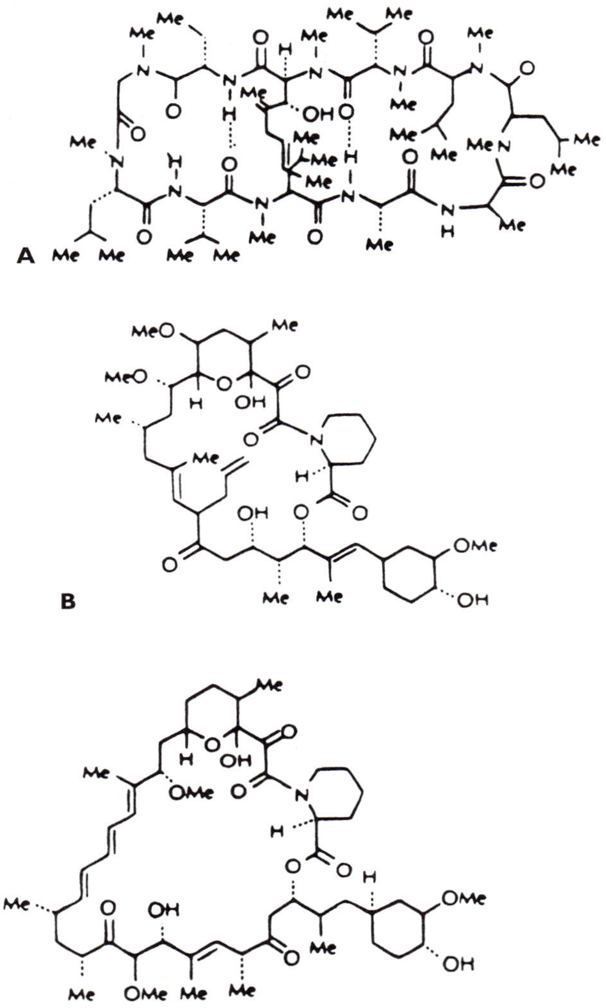

Figure 6-1. Chemical structures of immunosuppressant drugs. (A) Cyclosporine, a cyclic undecapeptide (1203 D). (B) Tacrolimus (FK506, Prograf), a macrolide antibiotic (822 D). (C) Rapamycin, a macrolide antibiotic (914 D). Me = methyl group; O = oxygen; H = hydrogen.

Table 6-1. Mammalian FK506-Binding Proteins

FKBP[a]	Molecular Weight (kD)	FK506 Affinity (K_d, nM)	Subcellular Localization
FKBP12[b]	12	1.7	Cytosol
FKBP12.6[b]	12	ND	Cytosol
FKBP13	13	55	ER
FKBP23[c]	23	ND	ER
FKBP25	25	160	Nucleus
FKBP38[d]	38	ND	ND
FKBP51[b,e]	51	ND	Cytosol
FKBP52[b,f]	52	10	Nucleus/cytosol
FKBP65[g]	65	45	Membrane[h]
FKBP6[i]	–	ND	ND
IPBP12[j]	–	ND	Membrane

[a] All FK506-binding proteins (FKBPs) exhibit peptidyl-prolyl isomerase (rotamase) activity.
[b] Family member known to inhibit the phosphatase activity of calcineurin.
[c] Contains an EF hand high-affinity calcium-binding motif and is glycosylated.
[d] Has a leucine zipper, a tetratricopeptide repeat domain, and a putative calmodulin-binding domain.
[e] Also known as FKBP54 and contains a carboxy terminal calmodulin-binding domain and a tetratricopeptide repeat domain.
[f] Also known as FKBP59, hsp56, HBI, and contains a tetratricopeptide repeat domain.
[g] Glycosylated and phosphorylated.
[h] Localization has yet to be established.
[i] Deleted in Williams syndrome.
[j] Is tyrosine phosphorylated and binds to IP$_3$ and IP$_4$.

phosphatase activity than cyclosporine on a molar basis, the two drugs share similar toxicity profiles, making it likely that immunosuppression and toxicity are related to calcineurin inhibition. Administration of either drug can be associated with serious side effects, including renal and central nervous system toxicity. A better understanding of immunophilin-interacting proteins and calcineurin substrates in tissues affected by toxicity may point to future compounds with wider therapeutic windows.

Rapamycin (sirolimus, Rapamune), a third immunosuppressant known to inhibit the proliferation of T cells, was isolated from the fermentation broth of *Streptomyces hygroscopicus* in 1975 (see Fig. 6-1). It has recently been approved for use by the FDA for prevention of acute renal transplant rejection.

Rapamycin shares structural similarity with, and binds to, the same family of intracellular receptors as tacrolimus, but acts to inhibit T-lymphocyte activation by a distinct mechanism (2,3,15). Rapamycin binding to FKBPs was shown to result in inhibition of another intracellular protein—mammalian target of rapamycin, or mTOR. Inhibition of mTOR results in a different pattern of biologic properties than that observed for tacrolimus or CsA (16). In T cells, rapamycin inhibits lymphokine-dependent (e.g., interleukin-2-dependent) proliferation without affecting lymphokine gene transcription (17,18). This chapter discusses the current understanding of the known biologic effects of the immunosuppressants tacrolimus, CsA, and rapamycin and how they interact with immune and nonimmune cell regulatory elements. An understanding of their molecular mechanisms of action and of the role of their targets in normal cellular functioning may improve our ability not only to anticipate and prevent unwanted side effects, but ultimately to design therapeutic regimens that minimize toxicity.

Calcineurin: A Central Intermediate

Calcineurin and T-Cell Activation

T-lymphocyte activation involves numerous signal transduction molecules and second messengers. Surface receptor engagement

Table 6-2. Mammalian Cyclophilins

Cyclophilin	Molecular Weight (kD)	CsA Affinity (K_d, nM)	Subcellular Localization	Functional Data
CyPA*	18	6	Cytosol	Inhibits calcineurin when bound to CsA; HIV cofactor
CyPB*	21	9	ER, secreted	Protein folding (?); interaction with CAML may regulate Ca^{2+} homeostasis
CyPC*	22	6	Cytosolic vesicles, secreted	Interacts with Cycap (Mac2 binding protein); LPS response modulator (?)
CyPD*	18	3.6 (K_i for PPIase)	Mitochondria	Chaperone (?); involved in opening of mitochondrial pore in apoptosis
CyP-40*	40	300	Cytosol	Component of glucocorticoid receptor; regulator of heat shock response
CyP-60	60	Unknown	Nucleus	Unknown
Nup-358	358	Unknown	Nuclear pore	Chaperone (?); modifies red/green opsin
NK-TR 150*	150	Unknown	Cell membrane (?), nucleus	Tumor recognition (?); RNA splicing cofactor (?)
CARS-cyp/ Matrin CYP*	89	Unknown	Nucleus, nuclear speckles(?)	RNA splicing (?)
Snu-cyp 20	20	Unknown	Nucleus, nuclear speckles	RNA splicing(?)
PPIE	33 (predicted)	Unknown	Unknown	Coamplified with L-myc in small cell lung cancer

Both human and murine counterparts for CyPA, CyPB, CyPC, CyPD, CyP-40, and NK-TR 150 have been described, whereas PPIE (223), CyP-60, Snu-cyp 20 (224), Nup-358, and CARS-cyp were isolated from human cells, and Matrin CYP from rat cells. Although not all cyclophilins have been tested for rotamase activity, those that have been tested exhibit activity that is inhibitable by CsA. The predominant subcellular localization for each protein is listed, along with speculation as to function derived from studies of protein-protein interactions and localization data.
*Exhibits rotamase activity.

and cross-linking results in the generation of two important second messengers, diacylglycerol (DAG) and inositol-1,4,5-trisphosphate (IP_3) (Fig. 6-2). DAG is important in the activation of classical protein kinase C isoenzymes, whereas IP_3 is a critical second messenger in the release of calcium from the endoplasmic reticulum into the cytoplasm. The elevation of intracellular calcium concentrations and subsequent activation of calcium-responsive proteins is central to lymphokine gene activation and cytokine production (19,20). The transcriptional activation of interleukin-2 (IL-2) in T lymphocytes has been well characterized. The production of IL-2 requires the coordinated actions of the calcium- and calmodulin-activated serine/threonine protein phosphatase, calcineurin (PP2B) (21) and the nuclear transcription factor, NFAT (14,22). Calcium binding to calmodulin results in its ability to bind to, and in turn activate, calcineurin, leading to the subsequent dephosphorylation of NFAT (23). Dephosphorylation of NFAT is required for its translocation from the cytoplasm to the nucleus (24) and its ability to bind to multiple sites in the IL-2 promoter as a multimeric complex with AP-1 family members (e.g., fos and jun) (25). Calcineurin/NFAT signaling pathways control expression not only of IL-2, but also a wide variety of cytokines (IL-4, IFN-γ, GM-CSF, IL-3, IL-13, and TNF-α) (14) and surface receptors (Fas ligand, CD40 ligand, CD69, and IL-2 receptor α chain) (14,26). Although the regulation of NFAT transcriptional activation by calcineurin is common, the biologic outcomes depend on the specific targets of calcineurin in specialized tissues.

Calcineurin Structure

Calcineurin is composed of a catalytic subunit, calcineurin A, and a regulatory subunit, calcineurin B; the latter is required not only for maximal phosphatase activity but also for the proper folding of the heterodimer (27) (Fig. 6-3). In mammals, three isoforms of the catalytic subunit (α, β, and γ) share approximately 75% to 80% primary sequence homology (28). Calcineurin Aα and Aβ are ubiquitously expressed, whereas Aγ is a testis-specific isoform of calcineurin (29). All three isoforms, however, can exist in multiple alternatively spliced forms resulting in divergent carboxy terminal sequences (28). There are two mammalian genes that encode calcineurin B: a form ubiquitously expressed and a testis-specific form (30). Calcineurin B is very similar to calmodulin, containing four high-affinity, low-capacity EF hand calcium-binding motifs, each capable of binding one mole of calcium per mole of protein (30). In contrast to calmodulin, the calcium-binding sites on calcineurin B serve a structural role, allowing calcineurin B to fold around the calcineurin B–binding helix on calcineurin A (31).

Maximal activation of calcineurin is a consequence of immune activation events that result in calcium influx into the cytosol and the subsequent activation of calmodulin and its binding to calcineurin. The binding of calcium-bound calmodulin to the calmodulin binding site within the carboxy terminus of calcineurin A appears to result in the displacement of the carboxy terminal autoinhibitory domain from the active site (32) (see Fig.

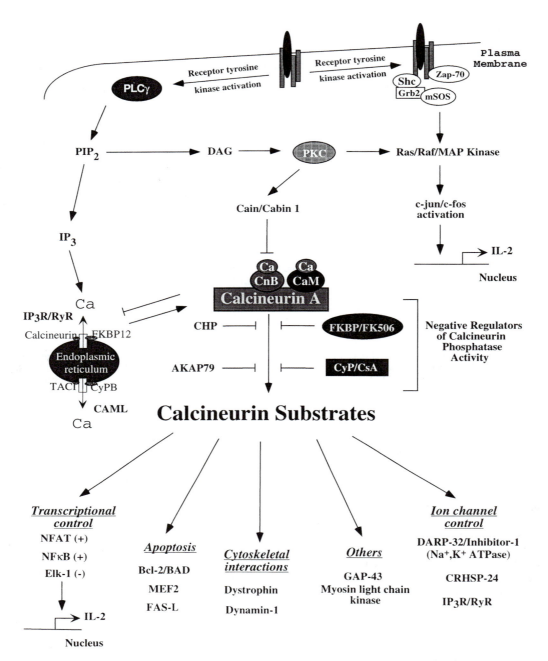

Figure 6-2. Simplified model of T-cell receptor (TCR)–mediated signal transduction events leading to activation of calcineurin. TCR engagement and co-cross-linking result in activation of receptor tyrosine kinases, leading to activation of PLCγ and generation of the second messengers, IP_3 and DAG. IP_3 results in calcium release from the internal stores of the endoplasmic reticulum; DAG activates PKC and downstream effectors of PKC. Calcium release from the cytoplasm results in activation of calcineurin and regulated phosphorylation of downstream effectors (calcineurin substrates). FK506 binds to its cognate binding protein, FKBP; cyclosporin A (CsA) binds to its cognate receptors, the cyclophilins (CyPs). CHP: calcineurin homologous protein; AKAP79: A kinase anchor protein of molecular weight 79kD; Cain/Cabin 1: endogenous negative regulators of calcineurin phosphatase activity; Shc/Grb2/mSOS/Zap-70: signaling intermediates that carry signals from surface activation to the nucleus. See "Calcineurin Substrates and Binding Proteins" for descriptions of all calcineurin substrates. Activation pathway: →; inhibitory pathway: —|; "+": positive influence on transcription; "–": negative influence on transcription.

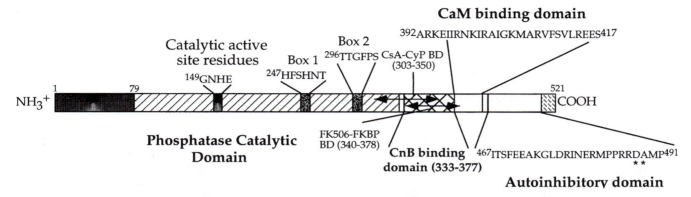

Figure 6-3. Calcineurin structure. The structure of human calcineurin Aα (accession number: J05480) is shown. The sequences of important regulatory regions are indicated. CaM: calmodulin; CnB: calcineurin B; CsA-CyP BD: cyclosporin A/cyclophilin-binding domain; FK506-FKBP BD: FK506/FK506 binding protein binding domain. Box 1 and Box 2: divergent sequences from the phosphatase catalytic domain of protein phosphatase 1 that may govern substrate specificity to calcineurin. Sequences important for the carboxyl terminal autoinhibitory domain are indicated by asterisks.

6-3) and a 10- to 20-fold increase in the phosphatase activity of the enzyme. It is the activated form of calcineurin that is the main target of drug/immunophilin complexes. These complexes sterically block access of substrates to the catalytic binding pocket, resulting in the loss of 80% to 90% of the calcium-activated phosphatase activity of calcineurin. The ability of immunophilins to inhibit calcineurin activity requires that they be bound to their cognate drugs (either tacrolimus or CsA), supporting a "gain of function" model for calcineurin inhibition. However, weak interactions between immunophilins and calcineurin can be detected in the absence of CsA or tacrolimus, suggesting that physiologically relevant interactions may occur in the absence of drug (33). Both the structure and the biologic function of drug-independent calcineurin associations remain to be determined.

Calcineurin Substrates and Binding Proteins

The central role of calcineurin in T-cell activation involves its interaction with NFAT family members. Calcineurin has also been demonstrated to regulate the transcriptional abilities of Elk1 (34), NFκB (35), and AP1 family members (36). In addition to calmodulin, other binding proteins have been demonstrated to regulate the phosphatase activity of calcineurin (see Fig. 6-2). Superoxide dismutase (37) was demonstrated to interact with calcineurin and protect its Fe-Zn catalytic center from the damaging effects of a changed redox environment. Cabin 1 (38) and Cain (39) were both shown to inhibit noncompetitively the catalytic function of calcineurin with an IC_{50} of $0.5\,\mu M$ (in comparison, tacrolimus/FKBP12 was observed to have an IC_{50} of $7.9\,nM$). Similarly, CHP (40) and AKAP79 (41) were also demonstrated to inhibit the phosphatase activity of calcineurin by binding to a site distinct from the immunophilin binding region. While a number of proteins have been identified that regulate the phosphatase activity of calcineurin, calcineurin has also been demon-

strated to modulate ER store driven calcium release (via the IP_3 receptor and ryanodine receptor) (42); control amylase secretion in rat pancreatic acinar cells (CRHSP-24) (43); control the interaction with the cytoskeletal matrix (dystrophin) (44); modulate synaptic vesicle endocytosis (dynamin) (45) (Mukerjee, Li, and Bierer, unpublished results); regulate degranulation of mast cells and basophils (46); control neuronal signaling elements such as GAP-43 (47) and ACtp10 (48); and influence muscle contraction (myosin light chain kinase) (49). Recently, a role for both calcineurin and NFAT was defined in a signaling pathway regulating skeletal (50) and cardiac (51) muscle hypertrophy. It was demonstrated that, under conditions of ischemia and cardiac damage within the heart, calcineurin becomes activated, resulting in the nuclear translocation of NFAT and the formation of an active transcriptional complex with GATA4 (51,52). Furthermore, the inhibition of calcineurin with the immunosuppressive drugs tacrolimus and CsA prevented the development of hypertrophy (51). Whether this approach will become clinically applicable remains to be examined.

The prevention of cellular death or apoptosis in the presence of either tacrolimus or CsA was demonstrated to correlate with the inhibition of the phosphatase activity of calcineurin (53,54). Recently, the potential targets of calcineurin in the cell death pathway have been characterized. Calcineurin is thought to control cellular apoptosis by several mechanisms, including NFAT-dependent control of Fas ligand (FasL) expression (55), calcineurin-regulated MEF2 control of Nur77 expression (56), and calcineurin-dependent regulation of the dephosphorylation of the Bcl-x_L binding protein BAD, facilitating the dissociation of BAD from cytosolic 14-3-3 proteins. The dissociation of BAD from 14-3-3 proteins would allow BAD binding to Bcl-x_L, thus interfering with the protective effects of Bcl-x_L (57). These studies illustrate the complex nature of apoptotic signaling pathways and the role calcineurin may play in the regulation of multiple signal transduction pathways leading to cell death.

Solution Structure of Tacrolimus/FKBP12 Complexed to Calcineurin

The solution structure of tacrolimus/FKBP12 (58), CsA/CyPA (59), and the composite structure of calcineurin A/calcineurin B/tacrolimus/FKBP12 (31,60), have been solved. The structure of calcineurin A/calcineurin B/tacrolimus/FKBP12 revealed that the complex of tacrolimus/FKBP12 makes intimate contacts with both the A and B chains of calcineurin at a location 10 Å away from the catalytic pocket. The interface of calcineurin with the tacrolimus/FKBP12 complex includes areas obtained from both calcineurin A and calcineurin B and also include surfaces obtained from both tacrolimus and FKBP12. Contact regions defining CsA/cyclophilin interactions with calcineurin have not yet been structurally determined, but deletional analysis (59) and molecular modeling (61) suggest that the CsA/cyclophilin-binding area resides in close proximity to the docking site of tacrolimus/FKBP12 (see Fig. 6-3). Drug/immunophilin complexes can thus prevent the entry of large protein substrates into the catalytic site by sterically inhibiting the entrance of substrates. However, the catalysis of a limited number of small molecule substrates, such as para-nitrophenyl phosphate (pNPP), is not affected by the binding of drug/immunophilin complexes. As the potential number of substrates for calcineurin increases, it will be important to determine whether there are small endogenous protein substrates of calcineurin that enter into the catalytic site and can be dephosphorylated even in the presence of drug/immunophilin complexes.

Tacrolimus Binding Proteins (FKBPs) and Associated Proteins

FK506 binding protein (FKBP) refers to proteins that bind both tacrolimus (FK506) and rapamycin, but not cyclosporine. Although not structurally similar to cyclophilins, FKBPs have an evolutionarily conserved enzymatic rotamase activity similar to that present within the cyclophilin family. Currently, 11 eukaryotic members of the tacrolimus binding protein family have been characterized (see Table 6-1), of which only FKBP12, FKBP12.6, and FKBP51 have been shown to interact with and inhibit the phosphatase activity of calcineurin (9); both FKBP12 and FKBP12.6 have also been demonstrated to affect the translocation of NFAT (13,62). The following subsection discusses the possible functions of the FKBPs and how they may interact with elements in order to maintain cellular homeostasis.

Tacrolimus Binding Proteins: Potential Modulators of Calcium Signaling

FKBP12 is a prototypical member of the FKBP family of proteins. It is an abundant protein in tissues, with the exception of primary mast cells and mast cell lines, in which FKBP12 expression is low (63,64). A physiologic cellular role for this immunophilin (in the absence of tacrolimus) still remains to be determined. However, a clue to the role of FKBP12 in cellular regulation is observed in its association (in the absence of tacrolimus) with two key intracellular sarcoplasmic/endoplasmic reticulum (ER) calcium channel proteins, the ryanodine receptor (65,66) and the inositol-1,4,5-trisphosphate (IP$_3$) receptor (42). Receptor association with FKBP12 was found to stabilize their conformation and induce tighter control of the opening potential of these channels (42,67). Forming a ternary complex, calcineurin was shown to interact with FKBP12 and a tetrapeptide stretch within the primary amino acid sequence of the IP$_3$ receptor (68). This sequence was shown to resemble the interaction surface of tacrolimus with FKBP12, suggesting that the interaction of FKBP12 with the IP$_3$ receptor may allow calcineurin to be targeted to the IP$_3$ receptor. Calcineurin is thought to function in closing the channel by dephosphorylation of a protein kinase C site on the IP$_3$ receptor. Calcium oscillations originating from the IP$_3$ receptor are thus thought to occur by a cycle of phosphorylation events, mediated primarily by PKC and resulting in calcium influx into the cytosol, and dephosphorylation events, possibly mediated by calcineurin and resulting in the inhibition of calcium influx into the cytosol. By bringing calcium-activated calcineurin to the IP$_3$ receptor, FKBP12 may prevent the depletion of IP$_3$-sensitive ER calcium stores. In addition to controlling IP$_3$ receptor phosphorylation levels, calcineurin has also been demonstrated to regulate IP$_3$ receptor mRNA expression (69) and thus appears to control calcium oscillations transcriptionally as well as by post-translational modification. Calcineurin and tacrolimus binding proteins appear not only to regulate translocation of transcription factors important for immune and other functions, but also to be important regulators of ion currents within the cell.

A clinical correlate of the biochemical associations between FKBP12 and the IP$_3$ receptor was demonstrated in mice lacking FKBP12. FKBP12-deficient mice developed severe dilated cardiomyopathy and ventricular septal defects that mimicked a human congenital heart disorder (70), supporting the role played by FKBP12 in cardiac muscle function and development. Interestingly, one study showed that five pediatric organ transplant recipients who received high doses of tacrolimus developed hypertrophic cardiomyopathy and heart failure, symptoms that resolved when the immunosuppressive regimen was changed to cyclosporine (71). If substantiated, these observations suggest that 1) inhibition of calcineurin does not alone explain the clinical observations, 2) FKBPs appear to have a unique effect on cardiac dynamics that is not mimicked by cyclophilins, and 3) the choice and administration of drug must be carefully monitored. A tightly regulated balance must be achieved between the desired immunosuppressive drug effect, contingent on inhibition of calcineurin phosphatase activity, and the modulation of calcium channel function and other possible functions of FKBP12.

In addition to FKBP12 and calcineurin emerging as new elements in the control of cellular calcium homeostasis, four other tacrolimus binding proteins may prove to influence calcium signaling. Human FKBP38 contains a calmodulin binding domain at the carboxy termini and two protein-protein interaction motifs—a leucine zipper and a tetratricopeptide repeat domain (72). Murine FKBP51 also contains a calmodulin binding domain at its carboxy termini and shares a 53% identity overall with a previously isolated and sequenced 52-kD tacrolimus binding protein (73). In addition, both FKBP51 and FKBP52 have tetratricopeptide repeat domains that bind to heat shock protein 90 (hsp90). Interestingly, FKBP51 does not appear to depend on its calmodulin-binding domain for interaction with calcineurin and has been demonstrated to bind to calcineurin in a tacrolimus-dependent and -independent manner (Li and Bierer, unpublished observations). In the presence of tacrolimus, the serine/threonine phosphatase activity of calcineurin is weakly inhibited by FKBP51 with an IC_{50} of $5\,\mu M$ [compared with $7.9\,nM$ for FKBP12/tacrolimus (73)]. FKBP51, however, appears to have a higher binding affinity for rapamycin than that of tacrolimus (IC_{50} of $29\,nM$ and $41\,nM$, respectively; FKBP12, by comparison, has values of rapamycin and tacrolimus binding of $14\,nM$ and $2\,nM$, respectively).

A recently cloned tacrolimus binding protein, FKBP23, is a glycoprotein localized to the endoplasmic reticulum and contains two high-affinity calcium binding EF hand motifs capable of binding calcium (74). FKBP23 was shown to have a limited tissue distribution with high levels in the heart, lung, and testis. Lastly, another recently cloned immunophilin, a 12-kD inositol phosphate binding protein, was shown to exhibit *cis-trans* isomerase activity that was inhibitable by tacrolimus, rapamycin, and nanomolar concentrations of the second messenger IP_3 and inositol-1,3,4,5-tetrakisphosphate (IP_4) (75). In addition, this new inositol phosphate FK506 binding protein (IPBP12) is tyrosine phosphorylated and is recognized by an anti-FKBP12 antibody, indicating a strong degree of similarity to FKBP12. It will be interesting to determine what role IPBP12 may play in control of calcium movements within the cell.

FKBP12: a Modulator of TGF-β Signaling

Transforming growth factor β (TGF-β) is a multifunctional cytokine that has diverse roles in the pathogenesis of wound healing, transcriptional regulation, and growth control (76). TGF-β type I and type II receptors contain a single transmembrane segment with a cytoplasmic serine/threonine kinase domain critical for mediating TGF-β signaling. The type II receptor is a constitutively active kinase that can bind TGF-β independently but cannot signal without the type I receptor (77,78). The type I receptor can bind TGF-β only in the presence of the type II receptor and requires phosphorylation by the associated type II receptor to initiate downstream signaling events. The TGF-β type I receptor was found to interact with the immunophilin FKBP12 and to inhibit TGF-β signaling (77). Tacrolimus reversed the inhibitory effects of FKBP12, possibly by competing FKBP12 from the complex of FKBP12/TGF-β type I receptor. Furthermore, it was demonstrated that the displacement of FKBP12 from the TGF-β type I receptor complex was essential for maximal TGF-β signaling. However, mutations within the FKBP12 recognition sequences on TGF-β type I receptors were shown to be dispensable for signal generation (79). Cells from wild type mice and mice rendered genetically deficient in FKBP12 did not display significant differences in TGF-β type I receptor signaling (70), again questioning the role of FKBP12 as a signal modulator in this system. Nevertheless, FKBP12 and the

TGF-β type I receptor are able to interact physically and have been cocrystallized (80).

The role of another immunosuppressant, cyclosporine, in TGF-β signaling has been recently characterized (81). Production of TGF-β by noninvasive cancerous cells was increased following prolonged exposure to cyclosporine. When exposed to cyclosporine in vitro, a human pulmonary adenocarcinoma cell line (A-549) became invasive and was more likely to divide, move, and spread. The remarkable phenotypic changes were reversed by the addition of anti–TGF-β antibodies (81). While the molecular basis remains to be clarified, increased TGF-β production by certain malignant cells may contribute to the aggressiveness of tumors; immunosuppressive therapy should, therefore, be administered with caution to patients with malignancies. Whether TGF-β production contributes to the increased incidence of certain malignancies following transplantation remains to be shown.

Functions of Other FKBP Family Members

FKBP13 is a membrane-associated immunophilin localized to the endoplasmic reticulum by an ER retention sequence (RTEL) at its carboxy terminus (82). It is present in both B and T cells, has peptidyl-prolyl *cis-trans* isomerase activity that is inhibited by both tacrolimus and rapamycin, and is a very weak inhibitor of calcineurin. FKBP13 shares 43% overall identity with FKBP12, most divergent at its amino terminus. It was recently shown that FKBP13 interacted with a novel homologue of the erythrocyte membrane cytoskeletal protein 4.1, suggesting that the role of FKBP13 is not limited to the ER (83). A cellular role for this immunophilin is currently unknown, but recent data suggest that it may function as a scaffolding protein.

FKBP25 is an immunophilin localized to the nucleus and contains several potential casein kinase II phosphorylation sites (84). A fusion protein of FKBP25 was able to associate physically with casein kinase II and nucleolin, a major substrate for casein kinase II. FKBP25 has been hypothesized to be a component of a macromolecular complex that carries casein kinase II to the nucleus on activation (84). This role for FKBP25 exemplifies the growing appreciation of the role played by immunophilins in protein folding and subcellular targeting and movement of bound proteins.

FKBP52 shares 53% overall identity with FKBP51 and is part of the glucocorticoid receptor complex, binding to calmodulin, hsp90 and hsp70, and the glucocorticoid receptor in the absence of tacrolimus or rapamycin (85). Physiologically, the association of FKBP52 with the glucocorticoid receptor may be very similar to the role played by FKBP25 in localizing casein kinase II to the nucleus. The presence of FKBP52 in the steroid receptor complex may indicate a need for the correct folding of the glucocorticoid receptor and possibly, together with hsp90, may allow trafficking of the receptor complex within the cell. Similar to the role of FKBP52 within the inactive steroid complex is the interaction of FKBP52 with the peroxisomal enzyme phytanoyl-CoA α-hydroxylase (PAHX) (86). Identified using a yeast two-hybrid system, the interaction of PAHX was specific for FKBP52 and was maintained in the presence of tacrolimus. PAHX is a peroxisomal enzyme catalyzing the first step in phytanic acid oxidation: the α-oxidation of phytanoyl-CoA to α-hydroxyphytoyl-CoA (86). Inactivation of this enzyme in humans results in Refsum disease characterized by accumulation of phytanic acid, a fatty acid derived from the diet, resulting in peripheral neuropathy, retinitis pigmentosa, and cerebellar ataxia (86). PAHX is identical to mouse lupus nephritis protein 1 (LN1), a protein involved in the progression of lupus nephritis. It is tempting to speculate that FKBP52 may be involved in trafficking PAHX to its point of action. In addition to PAHX interaction with FKBP52, FAP48 (FK506-associated protein of 48 kD) was also identified as binding not only to FKBP52 but also to FKBP12 (87). A physiologic role for this interaction remains to be determined, but it does suggest that endogenous ligands for the immunophilins may be found that carry out important cellular functions.

FKBP65 is a 65-kD phospho- and glycoprotein present in the lung, spleen, brain, and testis but absent from the liver (88). It is highly similar to FKBP12 and FKBP13 and less so to FKBP25 and FKBP52. Sequence alignment with FKBP12 revealed the presence of four peptidyl-prolyl isomerase domains and conservation of the identified binding residues for tacrolimus. Recently, FKBP65 was shown to interact with the amino terminal region of c-Raf kinase in association with hsp90 (89). FKBP65 also contains a potential endoplasmic reticulum–retention sequence (HEEL), and subcellular localization revealed that FKBP65 might be a membrane-associated protein.

Williams syndrome (WS) is a developmental disorder characterized by congenital cardiovascular defects, growth deficiency, infantile hypercalcemia, dysmorphic facial features, mental retardation, and a unique cognitive profile (90). It has been shown to result from haploinsufficiency of genes at chromosome 7q11.23 (91). FKBP6 was discovered as a gene completely deleted within the common WS deletional region (92). It is a distinct 38-kD protein containing a putative amino terminal tacrolimus binding and peptidyl-prolyl isomerase domains and an imperfect carboxy terminal tetratricopeptide repeat domain. Northern blot analysis revealed that the highest levels of FKBP6 were present in the heart, skeletal muscle, liver, and testis (92), a distribution very similar to the expression pattern of FKBP51 and FKBP52. The genes within region 7q11.23 have not been exhaustively characterized but include genes coding for the human homologue of the putative Drosophilia frizzled Wnt receptor gene FZD3 (93), an important neurotransmitter release gene (the syntaxin gene STX1A), the replication factor C subunit 2 gene (RFC2), a gene containing an RNA-binding motif (WSCR1), and a gene similar to restin (WSCR4) (92).

Cyclosporine Binding Proteins and Associated Proteins

The family of cyclosporine binding proteins (the cyclophilins, or CyPs) share a highly homologous 165 amino acid domain conferring the ability to bind to cyclosporine. Like the FKBPs, cyclophilins exhibit an intrinsic peptidyl-prolyl isomerase (rotamase) activity that is inhibited on binding of CsA. Cyclophilin homologues are present in all species examined to date, suggesting that they subserve a vital and evolutionarily conserved biochemical function. They are highly expressed in eukaryotic cells and can be found in all subcellular compartments and as secreted proteins (see Table 6-2). The intrinsic isomerase activities of cyclophilins have been demonstrated to mediate certain protein folding processes and to exhibit chaperone-like activities toward specific protein substrates. The mammalian cyclophilins are a diverse group of proteins with regard to size, intracellular localization, tissue-specific expression, and putative function. While no obvious unifying function for these molecules has been demonstrated, it seems likely that they are cofactors in the transport of proteins from one cellular compartment to another and constitute an integral component of the protein folding machinery.

Solution Structure of Cyclophilin/CsA

The structures of the cyclophilins have been solved in the presence (94) and absence (95) of CsA. Cyclophilin/CsA assumes a beta barrel structure characterized by eight antiparallel beta strands, two pairs of alpha helices above and below the barrel, and a highly conserved loop between strands B6 and B7 that forms part of the CsA-binding site. The crystal structures of cyclophilin A, cyclophilin B (96), and cyclophilin C (97) bound to CsA demonstrated that the same 13 highly conserved amino acids make contact with the CsA molecule, forming a hydrophobic pocket that interacts with one face of the CsA molecule. Structural data and biochemical studies with CsA analogues and cyclophilin mutants suggest that CsA is a bifunctional molecule, with one face mediating tight binding to the hydrophobic pocket of the cyclophilin molecule and the other face oriented to allow for interaction with calcineurin (98,99).

Mammalian Cyclophilins

Cyclophilin A (CyPA) was the first CsA binding protein identified in eukaryotes and was found to be a ubiquitous 18-kD cytosolic protein binding to CsA with high affinity (100). It was demonstrated to inhibit the function of calcineurin in T lymphocytes (101) and also catalyzed the rates of folding of ribonuclease T1 (102) and calcitonin (103). In addition, CyPA was found to reduce the aggregation of incompletely folded carbonic anhydrase polypeptides in a CsA-inhibitable manner (104). However, there is no evidence of an obligatory role for CyPA (or for any other immunophilin) in protein folding in vivo, because yeast deficient in all immunophilins as well as cell lines deficient in CyPA are viable (105).

Several proteins have been shown to interact with CyPA in the absence of CsA. AOP-1, a thiol-specific antioxidant protein (106), was demonstrated to bind to CyPA in a CsA-insensitive manner and this appears to stimulate the ability of AOP-1 to preserve the activity of glutamine synthetase during oxidative challenge. CyPA and CyPB have also been isolated as HIV-1 gag (pr55) binding proteins in a yeast two-hybrid screen, and CyPA is thought to become incorporated into HIV virions (107). Certain strains of HIV require CyPA binding for infectivity by facilitating HIV uncoating following entry into target cells (108,109). In vitro studies demonstrate that the replication of certain strains of HIV can be inhibited by CsA and CsA analogues, and this is thought to inhibit the CyPA/gag interaction (110). However, CyPA-mediated uncoating is not required for all strains of HIV, and the importance of this interaction as a determinant of the pathophysiology of HIV or as a potential therapeutic target is currently uncertain.

Cyclophilin B (CyPB) is a widely expressed 21-kD protein localized to the endoplasmic reticulum (ER) (111). CyPB has an amino terminal signal sequence targeting it to the ER, and a carboxy terminal extension allowing it to bind to another ER protein, CAML (112) (see below). CyPB can also be detected in extracellular fluids and has been proposed to play a role as a mediator of inflammation (113). Two classes of CyPB-binding sites have been described on T-cell membranes (114), and binding of CyPB to T cells is followed by internalization and degradation of the protein. CyPB binding to platelets has also been described (115), and in this context CyPB appears to initiate calcium flux in platelets and thus facilitate an increase in their adhesion to collagen.

Cyclophilin C (CyPC) is a membrane-bound 23-kD protein localized in cytosolic vesicles and secreted in a CsA-sensitive manner (12). Human CyPC appears to be widely expressed (116), while murine CyPC has a restricted tissue expression profile abundant in the kidney, bone marrow stroma, testis, and ovary (117). CyPC has been found to bind to a 77-kD glycoprotein (cycap or Mac2 binding protein) in a CsA-sensitive manner (118). Mice carrying a targeted disruption of the CyPC gene display increased sensitivity to the nephrotoxic and hepatotoxic side effects of CsA, and have altered metabolism of the drug (Friedman and Burakoff, unpublished observations). Cycap knockout animals are reported to show increased sensitivity to LPS-mediated cellular responses demonstrating increases in TNF-α, IL-12, and IFN-γ production in vitro and a lower LD_{50} following LPS challenge in vivo (119).

CyPD is a 19-kD mitochondrial matrix protein (120) that has been demonstrated to bind the adenine nucleotide translocase (ANT) in a CsA-sensitive manner (121). In addition, CyPD is thought to be involved in the opening of the mitochondrial permeability transition pore following proapoptotic stimuli (122,123). CsA can inhibit the opening of this mitochondrial pore and thus prevent the release of cytochrome C from the mitochondrial matrix upon apoptotic stimulation (123,124).

Several large molecular weight proteins with cyclophilin domains have been identified in mammalian cells. NK-TR 150 was originally isolated from natural killer cells as a component of a cell surface tumor recognition complex (125). In addition to a CyP domain, NK-TR 150 has a hydrophobic amino-terminal domain, three repeated domains homologous to Nopp 140, and three serine-arginine (SR)–rich repeat regions. Nopp 140 domains are thought to recognize nuclear localization signals, which suggests that NK-TR 150 may have a role in nuclear impor-

tation. SR domain proteins are thought to function in RNA splicing and also to localize to the nucleus (126). NK-TR 150 expression in HL-60 cells appears to be required for progression to a differentiated phenotype following induction by dimethyl sulfoxide (DMSO) or phorbol myristate acetate (PMA) (127). Antisense suppression of NK-TR 150 expression in a human T-cell line and in rat large granular lymphocyte (LGL) cells inhibits the ability of these cells to lyse targets, suggesting a role for NK-TR 150 in cytolysis (128,129). Clk-associating RS-cyclophilin (CARS-cyp) is a structurally similar but distinct arginine: serine (RS) cyclophilin isolated in a yeast two-hybrid screen from murine and human cDNA libraries via binding to Clk (CDC28/cdc2-like kinase) (130). CARS-cyp cDNA encodes a protein with a predicted molecular weight of 89kD that contains a cyclophilin domain, two Nopp 140 domains, and a large RS domain. Human CARS-cyp shares 93% amino acid identity with a rat protein (Matrin CYP) with an apparent molecular weight of 106kD. Matrin CYP is enriched in the nuclear fraction of cultured cells and appears to colocalize with splicing factors within nuclear speckles (131).

CyP-60 is a widely expressed 60-kD nuclear protein isolated in a yeast two-hybrid screen by its ability to interact with the serine proteinase inhibitor eglin C (132). CyP-40 is a 40-kD cytosolic protein that exists in mammalian cells as a component of the unliganded glucocorticoid receptor complex (133,134). CyP-40 binds to hsp90 in a CsA-insensitive manner through a tetratricopeptide repeat domain (TPR) homologous to the TPR domain of FKBP52, another component of the unliganded glucocorticoid receptor (135). CyP-40 has been postulated to facilitate signaling through the glucocorticoid receptor by maintaining the receptor in a signaling competent configuration (136). CyP-40 also appears to be involved in the regulation of the heat shock response in yeast, since CyP-40 mutants show increased heat shock transcription factor activity both constitutively and following a heat shock stimulus (137).

Ran BP2/Nup-358 is a large protein containing a cyclophilin domain, originally identified as a component of the nuclear pore (138). The cyclophilin domain of this protein interacts with an adjacent domain (RBD4 domain) to act as a chaperone for red/green opsin, and is thought to induce a conformational change in opsin allowing enhanced photoreceptor activity (139,140).

Cyclophilins: Potential Modulators of Calcium Signaling

In addition to a putative role in protein folding of specific substrates, cyclophilins and the FKBPs have been implicated in various aspects of lymphocyte signaling initiated by intracellular calcium release. A calcium-signal modulating cyclophilin B ligand (CAML) has been characterized and found to be a widely expressed integral membrane protein localized to cytoplasmic vesicles (112). It was found to colocalize with the sarcoplasmic/endoplasmic reticulum calcium ATPase-2 and calreticulin, a resident endoplasmic reticulum calcium storage protein (141). The amino terminal domain of CAML is directed toward the cytoplasm with the carboxy terminus forming two to three predicted membrane-spanning regions. The last two transmembrane segments appear to be important in forming a calcium channel and thus regulate the influx of calcium into the cytosol and subsequent activation of downstream calcium-sensitive transcriptional elements, such as NFAT (141). Expression studies in Src kinase (Fyn or Lck) negative cell lines revealed that CAML functions downstream of the T-cell receptor (TCR)–dependent Fyn/Lck activation events (112). Interestingly, CAML required exogenous stimulation of protein kinase C (PKC) by PMA in order to achieve the same degree of activation resulting from the activation of TCR, indicating that CAML effects are downstream of the TCR and phospholipase Cγ activation. Furthermore, both tacrolimus and CsA inhibited the activation of NFAT via CAML overexpression, placing CAML upstream of calcineurin activation (112). Further complicating the understanding of the role of CAML in T-cell signaling was the observation that extracellular levels of calcium also regulated the influence of CAML in NFAT-driven transcription (142). CAML may be important in calcium influx from the extracellular environment, with influx occurring after immediate early events in TCR activation (142). How initial emptying of the intracellular endoplasmic reticulum stores, triggered by TCR activation, communicates with the plasma membrane to allow influx of calcium from the extracellular milieu (capacitance calcium influx) remains poorly understood.

A lymphocyte-specific binding protein for CAML, transmembrane activator, and CAML-interactor or TACI (143) has been identified (see Fig. 6-2). TACI is a type III transmembrane protein with an extracellular amino terminus and is a member of the tumor necrosis factor receptor (TNFR) superfamily. Protein interaction studies revealed that the carboxyl terminal 126 amino acids of TACI were sufficient to bind to the amino terminal 201 amino acids of CAML and that this interaction was sensitive to extracellular levels of calcium. Maximal activation of NFAT-driven transcription occurred when both CAML and TACI were overexpressed in Jurkat cells (AP-1 and NFκB elements were not affected by the coexpression of CAML and TACI). These results suggest synergy between CAML and TACI, allowing the sustained activation of the TCR by maximizing the levels of calcium within the cytosol. The close proximity of the membrane network of the endoplasmic reticulum with that of the plasma membrane would allow the amino terminus of CAML to communicate with the carboxy terminus of TACI, allowing TACI to regulate calcium flow either directly or indirectly within the endoplasmic reticulum stores (144).

Cyclophilins have also been reported to have altered enzymatic properties in the presence of increased calcium levels. CyPA, CyPB, and CyPC have been found to exhibit a calcium-dependent (and magnesium-dependent) nuclease activity that may be involved in fragmentation of high-molecular-weight DNA after initiation of apoptosis (145). CyPD has been shown to be involved in the opening of the mitochondrial permeability transition pore (MPTP) following proapoptotic stimuli that increase mitochondrial calcium concentration (146). There is no indication at present that all the multidomain proteins that have CyP domains regulate calcium-dependent signaling pathways.

Rather, the limited data available suggest that these proteins perform predominantly chaperonin or protein folding functions on only a subset of specific substrates.

Rapamycin and Related Binding Proteins

Rapamycin was originally identified as an antifungal agent isolated from the fermentation culture broths of *Streptomyces hygroscopicus*. Both tacrolimus and rapamycin can bind to FKBP12, but it is only the complex of FKBP12/tacrolimus that mediates the inhibition of calcineurin and thereby early events in T-cell activation. Rapamycin was demonstrated to have a different molecular target when bound to FKBP12 and was found to target elements involved in G1/S progression of hematopoeitic and nonhematopoietic cells (Fig. 6-4) (147,148). Rapamycin appears to impair the response to mitogenic stimuli leading to proliferation; the identity and regulation of downstream molecular targets are still being determined. Calcineurin phosphatase activity, mitogen-activated kinase activity, and STAT5 transcriptional activity were all shown to be insensitive to the inhibitory effects of rapamycin (149). Rapamycin was, however, demonstrated to inhibit members of the family of S6 kinases (150) that are responsible for mediating the phosphorylation of the 40S ribosomal subunit, S6. Two families of S6 kinases have been identified: the p70 S6 kinase family and the p85 (rsk) S6 kinase family. The activity of p70 S6 kinase, but not of p85 S6 kinase, was inhibited by rapamycin (150), and in T cells, inhibition of activity of p70 S6 kinase correlated with inhibition of cellular proliferation (151). However, the correlation was not absolute: several cell lines have been identified in which inhibition of p70 S6 kinase activity by rapamycin does not correlate with inhibition of cellular proliferation (18,152). These observations suggest that p70 S6 kinase may not be an absolute requirement for normal cellular proliferation.

Rapamycin Targets: Cyclins and Cyclin-dependent Kinases

The immunosuppressive drugs tacrolimus and CsA block cellular activation at the G0/G1 transition stage by interfering with TCR-mediated signal transduction pathways (see Fig. 6-2). Rapamycin was shown to block the subsequent G1/S phase transition (see Fig. 6-4) and, in some cell systems, could be added up to 12 hours after growth-factor serum stimulation and still cause G1 arrest (153). The ability of rapamycin to induce G1 arrest in certain cell systems has prompted an examination of the targets of rapamycin action. The eukaryotic cell cycle is controlled by a complex interplay of kinases and phosphatases that control the actions of cell cycle suppressor elements. These elements include the retinoblastoma tumor suppressor (p110^{Rb}) and related family members (p107/p130) and the p53/p73/p63 family members. The function of the retinoblastoma family of proteins are regulated by cyclin-dependent kinases (CDKs) and their associated cyclins and cyclin-dependent kinase inhibitors (CKIs) (154). Rapamycin

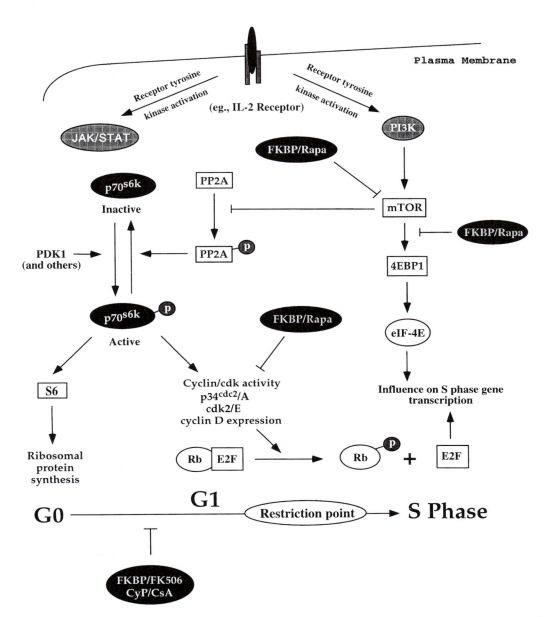

Figure 6-4. Simplified model of growth factor receptor signal transduction events leading to the cell cycle progression (IL-2 receptor mediated events are used to illustrate downstream events). IL-2 receptor engagement results in the activation of receptor tyrosine kinases leading to the activation of multiple pathways including the Janus kinases (JAK)/STAT pathway of signal transducers and the phosphatidylinositol (PI) 3-kinase activation pathway. PI 3-kinase is thought to link to the activation of mTOR (FRAP/RAFT1) that in turn activates p70[s6k] and 4EBP1, two important elements governing the G1/S phase progression, as illustrated. Rapamycin (Rapa) binds to its cognate binding protein, FKBP. PP2A: protein phosphatase 2A; PDK1: proline-directed kinase 1; Rb: retinoblastoma tumor suppressor protein (p110); E2F: S phase transcription factor; p: phosphorylation event. Activation pathway: →; inhibitory pathway: —|.

was shown to affect the kinase activity of both p34[cdc2] and p33[cdk2] by regulating the amount of cyclin A and cyclin E that associated with its kinase counterpart (153). In addition, rapamycin was demonstrated to affect the mRNA stability of cyclin D1 (155,156), D2, and D3 (157) and directly inhibit G1/S progression. Rapamycin has also been shown to inhibit the IL-2–dependent loss of the cyclin-dependent inhibitor p27[KIP1] (158); to inhibit the phosphorylation of at least two Rb-related tumor suppressor elements, p130 and p100 (157); and to affect the stability of E2F transcriptional DNA complexes (157). The molecular details of rapamycin regulation of cell cycle progression remain to be determined.

Rapamycin Targets: the TOR Proteins

In yeast, targets of FKBP12/rapamycin have been identified as the targets of rapamycin (TOR) proteins. Two gene loci, TOR1 (DRR1) and TOR2 (DRR2), have been identified coding for a protein of approximately 280 kD that, when mutated (S1975I) or deleted, confers rapamycin resistance (159). The amino terminal domains of TOR1 and TOR2 are 67% identical and contain sequences that may promote nuclear localization. The carboxy termini of both TOR1 and TOR2 are 77% homologous and share significant homology with the catalytic domain of phosphatidylinositol (PI) kinases and with the vacuolar sorting protein VPS34 (148). Gene disruption studies revealed that TOR1 is a nonessential protein, whereas disruption of TOR2 is lethal, suggesting that it is an essential component of a signaling pathway regulating cell cycle progression in yeast.

Signaling cascades initiated by growth-factor stimulation involve numerous effector pathways such as the Ras effector pathway (160), the JAK/STAT pathway (161), and the phosphoinositide 3-kinase (PI 3-kinase)/protein kinase B (Akt) pathway (149). The role of phosphoinositides (PIs) in signal transduction has been well established in certain cellular processes (162). As reviewed previously, the generation of diacylglycerol and IP_3 from the action of phospholipase C (PLC) on $PI4, 5P_2$ (PIP2) is critical for the triggering of intracellular calcium release from internal endoplasmic reticulum IP_3-sensitive calcium pools. Vesicular secretion by lipid kinases, such as VPS34, has also been shown to require PI metabolites (163,164). TOR2 was found to contain an intrinsic PI4-kinase activity that was not inhibited by the complex of FKBP12/rapamycin (20). However, FKBP12/rapamycin binding to either TOR1 or TOR2 resulted in the disappearance of TOR from the yeast vacuolar surface, resulting in physical separation of TOR2 from its in vivo substrates and the formation of large vacuoles. Vacuolar formation is necessary for acidification and thus the degradation of endocytosed proteins and for storage of ions, metabolites, and nutrients (165). It is thought that the lipid kinase activity of TOR may function in the generation of PI metabolites in response to extracellular conditions and hence regulate cell cycle progression.

The mammalian homologue of yeast TOR (mTOR) is also inhibited when complexed to FKBP12/rapamycin. However, the effect of rapamycin is not uniform and appears to vary with cell type. Mammalian TOR, also known as FKBP12/rapamycin-associated protein (FRAP) (166) or rapamycin and FKBP12 target 1 RAFT1 (167), is a 289-kD protein related to the novel family of phosphatidylinositol kinase–related kinases. Mammalian TOR has a carboxy terminal kinase domain that appears to phosphorylate p70 S6 kinase (168), an eIF4E binding protein (4EBPI) (169), and the autophosphorylation of mTOR itself (all of which are inhibitable by nanomolar concentrations of rapamycin; $IC_{50} = 10–15$ nM for the inhibition of the autophos-

phorylation of mTOR) (166). The inhibition of p70 S6 kinase activity by mTOR/rapamycin/FKBP12 results in the failure of p70 S6 kinase to phosphorylate the 40S ribosomal protein S6 (170). S6 functions to regulate the family of mRNAs containing an oligopyrimidine tract at their transcriptional start site (171,172). In a similar fashion, mTOR controls eukaryotic transcription by the phosphorylation of 4E-BP1, a repressor of the eukaryotic initiation factor 4E (eIF4E) (see Fig. 6-4). Phosphorylation of 4E-BP1 releases 4E-BP1 binding to eIF4E and allows the initiation factor to form a productive mRNA cap binding complex. The antiproliferative effects of rapamycin with respect to p70 S6 kinase activity destabilize the formation of active transcriptional complexes and thus prevent the entry into the DNA synthesis (S) phase of the cell cycle.

Several critical residues have been described that demonstrate the mode of action of mTOR. A critical serine residue, serine-2035, has been shown to disrupt mTOR binding to rapamycin/FKBP12 (173), while mutations at aspartic acids 2338 and 2357 influence TOR autophosphorylation, but not the ability to bind to FKBP12/rapamycin (166). Mutation of the ATP-binding site (tryptophan-2027) results in a dominant negative effect inhibiting the autophosphorylation of mTOR and mTOR-dependent phosphorylation of 4E-BP1 (174). The binding domain for rapamycin/FKBP12 (FRB) was localized to an 11-kD segment immediately adjacent to the kinase domain (amino acids 2015–2114) (174). Both the FRB domain and the kinase domain are highly conserved in the yeast homologues of TOR1 and TOR2. However, whereas TOR1 has a G1 function that is sensitive to rapamycin (regulation of p70 S6 activity), TOR2 has an additional actin cytoskeletal function that still requires kinase activity but is insensitive to rapamycin (175). The crystal structure of the FRB domain of mTOR indicates a defined four-helical bundle with its amino and carboxy termini close together (176,177), implying a potential role as a functional module.

Although mTOR is a target for rapamycin/FKBP12, it is puzzling that, in vitro, micromolar concentrations of rapamycin are required to inhibit mTOR kinase activity toward p70 S6 kinase compared with nanomolar concentrations of rapamycin needed in vivo. It has been difficult to observe an endogenous p70 S6 kinase activity in mTOR immunoprecipitates. Furthermore, in response to mitogens, p70 S6 kinase can be readily phosphorylated at the rapamycin-sensitive threonine-229 site in vivo even in the presence of rapamycin (178). Analysis of embryonic stem cells containing a targeted deletion of p70 S6 kinase demonstrated that a second isoform of this enzyme (70^{s6k2}) may exist, providing a potential explanation for the rapamycin sensitivity in the mice genetically deficient in p70 S6 kinase (179). These observations prompted a reevaluation of the effects of rapamycin treatment. Recently, it was demonstrated that the calyculin-sensitive serine/threonine phosphatase PP2A was associated with and regulated by mTOR (analogous to FKBP12/tacrolimus inhibition of calcineurin), and suggested that PP2A negatively regulated p70 S6 kinase activity by dephosphorylation of serine/threonine residues on the active p70 S6 kinase complex (180). Inhibition of mTOR activity by rapamycin would result in the removal of the inhibitory effect of mTOR on PP2A (by either a direct phosphorylation effect or a selective increase in the amount of unbound PP2A). Consequently, the active dephosphorylation of p70 S6 kinase by PP2A would result in G0/G1 arrest. The mTOR/PP2A interaction is thought to regulate mitogen-activated p70 S6 kinase (and 4E-BP1 kinase) by promoting the rapid PP2A-dependent dephosphorylation of multiple serine/threonine sites on p70 S6 kinase (and 4E-BP1) rather than inhibiting the multiple kinases that are responsible for their activation (180). In this way, mTOR may act as an intracellular sensor that can transmit signals and also function in halting the cell cycle machinery. A more detailed study of how mTOR controls PP2A activity is warranted.

Clinical Applications of Immunosuppressive Therapy

The introduction of cyclosporine to the clinical field of transplantation approximately 25 years ago revolutionized solid organ and stem cell transplantation by dramatically decreasing the incidence of graft rejection and graft-versus-host disease (GVHD). This agent is now used for treating a variety of autoimmune and other disorders, including acquired disorders of hematopoiesis. Tacrolimus has been approved for solid organ (liver and kidney) transplantation and is also widely used in stem cell transplantation. Both agents, however, have narrow therapeutic windows and similar spectra of toxicities, most likely owing to inhibition of calcineurin in target tissues. Chronic administration of either agent may be complicated by renal and nervous system toxicity, hyperglycemia, and hypertension, which limit their utility during prolonged therapy. Furthermore, maintenance of an immunosuppressed state for extended periods of time increases the likelihood that patients will experience serious, and at times fatal, infectious complications. These infections are typically those fought by the cellular arm of the immune system, consistent with the knowledge that these agents predominantly affect the function of T lymphocytes. Thus, although surgical techniques in solid organ transplantation have been refined over the past 30 years, the ability to prevent complications associated with the administration of immunosuppressive agents has lagged. Similarly, in allogeneic stem cell transplantation, life-threatening complications including infections associated with administration of immunosuppressive agents are far more common than graft rejection.

Many clinical trials have been conducted to determine and compare the efficacies of cyclosporine and tacrolimus in solid organ and stem cell transplantation, and an adequate review of all the reported trials is beyond the scope of this chapter. However, it should be noted that the early trials compared the efficacies and toxicities of regimens that are not those commonly used today, and therefore must be interpreted with caution. Microemulsion formulations of cyclosporine have changed the bioavailability and effective drug concentration significantly. Early trials of tacrolimus used a target therapeutic level for drug that was higher than that recommended today; therefore, the toxicity profiles (if toxicity relates to drug concentration) of early reports may be overestimated. The two reported, prospective, randomized multicenter trials comparing the efficacy of tacrolimus with that of cyclosporine in orthotopic liver transplantation are illustrative (181,182). Both enrolling more than 500 patients, the two studies had similar conclusions. In the trial conducted in the United States (181), administration of tacrolimus after liver transplantation was associated with an 82% rate of graft survival as compared with 79% in those receiving cyclosporine, demonstrating the equivalence of the two agents. Furthermore, the overall survival rate of 88% after 1 year was identical in the two cohorts. Importantly, at least two different dose schedules were used to treat the patients receiving tacrolimus, although the data were not stratified for dosage (Table 6-3). Higher incidences of neurotoxicity and renal insufficiency were noted in the group receiving tacrolimus compared with that receiving cyclosporine.

A second multicenter trial was simultaneously conducted in Europe (182). After 1 year, overall survival rates in the tacrolimus- and cyclosporine-treated groups were 82% and 77%, respectively. Rates of acute graft rejection were higher in those receiving cyclosporine as prophylaxis, and a greater proportion of these graft rejections were considered resistant to therapy. Higher rates of chronic rejection were also encountered in the group receiving cyclosporine. Those patients receiving tacrolimus required lower dosages of corticosteroids to control these complications and, accordingly, demonstrated a lower incidence of infectious complications. However, side effects from drug administration, such as renal and neural toxicity, were significantly more common in those treated with tacrolimus than in those receiving cyclosporine (see Table 6-3). Extrapolation of these results to current clinical practice is complicated because the target therapeutic levels for tacrolimus were higher than current recommendations, and because cyclosporine microemulsion was not available. While the results of both trials indicate that graft survival and overall patient survival were similar in the two treatment groups, the incidences of acute rejection refractory to treatment with corticosteroids and of chronic rejection were lower in those patients treated with tacrolimus. Long-term follow-up of patients receiving primary liver transplants has confirmed that actual 6-year patient and graft survival rates—68.1% and 62.5%, respectively—were excellent (183). Late rejection was rare, and outcome of pediatric patients was better than adults. The positive results in the trials of orthotopic liver transplantation are generally reflective of trials evaluating the efficacy of tacrolimus in prevention of rejection in renal, cardiac, lung, pancreatic, and small bowel transplantation (184–189). Furthermore, quality of life and the costs of post-transplantation care are not compromised and may even be improved by tacrolimus-based regimens (190,191).

The goal of immunosuppression in recipients of stem cell allografts is more complex than that in solid organ transplantation. Not only must rejection of the transplanted stem cell graft be prevented, but also the converse situation in which the graft reacts against donor antigens must be avoided. This condition, referred to

Table 6-3. Comparison of Toxicity Profiles of Tacrolimus and Cyclosporine from Two Large Trials in Liver Transplantation

	U.S. Study (181) (%) Tacrolimus (n = 250)	CBIR* (n = 250)	European Tacrolimus (n = 264)	Study (182) (%) CBIR (n = 265)
Hypertension	47	56	38	43
Nephrotoxicity	40	27	36	23
Nervous system:				
Headache	64	60	37	26
Tremor	56	46	48	32
Insomnia	64	68	32	23
Paresthesia	40	30	17	17
Gastrointestinal:				
Diarrhea	72	47	37	27
Nausea	46	37	32	27
LFT abnormal	36	30	6	5
Anorexia	34	24	7	5
Vomiting	27	15	14	11
Metabolic:				
Hyperkalemia	45	26	13	9
Hypokalemia	29	34	13	16
Hyperglycemia	47	38	33	22
Hypomagnesemia	48	45	16	9
Hematologic:				
Anemia	47	38	5	1
Leukocytosis	32	26	8	8
Thrombocytopenia	24	20	14	19
Miscellaneous:				
Abdominal pain	59	54	29	22
Pain	63	57	24	22
Fever	48	56	19	22
Pleural effusion	30	32	36	35
Dyspnea	29	23	5	4
Pruritus	36	20	15	7
Rash	24	19	10	4

*CBIR, cyclosporine-based immunosuppressive regimen.

as graft-versus-host disease (GVHD), represents a significant cause of morbidity and mortality in bone marrow transplant recipients. Cyclosporine has traditionally been used for both prophylaxis and treatment of GVHD but, as in solid organ transplantation, is associated with significant toxicity. Tacrolimus has now been used in several trials of both related and unrelated marrow transplantation. A phase III open-label, randomized trial of HLA-identical sibling bone marrow transplantation comparing tacrolimus/methotrexate and cyclosporine/methotrexate demonstrated that tacrolimus/methotrexate was superior in the prevention of both grade II–IV acute GVHD and extensive chronic GVHD (192). However, the apparent advantage of tacrolimus/methotrexate was offset by higher regimen-related toxicity and lower overall survival, the latter secondary to a greater number of patients with advanced disease assigned to the tacrolimus/methotrexate arm (193). Analysis of survival prognosis by comparison with a matched control population of patients from the

International Bone Marrow Transplant Registry demonstrated that the survival difference of the tacrolimus/methotrexate group was attributable to the assignment imbalance (193). Furthermore, early reports suggest that the source of stem cells (e.g., bone marrow versus growth-factor mobilized peripheral blood stem cells) may impact on outcome (194). Finally, studies of tacrolimus-based regimens for the prophylaxis of GVHD after marrow transplantation from unrelated donors are promising (195,196). Prospective comparative studies are underway.

Although the approval of tacrolimus for use in liver transplantation provides physicians with another option for the prevention and treatment of graft rejection, serious side effects are still commonly encountered with its administration. In addition, because cyclosporine and tacrolimus share a common intracellular target, combinations of these two agents are unlikely to improve efficacy and may significantly increase toxicity. Careful monitoring of therapeutic levels is warranted (197–199). Nevertheless, the consideration of other agents is often necessary because of dosage-limiting toxicity in the context of refractory rejection or GVHD.

Unlike cyclosporine and tacrolimus, rapamycin inhibits proliferation of nonhematopoietic as well as hematopoietic cells. This difference may result in wider applicability of rapamycin in the treatment of clinical problems. For instance, rapamycin has been shown to inhibit proliferation of vascular smooth muscle cells after balloon catheter injury (200–203) and may thus be useful in preventing restenosis after angioplasty. Rapamycin has been used extensively in solid organ transplantation, both as a single agent and in combination regimens, and demonstrates efficacy in both prophylactic and therapeutic settings. In animal models, it appears to interrupt rejection episodes and even to reverse chronic vascular disease (204) and to inhibit hepatic fibrosis (205). Rapamycin appears to be synergistic with cyclosporine in a murine model of kidney allograft rejection (206) and in a rat model of acute lung rejection (207). The observed synergy may relate to intragraft cytokine expression in this (208) and other transplant (209) settings. Rapamycin has recently been approved for use in prevention of acute renal transplant rejection, based on two large clinical trials that have yet to be published. It is recommended that rapamycin be used in combination with corticosteroids and cyclosporine. In adult renal transplantation, however, the addition of rapamycin to the armamentarium of agents used in preventing and treating rejection has been shown to permit reduction in cyclosporine and corticosteroid dosages and, in some settings, to allow complete steroid withdrawal (210–213). Importantly, its toxicity profile differs from that of cyclosporine, and therefore may be useful as adjunctive therapy (see, for example 214, 215). To date, rapamycin has not been shown to be neurotoxic, unlike cyclosporine and tacrolimus. The most prominent adverse side effects of rapamycin are hyperlipidemia, leukopenia, and thrombocytopenia (210,215); the molecular mechanisms of these toxicities are poorly understood.

The use of rapamycin in combination with other immunosuppressive agents may result in regimens more effective than those currently employed. Its use in combination with cyclosporine has been examined, and early trials have illuminated the importance of pharmacokinetic monitoring (216–218). Theoretically, rapamycin may be synergistic with tacrolimus despite both binding the FKBP family; the gain-of-function model of therapeutic action dictates that drug need bind only a fraction of FKBP protein for efficacy. Still other agents that target different pathways of lymphocyte function, such as purine and pyrimidine metabolism, are now being investigated. Rapamycin has been shown to be synergistic with mycophenolate mofetil in prevention and reversal of solid organ allograft rejection in the rat (219). The role of rapamycin in combination with agents that target T-cell costimulation pathways (220) including activation antigens (221) are being investigated. The availability of all these agents, of varying mechanism and with nonoverlapping side effect profiles, will enhance our ability to manipulate the immune systems of patients receiving allografts with optimal efficacy and minimal toxicity.

As outlined above, several pharmacologic agents are available that can prevent or dampen lymphocyte (specifically T-cell) activation. However, each of these agents remains a relatively blunt tool, inhibiting lymphocyte responses to pathogens as well as to engrafted tissue. The challenge to clinicians and immunologists is to develop strategies that allow for specific unresponsiveness (tolerance) to engrafted tissue while maintaining the ability to respond to infectious agents. New paradigms of graft tolerance are now in development. Some years ago, it was observed that some liver transplant recipients were able to discontinue immunosuppression for prolonged periods of time without rejecting their grafts (222). This state of graft tolerance resulted from a chimeric state in which donor and recipient immune cells coexisted, permitting maintenance of the graft in the absence of immunosuppressive therapy. If successfully developed, solid organ and stem cell transplantation from the same allogeneic donor may promote a state of mixed chimerism and specific tolerance of the host toward donor antigens. This approach, in combination with novel immunologic tools, would permit transplantation across histocompatibility barriers without the need for significant, nonspecific immunosuppressive therapy.

Summary

Cyclosporin A, tacrolimus, and rapamycin have been used successfully both in the clinic to prevent graft rejection and in the laboratory to further our understanding of lymphocyte signal transduction. Cyclosporin and tacrolimus share a common intracellular target, the serine/threonine phosphatase calcineurin. When complexed to their cognate receptors in T cells, cyclosporin A and tacrolimus inhibit the phosphatase activity of calcineurin toward the transcription factor NFAT, blocking the transcription of genes critical for T-cell activation. Rapamycin, which binds to the same intracellular receptors as tacrolimus, has a different mechanism of action. Rapamycin has been shown to inhibit the activity of $p70^{s6k}$ through interaction with mTOR or FRAP. This inhibition blocks mitogen-activated signals and prevents cell cycle progression in T cells.

Studies of cyclosporin A, tacrolimus, and rapamycin have opened novel avenues in cell biology by allowing delineation of critical T-cell signaling pathways and by revealing two families of receptor proteins, the FKBPs and the cyclophilins. Members of these families are expressed not only in T cells but throughout the body. We are just beginning to unravel the complex interactions between these immunophilins and a wide variety of cellular proteins. While there is no unifying theme in the interactions observed to date, these proteins are probably involved in regulation of calcium homeostasis and folding of specific protein substrates. Some of these interactions may be of importance when one considers potential drug interactions or toxicities associated with the use of immunophilin ligands.

The availability of cyclosporin A, tacrolimus, and now rapamycin will continue to facilitate a revolution in clinical transplantation. However, each of these agents carries a risk of life-threatening immunosuppression that cannot currently be separated from therapeutic efficacy. Improvements in understanding of the mechanism(s) by which immunosuppressive agents act will drive future progress in the field of clinical transplantation. This knowledge can be gained both from clinical studies and from laboratory research. It is hoped that, with such knowledge, the rational design of future regimens that enhance efficacy and reduce toxicity will be possible.

References

1. Shevach EM. The effects of cyclosporin A on the immune system. Annu Rev Immunol 1985;3:397–423.
2. Sigal NH, Dumont FJ. Cyclosporin A, FK-506, and rapamycin: pharmacological probes of lymphocyte signal transduction. Annu Rev Immunol 1992;10:519–560.
3. Bierer BE. Advances in therapeutic immunosuppression: biology, molecular actions, and clinical implications. Curr Opin Hematol 1993;1:149–159.
4. Schreiber SL. Chemistry and biology of the immunophilins and their immunosuppressive ligands. Science 1991;251:283–287.
5. Tacrolimus (FK506) for organ transplants. Med Lett 1994;36:82–83.
6. Tocci MJ, Matkovich DA, Collier KA, et al. The immunosuppressant FK506 selectively inhibits expression of early T cell activation genes. J Immunol 1989;143:718–726.
7. Bierer BE, Somers PK, Wandless TJ, et al. Probing immunosuppressant action with a nonnatural immunophilin ligand. Science 1990;250:556–559.
8. Handschumacher RE, Harding MW, Rice J, et al. Cyclophilin: a specific cytosolic binding protein for cyclosporin A. Science 1984;226:544–547.
9. Fruman DA, Burakoff SJ, Bierer BE. Immunophilins in protein folding and immunosuppression. Faseb J 1994;8:391–400.
10. Rosen MK, Standaert RF, Galat A, et al. Inhibition of FKBP rotamase activity by immunosuppressant FK506: twisted amide surrogate. Science 1990;248:863–866.
11. Bierer BE, Schreiber SL, Burakoff SJ. The effect of the immunosuppressant FK-506 on alternate pathways of T cell activation. Eur J Immunol 1991;21:439–445.
12. Friedman J, Weissman I. Two cytoplasmic candidates for immunophilin action are revealed by affinity for a new cyclophilin: one in the presence and one in the absence of CsA. Cell 1991;66:799–806.
13. Clipstone NA, Fiorentino DF, Crabtree GR. Molecular analysis of the interaction of calcineurin with drug-immunophilin complexes. J Biol Chem 1994;269:26431–26437.
14. Rao A, Luo C, Hogan PG. Transcription factors of the NFAT family: regulation and function. Annu Rev Immunol 1997;15:707–747.
15. Wood MA, Bierer BE. Rapamycin: biological and therapeutic effects, binding by immunophilins and molecular targets of action. Perspect Drug Disc Des 1994;2:163–184.
16. Bierer BE, Mattila PS, Standaert RF, et al. Two distinct signal transmission pathways in T lymphocytes are inhibited by complexes formed between an immunophilin and either FK506 or rapamycin. Proc Natl Acad Sci USA 1990;87:9231–9235.
17. Dumont FJ, Staruch MJ, Koprak SK, et al. Distinct mechanisms of suppression of murine T cell activation by the related macrolides FK-506 and rapamycin. J Immunol 1990;144:251–258.
18. Calvo V, Wood M, Gjertson C, et al. Activation of 70-kDa S6 kinase, induced by the cytokines interleukin-3 and erythropoietin and inhibited by rapamycin, is not an absolute requirement for cell proliferation. Eur J Immunol 1994;24:2664–2671.
19. Negulescu PA, Shastri N, Cahalan MD. Intracellular calcium dependence of gene expression in single T lymphocytes. Proc Natl Acad Sci USA 1994;91:2873–2877.
20. Cardenas ME, Heitman J. Role of calcium in T-lymphocyte activation. Adv Second Messenger Phosphoprotein Res 1995;30:281–298.
21. Klee CB, Ren H, Wang X. Regulation of the calmodulin-stimulated protein phosphatase, calcineurin. J Biol Chem 1998;273:13367–13370.
22. Crabtree GR. Generic signals and specific outcomes: signaling through Ca2+, calcineurin, and NF-AT. Cell 1999;96:611–614.
23. Northrop JP, Ho SN, Chen L, et al. NF-AT components define a family of transcription factors targeted in T-cell activation. Nature 1994;369:497–502.
24. Shibasaki F, Price ER, Milan D, et al. Role of kinases and the phosphatase calcineurin in the nuclear shuttling of transcription factor NF-AT4. Nature 1996;382:370–373.
25. Chen L, Glover JN, Hogan PG, et al. Structure of the DNA-binding domains from NFAT, Fos and Jun bound specifically to DNA. Nature 1998;392:42–48.
26. Hodge MR, Ranger AM, Charles de la Brousse F, et al. Hyperproliferation and dysregulation of IL-4 expression in NF-ATp-deficient mice. Immunity 1996;4:397–405.
27. Feng B, Stemmer PM. Interactions of calcineurin A, calcineurin B, and Ca2+. Biochemistry 1999;38:12481–12489.
28. McPartlin AE, Barker HM, Cohen PT. Identification of a third alternatively spliced cDNA encoding the catalytic subunit of protein phosphatase 2B beta. Biochim Biophys Acta 1991;1088:308–310.
29. Muramatsu T, Giri PR, Higuchi S, et al. Molecular cloning of a calmodulin-dependent phosphatase from murine testis: identification of a developmentally expressed nonneural isoenzyme [published erratum appears in Proc Natl Acad Sci USA 1992 May 15;89(10):4779]. Proc Natl Acad Sci USA 1992;89:529–533.
30. Guerini D, Krinks MH, Sikela JM, et al. Isolation and sequence of a cDNA clone for human calcineurin B, the Ca2+-binding subunit of the Ca2+/calmodulin-stimulated protein phosphatase. DNA 1989;8:675–682.
31. Griffith JP, Kim JL, Kim EE, et al. X-ray structure of calcineurin inhibited by the immunophilin-immunosuppressant FKBP12-FK506 complex. Cell 1995;82:507–522.
32. Sagoo JK, Fruman DA, Wesselborg S, et al. Competitive inhibition of calcineurin phosphatase activity by its autoinhibitory domain. Biochem J 1996;320:879–884.
33. Breuder T, Hemenway CS, Movva NR, et al. Calcineurin is essential in cyclosporin A- and FK506-sensitive yeast strains. Proc Natl Acad Sci USA 1994;91:5372–5376.
34. Tian J, Karin M. Stimulation of Elk1 transcriptional activity by mitogen-activated protein kinases is negatively regulated

by protein phosphatase 2B (calcineurin). J Biol Chem 1999; 274:15173–15180.

35. Trushin SA, Pennington KN, Algeciras-Schimnich A, et al. Protein kinase C and calcineurin synergize to activate IkappaB kinase and NF-kappaB in T lymphocytes. J Biol Chem 1999;274:22923–22931.

36. Werlen G, Jacinto E, Xia Y, et al. Calcineurin preferentially synergizes with PKC-theta to activate JNK and IL-2 promoter in T lymphocytes. Embo J 1998;17:3101–3111.

37. Wang X, Culotta VC, Klee CB. Superoxide dismutase protects calcineurin from inactivation. Nature 1996;383:434–437.

38. Sun L, Youn HD, Loh C, et al. Cabin 1, a negative regulator for calcineurin signaling in T lymphocytes. Immunity 1998;8:703–711.

39. Lai MM, Burnett PE, Wolosker H, et al. Cain, a novel physiologic protein inhibitor of calcineurin. J Biol Chem 1998;273:18325–18331.

40. Xin L, Sikkink RA, Rusnak F, et al. Inhibition of calcineurin phosphatase activity by a calcineurin B homologous protein. J Biol Chem 1999;274:36125–36131.

41. Kashishian A, Howard M, Loh C, et al. AKAP79 inhibits calcineurin through a site distinct from the immunophilin-binding region. J Biol Chem 1998;273:27412–27419.

42. Cameron AM, Steiner JP, Roskams AJ, et al. Calcineurin associated with the inositol 1,4,5-trisphosphate receptor-FKBP12 complex modulates Ca2+ flux. Cell 1995;83:463–472.

43. Groblewski GE, Yoshida M, Bragado MJ, et al. Purification and characterization of a novel physiological substrate for calcineurin in mammalian cells. J Biol Chem 1998;273:22738–22744.

44. Walsh MP, Busaan JL, Fraser ED, et al. Characterization of the recombinant C-terminal domain of dystrophin: phosphorylation by calmodulin-dependent protein kinase II and dephosphorylation by type 2B protein phosphatase. Biochemistry 1995;34:5561–5568.

45. Lai MM, Hong JJ, Ruggiero AM, et al. The calcineurin-dynamin 1 complex as a calcium sensor for synaptic vesicle endocytosis. J Biol Chem 1999;274:25963–25966.

46. Fruman DA, Wood MA, Gjertson CK, et al. FK506 binding protein 12 mediates sensitivity to both FK506 and rapamycin in murine mast cells. Eur J Immunol 1995;25:563–571.

47. Lyons WE, George EB, Dawson TM, et al. Immunosuppressant FK506 promotes neurite outgrowth in cultures of PC12 cells and sensory ganglia. Proc Natl Acad Sci USA 1994;91:3191–3195.

48. Paterson JM, Smith SM, Harmar AJ, et al. Control of a novel adenylyl cyclase by calcineurin. Biochem Biophys Res Commun 1995;214:1000–1008.

49. Hathaway DR, Adelstein RS, Klee CB. Interaction of calmodulin with myosin light chain kinase and cAMP-dependent protein kinase in bovine brain. J Biol Chem 1981;256:8183–8189.

50. Musaro A, McCullagh KJ, Naya FJ, et al. IGF-1 induces skeletal myocyte hypertrophy through calcineurin in association with GATA-2 and NF-ATc1. Nature 1999;400:581–585.

51. Molkentin JD, Lu JR, Antos CL, et al. A calcineurin-dependent transcriptional pathway for cardiac hypertrophy. Cell 1998;93:215–228.

52. Sussman MA, Lim HW, Gude N, et al. Prevention of cardiac hypertrophy in mice by calcineurin inhibition. Science 1998;281:1690–1693.

53. Fruman DA, Mather PE, Burakoff SJ, et al. Correlation of calcineurin phosphatase activity and programmed cell death in murine T cell hybridomas. Eur J Immunol 1992;22:2513–2517.

54. Shibasaki F, Kondo E, Akagi T, et al. Suppression of signalling through transcription factor NF-AT by interactions between calcineurin and Bcl-2. Nature 1997;386:728–731.

55. Toth R, Szegezdi E, Molnar G, et al. Regulation of cell surface expression of Fas (CD95) ligand and susceptibility to Fas (CD95)-mediated apoptosis in activation-induced T cell death involves calcineurin and protein kinase C, respectively. Eur J Immunol 1999;29:383–393.

56. Youn H-K, Sun L, Prywes R, Liu JO. Apoptosis of T cells mediated by Ca2+-induced release of the transcription factor MEF2. Science 1999;286:790–793.

57. Wang HG, Pathan N, Ethell IM, et al. Ca2+-induced apoptosis through calcineurin dephosphorylation of BAD. Science 1999;284:339–343.

58. Moore JM, Peattie DA, Fitzgibbon MJ, et al. Solution structure of the major binding protein for the immunosuppressant FK506. Nature 1991;351:248–250.

59. Braun W, Kallen J, Mikol V, et al. Three-dimensional structure and actions of immunosuppressants and their immunophilins. Faseb J 1995;9:63–72.

60. Kissinger CR, Parge HE, Knighton DR, et al. Crystal structures of human calcineurin and the human FKBP12-FK506-calcineurin complex. Nature 1995;378:641–644.

61. Ivery MT. A proposed molecular model for the interaction of calcineurin with the cyclosporin A-cyclophilin A complex. Bioorg Med Chem 1999;7:1389–1402.

62. Wesselborg S, Fruman DA, Sagoo JK, et al. Identification of a physical interaction between calcineurin and nuclear factor of activated T cells (NFATp). J Biol Chem 1996;271:1274–1277.

63. Kaye RE, Fruman DA, Bierer BE, et al. Effects of cyclosporin A and FK506 on Fc epsilon receptor type I-initiated increases in cytokine mRNA in mouse bone marrow-derived progenitor mast cells: resistance to FK506 is associated with a deficiency in FK506-binding protein FKBP12. Proc Natl Acad Sci USA 1992;89:8542–8546.

64. Hultsch T, Albers MW, Schreiber SL, et al. Immunophilin ligands demonstrate common features of signal transduction leading to exocytosis or transcription. Proc Natl Acad Sci USA 1991;88:6229–6233.

65. Brillantes AB, Ondrias K, Scott A, et al. Stabilization of calcium release channel (ryanodine receptor) function by FK506-binding protein. Cell 1994;77:513–523.

66. Xin HB, Rogers K, Qi Y, et al. Three amino acid residues determine selective binding of FK506-binding protein 12.6 to the cardiac ryanodine receptor. J Biol Chem 1999; 274:15315–15319.

67. Qi Y, Ogunbunmi EM, Freund EA, et al. FK-binding protein is associated with the ryanodine receptor of skeletal muscle in vertebrate animals. J Biol Chem 1998;273:34813–34819.

68. Cameron AM, Nucifora FC Jr, Fung ET, et al. FKBP12 binds the inositol 1,4,5-trisphosphate receptor at leucine-proline (1400–1401) and anchors calcineurin to this FK506-like domain. J Biol Chem 1997;272:27582–27588.

69. Genazzani AA, Carafoli E, Guerini D. Calcineurin controls inositol 1,4,5-trisphosphate type 1 receptor expression in neurons. Proc Natl Acad Sci USA 1999;96:5797–5801.

70. Shou W, Aghdasi B, Armstrong DL, et al. Cardiac defects and altered ryanodine receptor function in mice lacking FKBP12. Nature 1998;391:489–492.

71. Atkison P, Joubert G, Barron A, et al. Hypertrophic cardiomyopathy associated with tacrolimus in paediatric transplant patients. Lancet 1995;345:894–896.

72. Lam E, Martin M, Wiederrecht G. Isolation of a cDNA encoding a novel human FK506-binding protein homolog containing leucine zipper and tetratricopeptide repeat motifs. Gene 1995;160:297–302.

73. Baughman G, Wiederrecht GJ, Chang F, et al. Tissue distribution and abundance of human FKBP51, and FK506-binding protein that can mediate calcineurin inhibition. Biochem Biophys Res Commun 1997;232:437–443.

74. Nakamura T, Yabe D, Kanazawa N, et al. Molecular cloning, characterization, and chromosomal localization of FKBP23, a novel FK506-binding protein with Ca2+-binding ability. Genomics 1998;54:89–98.

75. Cunningham EB. The human erythrocyte membrane contains a novel 12-kDa inositolphosphate-binding protein that is an immunophilin. Biochem Biophys Res Commun 1995;215:212–218.

76. Kingsley DM. The TGF-beta superfamily: new members, new receptors, and new genetic tests of function in different organisms. Genes Dev 1994;8:133–146.

77. Wang T, Danielson PD, Li BY, et al. The p21 (RAS) farnesyltransferase alpha subunit in TGF-beta and activin signaling. Science 1996;271:1120–1122.

78. Wrana JL, Attisano L, Carcamo J, et al. TGF beta signals through a heteromeric protein kinase receptor complex. Cell 1992;71:1003–1014.

79. Charng MJ, Kinnunen P, Hawker J, et al. FKBP-12 recognition is dispensable for signal generation by type I transforming growth factor-beta receptors. J Biol Chem 1996;271:22941–22944.

80. Huse M, Chen YG, Massague J, et al. Crystal structure of the cytoplasmic domain of the type I TGF beta receptor in complex with FKBP12. Cell 1999;96:425–436.

81. Hojo M, Morimoto T, Maluccio M, et al. Cyclosporine induces cancer progression by a cell-autonomous mechanism. Nature 1999;397:530–534.

82. Jin YJ, Albers MW, Lane WS, et al. Molecular cloning of a membrane-associated human FK506- and rapamycin-binding protein, FKBP-13. Proc Natl Acad Sci USA 1991;88:6677–6681.

83. Walensky LD, Gascard P, Fields ME, et al. The 13-kD FK506 binding protein, FKBP13, interacts with a novel homologue of the erythrocyte membrane cytoskeletal protein 4.1. J Cell Biol 1998;141:143–153.

84. Jin YJ, Burakoff SJ, Bierer BE. Molecular cloning of a 25-kDa high affinity rapamycin binding protein, FKBP25. J Biol Chem 1992;267:10942–10945.

85. Tai PK, Chang H, Albers MW, et al. P59 (FK506 binding protein 59) interaction with heat shock proteins is highly conserved and may involve proteins other than steroid receptors. Biochemistry 1993;32:8842–8847.

86. Chambraud B, Radanyi C, Camonis JH, et al. Immunophilins, Refsum disease, and lupus nephritis: the peroxisomal enzyme phytanoyl-COA alpha-hydroxylase is a new FKBP-associated protein. Proc Natl Acad Sci USA 1999;96:2104–2109.

87. Chambraud B, Radanyi C, Camonis JH, et al. FAP48, a new protein that forms specific complexes with both immunophilins FKBP59 and FKBP12. Prevention by the immuno-suppressant drugs FK506 and rapamycin. J Biol Chem 1996;271:32923–32929.

88. Coss MC, Winterstein D, Sowder RC 2nd, et al. Molecular cloning, DNA sequence analysis, and biochemical characterization of a novel 65-kDa FK506-binding protein (FKBP65). J Biol Chem 1995;270:29336–29341.

89. Coss MC, Stephens RM, Morrison DK, et al. The immunophilin FKBP65 forms an association with the serine/threonine kinase c-Raf-1. Cell Growth Differ 1998;9:41–48.

90. Lenhoff HM, Wang PP, Greenberg F, et al. Williams syndrome and the brain. Sci Am 1997;277:68–73.

91. Ewart AK, Morris CA, Atkinson D, et al. Hemizygosity at the elastin locus in a developmental disorder, Williams syndrome. Nat Genet 1993;5:11–16.

92. Meng X, Lu X, Morris CA, et al. A novel human gene FKBP6 is deleted in Williams syndrome. Genomics 1998;52:130–137.

93. Wang YK, Samos CH, Peoples R, et al. A novel human homologue of the Drosophila frizzled wnt receptor gene binds wingless protein and is in the Williams syndrome deletion at 7q11.23. Hum Mol Genet 1997;6:465–472.

94. Kallen J, Spitzfaden C, Zurini M, et al. Structure of human cyclophilin and its binding site for cyclosporin A determined by x-ray crystallography and NMR spectroscopy. Nature 1991;353:276–279.

95. Ke H, Zydowsky L, Liu J, Walsh C. Crystal structure of recombinant human T-cell cyclophilin A at 2.5 Å resolution. Proc Natl Acad Sci USA 1991;88:9483–9487.

96. Mikol V, Kallen J, Walkinshaw MD. X-ray structure of a cyclophilin B/cyclosporin complex: comparison with cyclophilin A and delineation of its calcineurin-binding domain. Proc Natl Acad Sci USA 1994;91:5183–5186.

97. Ke H, Zhao Y, Luo F, et al. Crystal structure of murine cyclophilin C complexed with immunosuppressive drug cyclosporin A. Proc Natl Acad Sci USA 1993;90:11850–11854.

98. Kallen J, Mikol V, Taylor P, et al. X-ray structures and analysis of 11 cyclosporin derivatives complexed with cyclophilin A. J Mol Biol 1998;283:435–449.

99. Mikol V, Kallen J, Pflugl G, et al. X-ray structure of a monomeric cyclophilin A-cyclosporin A crystal complex at 2.1 A resolution. J Mol Biol 1993;234:1119–1130.

100. Fischer G, Wittmann-Liebold B, Lang K, et al. Cyclophilin and peptidyl-prolyl cis-trans isomerase are probably identical proteins. Nature 1989;337:476–478.

101. Bram RJ, Hung DT, Martin PK, et al. Identification of the immunophilins capable of mediating inhibition of signal transduction by cyclosporin A and FK506: roles of calcineurin binding and cellular location. Mol Cell Biol 1993;13:4760–4769.

102. Schonbrunner E, Mayer S, Tropschug M, et al. Catalysis of protein folding by cyclophilins from different species. J Biol Chem 1991;266:3630–3635.

103. Kern D, Drakenberg T, Wikstrom M, et al. The cis/trans interconversion of the calcium regulating hormone calcitonin is catalyzed by cyclophilin. FEBS Lett 1993;323:198–202.

104. Kern G, Kern D, Schmid FX, et al. A kinetic analysis of the folding of human carbonic anhydrase II and its catalysis by cyclophilin. J Biol Chem 1995;270:740–745.

105. Dolinski K, Muir S, Cardenas M, et al. All cyclophilins and FK506 binding proteins are, individually and collectively, dispensable for viability in Saccharomyces cerevisiae. Proc Natl Acad Sci USA 1997;94:13093–13098.

106. Jaschke A, Mi H, Tropschug M. Human T cell cyclophilin 18 binds to thiol-specific antioxidant protein Aop1 and stimulates its activity. J Mol Biol 1998;277:763–769.

107. Luban J, Bossolt KL, Franke EK, et al. Human immunodeficiency virus type 1 Gag protein binds to cyclophilins A and B. Cell 1993;73:1067–1078.

108. Franke EK, Luban J. Cyclophilin and gag in HIV-1 replication and pathogenesis. Adv Exp Med Biol 1995;374:217–228.

109. Braaten D, Franke EK, Luban J. Cyclophilin A is required for an early step in the life cycle of human immunodeficiency virus type 1 before the initiation of reverse transcription. J Virol 1996;70:3551–3560.

110. Franke EK, Luban J. Inhibition of HIV-1 replication by cyclosporine A or related compounds correlates with the ability to disrupt the Gag-cyclophilin A interaction. Virology 1996;222:279–282.

111. Price ER, Zydowsky LD, Jin MJ, et al. Human cyclophilin B: a second cyclophilin gene encodes a peptidyl-prolyl isomerase with a signal sequence. Proc Natl Acad Sci USA 1991;88:1903–1907.

112. Bram RJ, Crabtree GR. Calcium signalling in T cells stimulated by a cyclophilin B-binding protein. Nature 1994;371:355–358.

113. Mariller C, Allain F, Kouach M, et al. Evidence that human milk isolated cyclophilin B corresponds to a truncated form. Biochim Biophys Acta 1996;1293:31–38.

114. Carpentier M, Allain F, Haendler B, et al. Two distinct regions of cyclophilin B are involved in the recognition of a functional receptor and of glycosaminoglycans on T lymphocytes. J Biol Chem 1999;274:10990–10998.

115. Allain F, Durieux S, Denys A, et al. Cyclophilin B binding to platelets supports calcium-dependent adhesion to collagen. Blood 1999;94:976–983.

116. Schneider H, Charara N, Schmitz R, et al. Human cyclophilin C: primary structure, tissue distribution, and determination of binding specificity for cyclosporins. Biochemistry 1994;33:8218–8224.

117. Friedman J, Weissman I, Alpert S. An analysis of the expression of cyclophilin C reveals tissue restriction and an intriguing pattern in the mouse kidney. Am J Pathol 1994;144:1247–1256.

118. Friedman J, Trahey M, Weissman I. Cloning and characterization of cyclophilin C-associated protein: a candidate natural cellular ligand for cyclophilin C. Proc Natl Acad Sci USA 1993;90:6815–6819.

119. Trahey M, Weissman IL. Cyclophilin C-associated protein: a normal secreted glycoprotein that down-modulates endo-

120. Connern CP, Halestrap AP. Purification and N-terminal sequencing of peptidyl-prolyl cis-trans-isomerase from rat liver mitochondrial matrix reveals the existence of a distinct mitochondrial cyclophilin. Biochem J 1992;284:381–385.

121. Woodfield K, Ruck A, Brdiczka D, et al. Direct demonstration of a specific interaction between cyclophilin-D and the adenine nucleotide translocase confirms their role in the mitochondrial permeability transition. Biochem J 1998;336:287–290.

122. Hortelano S, Dallaporta B, Zamzami N, et al. Nitric oxide induces apoptosis via triggering mitochondrial permeability transition. FEBS Lett 1997;410:373–377.

123. Halestrap AP, Connern CP, Griffiths EJ, et al. Cyclosporin A binding to mitochondrial cyclophilin inhibits the permeability transition pore and protects hearts from ischaemia/reperfusion injury. Mol Cell Biochem 1997;174:167–172.

124. Bernardi P. The permeability transition pore. Control points of a cyclosporin A-sensitive mitochondrial channel involved in cell death. Biochim Biophys Acta 1996;1275:5–9.

125. Anderson SK, Gallinger S, Roder J, et al. A cyclophilin-related protein involved in the function of natural killer cells. Proc Natl Acad Sci USA 1993;90:542–546.

126. Simons-Evelyn M, Young HA, Anderson SK. Characterization of the mouse Nktr gene and promoter. Genomics 1997;40:94–100.

127. Giardina SL, Coffman JD, Young HA, et al. Association of the expression of an SR-cyclophilin with myeloid cell differentiation. Blood 1996;87:2269–2274.

128. Giardina SL, Anderson SK, Sayers TJ, et al. Selective loss of NK cytotoxicity in antisense NK-TR1 rat LGL cell lines. Abrogation of antibody-independent tumor and virus-infected target cell killing. J Immunol 1995;154:80–87.

129. Chambers CA, Gallinger S, Anderson SK, et al. Expression of the NK-TR gene is required for NK-like activity in human T cells. J Immunol 1994;152:2669–2674.

130. Nestel FP, Colwill K, Harper S, et al. RS cyclophilins: identification of an NK-TR1-related cyclophilin. Gene 1996;180:151–155.

131. Mortillaro MJ, Berezney R. Matrin CYP. An SR-rich cyclophilin that associates with the nuclear matrix and splicing factors. J Biol Chem 1998;273:8183–8192.

132. Wang BB, Hayenga KJ, Payan DG, et al. Identification of a nuclear-specific cyclophilin which interacts with the proteinase inhibitor eglin c. Biochem J 1996;314:313–319.

133. Kieffer LJ, Seng TW, Li W, et al. Cyclophilin-40, a protein with homology to the P59 component of the steroid receptor complex. Cloning of the cDNA and further characterization. J Biol Chem 1993;268:12303–12310.

134. Kieffer LJ, Thalhammer T, Handschumacher RE. Isolation and characterization of a 40-kDa cyclophilin-related protein. J Biol Chem 1992;267:5503–5507.

135. Hoffmann K, Handschumacher RE. Cyclophilin-40: evidence for a dimeric complex with hsp90. Biochem J 1995;307:5–8.

136. Duina AA, Chang HC, Marsh JA, et al. A cyclophilin function in Hsp90-dependent signal transduction. Science 1996;274:1713–1715.

137. Duina AA, Kalton HM, Gaber RF. Requirement for Hsp90

and a CyP-40-type cyclophilin in negative regulation of the heat shock response. J Biol Chem 1998;273:18974–18978.

138. Wu J, Matunis MJ, Kraemer D, et al. Nup358, a cytoplasmically exposed nucleoporin with peptide repeats, Ran-GTP binding sites, zinc fingers, a cyclophilin A homologous domain, and a leucine-rich region. J Biol Chem 1995;270: 14209–14213.

139. Ferreira PA, Nakayama TA, Pak WL, et al. Cyclophilin-related protein RanBP2 acts as chaperone for red/green opsin. Nature 1996;383:637–640.

140. Ferreira PA, Nakayama TA, Travis GH. Interconversion of red opsin isoforms by the cyclophilin-related chaperone protein Ran-binding protein 2. Proc Natl Acad Sci USA 1997;94:1556–1561.

141. Holloway MP, Bram RJ. Co-localization of calcium-modulating cyclophilin ligand with intracellular calcium pools. J Biol Chem 1998;273:16346–16350.

142. Serafini AT, Lewis RS, Clipstone NA, et al. Isolation of mutant T lymphocytes with defects in capacitative calcium entry. Immunity 1995;3:239–250.

143. von Bulow GU, Bram RJ. NF-AT activation induced by a CAML-interacting member of the tumor necrosis factor receptor superfamily. Sciene 1997;278:138–141.

144. Parekh AB, Penner R. Store depletion and calcium influx. Physiol Rev 1997;77:901–930.

145. Montague JW, Hughes FM Jr, Cidlowski JA. Native recombinant cyclophilins A, B, and C degrade DNA independently of peptidylprolyl cis-trans-isomerase activity. Potential roles of cyclophilins in apoptosis. J Biol Chem 1997;272:6677–6684.

146. Tanveer A, Virji S, Andreeva L, et al. Involvement of cyclophilin D in the activation of a mitochondrial pore by Ca2+ and oxidant stress. Eur J Biochem 1996;238:166–172.

147. Dumont FJ, Melino MR, Staruch MJ, et al. The immunosuppressive macrolides FK-506 and rapamycin act as reciprocal antagonists in murine T cells. J Immunol 1990;144: 1418–1424.

148. Kunz J, Henriquez R, Schneider U, et al. Target of rapamycin in yeast, TOR2, is an essential phosphatidylinositol kinase homolog required for G1 progression. Cell 1993;73:585–596.

149. Brennan P, Babbage JW, Burgering BM, et al. Phosphatidylinositol 3-kinase couples the interleukin-2 receptor to the cell cycle regulator E2F. Immunity 1997;7:679–689.

150. Chung J, Kuo CJ, Crabtree GR, et al. Rapamycin-FKBP specifically blocks growth-dependent activation of and signaling by the 70kd S6 protein kinases. Cell 1992;69:1227–1236.

151. Terada N, Takase K, Papst P, et al. Rapamycin inhibits ribosomal protein synthesis and induces G1 prolongation in mitogen-activated T lymphocytes. J Immunol 1995; 155:3418–3426.

152. Terada N, Franklin RA, Lucas JJ, et al. Failure of rapamycin to block proliferation once resting cells have entered the cell cycle despite inactivation of p70 S6 kinase. J Biol Chem 1993;268:12062–12068.

153. Morice WG, Wiederrecht G, Brunn GJ, et al. Rapamycin inhibition of interleukin-2-dependent p33cdk2 and p34cdc2 kinase activation in T lymphocytes. J Biol Chem 1993;268: 22737–22745.

154. Morgan DO. Principles of CDK regulation. Nature 1995; 374:131–134.

155. Hashemolhosseini S, Nagamine Y, Morley SJ, et al. Rapamycin inhibition of the G1 to S transition is mediated by effects on cyclin D1 mRNA and protein stability. J Biol Chem 1998;273:14424–14429.

156. Takuwa N, Fukui Y, Takuwa Y. Cyclin D1 expression mediated by phosphatidylinositol 3-kinase through mTOR-p70(S6K)-independent signaling in growth factor-stimulated NIH 3T3 fibroblasts. Mol Cell Biol 1999;19: 1346–1358.

157. Brennan P, Babbage JW, Thomas G, et al. p70(s6k) integrates phosphatidylinositol 3-kinase and rapamycin-regulated signals for E2F regulation in T lymphocytes. Mol Cell Biol 1999;19:4729–4738.

158. Nourse J, Firpo E, Flanagan WM, et al. Interleukin-2-mediated elimination of the p27Kip1 cyclin-dependent kinase inhibitor prevented by rapamycin. Nature 1994;372: 570–573.

159. Heitman J, Movva NR, Hall MN. Targets for cell cycle arrest by the immunosuppressant rapamycin in yeast. Science 1991;253:905–909.

160. Izquierdo Pastor M, Reif K, Cantrell D. The regulation and function of p21ras during T-cell activation and growth. Immunol Today 1995;16:159–164.

161. Heim MH. The Jak-STAT pathway: cytokine signalling from the receptor to the nucleus. J Recept Signal Transduct Res 1999;19:75–120.

162. Duronio V, Scheid MP, Ettinger S. Downstream signalling events regulated by phosphatidylinositol 3-kinase activity. Cell Signal 1998;10:233–239.

163. Schu PV, Takegawa K, Fry MJ, et al. Phosphatidylinositol 3-kinase encoded by yeast VPS34 gene essential for protein sorting. Science 1993;260:88–91.

164. Hay JC, Fisette PL, Jenkins GH, et al. ATP-dependent inositide phosphorylation required for Ca(2+)-activated secretion. Nature 1995;374:173–177.

165. Klionsky DJ, Herman PK, Emr SD. The fungal vacuole: composition, function, and biogenesis. Microbiol Rev 1990; 54:266–292.

166. Brown EJ, Beal PA, Keith CT, et al. Control of p70 s6 kinase by kinase activity of FRAP in vivo [published erratum appears in Nature 1995 Dec 7;378(6557):644]. Nature 1995; 377:441–446.

167. Sabatini DM, Erdjument-Bromage H, Lui M, et al. RAFT1: a mammalian protein that binds to FKBP12 in a rapamycin-dependent fashion and is homologous to yeast TORs. Cell 1994;78:35–43.

168. Dennis PB, Fumagalli S, Thomas G. Target of rapamycin (TOR): balancing the opposing forces of protein synthesis and degradation. Curr Opin Genet Dev 1999;9:49–54.

169. Beretta L, Gingras AC, Svitkin YV, et al. Rapamycin blocks the phosphorylation of 4E-BP1 and inhibits cap-dependent initiation of translation. EMBO J 1996;15:658–664.

170. Thomas G, Hall MN. TOR signalling and control of cell growth. Curr Opin Cell Biol 1997;9:782–787.

171. Jefferies HB, Fumagalli S, Dennis PB, et al. Rapamycin suppresses 5′TOP mRNA translation through inhibition of p70s6k. EMBO J 1997;16:3693–3704.

172. Levy S, Avni D, Hariharan N, et al. Oligopyrimidine tract at the 5′ end of mammalian ribosomal protein mRNAs is required for their translational control. Proc Natl Acad Sci USA 1991;88:3319–3323.

173. Chen J, Zheng XF, Brown EJ, et al. Identification of an 11-kDa FKBP12-rapamycin-binding domain within the 289-kDa FKBP12-rapamycin-associated protein and characterization of a critical serine residue. Proc Natl Acad Sci USA 1995;92:4947–4951.

174. Vilella-Bach M, Nuzzi P, Fang Y, et al. The FKBP12-rapamycin-binding domain is required for FKBP12-rapamycin-associated protein kinase activity and G1 progression. J Biol Chem 1999;274:4266–4272.

175. Schmidt A, Bickle M, Beck T, et al. The yeast phosphatidylinositol kinase homolog TOR2 activates RHO1 and RHO2 via the exchange factor ROM2. Cell 1997;88: 531–542.

176. Choi J, Chen J, Schreiber SL, et al. Structure of the FKBP12-rapamycin complex interacting with the binding domain of human FRAP. Science 1996;273:239–242.

177. Liang J, Choi J, Clardy J. Refined structure of the FKBP12-rapamycin-FRB ternary complex at 2.2 A resolution. Acta Crystallogr D Biol Crystallogr 1999;55:736–744.

178. Dennis PB, Pullen N, Kozma SC, et al. The principal rapamycin-sensitive p70(s6k) phosphorylation sites, T-229 and T-389, are differentially regulated by rapamycin-insensitive kinase kinases. Mol Cell Biol 1996;16:6242–6251.

179. Kawasome H, Papst P, Webb S, et al. Targeted disruption of p70(s6k) defines its role in protein synthesis and rapamycin sensitivity. Proc Natl Acad Sci USA 1998;95:5033–5038.

180. Peterson RT, Desai BN, Hardwick JS, et al. Protein phosphatase 2A interacts with the 70-kDa S6 kinase and is activated by inhibition of FKBP12-rapamycin-associated protein. Proc Natl Acad Sci USA 1999;96:4438–4442.

181. U.S. Multicenter FK506 Liver Study Group. A comparison of tacrolimus (FK506) and cyclosporine for immunosuppression in liver transplantation. New Engl J Med 1994; 331:1110–1115.

182. European FK506 Multicentre Liver Study Group. Randomised trial comparing tacrolimus (FK506) and cyclosporin in prevention of liver allograft rejection. Lancet 1994;344:423–428.

183. Jain A, Reyes J, Kashyap R, et al. What have we learned about primary liver transplantation under tacrolimus immunosuppression? Long-term follow-up of the first 1000 patients. Ann Surg 1999;230:441–448.

184. Gruessner RW. Tacrolimus in pancreas transplantation: a multicenter analysis. Tacrolimus Pancreas Transplant Study Group. Clin Transplant 1997;11:299–312.

185. Henry ML. Cyclosporine and tacrolimus (FK506): a comparison of efficacy and safety profiles. Clin Transplant 1999; 13:209–220.

186. Benfield MR, Stablein D, Tejani A. Trends in immunosuppressive therapy: a report of the North American Pediatric Renal Transplant Cooperative Study (NAPRTCS). Pediatr Transplant 1999;3:27–32.

187. Taylor DO, Barr ML, Radovancevic B, et al. A randomized, multicenter comparison of tacrolimus and cyclosporine immunosuppressive regimens in cardiac transplantation: decreased hyperlipidemia and hypertension with tacrolimus. J Heart Lung Transplant 1999;18:336–345.

188. Ghasemian SR, Light JA, Currier C, et al. Tacrolimus vs Neoral in renal and renal/pancreas transplantation. Clin Transplant 1999;13:123–125.

189. Knoll GA, Bell RC. Tacrolimus versus cyclosporin for immunosuppression in renal transplantation: meta-analysis of randomised trials. Br Med J 1999;318:1104–1107.

190. Shield CF III, McGrath MM, Goss TF. Assessment of health-related quality of life in kidney transplant patients receiving tacrolimus (FK506)-based versus cyclosporine-based immunosuppression. FK506 Kidney Transplant Study Group. Transplantation 1997;64:1738–1743.

191. Neylan JF, Sullivan EM, Steinwald B, et al. Assessment of the frequency and costs of posttansplantation hospitalizations in patients receiving tacrolimus versus cyclosporine. Am J Kidney Dis 1998;32:770–777.

192. Ratanatharathorn V, Nash RA, Przepiorka D, et al. Phase III study comparing methotrexate and tacrolimus (prograf, FK506) with methotrexate and cyclosporine for graft-versus-host disease prophylaxis after HLA-identical sibling bone marrow transplantation. Blood 1998;92:2303–2314.

193. Horowitz MM, Przepiorka D, Bartels P, et al. Tacrolimus vs. cyclosporine immunosuppression: results in advanced-stage disease compared with historical controls treated exclusively with cyclosporine. Biol Blood Marrow Transplant 1999;5:180–186.

194. Przepiorka D, Ippoliti C, Khouri I, et al. Allogeneic transplantation for advanced leukemia: improved short-term outcome with blood stem cell grafts and tacrolimus. Transplantation 1996;62:1806–1810.

195. Nash RA, Pineiro LA, Storb R, et al. FK506 in combination with methotrexate for the prevention of graft-versus-host disease after marrow transplantation from matched unrelated donors. Blood 1996;88:3634–3641.

196. Devine SM, Geller RB, Lin LB, et al. The outcome of unrelated donor bone marrow transplantation in patients with hematologic malignancies using tacrolimus (FK506) and low dose methotrexate for graft-versus-host disease prophylaxis. Biol Blood Marrow Transplant 1997;3:25–33.

197. Boswell GW, Bekersky I, Fay J, et al. Tacrolimus pharmacokinetics in BMT patients. Bone Marrow Transplant 1998;21: 23–28.

198. Wingard JR, Nash RA, Przepiorka D, et al. Relationship of tacrolimus (FK506) whole blood concentrations and efficacy and safety after HLA-identical sibling bone marrow transplantation. Biol Blood Marrow Transplant 1998;4:157–163.

199. Przepiorka D, Nash RA, Wingard JR, et al. Relationship of tacrolimus whole blood levels to efficacy and safety outcomes after unrelated donor marrow transplantation. Biol Blood Marrow Transplant 1999;5:94–97.

200. Akselband Y, Harding MW, Nelson PA. Rapamycin inhibits spontaneous and fibroblast growth factor β-stimulated proliferation of endothelial cells and fibroblasts. Transplant Proc 1991;23:2833–2836.

201. Gregory CR, Morris RE, Pratt R, et al. The use of new antiproliferative immunosuppressants is a novel and highly effective strategy for the prevention of vascular occlusive disease. J Heart Lung Transplant 1992;11:197.

202. Gregory CR, Huie P, Billingham MB, et al. Rapamycin inhibits arterial intimal thickening caused by both alloimmune and mechanical injury: its effect on cellular, growth factor, and cytokine response in injured vessels. Transplantation 1993;55:1409–1418.

203. Gregory CR, Pratt RE, Huie P, et al. Effects of treatment with cyclosporine, FK 506, rapamycin, mycophenolic acid, or

deoxyspergualin on vascular muscle proliferation in vitro and in vivo. Transplant Proc 1993;25:770–771.

204. Poston RS, Billingham M, Hoyt EG, et al. Rapamycin reverses chronic graft vascular disease in a novel cardiac allograft model. Circulation 1999;100:67–74.

205. Zhu J, Wu J, Frizell E, et al. Rapamycin inhibits hepatic stellate cell proliferation in vitro and limits fibrogenesis in an in vivo model of liver fibrosis. Gastroenterology 1999;117: 1198–1204.

206. Qi S, Xu D, Peng J, et al. Synergistic effect of rapamycin and cyclosporine in prevention of acute kidney allograft rejection in the mouse. Microsurgery 1999;19:344–347.

207. Hausen B, Boeke K, Berry GJ, et al. Coadministration of neoral and the novel rapamycin analog, SDZ RAD, to rat lung allograft recipients: potentiation of immunosuppressive efficacy and improvement of tolerability of staggered versus simultaneous treatment. Transplantation 1999;67: 956–962.

208. Saggi BH, Fisher RA, Naar JD, et al. Intragraft cytokine expression in tolerant rat renal allografts with rapamycin and cyclosporin immunosuppression. Clin Transplant 1999; 13:90–97.

209. Blazar BR, Taylor PA, Panoskaltsis-Mortari A, et al. Rapamycin inhibits the generation of graft-versus-host disease- and graft-versus-leukemia-causing T cells by interfering with the production of Th1 or Th1 cytotoxic cytokines. J Immunol 1998;160:5355–5365.

210. Kahan BD, Podbielski J, Napoli KL, et al. Immunosuppressive effects and safety of a sirolimus/cyclosporine combination regimen for renal transplantation. Transplantation 1998;66:1040–1046.

211. Kahan BD, Julian BA, Pescovitz MD, et al. Sirolimus reduces the incidence of acute rejection episodes despite lower cyclosporine doses in Caucasian recipients of mismatched primary renal allografts: a phase II trial. Rapamune Study Group. Transplantation 1999;68:1526–1532.

212. Watson CJ, Friend PJ, Jamieson NV, et al. Sirolimus: a potent new immunosuppressant for liver transplantation. Transplantation 1999;67:505–509.

213. Kahan BD. The potential role of rapamycin in pediatric transplantation as observed from adult studies. Pediatr Transplant 1999;3:175–180.

214. Murgia MG, Jordan S, Kahan BD. The side effect profile of sirolimus: a phase I study in quiescent cyclosporine-prednisone-treated renal transplant patients. Kidney International 1996;49:209–216.

215. Groth CG, Backman L, Morales JM, et al. Sirolimus (rapamycin)-based therapy in human renal transplantation: similar efficacy and different toxicity compared with cyclosporine. Sirolimus European Renal Transplant Study Group. Transplantation 1999;67:1036–1042.

216. Yatscoff RW. Pharmacokinetics of rapamycin. Transplant Proc 1996;28:970–973.

217. Kaplan B, Meier-Kriesche HU, Napoli KL, et al. The effects of relative timing of sirolimus and cyclosporine microemulsion formulation coadministration on the pharmacokinetics of each agent. Clin Pharmacol Ther 1998;63:48–53.

218. Kahan BD, Wong RL, Carter C, et al. A phase I study of a 4-week course of SDZ-RAD (RAD) quiescent cyclosporine-prednisone-treated renal transplant recipients. Transplantation 1999;68:1100–1106.

219. Vu MD, Qi S, Xu D, et al. Synergistic effects of mycophenolate mofetil and sirolimus in prevention of acute heart, pancreas, and kidney allograft rejection and in reversal of ongoing heart allograft rejection in the rat. Transplantation 1998;66:1575–1580.

220. Li Y, Zheng XX, Li XC, et al. Combined costimulation blockade plus rapamycin but not cyclosporine produces permanent engraftment. Transplantation 1998;66:1387–1388.

221. Hong JC, Kahan BD. Use of anti-CD25 monoclonal antibody in combination with rapamycin to eliminate cyclosporine treatment during the induction phase of immunosuppression. Transplantation 1999;68:701–704.

222. Starzl TE, Demetris AJ, Murase N, et al. Cell migration, chimerism, and graft acceptance. Lancet 1992;339:1579–1582.

223. Kim JO, Nau MM, Allikian KA, et al. Co-amplification of a novel cyclophilin-like gene (PPIE) with L-myc in small cell lung cancer cell lines. Oncogene 1998;17:1019–1026.

224. Teigelkamp S, Achsel T, Mundt C, et al. The 20kD protein of human [U4/U6.U5] tri-snRNPs is a novel cyclophilin that forms a complex with the U4/U6-specific 60kD and 90kD proteins. RNA 1998;4:127–141.

Chapter 7

Glucocorticoid Action

Jeffrey N. Miner
Myles Brown

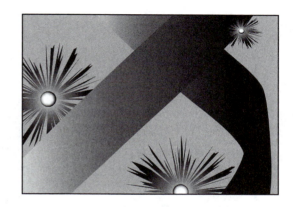

Glucocorticoids are used in the treatment of a wide variety of inflammatory disorders. Since their discovery in the middle of the twentieth century and the observation that "compound E" (cortisone) was an effective treatment for rheumatoid arthritis (1), glucocorticoids have become one of the most widely used of all classes of therapeutics. While these agents are highly effective, serious systemic side effects often limit their use. This chapter will review the current state of knowledge of glucocorticoid action at a molecular level and will outline the mechanistic bases for several clinical uses and for important side effects. In addition, it will point to the possibility that advances in the understanding of the molecular mechanisms underlying the beneficial effects of glucocorticoids hold the promise of finding selective glucocorticoid receptor (GR) modulators that eliminate some of the most serious side effects.

Physiology

The sex hormones, mineralocorticoids, and glucocorticoids are all produced by the adrenal cortex from cholesterol. Physiologic glucocorticoid production is primarily under the control of the hypothalamic-pituitary-adrenal (HPA) axis. Corticotropin-releasing hormone (CRH) and arginine vasopressin (AVP) are produced by the hypothalamus and regulate the pituitary production of corticotropin (ACTH). ACTH in turn acts on the adrenal to regulate the production and secretion of cortisol. Cortisol acts on the pituitary and hypothalamus to decrease production of both CRH and ACTH in a prototypical feedback loop. In response to stress, such as starvation, glucocorticoid levels increase. This evolutionarily conserved stress response probably explains the pleiotropic effects of glucocorticoids on a wide range of functions including regulation of metabolism, anti-inflammatory and immunosuppressive actions, and effects on mood and cognitive functions. These adaptive actions of glucocorticoids in response to stress are the basis of both the therapeutic effects and many of the side effects of chronic glucocorticoid use (2).

Pharmacology

The effects of glucocorticoids are regulated at multiple levels. For example, cortisone requires metabolic activation in the liver, and to a lesser extent in other tissues, to its active metabolite, cortisol. This is also the case for prednisone that must be converted to prednisolone in order to bind the glucocorticoid receptor efficiently. Traditional medicinal chemistry has led to the development of glucocorticoids with altered pharmacokinetics and receptor binding affinity. These approaches, as pointed out below, have been effective in the development of potent glucocorticoids that either are not absorbed well systemically or have short systemic half-lives for topical uses on the skin and in the lungs and gastrointestinal tract (3). In the circulation, glucocorticoids are highly protein bound, and once they reach target tissues they are under metabolic control. This is necessary because cortisol actually has a higher affinity for the mineralocorticoid receptor (MR) than it has for the GR. To avoid exerting mineralocorticoid effects in the kidneys, cortisol is degraded through the action of 11β-hydroxysteroid dehydrogenase (11β-HSD).

Molecular Biology

General Mechanism of Steroid Hormone Action

Glucocorticoids exert their effects, like other steroids, by binding to specific intracellular receptors. The glucocorticoid receptor (GR) is a member of a family of transcription factors that regulate gene expression in response to ligand binding. Cloning of GR and the other members of the nuclear receptor family has led to a detailed molecular understanding of many of the aspects of glucocorticoid action. While not all effects of steroid hormones are explained by their interactions with this class of receptors, these effects are the best understood. The genetic manipulation of these receptors through targeted gene disruption in the mouse should allow the more complete definition of the so far elusive non-receptor-mediated effects of steroid hormones. This chapter will focus exclusively on effects of glucocorticoids mediated by intracellular steroid hormone receptors.

While all of the details of the mechanism of transcriptional regulation remain to be worked out, there is now a general understanding of the broad outlines of the pathway [Fig. 7-1; for review, see (4)]. Glucocorticoids are small lipophilic molecules that freely cross plasma membranes, and thus their receptors do not require an extracellular domain. In the absence of glucocorticoids, the

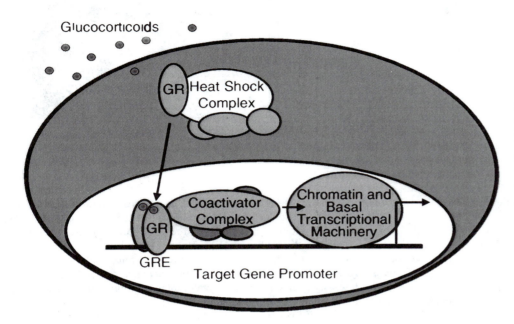

Figure 7-1. Model of glucocorticoid receptor function. Glucocorticoids enter the cell by diffusion and bind the glucocorticoid receptor (GR) in the cytoplasm where it exists in a heat shock protein containing chaperone complex. Hormone binding stimulates receptor dimerization, translocation of the receptor into the nucleus, and specific DNA binding to the glucocortiocoid responsive element (GRE) in target genes. Following DNA binding, the receptor recruits a coactivator complex with histone acetyltransferase activity to relieve the general repressive effects of chromatin and to stimulate the activity of the basal transcriptional machinery.

GR is held in the cytoplasm by a chaperone complex of heat shock proteins in an inactive but hormone-receptive state. This complex contains hsp90, hsp70, and smaller heat shock proteins including the cyclophilins (5). Once hormone binds, these chaperones are released, and the receptor translocates to the nucleus, dimerizes, associates, and binds tightly to specific palindromic DNA sequences termed glucocorticoid responsive elements (GRE) found in the promoters of target genes. Once bound to promoter sequences, the hormone-bound receptor recruits a complex of proteins, termed the coactivator complex (see below). This complex acts in two ways: first, by directly contacting and stabilizing components of the core transcriptional machinery; and second, by utilizing potent histone acetyltransferase activity carried by components of the complex to loosen the nucleosomal structure of the promoter, allowing better access by transcription factors. This model explains the ability of GR to activate directly the transcription of target genes. Less well understood, but also important for GR action, is its ability to regulate directly and negatively the expression of certain target genes.

Receptor Structure

Cloning of GR and the other members of the nuclear receptor family has led to important insights into both the physiology mediated by steroid hormones and the possible approaches to improving their use as therapeutics through increasing their selectivity. The human glucocorticoid receptor is a 777 amino acid protein. Functional studies and comparisons with other family members have revealed that these transcription factors are made up of several discrete and identifiable structural and functional domains (Fig. 7-2). The N-terminus of the molecule contains a ligand-independent transactivation domain, AF1 or τ1. The

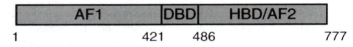

Figure 7-2. Domain structure of the glucocorticoid receptor. Numbers represent amino acid positions. AF1, constitutive activation domain (also known as τ1); DBD, DNA-binding domain; HBD, hormone-binding domain; AF2, ligand-dependent activation domain (also known as τ2).

central portion of the receptor contains the DNA-binding domain. This domain is characterized by two zinc nucleated alpha helices. The first of these helices makes specific contacts in the major groove of DNA while the second serves both to buttress this domain and as a dimerization interface. These details are understood at the atomic level, because an x-ray crystal structure of the DNA-binding domain has been solved (6). The C-terminal portion of the molecule contains the hormone-binding domain and a ligand-dependent activation function, AF2 or τ2. While the detailed structure of this domain has not been reported for GR, the hormone-binding domain of closely related receptors including estrogen receptor (ER) and progesterone receptor have been solved. This domain consists of a series of 12 alpha helices that form a hydrophobic core into which the ligand is entirely submerged. The most significant findings come from the comparison of agonist- and antagonist-bound receptors. These comparisons reveal significant structural differences between the complexes, most notably in the repositioning of helix 12. For example, when ER is bound to the antagonist 4-hydroxytamoxifen (4-OHT), helix 12 assumes a position that prevents binding of coactivators (see below). In contrast, binding of agonists such as estradiol and diethylstilbestrol (DES) allows helix 12 of ER to assume a posi-

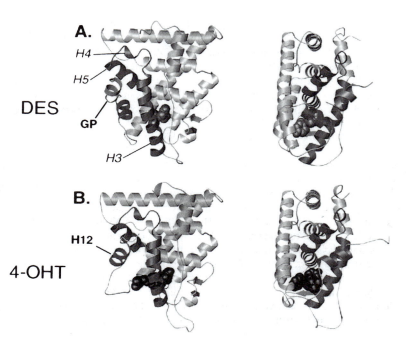

Figure 7-3. Structural basis for differential activity of steroid receptor ligands. Front and side views of the structure of the estrogen receptor (ER) hormone-binding domain bound (A) to the agonist diethyl-stilbesterol (DES) and the GRIP1 receptor interaction domain peptide and (B) to the antagonist 4-hydroxytamoxifen (4-OHT). The hormone-binding domain and GRIP1 peptide are shown as ribbon diagrams. The ligands are shown as space-filling models. Helices 3(*H3*), 4(*H4*), and 5(*H5*) of the hormone-binding domains are shown in black. Helix 12(*H12*) is shown in gray. The GRIP1 peptide (*GP*) is shown in gray. The remainder of the hormone-binding domain is shown in light gray. (Reproduced with permission from Shiau AK, Barstad D, Loria PM, et al. The structural basis of estrogen receptor/coactivator recognition and the antagonism of this interaction by tamoxifen. Cell 1998;95(7):927–937.)

tion in which a hydrophobic groove is formed in conjunction with other residues within the hormone-binding domain to facilitate binding by coactivators (7) (see Fig. 7.2).

Coactivators

As noted above, ligand binding activates the AF2/τ2 function of GR. A combination of approaches has identified a number of coregulatory molecules involved in nuclear receptor function [for a review, see (8)]. Although we now have an overview of these pathways, the details of which coregulators mediate which functions of individual receptors remain to be filled in. These coregulators fall into several classes. The p160 coactivators were first identified biochemically as factors that could interact with ER and other receptors dependent on agonist binding. This family includes at least three genes in humans: SRC-1 (or NcoA-1), TIF2 (or GRIP1, NcoA-2), and AIB1 (or ACTR, RAC3, p/CIP, TRAM). These factors make direct contacts with the receptor, and detailed structural data is available concerning these interactions (Fig. 7-3). It is likely that differential usage of the various members of this family of coactivators may impart both tissue- and promoter-specific activities to the receptor. There is currently no detailed description of the pattern of expression of these factors in the cells targeted by the anti-inflammatory effects of glucocorticoids.

Two highly related coactivators, CREB Binding Protein (CBP) and p300, also are likely to play important roles in modulating GR signaling. This class of coactivators has been implicated in the functioning of a very wide variety of transcription factors that mediate the effects of a multitude of signaling pathways. CBP and p300 have been postulated to serve an integrative

function through interactions with multiple signaling pathways. CBP and p300 exhibit a potent histone acetyltransferase activity that is critical for their ability to mediate steroid receptor signaling. In terms of immune function, p300 and CBP are involved in signaling by AP-1, NFκB, NFAT, and STAT pathways. GR and the other steroid receptors are thought to interact primarily with CBP/p300 indirectly. This interaction is mediated through a direct interaction of the receptors with p160 family members, which in turn interact directly with p300 or CBP. In addition, the other transcription factors, such as AP-1, target distinct regions of p300 or CBP. Although not yet established, p300 or CBP may serve in some cases to mediate the crosstalk between GR and these other pathways involved in immune modulation.

Various other factors have also been implicated in steroid receptor function. These include the p300/CBP-associated factor, P/CAF. This factor is the mammalian homolog of the yeast protein GCN5 and is, like CBP and p300, a histone acetyltransferase. Another enzyme implicated in GR-mediated activation is CARM1, an H3 histone methyltransferase (9). Under which conditions each of these coregulators plays a role in GR function remains to be sorted out. This complexity raises the possibility that there may be opportunities to develop new GR ligands that have unique partial agonist activity based on favoring the interaction of GR with one or another of these coregulators.

Crosstalk with Other Pathways

Surprisingly, given the general model of steroid receptor function, relatively few target genes containing GREs in their promoters have been found. This is especially true for genes involved in regulating immune responses. GR is able both to stimulate and to inhibit gene expression in response to hormone binding and direct promoter binding. The best example of this is the negative regulation of the pro-opiomelanocortin (POMC) gene through direct interaction of GR with a negative GRE (nGRE) located in the POMC promoter (10).

Other genes are negatively regulated by a GR in the absence of direct binding of the receptor to GRE sequences. These effects mediated by liganded GR interfere with the activity of a variety of regulatory pathways, including the cAMP-responsive transcription factor CREB, and AP-1. Significantly, AP-1 activity is stimulated by a wide variety of extracellular signals, including many proinflammatory cytokines.

Several transcription factors are now thought to be regulators of genes critical to the inflammatory response. These factors include members of the AP-1, NFκB, NFAT, and STAT families. There is evidence to suggest crosstalk between GR and each of these pathways. While the exact mechanisms are not fully appreciated, this suggests that a solution to the paradox of a lack of critical direct GRE containing target genes is that GR is able to regulate genes through an indirect mechanism involving interactions with other transcription factors (11). GR-mediated inhibition of AP-1 and NFκB are thought to play central roles in the anti-inflammatory effects of glucocorticoids. AP-1 activity is stimulated by many proinflammatory cytokines. Inhibition of AP-1 activity by GR does not require GR-DNA binding.

Central to the effects of glucocorticoids on the immune system is its ability to inhibit activation of critical target genes by NFκB. These genes include many immune modulatory molecules such as cytokines and chemokines. Two models have been proposed to explain the mechanism by which glucocorticoids inhibit NFκB activity. The first is the ability of glucocorticoids to induce IκB, the NFκB inhibitor. Perhaps more importantly, GR may directly inhibit the ability of NFκB to activate target genes. In this model, GR acts without DNA binding to repress NFκB-dependent gene expression (Fig. 7-4). What factors other than GR are required for this effect remains to be determined. There is evidence to suggest that there is a direct interaction between GR and the NFκB subunits p65 and p50. The zinc finger domain of GR is necessary for the inhibition of both NFκB and AP-1 although DNA binding per se is not required (12). This lack of a requirement for GR-DNA binding is supported by work done on mice. Reichardt and coworkers have "knocked-in" a mutant allele of GR that is unable to dimerize and therefore is severely defective in GRE binding (13). In these mice, direct GR target genes such as tyrosine aminotransferase (TAT) cannot be regulated by glucocorticoids, nor can directly negatively regulated genes such as POMC. In contrast to the postnatal lethal phenotype of mice harboring two null alleles of GR, mice containing the DNA binding/dimerization defective allele are relatively healthy in the absence of stress. Importantly, these mice are not defective in the ability of GR to regulate negatively AP-1 and NFκB target genes. Thus, in the current model of the mechanism by which glucocorticoids influence immune function, NFκB, AP-1, and GR interact in a complex regulatory network that results in glucocorticoid-mediated repression of cytokine transcription.

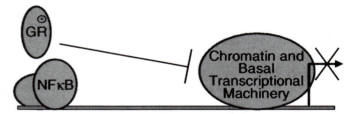

NFκB Target Gene Promoter

Figure 7-4. Model of ligand-dependent transrepression of NFκB action by glucocorticoids. Ligand-bound glucocorticoid receptor (GR) inhibits the ability of NFκB to activate target genes such as cytokines in the absence of direct GR-DNA binding.

Modulation of Cytokine Function by Glucocorticoids

Glucocorticoids inhibit the production of a wide variety of proinflammatory cytokines, including IL-1α, IL-1β, IL-2, IL-3, IL-5, IL-6, IL-8, IL-12, IFN-γ, TNF-α, and GM-CSF [for a review, see (14)]. These effects have been postulated to be the basis of the anti-inflammatory effects of glucocorticoids. Somewhat paradoxically, it has been reported that many of these same cytokines' receptors are actually increased by glucocorticoids. These include the IL-1 receptor (IL-1R) and the gp130 common subunit of IL-6R and IL-11R, among others. At present, there is no comprehensive picture of the overall effects of glucocorticoids on any of these pathways. However, these opposing effects of glucocorticoids may explain the lack of efficacy of glucocorticoids under conditions such as sepsis, in which down-regulation of cytokines such as TNF-α might be expected to be beneficial. A full understanding of the effects of glucocorticoids, both in different cell types and over time, will be required in order to predict under which scenarios glucocorticoids might be most effective. In addition, the differential mechanisms involved in GR-mediated activation and repression offer the possibility of developing novel GR ligands with selective properties.

General Aspects of Glucocorticoid Therapy

Glucocorticoids are used in several different clinical settings: in replacement therapy for various adrenal insufficiency syndromes (15), in anti-inflammatory therapy for rheumatoid arthritis and asthma, and in immunosuppressive therapy for transplant rejection and autoimmune disorders (16). Glucocorticoids are also used therapeutically for treatment of various lymphomas and leukemias and palliatively during treatment of certain solid tumors and late-stage metastatic cancers. This chapter will concentrate on the anti-inflammatory and immunomodulatory aspects of glucocorticoid therapy, analyzing the mechanisms of efficacy and of the adverse sequelae that occur when glucocorticoids are used.

Risk Versus Benefit

Glucocorticoids are among the most effective agents available to the clinician for treatment of inflammation. However, after the decision has been made to place a patient on glucocorticoid therapy, the primary challenge for the physician is balancing efficacy against side effects. The longer patients are exposed to glucocorticoids, the more the side effects become apparent (17–19). This balancing act between risk and benefit, while problematic for many drugs, is especially pronounced for glucocorticoids because of the exceptional efficacy of these molecules. Even the cessation of glucocorticoid therapy is complicated by the need to taper the dosage. Reduction in endogenous cortisol production by the adrenal glands secondary to suppression of the hypothalamic-pituitary-adrenal (HPA) axis occurs rapidly after exogenous steroid administration (17). Tapering the steroid dosage allows time for the production of endogenous cortisol to resume, reducing the chance of adrenal insufficiency. In addition, removing steroids abruptly can cause a significant flare in the inflammatory disease being treated, perhaps owing to a sudden increase in prostaglandin production (15,17). For these reasons, patients are typically weaned off steroids slowly.

Structure Activity Relationship

Currently used steroids are believed to differ from each other at the receptor only in their affinity for the glucocorticoid receptor. There are differences in biologic half-life, but generally the anti-inflammatory activity of a given steroid and its side effects are directly related to its affinity for the receptor (e.g., dexamethasone > prednisolone > cortisol) (20). This apparent linkage has hindered the development of new and more selective steroids (21). There are differences, however, in the relative cross-reactivity with the mineralocorticoid receptor; several of the synthetic glucocorticoids (dexamethasone and prednisolone) have less interaction with MR than the endogenous glucocorticoid cortisol (22).

Pharmacokinetics

Significant patient-to-patient variation exists in relative exposure for a given dosage of glucocorticoids. This variation is due in part to differences in the conversion of certain pro-drug steroids (e.g., prednisone and cortisone) into active forms (e.g., prednisolone and cortisol) (23,24). In addition, differences in either the amount or the capacity of corticosteroid-binding proteins in the serum may play a role in variable patient responses (25–27). Steroids are available in oral, topical, and intravenous formulations. Topical administration is almost always preferred when appropriate because of the potential reduction in side effects, but even topical administration is not without its complications (28–30). In addition, administration of other drugs together with steroids can produce either more or less exposure to the glucocorticoid as a result of changes in steroid elimination and metabolism or changes in parallel inhibitory or synergistic physiologic processes (22). Faced with this problem, it is essential that physicians monitor closely both the efficacy and side effects of a particular dosage regimen in each patient. In fact, although it has rarely been done, some have recommended the monitoring of serum corticosteroid concentrations during therapy (31).

Examples of Clinical Uses

The anti-inflammatory and immunomodulatory uses for corticosteroids include, but are not limited to, asthma, allergy, various dermatological disorders, rheumatoid arthritis, inflammatory bowel disease, and organ and tissue transplantation. The description that follows compares and contrasts the specific issues and mechanisms associated with glucocorticoid use for each disorder.

Asthma

Bronchial asthma is characterized by the development of significant pathologic airway inflammation. Triggers for this phenomenon can be either immune (allergens) or nonimmune (exercise, cold air inhalation, or chemical exposure). Exposure to these inducers leads to hyperplasia of bronchial smooth muscle, significant infiltration of eosinophils and neutrophils into lung tissue, degranulation of these cells resulting in inappropriate deposition of cellular proteins at sites of injury, and a buildup of thick protein-containing mucus in the airway itself (30). It is this accumulation that causes the blockage of airways characteristic of severe asthma. The release of inflammatory mediators in the lung in response to various triggers is a factor in the progression of the disease. These mediators conspire to constrict both peripheral airways and pulmonary vasculature, as well as increasing the permeability of airway microvasculature. This causes increased edema, mucus secretion, and eventual damage to lung epithelium (32,33). In excess of 50 different inflammatory mediators have been identified (34), many of which are redundant, which perhaps explains why therapeutic approaches targeting any single mediator have not shown significant efficacy.

A typical asthmatic response consists of two components: early and late. The early response to antigen begins within 10 minutes of antigen exposure and ends between 1 and 3 hours later. This particular response is thought to result from mediators released by mast cells (35). For steroids to be effective at this stage, patients must have been previously dosed 1 to 4 weeks prior to exposure to antigen (36). Dosing with steroid just prior to or during challenge is ineffective; adrenergics, however, are effective inhibitors at this stage (37). In contrast, the late asthmatic response is considerably more responsive to steroid treatment and begins approximately 3 hours after the early response has ended and lasts for about 12 hours. This stage of inflammation is quite complex, and exactly which inflammatory cells participate depends on the type of inducer that triggered it. However, the significant influx of eosinophils and/or neutrophils into lung tissue clearly is a precipitating event (38,39).

Glucocorticoids act on this disease at multiple points. The ability of glucocorticoids to inhibit the influx, activation, and degranulation of eosinophils and neutrophils in lung tissue probably explains the effectiveness of glucocorticoids in the treatment of the late asthmatic response (30). They inhibit cytokine-mediator production by several cell types involved in asthma, including mast cells, eosinophils, and lymphocytes—in particular, Th2 CD4 positive T cells. Inflammatory cytokines inhibited by glucocorticoids include both TNF-α and IL-1, among others (40). Glucocorticoids also decrease the synthesis of a number of small molecule inflammatory mediators such as histamine, platelet activating factor, and derivatives of arachidonic acid (prostaglandins, leukotrienes, and thromboxanes), the levels of which are correlated with the severity of the disease (41).

The incidence of both adult and pediatric asthma is apparently on the rise in the industrialized world (34), and many novel pharmacologic approaches to this disease are currently in clinical trials. Nevertheless, the mainstay of treatment remains the inhalation of corticosteroids. The use of inhaled formulation allows direct delivery of the steroid to affected tissue, both rapid and sustained action when used with beta-agonist bronchodilators such as albuterol (Ventolin), and a relatively safe side effect profile (42). The side effects associated with this form of treatment are usually oralpharyngeal candidiasis and dysphonia. There is some evidence for transient and reversible HPA suppression and growth suppression at high dosages, but other studies at lower but still efficacious dosages have shown no effects on these parameters (43–45).

Chronic Obstructive Pulmonary Disease (COPD)

Chronic obstructive pulmonary disease is a persistent reduction in the volume and force of exhalation resulting from any of several causes. Patients with a long history of asthma have an increased risk of developing COPD, although the bronchitis and emphysema brought on by smoking are more commonly associated with this disorder. Although they are often prescribed, it is not clear that glucocorticoids are effective at reducing treatment failure rate in patients hospitalized with exacerbations of COPD. The results from the Systemic Corticosteroids in Chronic Obstructive Pulmonary Disease Exacerbations Trial, or SCCOPE trial, have begun to answer this question (46–48). This and other trials are testing the impact of both long- and short-term corticosteroid use on treatment failure rate in hospitalized COPD patients. The results indicate that the impact of corticosteroids in this setting is "quite limited" in comparison with the results found in the treatment of asthma. The reason for this difference is not known, but several authors have speculated that it may lie in the types of cells that mediate the two diseases. In contrast to asthma (see above), inflammatory cells mediating COPD may be more resistant to glucocorticoid action. These cells include neutrophils and type 1 helper T cells responding to and producing the chemoattractant IL-8. There would need to be a tissue-specific reason for the poor activity of glucocorticoids in COPD because neutrophils and IL-8 are well-characterized targets for these drugs in rheumatoid arthritis (15,49–52). The mechanism notwithstanding, the use of glucocorticoids in COPD flares does

indeed have value—at least during the first few weeks of administration (48,53).

Allergy

Seasonal allergic rhinitis or hay fever and perennial rhinitis are both responsive to glucocorticoids. These ailments are characterized by the same types of inflammatory responses described for asthma. Inhaled allergens (hay fever) and other events (perennial rhinitis) trigger local edema, mucus production, mediator release, and inflammatory cell influx into the nasal cavity. Glucocorticoids inhibit all of these events. Although oral steroids are used for these indications, inhaled formulations have gained widespread acceptance (54–58). The use of inhaled steroids is reasonable given data suggesting that the allergic response actually originates in the epithelial tissues on the surface of the nasal mucosa itself. Injection of histamine (an inflammatory mediator) into the nasal mucosa causes only minor local edema, but spraying histamine onto the surface of the nasal mucosa results in all the symptoms of allergic rhinitis (59).

Dermatologic Disorders

Topical steroid treatment has revolutionized dermatology. The clinician can effectively halt the progression of a number of allergen- and autoimmune-mediated skin diseases. These diseases include atopic dermatitis, psoriasis, and seborrheic dermatitis, all of which are responsive to topical formulations of glucocorticoid (60). A key advance in the development of active compounds for these topical indications was the discovery that certain chemical modifications of the steroid backbone (including fluorination) enhanced topical potency, which led to the development of drugs such as betamethasone dipropionate (Diprosone) and fluocinonide (Lidex, Topsyn). Chronic use can lead to skin atrophy, however (3). As with any glucocorticoid, efficacy must be balanced against the potential for adverse side effects, which increase with both dosage and potency.

Rheumatoid Arthritis (RA)

This autoimmune disease most commonly affects women between the ages of 30 and 40, although men, teens, and children are also susceptible, resulting in a total U.S. incidence of 3%. These patients experience progressively worsening inflammation of synovial tissues with joint pain, joint degradation, and edema. One model for the initiation of RA suggests that bacterial infections (streptococcus and mycoplasma) can trigger autoimmune responses in dormant, self-recognizing T cells as a result of short regions of homology between bacterial proteins and human "self" peptides. Patients are initially treated with nonsteroidal anti-inflammatory drugs (NSAIDs). These drugs inhibit a key enzyme in the pathway for prostaglandin synthesis (cyclooxygenase and/or prostaglandin synthase). There are two isoforms of this protein, COX1 and COX2. COX2 mediates inflammation and COX1 acts in the gut. Inhibition of COX1 results in increased risk of gastropathy, and thus significant efforts have gone into preparing COX2-selective agents. The recent introduction of selective COX2 inhibitors will likely help reduce the gastric disturbance associated with the use of NSAIDs (61). Although treatment with NSAIDs provides significant benefit, the often inexorable progression of the RA eventually leads to the use of glucocorticoids. Steroids have been shown to be very effective at inhibiting signs and symptoms of the inflammation associated with RA, but unfortunately have little effect on structural damage that has already occurred in the joints. Furthermore, steroids do not necessarily prevent ongoing joint erosion, but merely slow the progression of the disease. RA patients on glucocorticoids for any length of time can experience significant rebound effects of the disease if taken off the therapy (62).

The mechanism of glucocorticoid action again involves diverse impacts on both immune and inflammatory processes. Glucocorticoids inhibit the production of both inflammatory cytokines and immunoglobulins as well as preventing the adhesion and transmigration of leukocytes into the affected joints (15,49–52). The tissue damage associated with RA has been tied to the degradative actions of neutrophils on bone and cartilage (49). These cells are found in high concentrations within the synovial effusion from inflamed joints (63). Glucocorticoids attack and inhibit practically every activity exhibited by activated neutrophils, including adhesion (16,64), phagocytosis, (65,66) chemokine release (67), eicosanoid release (16,68,69), nitric oxide release (68,70,71), apoptosis (72,73), chemotaxis (74–76), and degranulation (16,49,77). Glucocorticoids also induce the production of immunomodulatory proteins, such as annexin 1 (lipocortin), that act to reduce neutrophil activity (49,78). Thus, glucocorticoids inhibit key cellular and molecular factors that mediate the arthritic process; however, as will be discussed in subsequent sections, use of these compounds is not without significant risk.

Transplantation

Glucocorticoids have been used in organ transplantation for decades. They inhibit the immune system's response to transplantation by several mechanisms, including the induction of lipocortin, an inhibitor of phospholipase A2 activity, which is critical for the release of the inflammatory mediator arachidonic acid. Glucocorticoids also prevent key steps in T-cell activation, leukocyte adhesion, and cytokine production (79–81). Glucocorticoids preferentially inhibit the Th1 pathway, resulting in a Th2 cytokine secretion profile. This results in a reduction in the immune response that lingers after the glucocorticoids have been discontinued (79).

The development of acute and chronic graft-versus-host disease is a major problem following allogeneic bone marrow transplantation. It plays a major role in the success or failure of marrow transplantation. Glucocorticoids are extremely useful in treating this disease; other therapeutics are used only for steroid-resistant disease (82).

Immunosuppressive therapy in renal transplantation often utilizes cyclosporin as the key agent. High-dose glucocorticoids are used to suppress rejection crises. Induction immunosuppression also uses high intravenous doses of steroid—usually prednisone or prednisolone. This is followed by single oral daily doses for maintenance. Glucocorticoids can be withdrawn from renal transplant patients successfully under certain conditions (83–85). The development of other immunosuppressive drugs such as cyclosporin A has reduced the dependence on glucocorticoids. Steroids can also apparently be withdrawn after liver transplantation without adverse effects (86).

Inflammatory Bowel Disease (IBD)

Ulcerative colitis (UC) and Crohn's disease (CD) are thought to be autoimmune disorders, but their precise etiologies remain controversial (87). There are several reasons to associate these diseases with autoimmune malfunction, including immune-related damage to the gut wall, the presence of antibodies recognizing colonic mucosa in IBD, as well as autoimmune-like symptoms in other parts of the body, including uveitis, iritis, and polyarthritis. These diseases are effectively and routinely treated with glucocorticoids. However, the chronic nature of these diseases makes the use of oral systemic steroids a significant problem. Therefore, novel preparations have been used in attempts to reduce systemic impact. The general principle is to expose the gut wall to pharmacologic doses of a steroid that is subject to extensive first-pass metabolism without allowing systemic distribution. For example, budesonide, which is a very potent glucocorticoid used in Rinocort (Astra USA, Inc.) and Pulmocort (Astra USA, Inc.), is subject to extensive first-pass liver metabolism resulting in a bioavailability of only about 10% (88,89). This compound is used in both oral and enema preparations and has been shown to be effective in treating IBD without the concomitant HPA suppression found with other more bioavailable glucocorticoids (90,91). Rectal delivery of both stable and metabolically labile glucocorticoids is often used in treating UC, which frequently involves the distal colon (92–94). Unfortunately, this approach reaches only the lower regions of the colon (95,96), and many patients suffer from proximal disease. Delivering the steroid to the lower intestine without prior absorption presents a significant challenge, complicated by the fact that UC typically involves only the large intestine, while CD can affect both the large and small intestines. Thus, controlled release formulations, biodegradable coatings, and coatings sensitive to the more alkaline pH of the lower intestine have been used to increase the localization of the steroid to the afflicted area. This area is still fertile ground for additional improvements in the therapeutic ratio of glucocorticoids given the unique physical environment of the intestine (97).

Side Effects of Steroid Treatment

The side effects of glucocorticoid therapy are as extensive as their therapeutic activity, due in large part to the many systems in which glucocorticoids play a physiologic role. It has been suggested by some authors that pharmacologic dosages of glucocorticoid mimic the stress response in which the adrenals produce high serum cortisol concentrations. Complications can occur acutely with very high dosages, or more slowly with chronic exposure. The side effects of glucocorticoids have been shown to be strictly dosage-dependent, and thus, as the dosage is escalated to improve efficacy, the side effects also increase. A major goal of research in this area is to determine if some or all of these side effects can be reduced using the recent molecular discoveries described above. This section will discuss a specific subset of glucocorticoid-mediated side effects, their postulated mechanism, and available therapeutic approaches to reduce their impact on patient health.

Osteoporosis

Osteoporosis is one of the most debilitating effects of long-term glucocorticoid treatment. Patient susceptibility to fracture and aseptic necrosis of the femoral head increases soon after commencement of glucocorticoid therapy (17,98). Multiple studies have demonstrated inhibitory effects of glucocorticoids on bone density (99). In particular, long-term systemic steroid use is associated with progressive degradation of trabecular bone and is correlated with an increase in fracture rate (28,99,100). There is evidence for this side effect occurring in several disease settings, including but not limited to RA (101), COPD (28), asthma (102), and transplantation (103,104). The evidence indicates that the effect of glucocorticoids on bone density is directly related to dosage and duration. The impact of corticosteroid use on bone parameters correlates with the fracture data, with bone loss being highest in the first 6 months of therapy and then tapering off somewhat. Thus, patients treated for years with glucocorticoids continue to lose bone during that time. Fortunately, many patients at least partially regain bone when taken off steroids (99,105).

Glucocorticoids act by three distinct pathways to cause bone loss. First, glucocorticoids inhibit calcium uptake and increase calcium excretion, resulting in lower serum calcium levels. Patients taking glucocorticoids have a reduced calcium absorption in the intestine due to the inhibitory effect of glucocorticoids on the activity of 1,25-dihydroxyvitamin D, which mediates calcium uptake (106). Glucocorticoids have direct effects on kidney reabsorption, enhancing calcium and phosphate transport and excretion (98). This "double jeopardy" not only reduces the serum calcium that is available to form new bone, but also induces the bone-resorptive peptide parathyroid hormone (98,99). Bone integrity and strength are maintained by continuous bone remodeling, a dynamic process that balances bone resorption and bone formation. Increased parathyroid hormone levels in response to lower calcium enhances bone resorption, swinging the balance toward bone degradation.

Second, glucocorticoids inhibit bone formation by acting directly on osteoblasts—the cells responsible for laying down new bone. Glucocorticoids decrease osteoblast growth and enhance apoptosis (107). They activate the endogenous osteoblast glucocorticoid receptor to directly suppress osteocalcin, certain growth factors, and matrix production (98,108–111).

Third, glucocorticoids have effects on anabolic hormones that help maintain bone density. Males taking prednisone for RA have significantly decreased testosterone levels (112), a consequence of decreased adrenal and gonadal production in response to glucocorticoid treatment. Inhibition of testosterone produc-

tion could be one mechanism for glucocorticoid-induced catabolic effects on muscle and bone.

Several options are now available for the management of corticosteroid-induced osteoporosis. In particular, certain patients can significantly reduce their risk of fracture if bone-protective therapy is begun at the same time corticosteroid therapy is initiated. Obviously, a primary goal of any clinician using glucocorticoids is to reduce the dosage and duration of glucocorticoid exposure. In addition, patients have been treated with calcium and vitamin D (113,114), calcitonin (115), and sodium fluoride (116). The overall results of trials with these agents have been disappointing (117,118). Vitamin D, calcium, and calcitonin have little or no effect. Sodium fluoride will increase bone mineral density, but the bone that is produced is structurally distinct from normal bone and may not be as strong.

Supplementation with androgens increases bone density, decreases fat mass, and increases lean mass in men treated with glucocorticoids for asthma (102). Inhaled steroids are often touted as having little or no in effect on bone, but several studies of patients on high-dosage inhaled steroids have shown negative effects on osteocalcin, a bone formation marker (119), and on bone mineral density (120). Nevertheless, inhaled steroids are preferable to systemic steroids in this regard. As described above, anabolic steroids and hormone replacement therapy appear to be helpful in corticosteroid-treated patients with low sex hormone levels (102). Recent data on the activity of the bisphosphonate class of antiresorptive drugs in corticosteroid-treated patients indicate that they may be an appropriate addition to treatment regimes. These drugs have demonstrated benefits on both bone mineral density and the risk of vertebral fractures (121). The FDA has recently approved the use of the bisphosphonate drug Alendronate for the treatment of corticosteroid-induced osteoporosis.

Wound Healing

Glucocorticoids impair wound healing and increase the risk of infection by several fold (122). The dosage and timing of glucocorticoid administration significantly affects both natural and surgical wounds. Pre- and postoperative treatment with steroids has a greater effect on wound healing than postoperative treatment alone (123). Small doses of glucocorticoids (<10 mg prednisone) have little or no effect, but above this dose level, significant effects have been noted on both wound repair time and strength (124–126). Glucocorticoids can affect wound healing by several mechanisms. First, inflammation itself is a natural and critical part of the wound healing process. Thus, the anti-inflammatory effects of glucocorticoids are detrimental to wound repair (127). Second, glucocorticoid-mediated inhibition of collagen synthesis and cross-linking directly affects wound strength (128,129). Third, wound contracture and epithelialization are significantly reduced, possibly as a result of the inhibition of keratinocyte proliferation and growth factor secretion (130,131). These effects are of importance for patients undergoing surgery while being treated with glucocorticoids, because of the additional pain, infection risk, and overall morbidity associated with steroid use. There are reports that retinoids may be beneficial in treating this problem, although more work needs to be done to confirm this

(127). The possibility of finding selective glucocorticoid receptor modulators that separate anti-inflammatory activity from inhibition of wound healing seems remote because of the tight link between the inflammatory process and wound repair.

Behavioral Effects

At dosages of glucocorticoid greater than 40 mg prednisone daily, the Boston Collaborative Drug Surveillance Program found that approximately 5% of patients experience some degree of inappropriate euphoria or psychosis (132). Other retrospective studies have indicated that the incidence may be somewhat lower than 5% for this complication (133,134). However, all data indicate that at very high dosages (>80 mg prednisone daily) this complication becomes a significant factor. There is evidence that some aspects of the effects of these compounds in brain are due to cross-reactivity on the mineralocorticoid receptor. The involvement of MR in various behaviors associated with exogenous glucocorticoids is well documented in rodents (135–138). The hippocampus, a key brain region involved in modulation of behavior, expresses relatively high levels of MR and GR. The ratio of GR to MR may be critical in stress response and behavioral adaptation (139). The steroids prednisolone (prednisone) and dexamethasone will bind and activate the mineralocorticoid receptor, although with less potency than the endogenous steroid cortisol. Glucocorticoids with less cross-reactivity for MR may reduce this type of side effect.

Myopathy

Glucocorticoids generally act as catabolic hormones. They induce the production of substrates for the gluconeogenic pathway in the liver through the breakdown of fats (lipolysis) and muscle protein. Histologic analysis of corticosteroid-treated muscle from human and animal studies reveals atrophy of certain fast twitch fibers (140–142). The tendency for high-dosage glucocorticoids to decrease muscle mass and strength, thereby increasing the chance of falls, is especially troublesome for patients already at risk for fractures owing to corticosteroid-induced osteoporosis. Two key players in maintaining both muscle and bone mass are the sex steroids estrogen and testosterone. Glucocorticoid-mediated decreases in gonadal production of both of these anabolic hormones could contribute to loss of bone and muscle (143,144). Several case studies comparing asthmatics being treated with systemic corticosteroids with sedentary, age-matched healthy volunteers have noted an association between steroid use and myopathy (145,146). However, this type of study cannot distinguish muscle effects resulting from the asthma itself. Other studies have examined the effect of low-dosage glucocorticoids (~10 mg daily) on respiratory muscle strength in asthmatics compared with untreated asthmatics. No significant effects on muscle strength were detected in these relatively small studies (147–149).

Diabetes

The effects of glucocorticoids on glycemic control are thought to be primarily the result of targeting insulin signaling (150–152).

Glucocorticoids cause decreases in key insulin receptor signaling molecules; increase hepatic glucose output by increasing the rate-limiting and insulin-inhibited enzyme in gluconeogenesis, phosphoenolpyruvate carboxykinase (PEPCK) (153–155); and, finally, inhibit insulin-mediated increases in blood flow to muscles (156,157). Thus, glucocorticoids act both to enhance glucose production and to prevent efficient glucose uptake, utilization, and disposal. These effects act in concert to increase circulating glucose levels, which, during an acute stress response, is appropriate, but in the context of patients on either high-dosage or long-term corticosteroids, insulin resistance and frank diabetes are significant clinical issues (15,28,133). Insulin sensitizers (158) may represent a viable approach to patients with corticosteroid-induced glucose control difficulties.

Fat Redistribution/Cushingoid Habitus

High levels of glucocorticoids induce a characteristic type of fat redistribution and accumulation in which fat is shed from limbs and accumulates in truncal and visceral areas. Certain fat depots in the face and in the supraclavical and posterior cervical areas are particularly sensitive to glucocorticoids, resulting in the moon face and buffalo hump characteristic of long-term glucocorticoid treatment. This fat redistribution and the associated generalized truncal obesity significantly affect the quality of life for glucocorticoid-treated patients (159). These side effects occur frequently, up to four times more frequently than in placebo-treated patients (134). Moon face occurs in about 13% of patients treated with less than 12 mg daily for 60 days and in 66% of patients on steroids for more than 5 years. Patients on glucocorticoids often experience weight gain and a loss of lean body mass (15,160–162). However, improvement of the underlying disease condition itself may result in weight gain (133). These effects are probably caused by the impact of glucocorticoids on lipid metabolism and insulin resistance. As described above, glucocorticoids decrease insulin sensitivity, resulting in increased production of insulin by the pancreas. The combination of high glucocorticoid and high insulin is a powerful energy storage signal (163,164). Furthermore, the physiologic responses to glucocorticoids also include increased food intake (specifically fat) (163,165) and stimulated adipose tissue development (166). The reason for the high sensitivity of the fat depots in the face, trunk, and upper back is not known, but probably involves cell-type-specific responses to glucocorticoid and insulin action. Management of corticosteroid-induced weight gain usually involves careful attention to diet, but it is possible that weight-loss drugs and insulin sensitizers may be useful in extreme cases (158,159,163,164).

Summary and Future Perspectives

Glucocorticoids are unquestionably the most effective anti-inflammatory agents known. However, their use is severely limited because of significant side effects. Many of the side effects of glucocorticoids are apparently not related to their anti-inflammatory effects. Specifically, the effects on metabolism of muscle, skin, fat, and bone and the effects on behavior may be due to effects of the glucocorticoid receptor on pathways that are distinct from anti-inflammatory pathways. Screening for novel glucocorticoid receptor modulators that induce some, but not all of the activities of the receptor may provide a novel approach to identification of selective glucocorticoid modulators that retain the anti-inflammatory activity but lack certain side effects. Precedents for this effort can be found in the selective estrogen receptor modulators (167–169), which have been fashioned to have less negative impacts on breast and uterus than estrogen while maintaining the beneficial effects in bone and heart. Ligands that separate transcriptional activation from transcriptional repression offer one avenue to glucocorticoids with improved therapeutic profiles (13,170,171). Alternatively, ligands that modulate the receptor structure to allow subsets of coactivators and corepressors to bind could generate beneficial tissue and/or promoter selectivity. The development of novel glucocorticoids that have an improved therapeutic profile is currently a major area of research, and success in this area will be a boon to patients enduring the adverse consequences of chronic glucocorticoid use.

References

1. Hench PS, Boland EW. Potential reversibility of rheumatoid arthritis. Proc Staff Mtg Mayo Clin 1949;24:167–168.
2. Baxter JD. Advances in glucocorticoid therapy. Adv Intern Med 2000;45:317–349.
3. Schafer-Korting M, Schmid MH, Korting HC. Topical glucocorticoids with improved risk-benefit ratio. Rationale of a new concept. Drug Saf 1996;14(6):375–385.
4. Mangelsdorf DJ, Thummel C, Beato M, et al. The nuclear receptor superfamily: the second decade. Cell 1995;83(6):835–839.
5. Silverstein AM, Galigniana MD, Kanelakis KC, et al. Different regions of the immunophilin FKBP52 determine its association with the glucocorticoid receptor, hsp90, and cytoplasmic dynein. J Biol Chem 1999;274(52):36980–36986.
6. Luisi BF, Xu WX, Otwinowski Z, et al. Crystallographic analysis of the interaction of the glucocorticoid receptor with DNA [see comments]. Nature 1991;352(6335):497–505.
7. Shiau AK, Barstad D, Loria PM, et al. The structural basis of estrogen receptor/coactivator recognition and the antagonism of this interaction by tamoxifen. Cell 1998;95(7):927–937.
8. Glass CK, Rosenfeld MG. The coregulator exchange in transcriptional functions of nuclear receptors [In Process Citation]. Genes Dev 2000;14(2):121–141.
9. Chen D, Ma H, Hong H, et al. Regulation of transcription by a protein methyltransferase. Science 1999;284(5423):2174–2177.
10. Drouin J, Sun YL, Chamberland M, et al. Novel glucocorticoid receptor complex with DNA element of the hormone-repressed POMC gene. Embo J 1993;12(1):145–156.
11. Karin M. New twists in gene regulation by glucocorticoid receptor: is DNA binding dispensable? [comment]. Cell 1998;93(4):487–490.
12. Scheinman RI, Gualberto A, Jewell CM, et al. Characterization of mechanisms involved in transrepression of NF-kappa B by activated glucocorticoid receptors. Mol Cell Biol 1995;15(2):943–953.
13. Reichardt HM, Kaestner KH, Tuckermann J, et al. DNA binding of the glucocorticoid receptor is not essential for survival [see comments]. Cell 1998;93(4):531–541.
14. Wiegers GJ, Reul JM. Induction of cytokine receptors by glucocorticoids: functional and pathological significance. Trends Pharmacol Sci 1998;19(8):317–321.
15. Boumpas DT, Chrousos GP, Wilder RL, et al. Glucocorticoid therapy for immune-mediated diseases: basic and clinical correlates. Ann Intern Med 1993;119(12):1198–1208.
16. Schleimer RP, Freeland HS, Peters SP, et al. An assessment of the effects of glucocorticoids on degranulation, chemotaxis, binding to vascular endothelium and formation of leukotriene B4 by purified human neutrophils. J Pharmacol Exp Ther 1989:250(2):598–605.
17. Axelrod L. Glucocorticoids. In: Kelley WN, Harris ED, Ruddy S, Sledge CB, eds. Textbook of rheumatology. Philadelphia: WB Saunders, 1989.
18. Axelrod L. Glucocorticoid therapy. Medicine (Baltimore) 1976;55(1):39–65.
19. Axelrod L. Adrenal corticosteroids. In: Miller RR, Greenblatt J, eds. Handbook of drug therapy. Amsterdam: Elsevier, 1979:809–840.
20. Rousseau GG, Baxter JD, Tomkins GM. Glucocorticoid receptors: relations between steroid binding and biological effects. J Mol Biol 1972;67(1):99–115.
21. Markham A, Bryson HM. Deflazacort. A review of its pharmacological properties and therapeutic efficacy. Drugs 1995;50(2):317–333.
22. Szefler SJ. General pharmacology of glucocorticoids. In: Schleimer RP, Claman HN, Oronsky AL, eds. Anti-inflammatory steroid action. Basic and clinical aspects. San Diego: Academic Press, 1989:353–376.
23. Jenkins JS, Sampson PA. Conversion of cortisone to cortisol and prednisone to prednisolone. Br Med J 1967;2(546):205–207.
24. Powell LW, Axelsen E. Corticosteroids in liver disease: studies on the biological conversion of prednisone to prednisolone and plasma protein binding. Gut 1972;13(9):690–696.
25. Rocci ML Jr, D'Ambrosio R, Johnson NF, Jusko WJ. Prednisolone binding to albumin and transcortin in the presence of cortisol. Biochem Pharmacol 1982;31(3):289–292.
26. Rose JQ, Nickelsen JA, Ellis EF, et al. Prednisolone disposition in steroid-dependent asthmatic children. J Allergy Clin Immunol 1981;67(3):188–193.
27. Rose JQ, Yurchak AM, Jusko WJ. Dose dependent pharmacokinetics of prednisone and prednisolone in man. J Pharmacokinet Biopharm 1981;9(4):389–417.
28. McEvoy CE, Ensrud KE, Bender E, et al. Association between corticosteroid use and vertebral fractures in older men with chronic obstructive pulmonary disease. Am J Respir Crit Care Med 1998;157(3 Pt 1):704–709.
29. Patel L, Clayton PE, Addison GM, et al. Linear growth in prepubertal children with atopic dermatitis. Arch Dis Child 1998;79(2):169–172.
30. Toogood JH. Bronchial asthma and glucocorticoids. In: Schleimer RP, Claman HN, Oronsky AL, eds. Anti-inflammatory steroid action. Basic and clinical aspects. San Diego: Academic Press, 1989:423–468.
31. Ball BD, Hill M, Harbeck RJ, Szefler SJ. Application of corticosteroid pharmacokinetics to severe steroid-requiring asthmatics. J Allergy Clin Immunol 1988;81:316.
32. Lewis RA, Austen KF. The biologically active leukotrienes.

Biosynthesis, metabolism, receptors, functions, and pharmacology. J Clin Invest 1984;73(4):889–897.

33. Morris HG. Mechanisms of action and therapeutic role of corticosteroids in asthma. J Allergy Clin Immunol 1985;75(1 Pt 1):1–13.

34. Adcock IM, Matthews JG. New drugs for asthma. Drug Disc Today 1998;3(9):395–399.

35. Durham SR, Carroll M, Walsh GM, Kay AB. Leukocyte activation in allergen-induced late-phase asthmatic reactions. N Engl J Med 1984;311(22):1398–1402.

36. Burge PS, Efthimiou J, Turner-Warwich M, Nelmes PT. Double-blind trials of inhaled beclomethasone diproprionate and fluocortin butyl ester in allergen-induced immediate and late asthmatic reactions. Clin Allergy 1982;12(6):523–531.

37. Booij-Noord H, Vries KD, Sluiter HJ, Orie NG. Late bronchial obstructive reaction to experimental inhalation of house dust extract. Clin Allergy 1972;2(1):43–61.

38. De Monchy JG, Kauffman HF, Venge P, et al. Bronchoalveolar eosinophilia during allergen-induced late asthmatic reactions. Am Rev Respir Dis 1985;131(3):373–376.

39. Boschetto P, Fabbri LM, Zocca E, et al. Prednisone inhibits late asthmatic reactions and airway inflammation induced by toluene diisocyanate in sensitized subjects [published erratum appears in J Allergy Clin Immunol 1988 Fed;81(2):454]. J Allergy Clin Immunol 1987;80(3 Pt 1):261–267.

40. Kunicka JE, Talle MA, Denhardt GH, et al. Immunosuppression by glucocorticoids: inhibition of production of multiple lymphokines by in vivo administration of dexamethasone. Cell Immunol 1993;149(1):39–49.

41. Flint KC, Leung KB, Hudspith BN, et al. Bronchoalveolar mast cells in extrinsic asthma: a mechanism for the initiation of antigen specific bronchoconstriction. Br Med J (Clin Res Ed) 1985;291(6500):923–926.

42. Simons FE. Inhaled glucocorticoids in children: a favourable therapeutic index. Can Respir J 1999;6(2):175–178.

43. Utiger RD. Differences between inhaled and oral glucocorticoid therapy [editorial; comment]. N Engl J Med 1993;329(23):1731–1733.

44. Volovitz B, Amir J, Malik H, et al. Growth and pituitary-adrenal function in children with severe asthma treated with inhaled budesonide [see comments]. N Engl J Med 1993;329(23):1703–1708.

45. Hughes JA, Conry BG, Male SM, Eastell R. One year prospective open study of the effect of high dose inhaled steroids, fluticasone propionate, and budesonide on bone markers and bone mineral density. Thorax 1999;54(3):223–229.

46. Erbland ML, Deupree RH, Niewoehner DE. Systemic Corticosteroids in Chronic Obstructive Pulmonary Disease Exacerbations (SCCOPE): rationale and design of an equivalence trial. Veterans Administration Cooperative Trials SCCOPE Study Group. Control Clin Trials 1998;19(4):404–417.

47. Boushey HA. Glucocorticoid therapy for chronic obstructive pulmonary disease [editorial; comment]. N Engl J Med 1999;340(25):1990–1991.

48. Niewoehner DE, Erbland ML, Deupree RH, et al. Effect of systemic glucocorticoids on exacerbations of chronic obstructive pulmonary disease. Department of Veterans Affairs Cooperative Study Group [see comments]. N Engl J Med 1999;340(25):1941–1947.

49. Goulding NJ, Euzger HS, Butt SK, Perretti M. Novel pathways for glucocorticoid effects on neutrophils in chronic inflammation. Inflamm Res 1998;47(suppl 3):S158–S165.

50. Danning CL, Boumpas DT. Commonly used disease-modifying antirheumatic drugs in the treatment of inflammatory arthritis: an update on mechanisms of action. Clin Exp Rheumatol 1998;16(5):595–604.

51. Kern JA, Lamb RJ, Reed JC, et al. Dexamethasone inhibition of interleukin 1 beta production by human monocytes. Posttranscriptional mechanisms. J Clin Invest 1988;81(1):237–244.

52. Fessler BJ, Paliogianni F, Hama N, et al. Glucocorticoids modulate CD28 mediated pathways for interleukin 2 production in human T cells: evidence for posttranscriptional regulation. Transplantation 1996;62(8):1113–1118.

53. Pauwels RA, Lofdahl CG, Laitinen LA, et al. Long-term treatment with inhaled budesonide in persons with mild chronic obstructive pulmonary disease who continue smoking. European Respiratory Society Study on Chronic Obstructive Pulmonary Disease [see comments]. N Engl J Med 1999;340(25):1948–1953.

54. Mygind N. Local effect of intranasal beclomethasone dipropionate aerosol in hay fever. Br Med J 1973;4(890):464–466.

55. Rudolph R, Kunkel G, Staud RD, Koennecke R. The nasal application of beclomethasone diproprionate (Beconase) in allergic rhinitis. Clin Otolaryngol 1976;1(4):315–323.

56. Turkeltaub PC, Norman PS, Crepea S. Treatment of ragweed hay fever with an intranasal spray containing fluinsolide, a new synthetic corticosteroid. J Allergy Clin Immunol 1976;58(5):597–606.

57. Pipkorn U, Rundcrantz H, Lindqvist N. Budesonide—a new nasal steroid. Rhinology 1980;18(4):171–175.

58. Siegel SC, Katz RM, Rachelefsky GS, et al. Multicentric study of beclomethasone dipropionate nasal aerosol in adults with seasonal allergic rhinitis. J Allergy Clin Immunol 1982;69(4):345–353.

59. Okuda M, Otsuka H. Basophilic cells in allergic nasal secretions. Arch Otorhinolaryngol 1977;214(4):283–289.

60. Robertson DB, Maibach HI. Topical glucocorticoids. In: Schleimer RP, Claman HN, Oronsky AL, eds. Anti-inflammatory steroid action. Basic and clinical aspects. San Diego: Academic Press, 1989:494–524.

61. Simon LS. The evolution of arthritis antiinflammatory care: where are we today? J Rheumatol 1999;26(suppl 56):11–17.

62. Hickling P, Jacoby RK, Kirwan JR. Joint destruction after glucocorticoids are withdrawn in early rheumatoid arthritis. Arthritis and Rheumatism Council Low Dose Glucocorticoid Study Group. Br J Rheumatol 1998;37(9):930–936.

63. Bromley M, Woolley DE. Histopathology of the rheumatoid lesion. Identification of cell types at sites of cartilage erosion. Arthritis Rheum 1984;27(8):857–863.

64. Yoshida N, Yoshikawa T, Nakamura Y, et al. Methylprednisolone inhibits neutrophil-endothelial cell interactions induced by interleukin-1 beta under flow conditions. Life Sci 1997;60(25):2341–2347.

65. Petroni KC, Shen L, Guyre PM. Modulation of human polymorphonuclear leukocyte IgG Fc receptors and Fc receptor-mediated functions by IFN-gamma and glucocorticoids. J Immunol 1988;140(10):3467–3472.

66. Direnzo M, Pasqui AL, Chiarion C, et al. The in-vitro effect of 2 glucocorticoids on some lymphomonocyte and neutrophil functions. Int J Immunother 1994;10:103–112.

67. Wertheim WA, Kunkel SL, Standiford TJ, et al. Regulation of neutrophil-derived IL-8: the role of prostaglandin E2, dexamethasone, and IL-4. J Immunol 1993;151(4):2166–2175.

68. Paya M, Garcia Pastor P, Coloma J, Alcaraz MJ. Nitric oxide synthase and cyclo-oxygenase pathways in the inflammatory response induced by zymosan in the rat air pouch. Br J Pharmacol 1997;120(8):1445–1452.

69. Fradin A, Rothhut B, Poincelot-Canton B, et al. Inhibition of eicosanoid and PAF formation by dexamethasone in rat inflammatory polymorphonuclear neutrophils may implicate lipocortin "s". Biochim Biophys Acta 1988;963(2):248–257.

70. Kolls J, Xie J, LeBlanc R, et al. Rapid induction of messenger RNA for nitric oxide synthase II in rat neutrophils in vivo by endotoxin and its suppression by prednisolone. Proc Soc Exp Biol Med 1994;205(3):220–229.

71. McCall TB, Palmer RM, Moncada S. Induction of nitric oxide synthase in rat peritoneal neutrophils and its inhibition by dexamethasone. Eur J Immunol 1991;21(10):2523–2527.

72. Liles WC, Dale DC, Klebanoff SJ. Glucocorticoids inhibit apoptosis of human neutrophils. Blood 1995;86(8):3181–3188.

73. Cox G, Austin RC. Dexamethasone-induced suppression of apoptosis in human neutrophils requires continuous stimulation of new protein synthesis. J Leukoc Biol 1997;61(2):224–230.

74. Hirasawa N, Watanabe M, Mue S, et al. Induction of neutrophil infiltration by rat chemotactic cytokine (CINC) and its inhibition by dexamethasone in rats. Inflammation 1992;16(2):187–196.

75. Llewellyn-Jones CG, Hill SL, Stockley RA. Effect of fluticasone propionate on neutrophil chemotaxis, superoxide generation, and extracellular proteolytic activity in vitro. Thorax 1994;49(3):207–212.

76. Salak JL, McGlone JJ, Lyte M. Effects of in vitro adrenocorticotrophic hormone, cortisol and human recombinant interleukin-2 on porcine neutrophil migration and luminol-dependent chemiluminescence. Vet Immunol Immunopathol 1993;39(4):327–337.

77. Joseph BZ, Beam R, Martin RJ, Borish L. Prednisone inhibits leukocyte granule secretion into the asthmatic airway. Int J Immunopathol Pharmacol 1995;8:23–30.

78. Perretti M, Flower RJ. Measurement of lipocortin 1 levels in murine peripheral blood leukocytes by flow cytometry: modulation by glucocorticoids and inflammation. Br J Pharmacol 1996;118(3):605–610.

79. Almawi WY, Hess DA, Rieder MJ. Multiplicity of glucocorticoid action in inhibiting allograft rejection. Cell Transplant 1998;7(6):511–523.

80. Dupont E, Huygen K, Schandene L, et al. Depressed natural killer function in transplant recipients: an analysis. Transplant Proc 1984;16(6):1506–1508.

81. Dupont E, Vandercruys M, Wybran J. Deficient natural killer function in patients receiving immunosuppressive drugs: analysis at the cellular level. Cell Immunol 1984;88(1):85–95.

82. Deeg HJ, Henslee-Downey PJ. Management of acute graft-versus-host disease. Bone Marrow Transplant 1990;6(1):1–8.

83. Bry W, Warvariv V, Bohannon L, et al. Cadaveric renal transplant without prophylactic prednisone therapy. Transplant Proc 1991;23(1 Pt 2):994–996.

84. Salaman JR. Renal transplantation without steroids. Pediatr Nephrol 1991;5(1):105–107.

85. Salaman JR. Monitoring of rejection in renal transplantation. Immunol Lett 1991;29(1–2):139–142.

86. Everson GT, Trouillot T, Wachs M, et al. Early steroid withdrawal in liver transplantation is safe and beneficial. Liver Transpl Surg 1999;5:S48–S57.

87. Routes J, Claman HN. Corticosteroids in inflammatory bowel disease. A review. J Clin Gastroenterol 1987;9(5):529–535.

88. Edsbacker S, Jonsson S, Lindberg C, et al. Metabolic pathways of the topical glucocorticoid budesonide in man. Drug Metab Dispos 1983;11(6):590–596.

89. Ryrfeldt A, Andersson P, Edsbacker S, et al. Pharmacokinetics and metabolism of budesonide, a selective glucocorticoid. Eur J Respir Dis Suppl 1982;122:86–95.

90. Spencer CM, McTavish D. Budesonide. A review of its pharmacological properties and therapeutic efficacy in inflammatory bowel disease. Drugs 1995;50(5):854–872.

91. Brogden RN, McTavish D. Budesonide. An updated review of its pharmacological properties, and therapeutic efficacy in asthma and rhinitis [published errata appear in Drugs 1992 Dec;44(6):1012 and 1993 Jan;45(1):130]. Drugs 1992;44(3):375–407.

92. Halpern Z, Sold O, Baratz M, et al. A controlled trial of beclomethasone versus betamethasone enemas in distal ulcerative colitis. J Clin Gastroenterol 1991;13(1):38–41.

93. Lee DA, Taylor M, James VH, Walker G. Rectally administered prednisolone—evidence for a predominantly local action. Gut 1980;21(3):215–218.

94. Kumana CR, Seaton T, Meghji M, et al. Beclomethasone dipropionate enemas for treating inflammatory bowel disease without producing Cushing's syndrome or hypothalamic pituitary adrenal suppression. Lancet 1982;1(8272):579–583.

95. Nyman-Pantelidis M, Nilsson A, Wagner ZG, Borga O. Pharmacokinetics and retrograde colonic spread of budesonide enemas in patients with distal ulcerative colitis. Aliment Pharmacol Ther 1994;8(6):617–622.

96. Campieri M, Corbelli C, Gionchetti P, et al. Spread and distribution of 5-ASA colonic foam and 5-ASA enema in patients with ulcerative colitis. Dig Dis Sci 1992;37(12):1890–1897.

97. Hamedani R, Feldman RD, Feagan BG. Review article: drug development in inflammatory bowel disease: budesonide—a model of targeted therapy. Aliment Pharmacol Ther 1997;11(suppl 3):98–107.

98. Lukert BP, Kream BE. Clinical and basic aspects of glucocorticoid action in bone. In: Principles of bone biology. San Diego: Academic Press, 1996.

99. Ralston SH. Pathogenesis and management of corticosteroid-induced osteoporosis. Curr Opin Onc Endo Metab Invest Drugs 1999;1(1):25–30.

100. Adinoff AD, Hollister JR. Steroid-induced fractures and bone loss in patients with asthma. N Engl J Med 1983;309(5):265–268.

101. Lane NE, Goldring SR. Bone loss in rheumatoid arthritis: what role does inflammation play? [editorial; comment]. J Rheumatol 1998;25(7):1251–1253.

102. Reid IR, Wattie DJ, Evans MC, Stapleton JP. Testosterone

therapy in glucocorticoid-treated men [see comments]. Arch Intern Med 1996;156(11):1173–1177.

103. Shane E, Rodino MA, McMahon DJ, et al. Prevention of bone loss after heart transplantation with antiresorptive therapy: a pilot study. J Heart Lung Transplant 1998;17(11):1089–1096.

104. Shane E, Papadopoulos A, Staron RB, et al. Bone loss and fracture after lung transplantation. Transplantation 1999;68(2):220–227.

105. Axelrod L. Side effects of glucocorticoid therapy. In: Schleimer RP, Claman HN, Oronsky AL, eds. Anti-inflammatory steroid action. Basic and clinical aspects. San Diego: Academic Press, 1989:377–408.

106. Hahn TJ, Halstead LR, Baran DT. Effects of short term glucocorticoid administration on intestinal calcium absorption and circulating vitamin D metabolite concentrations in man. J Clin Endocrinol Metab 1981;52(1):111–115.

107. Weinstein RS, Jilka RL, Parfitt AM, Manolagas SC. Inhibition of osteoblastogenesis and promotion of apoptosis of osteoblasts and osteocytes by glucocorticoids. Potential mechanisms of their deleterious effects on bone. J Clin Invest 1998;102(2):274–282.

108. Canalis E. Effect of glucocorticoids on type I collagen synthesis, alkaline phosphatase activity, and deoxyribonucleic acid content in cultured rat calvariae. Endocrinology 1983;112(3):931–939.

109. Beresford JN, Gallagher JA, Poser JW, Russell RG. Production of osteocalcin by human bone cells in vitro. Effects of 1,25(OH)2D3, 24,25(OH)2D3, parathyroid hormone, and glucocorticoids. Metab Bone Dis Relat Res 1984;5(5):229–234.

110. Haussler MR, Manolagas SC, Deftos LJ. Glucocorticoid receptor in clonal osteosarcoma cell lines: a novel system for investigating bone active hormones. Biochem Biophys Res Commun 1980;94(1):373–380.

111. Manolagas SC, Anderson DC. Detection of high-affinity glucocorticoid binding in rat bone. J Endocrinol 1978;76(2):379–380.

112. Martens HF, Sheets PK, Tenover JS, et al. Decreased testosterone levels in men with rheumatoid arthritis: effect of low dose prednisone therapy. J Rheumatol 1994;21(8):1427–1431.

113. Adachi JD, Bensen WG, Bianchi F, et al. Vitamin D and calcium in the prevention of corticosteroid induced osteoporosis: a 3 year followup [see comments]. J Rheumatol 1996;23(6):995–1000.

114. Bernstein CN, Seeger LL, Anton PA, et al. A randomized, placebo-controlled trial of calcium supplementation for decreased bone density in corticosteroid-using patients with inflammatory bowel disease: a pilot study. Aliment Pharmacol Ther 1996;10(5):777–786.

115. Luengo M, Pons F, Martinez de Osaba MJ, Picado C. Prevention of further bone mass loss by nasal calcitonin in patients on long term glucocorticoid therapy for asthma: a two year follow up study. Thorax 1994;49(11):1099–1102.

116. Rizzoli R, Chevalley T, Slosman DO, Bonjour JP. Sodium monofluorophosphate increases vertebral bone mineral density in patients with corticosteroid-induced osteoporosis. Osteoporos Int 1995;5(1):39–46.

117. Sambrook P, Birmingham J, Kelly P, et al. Prevention of corticosteroid osteoporosis. A comparison of calcium, calcitriol, and calcitonin [see comments]. N Engl J Med 1993;328(24):1747–1752.

118. Meunier PJ. Is steroid-induced osteoporosis preventable? [editorial; comment]. N Engl J Med 1993;328(24):1781–1782.

119. Jennings BH, Andersson KE, Johansson SA. Assessment of systemic effects of inhaled glucocorticosteroids: comparison of the effects of inhaled budesonide and oral prednisolone on adrenal function and markers of bone turnover. Eur J Clin Pharmacol 1991;40(1):77–82.

120. Wisniewski AF, Lewis SA, Green DJ, et al. Cross sectional investigation of the effects of inhaled corticosteroids on bone density and bone metabolism in patients with asthma. Thorax 1997;52(10):853–860.

121. Saag KG, Emkey R, Schnitzer TJ, et al. Alendronate for the prevention and treatment of glucocorticoid-induced osteoporosis. Glucocorticoid-Induced Osteoporosis Intervention Study Group. N Engl J Med 1998;339(5):292–299.

122. Diethelm AG. Surgical management of complications of steroid therapy. Ann Surg 1977;185(3):251–263.

123. Sanberg N. Time relationship between administration of cortisone and wound healing in rats. Acta Chir Scand 1964;127:446–455.

124. Pollack SV. Wound healing: a review. IV. Systemic medications affecting wound healing. J Dermatol Surg Oncol 1982;8(8):667–672.

125. DiPasquale G, Steinetz BG. Relationship of food intake on the effect of cortisone acetate on skin wound healing. Proc Soc Exp Biol Med 1964;117:118–120.

126. Oxlund H, Fogdestam I, Viidik A. The influence of cortisol on wound healing of the skin and distant connective tissue response. Surg Gynecol Obstet 1979;148(6):876–880.

127. Anstead GM. Steroids, retinoids, and wound healing. Adv Wound Care 1998;11(6):277–285.

128. Autio P, Oikarinen A, Melkko J, et al. Systemic glucocorticoids decrease the synthesis of type I and type III collagen in human skin in vivo, whereas isotretinoin treatment has little effect. Br J Dermatol 1994;131(5):660–663.

129. Slavin J, Unemori E, Hunt TK, Amento E. Transforming growth factor beta (TGF-beta) and dexamethasone have direct opposing effects on collagen metabolism in low passage human dermal fibroblasts in vitro. Growth Factors 1994;11(3):205–213.

130. Lenco W, McKnight M, Macdonald AS. Effects of cortisone acetate, methylprednisolone and medroxyprogesterone on wound contracture and epithelization in rabbits. Ann Surg 1975;181(1):67–73.

131. Brauchle M, Fassler R, Werner S. Suppression of keratinocyte growth factor expression by glucocorticoids in vitro and during wound healing. J Invest Dermatol 1995;105(4):579–584.

132. TBCDS. Acute adverse reactions to prednisone in relation to dosage. Clin Pharmacol Ther 1972;13(5):694–698.

133. Smyllie HC, Connolly CK. Incidence of serious complications of corticosteroid therapy in respiratory disease. A retrospective survey of patients in the Brompton hospital. Thorax 1968;23(6):571–581.

134. Conn HO, Poynard T. Corticosteroids and peptic ulcer: meta-analysis of adverse events during steroid therapy [see comments]. J Intern Med 1994;236(6):619–632.

135. Bitran D, Shiekh M, Dowd JA, et al. Corticosterone is permissive to the anxiolytic effect that results from the block-

ade of hippocampal mineralocorticoid receptors. Pharmacol Biochem Behav 1998;60(4):879–887.

136. Smythe JW, Murphy D, Timothy C, Costall B. Hippocampal mineralocorticoid, but not glucocorticoid, receptors modulate anxiety-like behavior in rats. Pharmacol Biochem Behav 1997;56(3):507–513.

137. Meijer OC, Kortekaas R, Oitzl MS, de Kloet ER. Acute rise in corticosterone facilitates 5-HT(1A) receptor-mediated behavioural responses. Eur J Pharmacol 1998;351(1):7–14.

138. Lopez JF, Chalmers DT, Little KY, Watson SJ. A.E. Bennett Research Award. Regulation of serotonin1A, glucocorticoid, and mineralocorticoid receptor in rat and human hippocampus: implications for the neurobiology of depression. Biol Psychiatry 1998;43(8):547–573.

139. de Kloet ER, Sutanto W, van den Berg DT, et al. Brain mineralocorticoid receptor diversity: functional implications. J Steroid Biochem Mol Biol 1993;47(1–6):183–190.

140. Ruff R. Endocrine myopathies. In: Engel A, Banke B, eds. Myology. New York: McGraw-Hill; 1986:1871–1906.

141. Smith B. Histological and histochemical changes in the muscles of rabbits given the corticosteroid triamcinolone. Neurology 1964;14:857–863.

142. Wilcox PG, Hards JM, Bockhold K, et al. Pathologic changes and contractile properties of the diaphragm in corticosteroid myopathy in hamsters: comparison to peripheral muscle. Am J Respir Cell Mol Biol 1989;1(3):191–199.

143. Crilly R, Cawood M, Marshall DH, Nordin BE. Hormonal status in normal, osteoporotic and corticosteroid-treated postmenopausal women. J R Soc Med 1978;71(10):733–736.

144. Doerr P, Pirke KM. Cortisol-induced suppression of plasma testosterone in normal adult males. J Clin Endocrinol Metab 1976;43(3):622–629.

145. Bowyer SL, LaMothe MP, Hollister JR. Steroid myopathy: incidence and detection in a population with asthma. J Allergy Clin Immunol 1985;76(2 Pt 1):234–242.

146. Decramer M, Stas KJ. Corticosteroid-induced myopathy involving respiratory muscles in patients with chronic obstructive pulmonary disease or asthma. Am Rev Respir Dis 1992;146(3):800–802.

147. Mak VH, Bugler JR, Spiro SG. Sternomastoid muscle fatigue and twitch maximum relaxation rate in patients with steroid dependent asthma. Thorax 1993;48(10):979–984.

148. Picado C, Fiz JA, Montserrat JM, et al. Respiratory and skeletal muscle function in steroid-dependent bronchial asthma. Am Rev Respir Dis 1990;141(1):14–20.

149. Zanotti E, Corsico R, Rampulla C, et al. Effect of long-term therapy with oral steroids on respiratory muscle function and ventilatory drive. Monaldi Arch Chest Dis 1993;48(1):16–22.

150. Tappy L, Randin D, Vollenweider P, et al. Mechanisms of dexamethasone-induced insulin resistance in healthy humans. J Clin Endocrinol Metab 1994;79(4):1063–1069.

151. McMahon M, Gerich J, Rizza R. Effects of glucocorticoids on carbohydrate metabolism. Diabetes Metab Rev 1988;4(1);17–30.

152. Nosadini R, Del Prato S, Tiengo A, et al. Insulin resistance in Cushing's syndrome. J Clin Endocrinol Metab 1983;57(3):529–536.

153. Sutherland C, O'Brien RM, Granner DK. New connections in the regulation of PEPCK gene expression by insulin. Philos Trans R Soc London B Biol Sci 1996;351(1336):191–199.

154. Granner DK, Sasaki K, Chu D. Multihormonal regulation of phosphoenolpyruvate carboxykinase gene transcription. The dominant role of insulin. Ann N Y Acad Sci 1986;478:175–190.

155. Weber G. Hormonal control of gluconeogenesis. In: Bittar EE, Bittar N, eds. The biological basis of medicine. London: Academic Press, 1968:263–307.

156. Laakso M, Edelman SV, Brechtel G, Baron AD. Decreased effect of insulin to stimulate skeletal muscle blood flow in obese man. A novel mechanism for insulin resistance. J Clin Invest 1990;85(6):1844–1852.

157. Laakso M, Edelman SV, Olefsky JM, et al. Kinetics of in vivo muscle insulin-mediated glucose uptake in human obesity. Diabetes 1990;39(8):965–974.

158. Fonseca VA, Valiquett TR, Huang SM, et al. Troglitazone monotherapy improves glycemic control in patients with type 2 diabetes mellitus: a randomized, controlled study. The Troglitazone Study Group [see comments]. J Clin Endocrinol Metab 1998;83(9):3169–3176.

159. Baxter JD. The effects of glucocorticoid therapy. Hosp Pract (Off Ed) 1992;27(9):111–114, 5–8, 23 passim.

160. Kwong FK, Sue MA, Klaustermeyer WB. Corticosteroid complications in respiratory disease. Ann Allergy 1987;58(5):326–330.

161. Gallant C, Kenny P. Oral glucocorticoids and their complications. A review. J Am Acad Dermatol 1986;14(2 Pt 1):161–177.

162. Rimsza ME. Complications of corticosteroid therapy. Am J Dis Child 1978;132(8):806–810.

163. Brindley DN, McCann BS, Niaura R, et al. Stress and lipoprotein metabolism: modulators and mechanisms. Metabolism 1993;42(9 suppl 1):3–15.

164. Brindley DN. Role of glucocorticoids and fatty acids in the impairment of lipid metabolism observed in the metabolic syndrome. Int J Obes Relat Metab Disord 1995;19(suppl 1):S69–S75.

165. Dallman MF, Darlington DN, Suemaru S, et al. Corticosteroids in homeostasis. Acta Physiol Scand Suppl 1989;583:27–34.

166. Hauner H, Entenmann G, Wabitsch M, et al. Promoting effect of glucocorticoids on the differentiation of human adipocyte precursor cells cultured in a chemically defined medium. J Clin Invest 1989;84(5):1663–1670.

167. McDonnel DP, Clemm DL, Hermann T, et al. Analysis of estrogen receptor function in vitro reveals three distinct classes of antiestrogens. Mol Endocrinol 1995;9(6):659–669.

168. McDonnell DP, Norris JD. Analysis of the molecular pharmacology of estrogen receptor agonists and antagonists provides insights into the mechanism of action of estrogen in bone. Osteoporos Int 1997:7(suppl 1):S29–S34.

169. Tsai MJ, O'Malley BW. Molecular mechanisms of action of steroid/thyroid receptor superfamily members. Annu Rev Biochem 1994;63:451–486.

170. Gottlicher M, Heck S, Herrlich P. Transcriptional cross-talk, the second mode of steroid hormone receptor action [see comments]. J Mol Med 1998;76(7):480–489.

171. Vayssiere BM, Dupont S, Choquart A, et al. Synthetic glucocorticoids that dissociate transactivation and AP-1 transrepression exhibit antiinflammatory activity in vivo. Mol Endocrinol 1997;11(9):1245–1255.

Chapter 8

Cyclooxygenase Inhibitors

William L. Smith
David L. DeWitt

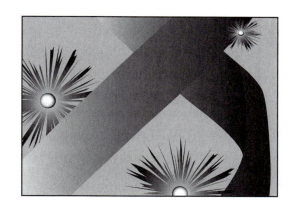

Nonsteroidal anti-inflammatory drugs (NSAIDs) inhibit the cyclooxygenase activities of prostaglandin endoperoxide H synthases (PGHSs), thereby blocking the biosynthesis of prostanoids (Fig. 8-1) (1–10). Prostanoids are oxygenated fatty acids most commonly derived from arachidonic acid and include the prostaglandins and thromboxanes (11,12). There are two PGHS isozymes, which are properly called PGH synthase-1 and -2 (PGHS-1 and PGHS-2) but are also known as cyclooxygenase-1 and -2 (COX-1 and COX-2). Both isozymes are capable of catalyzing the first step in prostanoid biosynthesis.

In intact cells, prostanoid biosynthesis occurs in three stages (see Fig. 8-1) (11): 1) release of arachidonic acid from phospholipid precursors catalyzed by various phospholipase A_2s (13–15); 2) oxygenation of arachidonic acid to prostaglandin endoperoxide H_2 (PGH$_2$) catalyzed by PGHSs; and 3) conversion of PGH$_2$ to a biologically active end product (PGD$_2$, PGE$_2$, PGF$_{2\alpha}$, prostacyclin (PGI$_2$) or thromboxane A$_2$ (TXA$_2$) through the action of a synthase or reductase (12). Newly synthesized prostanoids can exit the parent cell, probably by carrier-mediated diffusion (16) and then act locally on the parent (autocrine) and/or neighboring (paracrine) cells through G protein-linked receptors (17–21). Alternatively, prostanoids may interact with nuclear receptors that are transcription factors, such as the peroxisomal proliferator activating receptors (PPAR) (22,23).

NSAIDs exhibit a variety of pharmacologic activities. They are antipyretic, analgesic, anti-inflammatory, and antithrombogenic. In addition, NSAIDs appear to diminish the incidence of colon cancer (24–27) and may slow the development of Alzheimer's disease (28). Major side effects of NSAIDs include their ulcerogenic and nephrotoxic activities. All commercially available NSAIDs inhibit both PGHS-1 and PGHS-2 (2–7). Recently, inhibitors that are relatively selective toward PGHS-2 have been developed and found to have analgesic, anti-inflammatory and anti-pyretic activities with minimal ulcerogenic activity (29–31). Thus, it is currently thought that NSAIDs exhibit their analgesic, anti-inflammatory and antipyretic effects by inhibiting PGHS-2, whereas the ulcerogenic activities of NSAIDs are caused by their inhibition of PGHS-1 (32,33). In contrast, the beneficial effect of aspirin as an antithrombogenic agent (34–37) results from its action on PGHS-1 in platelets (7,38). As discussed below, PGHS-2 is expressed in conjunction with cell replication, differentiation, and inflammation. Based on this and other evidence, it is likely that NSAIDs exert their palliative effects on colon cancer (24,39–41) and, perhaps, Alzheimer's disease (28) by acting on PGHS-2.

The intent of this chapter is to discuss the mechanisms of actions of NSAIDs primarily at the biochemical level. To provide the necessary background, we first describe the reactions catalyzed by PGHSs, the biochemical properties of these isozymes, and the regulation of expression of the genes for PGHS-1 and PGHS-2. In discussing the regulation of expression of PGHS-2, we also discuss the actions of anti-inflammatory steroids to inhibit increases in PGHS-2 protein levels.

Cyclooxygenase and Peroxidase Catalysis

Cyclooxygenase Catalysis

For the sake of simplicity in describing both the reactions catalyzed by PGHSs and the enzymology of PGHSs, we treat the two isozymes as if they are the same. This is a reasonable approach because the deduced amino acid sequences of the two isozymes within a species are 60% identical, all amino acids identified as important for catalysis by PGHS-1 are conserved in PGHS-2, and the kinetic properties of the reactions catalyzed by the two isozymes are very similar. Nonetheless, much of what is known about the enzymology of PGHS isozymes actually comes from studies of ovine PGHS-1, and it is clear that there are some subtle biochemical differences between the two isoenzymes that may have important kinetic, and hence, physiologic consequences (42–46).

PGHSs catalyze two separate reactions (see Fig. 8-1): 1) a cyclooxygenase reaction in which arachidonic acid is converted to PGG$_2$ and 2) a peroxidase reaction in which PGH$_2$ undergoes a two-electron reduction to PGH$_2$ (3,45,47). Indeed, as discussed in further detail below, there are separate but interacting cyclooxygenase and peroxidase active sites on the enzymes.

In the first step of the cyclooxygenase reaction, PGHSs abstract the pro$S$ hydrogen from C-13 of arachidonic acid, generating an arachidonic acid radical (48–50). A molecule of O$_2$ is then added at C-11 from the side opposite that of the hydrogen abstraction. Serial cyclization of the incipient 11-peroxyl radical yields an endoperoxide with aliphatic chains *trans* to one another. A second O$_2$ is then added at C-15 to form PGG$_2$.

The two best fatty acid substrates for the cyclooxygenase activities of both PGHS-1 and PGHS-2 are arachidonic acid (20:4

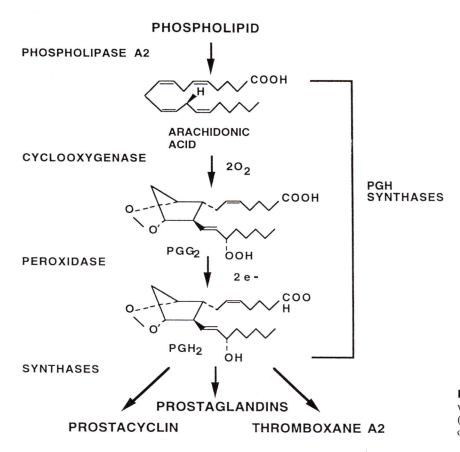

Figure 8-1. Prostanoid biosynthetic pathway. Nonsteroidal anti-inflammatory drugs (NSAIDs) inhibit the cyclooxygenase activities of the PGH synthases.

ω6) and dihomo-γ-linolenic acid (20:3 ω6). The K_m values for both substrates are about $5\,\mu M$ (51). PGHS-1 and PGHS-2 are also capable of catalyzing the oxygenation of 5,8,11,14,17-eicosapentaenoic acid (EPA), γ-linolenic acid, α-linolenic acid, and linoleic acid. EPA is converted to PGH₃, whereas the 18-carbon fatty acids are converted to monohydroxy acids (51). These latter substrates are more efficiently oxygenated by PGHS-2 than PGHS-1. For example, α-linolenic acid is oxygenated by PGHS-2 at about 20 times the rate observed with PGHS-1. Although ω3 and ω9 polyunsaturated fatty acids containing 18 to 22 carbons are poor substrates for PGHS-1, they are efficient, competitive inhibitors of the oxygenation of arachidonic acid PGHS-1 (52). Docosahexaenoic acid (22:6 ω3) is a competitive inhibitor of both PGHS-1 and PGHS-2 without being a substrate for either isozyme (3,51–53).

Peroxidase Catalysis

The peroxidase activity of PGHS-1 catalyzes reductions of PGG₂ and other hydroperoxides to their corresponding alcohols with concomitant oxidations of reducing cosubstrates (54,55). A convenient spectrophotometric assay for the peroxidase activity of PGHSs involves the use of H₂O₂ and guaiacol as the oxidizing and reducing substrates, respectively (56). PGHS-1 contains one heme per subunit, and this heme is required for both the perox-

idase and cyclooxygenase activities (12,57). The peroxidase activity of PGHS-1 forms two higher oxidation states that are spectroscopically analogous to compounds I and II of various peroxidases (12).

The peroxidase activity of PGHS-1 preferentially reduces primary and secondary alkyl hydroperoxides, is much less active toward H₂O₂, and is essentially inactive with tertiary hydroperoxides (54,55,58). As with most peroxidases, a wide variety of compounds can serve as reducing cosubstrates for PGHS-1 peroxidase (54,55). The identity of the physiologic reducing cosubstrate(s) is not known. PGHSs can also catalyze peroxidatic cooxidations of xenobiotics such as aromatic amines, polycyclic hydrocarbons, nitrofurans, mycotoxins, synthetic estrogens, bisulfite, phenols, heterocyclic amines, hydantoins, and indoles (59,60). These processes may be important in extrahepatic tissues having low levels of cytochrome P-450.

Cyclooxygenase–Peroxidase Interrelationships

The hydrogen abstracted from the 13-pro*S* position of arachidonic acid during the cyclooxygenase reaction is abstracted as a free radical (49,61). A radical enzyme species is required to affect this hydrogen abstraction, and there is now considerable evidence that

CYCLOOXYGENASE

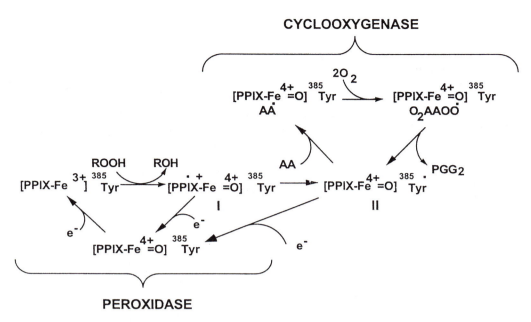

PEROXIDASE

Figure 8-2. Model for the mechanism of PGHS catalysis. Hydroperoxide-dependent heme oxidation leads to an intermediate I. An internal redox reaction produces intermediate II and an associated tyrosyl radical. This radical is proposed to be involved in abstraction of the 13-pro$S$ hydrogen from arachidonic acid. PPIX-Fe^{3+}, heme; AA, arachidonic acid. (Adapted from Deitz R, Nastaincyzk W, Ruf HH. Eur J Biochem 1988;171:321–328.)

this enzyme radical is a tyrosyl radical (49,62–64). Depicted in Fig. 8-2 is a model developed by Ruf and coworkers showing how a tyrosyl radical could be generated by the interaction of PGHS with an alkyl hydroperoxide (63). According to the model, two-electron oxidation of the heme group at the peroxidase active site of PGHSs by a hydroperoxide such as PGG$_2$ causes formation of intermediate I. Intermediate I has a two-electron oxidized heme in which the iron is in the 4+ state and the porphyrin group is oxidized to a radical cation (62,65). Intermediate I can abstract a hydrogen from the phenolic side chain of a neighboring protein tyrosine residue to produce an intermediate II with an associated protein tyrosyl radical. Intermediate II has a one-electron oxidized heme group in which the porphyrin is neutral and the iron is in its 4+ state (62,65). The tyrosyl radical associated with intermediate II was proposed by Ruf and coworkers to be the species that abstracts the 13-pro$S$ hydrogen from arachidonic acid, initiating the cyclooxygenase reaction (62).

The Ruf tyrosyl radical model (Fig. 8-2) is supported by the following observations. Alkyl hydroperoxides are required for cyclooxygenase activity (66), and treatment of PGHS-1 with alkyl hydroperoxides causes the formation of spectral intermediates I and II characteristic of heme peroxidases (62,65). Protein tyrosyl radicals are formed when PGHS-1 is incubated with hydroperoxides, and the formation of a tyrosyl radical and the heme spectral intermediate II occur concomitantly. A tyrosine residue, Tyr385, neighbors the heme group in the cyclooxygenase active site of PGH synthase and is required for cyclooxygenase (but not peroxidase) activity (8,10,67,68).

Structure of PGHS Active Sites

A model of the active site of ovine PGHS-1 is presented in Fig. 8-3 (12). An alkyl hydroperoxide is shown associated with the heme group bound to the peroxidase active site. The heme is liganded at the proximal position by His388 and at the distal position by His207 (8). An intramolecular electron transfer from a neighboring Tyr385 to an oxidized heme is envisioned to yield a tyrosyl radical centered on Tyr385. This tyrosyl radical may abstract the hydrogen atom from the arachidonic acid bound in the cyclooxygenase active site to initiate the cyclooxygenase reaction. Ser530, the site of aspirin acetylation (69–71), is shown in close proximity to the cyclooxygenase active site. Arg120 appears to be the counterion for the carboxyl group of arachidonic acid (72–74). The recent publication of the crystal structures of PGHS-1 and PGHS-2 (8–10) provides overall support for the model depicted in Figure 8-3. Additionally, these investigators have provided evidence that the arachidonic acid binding site takes the form of a hydrophobic channel in the core of what is observed as a globular protein.

Comparison of PGHS-1 and PGHS-2

Primary Structures of PGHS Isozymes

The deduced amino acid sequences of human PGHS-1 and PGHS-2 are compared in Figure 8-4. PGHS-1 was originally puri-

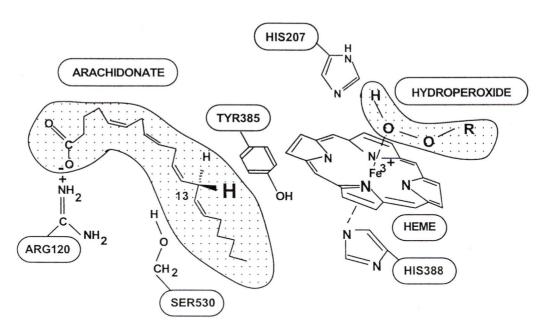

Figure 8-3. Model of the cyclooxygenase and peroxidase active sites of ovine PGHS-1. A hydroperoxide is shown bound to the heme group at the peroxidase active site. Arachidonic acid (arachidonate) is shown bound to the cyclooxygenase active site.

fied from ovine and bovine vesicular glands in the mid 1970s (75,76). cDNAs encoding murine (69), human (38), rat (77), and ovine (78–80) PGHS-1 have now been cloned.

PGHS-2 was originally described in 1991 as a v-*src*–inducible gene product from chicken fibroblasts (81) and as a phorbol ester–inducible, immediate, early gene product called TIS10 from mouse 3T3 cells (82). Human PGHS-2 has subsequently been cloned (83,84). Within a species there is about 60% amino acid identity between the deduced amino acid sequences of PGHS-1 and PGHS-2 (see Fig. 8-4). PGHS-2 differs significantly from PGHS-1 at positions before amino acid residue 30; processed PGHS-1 has 576 amino acids and an N-terminal sequence ADPGA as a result of the removal of a signal peptide with 25 amino acids (see Fig. 8-4). Mature PGHS-2 have the N-terminal sequence ANPCC (85), corresponding to cleavage of a 17-amino acid signal peptide from the N terminus of the deduced sequence. Most notably, PGHS-2 contains an 18-amino acid insert near the C terminus of the enzyme. This insert is absent from PGHS-1, and antibodies prepared against this peptide insert are specific for PGHS-2 (86). With the exclusion of the sequences near the N and C termini, the sequences of PGHS-1 and PGHS-2 are about 75% identical. All residues identified as essential for the catalytic activity of PGHS-1 are conserved in PGHS-2 (Figs. 8-4 and 8-5).

Physicochemical Properties of PGHS-1 and PGHS-2

PGHS-1 has a predicted subunit molecular weight of approximately 65,500, excluding the signal peptide; however, native PGHS-1 migrates on sodium dodecyl sulfate-polyacrylamide gel electrophoresis (SDS-PAGE) with a molecular weight of about 72,000 because of the presence of three high mannose oligosaccharides: one $Man_7(NAcGln)_2$ and two $Man_9(NAcGln)_2$ (87) located at Asn67, Asn143, and Asn409 of the human enzyme (Fig. 8-4) (88). The functional significance of glycosylation is not well understood, but glycosylation at Asn409 in PGHS-1 is required for enzyme activity (88).

In contrast to PGHS-1, PGHS-2 typically appears as a doublet on SDS-PAGE with molecular weights of 72,000 and 74,000 (88,89). The 72-kDa form contains three N-linked oligosaccharides, whereas the 74-kDa species contains four N-linked oligosaccharides (88). Asparagine residues homologous to those that are glycosylated in PGHS-1 are apparently glycosylated in PGHS-2; there is also a fourth site of N-glycosylation in PGHS-2 located near the C terminus (i.e., at Asn580 in human PGHS-2 [see Fig. 8-4]) that is glycosylated in about half of PGHS-2 molecules (88). Unlike PGHS-1, glycosylation of PGHS-2 is not critical for the folding of the enzyme in an active form, a fact that has facilitated its overexpression in baculovirus systems (9,10).

PGHS-1 and PGHS-2 are integral membrane proteins that appear to exist as dimers (8–10). Both PGHS-1 and PGHS-2 are located on the luminal surfaces of the endoplasmic reticulum and the inner and outer membranes of the nuclear envelope (88,90).

Differential Regulation of Expression of PGHS-1 and PGHS-2

PGHS-1 is considered to be the constitutive isoform and PGHS-2 the inducible isoform. PGHS-1 and PGHS-2 are encoded by

```
Human-2    MLARALLLCAVL----------------ALSHTANPCCSHPCQNRGVCMSVGFDQYKCD
Human-1    MSR-SLLLRFLLLLLLL-PPLP-VLLADPGAPTPVNPCCYYPCQHQGICVRFGLDRYQCD
               10        20        30        40        50

Human-2    CTRTGFYGENCSTPEFLTRIKFLLKPTPNTVHYILTHFKGFWNVVNNIPFLRNAIMSYVL
Human-1    CTRTGYSGPNCTIPGLWTWLRNSLRPSPSFTHFLLTHGRWFWEFVNAT-FIREMLMLLVL
               60        70        80        90       100       110

Human-2    TSRSHLIDSPPTYNADYGYKSWEAFSNLSYYTRALPPVPDDCPTPLGVKGKKQLPDSNEI
Human-1    TVRSNLIPSPPTYNSAHDYISWESFSNVSYYTRILPSVPKDCPTPMGTKGKKQLPDAQLL
              120       130       140       150       160       170

Human-2    VGKLLLRRKFIPDPQGSNMMFAFFAQHFTHQFFKTDHKRGPAFTNGLGHGVDLNHIYGET
Human-1    ARRFLLRRKFIPDPQGTNLMFAFFAQHFTHQFFKTSGKMGPGFTKALGHGVDLGHIYGDN
              180       190       200       210       220       230

Human-2    LARQRKIRLFKDGKMKYQIIDGEMYPPTVKDTQAEMIYPPQVPEHLRFAVGQEVFGLVPG
Human-1    LERQYQLRLFKDGKLKYQVLDGEMYPPSVEEAPVLMHYPRGIPPQSQMAVGQEVFGLLPG
              240       250       260       270       280       290

Human-2    LMMYATIWLREHNRVCDVLKQEHPEWGDEQLFQTSRLILIGETIKIVIDDYVQHLSGYHF
Human-1    LMLYATLWLREHNRVCDLLKAEHPTWGDEQLFQTTRLILIGETIKIVIEEYVQQLSGYFL
              300       310       320       330       340       350

Human-2    KLKFDPELLFNKQFQYQNRIAAEFNTLYHWHPLLPDTFQINDQKYNYQQFIYNNSILLEH
Human-1    QLKFDPELLFGVQFQYRNRIATEFNHLYHWHPLMPDSFKVGSQEYSYEQFLFNTSMLVDY
              360       370       380       390       400       410

Human-2    GITQFVESFTRQIAGRVAGGRNVPPAVQKVSQASIDQSRQMKYQSFNEYRKRFMLKPYES
Human-1    GVEALVDAFSRQIAGRIGGGRNMDHHILHVAVDVIRESREMRLQPFNEYRKRFGMKPYTS
              420       430       440       450       460       470

Human-2    FEELTGEKEMSAELEALYGDIDAVELYPALLVEKPRPDAIFGETMVEVGAPFSLKGLMGN
Human-1    FQELVGEKEMAAELEELYGDIDALEFYPGLLLEKCHPNSIFGESMIEIGAPFSLKGLLGN
              480       490       500       510       520       530

Human-2    VICSPAYWKPSTFGGEVGFQIINTASIQSLICNNVKGCPFTSFSVPDPELIKTVTINASS
Human-1    PICSPEYWKPSTFGGEVGFNIVKTATLKKLVCLNTKTCPYVSFRVPDASQDDGPAVE---
              540       550       560       570       580       590

Human-2    SRSGLDDINPTVLLKERSTEL
Human-1    --------------RPSTEL
                             599
```

Figure 8-4. Deduced amino acid sequences of human PGHS-1 and PGHS-2. Numbering refers to human PGHS-1 and begins with the methionine at the translation start site. Shown in bold letters are the signal peptides; asparagine residues, which are N-glycosylated; catalytically essential histidine and tyrosine residues; and the serine residue, which is acetylated by aspirin and the characteristic 18-amino-acid insert close to the C terminus of PGHS-2.

PGHS -1:

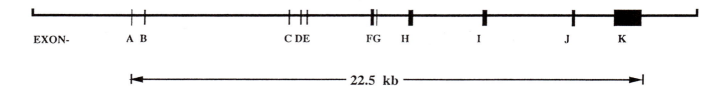

PGHS -2:

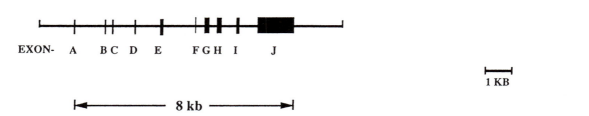

Figure 8-5. Structures of the genes encoding mouse PGHS-1 and PGHS-2. Exons are denoted with letters. The structures of the genes for PGHS-1 and -2 are from references (93) and (92), respectively. kb, kilobases.

separate genes (91–93) (see Fig. 8-5) located on human chromosomes 9 (38) and 1 (84), respectively. Apart from the first two exons, the intron/exon arrangements are the same, but the PGHS-2 gene (approximately 8 kilobases (kb)) is considerably smaller than the PGHS-1 gene (approximately 22 kb).

PGHS-1 is expressed more or less constitutively in almost all tissues (94). Apparently, cells use PGHS-1 to produce prostaglandins needed to regulate "housekeeping activities" that typically involve rapid responses to circulating hormones (see Fig. 8-1). The expression of PGHS-1 is controlled developmentally (95–97). However, PGHS-1 levels can be down-regulated in endothelial cells in response to acidic fibroblast growth factor (98) and up-regulated in mast cells treated with stem cell factor in combination with dexamethasone (99) and in seminal vesicles by testosterone (96). Typical of developmentally regulated "housekeeping" genes, the PGHS-1 gene lacks a TATA box. Little is known about the details of the regulation of PGHS-1 gene expression.

In contrast to PGHS-1, PGHS-2 apparently produces prostanoids, which function only during specific stages of cell differentiation or replication. Although there are a few exceptions (85,100–103), PGHS-2 does not appear to be expressed to any significant degree in unstimulated tissues (104). PGHS-2 has been detected *in vivo* after carrageenan injection in rat paw (104), in articular tissue during staphylococcal cell-wall or adjuvant-induced arthritis in rat (104), and in joints of humans with rheumatoid arthritis (105–107).

Much of what is known about the induction of PGHS-2 comes from studies with cultured fibroblasts and endothelial cells and purified macrophages. Typically, PGHS-2 is induced rapidly

(1 to 3 hours) and dramatically (20- to 80-fold). Growth factors, phorbol esters, v-*src*, and interleukin (IL)-1β induce PGHS-2 in fibroblasts and endothelial cells (84,108–114); lipopolysaccharide (LPS), IL-1, and tumor necrosis factor α (TNF-α) stimulate PGHS-2 expression ex vivo in monocytes, macrophages, and osteoblasts (115–119); and IL-1 stimulates PGHS-2 expression in mesangial cells (120,121). Although only a limited number of tissue and cell types have been examined, it is likely that PGHS-2 can be induced in almost any cell or tissue with the appropriate stimuli. Importantly, PGHS-2 expression, but not PGHS-1 expression, can be completely inhibited by anti-inflammatory glucocorticoids such as dexamethasone (92,105, 108–110,117,122).

The PGHS-2 promoter (Fig. 8-6), unlike the PGHS-1 promoter, contains a TATA box, typical of inducible genes. Experiments with reporter plasmids containing the PGHS-2 promoter and upstream 5′-flanking sequence have demonstrated that PGHS-2 is highly regulatable. Transcriptional activation of the PGHS-2 gene appears to be one important mechanism for increasing PGHS-2 expression (108,110). The transcription of PGHS-2 is unique in that it can be controlled by multiple signaling pathways, including the cyclic adenosine monophosphate (cAMP) pathway (123,124), by the protein kinase C pathway (phorbol esters) (82,83,106,112), by viral transformation (v-*src*) (108,114), and by other pleiotropic pathways such as those activated by platelet-derived growth factor (PDGF) and epidermal growth factor (EGF) (125), bacterial endotoxin (LPS) (77,83,84,115,117,118), inflammatory cytokines (IL-1) (77,84,106,107,121), and related lymphokines such as TNF-α (119).

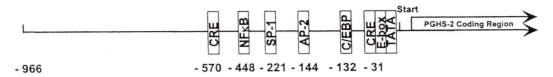

Figure 8-6. Structure of the promoter region of the mouse PGHS-2 gene showing putative transcriptional regulator elements. CRE, cyclic AMP responsive element; NFκB, nuclear factor κB; C/EBP, CAAT/enhancer binding protein.

The primary structures of the human (126), mouse (92), and rat (123,127) PGHS-2 genes and 5′-flanking regions have been determined (see Fig. 8-6). The complex analysis of *cis* elements responsible for the regulation of this gene are, as yet, rather incomplete. The transcriptional control elements necessary for activation of the mouse PGHS-2 gene by phorbol esters and serum are located within the first 371 nucleotides upstream of the mouse PGHS-2 transcription start site (92). Ongoing efforts designed to understand the multiple mechanisms that regulate PGHS-2 expression have identified several relevant enhancer sequences in the PGHS-2 gene promoter. In bovine endothelial cells, a CAAT/enhancer binding protein β (CEBPβ) site is responsible for the induction of PGHS-2 by LPS and tetramethyl phorbol acetate (TPA) (128), whereas the same site has been found to be responsible for TNF-α–mediated induction of PGHS-2 in MC3T3-E1 cells (119,129). An E-box sequence is essential for basal, luteinizing hormone (LH)- and gonadotropin-releasing hormone (GnRH)-stimulated transcription, and this element binds the USF transcription factor (130). A (CRE) mediates the effect of v-*src* on PGHS-2 expression in fibroblasts (114). c-Jun in combination with one of the ATF transcription factors appears to be important in IL-1β–, PDGF-, serum-, and v-*src*–mediated induction of PGHS-2 (114,121,131,132), and this appears to involve an interaction with the cyclic AMP responsive (CRE) element. Additional *cis*-acting DNA elements undoubtedly also participate in the many other effector pathways that regulate PGHS-2 expression.

The mechanisms underlying the inhibitory effect of glucocorticoids have still not been determined, but there appear to be both transcriptional (111) and post-transcriptional components (108,133).

Although PGHS-2 expression is regulated acutely by transcriptional activation, posttranscriptional regulation also occurs. PGHS-2 mRNA is unstable compared with PGHS-1 mRNA (110), a feature predicted from the presence of multiple RNA instability sequences (AUUUA) in its 3′-untranslated region. PGHS-2 mRNA is translated as soon as it is synthesized; therefore, the short mRNA half-life limits PGHS-2 production posttranscriptionally.

PGHS-2 protein is also much less stable in fibroblasts than is PGHS-1, a post-translational regulatory mechanism that limits PGHS-2 levels in fibroblasts (110). The factor(s) that account for the different protein stabilities of PGHS-1 and PGHS-2 are not known, but increased protein turnover of PGHS-2 may be mediated through the C-terminal protein sequences that are unique to PGHS-2.

Interactions of NSAIDs with PGHS-1 and PGHS-2

Vane first reported in 1971 that aspirin and indomethacin inhibit the biosynthesis of prostanoids (134). Shortly thereafter, Smith and Lands (135) established that these inhibitors specifically block the oxygenation of arachidonic acid (i.e., PGHS-1), and they noted that both aspirin and indomethacin are time-dependent inhibitors. In 1974, [1-^{14}C]acetyl-salicylate was found to cause the selective acetylation of a platelet protein with a molecular weight of about 70,000, now known to be PGHS-1 (136). At about the same time, careful kinetic studies by Rome and Lands (1) indicated that NSAIDs are competitive inhibitors of PGHS-1 (i.e., competitive with arachidonic acid) and that there are two types of inhibitors: (1) simple, competitive, and (2) competitive and time-dependent. After PGHS-1 was purified, it was recognized to have both cyclooxygenase and peroxidase activities, but only the cyclooxygenase activity was blocked by NSAIDs (53,137). During the 1980s numerous studies were performed to define the nature of the interactions of various NSAIDs with purified PGHS-1. The discovery of PGHS-2 in 1991 and evidence suggesting that this inducible isozyme is the actual target of NSAIDs acting in their anti-inflammatory capacities (33,138) led to numerous comparisons of the actions of NSAIDs on PGHS-1 and PGHS-2 (2–4,6,7,139). The goal was to develop PGHS-2 selective inhibitors. Beginning with work on DuP697 (140), it was soon recognized that this and other PGHS-2 selective inhibitors (COX-2 inhibitors) owed their selectivity to two factors: 1) they have somewhat higher affinities for the COX-2 versus the COX-1 active site, and 2) they are simple, competitive inhibitors of COX-1 but competitive, time-dependent inhibitors of COX-2. Indeed, all the COX-2 inhibitors developed commercially seem to share these biochemical characteristics, including DuP697 (140), NS398 (138,140), SC52125 (9), and L-745,337 (141,142). Two of these COX-2 inhibitors, Celebrex from Searle/Monsanto and Vioxx from Merck, are or will soon be available by prescription. Finally, COX-2 inhibitors have been developed that covalently modify PGHS-2 and, accordingly, cause a time-dependent but irreversible inhibition (143).

Comparisons of the reactivities of common NSAIDs for PGHS-1 and PGHS-2 (1–7) indicate that PGHS-1 and PGHS-2 are pharmacologically distinct and that the cyclooxygenase active site of PGHS-2 is somewhat larger than that of PGHS-1; this latter finding is consistent with analyses of the crystal structures of the two isozymes (8–10).

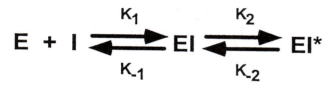

Figure 8-7. Interaction of PGHSs with nonsteroidal anti-inflammatory drugs. Class I inhibitors form EI complexes reversibly. Class II inhibitors form EI complexes, which rearrange to form EI* complexes; I can dissociate from EI*, but dissociation is normally quite slow. Class III inhibitors form EI* complexes through covalent modification of the protein, and $k_{-2} = 0$.

In the concluding section of this chapter, we summarize work on the classification of various NSAIDs and their interactions with PGHS-1 and PGHS-2. NSAIDs can be grouped into three broad classes based on their modes of inhibition of PGHSs (Fig. 8-7):

1. Class I—simple, competitive; for example, ibuprofen, mefenamic acid, flufenamic acid, piroxicam, sulindac sulfide, naproxen, and 6-methoxy-naphthyl-2-acetic acid (the active form of Relafen)
2. Class II—competitive, time-dependent, reversible; for example, indomethacin, meclofenamic acid, flurbiprofen diclofenac, DuP697, SC52125, NS398, and L745,337
3. Class III—competitive, time-dependent, irreversible; for example, aspirin, valeryl salicylate (144), and 2-(acetoxy phenyl)-hept-2-ynyl sulfide (143)

Class I inhibitors are typical reversible inhibitors that rapidly and reversibly form an EI complex only (i.e., $k_2 = 0$). Class II inhibitors form an EI complex and then cause a conformational change in the protein leading to an EI* complex; formation of EI* is relatively slow, as is the reversal of EI* to EI. No covalent modification occurs in forming EI*. Class III inhibitors form an EI* complex by covalent modification of the protein. Shown in Fig. 8-8 are the structures of some of the relevant inhibitors that will be discussed. Further details about COX-2–specific inhibitors are presented in two recent, excellent reviews (145,146).

Class I NSAIDs

Many of the common NSAIDs are simple, competitive inhibitors that compete reversibly with arachidonic acid for binding to the cyclooxygenase active site. Included in this class of compounds are piroxicam (147), flufenamate (1), sulindac sulfide (3), and naproxen and ibuprofen (1–3).

The relative affinities of NSAIDs for PGHS-1 and PGHS-2 can be determined conveniently by measuring the "instantaneous" inhibition of PGHS-1 and PGHS-2 in vitro (2,148) in the following ways. Substrate arachidonic acid (and O_2) and inhibitor are placed in an assay system, and O_2 consumption resulting from cyclooxygenase activity is measured immediately on the addition of PGHS preparations. Because there is no preincubation of inhibitor with enzyme and because k_2 values are much smaller

than k_1 values (see Fig. 8-7), the phenomenon of time-dependent inhibition can be circumvented with this protocol. In addition, the K_m values of PGHS-1 and PGHS-2 for arachidonic acid are identical (2). Therefore, the IC_{50} values can be compared directly to obtain an estimate of the relative affinities of any NSAID for either isozyme; it is not necessary to determine an absolute K_i value, which is a much more laborious procedure.

Most common NSAIDs have higher affinities for PGHS-1 than for PGHS-2 (2). Furthermore, whereas all of the common NSAIDs inhibit PGHS-1, some of these compounds (e.g., piroxicam, indomethacin, and phenylbutazone), which are relatively potent as NSAIDs, are inefficient instantaneous inhibitors of PGHS-2 ($IC_{50} \geq 100\,\mu M$). As discussed below, indomethacin, for example, causes time-dependent inhibition of cyclooxygenase activity. Accordingly, measurements of instantaneous inhibition understate the potencies of these NSAIDs as cyclooxygenase inhibitors.

It is now recognized that measurements of NSAID potencies are most appropriately conducted in intact cell systems in which endogenous arachidonic acid is used as the substrate (7,145).

Class II NSAIDs

Class II NSAIDs such as indomethacin, flurbiprofen, meclofenamate, and diclofenac and the new COX-2 selective inhibitors exhibit more complex kinetics than class I inhibitors. With class II NSAIDs, k_2 values are significant, and relatively stable EI* complexes are formed (see Fig. 8-7). Class II NSAIDs are time-dependent, competitive inhibitors of cyclooxygenase activity (1,2,140,145,149,150). These agents bind rapidly and reversibly in a first phase to form EI complexes, but, if retained for a sufficient time in the active site, cause a conformational change in the protein associated with tighter (but noncovalent) binding. Once bound in this tighter form, these time-dependent NSAIDs only slowly dissociate from the cyclooxygenase active site. There are differences in the k_{-2} values for different inhibitors (flurbiprofen~meclofenamate>>indomethacin) (2,148,150). In addition, the dissociation of flurbiprofen and meclofenamate from PGHS-2 is relatively rapid compared with their dissociation from PGHS-1 (2).

The nature of the interactions of class II NSAIDs with the cyclooxygenase active site is not clearly understood and probably differs somewhat for different time-dependent inhibitors. The formation of EI* results in a conformational change in PGHSs because, in the case of PGHS-1, the binding of either indomethacin and/or flurbiprofen causes the protein to become less susceptible to cleavage by proteases such as trypsin (151).

It is not yet possible to predict from examination of a chemical structure whether an inhibitor will cause a time-dependent inhibition of PGHS-1 or PGHS-2. Conversion of compounds like indomethacin or flurbiprofen to their methyl esters converts these compounds to class I reversible, competitive inhibitors (1). Moreover, replacement of the Arg120 of PGHS-1 or the homologous Arg106 of PGHS-2 with an uncharged glutamine residue yields mutant enzymes that do not bind 2-phenyl-propionate

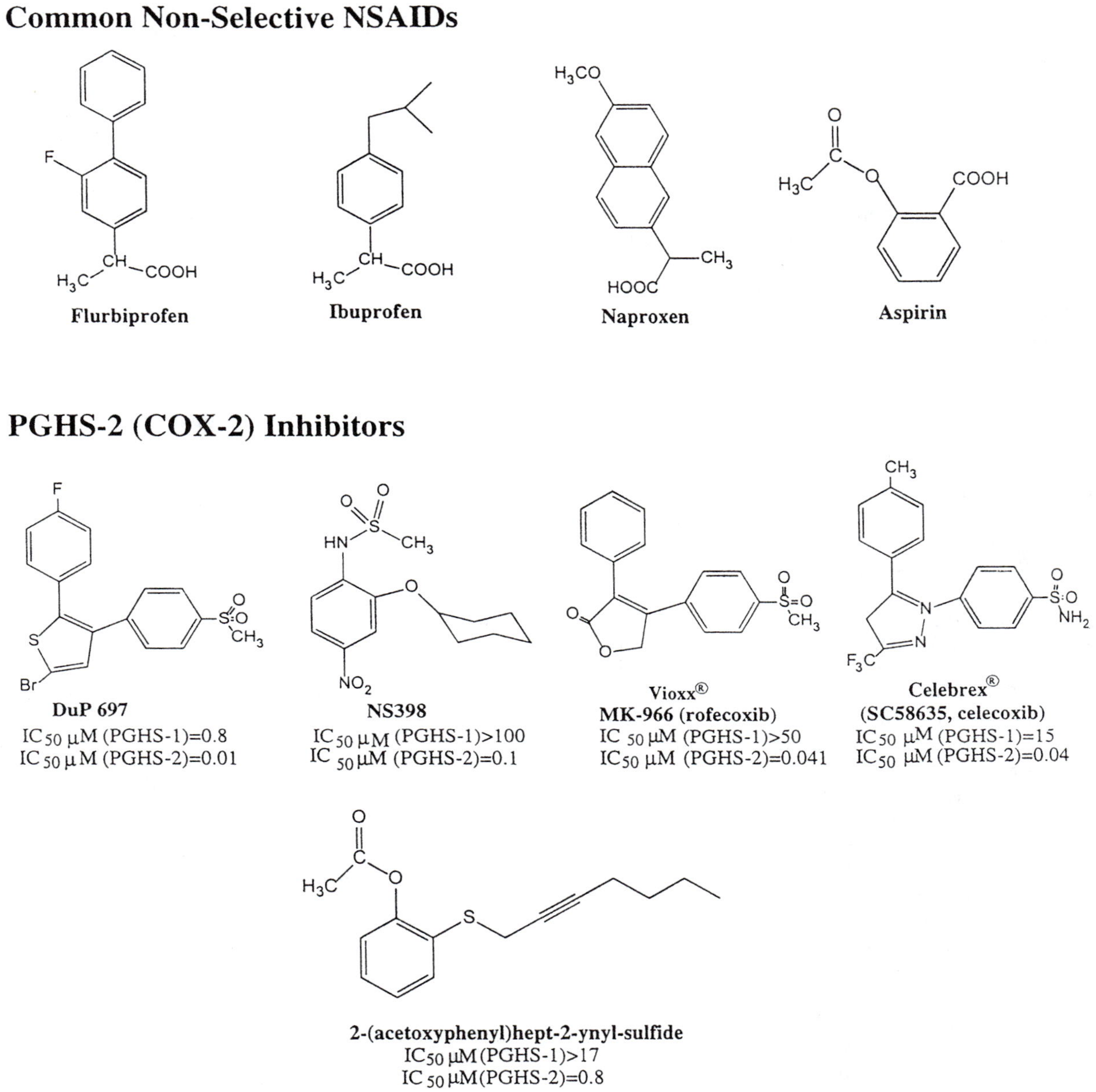

Common Non-Selective NSAIDs

Flurbiprofen   **Ibuprofen**   **Naproxen**   **Aspirin**

PGHS-2 (COX-2) Inhibitors

DuP 697
IC$_{50}$ μM (PGHS-1)=0.8
IC$_{50}$ μM (PGHS-2)=0.01

NS398
IC$_{50}$ μM (PGHS-1)>100
IC$_{50}$ μM (PGHS-2)=0.1

Vioxx®
MK-966 (rofecoxib)
IC$_{50}$ μM (PGHS-1)>50
IC$_{50}$ μM (PGHS-2)=0.041

Celebrex®
(SC58635, celecoxib)
IC$_{50}$ μM (PGHS-1)=15
IC$_{50}$ μM (PGHS-2)=0.04

2-(acetoxyphenyl)hept-2-ynyl-sulfide
IC$_{50}$ μM (PGHS-1)>17
IC$_{50}$ μM (PGHS-2)=0.8

Figure 8-8. Chemical structures of some common NSAIDs, including COX-2 specific inhibitors.

inhibitors such as flurbiprofen effectively, and these mutant enzymes no longer undergo time-dependent inhibition by this class of inhibitors. Those inhibitors that are time-dependent inhibitors of PGHS-1 (e.g., indomethacin, flurbiprofen, diclofenac, and meclofenamate) are uniformly time-dependent inhibitors of PGHS-2.

Two active site residues are of different degrees of importance in the time-dependent inhibition of PGHS-2 by class II NSAIDs. The first is Arg120. Replacement of this residue with a glutamine eliminates the time-dependent inhibition by 2-phenylpropionate inhibitors and NS398 but not by DuP697 or SC52125 (152). A second important residue is Val509 of PGHS-2, which is Ile523 in PGHS-1 and the only residue in the first shell of the cyclooxygenase active site that is different between PGHS-1 and PGHS-2 (153,154). A smaller residue in this position serves to open a "side pocket" in the cyclooxygenase active site of PGHS-2, which is important for binding and time-dependent inhibition by COX-2–specific inhibitors (9,10).

Class III NSAIDs

Aspirin is a unique NSAID because it is the only one known to covalently modify both PGHS-1 and PGHS-2. Aspirin binds to the cyclooxygenase active site of PGHSs, although with very low affinity ($K_i \sim 20\,mM$) (69). However, on binding to the cyclooxygenase active site, aspirin transfers its acetyl group from salicylate to a specific "active site" sersine residue (see Fig. 8-3) (69,71,155). In ovine PGHS-1, this acetylated serine is Ser530 (69,71). A homologous serine in human PGHS-2 (Ser516) is also acetylated (70).

Salicylic acid itself is not an effective inhibitor of PGHS-1 or PGHS-2(2).Like aspirin, this compound has a relatively high K_i (approximately 20 mM), but unlike aspirin salicylate fails to cause covalent modification of PGHSs. Indeed, the basis for the anti-inflammatory activity of salicylic acid remains a mystery.

Acetylation of PGHS-1 by aspirin causes complete inhibition of cyclooxygenase activity, but does not affect peroxidase activity (137,156). Acetylation of PGHS-2 by aspirin converts this isozyme to a form that still oxygenates arachidonic acid, but the product is 15R-hydroxyeicosatetraenoic acid (15R-HETE) instead of PGG$_2$ (4,70,157).

The so-called "active site" serine residue of PGHS-1 is not required for enzyme activity or arachidonic acid binding, because replacement of this residue with an alanine yields a mutant enzyme that is catalytically active and has a K_m for arachidonic acid that is very close to the K_m of the native enzyme (69,70). Substitution of Ser530 with a threonine yields a mutant that forms primarily PGG$_2$ but has a K_m for arachidonic acid of 45 μM, approximately eight times that of the native enzyme (69,158). Replacement of Ser530 with asparagine or leucine, both of which are approximately isosteric with an acetylated Ser530, completely blocks the cyclooxygenase activity of PGHS-1 without affecting peroxidase activity (69,158). These studies, along with the crystal structure of an aspirin-acetylated PGHS-1 (71), indicate that aspirin acetylation of PGHS-1 places a bulky group at Ser530 that prevents arachidonic acid from binding productively in the cyclooxygenase active site.

The effect of aspirin on PGHS-2 is somewhat more complex. In contrast to the results obtained with PGHS-1, replacement of the active site Ser516 of human PGHS-2 with asparagine (or alanine) does not affect enzyme activity (70). Only when the larger glutamine residue is used to replace Ser516 is the cyclooxygenase activity completely blocked (70). Although aspirin-acetylated PGHS-2 produces 15R-HETE instead of PGG$_2$, the K_m values for acetylated PGHS-2 and native PGHS-2 for arachidonic acid are the same (70). Accordingly, it is reasonable to conclude that arachidonic acid binds both native and aspirin-acetylated PGHS-2, but that arachidonic acid is oriented in the active site of the aspirin-acetylated PGHS-2 such that the 13-pro$R$ hydrogen instead of the 13-pro$S$ hydrogen is abstracted by the Tyr385 radical and consequently that the addition of O$_2$ to the resultant arachidonic acid radical yields 15R-HPETE (159).

Various acyl salicylates have been prepared and tested for their relative activities toward PGHS-1 and PGHS-2 (144). Acetyl- and propanoyl-salicylate are about equally effective inhibitors of PGHS-1 and PGHS-2. Acyl salicylates containing four carbons in the acyl chains (i.e., butanoyl, isobutanoyl, and cyclopropyl carboxyl) fail to inhibit either isozyme effectively. Somewhat surprisingly valeryl (pentanoyl) salicylate is a relatively selective inhibitor of PGHS-1, and valeryl salicylate, like aspirin, causes an acylation of Ser530 of PGHS-1 (144). Finally, heptanoyl salicylate inhibits both PGHS-1 and PGHS-2 effectively. Aspirin-like analogs (e.g., 2-[acetoxy phenyl]-hept-2-ynyl sulfide) have recently been developed that selectively inhibit the cyclooxygenase activity of PGHS-2 (146).

A general conclusion from studies with aspirin is that the cyclooxygenase active site of PGHS-2 is slightly larger than that of PGHS-1. This concept is consistent with the broader fatty acid substrate specificity of PGHS-2 and with the lower relative affinities of common NSAIDs for PGHS-2 as opposed to PGHS-1.

Acknowledgments

Studies in the authors' laboratories described in this chapter were supported in part by NIH grants GM57323 (WLS and DLD), DK22042 (WLS), and GM40713 (DLD).

References

1. Rome LH, Lands WEM. Structural requirements for time-dependent inhibition of prostaglandin biosynthesis by anti-inflammatory drugs. Proc Natl Acad Sci USA 1975;72: 4863–4865.
2. Laneuville O, Breuer DK, DeWitt DL, et al. Differential inhibition of human prostaglandin endoperoxide H synthases-1 and -2 by nonsteroidal anti-inflammatory drugs. J Pharmacol Exp Ther 1994;271:927–934.
3. Meade EA, Smith WL, DeWitt DL. Differential inhibition of prostaglandin endoperoxide synthase (cyclooxygenase) isozymes by aspirin and other non-steroidal anti-inflammatory drugs. J Biol Chem 1993;268:6610–6614.
4. O'Neill GP, Mancini JA, Kargman S, et al. Overexpression of human prostaglandin G/H synthase-1 and -2 by recombinant vaccinia virus: inhibition by nonsteroidal anti-inflammatory drugs and biosynthesis of 15-hydroxyeicosatetraenoic acid. Mol Pharmacol 1994;45:245–254.
5. Mitchell JA, Akarasereenont P, Thiemermann C, et al. Selectivity of nonsteroidal antiinflammatory drugs as inhibitors of constitutive and indicible cylooxygenase. Proc Natl Acad Sci USA 1993;90:11693–11697.
6. Barnett J, Chow J, Ives D, et al. Purification, characterization and selective inhibition of human prostaglandin G/H synthase 1 and 2 expressed in the baculovirus system. Biochim Biophys Acta 1994;1209:130–139.
7. Patrignani P, Panara MR, Greco A, et al. Biochemical and pharmacological characterization of the cyclooxygenase activity of human blood prostaglandin endoperoxide synthases. J Pharmacol Exp Ther 1994;271:1705–1712.
8. Picot D, Loll PJ, Garavito M. The X-ray crystal structure of the membrane protein prostaglandin H2 synthase-1. Nature 1994;367:243–249.
9. Kurumbail RG, Stevens AM, Gierse JK, et al. Structural basis for selective inhibition of cyclooxygenase-2 by anti-inflammatory agents. Nature 1996;384:644–648.
10. Luong C, Miller A, Barnett J, et al. Flexibility of the NSAID

binding site in the structure of human cyclooxygenase-2. Nature Structural Biology 1996;3:927–933.

11. Smith WL. The eicosanoids and their biochemical mechanisms of action. Biochem J 1989;259:315–324.

12. Smith WL, Garavito RM, DeWitt DL. Prostaglandin endoperoxide H synthases (cyclooxygenases)-1 and -2. J Biol Chem 1996;271:33157–33160.

13. Balsinde J, Balboa MA, Dennis EA. Functional coupling between secretory phospholipase A2 and cyclooxygenase-2 and its regulation by cytosolic group IV phospholipase A2. Pro Natl Acad Sci USA 1998;95:7951–7956.

14. Murakami M, Shimbara S, Kambe T, et al. The functions of five distinct mammalian phospholipase A2 in regulating arachidonic acid release. Type IIa and type V secretory phospholipase A2 are functionally redundant and act in concert with cytosolic phospholipase A2. J Biol Chem 1998;273:14411–14423.

15. Murakami M, Kambe T, Shimbara S, Kudo I. Functional coupling between various phospholipase A2s and cyclooxygenases in immediate and delayed prostanoid biosynthetic pathways. J Biol Chem 1999;274:3103–3115.

16. Chan BS, Satriano JA, Pucci M, Schuster VL. Mechanism of prostaglandin E2 transport across the plasma membrane of HeLa cells and Xenopus oocytes expressing the prostaglandin transporter "PGT." J Biol Chem 1998;273:6689–6697.

17. Narumiya S. Molecular diversity of prostanoid receptors; subtypes and isoforms of prostaglandin E receptor. Adv Exp Med Biol 1997;400A:207–213.

18. Murata T, Ushikubi F, Matsuoka T, et al. Altered pain perception and inflammatory response in mice lacking prostacyclin receptor. Nature 1997;388:678–682.

19. Sugimoto Y, Yamasaki A, Segi E, et al. Failure of parturition in mice lacking the prostaglandin F receptor. Science 1997;277:681–683.

20. Ushikubi F, Segi E, Sugimoto Y, et al. Impaired febrile response in mice lacking the prostaglandin E receptor subtype EP3. Nature 1998;395:281–284.

21. Segi E, Sugimoto Y, Yamasaki A, et al. Patent ductus arteriosus and neonatal death in prostaglandin receptor EP4-deficient mice. Biochem Biophys Res Commun 1998;246:7–12.

22. Forman BM, Tontonoz P, Chen J, et al. 15-Deoxy-delta-12,14-prostaglandin J2 is a ligand for the adipocyte determination factor PPAR-gamma. Cell 1995;83:803–812.

23. Lim H, Gupta RA, Paria BC, et al. Cyclooxygenase-2 derived prostacyclin mediates embryo implantation in the mouse via PPAR-delta. Cell 1999;13:1561–1574.

24. Levy GN. Prostaglandin H synthases, nonsteroidal anti-inflammatory drugs, and colon cancer. FASEB J 1997;11:234–247.

25. Tsujii M, Kawano S, Tsuji S, et al. Cyclooxygenase regulates angiogenesis induced by colon cancer cells. Cell 1998;93:705–716.

26. Thun MJ, Namboodiri MM, Heath CW. Aspirin use and reduced risk of fatal colon cancer. N Engl J Med 1991;325:1593–1596.

27. Thun MJ. NSAID use and decreased risk of gastrointestinal cancers. Gastroenterol Clin North Am 1996;25:333–348.

28. Breitner JC. Inflammatory processes and antiinflammatory drugs in Alzheimer's disease: a current appraisal. Neurobiol Aging 1996;17:789–794.

29. Riendeau D, Percival MD, Boyce S, et al. Biochemical and pharmacological profile of a tetrasubstituted furanone as a highly selective COX-2 inhibitor. Br J Pharmacol 1997;121:105–117.

30. Smith CJ, Zhang Y, Koboldt CM, et al. Pharmacological analysis of cyclooxygenase-1 in inflammation. Proc Natl Acad Sci USA 1998;95:13313–13318.

31. Zhang Y, Shaffer A, Portanova J, et al. Inhibition of cyclooxygenase-2 rapidly reverses inflammatory hyperalgesia and prostaglandin E2 production. J Pharmacol Exp Ther 1997;283:1069–1075.

32. Kargman S, Charleson S, Cartwright M, et al. Characterization of Prostaglandin G/H Synthase 1 and 2 in rat, dog, monkey, and human gastrointestinal tracts. Gastroenterology 1996;111:445–454.

33. Masferrer JL, Zweifel BS, Manning PT, et al. Selective inhibition of inducible cyclooxygenase 2 in vivo is antiinflammatory and nonulcerogenic. Proc Natl Acad Sci USA 1994;91:3228–3232.

34. Patrono C, Ciabattoni G, Davi G. Thromboxane biosynthesis in cardiovascular diseases. Stroke 1990;21(suppl 12):IV130–133.

35. Willard J, Lange RA, Hillis LD. The use of aspirin in ischemic heart disease. N Engl J Med 1992;327:175–181.

36. Oates JA, FitzGerald GA, Branch RA, et al. Clinical implications of prostaglandin and thromboxane A2 formation. N Engl J Med 1988;319:689–698.

37. Patrono C. Aspirin as an antiplatelet drug. N Engl J Med 1994;330:1287–1294.

38. Funk CD, Funk LB, Kennedy ME, et al. Human platelet/-erythroleukemia cell prostaglandin G/H synthase: cDNA cloning, expression, and gene chromosomal assignment. FASEB J 1991;5:2304–2312.

39. Sheng H, Shao J, Kirkland SC, et al. Inhibition of human colon cancer cell growth by selective inhibition of cyclooxygenase-2. J Clin Invest 1997;99:2254–2259.

40. Kargman SL, O'Neill GP, Vickers PJ, et al. Expression of prostaglandin G/H synthase-1 and -2 protein in human colon cancer. Cancer Res 1995;55:2556–2559.

41. Kutchera W, Jones DA, Matsunami N, et al. Prostaglandin H synthase 2 is expressed abnormally in human colon cancer: evidence for a transcriptional effect. Proc Natl Acad Sci USA 1996;93:4816–4820.

42. So O-Y, Scarafia LE, Mak AY, et al. The dynamics of prostaglandin H synthases. Studies with prostaglandin H synthase 2 Y355F unmask mechanisms of time-dependent inhibition and allosteric activation. J Biol Chem 1998;273:5801–5807.

43. Kulmacz RJ, Wang L-H. Comparison of hydroperoxide initiator requirements for the cyclooxygenase activities of prostaglandin H synthase-1 and -2. J Biol Chem 1995;270:24019–24023.

44. Capdevila JH, Morrow JD, Belosludtsev YY, et al. The catalytic outcomes of the constitutive and the mitogen inducible isoforms of prostaglandin H2 synthase are markedly affected by glutathione and glutathione peroxidase. Biochemistry 1995;34:3325–3337.

45. Landino LM, Crews BC, Gierse JK, et al. Mutational analysis of the role of the distal histidine and glutamine residues of prostaglandin-endoperoxide synthase-2 in peroxidase catalysis, hydroperoxide reduction, and cyclooxygenase activation. J Biol Chem 1997;272:21565–21574.

46. Kulmacz RJ. Cellular regulation of prostaglandin H synthase catalysis. FEBS Lett 1998;430:154–157.

47. Ohki S, Ogino N, Yamamoto S, Hayaishi O. Prostaglandin hydroperoxidase, an integral part of prostaglandin endoperoxide synthetase from bovine vesicular gland microsomes. J Biol Chem 1979;254:829–836.

48. Hamberg M, Samuelsson B. On the mechanism of the biosynthesis of prostaglandins E-1 and F-1-alpha. J Biol Chem 1967;242:5336–5343.

49. Tsai A, Kulmacz RJ, Palmer G. Spectroscopic evidence for reaction of prostaglandin H synthase-1 tyrosyl radical with arachidonic acid. J Biol Chem 1995;270:10503–10508.

50. Tsai A-L, Palmer G, Xiao G, et al. Structural characterization of arachidonyl radicals formed by prostaglandin H synthase-2 and prostaglandin H synthase-1 reconstituted with mangano protoporphyrin IX. J Biol Chem 1998;273:3888–3894.

51. Laneuville O, Breuer DK, Xu N, et al. Fatty acid substrate specificities of human prostaglandin endoperoxide H synthases-1 and -2. Formation of 12 hydroxy-(9Z, 13E/Z, 15Z)-octadecatrienoic acids from alpha-linolenic acid. J Biol Chem 1995;270:19330–19336.

52. Lands WEM, LeTellier PR, Rome LH, Vanderhoek JY. Inhibition of prostaglandin biosynthesis. Adv Biosci 1973;9:15–28.

53. Marshall PJ, Kulmacz RJ. Prostaglandin H synthase: distinct binding sites for cyclooxygenase and peroxidase substrates. Arch Biochem Biophys 1988;266:162–170.

54. Ogino N, Ohki S, Yamamoto S, Hayaishi O. Prostaglandin endoperoxide synthetase from bovine vesicular gland microsomes. Inactivation and activation by heme and other metalloporphyrins. J Biol Chem 1978;253:5061–5068.

55. Markey CM, Alward A, Weller PE, Marnett LJ. Quantitative studies of hydroperoxide reduction by prostaglandin H synthase. Reducing substrate specificity and the relationship of peroxidase to cyclooxygenase activities. J Biol Chem 1987;262:6266–6279.

56. Marnett LJ, Chen YN, Maddipati KR, et al. Functional differentiation of cyclooxygenase and peroxidase activities of prostaglandin synthase by trypsin treatment. Possible location of a prosthetic heme binding site. J Biol Chem 1988;263:16532–16535.

57. Smith WL, Marnett LJ. Prostaglandin endoperoxide synthases. In: Sigel H, Sigel A, eds. Metal ions in biological systems. Vol. 30. New York: Marcel Dekker, 1994:163–199.

58. Kulmacz RJ, Lands WE. Requirements for hydroperoxide by the cyclooxygenase and peroxidase activities of prostaglandin H synthase. Prostaglandins 1983;25:531–540.

59. Eling TE, Thompson DC, Foureman GL, et al. Prostaglandin H synthase and xenobiotic oxidation. Annu Rev Pharmacol Toxicol 1990;30:1–45.

60. Marnett LJ, Maddipati KR. Prostaglandin H synthase. In: Everse J, Everse K, Grisham M, eds. Peroxidases: chemistry and biology. Boca Raton, FL: CRC Press, 1991:293–334.

61. Kwok P-Y, Muellner FW, Fried J. Enzymatic conversion of 10,10-difluoroarachidonic acid with PGH synthase and soybean lipoxygenase. J Am Chem Soc 1987;109:3692–3698.

62. Dietz R, Nastainczyk W, Ruf HH. Higher oxidation states of prostaglandin H synthase. Rapid electronic spectroscopy detected two spectral intermediates during the peroxidase reaction with prostaglandin G2. Eur J Biochem 1988;171:321–328.

63. Karthein R, Dietz R, Nastainczyk W, Ruf HH. Higher oxidation states of prostaglandin H synthase. EPR study of a transient tyrosyl radical in the enzyme during the peroxidase reaction. Eur J Biochem 1988;171:313–320.

64. Gunther MR, Hsi LC, Curtis JF, et al. Nitric oxide trapping of the tyrosyl radical of prostaglandin H synthase-2 leads to tyrosine iminoxyl radical and nitrotyrosine formation. J Biol Chem 1997;272:17086–17090.

65. Lambeir AM, Markey CM, Dunford HB, Marnett LJ. Spectral properties of the higher oxidation states of prostaglandin H synthase. J Biol Chem 1985;260:14894–14896.

66. Hemler ME, Lands WEM. Evidence for a peroxide-initiated free radical mechanism of prostaglandin biosynthesis. J Biol Chem 1980;255:6253–6261.

67. Shimokawa T, Kulmacz RJ, DeWitt DL, Smith WL. Tyrosine 385 of prostaglandin endoperoxide synthase is required for cyclooxygenase catalysis. J Biol Chem 1990;265:20073–20076.

68. Kurumbail RG, personal communication, 1996.

69. DeWitt DL, El-Harith EA, Kraemer SA, et al. The aspirin and heme-binding sites of ovine and murine prostaglandin endoperoxide synthases. J Biol Chem 1990;265:5192–5198.

70. Lecomte M, Laneuville O, Ji C, et al. Acetylation of human prostaglandin endoperoxide synthase-2 (cyclooxygenase-2) by aspirin. J Biol Chem 1994;269:13207–13215.

71. Loll PJ, Picot D, Garavito RM. The structural basis of aspirin activity inferred from the crystal structure of inactivated prostaglandin H2 synthase. Nature Structural Biology 1995;2:637–643.

72. Bhattacharyya DK, Lecomte M, Rieke CJ, et al. Involvement of Arginine 120, Glutamate 524, and Tyrosine 355 in the binding of arachidonate and 2-phenylpropionic acid inhibitors to the cyclooxygenase active site of ovine prostaglandin endoperoxide H synthase-1. J Biol Chem 1996;271:2179–2184.

73. Mancini JA, Riendeau D, Falgueyret JP, et al. Arginine 120 of prostaglandin G/H synthase-1 is required for the inhibition by nonsteroidal anti-inflammatory drugs containing a carboxylic acid moiety. J Biol Chem 1995;270:29372–29377.

74. Greig GM, Francis DA, Falgueyret JP, et al. The interaction of arginine 106 of human prostaglandin G/H synthase-2 with inhibitors is not a universal component of inhibition mediated by nonsteroidal anti-inflammatory drugs. Mol Pharmacol 1997;52:829–838.

75. Hemler M, Lands WEM, Smith WL. Purification of the cyclooxygenase that forms prostaglandins. Demonstration of two forms of iron in the holoenzyme. J Biol Chem 1976;251:5575–5581.

76. Miyamoto T, Ogino N, Yamamoto S, Hayaishi O. Purification of prostaglandin endoperoxide synthetase from bovine vesicular gland microsomes. J Biol Chem 1976;251:2629–2636.

77. Feng L, Sun W, Xia Y, et al. Cloning two isoforms of rat cyclooxygenase: differential regulation of their expression. Arch Biochem Biophys 1993;307:361–368.

78. DeWitt DL, Smith WL. Primary structure of prostaglandin G/H synthase from sheep vesicular gland determined from

the complementary DNA sequence. Proc Natl Acad Sci USA 1988;85:1212–1216.

79. Merlie JP, Fagan D, Mudd J, Needleman P. Isolation and characterization of the complementary DNA for sheep seminal vesicle prostaglandin endoperoxide synthase (cyclooxygenase). J Biol Chem 1988;263:3550–3553.

80. Yokoyama C, Takai T, Tanabe T. Primary structure of sheep prostaglandin endoperoxide synthase deduced from cDNA sequence. FEBS Lett 1988;231:347–351.

81. Xie W, Chipman JG, Robertson DL, et al. Expression of a mitogen-responsive gene encoding prostaglandin synthase is regulated by mRNA splicing. Proc Natl Acad Sci USA 1991;88:2692–2696.

82. Kujubu DA, Fletcher BS, Varnum BC, et al. TIS10, a phorbol ester tumor promoter inducible mRNA from Swiss 3T3 cells, encodes a novel prostaglandin synthase/cyclooxygenase homologue. J Biol Chem 1991;266:12866–12872.

83. Hla T, Neilson K. Human cyclooxygenase-2 cDNA. Proc Natl Acad Sci USA 1992;89:7384–7388.

84. Jones DA, Carlton DP, McIntyre TM, et al. Molecular cloning of human prostaglandin endoperoxide synthase type II and demonstration of expression in response to cytokines. J Biol Chem 1993;268:9049–9054.

85. Simmons DL, Xie W, Chipman JG, Evett GE. Multiple cyclooxygenases: cloning of a mitogen-inducible form. In: Bailey JM, ed. Prostaglandins, leukotrienes, lipoxins, and PAF. New York: Plenum, 1991:67–78.

86. Otto JC, Smith WL. The orientation of prostaglandin endoperoxide synthases-1 and -2 in the endoplasmic reticulum. J Biol Chem 1994;269:19868–19875.

87. Mutsaers JH, van-Halbeek H, Kamerling JP, Vliegenthart JF. Determination of the structure of the carbohydrate chains of prostaglandin endoperoxide synthase from sheep. Eur J Biochem 1985;147:569–574.

88. Otto JC, DeWitt DL, Smith WL. N-glycosylation of prostaglandin endoperoxide synthases-1 and -2 and their orientations in the endoplasmic reticulum. J Biol Chem 1993;268:18234–18242.

89. Sirois J, Richards JS. Purification and characterization of a novel, distinct isoform of prostaglandin endoperoxide synthase induced by human chorionic gonadotropin in granulosa cells of rat preovulatory follicles. J Biol Chem 1992;267:6382–6388.

90. Spencer AG, Woods JW, Arakawa T, et al. Subcellular localization of prostaglandin endoperoxide H synthases-1 and -2 by immunoelectron microscopy. J Biol Chem 1998;273:9886–9893.

91. Yokoyama C, Tanabe T. Cloning of the human gene encoding prostaglandin endoperoxide synthase and primary structure of the enzyme. Biochem Biophys Res Commun 1989;165:888–894.

92. Fletcher BS, Kujubu DA, Perrin DM, Herschman HR. Structure of the mitogen-inducible TIS10 gene and demonstration that the TIS10-encoded protein is a functional prostaglandin G/H synthase. J Biol Chem 1992;267:4338–4344.

93. Kraemer SA, Meade SA, DeWitt DL. Prostaglandin endoperoxide synthase gene structure: identification of the transcriptional start site and 5′-flanking regulatory sequences. Arch Biochem Biophys 1992;293:391–400.

94. Smith WL. Localization of enzymes responsible for

prostaglandin formation. In: Willis AL, ed. CRC handbook of eicosanoids: prostaglandins and related lipids. Vol. 1. Boca Raton, FL: CRC Press, 1987:175–184.

95. Brannon TS, North AJ, Wells LB, Shaul PW. Prostacyclin synthesis in ovine pulmonary artery is developmentally regulated by changes in cyclooxygenase-1 gene expression. J Clin Invest 1994;93:2230–2235.

96. Silvia WJ, Brockman JA, Kaminski MA, et al. Prostaglandin endoperoxide synthase in seminal vesicles. Mol Androl 1994;6:197–207.

97. Ueda N, Yamashita R, Yamamoto S, Ishimura K. Induction of cyclooxygenase-1 in a human megakaryoblastic cell line (CMK) differentiated by phorbol ester. Biochim Biophys Acta 1997;1344:103–110.

98. Hla T, Maciag T. Cyclooxygenase gene expression is downregulated by heparin-binding (acidic fibroblast) growth factor-1 in human endothelial cells. J Biol Chem 1991;266:24059–24063.

99. Samet JM, Fasano MB, Fonteh AN, Chilton FH. Selective induction of prostaglandin G/H synthase I by stem cell factor and dexamethasone in mast cells. J Biol Chem 1995;270:8044–8049.

100. Harris RC, McKanna JA, Akai Y, et al. Cyclooxygenase-2 is associated with the macula densa of rat kidney and increases with salt restriction. J Clin Invest 1994;94:2504–2510.

101. McKanna JA, Zhang MZ, Wang JL, et al. Constitutive expression of cyclooxygenase-2 in rat vas deferens. Am J Physiol 1998;275:R227–233.

102. Yamagata K, Andreasson KI, Kaufmann WE, et al. Expression of a mitogen-inducible cyclooxygenase in brain neurons: regulation by synaptic activity and glucocorticoids. Neuron 1993;11:371–386.

103. Walenga RW, Kester M, Coroneos E, et al. Constitutive expression of prostaglandin endoperoxide G/H synthetase (PGHS)-2 but not PGHS-1 in human tracheal epithelial cells in vitro. Prostaglandins 1996;52:341–359.

104. Kargman S, Chan S, Evans J, et al. Tissue distribution of prostaglandin G/H synthase-1 and -2 (PGHS-1 and PGHS-2) using specific anti-peptide antibodies. J Cell Biochem Suppl 1994;18B:319. Abstract O109.

105. Sano H, Hla T, Maier JAM, et al. In vivo cyclooxygenase expression in synovial tissue of patients with rheumatoid arthritis and osteoarthritis and rats with adjuvant and streptococcal cell wall arthritis. J Clin Invest 1992;89:97–108.

106. Crofford LJ, Wilder RL, Ristimaki AP, et al. Cyclooxygenase-1 and -2 expression in rheumatoid synovial tissues. Effects of interleukin-1 beta, phorbol ester, and corticosteroids. J Clin Invest 1994;93:1095–1101.

107. Hulkower KI, Wertheimer SJ, Levin W, et al. Interleukin-1 beta induces cytosolic phospholipase A2 and prostaglandin H synthase in rheumatoid synovial fibroblasts. Evidence for their roles in the production of prostaglandin E2. Arthritis Rheum 1994;37:653–661.

108. Evett GE, Xie W, Chipman JG, et al. Prostaglandin G/H isoenzyme 2 expression in fibroblasts: regulation by dexamethasone, mitogens, and oncogenes. Arch Biochem Biophys 1993;306:169–177.

109. Kujubu DA, Herschman HR. Dexamethasone inhibits mitogen induction of the TIS10 prostaglandin synthase/cyclooxygenase gene. J Biol Chem 1992;267:7991–7994.

110. DeWitt DL, Meade EA. Serum and glucocorticoid regulation of gene transcription and expression of the prostaglandin H synthase-1 and prostaglandin H synthase-2 isozymes. Arch Biochem Biophys 1993;306:94–102.

111. Kujubu DA, Reddy ST, Fletcher BS, Herschman HR. Expression of the protein product of the prostaglandin synthase-2/TIS10 gene in mitogen-stimulated Swiss 3T3 cells. J Biol Chem 1993;268:5425–5430.

112. Pilbeam CC, Kawaguchi H, Hakeda Y, et al. Differential regulation of inducible and constitutive prostaglandin endoperoxide synthase in osteoblastic MC3T3-E1 cells. J Biol Chem 1993;268:25643–25649.

113. Han J, Sadowski H, Young DA, Macara IG. Persistant induction of cyclooxygenase in p60v-src-transformed 3T3 fibroblasts. Proc Natl Acad Sci USA 1990;87:3373–3377.

114. Xie W, Herschman HR. v-src Induces prostaglandin synthase 2 gene expression by activation of the c-Jun N-terminal kinase and the c-Jun transcription factor. J Biol Chem 1995;270:27622–27628.

115. O'Sullivan GM, Chilton FH, Huggins EM Jr, McCall CE. Lipopolysaccharide priming of alveolar macrophages for enhanced synthesis of prostanoids involves induction of a novel prostaglandin H synthase. J Biol Chem 1992;267:14547–14550.

116. O'Sullivan MG, Huggins EM Jr, Meade EA, et al. Lipopolysaccharide induces prostaglandin H synthase-2 in alveolar macrophages. Biochem Biophys Res Commun 1992;187:1123–1127.

117. Lee SH, Soyoola E, Chanmugam P, et al. Selective expression of mitogen-inducible cyclooxygenase in macrophages stimulated with lipopolysaccharide. J Biol Chem 1992;267:25934–25938.

118. Riese J, Hoff T, Nordhoff A, et al. Transient expression of prostaglandin endoperoxide synthase-2 during mouse macrophage activation. J Leukoc Biol 1994;55:476–482.

119. Yamamoto K, Arakawa T, Taketani Y, et al. TNF alpha-dependent induction of cyclooxygenase-2 mediated by NF kappa B and NF-IL6. Adv Exp Med Biol 1997;407:185–189.

120. Guan Z, Baier LD, Morrison AR. p38 mitogen-activated protein kinase down-regulates nitric oxide and up-regulates prostaglandin E2 biosynthesis stimulated by interleukin-1. J Biol Chem 1997;272:8083–8089.

121. Guan Z, Buckman SY, Pentland AP, et al. Induction of cyclooxygenase-2 by the activated MEKK1 → SEK1/MKK4 → p38 mitogen-activated protein kinase pathway. J Biol Chem 1998;273:12901–12908.

122. O'Banion MK, Winn VD, Young DA. cDNA Cloning and functional activity of a glucocorticoid-regulated inflammatory cyclooxygenase: induction with interleukin 1B in fibroblasts and monocytes. Proc Natl Acad Sci USA 1992;89:4888–4892.

123. Sirois J, Levy LO, Simmons DL, Richards JS. Characterization and hormonal regulation of the promoter of the rat prostaglandin endoperoxide synthase 2 gene in granulosa cells. Identification of functional and protein-binding regions. J Biol Chem 1993;268:12199–12206.

124. Tetradis S, Pilbeam CC, Liu Y, et al. Parathyroid hormone increases prostaglandin G/H synthase-2 transcription by a cyclic adenosine 3',5'-monophosphate-mediated pathway in murine osteoblastic MC3T3-E1 cells. Endocrinology 1997;138:3594–3600.

125. Xie W, Herschman HR. Transcriptional regulation of prostaglandin synthase 2 gene expression by platelet derived growth factor and serum. J Biol Chem 1996;271:31742–31748.

126. Appleby SB, Ristimaki A, Neilson K, et al. Structure of the human cyclo-oxygenase-2 gene. Biochem J 1994;302:723–727.

127. Sirois J, Richards JS. Transcriptional regulation of the rat prostaglandin endoperoxide synthase 2 gene in granulosa cells. J Biol Chem 1993;268:21931–21938.

128. Inoue H, Yokoyama C, Hara S, et al. Transcriptional regulation of human prostaglandin-endoperoxide synthase-2 gene by lipopolysaccharide and phorbol ester in vascular endothelial cells. J Biol Chem 1995;270:24965–24971.

129. Yamamoto K, Arakawa T, Ueda N, Yamamoto S. Transcriptional roles of nuclear factor kB and nuclear factor-interleukin-6 in the tumor necrosis factor alpha-dependent induction of cyclooxygenase-2 in MC3T3-E1 cells. J Biol Chem 1995;270:31315–31320.

130. Morris JK, Richards JS. An E-box region within the prostaglandin endoperoxide synthase-2 (PGS-2) promoter is required for transcription in rat ovarian granulosa cells. J Biol Chem 1996;271:16633–16643.

131. Xie W, Herschman HR. Transcriptional regulation of prostaglandin synthase 2 gene expression by platelet-derived growth factor and serum. J Biol Chem 1996;271:31742–31748.

132. Guan Z, Buckman SY, Miller BW, et al. Interleukin-1beta-induced cycloxygenase-2 expression requires activation of both c-Jun NH2-terminal kinase and p38 MAPK signal pathways in rat renal mesangial cells. J Biol Chem 1998;273:28670–28676.

133. Ristimaki A, Garfinkel S, Wessendorf J, et al. Induction of cyclooxygenase-2 by interleukin-1 alpha. Evidence for post-transcriptional regulation. J Biol Chem 1994;269:11769–11775.

134. Vane JR. Inhibition of prostaglandin synthesis as a mechanism of action for aspirin-like drugs. Nature New Biol 1971;231:232–235.

135. Smith WL, Lands WE. Stimulation and blockade of prostaglandin biosynthesis. J Biol Chem 1971;246:6700–6702.

136. Roth GJ, Stanford N, Majerus PW. Acetylation of prostaglandin synthase by aspirin. Proc Natl Acad Sci USA 1975;72:3073–3076.

137. Mizuno K, Yamamoto S, Lands WEM. Effects of non-steroidal anti-inflammatory drugs on fatty acid cyclo-oxygenase and prostaglandin hydroperoxidase activities. Prostaglandins 1982;23:743–757.

138. Futaki N, Takahishi S, Yokoyama M, et al. NS398, a new anti-inflammatory agent, selectively inhibits a novel prostaglandin G/H synthase/cyclooxygenase (COX-2) activity in vitro. Prostaglandins 1994;47:55–59.

139. Mitchell JA, Akarasereenont P, Thiemermann C, et al. Selectivity of nonsteroidal antiinflammatory drugs as inhibitors of constitutive and inducible cyclooxygenase. Proc Natl Acad Sci USA 1993;90:11693–11697.

140. Copeland RA, Williams JM, Giannaras J, et al. Mechanism of selective inhibition of the inducible isoform of prostaglandin G/H synthase. Proc Natl Acad Sci USA 1994;91:11202–11206.

141. Chan CC, Boyce S, Brideau C, et al. Pharmacology of a selective cyclooxygenase-2 inhibitor, L-745,337: a novel nonsteroidal anti-inflammatory agent with an ulcerogenic sparing effect in rat and nonhuman primate stomach. J Pharmacol Exp Ther 1995;274:1531–1537.

142. Riendeau D, Charleson S, Cromlish W, et al. Comparison of the cyclooxygenase-1 inhibitory properties of nonsteroidal anti-inflammatory drugs (NSAIDs) and selective COX-2 inhibitors, using sensitive microsomal and platelet assays. Can J Physiol Pharmacol 1997;75:1088–1095.

143. Kalgutkar AS, Crews BC, Rowlinson SW, et al. Aspirin-like molecules that covalently inactivate cyclooxygenase-21211 [see comments]. Science 1998;280:1268–1270.

144. Bhattacharyya DK, Lecomte M, Dunn J, et al. Selective inhibition of prostaglandin endoperoxide synthase-1 (cylooxygenase-1) by valerylsalicylic acid. Arch Biochem Biophys 1995;317:19–24.

145. DeWitt DL. COX-2 selective inhibitors—the new super aspirins. Mol Pharmacol 1999;55:625–631.

146. Marnett LJ, Kalgutkar AS. Cyclooxygenase-2 inhibitors: discovery, selectivity and the future. TIPS 1999;20:465–469.

147. Carty TJ, Stevens JS, Lombardino JG, et al. Piroxicam, a structurally novel anti-inflammatory compound. Mode of prostaglandin synthesis inhibition. Prostaglandins 1980;19:671–682.

148. Ondine HC, On-Yee S, Swinney DC. The kinetic factors that determine the affinity and selectivity for slow binding inhibition of human prostaglandin H synthase 1 and 2 by indomethacin and flurbiprofen. J Biol Chem 1996;271:3548–3554.

149. Kulmacz RJ, Lands WEM. Stoichiometry and kinetics of the interaction of prostaglandin H synthase with anti-inflammatory agents. J Biol Chem 1985;260:12572–12578.

150. Walenga RW, Wall SF, Setty BN, Stuart MJ. Time-dependent inhibition of platelet cyclooxygenase by indomethacin is slowly reversible. Prostaglandins 1986;31:625–637.

151. Kulmacz RJ. Topography of prostaglandin H synthase. Anti-inflammatory agents and the protease-sensitive arginine 253 region. J Biol Chem 1989;264:14136–14144.

152. Rieke CJ, Mulichak AM, Garavito RM, Smith WL. The role of Arg120 of prostaglandin endoperoxide H synthase-2 in the interaction with fatty acid substrates and inhibitors. J Biol Chem 1999;274:17109–17114.

153. Gierse JK, McDonald JJ, Hauser SD, et al. A single amino acid difference between cyclooxygenase-1 (COX-1) and -2 (COX-2) reverses the selectivity of COX-2 specific inhibitors. J Biol Chem 1996;271:15810–15814.

154. Guo Q, Wang LH, Ruan KH, Kulmacz RJ. Role of Val509 in time-dependent inhibition of human prostaglandin H synthase-2 cyclooxygenase activity by isoform-selective agents. J Biol Chem 1996;271:19134–19139.

155. Roth GJ, Machuga ET, Ozols J. Isolation and covalent structure of the aspirin-modified, active-site region of prostaglandin synthetase. Biochemistry 1983;22:4672–4675.

156. Van der Ouderaa FJ, Buytenhek M, Nugteren DH, VanDorp DA. Acetylation of prostaglandin endoperoxide synthetase with acetylsalicylic acid. Eur J Biochem 1980;109:1–8.

157. Holtzman MJ, Turk J, Shornick LP. Identification of a pharmacologically distinct prostaglandin H synthase in cultured epithelial cells. J Biol Chem 1992;267:21438–21445.

158. Shimokawa T, Smith WL. Prostaglandin endoperoxide synthase: the aspirin acetylation region. J Biol Chem 1992;267:12387–12392.

159. Xiao G, Tsai A-L, Palmer G, et al. Analysis of hydroperoxide-induced tyrosyl radicals and lipoxygenase activity in aspirin-treated human prostaglandin H synthase-2. Biochemistry 1997;36:1836–1845.

Chapter 9

Antileukotrienes (Leukotriene Modifiers) in the Treatment of Asthma

Jeffrey M. Drazen

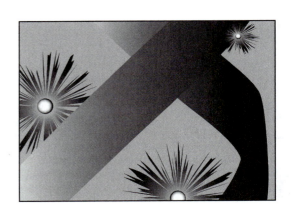

The leukotrienes are a family of bioactive fatty acids that were discovered more than 60 years ago by Australian investigators who were seeking to delineate the smooth muscle–stimulating constituents generated by anaphylaxis in guinea pig lungs (1). For 40 years after their biologic identification, these substances were know as slow-reacting substances because of the characteristic slow onset of contraction in isolated assay tissues compared with the onset of contraction achieved with histamine as the contractile agonist (2). In 1979 the chemical structure of the first member of the leukotriene family was elucidated (3), and within a few years thereafter, all the chemical constituents of the material known as slow-reacting substance of anaphylaxis (SRS-A) were identified (4,5). Shortly after the elucidation of the structure of SRS-A as the cysteinyl leukotrienes, experiments conducted in volunteers with and without asthma provided evidence that the leukotrienes were the most potent bronchoconstrictor substances ever identified (6–11). With the chemical structure in hand and the availability of molecules created by total chemical synthesis, the pharmaceutical industry launched a major effort to identify compounds with the capacity to inhibit the synthesis or action of the leukotrienes. The use of antileukotrienes (leukotriene modifiers) in the treatment of asthma represents the results of this endeavor. In this chapter, the biochemical pathways leading to the formation of the leukotrienes are briefly reviewed, and then the evidence that antileukotriene agents are safe and effective therapy in asthma is considered.

The Cysteinyl Leukotrienes

The members of the leukotriene family whose structure contains cysteine are referred to as cysteinyl leukotrienes. The three moieties in this family, leukotriene (LT) C_4, LTD_4, and LTE_4, derive from the metabolism of arachidonic acid, commonly found esterified in the *sn-2* position of membrane phospholipids. When cells containing the appropriate enzymatic apparatus are activated or when cells are in an inflammatory microenvironment, arachidonic acid (5,8,11,14-*cis*-eicosatetraenoic acid) is cleaved from either the perinuclear membrane or the external cell membrane (12,13). Current understanding of this process is that when a cell is activated to produce leukotrienes, the cytosolic form of phospholipase A_2 (PLA_2), an 85-kDa protein, capable of cleaving

arachidonic acid from membrane phospholipids at intercellular calcium concentrations and pH levels, is the most active moiety. Alternatively, arachidonic acid can derive from the action of a variety of enzymes, known collectively as secretory phospholipase A_2s, that cleave arachidonic acid from the *sn-2* position of plasmalemmal phospholipids (14,15). In this circumstance arachidonic acid localizes in an extracellular pool and is thought to diffuse into the cytosol. Regardless of its source, arachidonic acid becomes a substrate for the enzyme 5-lipoxygenase (Alox-5 or 5-LO), which is translocated to the perinuclear membrane (16,17) when cells are activated and performs two catalytic reactions on arachidonic acid in succession. The product of the first catalytic reaction is 5-hydroperoxyeicosatetraenoic acid (5-HPETE), and the product of the second is 5,6-oxido-7,9-*trans*-11,14-*cis*-eicosatetraneoic acid, also known as LTA_4 (Fig. 9-1). The arachidonic acid that derives from membrane phospholipids appears to be chaperoned by the 5-LO–activating protein (FLAP; Alox-5 AP), which binds arachidonic acid and presents it to 5-LO (18,19). LTA_4 then becomes a substrate for the enzyme LTC_4 synthase (LTC_4-S), which adducts the tripeptide glutathione at the C6 position of LTA_4 to form the first of the cysteinyl leukotrienes, LTC_4 (20,21). LTC_4, synthesized in the cell cytosol, is exported through the plasmalemma by a transport mechanism involving the multidrug resistance protein (22–26). Once outside of the cell, the glutamic acid moiety of LTC_4 is cleaved by the exo-enzyme, gammaglutamyl transpeptidase, to yield LTD_4, the 6-cysteinylglycyl analog of LTC_4. This molecule is a ligand for the cysteinyl leukotriene receptor type 1 ($CysLT_1$), which, when stimulated, produces the transduction of airway narrowing and vascular leak (27). LTD_4 is also a substrate for a variety of dipeptidases that cleave the glycine moiety to form the 6-cysteinyl analog of LTC_4, LTE_4.

All three cysteinyl leukotrienes have the capacity to stimulate the $CysLT_1$ receptor, although LTD_4 is the preferred agonist. LTE_4 may be acetylated, may undergo ω-oxidation and β-elimination to yield inactive products (28,29), or in the presence of hypochlorous acid and hydrogen peroxide may be converted to LTB_4 and LTE_4 sulfoxide (30). Each of these moieties is substantially less active with respect to signal transduction at the $CysLT_1$ receptor than the respective native molecule. Approximately 10% of the LTE_4 that becomes available in the lung is excreted as the authentic molecule in the urine (29,31–34).

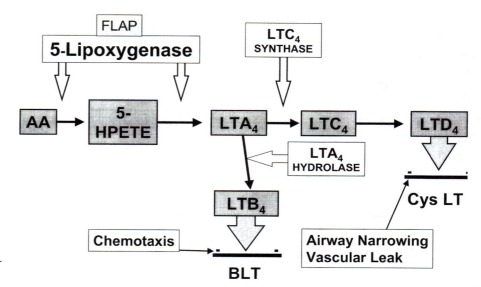

Figure 9-1. Schematic diagram of leukotriene synthesis. AA, arachidonic acid.

Leukotriene-Modifying Drugs

As of March 1999, four agents are available by prescription in various countries throughout the world that act at specific points in the 5-LO pathway (35,36). Zileuton (Zyflo™, Abbott Laboratories) directly inhibits the action of 5-LO, and, therefore, it inhibits the production of LTA_4 from arachidonic acid. Zileuton is the only biosynthetic inhibitor of the leukotriene pathway available for clinical use. The family of "... lukasts," consisting of montelukast (Singulair™, Merck), pranlukast (Onon™, Ono Pharmaceuticals) and zafirlukast (Accolate™, Zeneca Pharmaceuticals), all prevent signal transduction by the cysteinyl leukotrienes at the $CysLT_1$ receptor.

The efficacy of the "... lukasts" with respect to their primary action can be graded by ascertaining the extent their administration is associated with a loss of sensitivity to the bronchoconstrictor actions of inhaled LTD_4. At the usually administered clinical doses, pranlukast shifts the LTD_4 dose response curve by 30- to 50-fold (i.e., it takes 30- to 50-fold more LTD_4 to achieve the same degree of bronchoconstriction after the administration of pranlukast that it did before) (37). Montelukast (38) and zafirlukast (39) appear to be, at their clinically recommended doses, equally effective in shifting the leukotriene dose response curve by a factor of 100 or more.

The potency of the biosynthetic inhibitor zileuton has been measured in two ways. In the first, the capacity of mixed leukocytes, as found in whole blood, to produce LTB_4 (a dihydroxy derivative of LTA_4) in response to stimulation with the calcium ionophore A23187 is used. Zileuton, at the clinically recommended doses, inhibits the calcium ionophore A23187-initiated synthesis of LTB_4 in whole blood by 70% to 90% (40,41). In the second, the change in the rate of urinary LTE_4 excretion is examined in patients being treated on a chronic basis with these biosynthetic inhibitors (42). Clinically effective doses of zileuton are associated with a 35% to 45% decrease in the capacity of

humans to synthesize the cysteinyl leukotrienes, as measured by urinary excretion of LTE_4.

Because there are no direct comparisons of any of the agents in this family, the evidence for the use of leukotriene modifiers in the treatment of asthma will be presented as a class. Similarly, recommendations for the therapeutic use of these agents will be considered by class, rather than by specific agent.

Treatment of Induced Asthma

Exercise-Induced Asthma

Exercise-induced bronchospasm is a common manifestation of many forms of asthma. It has been estimated that 50% to 80% of patients who carry a physician's diagnosis of asthma will develop bronchospasm in the 5 to 10 minutes after the cessation of moderate or more strenuous exercise (43,44). Because many individuals (including children at play, as well as adults in the course of their vocation) need to exercise at a level severe enough to induce bronchoconstriction, adequate treatment for this form of induced asthma has substantial implications for the everyday treatment of patients with asthma.

The standard treatment for exercise-induced asthma is the administration of short-acting β-agonists such as albuterol or a long-acting β-agonist such as salmeterol in anticipation of the exercise event (43–45). The so-called "bronchoprotection" achieved by this treatment usually is sufficient for the patient to be able to complete the exercise task with minimally disruptive bronchoconstriction (46).

All the antileukotrienes available are effective in this regard. Montelukast, zafirlukast, and zileuton have all been shown in randomized, placebo-controlled, clinical trials to inhibit the bronchospasm that follows exercise (47–49). Treatment with any of these agents results in approximately a 50% decrease in

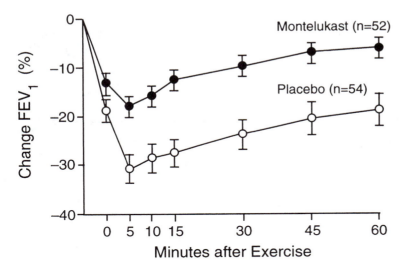

Figure 9-2. Mean (±SE) changes in FEV_1 after exercise challenge of patients treated for 12 weeks with montelukast or placebo. Treatment with montelukast was associated with a significant ($P = .002$) reduction in exercise-induced bronchoconstriction. (Reproduced with permission from Leff JA, Busse WW, Pearlman D, et al. Montelukast, a leukotriene-receptor antagonist, for the treatment of mild asthma and exercise-induced bronchoconstriction. N Engl J Med 1998;339:147–152. Copyright © 1998 Massachusetts Medical Society. All rights reserved.)

magnitude of the integrated area over the FEV_1 curve after exercise.

One of the major advantages of antileukotriene treatment of exercise-induced bronchospasm is the prolonged duration of the effect achieved in standard clinical dosing. For example, treatment with montelukast provides significant protection against bouts of exercise-induced bronchoconstriction, even 24 hours after the last dose (49) (Fig. 9-2). An even more compelling case is made for leukotriene receptor antagonists when one considers the loss of bronchoprotective effect that occurs with repeated treatment with inhaled β-agonist (45,50). In contrast, the bronchoprotective effect of treatment with montelukast, for periods as long as 12 weeks, does not wane. Simply put, the degree of bronchoprotection achieved after the first dose of montelukast is similar to that achieved after 12 weeks of continuous dosing with montelukast.

These data from multiple, randomized, placebo-controlled, clinical trials with a variety of antileukotriene agents provide strong evidence that the antileukotrienes are beneficial in the treatment of exercise-induced bronchoconstriction.

Aspirin-Induced Asthma

Between 1% and 5% of patients with asthma develop severe bronchoconstriction after the ingestion of aspirin or other non-steroidal anti-inflammatory agents that inhibit the action of cyclo-oxygenase type I (prostaglandin H-synthase type I [PGHS-1] or COX1). Data from a number of studies have shown that the bronchospasm that occurs in this setting results from the physiologic effects of leukotrienes at the $CysLT_1$ receptor. In randomized, placebo-controlled, clinical trials in which aspirin is administered to patients who are treated with either an active antileukotriene agent or a placebo, there is statistically and clinically significant protection from the bronchoconstriction (51–55).

Furthermore, in double-blind, placebo-controlled, randomized clinical trials with patients with aspirin-induced asthma who experience daily asthma symptoms even though they are not exposed to aspirin or related compounds, the administration of zileuton results in an improvement in lung function. Efficacy, as measured by the FEV_1; improvement in nasal function, as indicated by the sense of smell; and a reduction in daily asthma symptoms were observed in the patients receiving zileuton as compared with placebo (56).

It is important to realize that a leukotriene modifier does not necessarily provide protection against the adverse physiologic consequences of the ingestion of therapeutic doses of agents inhibiting PGHS-I (57). Indeed, in one case a patient with moderately severe aspirin-intolerant asthma who was being treated with zafirlukast in the clinically recommended dose developed an anaphylactic response after the ingestion of 400 mg of ibuprofen (57). In clinical trials in which the bronchoprotective effect of leukotriene-modifying agents on aspirin-induced asthma is studied, the dose of aspirin administered to an individual subject is increased by small amounts until the dose is found that induces a clinically and physiologically significant loss of lung function. Then, the efficacy of the antileukotriene treatment is studied by comparing the physiologic responses to aspirin ingestion in both the presence and the absence of pretreatment with the leukotriene-modifying agent. However, the amount of aspirin or other PGHS-I inhibitor that induces a physiologic response may be far below the clinically encountered dose. Thus, the protection in clinical trials cannot be directly translated to protection from bronchospasm induced by inadvertent aspirin ingestion. It is tempting to speculate that leukotriene-modifying agents may be useful in achieving "aspirin desensitization," which is commonly produced by administering increasingly large doses of aspirin until patients can tolerate the clinical symptoms. With the use of a leukotriene-receptor antagonist, it is possible that the desensitization protocol could be completed with much less inconvenience to the patient.

Taken together, these data indicate that leukotriene-modifying agents are important novel additions for the treatment of aspirin-induced asthma. When combined with aspirin avoidance, these agents can provide a level of control of aspirin-intolerant asthma that was not available before even with moderately high doses of corticosteroids.

Treatment of Chronic Persistent Asthma with Antileukotrienes

All of the antileukotrienes have a beneficial effect in the treatment of chronic persistent asthma. One of the major advances offered by antileukotriene therapy is the ability to treat patients with chronic persistent asthma with an orally administered controller agent that will improve lung function, enhance the quality of life, decrease asthma symptoms, and have a beneficial effect on pharmaco-economic outcomes.

Leukotriene Modifiers as First-Line Asthma Therapy

In a number of double-blind, randomized, placebo-controlled trials, patients with asthma have received montelukast, pranlukast, zafirlukast, or zileuton as their sole treatment, other than the intermittent use of an inhaled β-agonist (58–60). Over a period of 6 to 16 weeks, the patients treated with drug exhibited a significant improvement in FEV_1 (7% to 15%) compared with individuals being treated with placebo (Table 9-1). Moreover, the patients treated with a leukotriene modifier, when compared with those receiving placebo, had a significantly diminished need for rescue β-agonist use, decreased nighttime awakening due to asthma, improved daytime asthma symptoms, and a diminished need for oral corticosteroid rescue. Indeed, these treatments fulfill all the requirements outlined for an asthma treatment in the National Asthma Education and Prevention Program Expert Panel Report 2 (61).

Combination Therapy with Other Antiasthma Agents

Clinical trials have been conducted and reported in which a substantial fraction of the enrolled patients were receiving asthma

Table 9-1. Studies of Leukotriene Modifiers in Patients with Chronic Persistent Asthma*

	Zafirlukast	Montelukast	Pranlukast	Zileuton
No. of patients[a]	70	408	45	122
Length of study	6 weeks	12 weeks	6 weeks	6 months
Dose (oral)	20 mg bid	10 mg qd	337.5 mg bid	600 mg q.i.d.
Baseline FEV_1 (percent of predicted)	66	66	66	62
Trough[b] improvement in FEV_1 (L)	0.23L[c]	–	~0.31L[c]	0.34L
Trough[b] improvement in FEV_1 (percent)[d]	11 (13–14)[c]	–	~11.5[c,e]	15 (18)
Peak[f] improvement in FEV_1 (percent)[d]	–	13	–	20[g] (23)[c]
β-adrenergic agonist use reduction[d]	31%	27%[g]	NC	(30%)
Improvement in AM PEFR[d]	6%	6.1%	~5%[c]	7.1% (8.5%)
Treatment failure/Corticosteroid rescue therapy (treatment[i] vs. placebo)	2% vs 10%	–	–	8.3% vs 21.5%[c]
Decrease in symptoms: day/night (percent)	28/46	20/NC	NC/28	36/33

* Compared with pretreatment values. Only data from double-blind, randomized, placebo-controlled studies are included. The study chosen for display is representative of multiple reported studies with each drug. All values were statistically significant compared to placebo unless otherwise indicated. (Table modified, with permission, from Drazen JM, Israel E, O'Byrne PM. Treatment of asthma with drugs modifying the leukotriene pathway. N Engl J Med 1999;340:197–206. Copyright © 1999 Massachusetts Medical Society. All rights reserved.)

[a] Number of patients receiving active treatment at the dose indicated. Zafirlukast was administered at twice the currently recommended dose.

[b] Trough values—values immediately before next dose or those values not reported as obtained at times of expected peak plasma concentrations or effects.

[c] Derived from figures of statistics.

[d] Figures not in parentheses represent means over the study period or endpoint analyses. Figures in parentheses represent maximum effect among the study observation intervals reported.

[e] 225 mg dose.

[f] Values recorded at or near time of drug's expected peak plasma concentration or effects.

[g] Endpoint value. NS vs placebo at week 26.

[h] Percentage difference compared with placebo.

[i] Treatment failures for zafirlukast, corticosteroid rescue therapy for zileuton.

NC, significant change; PEFR, peak expiratory flow rate; –, data not available.

therapies other than antileukotrienes and short-acting inhaled β-agonists. One type of such trial is an antileukotriene addition trial. In these randomized, blinded, and placebo-controlled studies, patients with chronic stable asthma that is otherwise not optimally controlled are treated with a leukotriene modifiers or with placebo in addition to their regular asthma treatment regimen, and the outcomes of the two groups are compared. For example, in a recently published trial (59), montelukast or placebo was administered to a group of patients whose FEV_1 was between 50% and 85% of their predicted values, of whom approximately 25% were using concomitant inhaled corticosteroids. When compared with placebo, the administration of montelukast resulted in improvement in the FEV_1, the morning and evening peak flow rates, day-time asthma symptoms, and the need for β-agonist rescue treatments. Thus, the addition of antileukotrienes to the treatment regimen of patients with moderate-to-severe persistent asthma, even if they are receiving inhaled corticosteroids, can provide additional therapeutic effects.

In another trial design, studies are conducted of patients with chronic persistent asthma, who are receiving β-agonists as their sole treatment but whose asthma control is such that they could potentially benefit from additional asthma therapies. In these comparison trials, antileukotrienes were compared with theophylline (62) or to inhaled corticosteroids (63). Zileuton was equally effective with theophylline, and montelukast had weaker effect on the FEV_1 than inhaled beclomethasone. Inhaled corticosteroids produced a larger improvement in the FEV_1 than montelukast. One interpretation of these data is that inhaled corticosteroids are superior to leukotriene modifiers as treatment for asthma. However, in this trial the mean response to beclomethasone was driven by a small number of patients with a very large increase in the FEV_1, and the proportion of patients achieving a >10% improvement in the FEV_1 for the two groups was quite similar (63). For example, based on the data available, if 100 patients with mild-to-moderate asthma were treated with inhaled steroids, 50 of these patients would manifest an improvement in the FEV_1 of >11%, while 42 of the patients would manifest a response of this magnitude when treated with montelukast. Thus, although the mean percentage increase in FEV_1, compared with baseline, is almost twice as great with inhaled steroids as it is with antileukotrienes, the proportions of patients responding by this definition are similar for both groups.

The choice of treatment for persons with chronic persistent asthma must be based not only on the effectiveness of a therapy in clinical trials but also on the likelihood that patients actually encountered in practice will comply with the treatment regimen. Kelloway and coworkers (64) have studied the compliance of both adults and children with asthma with oral treatment regimens (i.e., theophylline) and with inhaled corticosteroids. The compliance rates were considerably greater for the oral therapy than for the inhaled therapy. Indeed, the difference in compliance rates over 3 months of therapy exceeds the difference in the proportion of patients having a beneficial response to montelukast compared with inhaled beclomethasone. Thus, if both the difference in proportion of responders and the likely difference in compliance are considered, these two forms of therapy are quite

similar, although the leukotriene-modifier therapy may have a slight advantage over inhaled corticosteroids.

In a third type of treatment trial, an antileukotriene agent or placebo is added to the treatment regimens of patients requiring moderately high doses of inhaled corticosteroids to maintain adequate asthma control. In these trials patients are stabilized on their asthma regimen, which includes high doses of inhaled corticosteroids, over a "run-in" period. Once the asthma is stabilized, an antileukotriene or placebo is added in a randomized, blinded, and placebo-controlled fashion, and the inhaled corticosteroid dose is decreased in a systematic fashion. For example, in a recent trial conducted by Tamaoki et al (65), patients receiving, on average, slightly less than 2000 μg/day of beclomethasone by inhalation reduced this dose by a factor of two while simultaneously adding pranlukast or placebo to their treatment regimen. The patients receiving pranlukast maintained their asthma control when their dose of corticosteroids was cut, while the group receiving placebo had significant reductions in morning peak flow rates (Fig. 9-3) FEV_1 and an increase in asthma symptoms (65).

Safety of Antileukotrienes

The leukotriene modifiers are safe and well tolerated. In the trials performed with all the receptor antagonists at the clinically recommended doses, there have been no differences between the active treatment groups and the placebo-treated groups with respect to symptoms perceived or laboratory abnormalities monitored. When higher-than-recommended doses of zafirlukast are administered chronically, a small fraction of patients develops reversible elevations in the serum alanine aminotransferase (ALT) level.

However, at the clinically recommended dose of zileuton, patients receiving zileuton plus their usual asthma care exhibit a 4.6% incidence of elevated ALT values compared with a 1.1% incidence of elevated ALT values in patients receiving standard care (66). Elevated ALT levels occur mostly within the first 3 months of zileuton therapy; after this time the case rate of elevated ALT levels falls to that of placebo. These observations have led to the recommendation for monitoring ALT values at the time of inception of zileuton treatment, monthly for the first 3 months, and periodically thereafter. Zileuton therapy should not be initiated if the ALT value is greater than three times the upper limit of normal. If the ALT values begin in the normal range and then increase to three times the upper limit of normal, monitoring every 2 weeks is recommended until the level either returns to the normal range or increases to greater than five times the upper limit of normal, in which case the zileuton therapy should be stopped. In all the cases that have been reported to date, the increased ALT levels have returned to normal, either with continued therapy or with cessation of therapy. There have been no reported cases of irreversible hepatic damage.

A rare systemic vasculitic syndrome that meets the diagnostic criteria for Churg-Strauss Syndrome has been reported in patients receiving montelukast or zafirlukast therapy for asthma (67–69). Examination of the incidence case rates in patients treated with

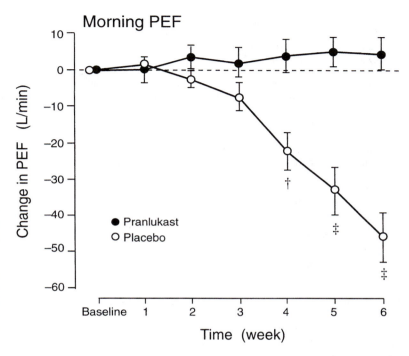

Figure 9-3. Changes in mean morning PEF during 6 weeks of treatment with ONO-1078 (*closed circles*) or placebo (*open circles*). After baseline period the dose of inhaled beclomethasone dipropionate was reduced to half in each patient. Values represent mean (±SEM) changes in weekly PEF $^\dagger P < .01$, $^\ddagger P < .001$, significantly different from baseline values. (Reproduced with permission from Tamaoki J, Kondo M, Sakai N, et al. Leukotriene antagonist prevents exacerbation of asthma during reduction of high-dose inhaled corticosteroid. Am J Respir Crit Care Med 1997;155: 1235–1240.)

montelukast and zafirlukast indicates that there are approximately six cases of Churg-Strauss Syndrome for 100,000 asthma-years of treatment. Thus, the appearance of this syndrome is an exceedingly rare event; that is, one case will occur in approximately 17,000 patient-years of treatment. More importantly, these cases have not occurred in patients who previously had mild asthma. Virtually all the cases have occurred in patients whose asthma could be categorized as severe, almost all of whom had required systemic corticosteroid therapy for the control of their asthma, or high-dose inhaled corticosteroid therapy within a year of the onset of symptoms. It is highly likely that these patients had a vasculitis which, because of its clinical presentation, had been recognized as severe asthma rather than as vasculitis. In this group of patients treatment with a leukotriene modifier blocked the bronchoconstrictor action of the leukotrienes and, hence, allowed reduction of corticosteriod therapy without the recurrence of airway narrowing. Thus, antileukotriene therapy likely unmasked a previously extant vasculitic syndrome. Patients who had previously required oral or substantial doses of inhaled corticosteroids for their asthma control and now have a substantial beneficial therapeutic effect from antileukotriene therapy, such that their dose of steroids can be substantially reduced, require special attention to the development of clinical signs or symptoms consistent with this systemic vasculitis.

Drug Interactions

A case has been reported of an individual in whom treatment with the combination of zafirlukast and theophylline produced an increase in blood theophylline levels (70). Indeed, this response is to be expected with this drug combination. Although general monitoring of theophylline levels above that which would normally be recommended for a patient receiving theophylline alone is not recommended when a leukotriene modifier is added to the treatment regimen, it is important to maintain cognizance of this drug-drug interaction.

The dose of zileuton need not be modified in patients with renal failure (71). Data are not available in the archival literature with respect to other leukotriene modifiers and renal failure.

Summary

Agents that inhibit the synthesis or action of the leukotrienes represent the first totally novel form of asthma therapy in more than 2 decades. These therapies were derived from knowledge of the primary pathobiology. Their beneficial effect for patients with all degrees of severity of persistent asthma, as well as for those with induced asthma, provides strong testimony to the importance of leukotrienes as critical mediators of the biology of asthma and to the usefulness of leukotriene modifiers in the treatment of this chronic syndrome.

Acknowledgments
In the period from 1994 to 1999, Dr. Drazen's laboratory has received grant support from each of the companies marketing antileukotrienes in the United States.

References

1. Kellaway CH, Trethewie ER. The liberation of a slow-reacting smooth muscle stimulating substance in anaphylaxis. Q J Exp Physiol 1940;30:121–145.
2. Brocklehurst WE. The release of histamine and the formation of a slow-reacting substance (SRS-A) during anaphylactic shock. J Physiol (Lond) 1960;151:416–435.
3. Murphy RC, Hammarstrom S, Samuelsson B. Leukotriene C: a slow-reacting substance from murine mastocytoma cells. Proc Natl Acad Sci USA 1979;76:4275–4279.
4. Samuelsson B. Leukotrienes: mediators of immediate hypersensitivity reactions and inflammation. Science 1983;220:568–575.
5. Samuelsson B, Dahlen SE, Lindgren JA, et al. Leukotrienes and lipoxins: structures, biosynthesis, and biological effects. Science 1987;237:1171–1176.
6. Holroyde MC, Altounyan RE, Cole M, et al. Bronchoconstriction produced in man by leukotrienes C and D. Lancet 1981;2:17–18.
7. Weiss JW, Drazen JM, Coles N, et al. Bronchoconstrictor effects of leukotriene C in humans. Science 1982;216:196–198.
8. Barnes NC, Piper PJ, Costello JF. Comparative effects of inhaled leukotriene C_4, leukotriene D_4, and histamine in normal human subjects. Thorax 1984;39:500–504.
9. Griffin M, Weiss JW, Leitch AG, et al. Effects of leukotriene D on the airways in asthma. N Engl J Med 1983;308:436–439.
10. Smith LJ, Greenberger PA, Patterson R, et al. The effect of inhaled leukotriene D_4 in humans. Am Rev Respir Dis 1985;131:368–372.
11. Adelroth E, Morris MM, Hargreave FE, O'Byrne PM. Airway responsiveness to leukotrienes C_4 and D_4 and to methacholine in patients with asthma and normal controls. N Engl J Med 1986;315:480–484.
12. Woods JW, Coffey MJ, Brock TG, et al. 5-lipoxygenase is located in the euchromatin of the nucleus in resting human alveolar macrophages and translocates to the nuclear envelope upon cell activation. J Clin Invest 1995;95:2035–2046.
13. Dennis EA, Ackermann EJ, Deems RA, Reynolds LJ. Multiple forms of phospholipase A_2 in macrophages capable of arachidonic acid release for eicosanoid biosynthesis. Adv Prostaglandin Thromboxane Leukot Res 1995;23:75–80.
14. Shamsuddin M, Anderson J, Smith LJ. Differential regulation of leukotriene and platelet-activating factor synthesis in rat alveolar macrophages. Am J Respir Cell Mol Biol 1995;12:697–704.
15. Shamsuddin M, Chen E, Anderson J, Smith LJ. Regulation of leukotriene and platelet-activating factor synthesis in human alveolar macrophages. J Lab Clin Med 1997;130:615–626.
16. Coffey M, Peters-Golden M, Fantone JC, Sporn PHS. Membrane association of active 5-lipoxygenase in resting cells—evidence for novel regulation of the enzyme in the rat alveolar macrophage. J Biol Chem 1992;267:570–576.
17. Peters-Golden M, McNish RW. Redistribution of 5-lipoxygenase and cytosolic phospholipase A_2 to the nuclear fraction upon macrophage activation. Biochem Biophys Res Commun 1993;196:147–153.
18. Dixon RA, Diehl RE, Opas E, et al. Requirement of a 5-lipoxygenase-activating protein for leukotriene synthesis. Nature 1990;343:282–284.
19. Miller DK, Gillard JW, Vickers PJ, et al. Identification and isolation of a membrane protein necessary for leukotriene production. Nature 1990;343:278–281.
20. Lam BK, Penrose JF, Freeman GJ, Austen KF. Expression cloning of a cDNA for human leukotriene C_4 synthase, an integral membrane protein conjugating reduced glutathione to leukotriene A_4. Proc Natl Acad Sci USA 1994;91:7663–7667.
21. Penrose JF, Spector J, Baldasaro M, et al. Molecular cloning of the gene for human leukotriene C_4 synthase—organization, nucleotide sequence, and chromosomal localization to 5q35. J Biol Chem 1996;271:11356–11361.
22. Lam BK, Owen WFJ, Austen KF, Soberman RJ. The identification of a distinct export step following the biosynthesis of leukotriene C_4 by human eosinophils. J Biol Chem 1989;264:12885–12889.
23. Gao M, Loe DW, Grant CE, et al. Reconstitution of ATP-dependent leukotriene C_4 transport by co-expression of both half-molecules of human multidrug resistance protein in insect cells. J Biol Chem 1996;271:27782–27787.
24. Loe DW, Almquist KC, Deeley RG, Cole SPC. Multidrug resistance protein (MRP)-mediated transport of leukotriene C_4 and chemotherapeutic agents in membrane vesicles—demonstration of glutathione-dependent vincristine transport. J Biol Chem 1996;271:9675–9682.
25. Nguyen T, Gupta S. Leukotriene C_4 secretion from normal murine mast cells by a probenecid-sensitive and multidrug resistance-associated protein-independent mechanism. J Immunol 1997;158:4916–4920.
26. Gao M, Yamazaki M, Loe DW, et al. Multidrug resistance protein—identification of regions required for active transport of leukotriene C_4. J Biol Chem 1998;273:10733–10740.
27. Lynch KR, O'Neill GP, Liu Q, et al. Characterization of the human cysteinyl-leukotriene $CysLT_1$ receptor. Nature 1999;399:789–793.
28. Stene DO, Murphy RC. Metabolism of leukotriene E_4 in isolated rat hepatocytes. Identification of beta-oxidation products of sulfidopeptide leukotrienes. J Biol Chem 1988;263:2773–2778.
29. Sala A, Voelkel N, Maclouf J, Murphy RC. Leukotriene E_4 elimination and metabolism in normal human subjects. J Biol Chem 1990;265:21771–21778.
30. Lee CW, Lewis RA, Corey EJ, et al. Oxidative inactivation of leukotriene C_4 by stimulated human polymorphonuclear leukocytes. Proc Natl Acad Sci USA 1982;79:4166–4170.
31. Hammarstrom S, Orning L, Bernstrom K, et al. Metabolism of leukotriene C_4 in rats and humans. Adv Prostaglandin Thromboxane Leukot Res 1985;15:185–188.
32. Hammarstrom S, Orning L, Bernstrom K. Metabolism of leukotrienes. Mol Cell Biochem 1985;69:7–16.
33. Orning L, Kaijser L, Hammarstrom S. In vivo metabolism of leukotriene C_4 in man: urinary excretion of leukotriene E_4. Biochem Biophys Res Commun 1985;130:214–220.
34. Hammarstrom S, Orning L, Bernstrom K. Metabolism and excretion of cysteinyl-leukotrienes. Adv Prostaglandin Thromboxane Leukot Res 1986;16:383–396.
35. O'Byrne PM, Israel E, Drazen JM. Antileukotrienes in the treatment of asthma. Ann Intern Med 1997;127:472–480.
36. Drazen JM, Israel E, O'Byrne PM. Treatment of asthma with drugs modifying the leukotriene pathway. N Engl J Med 1999;340:197–206.
37. O'Shaughnessy TC, Georgiou P, Howland K, et al. Effect of pranlukast, an oral leukotriene receptor antagonist, on leukotriene D_4 (LTD_4) challenge in normal volunteers. Thorax 1997;52:519–522.

38. De-Lepeleire I, Reiss TF, Rochette F, et al. Montelukast causes prolonged, potent leukotriene D_4-receptor antagonism in the airways of patients with asthma. Clin Pharmacol Ther 1997;61:83–92.

39. Smith LJ, Geller S, Ebright L, et al. Inhibition of leukotriene D_4-induced bronchoconstriction in normal subjects by the oral LTD_4 receptor antagonist ICI 204, 219. Am Rev Respir Dis 1990;141:988–992.

40. Israel E, Dermarkarian R, Rosenberg M, et al. The effects of a 5-lipoxygenase inhibitor on asthma induced by cold, dry air. N Engl J Med 1990;323:1740–1744.

41. Rubin P, Dube L, Braeckman R, et al. Pharmacokinetics, safety, and ability to diminish leukotriene synthesis by zileuton, an inhibitor of 5-lipoxygenase. Prog Inflamm Res Ther 1991;35:103–116.

42. Israel E, Rubin P, Kemp JP, et al. The effect of inhibition of 5-lipoxygenase by zileuton in mild to moderate asthma. Ann Intern Med 1993;119:1059–1066.

43. McFadden ER, Hejal R. Asthma. Lancet 1995;345:1215–1220.

44. Anderson SD. Asthma provoked by exercise, hyperventilation and the inhalation of non-isotonic aerosols. Asthma: basic mechanisms and clinical management. 3rd Ed. 1998;569–587.

45. Nelson JA, Strauss L, Skowronski M, et al. Effect of long-term salmeterol treatment on exercise-induced asthma. N Engl J Med 1998;339:141–146.

46. Adelroth E, Inman MD, Summers E, et al. Prolonged protection against exercise-induced bronchoconstriction by the leukotriene D_4-receptor antagonist cinalukast. J Allergy Clin Immunol 1997;99:210–215.

47. Meltzer SS, Hasday JD, Cohn J, Bleecker ER. Inhibition of exercise-induced bronchospasm by zileuton: a 5-lipoxygenase inhibitor. Am J Respir Crit Care Med 1996;153:931–935.

48. Dessanges JF, Prefaut C, Taytard A, et al. The effect of zafirlukast on repetitive exercise-induced bronchoconstrictions: The possible role of leukotrienes in exercise-induced refractoriness. J Allergy Clin Immunol 1999;104:1155–1161.

49. Leff JA, Busse WW, Pearlman D, et al. Montelukast, a leukotriene-receptor antagonist, for the treatment of mild asthma and exercise-induced bronchoconstriction [see comments]. N Engl J Med 1998;339:147–152.

50. Anderson SD, Rodwell LT, Dutoit J, Young IH. Duration of protection by inhaled salmeterol in exercise-induced asthma. Chest 1991;100:1254–1260.

51. Dahlen B, Margolskee DJ, Zetterstrom O, Dahlen SE. Effect of the leukotriene receptor antagonist MK-0679 on baseline pulmonary function in aspirin sensitive asthmatic subjects. Thorax 1993;48:1205–1210.

52. Nasser SM, Bell GS, Hawksworth RJ, et al. Effect of the 5-lipoxygenase inhibitor ZD2138 on allergen-induced early and late asthmatic responses. Thorax 1994;49:743–748.

53. Israel E, Fischer AR, Rosenberg MA, et al. The pivotal role of 5-lipoxygenase products in the reaction of aspirin-sensitive asthmatics to aspirin. Am Rev Respir Dis 1993;148:1447–1451.

54. Fischer AR, Rosenberg MA, Lilly CM, et al. Direct evidence for a role of the mast cell in the nasal response to aspirin in aspirin-sensitive asthma. J Allergy Clin Immunol 1994;94:1046–1056.

55. O'Sullivan S, Dahlen B, Dahlen SE, Kumlin M. Increased urinary excretion of the prostaglandin D_2 metabolite 9 alpha, 11 beta-prostaglandin $F_{2\alpha}$ after aspirin challenge supports mast cell activation in aspirin-induced airway obstruction. J Allergy Clin Immunol 1996;98:421–432.

56. Dahlen B, Nizankowska E, Szczeklik A, et al. Benefits from adding the 5-lipoxygenase inhibitor zileuton to conventional therapy in aspirin-intolerant asthmatics. Am J Respir Crit Care Med 1998;157:1187–1194.

57. Menendez R, Venzor J, Ortiz G. Failure of zafirlukast to prevent ibuprofen-induced anaphylaxis. Ann Allergy Asthma Immunol 1998;80:225–226.

58. Grossman J, Faiferman I, Dubb JW, et al. Results of the first U.S. double-blind, placebo-controlled, multicenter clinical study in asthma with pranlukast, a novel leukotriene receptor antagonist. J Asthma 1997;34:321–328.

59. Reiss TF, Chervinsky P, Dockhorn RJ, et al. Montelukast a once daily leukotriene receptor antagonist in the treatment of chronic asthma. Arch Int Med 1998;158:1213–1220.

60. Fish JE, Kemp JP, Lockey RF, et al. Zafirlukast for symptomatic mild-to-moderate asthma: a 13-week multicenter study. The Zafirlukast Trialists Group. Clin Ther 1997;19:675–690.

61. National Asthma Education Program. Guidelines for the diagnosis and treatment of asthma II. Bethesda, MD: National Institutes of Health. 1997.

62. Schwartz HJ, Petty T, Dube LM, et al. A randomized controlled trial comparing zileuton with theophylline in moderate asthma. Arch Intern Med 1998;158:141–148.

63. Montelukast Research and Marketing Team. Montelukast Package Insert. Rahway, NJ: Merck, 1998.

64. Kelloway JS, Wyatt RA, Adlis SA. Comparison of patient's compliance with prescribed oral and inhaled asthma medications. Arch Int Med 1994;154;1349–1352.

65. Tamaoki J, Kondo M, Sakai N, et al. Leukotriene antagonist prevents exacerbation of asthma during reduction of high-dose inhaled corticosteroid. Am J Respir Crit Care Med 1997;155:1235–1240.

66. Lazarus SC, Lee T, Kemp JP, et al. Safety and clinical efficacy of zileuton in patients with chronic asthma. Am J Manag Care 1998;4:841–848.

67. Wechsler ME, Garpestad E, Flier SR, et al. Pulmonary infiltrates, eosinophilia, and cardiomyopathy following corticosteroid withdrawal in patients with asthma receiving zafirlukast. JAMA 1998;279:455–457.

68. Holloway J, Ferriss J, Groff J, et al. Churg-Strauss syndrome associated with zafirlukast. J Am Osteopath Assoc 1998;98:275–278.

69. Knoell DL, Lucas J, Allen JN. Churg-Strauss syndrome associated with zafirlukast. Chest 1998;114:332–334.

70. Katial RK, Stelzle RC, Bonner MW, et al. A drug interaction between zafirlukast and theophylline. Arch Intern Med 1998;158:1713–1715.

71. Awni WM, Wong S, Chu SY, et al. Pharmacokinetics of zileuton and its metabolites in patients with renal impairment. J Clin Pharmacol 1997;37:395–404.

Chapter 10

Phosphodiesterase Inhibitors

Nicky Cooper
Mamidipudi Thirumala Krishna
Robert Gristwood
Stephen Holgate

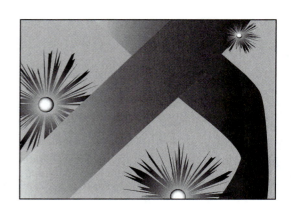

The cyclic nucleotides, namely cyclic 3′,5′-adenosine monophosphate (cAMP) and cyclic 3′,5′-guanosine monophosphate (cGMP), play an important role in the regulation of cell function, including mediating the bronchodilator action of β_2-adrenoceptor agonists. This effect is achieved by activation of receptor-linked adenylate cyclase, which subsequently catalyzes the conversion of adenosine triphosphate (ATP) to cAMP. cAMP mediates its effect by activating cAMP-dependent protein kinases, which selectively phosphorylate proteins to inhibit excitation-contraction coupling in smooth muscle. The cAMP is soon hydrolyzed by a magnesium-dependent enzyme termed phosphodiesterase (PDE) to adenosine 5′-monophosphate (AMP). Phosphodiesterases are widely distributed in body tissues, and so far nine different isoenzymes have been identified. Selective inhibitors of these isoenzymes increase the intracellular cyclic nucleotide levels, which leads to altered tissue function. This property has led to the development of a family of drugs called PDE inhibitors. The PDE inhibitors can be broadly divided into two groups: 1) standard nonspecific inhibitors of PDE activity such as theophylline and 3-isobutyl-1-methylxanthine (IBMX), and 2) inhibitors that are selective for individual PDE isoenzymes.

In this chapter the main focus is on theophylline and inhibitors of type IV PDE and their roles in the treatment of asthma.

Theophylline

Theophylline derives its name from Greek for "divine leaf" in tribute to the leaves of the tea plant Thea (camellia) Sinensis. It is a naturally occurring plant alkaloid, and structurally it is described as 1,3-dimethylxanthine. Its structure is closely related to that of two other plant alkaloids, caffeine and theobromine. The use of xanthines in the treatment of asthma dates back to 1859, when it was first reported in the *Edinburgh Medical Journal* that strong, black coffee was the most common and best remedy for attacks of asthma (1). In 1888 the active agent was extracted from tea leaves and named theophylline. In 1962 Butcher and Sutherland (2) hypothesized that the bronchodilator action of theophylline was related to its PDE inhibitor activity. However, other pharmacologic functions of theophylline have been identi-

fied that help in the symptomatic relief of asthma and chronic obstructive pulmonary disease (COPD), although the exact mechanism of action is not clear.

Clinical Pharmacology

Theophylline has multiple recognized pharmacologic effects, as are discussed below.

Bronchodilation

Inhibition of PDE Activity. Polson et al (3) showed that at therapeutic concentrations theophylline could inhibit only 10% to 12% of PDE activity. Therefore, the mode of action of theophylline cannot be entirely attributed to its PDE inhibition.

Adenosine Antagonism. When administered by inhalation, adenosine causes bronchoconstriction in patients with asthma. In vitro studies have shown that adenosine is released from lung tissue in response to antigen challenge, ischemia, or hypoxia (4). Adenosine mediates its effects by stimulating specific receptors, A_1 and A_2, which inhibit and stimulate adenylate cyclase, respectively (5). Theophylline at therapeutic concentrations competitively inhibits the effects of adenosine at A_1 and A_2 receptors (6). Adenosine antagonism may account for some of the side effects of theophylline such as central nervous system stimulation, gastric hypersecretion, gastroesophageal reflux, cardiotoxicity, and diuresis. Because adenosine is a bronchoconstrictor released in asthma, part of the therapeutic action of theophylline may be mediated through adenosine antagonism.

Other Actions

Stimulation of Mucociliary Clearance. Although theophylline stimulates mucociliary clearance, the clinical significance of this effect is unclear because of the epithelial desquamation and loss of cilia that result from the underlying mucosal inflammation in asthma (7).

Anti-inflammatory Effects. Several studies have highlighted the anti-inflammatory potential of theophylline at subtherapeutic concentrations (<10 μg/mL). Theophylline stabilizes and inhibits a variety of inflammatory cells implicated in the pathogenesis of asthma, including mast cells, macrophages, basophils, neutrophils, and thrombocytes (8–13). This anti-inflammatory action is related to the PDE inhibition. Fink et al noted (14) quantitative, as well as qualitative, immunologic alterations with an increase in the number and activity of suppressor T cells in patients with asthma who were treated with theophylline. Moreover, when serum from theophylline-treated patients was administered to immunosuppressed rats, the graft-versus-host response was impaired. Nelson et al (15) reported that in mice theophylline reduced the inflammatory response of the polymorphonuclear neutrophils after a bacterial challenge. Pauwels et al (16) reported that at plasma levels of 10 μg/mL theophylline suppressed the late-phase bronchoconstrictor response in atopic patients with asthma. Sullivan et al (17) showed that low-dose oral theophylline administered to atopic patients with asthma for 6 weeks attenuated the airway inflammatory response to allergen inhalation. At subtherapeutic concentrations, there was a significant reduction in both the number of EG2$^+$ (activated) eosinophils and the total number of eosinophils beneath the bronchial epithelial basement membrane (17). Withdrawal of chronic oral theophylline treatment from patients with asthma is associated with clinical deterioration, and this is accompanied by an increase in lymphocytic infiltration in the bronchial mucosa (18). This observation is further supported by a recent study (19) in patients with moderately severe asthma who were being treated with a combination of low-dose theophylline (400 mg/day) and inhaled beclomethasone dipropionate (400 to 800 μg/day). Withdrawal of theophylline resulted in a worsening of asthma symptoms, a small but significant decrease in peak expiratory flow rates, and an increase in total and activated eosinophils in the sputum. In addition, our study (20) showed that treatment with theophylline for 6 weeks reduces the number of mucosal mast cells expressing interleukin (IL)-4 and IL-5, cytokines critically involved in isotype switching of B cells to IgE; the up-regulation of vascular cell adhesion molecule-1 (VCAM-1); the maintenance of TH$_2$-CD4$^+$ lymphocytes (IL-4), and the differentiation, migration, priming, and activation of eosinophils (IL-5). Wright and coworkers (21) determined that theophylline may also be exerting its effects by acting directly on the bronchial epithelium. Using reverse transcriptase-polymerase chain reaction, they demonstrated that A549 cells and human airway epithelial cells mainly expressed type IV PDE (PDE IV) and to a lesser extent types I, III, and V PDE (PDE I, III, and V). Inhibition of PDE IV and III reduced secretion from these cells. Overall, these studies support the view that theophylline has an anti-inflammatory action in addition to its bronchodilator action.

Effect on the Diaphragm.   Theophylline has a potent and long-lasting effect on diaphragmatic strength and fatigue in patients with fixed airway obstruction (22). The mechanism is not well understood, although it has been suggested that it could be related to its property of inhibiting the cyclic nucleotide PDEs. Because voltage-dependent calcium channel blockers inhibit this effect (23), it seems likely that theophylline acts via an influx of Ca^{2+} through the slow Ca^{2+} channels of the sarcolemma and that

this mechanism is probably dependent on the activation of adenosine receptors (24).

Effect on Adrenal Medulla.   Theophylline stimulates the release of catecholamines from the adrenal medulla (25), thereby adding to its bronchodilator effect.

Decreases Sensation of Dyspnea.   Sustained-release theophylline reduces the sensation of dyspnea in patients with COPD (26) and reduces the work of breathing at a given minute ventilation (27).

Increase in Respiratory Drive.   Theophylline stimulates respiratory drive in patients with COPD by stimulating the medullary respiratory center (28). It also reduces the O$_2$ desaturation and arrhythmias in these patients (29), and thus has been used in the treatment of sleep apnea (30).

Cardiac Output.   Theophylline increases the right ventricular ejection fraction in patients with cor pulmonale (31).

Miscellaneous.   When administered intravenously to normal humans, theophylline stimulates the central nervous system, decreases blood pressure, increases heart rate and gastric acid output, and produces a transient diuresis (32).

Pharmacokinetics

Theophylline is well absorbed from the gastrointestinal tract, although food delays its absorption. After intravenous administration, it is rapidly and readily distributed in all body compartments. It crosses the placenta and passes into breast milk. The drug is 60% bound to plasma proteins, and its plasma half-life ranges between 1.4 and 12.8 hours. Theophylline is principally (90%) metabolized in the liver by oxidation and demethylation to 3-methylxanthine, 1,3-dimethyluric acid, and 1-methyluric acid, and 10% of the drug is excreted unchanged in the urine. Its half-life in healthy individuals varies considerably, and the factors affecting the clearance of theophylline are summarized in Table 10-1. Theophylline clearance is decreased in individuals with cirrhosis, but remains unaffected in those with acute hepatitis or cholestasis (32). However, viral infections, particularly influenza B, predispose individuals to toxicity (33). In most individuals

Table 10-1. Factors Affecting Clearance of Theophylline

Factors Decreasing Clearance	Factors increasing Clearance
Cirrhosis, heart failure, hypoxia, hypercapnia, acidosis	Smoking
	Drugs: phenytoin, carbamazepine, rifampicin, barbiturates
Drugs: cimetidine, erythromycin, allopurinol, ciprofloxacin	

plasma concentrations of between 10 and 20 mg/L are required for satisfactory bronchodilatation.

Dosage

Theophylline is administered orally, either as rapid-release preparations or sustained-release preparations. Because of their rapid absorption and high incidence of systemic side effects, the rapid-release preparations have become less popular. Sustained-release formulations are able to produce adequate plasma levels for up to 12 hours and are therefore particularly useful in controlling nocturnal asthma (34) and early morning wheezing. Theophylline can be administered intravenously and rectally as aminophylline (combination of theophylline and ethylenediamine, 20 times more soluble than theophylline alone [35]). Dosage and treatment regimens are summarized in Table 10-2. Aminophylline suppositories are no longer recommended because they cause proctitis and, as a result of erratic drug absorption, they produce an unpredictable therapeutic response. The intramuscular route is too irritating and hence is not recommended.

Although theophylline is used widely in the treatment of both acute and chronic asthma, its role in guidelines for asthma treatment remains controversial. Clinical studies of its use in the treatment of acute asthma have been hampered by poor trial design and small numbers of subjects. Because of these limitations, no definite advantage of theophylline has been demonstrated. Nevertheless, treatment with theophylline reduces the steroid dosage requirement in steroid-dependent patients with asthma (36). Although few studies have shown clear advantage to its use, it does seem to have a role, especially in the treatment of patients with more long-standing, chronic asthma and fixed airways obstruction.

Adverse Effects

Theophylline toxicity is dose related. Side effects can occur with concentrations below 20 mg/L, but are more common at concentrations greater than 30 to 40 mg/L (35). Tachycardia, palpitations, tremors, nausea, gastrointestinal disturbances, headache, and insomnia are among the common adverse effects. Theophylline therapy can sometimes produce potentially life-threatening cardiac arrhythmias and seizures. The seizures are usually focal in onset and soon may become generalized and tonic-clonic in type (37). The electroencephalogram characteristically shows periodic, lateralized epileptiform discharges. Theophylline-induced seizures are difficult to treat and are associated with a mortality rate of approximately 29% (37), which is directly related to the age of the patient. The underlying mechanism for these seizures is unclear. Seizures may respond to intravenous diazepam, phenobarbital, or a combination of both, but not to phenytoin (37). Among the cardiac arrhythmias, premature atrial and ventricular contractions, atrial fibrillation, supraventricular tachycardia, and multifocal atrial tachycardia have been reported (37). Supraventricular tachycardias respond to verapamil, and the ventricular tachycardias and ectopics respond to propranolol and procainamide (37).

Table 10-2. Theophylline Dosage

Variable	Description (35)
Oral preparations	Dosage of sustained-release preparations depends on the brand. Plasma theophylline concentration for optimal response is 10–20 mg/L.
Intravenous preparations	Aminophylline: slow intravenous injection (over 20 min.) of 250–500 mg (5 mg/kg) when necessary; for maintenance, slow i.v infusion of 500 micrograms/kg/hour (for patients not previously on theophylline).
Children	Aminophylline: slow intravenous injection (over 20 min.) of 5 mg/kg; for maintenance, slow intravenous infusion of 1 mg/kg/hour for children age 6 months to 9 years and 800 micrograms/kg/hour for children age 10–16 years (for patients not previously on theophylline).

Selective PDE Inhibitors

Classification of PDE Isoforms

Among the nine biochemically distinct families of PDEs that exist, at least seven have been extensively characterized (Table 10-3). Each family of proteins is encoded by a single gene or by a series of closely related genes, and further diversity in enzyme structure occurs through alternative splicing and posttranslation modification.

The PDEs are classified by their substrate specificity, cofactor dependence, and sensitivity to inhibitors. The type I PDEs are dependent on calcium and calmodulin for activation. The cAMP hydrolytic activity of type II PDEs is stimulated by cGMP, whereas type III PDEs are inhibited by cGMP. The low-Km, cAMP-specific PDEs that are not affected by cGMP are classified as type IV and are further identified by potent and selective inhibitors such as rolipram. The type V PDEs are cGMP specific, and type VI isoforms are the products of three distinct genes associated with the photoreceptor. The type VII PDEs are similar to the type IV PDEs in that they are cGMP insensitive and cAMP specific, but they have a higher affinity for cAMP and are insensitive to the selective inhibitors such as rolipram. The type VIII PDEs (38) are also very similar to the type IV PDEs, with a high affinity for cAMP and insensitivity to cGMP and IBMX. The type IX PDEs are highly specific for cGMP and have a Km 40–70 times lower than that of PDE V and PDE VI, respectively (39).

Table 10-3. Phosphodiesterase Gene Families*

Enzyme	Gene Family	No. of Genes	Splice Variants
PDE I	Calcium and calmodulin dependent	3	9+
PDE II	cGMP-stimulated	1	2
PDE III	cGMP-inhibited	2	2+
PDE IV	cAMP-specific	4	15+
PDE V	cGMP-specific	2	2
PDE VI	Photoreceptor	3	2
PDE VII	cAMP-specific, high infinity	1	1
PDE VIII	cAMP-specific IBMX-insensitive	1	1
PDE IX	cGMP-specific (not fully classified)	1	?

*This information is based on currently available publications, some of which report preliminary data that may change with more extensive investigation. Subsequently cited PDEX and PDEXII, see references 83 and 84.

The structure, regulation, and inhibition of PDEs have been comprehensively reviewed by Beavo (40) and Houslay and Milligan (41).

All mammalian PDEs contain a large region close to the carboxyl terminus that is highly conserved within subtypes (60% amino acid homology) but that has less homology between different subtypes. There is evidence that this region contains the catalytic domain, although distinct cyclic nucleotide binding regions have been found in different domains of the same isoenzyme. Similarly, selective inhibitors of PDEs, notably the PDE IV inhibitor rolipram, interact with the enzyme at different sites (42). PDE IV isoforms have a high-affinity rolipram-binding site (HARBS), which is a second catalytic site on the PDE IV enzyme; this site is characterized by its increased affinity for rolipram specifically, but it also has affinity for a variety of other PDE IV inhibitors (43,44). The low-affinity catalytic site and the HARBS co-exist on at least 2 long-form splice variants of PDE IV. Inhibitors with selectivity for the PDE IV isozyme with different affinities for the two sites have been used in attempts to determine why the two sites exist. PDE IV inhibitors have a range of functional responses, some beneficial and others detrimental. Correlations exist between the former and the low-affinity catalytic site and between the latter and the HARBS (Table 10-4) (45). The biochemical characterization and molecular cloning of PDE isoforms have enabled PDE distribution to be assessed in different tissues, although this process is at an early stage (Table 10-5). A number of organs contain mixtures of PDE isoenzymes, but there are also tissues that appear to contain predominantly one PDE isoenzyme.

Most of the information currently at hand about the selective PDE inhibitors derives primarily from animal experiments and in vitro studies with human tissues; however, clinical data are becoming available. The wide-spread distribution of the PDE isoenzymes makes their selective inhibition a therapeutic target. Inhibitors of PDE IV are of particular interest because these agents possess anti-inflammatory activity that could prove useful in the treatment of asthma, atopic dermatitis, rheumatoid arthri-

Table 10-4. Association of Functional Response of PDE IV Inhibitors with Active Site Selectivity

Low-Affinity Catalytic Site	HARBS
Inhibition of TNF-α release from monocytes	Nausea and emesis
Inhibition of *Staphylococcus aureus* enterotoxin A–induced IL-2 production	Inhibition of histamine-induced contraction in guinea pig trachea
Potentiation of PGE$_2$-induced cAMP in monocytes	Acid secretion in parietal cells

TNF-α, tumor necrosis factor α; PGE$_2$, prostaglandin E$_2$.

Table 10-5. PDE Isoenzyme Profiles of Respiratory Smooth Muscle

Species	Tissue	PDE Isoenzymes	References
Guinea pig	Trachealis	III, IV	51
Canine	Trachealis	I, II, III, IV, V	52
Bovine	Trachealis	I, II, IV, V	53
Human	Bronchus	I, II, IV, V	54
	Bronchus	I, II, (III*), IV, V	55
	Trachealis	I, II, III, IV, V	56

*Detected in small quantities.

tis, inflammatory bowel disease, and septic shock. Because of their bronchodilator properties, inhibitors of PDE I, III, IV, and V may be useful in the treatment of asthma (46). The anti-inflammatory property of PDE IV inhibitors and the ability of PDE V inhibitors to attenuate the release of histamine from the mast cells make them potential agents for use in the prophylaxis of asthma (47). Animal studies have revealed that the PDE III inhibitors inhibit platelet aggregation in addition to their bronchodilator action. PDE III inhibitors are used clinically for the acute treatment of congestive heart failure.

A new class of inhibitor, that of PDE V, has now overtaken the PDE III inhibitor family in terms of number of patients treated. The PDE V inhibitor class is exemplified by sildenafil (Viagra) (48), which is currently used in the treatment of male erectile dysfunction. In human corpus cavernosum the release of nitric oxide stimulates guanylyl cyclase, thereby increasing levels of cGMP. The increase in intracellular cGMP modulates levels of intracellular calcium and thereby regulates smooth-muscle contractility and erectile function. By inhibiting PDE V cGMP hydrolytic activity, sildenafil promotes penile erection through increased cGMP levels. The inhibition of PDE IX may also be implicated in the actions of sildenafil (49).

Inhibitors of PDE IV

A key event in the history of PDE IV inhibitors was the report in 1987 on the identification of a new, cyclic nucleotide PDE activity in guinea pig and human cardiac ventricle (PDE IV) and on the finding that two known compounds, rolipram (Fig. 10-1*A*) and RO-201724 (Fig. 10-1*B*), are potent, selective inhibitors of this enzyme (50). Another known compound, denbufylline (Fig. 10-1*C*), was also identified as a selective PDE IV inhibitor. The most striking aspects of the inhibitors of type IV PDEs are their anti-inflammatory and bronchodilator actions, and these properties have prompted researchers to test their usefulness in the treatment of asthma. It is clear that in a number of tissues and cells involved in inflammation in asthma (such as airway smooth muscle, mast cells, inflammatory leukocytes, and sensory neurones) PDE IV is an important regulator of cAMP.

Biochemical assay of the PDE isoenzyme profile of airways smooth muscle has been carried out with tissue obtained from a number of species, including humans. As indicated in Table 10-4, PDE IV is consistently present in this tissue (51–56). In human bronchus, PDE IV is the major isoform present, having greater than 50% of the total cAMP hydrolytic activity (54). PDE IV is characterized in Table 10-6.

Type IV PDE activity has been detected in human inflammatory leukocytes (57), and, with the exception of lymphocytes, PDE IV is the predominant subtype. Inhibition of PDE IV in neutrophils, monocytes, basophils, and mast cells results in suppression of mediator release. Similarly, the respiratory burst and superoxide production by neutrophils and eosinophils are reduced by PDE inhibitors. This effect correlates with an elevation of intracellular cAMP.

In general, the elevation of cAMP leads to down-regulation of inflammatory cell activity, although the mechanism(s) accounting for this effect is not clearly understood. It is possible that cAMP modulates the free cytosolic calcium concentration that is mobilized during cell activation. PDE IV inhibitors reduce the release of cytokines from activated peripheral blood monocytes (58), perhaps because there is a cAMP response element in the transcription of cytokine genes. Certainly any inhibition of the synthesis or release of cytokines such as tumor necrosis factor-

Table 10-6. Characterization of PDE IV from Human Bronchial Smooth Muscle

Enzyme Characteristics	Activity
Km cyclic AMP	$1.5\,\mu M$
Km cyclic GMP	$>500\,\mu M$
Calcium and calmodulin activation	None
Cyclic GMP activation	None
Molecular weight	82.3 KD
Zaprinast IC_{50}	$61\,\mu M$
SK&F 94120 IC_{50}	$>500\,\mu M$
Theophylline IC_{50}	$151\,\mu M$
Denbufylline IC_{50}	$0.46\,\mu M$
Rolipram IC_{50}	$0.62\,\mu M$

Data from Cortijo J, Bou J, Beleta J, et al. Investigation into the role of phosphodiesterase IV in bronchorelaxation, including studies with human bronchus. Br J Pharmacol 1993;108:562–568.

α or IL-1, would provide a plausible mechanism for anti-inflammatory activity. Lymphocytes have both PDE III and PDE IV activity, and reports suggest that they also contain a distinct PDE activity classified as PDE VII (59). There is evidence that elevation of cAMP in lymphocytes suppresses cytotoxicity, IgE formation, cytokine synthesis, and blastogenesis (57).

The synthesis of IL-5 by allergen-specific T lymphocytes in the lungs of persons with asthma is thought to be a key factor in the recruitment of eosinophils (60). The participation of eosinophils in allergic asthma could, therefore, be reduced by PDE inhibitors acting to inhibit both the generation of IL-5 and the activation and degranulation of the eosinophils themselves.

Important neuronal factors influence the control of bronchial smooth-muscle tone and reactivity. It has been suggested that the elevation of cAMP in the sensory neurones by sympathomimetic drugs like salmeterol contributes to the control of airway dynamics by these drugs (61). The elevation of cAMP in a neuronal cell line is augmented by rolipram, indicating that a PDE IV is present. Bronchial tone is also regulated by non-adrenergic, noncholinergic (NANC) control mechanisms. NANC bronchoconstriction is mediated by the release of constrictor neurokinins such as neurokinin A from sensory nerve terminals. This release can be blocked by rolipram but not by specific inhibitors of PDE III or PDE V (62). Thus, the elevation of cAMP in sensory neurones prevents neuokinin release and explains why rolipram markedly reduces ozone-induced bronchial hyperreactivity in guinea pigs (63).

The most interesting inhibitors of PDE IV are considered below.

Xanthine Derivatives

The methylxanthines theophylline (Fig. 10-1*D*) and isobutyl-methylxanthine (IBMX) (Fig. 10-1*E*) are well known as nonselective PDE IV inhibitors. In 1987 denbufylline (BRL 30892) was reported to be a potent and selective inhibitor of PDE IV (64). At that time, the compound was under clinical development for the treatment of multi-infarct dementia, although development

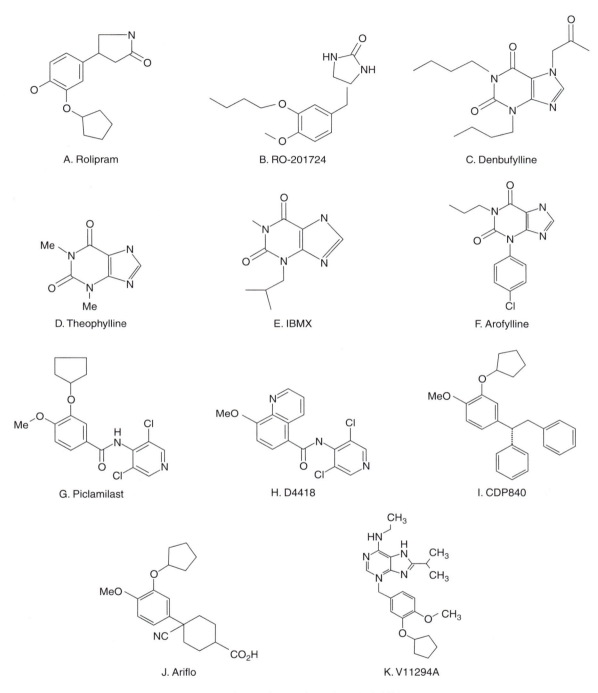

Figure 10-1. *A–K.* Chemical structures of nonselective and selective PDE IV inhibitors.

of the compound has now ceased. The evidence with denbufylline—that structural modification of xanthines could give rise to compounds having PDE IV selectivity—encouraged other groups to synthesize and test novel xanthine derivatives as selective PDE IV inhibitors. Laboratorios Almirall (Spain) has

patented a number of substituted xanthines that are claimed to be selective PDE IV inhibitors (65). One of these compounds, LAS 31025 (Fig. 10-1*F*), now known as arofylline, has been described as a selective PDE IV inhibitor (IC$_{50}$ 5.8 μM), as well as being an adenosine antagonist with similar affinities for A1

Table 10-7. Newer PDE IV Inhibitors

Compound	Indication	Phase Reached	Efficacy Marker	Refs
CDP840	Asthma	I (discontinued)	Inhibition of antigen bronchospasm	75
Piclamilast	Asthma	II (discontinued)	Inhibition of TNF-α release ex vivo	77
	Rheumatoid Arthritis	I	Improvement of tender joint counts Reduced C-reactive protein and IL-6 levels	76
Arofylline	Asthma	III	Bronchodilatation	78
Ariflo	Asthma	II	Exercise-induced asthma	79
	COPD	III	Bronchodilatation	80
D4418	Asthma	I (discontinued)	Inhibition of TNF-α release and elevation of cAMP ex vivo	71
V-11294A	Asthma	I	Inhibition of TNF-X release and PHA- stimulated mononuclear cell proliferation	81

PHA: phytohemagglutinin antigen

(3.7 μM) and A2 (7.2 μM) receptors (66). This compound was tested through the oral route as an antiasthmatic agent in phase III clinical trials.

Rolipram Analogs

Rolipram is a relatively old compound and was under development as an antidepressant agent. In addition to its own bronchodilator action, a marked synergistic bronchodilatory effect has been observed with inhibitors of PDE III (67). This finding suggests that a dual PDE III and PDE IV inhibitor may prove to be the most effective inhibitor of asthmatic bronchoconstriction. Synergy has also been demonstrated between rolipram and the bronchodilator β_2-adrenoceptor agonist isoproterenol (67), which elevates smooth muscle cAMP by a different molecular mechanism from that of the PDE inhibitors. The β_2 receptor activates adenylate cyclase to produce more cAMP. The bronchodilator potency of isoproterenol is enhanced by rolipram but not by the PDE III inhibitor siguazodan. This finding has led to the suggestion that the β_2 receptor is linked to PDE IV (67). A number of rolipram analogs have been reported from Pfizer (68) and Smith Kline Beecham (69), although the development status of these is not clear.

RP 73401

RP 73401, also known as piclamilast (Fig. 10-1*G*), is particularly potent against PDE IV, with an IC_{50} value of 1 nM on PDE IV enzyme from pig aorta, and is about 1000 times more potent than rolipram (70).

D4418

D4418 (Fig. 10-1*H*), a Chiroscience compound, shows high selectivity for PDE IV over the other PDE isoenzymes and a wide therapeutic index (71). The compound significantly inhibits eosinophilia and early- and late-phase bronchoconstriction when administered at a dose of 10 mg/kg orally in an allergic guinea pig model. At an oral dose of 60 mg/kg no nausea or emesis was observed in either ferrets or dogs.

CDP 840

Like piclamilast and D4418, CDP840 (Fig. 10-1*I*) is claimed to have a favorable catalytic-to-HARBS selectivity ratio. In sensitized guinea pigs with antigen-induced bronchoconstriction, CDP840 decreased the mean inflation pressure and reduced eosinophil numbers in bronchoalveolar lavage fluid. CDP840 did not, however, change the bronchoconstrictor response to histamine (72).

SB 207499

Also known as Ariflo, SB 207499 (Fig. 10-1*J*) is claimed to have an improved therapeutic index over first-generation PDE IV inhibitors such as rolipram. An improved catalytic-to-HARBS potency ratio is believed to underlie this improvement. Ariflo is equipotent to rolipram against the catalytic site, but is 100-fold less potent against the HARBS (73).

V-11294A

V-11294A from NAPP Laboratories (Fig. 10-1*K*) inhibited the lipopolysaccharide-induced increase in plasma tumor necrosis factor-X in mice and antigen-induced eosinophil accumulation in bronchoalveolar lavage in guinea pigs after oral administration (74). It also was an effective relaxant of isolated tracheal smooth muscle in allergic guinea pigs. Oral doses well above the effective dose had no effects on the CNS, cardiovascular, gastrointestinal, or urinary systems.

Clinical Experience with PDE IV Inhibitors

Results from clinical phase 1 up to phase III studies have been reported for Arofylline, CDP840, ariflo, piclamilast, D4418, and V-11294A. Data from the studies along with indications of the current status of the compounds are indicated in Table 10-7.

Adverse Effects of PDE IV Inhibitors

Gastric disturbances (nausea and emesis) have been reported as secondary effects of the PDE IV inhibitors rolipram and denbufylline when administered orally to humans, although these effects may represent a high dose or an exaggerated pharmacologic phenomenon. Paradoxically, Puig et al (82) showed that rolipram and denbufylline have a gastric cytoprotective effect in the rat, inhibiting ethanol-induced gastric ulcers at low doses (ID$_{50}$ values of 0.05 and 0.25 mg/kg orally for rolipram and denbufylline, respectively). The selective PDE III inhibitor SK&F 94120 was only weakly active in this test.

Thus, it remains to be seen whether limiting side effects of PDE IV inhibitors will be of importance after oral administration in humans. If so, then it is possible that topical administration (dry powder or solution to the lungs) would overcome the problem.

Conclusion

The identification of so many ways that cyclic nucleotide PDEs vary in their expression in different cells and tissues provides strong evidence that specific inhibitors could be developed in relation to different diseases. Indeed, for the treatment of erectile dysfunction Viagra has recently been established as the largest selling new drug ever. Considerable progress has also been made with respect to the development of novel drugs for the treatment of asthma and COPD. With increased selectivity and potency of PDE inhibitors, an important future task will be to develop compounds with few systemic side effects, particularly nausea and vomiting in the case of PDE IV inhibitors. The recognition that these enzyme inhibitors are capable of down-regulating inflammatory pathways in asthma and other allergic diseases provides optimism that there will be a new generation of these drugs available to patients with common chronic diseases.

References
1. Salter H. On some points in the treatment and clinical history of asthma. Edinburgh Med J 1859;4:1109–1115.
2. Butcher RW, Sutherland EW. Adenosine 3′, 5′-phosphate in biological materials. J Biol Chem 1962;237:1244–1250.
3. Polson JB, Krzanowski JJ, Goldman AL, Scentivanyi A. Inhibition of human phosphodiesterase activity by therapeutic levels of theophylline. Clin Exp Pharmacol Physiol 1978;5:536–539.
4. Mentzer RM, Rubio R, and Berne RM. Release of adenosine by hypoxic canine lung tissue and its possible role in pulmonary circulation. Am J Physiol 1975;229:1625–1631.
5. Wolff J, Londos C, Cooper DMF. Adenosine receptors and the regulation of adenylate cyclase. Adv Cyclic Nucleotide Res 1981;14:199–214.
6. Cushley M, Holgate ST. The mechanisms of action of theophylline at cellular level. In: Buckle DR, Smith H, eds. Development of anti-asthma drugs. Kent, England: Butterworth, 1984:205–223.
7. Pavia D, Sutton PP, Lopez-Vidreiro MT, et al. Drug effects on muco-ciliary function. Eur J Respir Dis 1983;64(supp 128):304–317.
8. Persson CGA. Overview of effects of theophylline. J Allergy Clin Immunol 1986;78:780–787.
9. Persson CGA. Experimental lung actions of xanthines. In: Andersson KE, Persson CGA, eds. Anti-asthma xanthines and adenosine. Amsterdam: Excerpta Medica, 1985:61–82.
10. Lichtenstein LM, Margolis S. Histamine release in vitro: inhibition by catecholamines and methylxanthines. Science 1968;161:902.
11. Kaliner M, Austen KF. Cyclic nucleotides and modulation of effector systems of inflammation. Biochem Pharmacol 1974;23:763–771.
12. Weissmann G, Dukor B, Zarier RB. Effect of cyclic AMP on release of lysosomal enzymes from phagocytes. Nature 1971;231:131–135.
13. Bussolino F, Benveniste J. Pharmacologic modulation of platelet activating factor (PAF) release from rabbit phagocytes. Immunology 1980;49:367–376.
14. Fink G, Mittleman M, Shohat B, Spitzer SA. Theophylline-induced alterations in cellular immunity in asthmatic patients. Clin Allergy 1987;17:313–316.
15. Nelson S, Summer WR, Jakab GJ. Aminophylline-induced suppression of pulmonary antibacterial defenses. Am Rev Respir Dis 1985;131:923–927.
16. Pauwels R, Van Reuterghem D, Van Der Straeten M, et al. The effect of theophylline and enprofylline on allergen-induced bronchoconstriction. J Allergy Clin Immunol 1985;76:583–590.
17. Sullivan P, Bekir S, Jaffar Z, et al. Anti-inflammatory effects of low dose oral theophylline in atopic asthma. Lancet 1994;343:1006–1008.
18. Kidney JC, Dominguez M, Rose M, et al. Withdrawing chronic theophylline treatment increases airway lymphocytes in asthma. Thorax 1994;49:396.
19. Minoguchi K, Kohno Y, Oda N, et al. Effect of theophylline withdrawal on airway inflammation in asthma. Clin Exp Allergy 1998;68:57–63.
20. Finnerty JP, Lee C, Wilson S, et al. Effects of theophylline on inflammatory cells and cytokines in asthmatic subjects: a placebo-controlled parallel group study. Eur Respir J 1996;9:1672–1677.
21. Wright LC, Seybold J, Robichaud A, et al. Phosphodiesterase

expression in human epithelial cells. Am J Physiol 1998;275: L694–700.

22. Murciano D, Aubier M, Lecocguic Y, Pariente R. Effect of theophylline on diaphragmatic strength and fatigue in patients with chronic obstructive pulmonary disease. N Engl J Med 311;6:349–353.

23. Aubier M, Murciano D, Viires N, et al. Diaphragmatic contractility enhanced by aminophylline: role of extra cellular calcium. J Appl Physiol 1983;54:460–464.

24. Sanchez JA, Stefani E. Inward calcium current in twitch muscle fibres of the frog. J Physiol (Lond) 1978;283:197–209.

25. Persson CGA. Overview of effects of theophylline. J Allergy Clin Immunol 1986;78:780–787.

26. Mahler OA, Matthay RA, Synder FE, et al. Sustained release theophylline reduces sensation of dyspnoea in nonreversible obstructive airway disease. Am Rev Respir Dis 1985;131: 22–25.

27. Jenne JW, Siever JR, Druz WS, et al. The effect of maintenance theophylline therapy on lung work in severe chronic obstructive pulmonary disease while standing and walking. Am Rev Respir Dis 1984;130:600–605.

28. Poe RH, Utell MJ. Theophylline in asthma and COPD: changing perspectives and controversies. Geriatrics 1991;46: 4:55–65.

29. Fleetham JA, Fera T, Edgell FG. The effect of theophylline in sleep disorders in COPD patients. Am Rev Respir Dis 1983;127(suppl):A85.

30. Mayer J, Fuchs E, Hugens M. Long-term sleep therapy in sleep apnea syndrome. Am Rev Respir Dis 1984;129(suppl): A252.

31. Hendeles L, Weinberger M. Theophylline. A "state of art" review. Pharmacotherapy 1983;3:2–44.

32. Staib AH, Schuppan D, Lissner R, et al. Pharmacokinetics and metabolism of theophylline in patients with liver diseases. Int J Clin Pharmacol Ther Toxicol 1980;18:500–502.

33. Kraemer MJ, Furukawa CT, Koup JR, et al. Altered theophylline clearance during an influenza B outbreak. Paediatrics 1982;69:476–480.

34. Zwillich CW, Neagey SR, Ciccutu L, et al. Nocturnal asthma therapy: inhaled bitolterol versus sustained-release theophylline. Am Rev Respir Dis 1989;139:470–474.

35. British National Formulary. September 1993;Number 26.

36. Nassif EG, Weinberger M, Thompson R, Huntly W. The value of maintenance theophylline in steroid-dependent asthma. N Engl J Med 1981;304:71–75.

37. Kelly HW. Theophylline toxicity. In: Jenne J, Murphy S, eds. Drug therapy for asthma: research and clinical practice. New York: Marcel Dekker, 1987:925–951.

38. Fisher DA, Smith JF, Pillar JS, et al. Isolation and characterization of PDE8A, a novel human cAMP-specific phosphodiesterase. Biochem Biophys Res Commun 1998;246: 570–577.

39. Soderling SH, Bayuga SJ, Beavo JA. Identification and characterization of a novel family of cyclic nucleotide phosphodiesterases. J Biol Chem 1998;273:15553–15558.

40. Beavo JA. Cyclic nucleotide phosphodiesterases: functional implications of multiple isoforms. Physiol Rev 1995;75:725–748.

41. Houslay MD, Milligan G. Tailoring cAMP-signalling responses through isoform multiplicity. Trends Biochem Sci 1997;22:217–224.

42. Torphy TJ, Stadel JM, Burman M, et al. Coexpression of human cAMP specific phosphodiesterase activity and high-affinity rolipram binding in yeast. J Biol Chem 1992;267: 1798–1804.

43. Harris AL, Connell MJ, Furguson EW, et al. Role of low Km cyclic AMP phosphodiesterase inhibition in tracheal relaxation and bronchodilation in guinea pig. J Pharm Exp Ther 1989;251:199–206.

44. Schudt C, Dent G, Rabe KF. Handbook of immunopharmacology. San Diego: Academic Press, 1996.

45. Souness JE, Sudha R. Proposal for pharmacologically distinct cAMP phosphodiesterases. Cell Signal 1997;9:227–236.

46. Reeves ML, Leigh BK, England PJ. The identification of a new cyclic nucleotide phosphodiesterase in human and guinea pig cardiac ventricle. Implications for the mechanism of action of selective phosphodiesterase inhibitors. Biochem J 1987;241:535–541.

47. Nicholson CD, Challis RAJ, Shahid M. Differential modulation of tissue function and therapeutic potential of selective inhibitors of cyclic nucleotide phosphodiesterase enzymes. Trends Pharmacol Sci 1991;12:19–27.

48. Hall IP. Isoenzyme selective phosphodiesterase inhibitors: potential clinical uses. Br J Clin Pharmacol 1993;35:1–7.

49. Moreland RB, Goldstein I, Traish A. Sildenafil, a novel inhibitor of phosphodiesterase type 5 in human corpus cavernosum smooth muscle cells. Life Sci 1998;62:309–318.

50. Fisher DA, Smith JF, Pillar JS, et al. Isolation and characterization of PDE9A, a novel human cGMP-specific phosphodiesterase. J Biol Chem 1998;273:15559–155564.

51. Silver PJ, Hammel LT, Perrone MH, et al. Differential pharmacologic sensitivity of cyclic nucleotide phosphodiesterase isozymes isolated from cardiac muscle, arterial and airway smooth muscle. Eur J Pharmacol 1988;150:85–94.

52. Torphy TJ, Cieslinski LB. Characterization and selective inhibition of cyclic nucleotide phosphodiesterase isozymes in canine tracheal smooth muscle. Mol Pharmacol 1990;37: 206–214.

53. Nicholson CD, Shahid M, van Amderstand RGM, Zaagsma J. Cyclic nucleotide phosphodiesterase (PDE) isoenzymes in bovine tracheal smooth muscle, their inhibition and the ability of isoenzyme inhibitors to relax preconstricted preparations. Eur J Pharmacol 1990;183:1097–1098.

54. Cortijo J, Bou J, Beleta J, et al. Investigation into the role of phosphodiesterase IV in bronchorelaxation, including studies with human bronchus. Br J Pharmacol 1993;108:562–568.

55. de Boer J, Philpott AJ, van Amsterdam AGM, et al. Human bronchial cyclic nucleotide phosphodiesterase isoenzymes: biochemical and pharmacological analysis using selective inhibitors. Br J Pharmacol 1992;106:1028–1034.

56. Torphy TJ, Undem BJ, Cieslinsky LB, et al. Identification, characterization and functional role of phosphodiesterase isozymes in human airway smooth muscle. J Pharmacol Exp Ther 1993;265:1213–1223.

57. Torphy TJ, Undem BJ. Phosphodiesterase inhibitors: new opportunities in the treatment of asthma. Thorax 1991;46: 512–523.

58. Molnar-Kimber KL, Yonno L, Heaslip RJ, Weichman BM. Differential regulation of TNF-α and IL-1β production from endotoxin-stimulated human monocytes by phosphodiesterase inhibitors. Mediators Inflamm 1992;1:411–417.

59. Ichimura M, Kase H. A new cyclic nucleotide phosphodiesterase isoenzyme expressed in the T lymphocyte cell line. Biochem Biophys Res Commun 1993;193:985–990.
60. Corrigan CJ, Kay AB. CD4 T-lymphocyte activation in acute severe asthma. Relationship to disease severity and atopic status. Am Rev Respir Dis 1990;141:970–977.
61. McCrea KE, Hill SJ. Salmeterol, a long-acting β_2-adrenoceptor agonist mediating cyclic AMP accumulation in a neuronal cell line. Br J Pharmacol 1993;110:619–626.
62. Qian Y, Girard V, Martin CAE, et al. Rolipram, but not siguazodan or zaprinast, inhibits the excitatory noncholinergic neurotransmission in guinea pig bronchi. Eur Respir J 1994;7:306–310.
63. Holbrook M, Hughes B. The effect of rolipram and SK&F 94120 on ozone-induced bronchial hyperreactivity to inhaled histamine in guinea pigs. Br J Pharmacol 1992;107:254P.
64. Nicholson CD, Wilke R. The selective inhibition of a low Km cyclic AMP phosphodiesterase from rat cerebral cortex by denbufylline. Br J Pharmacol 1987;92:680.
65. Noverola AV, Sota JMP, Mauri JM, Gristwood RW. Xanthine compounds and compositions and methods of using them. US patent 5 233 504. June 29, 1993.
66. Beleta J, Bou J, Miralpeix M, et al. LAS 31025, a new compound with selective phosphodiesterase IV inhibitory activity. Presented at the Third International Conference on Cyclic Nucleotide Phosphodiesterases: From Genes to Therapies, Glasgow, Scotland, July 1996.
67. Qian Y, Naline E, Karlsson JA, et al. Effect of rolipram and siguazodan on the human isolated bronchus and their interaction with isoprenaline and sodium nitroprusside. Br J Pharmacol 1993;109:774–778.
68. Koe BK, Lebel LA, Nelson JA, et al. Effects of novel catechol ether imidazolidinones on calcium-independent phosphodiesterase activity, ^{3}H rolipram binding and reserpine-induced hypothermia in mice. Drug Dev Res 1990;21:135–142.
69. Pinto LL, Buckle DR, Readshaw SA, Smith DG. The selective inhibition of phosphodiesterase IV by benzopyran derivatives of rolipram. Bioorg Med Chem Lett 1993;8:1743–1746.
70. Raeburn D, Underwood SL, Lewis SA, et al. Anti-inflammatory and bronchodilator properties of RP 73401, a novel and selective phosphodiesterase type IV inhibitor. Br J Pharmacol 1994;113:1423–1431.
71. Montana J, Cooper N, Dyke H, et al. Activity of D4418, a novel phosphodiesterase inhibitor IV (PDE IV). Effects in cellular and animal models of asthma and early clinical studies. Am J Respir Crit Care Med 1999;159:A624.
72. Hughes B, Howat D, Lisle H, et al. The inhibition of antigen-induced eosinophilia and bronchoconstriction by CDP840, a novel stereo-selective inhibitor of phosphodiesterase type 4. Br J Pharmacol 1996;118:1183–1191.
73. Barnette MS, Christiansen SB, Essayan DM, et al. SB 207499 (Ariflo), a potent and selective second-generation phosphodiesterase 4 inhibitor: in vitro anti-inflammatory actions. J Pharmacol Exp Ther 1998;284:420–426.
74. Cavalla D, Gale DD, Spina D, et al. Activity of V11294A, a novel phosphodiesterase 4 (PDE4) inhibitor, in cellular and animal models of asthma. Am J Crit Care Med 1997;155:A660.
75. Harbinson PL, MacLeod D, Hawksworth R, et al. The effect of a novel orally active selective PDE4 isoenzyme inhibitor (CDP840) on allergen-induced responses in asthmatic subjects. Eur Respir J 1997;10:1008–1014.
76. Chikanza IC, Jawed SJ, Blake DR, et al. Treatment of patients with rheumatoid arthritis with RP73401 phosphodiesterase type IV inhibitor. Arthritis Rheum 1996;39(suppl):282.
77. Souness JE. Conformers of phosphodiesterase 4. Presented at Conquering Airway Inflammation in the 21st Century. Imperial College School of Medicine. National Heart and Lung Institute, London, September 1997.
78. Ferrer P, Dihn Xuan T, Chanal I, et al. Bronchodilator activity of LAS 31025, a new selective phosphodiesterase IV inhibitor. Am J Respir Crit Care Med 1997;155(4):A660.
79. Neiman RB, Fischer BD, Amit O, Dockhorn RJ. SB 207499 (Airflo™), a second generation, selective phosphodiesterase type 4 (PDE 4) inhibitor, attenuates exercise-induced bronchoconstriction in patients with asthma. Am J Respir Crit Care Med 1998;157:A413.
80. Torphy TJ. Phosphodiesterase 4 inhibitors: from concept to clinic. Presented at Conquering Airway Inflammation in the 21st Century. Imperial College School of Medicine. National Heart and Lung Institute, London, September 1998.
81. Landells LJ, Jensen MW, Spina D. Oral administration of the phosphodiesterase (PDE) 4 inhibitor V11294A inhibits the ex-vivo agonist-induced cell activation. Eur Respir J 1998;12(suppl 28):2393. Abstract.
82. Puig J, Fernandez AG, Beleta J, Gristwood RW. Rolipram and denbufylline, two phosphodiesterase inhibitors, induce gastric cytoprotective effects in the rat. Farm Clin Exp 1992(Sept):290.
83. Soderling SH, Bayuga SJ, Beavo JA. Isolation and characterization of a dual-substrate phosphodiesterase gene family: 10A. Proc Natl Acad Sci 1999;12:7071–7076.
84. Fawcett L, Baxendale R, Stacey P, et al. Molecular cloning and characterization of a distinct human phosphodiesterase gene family: PDE11A. Proc Natl Acad Sci 2000;97:3702–3707.

Chapter 11

Tryptase Inhibitors

Andrew F. Walls

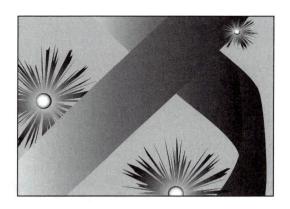

Mast cells have long been recognized as having a key role in the pathogenesis of inflammatory disease. These cells are ubiquitous in distribution, although they are particularly abundant at the portals of entry to the body, at mucosal surfaces in the respiratory and intestinal tracts, and in the skin. The mast cell plays an important role in the initiation of allergic responses, and increasingly this cell is being seen as a participant in processes of chronic inflammation and fibrosis. The cross-linking of membrane-bound IgE receptors by specific allergens or the direct action of a range of stimuli can trigger the explosive release from these cells of proteases, histamine, proteoglycans, arachidonic acid metabolites such as prostaglandin D_2 and leukotriene C_4, and various inflammatory cytokines (1,2). Mast cell–derived mediators have attracted attention for their potent pharmacologic actions, and several have become targets for therapeutic intervention.

The proteases have until recently received relatively little attention as mediators of disease. This fact is surprising in some respects, as the presence of tryptic (3,4) and chymotryptic enzymes (5–7) in mast cells has been recognized since the development of histochemical substrates for such proteases in the 1950s. Moreover, the proteases are the most abundant products of human mast cell activation, with a cumulative total of up to 60 pg stored in human mast cells (8). This amount compares with the presence of just 1 or 2 pg histamine in these cells.

The serine protease tryptase (EC3.4.21.59) is stored in quantities of about 10 to 35 pg in human mast cells (9). Greater amounts of tryptase are present in cells in the skin than in the lung, and there is more in the cells of adults than of infants (9). Other proteases stored in human mast cells include chymase (0 to 4.5 pg/cell [9]), carboxypeptidase (0 to 16 pg/cell [10,11]), cathepsin G (0.1 to 0.7 pg [12,13]), elastase (0 to 0.3 pg/cell [12]), and tissue type plasminogen activator (14). Of the proteases identified, tryptase alone appears to be present in all human mast cell populations (15,16). Chymase has been localized to a subpopulation of mast cells that occurs predominantly, though not exclusively in connective tissues, and has been designated MC_{TC} to denote the presence of both tryptase and chymase (17). The MC_T subset, which contains tryptase but not chymase, predominates in normal mucosal tissues. Carboxypeptidase (11) and cathepsin G (13) both appear to be selectively present in the MC_{TC} population. There have been suggestions that certain mast cells may contain chymase but not tryptase (MC_C) (18,19); but the proportion of cells of this phenotype, if seen at all, appears to depend on the sensitivity of the detection system for tryptase and can be affected to a large degree by the length of incubation periods used in immunocytochemistry (20).

Mast cells are the major cellular stores of tryptase. This protease has not been convincingly demonstrated to exist in any other cell type except for basophils, which have been calculated to contain just 0.4% of the quantity of tryptase in normal tissue mast cells (21). Increased amounts of tryptase may be stored in peripheral-blood basophils of individuals with asthma or other allergic conditions (22), but tryptase is predominantly a mast-cell product and has received widespread acceptance as a unique marker for mast cells.

An appreciation of the value of tryptase as a cell-specific marker preceded an understanding of its function. In recent years, however, studies with purified tryptase have provided some compelling evidence that tryptase may be a potent mediator of inflammation and tissue remodeling. The development of inhibitors of tryptase is now beginning to provide confirmation of the key mediator role of tryptase, as well as to point to a potential new treatment for mast cell–mediated disease.

Molecular Properties and the Regulation of Tryptase Activity

Tryptase was named after its ability to cleave certain histochemical chromogenic substrates of trypsin (4). It is a serine endopeptidase that preferentially cleaves peptide and ester bonds on the carboxyl side of basic amino acids (23), but, unlike trypsin, tryptase displays a considerable degree of selectivity in the cleavage of protein substrates. The structure is unusual, being a tetramer of about 130 kDa with variably glycosylated subunits of some 28 to 38 kDa (15,24–26). Two cDNA molecules for tryptase, termed α and β, have been cloned from a human lung mast-cell library (27,28); and three, termed I, II, and III, have been cloned from a skin library (29). The β tryptase gene encodes a catalytic region of the molecule with 90% amino acid sequence identity with α-tryptase and 98% to 100% identity with tryptase I, II, and III, and a prepro region that displays 87% homology with α-tryptase and 100% with tryptases I, II, and III. Derived molecular-mass values have all been approximately 27.5 kDa for the catalytic portions and 3.0 kDa for the prepro regions.

Early attempts to express active α-tryptase in an insect expression system were unsuccessful, prompting the suggestion that the pre-enzyme is not susceptible for further processing within the mast cell but is secreted constitutively in an inactive form (30,31). However, subsequent studies in other laboratories have indicated that functionally active α-tryptase may be obtained from insect (32) and COS cell expression systems (33). A single amino acid sequence difference in a surface loop that forms the substrate-binding cleft appears to be responsible for α-tryptase having a more restricted substrate specificity than β-tryptase (32).

Crystalization of a preparation of tryptase purified from human lung tissue (found to have the sequence of β-tryptase, or tryptase II) has provided some explanations at the structural level for the unusual properties of this protease (34). The four subunits are arranged in a flat ring structure, with the catalytic site of each directed toward an oval central pore. This arrangement is likely to restrict access of both substrates and inhibitors to the active sites. An elongated, positively charged patch spanning adjacent pairs of monomers has been suggested to provide a means by which heparin can stabilize the complex.

Despite investigations spanning 2 decades, an effective endogenous inhibitor of tryptase has yet to be identified. Inhibitory effects have not been found for the circulating inhibitors α_1-antitrypsin, α_2-macroglobulin, and C_1-esterase inhibitor, nor for various inhibitors isolated from human tissues, including low-molecular-weight elastase inhibitor and bikunin (24,25,35–38). Secretory leukoprotease inhibitor (SLPI, also known as antileukoprotease) has been discounted as a tryptase inhibitor (36), but recent studies have suggested that there may be conditions when this broad-spectrum inhibitor may indeed inhibit the actions of tryptase (39).

Factors that influence the enzymatic stability of tryptase could be of more importance in the regulation of activity than protease inhibitors. Purified tryptase is highly unstable in physiologic buffers, and the calculated half-life can be as short as 3 minutes or less (40). There appears to be conversion of the active tetrameric molecule into inactive monomers (41–43). This process is markedly reduced in the presence of heparin or other proteoglycans, the effectiveness of stabilization being dependent on the negative charge density of the glycosaminoglycans (40). Tryptase has little enzymatic activity when maintained in high ionic-strength buffers, which disrupt the interaction with proteoglycans. Divalent cations such as calcium and magnesium (44) are competitive inhibitors of tryptase; and histamine, at least in millimolar concentrations, can shift the substrate dose-response curve to the right and induce allosteric behavior (44). Heparin-binding proteins such as antithrombin III (35), and the neutrophil granule proteins lactoferrin (45) and myeloperoxidase (46) can compete with tryptase for heparin and by this means reduce the enzymatic activity.

Tryptase in Nonhuman Species

All mammalian species examined to date appear to possess mast cells that contain tryptase. With histochemical substrates, tryptic activity has been detected in the mast cells of the rat, mouse, guinea pig, gerbil, dog, cow, and monkey (4,47–52). In some early studies tryptase was not detected in the mast cells of certain species such as the guinea pig and mouse (3), but subsequent application of more sensitive substrates has allowed tryptase to be identified in the mast cells of these species (52,53). In the rat, immunohistochemistry with a rat tryptase–specific antibody has suggested that the presence of tryptase is restricted to a subpopulation of connective tissue–type mast cells (54). In the mouse, immunostaining for tryptases may be transiently acquired in mast cells located in the lamina propria during *Trichinella* infection of the gut (55).

There is considerable variation between species in the physicochemical and enzymatic properties of the tryptases identified. Tryptase has now been purified or partially purified from tissues of the mouse, rat, guinea pig, cow, sheep, and monkey (52–61); and cDNA sequences have been derived for two tryptases in the rat (62), two in the mouse (63,64), two in the sheep (60), and one in the dog (50). Like human tryptase (24), those of the rat, mouse, sheep, and monkey are tetramers of 120 to 140 kDa, composed of equally sized glycosylated subunits of 30 to 40 kDa. In contrast, tryptase isolated from bovine tissues is some 360 kDa (56) and that from guinea pig tissues has an estimated molecular mass of 860 kDa, indicative of a massive structure with 20 to 22 subunits (52). Most of the nonhuman tryptases characterized to date bind readily to heparin and are not inhibited by circulating inhibitors of serine proteases. However, in these respects the isolated rat tryptase is an exception in that it fails to bind to heparin in physiologic buffers and is inhibited by α_1-antitrypsin, as well as several other protease inhibitors that are without effect on human tryptase, including soybean trypsin inhibitor, antipain, and aprotinin (53–55).

Studies with nonhuman tryptases have yielded useful insights into the expression and contribution of mast-cell proteases in health and disease. Nonetheless, major differences in their distribution and in their physicochemical and enzymatic properties would suggest that tryptases fulfill different functions in different mammalian species. Therefore, caution is called for when animal models of human disease are used in investigations of the therapeutic potential of tryptase inhibitors.

Tryptase Secretion in Disease

The value of tryptase as a marker of mast-cell activation depends not only on its selective presence in mast cells but also on its relative stability in an immunoreactive form in biologic fluids. In this regard, tryptase offers major advantages over histamine and prostaglandin D_2, and the measurement of tryptase has provided useful information on the extent of mast-cell activation in clinical disease.

Inevitably, assays for tryptase have been applied in particular to biologic fluids collected from patients with allergic disease. Increased levels of tryptase have been detected in bronchoalveolar lavage (BAL) fluids of patients with asthma, even in asymptomatic periods (65–67). However, at least in childhood asthma, strong correlations have been noted with bronchial hyperresponsiveness as assessed by PC_{20} measurements (68). BAL fluid concentrations of tryptase of 10 ng/mL or more have been detected, which, assuming a dilution factor in the region of 100, would indicate that concentrations in the lung lining fluid can reach high levels. Introduction of allergen into the lower airways of atopic individuals with asthma can stimulate further elevations in BAL fluid tryptase concentration within minutes (69,70). Altered tryptase levels have not been detected 24 hours after allergen challenge (71); and exercise (72,73) and local challenge with hypertonic saline (74) both fail to induce increases in BAL fluid tryptase concentration, suggesting that the bronchoconstriction observed in these models is not mast cell dependent. A short course of inhaled steroids is associated with a marked decrease in BAL fluid tryptase levels in atopic individuals with asthma, in parallel with a decline in mast cell numbers in BAL fluid and in the bronchial mucosa (75,69), whereas treatment with a β_2-adrenoceptor agonist appears to leave tryptase concentrations and mast cell numbers unaffected (76).

Observations of altered tryptase levels in the lower airways of individuals with asthma have some parallels with findings in other biologic fluids from persons with various other allergic conditions. In patients with rhinitis, provocation with allergen or with cold dry air is associated with the rapid release into nasal lavage fluid of tryptase, as well as other mast cell derived mediators (77–79). Allergen challenge in the skin stimulates increased tryptase levels in skin blister fluid in atopic individuals (80) and in the eye can provoke elevated tryptase concentrations in tears (81). Increased concentrations of tryptase are rare in serum, except in patients with systemic anaphylaxis or mastocytosis (31,82).

Tryptase at quite high levels has been detected in biologic fluids from patients with conditions in which the contribution of the mast cell has received relatively little attention. Increased tryptase concentrations have been detected in BAL fluid from patients with interstitial lung disease or bronchial carcinoma (83), as well as from people who smoke (84). Tryptase has been detected also in synovial fluid from patients with rheumatoid arthritis, osteoarthritis, and seronegative spondyloarthritis (85), and in urine from individuals with interstitial cystitis (86).

In immunoassays for tryptase used to date, antibodies are employed that bind equally well to α and β tryptase or that react preferentially with β-tryptase. When comparisons have been made between the results of these assays applied to measure tryptase in the same sample, the β form of tryptase predominates in the serum from patients with anaphylaxis and the α form in that from normal individuals or patients with mastocytosis (31). The α form is the major form detected in the synovial fluid from patients with rheumatoid arthritis or osteoarthritis (85). The relative amounts of each form of tryptase in other diseases and the biologic significance remain to be established.

Substrates of Tryptase

The list of naturally occurring peptide and protein substrates identified for tryptase is quite limited (Table 11-1). A role for

Table 11-1. Extracellular Substrates of Tryptase

Substrate	Action of Tryptase
Vasoactive intestinal peptide (VIP)	Degradation
Peptide histidine methionine (PHM)	Degradation
Calcitonin gene-related peptide (CGRP)	Degradation
Fibrinogen	Inactivation
Fibronectin	Cleavage
Type VI collagen	Cleavage
Kininogens	Generation of kinins
Prekallikrein	Activation
ProMMP-3	Activation
Pro-urokinase	Activation
Matrix metalloprotease 9 (MMP-9)	Cleavage
Protease activated receptor 2 (PAR-2)	Activation

tryptase in mediating neurogenic inflammation has been suggested by the efficient cleavage by this protease of the neuropeptides, vasoactive intestinal peptide (VIP), peptide histidine methionine (PHM) (87), and calcitonin gene-related peptide (CGRP) (88). Both VIP and PHM are potent relaxants of bronchial muscle, and their cleavage could contribute to bronchoconstriction in asthma, while CGRP is a vasodilator.

The ability of tryptase to generate kinins from either low- (89,90) or high-molecular-weight kininogen (90,91) further supports a role for this enzyme as a mediator of inflammation. Tryptase can also activate prekallikrein (91) and act cooperatively with neutrophil elastase to generate bradykinin with a yield comparable to that of plasma kallikrein (92). Inactivation of fibrinogen by tryptase could serve to limit the clotting reaction in the vicinity of degranulating mast cells (93–95).

Tryptase could participate in processes of tissue degradation by cleaving several components of the extracellular matrix, including matrix metalloprotease 9 (MMP-9) and to some extent fibronectin (96) and type VI collagen (97). Also relevant in this context could be the observations that tryptase can activate pro-urinary plasminogen activator (pro-urokinase) (98) and promatrix metalloprotease 3 (proMMP-3) (99).

Cellular Targets of Tryptase

The demonstration of defined natural substrates for tryptase has long been a challenge. In recent years, however, it has become apparent that tryptase can have profound actions on a number of human cell types (Table 11-2). Cells at sites of mast cell degranulation are likely to be exposed to high concentrations of tryptase, and the ability to modulate cell function may well prove the key to understanding the primary functions of this major mast-cell product.

Human tryptase is a potent mitogen for fibroblasts, as well as a chemoattractant, and can stimulate the synthesis of collagen type I and the release of collagenase from these cells (100–102). Such findings, coupled with the observation that tryptase can induce airway smooth muscle mitogenesis (103),

Table 11-2. Actions of Tryptase on Human Cells and Tissues in Vitro

Target	Action of Tryptase
Fibroblast	Proliferation Collagen synthesis and release Secretion of collagenase Chemotaxis
Epithelial cell	Proliferation Synthesis and secretion of IL-6, IL-8, and GM-CSF Up-regulation of ICAM-1
Airway smooth-muscle cells	Proliferation
Endothelial cells	Proliferation (for microvascular cells but not for human umbilical vein endothelial cells) Induction of mRNA for IL-1β and IL-8 Secretion of IL-8
Mast cell	Histamine release
Eosinophil	Chemotaxis Secretion of eosinophil cationic protein (ECP)
Neutrophil	Chemotaxis
Airway tissue	Induction of smooth-muscle hyperresponsiveness

Table 11-3. Actions of Human Tryptase in Vivo

Site	Action of Tryptase
Guinea pig skin	Microvascular leakage Accumulation of neutrophils and eosinophils
Mouse peritoneum	Accumulation of neutrophils, eosinophils, macrophages and lymphocytes
Sheep skin	Microvascular leakage
Sheep airways	Bronchoconstriction

underscores the potential for tryptase to contribute to tissue remodeling.

Proinflammatory actions have been demonstrated with several cell types when tryptase has been added. As well as inducing the proliferation of airway epithelial cells, tryptase can stimulate the synthesis and release of interleukins (IL) 6 and 8 and granulocyte macrophage colony-stimulating factor (GM-CSF) and can up-regulate expression of intercellular adhesion molecule 1 (ICAM-1) (104,105). Endothelial cells can be stimulated by tryptase to secrete IL-8 and up-regulate expression of mRNA for IL-8 and IL-1β (106). Perhaps related to this action, incubation of endothelial cells with tryptase releases a factor that can promote neutrophil transendothelial cell migration (107). Human eosinophil and neutrophil chemotaxis is stimulated directly by tryptase, and eosinophils may be induced to secrete eosinophil cationic protein (108). Tryptase can also stimulate the degranulation of both guinea pig (109) and certain populations of human mast cells in vitro (110), and this action may represent an amplification mechanism in allergic disease. In keeping with this finding, inhibitors of tryptase have proved potent as mast cell–stabilizing agents (110).

The precise mechanisms by which tryptase can alter cell function remain to be determined. The cloning and characterization of a receptor for thrombin (111), now termed protease-activated receptor 1 (PAR-1), has opened the way for the identification of a series of related receptors. These receptors possess seven transmembrane loops, and activation involves the binding of a "tethered ligand" on the receptor, which is exposed by proteolysis. PAR-2, PAR-3, and PAR-4 have now been cloned (112), and it seems likely that further members of this family will be identified. Tryptase has been reported to activate PAR-1 when it is expressed on COS-1 cells, but not when expressed on human endothelial cells (113). The activation of PAR-2 by tryptase could be of greater significance, though tryptase is less effective in this reaction than trypsin (113,114). PAR-3 and PAR-4 can be activated by both thrombin and trypsin (112), and it remains to be determined if these receptors could represent another means by which tryptase can interact with cells.

Actions of Tryptase on Tissues

Ethical considerations have prevented direct investigation of the actions of tryptase in vivo in humans. However, several studies involving the transfer of human tryptase into animal models have provided striking evidence that tryptase may be an important mediator of inflammation (Table 11-3). Some of the findings have been consistent with what would be predicted on the basis of studies in vitro with human cells.

The injection of tryptase into the skin of guinea pigs provokes a prolonged increase in microvascular permeability at the injection sites (109). Tryptase-induced microvascular leakage was abolished by pretreating guinea pigs with histamine antagonists, suggesting that the effect may be mediated by tryptase-induced mast-cell degranulation. Similarly, cutaneous reactions induced in sheep (115) and bronchoconstriction induced by administration of aerosolized tryptase into sheep airways (116) are both blocked by treatment with antihistamine. Human tryptase fails by itself to induce contraction in isolated human bronchial tissue, but it potentiates contractile responses to histamine in vitro, an alteration associated with a change in mast-cell distribution in these tissues (117).

A neutrophil- and eosinophil-rich inflammatory infiltrate occurs within 6 hours at sites of tryptase injection into guinea pig skin (118). Parallel experiments in which human tryptase was injected into the mouse peritoneum also provoked a massive accumulation of neutrophils and eosinophils, as well as small, but significant increases in numbers of macrophages and lymphocytes in peritoneal washings (118). Co-injection of tryptase with histamine provoked a selective eosinophilia, suggesting that the actions of tryptase are modified by other mediators in vivo.

Therapeutic Potential of Tryptase Inhibitors

The range of potent actions demonstrated for tryptase and the increases in levels that occur in both allergic and "nonallergic" conditions provide a strong case for considering this protease an important mediator of inflammation and fibrosis. A consistent finding with both in vitro and in vivo experimental models has been that the biologic actions of tryptase are dependent on an intact catalytic site and can be inhibited by protease inhibitors. There have been relatively few investigations of the ability of tryptase inhibitors to modulate disease processes, and the primary focus of studies reported to date has been on the modulation of acute airway responses. For the species selected as animal models, the sheep and the guinea pig, little is known of the nature of the tryptases present, or even of the extent to which their activity may be controlled by the protease inhibitors administered. Nevertheless, the data collected from such models and the limited information available from clinical trials have been encouraging (Table 11-4).

The synthetic tryptase inhibitors APC-366 and BABIM have shown remarkable efficacy in a naturally sensitized sheep model of allergic airways disease (119). Their administration into the airways significantly reduced early-phase bronchoconstriction, provided almost complete protection against late-phase responses to allergen, and blocked acquired airway hyperresponsiveness to carbachol. APC-366 also inhibited the increase in microvascular leakage as assessed by albumin concentration in BAL fluid and reduced the extent of eosinophil accumulation. The administration of lactoferrin, a destabilizer of tryptase activity, in the same sheep model had relatively little effect on the early response, but once again abolished both late-phase airway reactivity and airway hyperresponsiveness (45).

The properties of SLPI as an inhibitor of tryptase, in addition to its well-established function as an inhibitor of neutrophil elastase and various other proteases, require further clarification. However, SLPI instilled into the trachea of sensitized guinea pigs before allergen challenge has a protective effect on airway hyperresponsiveness to histamine, and this effect has been attributed to the inhibition of tryptase by SLPI (120). The inhibitory properties of SLPI for a number of proteases are enhanced in the presence of heparin, and coadministration of SLPI and heparin in the allergic sheep model reduced early- and late-phase bronchoconstriction, as well as allergen-induced hyperresponsiveness (121).

Recently, the results have been reported of a phase II clinical trial in which the tryptase inhibitor APC-366 was administered by inhalation to 16 patients with mild-to-moderate asthma in a randomized crossover study (122). As in the sheep model, late-phase bronchoconstriction to allergen was significantly reduced, with the area under the curve for FEV_1 32% less with APC-366 administration than with placebo. There was a trend also for protection against early-phase allergen-induced bronchoconstriction, although this failed to reach significance, and the acquired increase in airway responsiveness to histamine was not affected by APC-366.

The finding that short-term treatment with APC-366 can reduce allergen-induced, late-phase bronchoconstriction in individuals with asthma provides further evidence for a key role for tryptase in mediating late-phase responses in asthma and must encourage further investigation of tryptase inhibitors as a new form of therapy. The efficacy of this first-generation tryptase inhibitor in humans with asthma was rather less impressive than in the sheep model, but it will be important to examine the actions of the more potent inhibitors now available and to study their ability to modulate inflammatory responses, as well as to alter airway physiology. The potential for tryptase to participate in fibrosis and tissue remodeling also calls for investigations of the ability of inhibitors of tryptase to control these processes. Future approaches could involve the administration of new, small

Table 11-4. Pharmacologic Actions of Compounds with the Potential to Inhibit Tryptase Activity on Airway Responses to Allergen

Compound	Model	Protection from Airway Response		
		Early	*Late*	*Hyper-responsiveness*
BABIM	Allergic sheep	+	++	++
APC-366	Allergic sheep	+	++	++
Lactoferrin	Allergic sheep	±	++	++
SLPI + heparin	Allergic sheep	+	+	+
SLPI	Allergic guinea pigs	NR	NR	++
APC-366	Humans with mild/moderate asthma	±	+	−

− No effect.
± Trend (but not significant).
+ Significant protection.
++ Almost complete protection.
NR Not reported.

molecule inhibitors that are highly selective for tryptase or polypeptide protease broad-spectrum inhibitors (produced in recombinant expression systems or in transgenic animals). Developments in these areas could lead soon to the provision of a new class of anti-inflammatory drug that could be effective in the treatment of both acute and chronic disease.

References

1. Bradding P, Walls AF, Church MK. Mast cells and basophils: their role in initiating and maintaining inflammatory responses. In: Holgate ST, ed. Immunology of the respiratory system. London: Academic Press, 1995:53–84.
2. Church MK, Holgate ST, Shute JK, et al. Mast cell-derived mediators. In: Middleton E, Reed CE, Ellis E, et al, eds. Allergy: principles and practice. 5th ed. St Louis: Mosby, 1988:146–167.
3. Glenner GG, Cohen LA. Histochemical demonstration of a species specific trypsin-like enzyme in mast cells. Nature 1960;185:846–847.
4. Lagunoff D, Benditt EP. Proteolytic enzymes of mast cells. Ann NY Acad Sci 1963;103:184.
5. Gomori G. Chloroacetyl esters as histochemical substrates. J Histochem Cytochem 1953;1:469.
6. Benditt EP, Arase M. An enzyme in mast cells with properties like chymotrypsin. J Exp Med 1959;110:451–460.
7. Lagunoff D, Benditt EP. Histochemical examinations of a chymotrypsin-like esterase. Nature 1961;192:1198–1199.
8. Walls AF. The roles of neutral proteases in asthma and rhinitis. In: Busse WW, Holgate ST, eds. Asthma and rhinitis. Boston: Blackwell, 2000:968–998.
9. Schwartz LB, Irani AA, Roller K, et al. Quantitation of histamine, tryptase, and chymase in dispersed human T and TC mast cells. J Immunol 1987;138:2611–2615.
10. Goldstein SM, Kaempfer CE, Kealey JT, Wintroub BU. Human mast cell carboxypeptidase. Purification and characterisation. J Clin Invest 1989;83:1630–1636.
11. Irani AA, Goldstein SM, Wintroub BU, et al. Human mast cell carboxypeptidase. Selective localisation to MC$_{TC}$ cells. J Immunol 1991;147:247–253.
12. Meier HL, Heck LW, Schulman ES, MacGlashan DW. Purified human mast cells and basophils release human elastase and cathepsin G by an IgE-mediated mechanism. Int Arch Allergy Appl Immunol 1985;77:179–183.
13. Schechter NM, Irani AA, Sprows JL, et al. Identification of a cathepsin G-like proteinase in the MC$_{TC}$ type of human mast cell. J Immunol 1990;145:2652–2661.
14. Sillaber C, Baghestanian M, Bevec D, et al. The mast cell as a site of tissue type plasminogen activator (tPA) expression and fibrinolysis. J Immunol 1999;162:1032–1041.
15. Walls AF, Bennett AR, McBride HM, et al. Production and characterisation of monoclonal antibodies specific for human mast cell tryptase. Clin Exp Allergy 1990;20:581–589.
16. Craig SS, De Blois G, Schwartz LB. Mast cells in human keloid, small intestine and lung by an immunoperoxidase technique using a murine antibody against tryptase. Am J Pathol 1986;124:427–435.
17. Irani AA. Tissue and developmental variation of protease expression in human mast cells. In: Caughey GH, ed. Mast cell proteases in immunology and biology. New York: Marcel Dekker, 1995:127–143.
18. Weidner N, Austen KF. Heterogeneity of mast cells at multiple body sites. Florescent determination of avidin binding and immunofluorescent determination of chymase, tryptase and carboxypeptidase content. Pathol Res Pract 1993;189:156–162.
19. Kleinjan A, Godthelp T, Blom HM, Fokkens WJ. Fixation with Carnoy's fluid reduces the number of chymase-positive mast cells: not all chymase-positive mast cells are also positive for tryptase. Allergy 1996;51:614–620.
20. Beil WJ, Schultz M, McEuen AR, et al. Number, fixation properties, dye binding and protease expression of duodenal mast cells: comparisons between healthy subjects and patients with gastritis or Crohn's disease. Histochem J 1997;29:1–15.
21. Castells MC, Irani AA, Schwartz LB. Evaluation of human peripheral blood leukocytes for mast cell tryptase. J Immunol 1987;138:2184–2189.
22. Li L, Li Y, Reddel SW, et al. Identification of basophilic cells that express mast cell granule proteases in the peripheral blood of asthma, allergy and drug reactive patients. J Immunol 1998;161:3079–3086.
23. Tanaka T, McRae BJ, Cho K, et al. Mammalian tissue trypsin-like enzymes. Comparative reactivities of human skin tryptase, human lung tryptase, and bovine trypsin with peptide 4-nitroaniclide and thioester substrates. J Biol Chem 1983;258:13552–13557.
24. Schwartz LB, Lewis RA, Austen KF. Tryptase from human pulmonary mast cells. Purification and characterisation. J Biol Chem 1981;256:11939–11943.
25. Smith TJ, Hougland MW, Johnson DA. Human lung tryptase. Purification and characterisation. J Biol Chem 1984;259:11046–11051.
26. Benyon CR, Enciso JA, Befus AD. Analysis of human skin mast cell proteins by two-dimensional gel electrophoresis. Identification of tryptase as a sialylated glycoprotein. J Immunol 1993;151:2699–2706.
27. Miller JS, Moxley G, Schwartz LB. Cloning and characterisation of a second complementary DNA for human tryptase. J Clin Invest 1990;86:864–870.
28. Miller JS, Westin EH, Schwartz LB. Cloning and characterisation of complementary DNA for human tryptase. J Clin Invest 1989;84:1188–1195.
29. Vanderslice P, Ballinger SM, Tam EK, et al. Human mast cell tryptase: multiple cDNAs and genes reveal a multigene serine protease family. Proc Nat Acad Sci USA 1990;87:3811–3815.
30. Sakai K, Ren S, Schwartz LB. A novel heparin-dependent processing pathway for human tryptase: autocatalysis followed by activation by dipeptidyl peptidase I. J Clin Invest 1996;97:988–995.
31. Schwartz LB, Sakai K, Bradford TR, et al. The α form of human tryptase is the predominant form present in blood at baseline in normal subjects and is elevated in those with systemic mastocytosis. J Clin Invest 1995;96:2702–2710.
32. Mirza H, Schmidt VA, Derian CK, et al. Mitogenic responses mediated through the protease-activated receptor-2 are induced by expressed forms of mast cell α- or β-tryptases. Blood 1997;90:3914–3922.
33. Huang C, Li L, Krilis SA, et al. Human tryptases α and β/II are functionally distinct due, in part, to a single amino acid

difference in one of the surface loops that forms the substrate-binding cleft. J Biol Chem 1999;274:19670–19676.

34. Pereira PJ, Bergner A, Macedo Ribeiro S, et al. Human β-tryptase is a ring-like tetramer with active sites facing a central pore. Nature 1998;392:306–311.

35. Alter SC, Kramps JA, Janoff A, Schwartz LB. Interactions of human mast cell tryptase with biological protease inhibitors. Arch Biochem Biophys 1990;276:26–31.

36. Hochstrasser K, Gebhard W, Albrecht G, et al. Interaction of human mast cell tryptase and chymase with low-molecular-mass serine proteinase inhibitors from the human respiratory tract. Eur Arch Otorhinolaryngol 1993;249:455–458.

37. Sommerhoff CP, Söllner C, Mentele R, et al. A Kazal-type inhibitor of human mast cell tryptase: isolation from the medicinal leech Hirudo medicinalis, characterisation and sequence analysis. Biol Chem Hoppe-Seyler 1994;375:685–694.

38. Kido H, Katunuma N. Control of tryptase and chymase activity by protease inhibitors. In: Caughey GH, ed. The biology of mast cell proteases. New York: Marcel Dekker, 1995:145–167.

39. Robinson T, Delavia K, Harris P, et al. Secretory leukoprotease inhibitor of mast cell tryptase. Am J Respir Crit Care Med 1996:A399.

40. Alter SC, Metcalfe DD, Bradford TR, Schwartz LB. Stabilisation of human mast cell tryptase: effects of enzyme concentration, ionic strength and the structure and negative charge density of polysaccharides. Biochem J 1987;248:821–827.

41. Schwartz LB, Bradford TR. Regulation of tryptase from human lung mast cells by heparin. Stabilisation of the active tetramer. J Biol Chem 1986;261:7372–7379.

42. Schwartz LB, Bradford TR, Lee DC, Chlebowski JF. Immunologic and physicochemical evidence for conformation changes occurring on conversion of human mast cell tryptase from active tetramer to inactive monomer. Production of monoclonal antibodies recognising active tryptase. J Immunol 1990;144:2304–2311.

43. Schechter NM, Eng GY, McCaslin DR. Human skin tryptase: kinetic characterisation of its spontaneous inactivation. Biochemistry 1993;32:2617–2625.

44. Alter SC, Schwartz LB. Effect of histamine and divalent cations on the activity and stability of tryptase from human mast cells. Biochem Biophys Acta 1989;991:426–430.

45. Elrod KC, Moore WR, Abraham WM, Tanaka RD. Lactoferrin, a potent tryptase inhibitor, abolishes late phase airway responses in allergic sheep. Am J Respir Crit Care Med 1997;156:375–381.

46. Cregan L, Elrod KC, Putnam D, Moore WR. Neutrophil myeloperoxidase is a potent and selective inhibitor of mast cell tryptase. Arch Biochem Biophys 1999;366:125–130.

47. Chiu H, Lagunoff D. Histochemical comparison of vertebrate mast cells. Histochem J 1972;4:135–140.

48. Nawa Y, Horii Y, Okada M, Arizono N. Histochemical and cytological characterisations of mucosal and connective tissue mast cells of Mongolian gerbils (meriones unguiculatus). Int Arch Allergy Immunol 1994;104:249–254.

49. Welle MM, Proske SM, Harvima IT, Schechter NM. Demonstration of tryptase in bovine cutaneous and tumor mast cells. J Histochem Cytochem 1995;43:1139–1144.

50. Vanderslice P, Craik CS, Nadel JA, Caughey GH. Molecular cloning of a dog mast cell tryptase and a related protease. Structural evidence of a unique mode of serine protease activation. Biochemistry 1989;28:41–48.

51. Glenner GG, Cohen LA. Histochemical demonstration of a species-specific trypsin-like enzyme in mast cells. Nature 1960;185:846–847.

52. McEuen AR, He S, Brander ML, Walls AF. Guinea pig lung tryptase. Localisation to mast cells and characterisation of the partially purified enzyme. Biochem Pharmacol 1996;52:331–340.

53. Valchanov KP, Proctor GB. Enzyme histochemistry of tryptase in the stomach mucosal mast cells of the mouse. J Histochem Cytochem 1999;47:617–622.

54. Chan Z, Irani AA, Bradford TR, et al. Localisation of rat tryptase to a subset of the connective tissue type of mast cell. J Histochem Cytochem 1993;41:961.

55. Friend DS, Ghildyal N, Gurish MF, et al. Reversible expression of tryptases and chymases in the jejunal mast cells of mice infected with Trichinella spiralis. J Immunol 1998;160:5537–5545.

56. Katunuma N, Kido H. Recent advances in research on tryptases and endogenous tryptase inhibitors. In: Schwartz LB, ed. Neutral proteases of mast cells. Monogr Allergy. Basel: Karger, 1990;27:51–66.

57. Lagunoff D, Rickard A, Marquart C. Rat mast cell tryptase. Arch Biochem Biophys 1991;291:52–58.

58. Braganza VJ, Simmons WH. Tryptase from rat skin: purification and properties. Biochemistry 1991;30:4997–5007.

59. Fiorucci L, Erba F, Ascoli F. Bovine tryptase: purification and characterisation. Biol Chem Hoppe-Seyler 1992;373:483–490.

60. Pemberton AD, McAleese SM, Huntley JF, et al. cDNA sequence of two sheep mast cell tryptases and the differential expression of tryptase and sheep mast cell proteinase-1 in lung, dermis and gastrointestinal tract. Clin Exp Allergy 2000;30:818–832.

61. Robinson TL, Muller DK. Purification and characterisation of cynomolgus monkey tryptase. Comp Biochem Physiol 1997;118B:783–792.

62. Lutzelschwab C, Pejler G, Aveskogh M, Hellman L. Secretory granule proteases in rat mast cells. Cloning of 10 different serine proteases and a carboxypeptidase A from various rat mast cell populations. J Exp Med 1997;185:13–29.

63. Reynolds DS, Gurley DS, Austen KF, Serafin WE. Cloning of the cDNA and gene of mouse mast cell protease-6. Transcription by progenitor mast cells and mast cells of the connective tissue subclass. J Biol Chem 1991;266:3845–3853.

64. McNeil HP, Reynolds DS, Schiller V. Isolation, characterisation, and transcription of the gene encoding mouse mast cell protease 7. Proc Nat Acad Sci USA 1992;89:11174–11178.

65. Walls AF, Djukanovic R, Walters C, et al. Mast cell, eosinophil and neutrophil activation in the lungs of asthmatic patients. Am J Respir Crit Care Med 1995;151:A38.

66. Broide DH, Gleich GJ, Cuomo AJ, et al. Evidence of ongoing mast cell and eosinophil degranulation in symptomatic asthma airway. J Allergy Clin Immunol 1991;88:637–648.

67. Jarjour NN, Calhoun WJ, Schwartz LB, Busse WW. Elevated bronchoalveolar lavage fluid histamine levels in allergic

asthmatics are associated with increased airway obstruction. Am Rev Respir Dis 1991;144:83–87.

68. Ferguson AC, Whitelaw M, Brown H. Correlation of bronchial eosinophil and mast cell activation with bronchial hyperresponsiveness in children with asthma. J Allergy Clin Immunol 1992;90:601–613.

69. Wenzel SE, Fowler AA, Schwartz LB. Activation of pulmonary mast cells by bronchoalveolar allergen challenge. In vivo release of histamine and tryptase in atopic subjects with and without asthma. Am Rev Respir Dis 1988;137:1002–1008.

70. Salmonsson P, Gronneberg R, Gilljam H, et al. Bronchial exudation of bulk plasma at allergen challenge in allergic asthma. Am Rev Respir Dis 1992;146:1535–1542.

71. Frew AJ, St Pierre J, Teran LM, et al. Cellular and mediator responses twenty four hours after local endobronchial allergen challenge of asthmatic airways. J Allergy Clin Immunol 1996;98:133–143.

72. Broide DH, Eisman S, Ramsdell JW, et al. Airway levels of mast cell-derived mediators in exercise-induced asthma. Am Rev Respir Dis 1990;141:563–568.

73. Jarjour NN, Calhoun WJ, Stevens CA, Salisbury SM. Exercise induced asthma is not associated with mast cell activation or airway inflammation. J Allergy Clin Immunol 1992;89:60–68.

74. Makker HK, Walls AF, Goulding D, et al. Local airway challenge with hypertonic saline in asthma: Effect on airway size, mast cell mediator release and epithelial structure. Am Rev Respir Crit Care Med 1994;149:1012–1019.

75. Djukanović R, Wilson JW, Britten KM, et al. Effect of an inhaled corticosteroid on airway inflammation and symptoms in asthma. Am Rev Respir Dis 1992;145:669–674.

76. Roberts JA, Bradding P, Britten KM, et al. The effect of long-acting inhaled β_2 agonist salmeterol xinafoate on indices of airway inflammation in asthma. Eur Respir J 1999;14:275–282.

77. Castells M, Schwartz LB. Tryptase levels in nasal-lavage fluid as an indicator of the immediate allergic response. J Allergy Clin Immunol 1988;82:348–355.

78. Juliusson S, Holmberg K, Baumgarten CR, et al. Tryptase in nasal lavage fluid after local allergen challenge. Relationship to histamine levels and TAME-esterase activity. Allergy 1991;46:459–465.

79. Proud D, Bailey GS, Naclerio RM, et al. Tryptase and histamine as markers to evaluate mast cell activation during the responses to nasal challenge with allergen, cold, dry air, and hyperosmolar solutions. J Allergy Clin Immunol 1992;89:1098–1110.

80. Shalit M, Schwartz LB, Golzar N, et al. Release of tryptase in vivo after prolonged cutaneous challenge with allergen in humans. J Immunol 1988;141:821–826.

81. Befus SI, Ochsner KI, Abelson MB, Schwartz LB. The level of tryptase in human tears. An indicator of activation of human mast cells. Ophthalmology 1990;97:1678–1683.

82. Schwartz LB, Metcalfe DD, Miller JS, et al. Tryptase levels as an indicator of mast cell activation in systemic anaphylaxis and mastocytosis. N Engl J Med 1987;316:1622–1626.

83. Walls AF, Bennett AR, Godfrey RC, et al. Mast cell tryptase and histamine concentrations in bronchoalveolar lavage fluid from patients with interstitial lung disease. Clin Sci 1991;81:183–188.

84. Kalenderian R, Raju L, Roth W, et al. Elevated histamine and tryptase levels in smokers' bronchoalveolar lavage fluid. Do lung mast cells contribute to smokers' emphysema? Chest 1988;94:119–123.

85. Buckley MG, Walters C, Wong WM, et al. Mast cell activation in arthritis: detection of α and β tryptase, histamine and eosinophil cationic protein in synovial fluid. Clin Sci 1997;93:363–370.

86. Boucher W, El-Mansoury M, Pang X, et al. Elevated mast cell tryptase in the urine of patients with interstitial cystitis. Br J Urol 1995;76:94–100.

87. Tam EK, Caughey GH. Degradation of airway neuropeptides by human lung tryptase. Am Rev Respir Cell Mol Biol 1990;3:27–32.

88. Walls AF, Brain SD, Jose PJ, et al. Human mast cell tryptase attenuates the vasodilator activity of calcitonin gene-related peptide (CGRP). Biochem Pharmacol 1992;43:1243–1248.

89. Proud D, Siekierski ES, Bailey GS. Identification of human lung mast cell kininogenase as tryptase and relevance of tryptase kininogenase activity. Biochem Pharmacol 1988;37:1473–1480.

90. Walls AF, Bennett AR, Suieras-Diaz J, Olsson H. The kininogenase activity of human mast cell tryptase. Biochem Soc Trans 1992;20:260S.

91. Imamura T, Dubin A, Moore W, et al. Induction of vascular permeability enhancement by human tryptase: dependence on activation of prekallikrein and direct release of bradykinin from kininogens. Lab Invest 1996;74:861–870.

92. Kozik A, Moore RB, Potempa J, et al. A novel mechanism for bradykinin production at inflammatory sites. Diverse effects of a mixture of neutrophil elastase and mast cell tryptase versus tissue and plasma kallikreins on native and oxidised kininogens. J Biol Chem 1998;273:33224–33229.

93. Schwartz LB, Bradford TR, Littman BH, Wintroub BU. The fibrinogenolytic activity of purified tryptase from human lung mast cells. J Immunol 1985;135:2762–2767.

94. Ren S, Lawson AE, Carr M, et al. Human tryptase fibrinogenolysis is optimal at acid pH and generates anticoagulant fragments in the presence of the anti-tryptase monoclonal antibody. J Immunol 1997;159:3540–3548.

95. Thomas VA, Wheeless CJ, Stack MS, Johnson DA. Human mast cell tryptase fibrinogenolysis: Kinetics, anticoagulation mechanism and cell adhesion disruption. Biochemistry 1998;37:2291–2298.

96. Lohi J, Harvima I, Keski-Oja J. Pericellular substrates of human mast cell tryptase: 72,000 Dalton gelatinase and fibronectin. J Cell Biochem 1992;50:337–349.

97. Kielty CM, Lees M, Shuttleworth CA, Woolley D. Catabolism of intact type VI collagen microfibrils: susceptibility to degradation by serine proteases. Biochem Biophys Res Commun 1993;191:1230–1236.

98. Stack MS, Johnson DA. Human mast cell tryptase activates single-chain urinary-type plasminogen activator (pro-urokinase). J Biol Chem 1994;269:9416–9419.

99. Gruber BL, Marchese MJ, Suziki K, et al. Synovial procollagenase activation by human mast cell tryptase. Dependence upon matrix metalloproteinase 3 activation. J Clin Invest 1989;84:1657–1662.

100. Hartmann T, Ruoss SJ, Raymond WW, et al. Human tryptase as a potent, cell-specific mitogen: role of signalling pathways

in synergistic responses. Am J Physiol 1992;262(Lung Cell Mol Physiol 6):L528–L534.

101. Cairns JA, Walls AF. Mast cell tryptase stimulates the synthesis of type I collagen in human lung fibroblasts. J Clin Invest 1997;99:1313–1321.

102. Gruber BL, Kew RR, Jelaska A, et al. Human mast cells activate fibroblasts. J Immunol 1997;158:2310–2317.

103. Thabrew H, Cairns JA, Walls AF. Mast cell tryptase is a growth factor for human airway smooth muscle. J Allergy Clin Immunol 1996;97:969.

104. Cairns JA, Walls AF. Mast cell tryptase is a mitogen for epithelial cells. Stimulation of IL-8 production and intercellular adhesion molecule-1 expression. J Immunol 1996;156:275–283.

105. Perng D-W, Leir S-H, Compton SJ, et al. Mast cell tryptase stimulates cytokine synthesis and secretion from bronchial epithelial cells: a role for protease activated receptor 2 (PAR-2). Am J Respir Crit Care Med 1999;159:A336.

106. Compton SJ, Cairns JA, Holgate ST, Walls AF. The role of mast cell tryptase in regulating endothelial cell proliferation, cytokine release and adhesion molecule expression: tryptase induces expression of mRNA for IL-1β and IL-8 and stimulates the selective release of IL-8 from human umbilical vein endothelial cells. J Immunol 1998;161:1939–1946.

107. Compton SJ, Cairns JA, Holgate ST, Walls AF. Interaction of human mast cell tryptase with endothelial cells to stimulate inflammatory cell recruitment. Int Arch Allergy Immunol 1999;200–205.

108. Walls AF, He S, Teran L, et al. Granulocyte recruitment by human mast cell tryptase. Int Arch Allergy Immunol 1995;107:372–373.

109. He S, Walls AF. Human mast cell tryptase: A stimulus of microvascular leakage and mast cell activation. Eur J Pharmacol 1997;328:89–97.

110. He S, Gaça MDA, Walls AF. A role for tryptase in the activation of human mast cells: modulation of histamine release by tryptase and inhibitors of tryptase. J Pharmacol Exp Ther 1998;286:289–297.

111. Vu T-K, Hung DT, Wheaton VI, Coughlin SR. Molecular cloning of a functional thrombin receptor reveals a novel proteolytic mechanism of receptor activation. Cell 1991;64:1057–1068.

112. Déry O, Bunnett NW. Proteinase activated receptors: a growing family of heptahelical receptors for thrombin, trypsin and tryptase. Biochem Soc Trans 1999;27:246–254.

113. Molino M, Barnathan ES, Numerof R, et al. Interactions of mast cell tryptase with thrombin receptors and PAR-2. J Biol Chem 1997;272:4043–4049.

114. Mirza H, Schmidt VA, Derian CK, et al. Mitogenic responses mediated through the proteinase activated receptor –2 are induced by expressed forms of mast cell α- or β-tryptases. Blood 1997;90:3914–3922.

115. Molinari JF, Moore WR, Clark J, et al. Role of tryptase in immediate cutaneous responses in allergic sheep. J Appl Physiol 1995;79:1966–1973.

116. Molinari JF, Scuri M, Moore WR, et al. Inhaled tryptase causes bronchoconstriction in sheep via histamine release. Am J Respir Crit Care Med 1996;154:649–653.

117. Berger P, Compton SJ, Molimard M, et al. Mast cell tryptase as a mediator of hyperresponsiveness in human isolated bronchi. Clin Exp Allergy 1999;29:804–812.

118. He S, Peng Q, Walls AF. Potent induction of a neutrophil and eosinophil-rich infiltrate *in vivo* by human mast cell tryptase: selective enhancement of eosinophil recruitment by histamine. J Immunol 1997;159:6216–6225.

119. Clark JM, Abraham WM, Fishman CE, et al. Tryptase inhibitors block allergen induced airway and inflammatory responses in allergic sheep. Am J Respir Crit Care Med 1995;152:2076–2083.

120. Havill AM, Middleton S, Lyons D, Wright C. Secretory leukocyte protease inhibitor (SLPI) prevents the development of airway hyperresponsiveness (AWHR) in allergen challenged guinea pigs. Am J Respir Crit Care Med 1997;155:A654.

121. Fath MA, Wu X, Hilemam RE, et al. Interaction of secretory leukoprotease inhibitor with heparin inhibits proteases involved in asthma. J Biol Chem 1998;273:13563–13569.

122. Krishna TK, Chauham AJ, Little L, et al. Effect of inhaled APC-366 on allergen-induced bronchoconstriction and airway hyperresponsiveness to histamine in atopic asthmatics. Am J Respir Crit Care Med 1998;157:A456.

Chapter 12

5-Aminosalicylic Acid (Mesalamine) and Sulfasalazine

Richard P. MacDermott

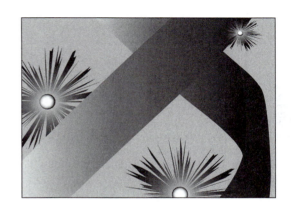

5-aminosalicylic acid (5-ASA) is an anti-inflammatory agent with proven efficacy in the treatment of inflammatory bowel disease (IBD). Because 5-ASA can inhibit many pathways of intestinal inflammation, it is particularly useful in the treatment of patients with IBD. Although the precise mechanism of action responsible for the clinical efficacy of 5-ASA is not known, a wide range of anti-inflammatory and immunosuppressive properties of 5-ASA have been identified in vitro. Recently, 5-ASA has been demonstrated to inhibit tumor necrosis factor-α (TNF-α)–stimulated nuclear factor-κB (NF-κB) activation, NF-κB nuclear translocation, and inhibitory κBα (IκBα) degradation, which may provide a common mechanism that could explain many of the actions of 5-ASA. The purpose of this chapter is to review the clinical use of 5-ASA, the current understanding of the pathways of inflammation involved in IBD, and the pathways of inflammation that are inhibited by 5-ASA.

Sulfasalazine

5-ASA was combined with sulfapyridine by Svartz and Willstedt to form salicylazosulfapyridine in the 1930s as a treatment for rheumatoid arthritis and ulcerative colitis (1,2). Salicylazosulfapyridine was designed to attain high concentrations of 5-ASA (as an anti-inflammatory) and sulfapyradine (as an antibiotic) in inflamed joint synovial tissue and intestinal mucosa. Since its introduction, salicylazosulfapyridine (now termed sulfasalazine and marketed as Azulfidine) has been a mainstay of outpatient medical management for patients with mild to moderately active ulcerative colitis.

Sulfasalazine is minimally absorbed in the jejunum; the majority is excreted intact into bile and delivered back to the intestinal lumen. On reaching the large intestine, sulfasalazine is reduced by the bacterial enzyme azoreductase to 5-ASA and sulfapyridine (3). The 5-ASA moiety is poorly absorbed from the colon and acts topically at the site of mucosal inflammation. Sulfapyridine is rapidly absorbed from the colon, metabolized by the liver, and excreted in the urine, with only small amounts remaining in the stool (4). The sulfapyridine moiety thus serves as a carrier molecule to topically deliver 5-ASA to the mucosal surface of the colon.

Clinical Use in Ulcerative Colitis

Sulfasalazine has been proven to be efficacious in the treatment of active ulcerative colitis (5,6). The effective dose range of 3 to 4 g/day induces a remission in 50% to 80% of patients. Sulfasalazine has also proven to be effective in the maintenance of remission in patients with ulcerative colitis (7–10).

For mild to moderately active ulcerative colitis, proctosigmoiditis, or proctitis, sulfasalazine therapy is initiated with a low dose of 1 g (one 500 mg tablet, two times per day), followed by a gradual increase in dosage over several days to 4 g per day. To maintain optimum levels, two 500-mg tablets given four times per day is preferred. Sulfasalazine often takes 4 to 6 weeks to begin to effectively control colonic inflammation. After 5 to 6 months of therapy, when the ulcerative colitis is in remission, a maintenance dose of 3 to 4 g per day (two 500-mg tablets three to four times per day) is used. Folic acid supplementation is recommended because sulfasalazine can block dietary folic acid absorption.

Side Effects

Commonly observed side effects in patients being treated with sulfasalazine include nausea, headache, and anorexia, all of which usually resolve when the dose is lowered. Heartburn, dyspepsia, and abdominal pain can be reduced with the use of enteric-coated sulfasalazine tablets. Other more serious side effects such as persistent fever, severe rash, worsening of colitis, bone marrow toxicity, hepatitis, pancreatitis, pneumonitis, and pericarditis require discontinuation of the sulfasalazine. Infertility in males, as a result of decreased sperm count and impaired sperm motility, reverses when sulfasalazine is discontinued.

5-Aminosalicylic Acid (5-ASA)

Clinical research studies have revealed that the active moiety in sulfasalazine is 5-ASA. The sulfapyridine carrier molecule is absorbed and is responsible for many, but not all, of the side effects observed with sulfasalazine. Because these side effects of sulfapyridine have limited the use of sulfasalazine in up to 20% of patients, new 5-ASA preparations without sulfapyridine have been developed to permit site-specific targeted delivery of higher doses of 5-ASA. With different formulations (azo bond, delayed release, or continuous release) and the development of enema and suppository formulations, the new 5-ASA (mesalamine) drugs can target specific sites in the intestine for maximal 5-ASA topical delivery.

Because 5-ASA is rapidly absorbed in the jejunum after oral ingestion, delayed release formulations were developed to deliver the drug to diseased small bowel and colonic sites for the treatment of IBD. In these formulations 5-ASA is coated with acrylic resins or encapsulated in ethylcellulose microgranules. The acrylic-base resin (Eudragit) dissolves at a pH greater than 6, whereas the ethylcellulose is a semipermeable membrane allowing the time-dependent release of 5-ASA as it traverses the intestinal tract. Two 5-ASA dimers are olsalazine (Dipentum) and balsalazine (Colazide). Olsalazine is two 5-ASAs joined together by an azo bond, whereas balsalazide is one 5-ASA linked to an inert, unabsorbed carrier molecule. As with sulfasalazine, both drugs require colonic bacteria to cleave the azo bond and release the 5-ASA moiety and therefore are mainly active at colonic sites of disease. 5-ASA has also been formulated in enema and suppository forms.

Clinical Use of Topical 5-ASA in Ulcerative Proctitis and Proctosigmoiditis

Controlled trials have confirmed the efficacy of 4-g 5-ASA enemas in patients with active ulcerative proctitis or proctosigmoiditis (11,12). 5-ASA enemas are also useful for maintaining remission in patients with ulcerative proctitis and ulcerative proctosigmoiditis (13,14). 5-ASA suppositories (500-mg) can be very effective for distal ulcerative proctitis and are also useful for maintenance therapy.

For mild to moderately active ulcerative proctitis, 500-mg 5-ASA suppositories can be given twice daily. Although symptomatic improvement and a decrease in bleeding are apparent within a few days, complete healing usually takes 4 to 6 weeks or longer. For patients with mild to moderately active proctosigmoiditis, in addition to 5-ASA suppositories, 4-g 5-ASA enemas can be given twice daily, continued for 6 to 8 weeks, and then gradually tapered to a maintenance regimen of one each night and then to one every other night. 5-ASA enemas and/or suppositories are the therapy of choice for proctitis and proctosigmoiditis because of their ability to both induce and maintain remission. In the future, 1-g 5-ASA enemas may be able to be used, because the efficacy of 1-g or 2-g enemas is almost equal to that of 4-g 5-ASA enemas.

Clinical Use of Oral 5-ASA in Ulcerative Colitis

Asacol is composed of 5-ASA (mesalamine) coated in a pH-dependent acrylic resin, which dissolves as the pH of the intestinal fluid rises above 6.0. This formulation results in the delayed release of the therapeutic agent, 5-ASA, in the distal ileum and colon. Pentasa contains microgranules of 5-ASA (mesalamine)

coated with ethylcellulose to form delayed-release beads that continuously release 5-ASA throughout the small intestine and colon.

Controlled trials have convincingly demonstrated the efficacy of oral forms of 5-ASA (mesalamine) in the treatment of mild to moderately active ulcerative colitis (15–17). Asacol and Pentasa also have proven to be of benefit in maintaining remission in ulcerative colitis. Neither Asacol nor Pentasa is significantly more effective for ulcerative colitis than sulfasalazine; their major advantage is their much lower side-effect profile.

For patients with mild to moderately active ulcerative colitis, the oral mesalamine agents need to be used in high doses to achieve maximal effect. The effective daily dose ranges usually are 3.6 to 4.8 g for Asacol (400 mg) and 3 to 4 g for Pentasa (250 mg) given in three to four divided doses per day. Once a successful therapeutic effect has been achieved, usually in 6 to 8 weeks, the dosage used to achieve remission should be continued in the optimal range to maintain remission. Tapering the 5-ASA dose below 3 to 3.6 g per day may lead to earlier relapse. In patients with severe left-sided ulcerative colitis, severe proctosigmoiditis, or severe proctitis, optimal doses of oral mesalamine used in combination with 5-ASA enemas and/or suppositories are usually needed to provide maximal, topical 5-ASA delivery throughout the colon.

Clinical Use of Oral 5-ASA in Crohn's Disease

Trials of oral 5-ASA agents support their use for both active and quiescent Crohn's disease. Mesalamine has moderate efficacy in the treatment of active Crohn's disease (18). The oral 5-ASA preparations are more effective in small bowel (ileal) Crohn's disease than large bowel Crohn's disease. Clinical efficacy with mesalamine for maintenance of medically induced remission for Crohn's disease has been modest at best (19). Oral 5-ASA agents are not as clearly effective in Crohn's disease as they are in ulcerative colitis, perhaps because oral mesalamine provides 5-ASA topically within the lumen for direct delivery to the mucosa. Crohn's disease is a full-thickness, inflammatory process, whereas ulcerative colitis is characterized by mucosal inflammation; and therefore the topical 5-ASA in the lumen is able to act directly at the site of inflammation in ulcerative colitis but not in Crohn's disease.

The future development of better delivery systems, which will allow penetration of 5-ASA through the full thickness of the inflamed bowel, may improve the ability of 5-ASA to be used in Crohn's disease. A novel approach to optimizing intestinal delivery of 5-ASA to inflamed intestinal tissue has employed anionic liposomes packaged with 5-ASA (20). 5-ASA packaged in liposomes delivers less drug systemically and leads to higher tissue levels of drug. In animal models of colitis, 5-ASA packaged in liposomes increased the tissue levels of 5-ASA, suggesting that liposomes were able to preferentially target 5-ASA to the mucosa and lead to the accumulation of 5-ASA in inflamed intestinal tissue (20).

Oral mesalamine agents delay both endoscopic and clinical recurrences of Crohn's disease after resection and anastomosis (21). The use of oral 5-ASA products to prevent the recurrence of Crohn's disease after surgical resection has been evaluated with both endoscopic and clinical end points. Mucosal aphthous ulcerations, consistent with early Crohn's disease, can be observed by colonoscopy in up to 90% of patients 1 year after surgical resection. Studies with oral 5-ASA products have convincingly demonstrated reduction in the endoscopic recurrence rate of Crohn's disease after surgery (22). More importantly, oral 5-ASA products have also decreased the clinical (symptomatic) recurrence rate, with the highest rate of prevention of clinical recurrence being in patients with either large bowel or small bowel plus large bowel Crohn's disease; less effect was seen in patients with disease of the small bowel only (23). Oral 5-ASA agents that are topically delivered to the mucosa appear to intervene more effectively in the early steps of the recurrence of Crohn's disease after surgical resection, in contrast to the modest results in the induction and maintenance of medically induced remission in patients with established Crohn's disease.

Side Effects of 5-ASA Agents

Although the newer 5-ASA formulations have a much lower rate of side effects than the 12% to 20% rate seen with sulfasalazine, side effects and adverse reactions occur with all 5-ASA preparations. Adverse 5-ASA–induced reactions include a colonic hypersensitivity reaction (severe colitis), anal irritation with the 5-ASA enemas (perhaps related to the sulfite carrier), rash and fever (serum sickness), hair loss, diarrhea, pancreatitis, hepatitis, pneumonitis, pericarditis, anemia, leukopenia, thrombocytopenia, and nephritis (24–29). Unlike sulfasalazine, the 5-ASA agents do not cause male infertility.

Mechanisms of Action of 5-ASA in IBD

The roles of intestinal bacteria, the mucosal immune system, and inflammatory mediators in initiating IBD have become better clarified in recent years (30,31). Stimulatory molecules in the gut lumen include bacterial cell-wall products such as peptidoglycanpolysaccharide (PGPS) and lipopolysaccharide (LPS), which highly activate macrophages to synthesize and secrete proinflammatory cytokines, including tumor necrosis factor-α (TNF-α), interleukin (IL)-1, and IL-6. TNF-α and IL-1 activate epithelial cells, endothelial cells, macrophages, and fibroblasts to secrete potent chemotactic cytokines (chemokines) such as IL-8, monocyte chemoattractant protein-1 (MCP-1), and epithelial cell–derived neutrophil activator-78 (ENA-78). TNF-α and IL-1 also increase adhesion-molecule expression on circulating leukocytes and endothelial cells. Together, increased chemokine production and adhesion-molecule expression promote the movement of macrophages and granulocytes from the circulation into the inflamed mucosa of IBD. TNF-α, IL-1, IL-6, IL-8, MCP-1, and ENA-78 also activate epithelial cells, endothelial cells, and macrophages to produce reactive oxygen species (ROS), nitric

oxide, leukotrienes, and proteases, all of which mediate intestinal inflammation and injury. Activated Th-1 cells also participate in the up-regulation of inflammation in IBD. Th-1 cells are driven by IL-12 to produce proinflammatory cytokines, which leads to the further amplification and perpetuation of intestinal mucosal inflammation. The ability of 5-ASA to block many of the immune cellular responses and inflammatory pathways involved in the immunopathogenesis of IBD has been examined extensively and will be reviewed below.

T Cells

In both animal models of intestinal inflammation and in patients with IBD, bacterial product–initiated, IL-12–driven CD4+ T helper cell secretion of interferon-γ (IFN-γ), IL-1, and TNF-α is a central regulatory pathway. Sulfasalazine and 5-ASA inhibit T-cell proliferation by preventing DNA synthesis and entry into the S phase of the cell cycle. 5-ASA prevents the accumulation of steady-state transcript levels of IL-2 (32). Sulfasalazine and 5-ASA also inhibit the expression of major histocompatibility complex (MHC) class II molecules, which present processed antigen to CD4+ cells. MHC molecules are activated and up-regulated on intestinal epithelial cells in inflamed IBD tissue specimens (33,34). Sulfasalazine and 5-ASA interfere with MHC class II expression on intestinal epithelial cells and may thereby prevent intraepithelial T-cell recognition of antigens that could be presented by intestinal epithelial cells (35,36). Sulfasalazine and 5-ASA also inhibit T-cell and natural killer–cell cytotoxic effector cells (37–40).

B Cells

In patients with IBD, intestinal B cells secrete increased amounts of immunoglobulin (Ig) G1 (41). Heightened IgG1 serum levels reflect the increased proportion of IgG1-containing cells in the inflamed intestinal mucosa (42). IgG1 and IgG3 antibodies are potent complement pathway activators and opsonins. The heightened IgG1 secretion in Crohn's disease and the increased secretion of both IgG1 and IgG3 in ulcerative colitis may enhance complement activation and tissue injury (41,42). 5-Aminosalicylate inhibits antibody production by stimulated, peripheral-blood B cells in a dose-dependent manner (43). Therefore, 5-ASA inhibition of IgG1 synthesis and secretion may lead to inhibition of IgG1-induced phagocytosis and cytotoxicity.

Proinflammatory Cytokines

During chronic intestinal inflammation large amounts of the proinflammatory cytokines TNF-α, IL-1, and IL-6 are synthesized and secreted by highly activated mucosal lymphocytes and macrophages (44–46). Many of the systemic manifestations of active IBD are caused by the release of large amounts of these cytokines into the circulation from the inflamed intestine. TNF-α can lead to cachexia, fever, fatigue, myalgias, and hypercoagulability; it also can induce thrombosis by reducing the amount of thrombomodulin and increasing levels of procoagulant tissue factor. IL-1 leads to fever, malaise, and anorexia. IL-6 can contribute to hypercoagulability by increasing circulating platelets. All three cytokines induce leukocytosis and can cause decreased iron levels.

The biologic effects of TNF-α, IL-1, and IL-6 result in the amplification of immunologic and inflammatory processes. For example, TNF-α activates endothelial cells and can induce synthesis and secretion of IL-1 and IL-6. IL-1 stimulates acute-phase protein synthesis and initiates T-cell activation events. Proinflammatory cytokines and chemokines increase the expression of endothelial-cell adhesion molecules, which in turn enhances the influx of monocytes, granulocytes, and lymphocytes into areas of chronic inflammation. Proinflammatory cytokines are therefore of central importance in the initiation and perpetuation of intestinal inflammation in ulcerative colitis and Crohn's disease.

Sulfasalazine and 5-ASA both block the production of IL-1 by stimulated, peripheral-blood mononuclear cells (47) and mononuclear cells from inflamed intestinal tissues (48). 5-ASA inhibits IL-1β secretion from colonic biopsy specimens in a dose-dependent manner (49). TNF-α secretion was also inhibited by sulfasalazine (47). Sulfasalazine inhibits TNF-α binding with its receptor, thereby preventing signaling of subsequent inflammatory responses (50). 5-ASA does not appear to have a major effect on IL-6 production. Furthermore, IL-6 measurements in patients with IBD have not correlated with sulfasalazine or 5-ASA treatment. 5-ASA was capable of partially protecting a human, colonic, goblet-cell line against cellular injury caused by IFN-γ and TNF-α, as measured by morphometric and kinetic studies (51).

Granulocytes and Macrophages: Chemokines, Adhesion Molecules, and Chemotaxis

Chemokines are highly potent chemoattractants for and activators of monocytes, macrophages, neutrophils, lymphocytes, eosinophils, basophils, and mast cells. After their activation by proinflammatory cytokines or invasive infectious pathogens, many cells in the intestine, including lymphocytes, granulocytes, macrophages, epithelial cells, endothelial cells, smooth-muscle cells, and fibroblasts, rapidly synthesize and secrete chemokines. Thus, the gastrointestinal tract is a rich source of cell types capable of producing chemokines after stimulation and activation by TNF-α, IL-1, and IL-6 or infectious pathogens (52). Chemokines such as IL-8, MCP-1, and ENA-78 are involved in recruiting, stimulating, and activating subsets of leukocytes, which then mediate destructive and inflammatory processes in the intestine (52).

Adhesion molecules on endothelial cells play important roles in the perpetuation of mucosal inflammatory processes, as well as in the extraintestinal manifestations of IBD. In the intestine of patients with active IBD, neutrophils, lymphocytes, and monocytes continuously migrate from the circulation into the inflamed mucosa and then into the intestinal lumen. Proinflammatory cytokine and chemokine activation of endothelial cells and circulating leukocytes leads to the coordination of leukocyte attachment, rolling, and adhesion events followed by migration of macrophages, granulocytes, and lymphocytes between endothelial cells and then into the intestinal mucosa.

The sequence of events that explains reactive arthritis in IBD also involves adhesion molecules: antigens introduced by way of the gut are processed by intestinal macrophages, which migrate to the synovial microcirculation utilizing P-selectin. P-selectin is then up-regulated on endothelial cells by circulating cytokines from sites of intestinal inflammation. Increased macrophage-mediated inflammatory processes lead to enhanced synovial endothelial activation. Mucosal lymphoblasts, which have been sensitized by the same intestinal antigens, are then capable of migrating to and binding to synovial cells with vascular adhesion protein-1 (VAP-1). Macrophages and lymphoblasts, which then migrate into the synovium, produce large amounts of proinflammatory cytokines, chemotactic molecules, and destructive molecules, which lead to chronic reactive arthritis in patients with IBD (53). The ability of 5-ASA to inhibit adhesion-molecule activation and chemotaxis by granulocytes and macrophages may be important for both intestinal inflammation and reactive arthritis in IBD.

Neutrophil chemotaxis is markedly inhibited by sulfasalazine and 5-ASA in vitro (54–58). Similarly, chemotaxis and phagocytosis by monocytes are inhibited by sulfasalazine at concentrations achieved in the intestinal lumen (55). Neutrophil chemotaxis is also reduced by sulfasalazine and 5-ASA in a dose-dependent fashion, as are degranulation and release of lysozyme and β-glucuronidase by activated neutrophils. The activation of myeloperoxidase within neutrophils, a potent enzyme of the respiratory burst pathway, is inhibited by sulfasalazine and 5-ASA (58). In IL-1–stimulated, peripheral-blood mononuclear cells, sufasalazine suppressed IL-8 mRNA and protein production, whereas sulfapyridine had no effect (55). By blocking IL-8, sulfasalazine may decrease the influx of granulocytes into the mucosa.

Sulfasalazine inhibits the activation and expression of E-selectin and intercellular adhesion molecule-1 (ICAM-1) on endothelial cells. In addition, in both monocytes and granulocytes, sulfasalazine and 5-ASA reduced the TNF-α–stimulated expression of the adhesion molecule CD11b/CD18 (59). By impairing adhesion, sulfasalazine and 5-ASA may interfere with the rolling and binding of leukocytes to endothelial surfaces, preventing the diapedesis of neutrophils into tissues and thereby reducing inflammation. Therefore, both 5-ASA and the parent molecule sulfasalazine have a significant, in vitro, anti-inflammatory effect on macrophage and neutrophil function by impairing chemotaxis, adhesion, myeloperoxidase activity, and ROS production.

Eicosanoids

Because of its similar structure, 5-ASA was compared with acetylsalicylic acid (aspirin), a known inhibitor of cyclooxygenase within the arachidonic acid cascade. Sulfasalazine and 5-ASA both proved to be potent inhibitors of cyclooxygenase, whereas sulfapyridine was less effective. Subsequent studies with intestinal specimens confirmed this inhibitory action of sulfasalazine and 5-ASA on cyclooxygenase (60–62). Sulfasalazine and 5-ASA inhibited the induction of prostaglandin E_2 by 60% in inflamed intestinal specimens (63,64). Sulfasalazine also inhibited thromboxane synthetase, thereby decreasing the production of thromboxanes (65,66). Nonsteroidal, anti-inflammatory drugs (NSAIDs) that inhibit cyclooxygenase were therefore used in clinical trials of ulcerative colitis. Not only was there no clinical benefit, but some patients markedly worsened on NSAID therapy (67). NSAIDs are currently contraindicated in patients with IBD because they can exacerbate intestinal inflammation.

Mucosal levels of leukotriene B_4 (LTB_4) directly correlate with active intestinal inflammation in IBD. Sulfasalazine and 5-ASA inhibit the production of platelet-activating factor in IBD (68,69). Sulfasalazine and 5-ASA inhibit both 5-lipoxygenase and 5-lipoxygenase–activating protein (70,71), thereby blocking the production and chemotactic activity of leukotrienes. LTB_4-stimulated macrophage chemotaxis is blocked by sulfasalazine, 5-ASA, and the 5-ASA dimer olsalazine (72). Sulfasalazine also inhibits *N*-formyl-methionine-leucine-phenylanine (FMLP) binding to neutrophils (57).

Reactive Oxygen and Nitrogen Species

Both nitric oxide and reactive oxygen species are important mediators of mucosal inflammation and injury in IBD. Proinflammatory cytokines and chemokines stimulate the respiratory burst and increase the production of ROS by granulocytes and macrophages, which leads to further tissue destruction and intestinal inflammation. Free radicals are composed of partially reduced oxygen and nitrogen species with an odd number of electrons. In general, free radicals are reactive because of their propensity to acquire electrons from surrounding organic compounds. Oxygen-derived species oxidize proteins, carbohydrates, and sulfhydryls; degrade hyaluronic acid; are directly cytotoxic to many types of cells; and can cause tissue injury indirectly by inactivating protective proteins and enzymes.

At concentrations of 0.1 to 0.2 mmol, which are achieved within the intestinal mucosa, 5-ASA is one of the most potent, known, free-radical scavengers and antioxidants (73–76). Interaction with oxygen radicals results in the increased production of oxidized 5-ASA metabolites in the colonic mucosa and intestine (76). 5-ASA plays a direct role in scavenging potent neutrophil ROS. 5-ASA is also capable of preventing the generation of nitrosamine-reactive nitrogen species (77). Therefore, free-radical scavenging is an important anti-inflammatory capability of 5-ASA.

Signaling Pathways

The effect of sulfasalazine on signal transduction pathways has received limited study in leukocytes. When neutrophils were stimulated with FMLP, sulfasalazine blocked the production of phosphoinositol 1,4,5-phosphate (IP3) and thereby prevented an increase in cytosolic calcium. Sulfasalazine inhibited superoxide release from neutrophils when stimulated with guanosine 5-triphosphate (GTP), suggesting that sulfasalazine interrupted the signaling cascade between the GTP-binding protein and the production of IP3; phospholipase C is implicated as a possible target (78).

Nuclear Factor-κB (NF-κB)

Transcription factors play a central role in the regulation of immunologic and inflammatory processes. NF-κB is found in the cytoplasm of cells bound to the inhibitory protein IκBα, which prevents NF-κB from entering the nuclei (79–82). On cell activation, phosphorylation of IκBα by kinases leads to the degradation of IκBα, with the resultant release of NF-κB. NF-κB then moves into the nucleus, where it binds to κB sites in the promoter regions of target genes. NF-κB binding to specific promoter regions leads to increased expression of genes for many proinflammatory cytokines, chemokines, adhesion molecules, and inflammatory mediators (82). NF-κB, therefore, is a central transcription regulatory factor involved in mediating the initiation and perpetuation of inflammatory processes (79–82).

The kinases that phosphorylate IκBα are IκB kinase-α (IKK-α) and IκB kinase-β (IKK-β) (83–87). After the binding of TNF-α or IL-1 to the cell surface, IKK-β targets and sets the stage for the degradation of IκBα, leading to NF-κB activation. IKK-β plays a pivotal role in the inducible activation of NF-κB responsive genes involved in inflammatory responses. Therefore, IKK-β is an important target for proinflammatory stimuli (83–87).

The local administration of an antisense oligonucleotide targeted against the translation start site of NF-κB p65 inhibited both clinical and histologic colitis in IL-10 mice (88). Administration of antisense p65 to mice with 2,4,6-trinitrobenzene sulfonic acid–induced colitis resulted in a complete abrogation of intestinal inflammation 7 days later. Furthermore, macrophages isolated from the lamina propria of the p65 antisense–treated mice produced significantly lower amounts of IL-1, IL-6, and TNF-α mRNA (88). Therefore, NF-κB appears to play a central role in the transcriptional regulation of intestinal inflammation. Specific p65 antisense oligonucleotide therapy may inhibit colitis by reducing the local production of proinflammatory cytokines (89).

Activated NF-κB has been detected in increased amounts in inflamed mucosa from patients with Crohn's disease and ulcerative colitis. NF-κB activation was particularly increased in macrophages and epithelial cells (90). Analysis of nuclear extracts from lamina propria mononuclear cells and epithelial cells revealed strong activation of NF-κB with the presence of the p65 subunit (90). Therefore, the activation of NF-κB p65 is markedly increased in mucosal biopsies from patients with active Crohn's disease and ulcerative colitis (90).

Nuclear levels of NF-κB p65 were increased in extracts from colonic biopsies, as well as from isolated lamina propria mononuclear cells, from patients with active Crohn's disease (91). Examination of nuclear extracts from colonic biopsy samples from patients with active Crohn's disease before and after steroid therapy revealed a reduction in nuclear levels of NF-κB p65 after steroid treatment (91). By virtue of its ability to play a significant proinflammatory role in the induction of inflammation-associated gene expression, NF-κB p65 may be an important factor in the induction and perpetuation of inflammation in Crohn's disease (91).

Aspirin and sodium salicylate inhibit TNF-α–induced IκBα phosphorylation, IκBα degradation, and NF-κB activation (92). Aspirin and sodium salicylate also markedly inhibit IKK-β (93). Aspirin and sodium salicylate compete with ATP for binding to IKK-β (93). Therefore, inhibition of phosphorylation of IκB by aspirin and sodium salicylate prevents the degradation of IκB, which in turn prevents the activation of NF-κB (93).

Sulfasalazine induces a dose-dependent suppression of TNF-α–induced NF-κB activity (94) and decreases IκBα mRNA levels. Sulfasalazine also blocks nuclear translocation of NF-κB through inhibition of IκBα degradation (94) and interferes with phosphorylation of IκBα. Therefore, sulfasalazine is a potent inhibitor of NF-κB activation, suppresses NF-κB–dependent transcription, and prevents nuclear translocation of NF-κB due to inhibition of IκBα phosphorylation and subsequent degradation (94).

5-ASA inhibits TNF-α signaling events, including the activation of MAP kinase and NF-κB (95). 5-ASA inhibits both TNF-α–stimulated nuclear translocation of NF-κB and TNF-α–stimulated IκBα degradation (95). 5-ASA also inhibits IL-1–stimulated p65 phosphorylation without affecting IκBα degradation (96). Therefore, mesalamine may alter NF-κB activity by pathways distinct from IκB by modulating the phosphorylation by NF-κB proteins (96).

Conclusion

Recent progress has helped to clarify the mechanisms of action of 5-ASA. In the past, the ability of 5-ASA to inhibit multiple different inflammatory pathways was felt to be important for its effectiveness. It is now clear that a central mechanism for the inhibitory effects of 5-ASA may result from its effect on NF-κB. Many of the effects of 5-ASA can be explained by inhibition of activation of NF-κB. The ability of NF-κB to up-regulate proinflammatory cytokines, including TNF-α, IL-1, and IL-6, as well as chemokines such as IL-8 and MCP-1, leads to activation of an important proinflammatory cytokine feedback loop in IBD, which can be inhibited by 5-ASA. NF-κB activation leads to increased adhesion molecule expression, including ICAM-1 VCAM-1, and E-selectin in IBD. 5-ASA inhibition of adhesion molecule expression leads to decreased inflammatory cell recruitment into areas of chronic intestinal inflammation. NF-κB activation increases the production of oxygen radicals and leukotrienes, and 5-ASA inhibition of these pathways decreases these important effector molecules of inflammation and cell damage. Therefore, the ability of 5-ASA to inhibit specific tran-

scriptional regulation pathways has important implications for our understanding of the role of 5-ASA in the treatment of IBD.

References

1. Svartz N. Salazopyrin: a new sulfanilamide preparation. Acta Med Scand 1942;110:577–596.
2. Svartz N. Sulfasalazine II: some notes on the discovery and development of salazopyrin. Am J Gastroenterol 1988; 83:497–503.
3. Peppercorn MA, Goldman P. The role of intestinal bacteria in the metabolism of salicylazosulfapyridine. J Pharmacol Exp Ther 1972;181:555–562.
4. Peppercorn MA, Goldman P. Distribution studies of salicylazosulfapyridine and its metabolites. Gastroenterology 1973;64:240–245.
5. Baron JH, Connell PM, Lennard-Jones JE, et al. Sulphasalazine and salicylazosulphadimidine in ulcerative colitis. Lancet 1962;1:1094–1096.
6. Dick AP, Grayson MJ, Carpenter RG, et al. Controlled trial of sulphasalazine in the treatment of ulcerative colitis. Gut 1964;5:437–442.
7. Misiewicz JJ, Lennard-Jones JE, Connell AM. Controlled trial of sulphasalazine in maintenance for ulcerative colitis. Lancet 1965;1:185–188.
8. Dissanayake AS, Truelove SC. A controlled therapeutic trial of long-term maintenance treatment of ulcerative colitis with sulphasalazine (salazopyrin). Gut 1973;14:923–926.
9. Riis P, Anthonisen P, Wulff HR, et al. The prophylactic effect of salazosulphapyridine in ulcerative colitis during long-term treatment. A double-blind trial on patients asymptomatic for one year. Scand J Gastroenterol 1973;8:71–74.
10. Azad Khan AK, Howes DT, Piris J, Truelove SC. Optimum dose of sulphasalazine for maintenance treatment in ulcerative colitis. Gut 1980;21:232–240.
11. Willoughby CP, Piris J, Truelove SC. The effect of topical N-acetyl-5-aminosalicylic acid in ulcerative colitis. Scand J Gastroenterol 1980;15:715–719.
12. Campieri M, Lanfranchi GA, Bazzochi G, et al. Treatment of ulcerative colitis with high-dose 5-aminosalicylic acid enemas. Lancet 1981;2:270–271.
13. Griffin M, Miner P. Conventional drug therapy in inflammatory bowel disease. Gastroenterol Clin North Am 1995; 24:509–521.
14. Stotland B, Lichtenstein G. Newer treatments for inflammatory bowel disease. Gastroenterology 1996;23:577–608.
15. Riley SA, Mani V, Goodman MJ, et al. Comparison of delayed release 5-aminosalicylic acid (mesalazine) and sulphasalazine in the treatment of mild to moderate ulcerative colitis relapse. Gut 1988;29:669–674.
16. Schroeder KW, Tremaine WJ, Ilstrup DM. Coated oral 5-aminosalicylic acid therapy for mildly to moderately active ulcerative colitis. A randomized study. N Engl J Med 1987;317:1625–1629.
17. Sninsky CA, Cort DH, Shanahan F, et al. Oral mesalamine (Asacol) for mildly to moderately active ulcerative colitis. A multicenter study. Ann Intern Med 1991;115:350–355.
18. Singleton J, Hanauer SB, Gitnick GL, et al. Pentasa Crohn's Disease Study Group. Mesalamine capsules for the treatment of active Crohn's disease: results of a 16-week trial. Gastroenterology 1993;104:1293–1301.

19. Gendre JP, Mary JY, Florent C, et al. The Groupe d'Etudes Therapeutiques des Affections Inflammatoires Digestives. Oral mesalamine (Pentasa) as maintenance treatment in Crohn's disease: a multicenter placebo-controlled study. Gastroenterology 1993;104:435–439.
20. Zhou S, Fleisher D, Weiner N, et al. Lumenal liposomes preferentially target drugs to inflamed intestinal tissue. Gastroenterology 1996;116:A852.
21. Caprilli R, Andreoli A, Capurso L, et al. Gruppo Italiano per lo Studio del Colon e del Retto (GISC). Oral mesalamine (5-aminosalicylic acid; Asacol) for the prevention of post-operative recurrence of Crohn's disease. Aliment Pharmacol Ther 1994;8:35–43.
22. Florent C, Cartot A, Quandale P, et al. Placebo-controlled clinical trial of mesalazine in the prevention of early endoscopic recurrences after resection for Crohn's disease. Eur J Gastroenterol Hepatol 1996;8:229–233.
23. McLeod R. Is it possible to prevent recurrent Crohn's disease with medical or surgical interventions? Neth J Med 1996;48:68–70.
24. Jick H, Myers M, Dean A. The risk of sulfasalazine- and mesalazine-associated blood disorders. Pharmacotherapy 1995;15:176–181.
25. Kreisel W, Wolf L, Grotz W, et al. Renal tubular damage: an extraintestinal manifestation of chronic inflammatory bowel disease. Eur J Gastroenterol Hepatol 1996;8:461–468.
26. World M, Stevens P, Ashton M, et al. Mesalazine-associated interstitial nephritis. Nephrol Dial Transplant 1996;11:614–621.
27. Schreiber S, Hamling J, Zehnter E, et al. Renal tubular dysfunction in patients with inflammatory bowel disease treated with aminosalicylate. Gut 1997;40:761–766.
28. Hamling J, Raedler A, Helmchen U, et al. 5-Aminosalicylic acid–associated renal tubular acidosis with decreased renal function in Crohn's disease. Digestion 1997;58:304–307.
29. Sviri S, Gafanovich I, Kramer M, et al. Mesalamine-induced hypersensitivity pneumonitis. A case report and review of the literature. J Clin Gastroenterol 1997;24:34–36.
30. MacDermott RP. Etiology and pathogenesis of inflammatory bowel disease. Curr Opin Gastroenterol 1997;13:302–306.
31. MacDermott RP. Immunology of inflammatory bowel disease. Curr Opin Gastroenterol 1998;14:289–294.
32. Stevens C, Lipman M, Fabry S, et al. 5-Aminosalicylic acid abrogates T-cell proliferation by blocking interleukin-2 production in peripheral blood mononuclear cells. J Pharmacol Exp Ther 1995;272:399–406.
33. Selby WS, Janossy G, Mason DY, Jewell DP. Expression of HLA-DR antigens by colonic epithelium in inflammatory bowel disease. Clin Exp Immunol 1983;53:614–618.
34. Mayer L, Shlien R. Evidence for function of Ia molecules on gut epithelial cells in man. J Exp Med 1987;166:1471–1483.
35. Crotty B, Hoang P, Dalton H, et al. Salicylates used in inflammatory bowel disease and colchicine impair interferon-γ–induced HLA-DR expression. Gut 1992;33:59–64.
36. Chen D, Radford-Smith G, Diapolo M, et al. Cytokine gene transcription of human colonic intraepithelial lymphocytes costimulated with epithelial cells bearing HLA-DR and its inhibition by 5-aminosalicylic acid. J Clin Immunol 1996;16:237–241.
37. Aparicio-Pages MN, Verspaget HW, Hafkenscheid JC, et al. Inhibition of cell-mediated cytotoxicity by sulfasalazine: effect of in vivo treatment with 5-aminosalicylic acid and sulfasalazine on in vitro natural killer cell activity. Gut 1990;31:1030–1032.
38. Gibson PR, Jewell DP. Sulphasalazine and derivatives, natural killer activity and ulcerative colitis. Clin Sci 1985;69:177–184.
39. MacDermott RP, Kane MG, Steele LL, Stenson WF. Inhibition of cytotoxicity by sulfasalazine. I. Sulfasalazine inhibits spontaneous cell-mediated cytotoxicity by peripheral blood and intestinal mononuclear cells from control and inflammatory bowel disease patients. Immunopharmacology 1986;11:101–109.
40. Shanahan F, Niederlehner A, MacDermott RP, et al. Inhibition of cytotoxicity by sulfasalazine. II. Sulfasalazine and sulfapyridine inhibit different stages of the NK and NKCF lytic processes. Immunopharmacology 1986;11:111–118.
41. Scott MG, Nahm MH, Macke K, et al. Spontaneous secretion of IgG subclasses by intestinal mononuclear cells: differences between ulcerative colitis, Crohn's disease and controls. Clin Exp Immunol 1986;66:209–215.
42. MacDermott RP, Nash GS, Shlien R, et al. Alterations in serum immunoglobulin G subclasses in patients with ulcerative colitis and Crohn's disease. Gastroenterology 1989;96:764–768.
43. MacDermott RP, Schloemann SR, Bertovich MJ, et al. Inhibition of antibody secretion by 5-aminosalicylic acid. Gastroenterology 1989;96:442–448.
44. Mahida YR, Wu K, Jewell DP. Enhanced production of interleukin 1-beta by mononuclear cells isolated from mucosa with active ulcerative colitis or Crohn's disease. Gut 1989;30:835–838.
45. Stevens C, Walz G, Singaram C, et al. Tumor necrosis factor-alpha, interleukin 1 beta, and interleukin-6 expression in inflammatory bowel disease. Dig Dis Sci 1992;37:818–826.
46. Reinecker HC, Steffen M, Witthoeft T, et al. Enhanced secretion of tumour necrosis factor-alpha, IL-6, and IL-1β by isolated lamina propria mononuclear cells from patients with ulcerative colitis and Crohn's disease. Clin Exp Immunol 1993;94:174–181.
47. Cominelli F, Zipser CA, Dinarello CA. Sulfasalazine inhibits cytokine production in human mononuclear cells: a novel anti-inflammatory mechanism. Gastroenterology 1992;96:A96.
48. Rachmilewitz D, Karmeli F, Schwartz LW, et al. Effect of aminophenols (5-ASA and 4-ASA) on colonic interleukin-1 generation. Gut 1992;33:929–932.
49. Mahida Y, Lamming C, Gallagher A, et al. 5-aminosalicylic acid is a potent inhibitor of interleukin 1 beta production in organ culture of colonic biopsy specimens from patients with inflammatory bowel disease. Gut 1991;32:50–54.
50. Shanahan F, Niederlehner A, Carramanzana N, Anton P. Sulfasalazine inhibits the binding of TNF alpha to its receptor. Immunopharmacology 1990;20:217–224.
51. Jarry A, Muzeau F, Laboisse C. Cytokine effects in a human colonic goblet cell line. Cellular damage and its partial prevention by 5-aminosalicylic acid. Dig Dis Sci 1992;37:1170–1178.
52. MacDermott RP, Sanderson IR, Reinecker HC. The central role of chemokines (chemotactic cytokines) in the immunopathogenesis of ulcerative colitis and Crohn's disease. Inflamm Bowel Dis 1998;4:54–67.

53. Salmi M, Jalkanen S. Endothelial ligands and homing of mucosal leukocytes in extraintestinal manifestations of IBD. Inflamm Bowel Dis 1998;4:149–156.

54. Molin L, Stendahl O. The effect of sulfasalazine and its active components on human polymorphonuclear leukocyte function in relation to ulcerative colitis. Acta Med Scand 1979;206:451–457.

55. Deleuran B, Kristensen M, Paludan K, et al. The effect of second-line antirheumatic drugs on interleukin-8 mRNA synthesis and protein secretion in human endothelial cells. Cytokine 1992;4:403–409.

56. Axelsson LG, Ahlstedt S. Characteristics of immune-complex–induced chronic experimental colitis in rats with a therapeutic effect of sulphasalazine. Scand J Gastroenterol 1990;25:203–209.

57. Stenson WF, Mehta J, Spilberg I. Sulfasalazine inhibition of binding of *N*-formyl-methyonyl-leucyl-phenylanine (FMLP) to its receptor on human neutrophils. Biochem Pharmacol 1984;33:407–412.

58. Neal TM, Winterbourn CC, Vissers MC. Inhibition of neutrophil degranulation and superoxide production by sulfasalazine. Comparison with 5-aminosalicylic acid, sulfapyridine and olsalazine. Biochem Pharmacol 1987; 36:2765–2768.

59. Greenfield S, Hamblin A, Shakoor Z, et al. Inhibition of leucocyte adhesion molecule upregulation by tumour necrosis factor α: a novel mechanism of action of sulphasalazine. Gut 1993;34:252–256.

60. Collier HO, Francis AA, McDonald-Gibson WJ, et al. Inhibition of prostaglandin biosynthesis by sulfasalazine and its metabolites. Prostaglandins 1976;11:219–225.

61. Sharon P, Ligumsky M, Rachmilewitz D, et al. Role of prostaglandins in ulcerative colitis. Enhanced production during active disease and inhibition by sulfasalazine. Gastroenterology 1978;75:638–640.

62. Smith PR, Dawson DJ, Swan CHJ. Prostaglandin synthetase activity in active ulcerative colitis: effects of treatment with sulphasalazine, codeine phosphate and prednisolone. Gut 1978;20:802–805.

63. Sharon P, Stenson WF. Metabolism of arachidonic acid in acetic acid colitis in rats. Similarity to human inflammatory disease. Gastroenterology 1985;88:55–63.

64. Hawkey CJ, Boughton-Smith NK, Whittle BI. Modulation of human colonic arachidonic acid metabolism by sulfasalazine. Dig Dis Sci 1985;30:1161–1165.

65. Ligumsky M, Karmeli F, Sharon P, et al. Enhanced thromboxane A2 and prostacyclin production by cultured rectal mucosa in ulcerative colitis and its inhibition by steroids and sulfasalazine. Gastroenterology 1981;81:444–449.

66. Stenson WF, Lobos E. Inhibition of platelet thromboxane synthetase by sulfasalazine. Biochem Pharmacol 1983; 32:2205–2209.

67. Kaufman HJ, Taubin HL. Nonsteroidal anti-inflammatory drugs activate quiescent inflammatory bowel disease. Ann Intern Med 1987;107:513–516.

68. Eliakim R, Karmeli F, Razin R, et al. Role of platelet-activating factor in ulcerative colitis: enhanced production during active disease and inhibition by sulfasalazine and prednisolone. Gastroenterology 1988;95:1167–1172.

69. Capasso F, Tavares IA, Bennett A. Release of platelet-activating factor (PAF) from human colon mucosa and its inhibition by 5-aminosalicylic acid. Drugs Exp Clin Res 1991;17:351–353.

70. Stenson WF. Role of eicosanoids as mediators of inflammation in inflammatory bowel disease. Scand J Gastroenterol 1990;172(suppl):13–18.

71. Stenson WF, Lobos E. Sulfasalazine inhibits the synthesis of chemotactic lipids by neutrophils. J Clin Invest 1982; 69:494–497.

72. Wandall JH. Effects of sulphasalazine and its metabolites on neutrophil chemotaxis, superoxide production, degranulation and translocation of cytochrome b-245. Aliment Pharmacol Ther 1991;5:609–619.

73. Aruoma OI, Wasil M, Halliwell B, et al. The scavenging of oxidants by sulphasalazine and its metabolites. A possible contribution to their anti-inflammatory effect? Biochem Pharmacol 1987;36:3739–3742.

74. Dull BJ, Salata K, Van Langenhove AV, et al. 5-Aminosalicylate: oxidation by activated leukocytes and protection of cultured cells from oxidative damage. Biochem Pharmacol 1987;36:2467–2472.

75. Williams JG, Hallett MB. The reaction of 5-aminosalicylic acid with hypochlorite: implications for its actions by its mode of action in inflammatory bowel disease. Biochem Pharmacol 1989;38:149–154.

76. Ahnfelt-Ronne I, Nielsen OH, Christensen A, et al. Clinical evidence supporting the radical scavenger mechanism of 5-aminosalicylic acid. Gastroenterology 1990;98:1162–1169.

77. Pallapies B, Peskar BA, Peskar BM. 5-Aminosalicylic acid (5-ASA) inhibits the activity of nitric oxide (NO): contribution to its anti-inflammatory effects? Gastroenterology 1992; 96:A677.

78. Carlin G, Djursater R, Smedegard G. Sulphasalazine inhibition of human granulocyte activation by inhibition of second messenger compounds. Ann Rheum Dis 1992;51: 1230–1236.

79. Lenardo M, Baltimore D. NF-κB: A pleiotropic mediator of inducible and tissue-specific gene control. Cell 1989; 58:227–229.

80. Baeuerle P, Baltimore D. NF-κB: ten years after. Cell 1996; 87:13–20.

81. Siebenlist U, Granzoso G, Brown K. Structure, regulation and function of NK-κB. Annu Rev Cell Biol 1994;10:405–455.

82. Barnes P, Karin M. Nuclear factor-κB: a pivotal transcription factor in chronic inflammatory diseases. N Engl J Med 1997:1066–1071.

83. Zandi E, Rothwarf D, Delhase M, et al. The IκB kinase complex (IKK) contains two kinase subunits, IKKα and IKKβ, necessary for IκB phosphorylation and NF-κB activation. Cell 1997;91:243–252.

84. Manning A, Rao A, et al. IKK-1 and IKK-2: cytokine-activated IκB kinases essential for NF-κB activation. Science 1997;278:860–866.

85. DiDonato J, Hayakawa M, Rothwarf D, et al. A cytokine-responsive IκB kinase that activates the transcription factor NF-κB. Nature 1997;388:548–554.

86. Delhase M, Hayakawa M, Chen Y, et al. Positive and negative regulation of IκB kinase activity through IKKβ subunit phosphorylation. Science 1999;284:309–313.

87. May M, Ghosh S. IκB kinases: kinsmen with different crafts. Science 1999;284:271–273.

88. Neurath M, Pettersson S, Buschenfelde K, et al. Local administration of antisense phosphorothioate oligonucleotides to the p65 subunit of NF-κB abrogates established experimental colitis in mice. Nature Medicine 1996;2:998–1004.
89. Neurath M, Becker C, Barbulescu K. Role of NF-κB in immune and inflammatory responses in the gut. Gut 1998;43:856–860.
90. Rogler G, Brand K, Vogl D. Nuclear factor κB is activated in macrophages and epithelial cells of inflamed intestinal mucosa. Gastroenterology 1998;115:357–369.
91. Schreiber S, Nikolaus S, Hampe J. Activation of nuclear factor κB in inflammatory bowel disease. Gut 1998;42:477–484.
92. Kopp E, Ghosh S. Inhibition of NF-κB by sodium salicylate and aspirin. Science 1994;265:956–959.
93. Yin M, Yamamoto Y, Gaynor R. The anti-inflammatory agents aspirin and salicylate inhibit the activity of IκB kinase-β. Nature 1998;396:77–80.
94. Wahl C, Liptay S, Adler G, et al. Sufasalazine: a potent and specific inhibitor of nuclear factor kappa B. J Clin Invest 1998;5:1163–1174.
95. Kaiser G, Yan F, Polk D. Mesalamine blocks tumor necrosis factor growth inhibition and nuclear factor κB activation in mouse colonocytes. Gastroenterology 1999;116:602–609.
96. Egan L, McKean D, Mays D, et al. Mesalamine regulates nuclear factor kappa B (NF-κB) activity in intestinal epithelial cells by a novel mechanism: inhibition of inducible phosphorylation of rela (p65). Gastroenterology 1999;116: G3064.

Chapter 13

Antihistamines (H$_1$-Receptor Antagonists)

F. Estelle R. Simons

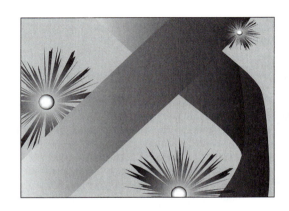

Histamine is an important chemical mediator of inflammation. It is produced and stored in cytoplasmic granules in tissue mast cells and basophils, from which it is released in large quantities by noncytotoxic mechanisms during the immediate hypersensitivity response. Acting at H$_1$-receptors on the postcapillary venules, histamine leads to vasodilation, increased vascular permeability, extravasation of fluid and cells, and edema. It also causes itching through stimulation of thin, nonmyelinated afferent C-fibers. Acting at H$_2$-receptors, histamine increases gastric acid secretion, increases vascular permeability, and has a variety of other effects. Acting at H$_3$-receptors located presynaptically on histaminergic nerve terminals, histamine controls its own synthesis and release in neurons; the H$_3$-receptor also functions as a heteroceptor and regulates the release of other neurotransmitters (1).

The molecular structures and signal-transduction mechanisms of the G-protein–coupled histamine H$_1$- and H$_2$-receptors have been elucidated. The molecular structure of the H$_3$-receptor has also been established. The intronless human H$_1$-receptor gene encodes a protein of 487 amino acids and maps to chromosome 3p24. The H$_1$-receptor shows approximately 45% homology with the muscarinic receptor and no homology with the H$_2$-receptor. A degenerate polymorphism identified in the human H$_1$-receptor gene may or may not provide one explanation as to why some patients fail to respond to H$_1$-receptor antagonists (1).

H$_1$-receptor antagonists, commonly known as antihistamines, comprise the largest and most pharmacologically diverse class of medications used in the treatment of allergic disorders. They play an especially prominent role in relieving symptoms in rhinoconjunctivitis and urticaria. During the past decade, new H$_1$-antagonists with improved safety profiles have been developed (1,2). The efficacy of H$_1$-antagonists depends primarily on their ability to produce histamine blockade at H$_1$-receptors on the vascular smooth muscle and decrease permeability, extravasation, and edema, and on their ability to block the effect of histamine at H$_1$-receptors on the afferent C-fibers and decrease itching and sneezing (1–3). Antiallergic and anti-inflammatory effects of H$_1$-antagonists, which occur independently of H$_1$-blockade, can be demonstrated after pretreatment with high doses and may contribute additional clinical benefits to those produced by H$_1$-blockade alone (4).

Clinical Pharmacology

H$_1$-antagonists differ considerably in their chemical structures and in their pharmacokinetic and pharmacodynamic profiles (Table 13-1) (1,2,5–11). In general, they are well absorbed after oral administration. They can be divided into two groups: those that are transformed into metabolites in the cytochrome P$_{450}$ system in the liver and gastrointestinal tract (e.g., acrivastine, azelastine, and loratadine) and those that are eliminated largely unchanged in the urine and/or feces and are not metabolized extensively in the cytochrome P$_{450}$ system (e.g., cetirizine, fexofenadine, and levocabastine). Terminal elimination half-life values of these H$_1$-antagonists range from 2 to more than 24 hours.

After oral administration, H$_1$-antagonists rapidly achieve peak tissue concentrations (1,2,5–11). Suppression of the histamine- or allergen-induced wheal and flare in the skin is a useful bioassay for defining dose response curves and for identifying clinically relevant differences in onset of H$_1$-antagonist activity, maximum activity, and offset of activity. Most orally administered H$_1$-antagonists produce significant H$_1$-receptor blockade within a few hours and have a duration of action of at least 24 hours after a single dose (Fig. 13-1) (5).

During long-term daily administration of an H$_1$-antagonist, there is no decrease in the amount of H$_1$-receptor blockade produced. In studies of 4 to 12 weeks' duration, no subsensitivity to the effect of new H$_1$-antagonists such as cetirizine and loratadine has been identified with objective monitoring of skin wheal-and-flare suppression (see Fig. 13-1) (5), nor has loss of efficacy been found with subjective monitoring of symptomatic relief in allergic rhinoconjunctivitis or urticaria (Figs. 13-2, 13-3, and 13-4) (12–14). The apparent subsensitivity to the antihistaminic effects of the H$_1$-antagonists reported years ago may have been the result of lack of compliance secondary to the relatively poor benefit-to-risk vatio of the earlier medications.

H$_1$-Receptor Antagonists in Allergic Rhinoconjunctivitis

After patients with allergic rhinitis are exposed to allergens, histamine concentrations in the nasal mucosa and secretions may be

Table 13-1. Practical Pharmacokinetics and Pharmacodynamics of Representative New H₁-Antagonists

H₁-Receptor Antagonist (Metabolite)	t_{max}* (hr) After a Single Dose	Terminal Elimination $t_{1/2}$ᵃ (hr)	% Eliminated Unchanged in the Urine/ Feces	Clinically Relevant Drug Interactions	Duration of Action (h)	Once-Daily Dosing Possible?	Population in Which Dose Adjustment is Required
Eliminated largely unchanged							
Cetirizine	1.0	7.4	60/0	Unlikely	24	Yes	G,R,H
Fexofenadine	2.6	14.4	12/80	Unlikely	24	Yes	G,Rᶜ
Extensively metabolized							
Acrivastine	1.4	1.7	59	Unlikely	8	No	Noneᶜ
Loratadineᵇ (descarboethoxyloratadine)	1.0 (1.5)	7.8–11.0 (17–24)	Trace	Unlikelyᵇ	24	Yes	R,H

Results are expressed as means.
* Time from oral intake to peak plasma concentration.
ᵃ Terminal elimination half-life.
ᵇ In the presence of CYP3A4 inhibition, loratadine is eliminated via the CYP2D6 metabolic pathway.
ᶜ No active metabolites identified.
na, information not available; bid, twice daily; G, geriatric; R, renal function impaired; H, hepatic function impaired.

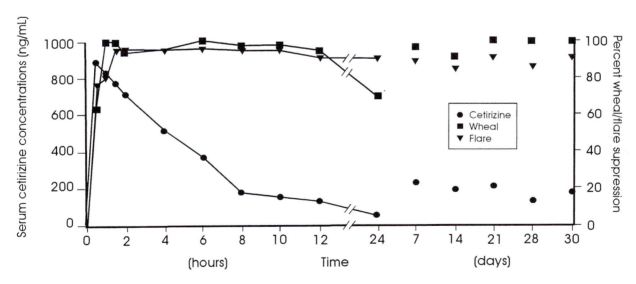

Figure 13-1. Relationship between H₁-receptor antagonist serum concentrations and peripheral H₁-blockade effect in the skin. In a prospective, randomized, double-blind, parallel-group study, serum concentrations of orally administered cetirizine were monitored concomitantly with the ability of the drug to suppress the skin wheals and flares induced by epicutaneous tests with histamine phosphate, 1 mg/mL. After a 10-mg dose of cetirizine, serum concentrations and percent suppression of the wheals and flares were monitored for 24 hours; in addition, during regular daily administration for several weeks, they were monitored 12 hours after a dose at weekly intervals. Peak wheal-and-flare suppression followed peak H₁-antagonist concentrations, and wheal-and-flare suppression continued after H₁-antagonist concentrations became negligible. This temporal relationship is characteristic of all H₁-antagonists in all populations studied with this method. (Adapted with permission from Watson WTA, Simons KJ, Chen XY, Simons FER. Cetirizine: a pharmacokinetic and pharmacodynamic evaluation in children with seasonal allergic rhinitis. J Allergy Clin Immunol 1989; 84:457–464.)

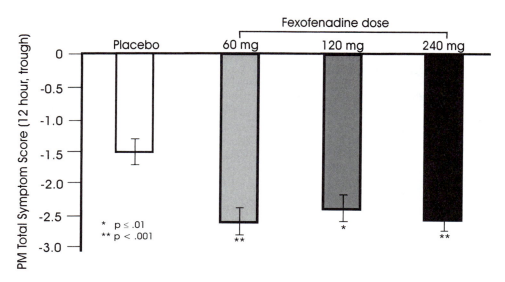

Figure 13-2. Effectiveness of H₁-antagonists in allergic rhinitis. In a double-blind, placebo-controlled, parallel, 2-week study in 570 patients with ragweed-induced rhinitis, fexofenadine HCl at doses of 60, 120, and 240 mg bid provided significant improvement compared with placebo in the 12-hour, reflective, total symptom score ($P \leq .003$) and in all individual nasal symptoms. No sedative effects or ECG abnormalities were detected. The frequency of adverse effects was similar in all treatment groups. (Reproduced with permission from Bernstein DI, Schoenwetter WF, Nathan RA, et al. Efficacy and safety of fexofenadine for treatment of seasonal allergic rhinitis. Ann Allergy Asthma Immunol 1997;79:443–448.)

elevated, and responsiveness to nasal challenge with histamine increases.

In seasonal or perennial allergic rhinitis, the efficacy of H₁-antagonists has been well documented in randomized, double-blind, placebo-controlled clinical trials (see Fig. 13-2) (1,2,6–13). They effectively reduce nasal itching, sneezing, and rhinorrhea, but are less effective in relieving nasal congestion. They also relieve concomitant itching, watering, and redness of the eye and itching of the throat and ear. In seasonal allergic rhinitis, they should be started before peak pollination and used regularly rather than "as needed."

Overall, H₁-antagonists have similar efficacy profiles (1,2). Topical application of levocabastine or azelastine to the nasal mucosa or conjunctivae may result in faster onset of relief than administration of oral H₁-antagonists such as acrivastine, cetirizine, fexofenadine, or loratadine; however, the topical formulations must be applied several times daily. Selection of an H₁-antagonist for the treatment of allergic rhinoconjunctivitis is based on considerations such as safety profile, cost, convenience of dose regimen, and patient preference for a particular formulation.

Although a dose-response effect may be noted for some symptoms, doubling the manufacturers' recommended dose of H₁-antagonist does not usually result in a further significant increase in overall symptom relief and may increase the likelihood of adverse effects. Although some individuals who do not respond to one H₁-antagonist may respond to another, these non-responders should generally be considered to be candidates for treatment with intranasal topical glucocorticoids.

H₁-antagonists are less effective than intranasal glucocorticoids for relief of nasal symptoms (15), have similar or greater efficacy for the alleviation of eye symptoms, and produce similar improvement in overall quality of life. They provide relief of allergic rhinoconjunctivitis symptoms comparable with or greater than that provided by intranasal sodium cromoglycate in a 4% solution administered topically four to six times daily or to nedocromil 2% solution administered topically. In initial studies, they also appear to have similar efficacy to that of leukotriene antagonists. To improve relief of nasal congestion, many H₁-antagonists are available in a fixed-dose combination with a decongestant, usually pseudoephedrine (6).

H₁-Receptor Antagonists in Other Upper Respiratory Tract Disorders

H₁-antagonists are less effective in the treatment of nonallergic rhinitis than in the treatment of allergic rhinitis. They are commonly used for the treatment of upper respiratory tract infections ("colds") (16). Although they are often administered to patients with sinusitis, acute otitis media, or otitis media with effusion, there is little evidence from randomized, controlled, double-blind studies that they are effective in these disorders.

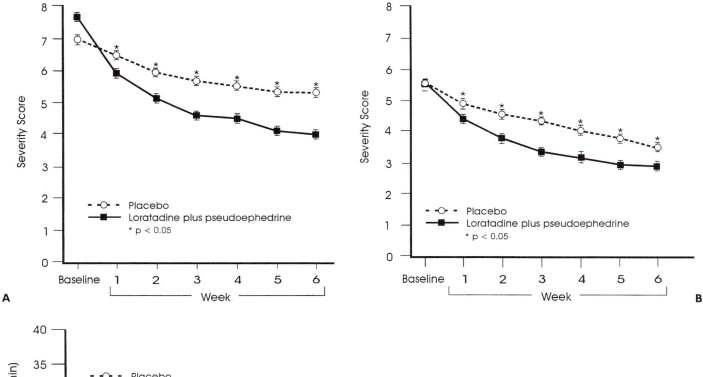

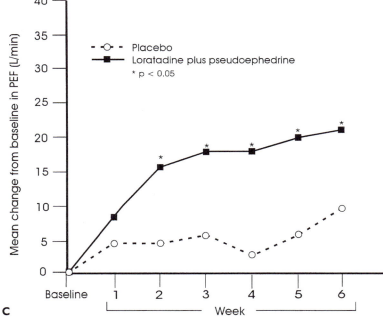

Figure 13-3. Effect of H_1-antagonists on upper and lower airway symptoms in patients with concomitant seasonal allergic rhinitis and mild persistent asthma. In a 6-week randomized, double-blind, placebo-controlled study of 193 subjects during the fall allergy season, loratadine (5 mg) plus pseudoephedrine (120 mg twice daily) decreased symptoms in the (*A*) upper and (*B*) lower airways and the use of albuterol. Morning peak expiratory flow rates (PEF) (*C*), FEV_1, and quality of life also improved significantly (not shown). (Reproduced with permission from Corren J, Harris AG, Aaronson D, et al. Efficacy and safety of loratadine plus pseudoephedrine in patients with seasonal allergic rhinitis and mild asthma. J Allergy Clin Immunol 1997;100:781–788.)

H_1-Receptor Antagonists in Asthma

H_1-antagonists protect against the early bronchoconstrictor response to inhaled allergen and have a synergistic response with leukotriene antagonists against both the early and late bronchoconstrictor response to inhaled allergen.

In mild, persistent asthma, H_1-antagonists relieve symptoms and have a small, dose-related bronchodilator effect. They are particularly useful in the treatment of patients with concomitant seasonal allergic rhinitis and asthma (see Fig. 13-3) (13). In moderate persistent asthma, H_1-antagonists may have a glucocorticoid-sparing

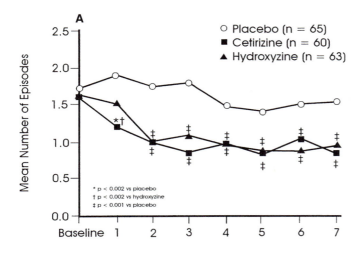

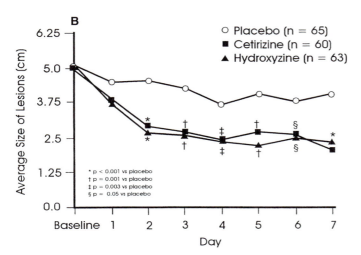

Figure 13-4. Efficacy of new and old H_1-antagonists in chronic urticaria. In a 4-week, randomized, double-blind, double-dummy, placebo-controlled study, 188 patients with chronic idiopathic urticaria were treated with either cetirizine (10 mg once daily), hydroxyzine (25 mg three times daily), or placebo. Cetirizine and hydroxyzine both significantly reduced (*A*) the number of episodes of urticaria and (*B*) the size of the urticarial lesions. The number of lesions and the severity of pruritus were also decreased (not shown). (Reproduced with permission from Breneman DL. Cetirizine versus hydroxyzine and placebo in chronic idiopathic urticaria. Ann Pharmacother 1996;30:1075–1079.)

effect. In severe persistent asthma, they have no significant beneficial effects, although they do no harm (1).

H_1-Receptor Antagonists in Urticaria

In urticarial lesions, skin tissue fluid histamine concentrations are elevated compared with histamine concentrations in surrounding uninvolved skin, and patients with chronic urticaria have a reduced clinical tolerance to histamine.

The efficacy of H_1-antagonists in the treatment of acute and chronic urticaria has been well documented, particularly for the symptomatic relief of itching, which is primarily mediated by the action of histamine at H_1-receptors (3), but also for reducing the number, size, and duration of urticarial lesions (see Fig. 13-4) (1,2,6,8,9,11,14). In chronic urticaria, H_1-antagonists should optimally be given on a regular basis, rather than as needed, to prevent urticarial lesions from appearing. Relief of the wheal-and-flare response may be incomplete because the underlying increased vascular permeability, vasodilation, and extravasation may also be mediated through the action of histamine at H_2-receptors and by other vasoactive mediators, including proteases, eicosanoids such as prostaglandin D_2, and neuropeptides such as substance P. The response to H_1-antagonist treatment in delayed-pressure urticaria and in urticarial vasculitis is often unsatisfactory.

Old, sedating H_1-antagonists are still used in the treatment of urticaria, despite their poor benefit-to-risk ratio. In time-honored tradition, they are often given three or four times daily; however, this regimen is unnecessary as most of them, e.g. hydroxyzine or chlorpheniramine have long elimination half-life values (1,2). Combinations of old H_1-antagonists (e.g., hydroxyzine plus cyproheptadine) or of old and new H_1-antagonists (e.g., cetirizine in the morning and hydroxyzine at night) are recommended on an empirical basis by some highly respected physicians. These regimens have not been rigorously tested in randomized, prospective, double-blind, placebo-controlled trials, and the administration of an old H_1-antagonist at hight places patients at increased risk for an antihistamine "hangover" (Fig. 13-5) (17). In prospective, controlled, double-blind studies, new H_1-antagonists have been found to be less sedating and as effective as old H_1-antagonists, although higher doses than those used to treat allergic rhinitis (Table 13-2) may be required.

H_1-Receptor Antagonists in Anaphylaxis

In patients with anaphylactic or anaphylactoid reactions, the initial treatment of choice is the physiologic agonist epinephrine. However, H_1-antagonists are useful for adjunctive relief of pruritus, urticaria, rhinorrhea, and other symptoms (1,2). Old H_1-antagonists such as chlorpheniramine, diphenhydramine, and hydroxyzine remain useful in the treatment of anaphylactic or anaphylactoid reactions. Unlike most of the new medications in this class, they have relatively high aqueous solubility and are available commercially in parenteral formulations for injection.

H_1-Receptor Antagonists in Atopic Dermatitis

In atopic dermatitis, histamine is the main pruritogen, and histamine concentrations may be elevated in the skin and plasma. In this disorder, relief of itching by H_1-antagonists is often incomplete. There is a perception that the old, sedating H_1-antagonists

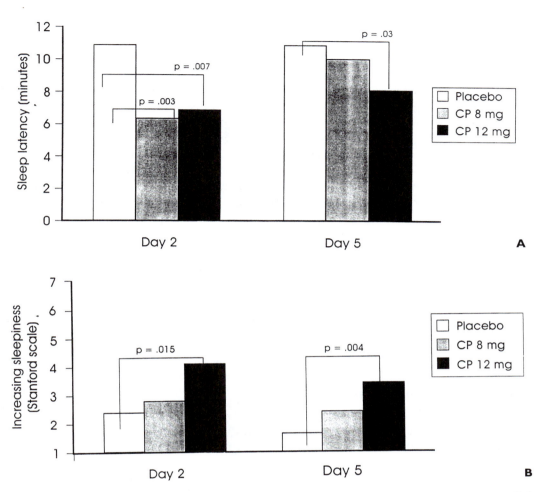

Figure 13-5. "Hangover" effect of old H_1-antagonists given at bedtime. A double-blind, placebo-controlled, parallel study was performed in 29 healthy subjects over 7 days. Subjects received an evening dose of chlorpheniramine (CP) (12 mg) with a morning dose of terfenadine (60 mg); or an evening dose of chlorpheniramine (8 mg) with a morning dose of terfenadine (60 mg); or a placebo both morning and evening. Multiple sleep latency tests and Stanford Sleepiness Scale test results showed (*A*) that an evening dose of chlorpheniramine increased daytime sleepiness and decreased alertness, with the most pronounced effects occurring in subjects who received the higher dose, and that (*B*) those who received an evening dose of chlorpheniramine also had more subjective carryover sedation. (Reproduced with permission from Kay GG, Plotkin KE, Quig MB, et al. Sedating effects of AM/PM antihistamine dosing with evening chlorpheniramine and morning terfenadine. Am J Man Care 1997;3:1843–1848.)

such as hydroxyzine and diphenhydramine, which relieve itching by central, as well as by peripheral, H_1-blockade mechanisms, are more effective for relief of pruritus than the new, nonsedating H_1-antagonists. New medications such as cetirizine and loratadine have been shown to relieve itching in atopic dermatitis; however, high doses may be required (1,2,8).

Infants with atopic dermatitis and/or elevated serum IgE levels and a family history of atopy are at increased risk for the development of asthma. In placebo-controlled studies of 1 to 3 years' duration, high doses of cetirizine or ketotifen significantly delayed the development of asthma in these high-risk infants by mechanisms that are not yet completely understood (18).

Adverse Effects

Old, first-generation H_1-antagonists potentially cause a wide variety of adverse effects, including anticholinergic effects (dry mouth and mucous membranes, difficulty in micturition, impotence, tachycardia, constipation, and other gastrointestinal symptoms) and antiserotonin effects (appetite stimulation and inappropriate weight gain) (1,2). Topical application to the skin may lead to somnolence and other central nervous system (CNS) effects and may also result in sensitization and contact dermatitis.

Table 13-2. Formulations and Dosages of Representative New H₁-Receptor Antagonists

New H₁-Antagonists	Formulation	Recommended Dose
Acristavine* (Semprex-D®)	Tablets 8 mg	Adult: 8 mg qd
Azelastine (Astelin®)	Nasal solution 0.1% (0.137 µg/spray)	Adult (intranasal): 2 sprays/nostril bid
Cetirizine (Reactine®, Zyrtec®)	Tablets 10 mg Syrup 5 mg/5 mL	Adult: 5–10 mg qd Pediatric (6–11 yrs): 5–10 mg qd (2–5 yrs): 2.5 mg qd or bid
Fexofenadine (Allegra®)	Tablets 60 mg, 120 mg	Adult: 60 mg bid or 180 mg qd Pediatric (6–11 yrs): 30 mg bid
Levocabastine (Livostin®)	Intranasal microsuspension 50 µg/spray Ophthalmic suspension 0.05% (0.5 mg/mL)	Adult (intranasal): 2 sprays/nostril bid–qid Adult (ophthalmic): 1 drop in each eye bid–qid
Loratadine* (Claritin®)	Tablets 10 mg RediTabs® 10 mg (rapidly disintegrating) Syrup 5 mg/5 mL	Adult: 10 mg qd Pediatric: (6–9 yrs) (<30 kg); 10 mg qd

*Available with pseudoephedrine; acristavine is *only* available in fixed dose combination with pseudoephedrine hydrochloride 120 mg.
qd, once daily; bid, twice daily; tid, three times daily.

Most new, second-generation H₁-antagonists are unlikely to cause dry mouth or other anticholinergic effects. More importantly, some new H₁-antagonists are free from both CNS effects and from cardiac toxicity (1,2,6–11).

Central Nervous System (CNS) Effects

In the CNS, histamine is stored in vesicles in histaminergic neurons, from which it is released to play a pivotal role in neurotransmission and maintenance of the waking state (1). The blood-brain barrier, which has evolved to provide a stable chemical environment for neurons, consists of astrocyte-encased CNS capillaries lined with endothelial cells characterized by tight junctions and no fenestrae. The physicochemical properties of the old H₁-antagonists readily permit penetration of this barrier, and in manufacturers' recommended doses, as demonstrated by positron emission tomography, they occupy a major fraction of the H₁-receptors in the frontal cortex, temporal cortex, hippocampus, and pons. Their CNS effects in humans, which appear to be mediated primarily by blockade of endogenous histamine (19), are similar to those produced by alcohol or major tranquilizers (20). They are widely used as inexpensive sedatives. Concomitant ingestion of alcohol or other CNS-active chemicals potentiates the adverse CNS effects of old H₁-antagonists. An overdose of an old H₁-antagonist can be fatal.

The use of the old, sedating H₁-antagonists is of concern in the treatment of any patient with allergic disorders, which themselves may cause CNS symptoms (1,19). Self-reporting of adverse CNS effects usually underestimates true CNS functional impairment, which can be documented even in the absence of symptoms. The true prevalence of the adverse CNS effects of old H₁-antagonists is unknown, but they have been reported in approximately 40% of unselected users after chlorpheniramine or brompheniramine. Furthermore, old H₁-antagonists remain sedating even when administered in fixed-dose combinations

with a CNS-stimulating decongestant. The warning contained in the package insert for the old antihistamines, "may cause drowsiness—avoid activities requiring mental alertness," is irrelevant in an era in which a high level of mental alertness and coordination is needed for most daily tasks.

In patients with allergic disorders, some physicians recommend giving old H₁-antagonists only at bedtime, as somnolence is of no concern during the night, and H₁-blockade may still be present the next morning. However, the day after taking an old H₁-antagonist at bedtime, the adverse CNS effects may not have disappeared (1,17,19) (Fig. 13-5). Other physicians advise regular daytime use, anticipating that tolerance will develop to the adverse CNS effects but not to the peripheral H₁-blockade. Although anecdotal and subjective reports of tolerance to the CNS effects of old antihistamines are common, tolerance may not be evident on objective testing (1,17,19) (Fig. 13-5). H₁-receptors in the CNS do not differ from H₁-receptors in the skin, where tolerance (decreased peripheral H₁-blockade over months of treatment) cannot be demonstrated (5).

The new H₁-antagonists do not cross the blood-brain barrier to the same degree that their predecessors did (1,19) and do not interfere with the important neurotransmitter and "waking" effects of histamine in the central nervous system (CNS). They differ slightly from each other in their ability to cause adverse CNS effects; however, compared with the old H₁-antagonists, they are all relatively free from these effects when administered in recommended doses. Also, in contrast to their predecessors, they do not potentiate the adverse CNS effects produced by alcohol or other CNS-active chemicals.

Cardiac Toxicity

The H₁-antagonists terfenadine and astemizole have been implicated in prolonging the QTc interval and, rarely, in causing torsade de pointes and other potentially fatal ventricular arrhythmias (21). Regulatory approval has been withdrawn for terfenadine and astemizole in most countries. The risk of prolonged QTc interval and ventricular arrhythmias from old, sedating H_1-antagonists and from new H_1-antagonists (with the exception of terfenadine and astemizole) is low.

The primary cellular event leading to arrhythmias is the inhibition of repolarization potassium channels, particularly the delayed rectifier potassium channel (I_K). This leads to prolonged duration of the action potential (QT interval on the surface electrocardiogram) and development of early after-depolarization, which triggers torsade de pointes. Other electrophysiologic changes, for example, blockade of the inward rectifier (I_{K1}) potassium channel or the transient outward (I_{TO}) potassium channel, may also lead to prolongation of the action potential. Before new H_1-antagonists enter clinical development, their potential arrhythmogenic effects can now be predicted in vitro in human ventricular tissue or in cloned human ion channels. The molecular target in the human ventricle for the potassium channel blockade of H_1-antagonists is HERG, the human ether-a-go-go–related gene on chromosone 7 that expresses the delayed rectifier I_{Kr} channel.

Host variables play an important role in the development of cardiac toxicity from terfenadine and astemizole. Factors that increase the risk include the following: a pre-existing cardiac disorder such as congenital or acquired prolonged QT syndrome or bradycardia; a metabolic problem such as hypokalemia, hypocalcemia, or hypomagnesemia; or the concomitant ingestion of another medication that is eliminated in the cytochrome P_{450} system.

Safety During Pregnancy and Lactation

H_1-antagonists cross the placenta. Most are classified as FDA Pregnancy Category C, meaning that there is inadequate information about their use in humans and either no information about their use in animals or documented teratogenicity in animals. These medications should be used during pregnancy only if the expected benefits to the mother exceed the unknown risks to the fetus. Prospective, controlled, observational studies of women taking H_1-antagonists during the first trimester of pregnancy are now being performed. Some H_1-antagonists such as cetirizine and loratadine are classified as lower-risk Pregnancy Category B, meaning that, although adequate studies have not been performed in humans, the drugs are documented to be safe in animals (22).

In infants whose mothers received large, therapeutic doses of old H_1-antagonists immediately before delivery, withdrawal symptoms, including tremulousness and irritability, may occur. In nursing infants whose mothers have ingested old H_1-antagonists, irritability or drowsiness have been reported.

Summary

H_1-antagonists play an important role in the symptomatic treatment of allergic rhinoconjunctivitis and urticaria and a less important role in the treatment of other allergic disorders. The potential benefits of each H_1-antagonist should be weighed against the potential risks. Although the rare, potentially fatal cardiovascular effects produced by two of the newer H_1-antagonists have recently been a major concern, attention should now be refocused on the common, subclinical, CNS adverse effects ubiquitously produced by the older H_1-antagonists.

References

1. Simons FER. Antihistamines. In: Middleton E Jr, Reed CE, Ellis EF, et al, eds. Allergy principles and practice. 5th ed. St. Louis: Mosby–Year Book, 1998:612–637.
2. Simons FER, Simons KJ. The pharmacology and use of H_1-receptor antagonist drugs. N Engl J Med 1994; 330:1663–1670.
3. Schmelz M, Schmidt R, Bickel A, et al. Specific C-receptors for itch in human skin. J Neurosci 1997;17:8003–8008.
4. Naclerio RM, Baroody FM. H_1-receptor antagonists: antiallergic effects in humans. In: Simons FER, ed. Histamine and H_1-receptor antagonists in allergic disease. New York: Marcel Dekker, 1996:145–174.
5. Watson WTA, Simons KJ, Chen XY, Simons FER. Cetirizine: a pharmacokinetic and pharmacodynamic evaluation in children with seasonal allergic rhinitis. J Allergy Clin Immunol 1989;84:457–464.
6. Brogden RN, McTavish D. Acristavine: a review of its pharmacological properties and therapeutic efficacy in allergic rhinitis, urticaria and related disorders. Drugs 1991;41:927–940.
7. McNeely W, Wiseman LR. Intranasal azelastine. A review of its efficacy in the management of allergic rhinitis. Drugs 1998;56:91–114.
8. Spencer CM, Faulds D, Peters DH. Cetirizine. A reappraisal of its pharmacological properties and therapeutic use in selected allergic disorders. Drugs 1993;46:1055–1080.
9. Markham A, Wagstaff AJ. Fexofenadine. Drugs 1998; 55:269–274.
10. Heykants J, Van Peer A, Van de Velde V, et al. The pharmacokinetic properties of topical levocabastine. A review. Clin Pharmacokinet 1995;29:221–230.
11. Haria M, Fitton A, Peters DH. Loratadine. A reappraisal of its pharmacological properties and therapeutic use in allergic disorders. Drugs 1994;48:617–637.
12. Bernstein DI, Schoenwetter WF, Nathan RA, et al. Efficacy and safety of fexofenadine hydrochloride for treatment of seasonal allergic rhinitis. Ann Allergy Asthma Immunol 1997;79:443–448.
13. Corren J, Harris AG, Aaronson D, et al. Efficacy and safety of loratadine plus pseudoephedrine in patients with seasonal allergic rhinitis and mild asthma. J Allergy Clin Immunol 1997;100:781–788.
14. Breneman DL. Cetirizine versus hydroxyzine and placebo in chronic idiopathic urticaria. Ann Pharmacother 1996; 30:1075–1079.
15. Weiner JM, Abramson MJ, Puy RM. Intranasal corticosteroids versus oral H_1 receptor antagonists in allergic rhinitis: systematic review of randomised controlled trials. Br Med J 1998;317:1624–1629.
16. D'Agostino RB Sr, Weintraub M, Russell HK, et al. The effectiveness of antihistamines in reducing the severity of

runny nose and sneezing: a meta-analysis. Clin Pharmacol Ther 1998;64:579–596.

17. Kay GG, Plotkin KE, Quig MB, et al. Sedating effects of AM/PM antihistamine dosing with evening chlorpheniramine and morning terfenadine. Am J Man Care 1997;3:1843–1848.

18. Wahn U, for the ETAC Study Group. Allergic factors associated with the development of asthma and the influence of cetirizine in a double-blind, randomised, placebo-controlled trial: first results of ETAC. Pediatr Allergy Immunol 1998;9:116–124.

19. Simons FER. H_1-receptor antagonists. Comparative tolerability and safety. Drug Saf 1994;10:350–380.

20. Roehrs T, Zwyghuizen-Doorenbos A, Roth T. Sedative effects and plasma concentrations following single doses of triazolam, diphenhydramine, ethanol and placebo. Sleep 1993;16:301–305.

21. Woosley RL. Cardiac actions of antihistamines. Annu Rev Pharmacol Toxicol 1996;36:233–252.

22. Schatz M, Petitti D. Antihistamines and pregnancy. Ann Allergy Asthma Immunol 1997;78:157–159.

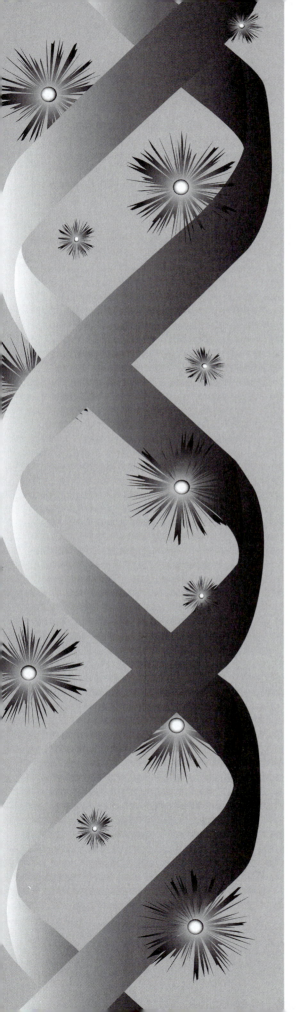

III

Biologic Agents

Cytokines

Macromolecules

Antibody-Based Therapy

Immunotherapy of Allergic Disease

Chimeric Protein

Vaccines and Peptide Therapy

177

Chapter 14

Hematopoietic Growth Factors

Colin A. Sieff

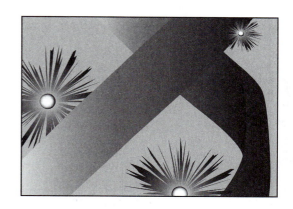

The family of glycoproteins known as the hematopoietic growth factors (HGFs) plays a major role in the proliferation, differentiation, and survival of primitive hematopoietic stem and progenitor cells, as well as in functional activation of some mature cells. These effects are mediated by high-affinity binding to specific receptors expressed on the surfaces of the target cells. Correction or amelioration of marrow failure by administration of HGFs has been and continues to be the major practical goal of research in hematopoiesis. This goal could not be achieved, however, without the early tissue culture work that led to the characterization of the HGF family, and without recombinant DNA technology, which provided the genes that allowed efficient production of the hormones to permit interpretable in vitro and in vivo investigations.

History

Beginning with the pioneering work in the early 1960s by Metcalf (1) and Sachs (2) and their coworkers, it has been recognized that normal and leukemic blood progenitor cells can be propagated in semisolid culture in the presence of soluble growth factors. These factors were originally termed colony-stimulating factors, or CSFs, based on their ability to support the formation of colonies of blood cells by bone marrow cells plated in semisolid medium (3,4). During the 1970s and 1980s, it was recognized that there exist multiple types of CSFs based on the different types of colonies that grow in the presence of the different factors, leading to the hypothesis that the growth and differentiation of blood cells are controlled, at least in part, by exposure of progenitor cells to CSFs having different lineage specificities (3–5). With the molecular cloning of the genes for many of these factors and their receptors during the 1980s and 1990s, it became possible to study in detail the structure, function, and biology of the recombinant CSFs as well as the molecular biology of their respective genes (4–7). This analysis, along with similar work on the regulation of cells in the immune system, led to the realization that there exists a large family of interacting regulatory molecules now generally known as cytokines or lymphohematopoietic cytokines that together serve to control the hematopoietic and immune systems and to integrate the responses of these systems with those of other systems (7–10). This interacting network of cytokines includes the interferons (11), interleukins (12), tumor necrosis factors (13), and hematopoietic growth factors (including the CSFs) (3,4) (Table 14-1). Over the past 15 years, the cDNAs and genes for the hematopoietic growth factors and their receptors have been cloned. This work has provided an incredible array of tools for analysis of the molecular and cellular biology of hematopoiesis beginning with molecular clones for analysis of the expression of the HGF and HGF receptor genes as well as recombinant proteins for evaluation of the biology of the various factors in vivo and in vitro (Fig. 14-1).

The discovery, cloning, and expression of the gene for murine interleukin 3 (IL-3) presented the first opportunity to evaluate hematopoietic growth factors in an unambiguous fashion (14,15). Sublethally irradiated mice were infused for 7 days with recombinant IL-3 or with control protein (16). The spleens of the multi-CSF treated marrow recipients were much larger than those of the controls, were more cellular, and contained more progenitors. The increase in progenitor cells affected erythroid and myeloid lineages. In contrast, bone marrow cellularity was unaffected and progenitor content was reduced. Metcalf et al (17) injected mice with purified bacterially synthesized IL-3 by the intraperitoneal route and obtained similar results. In addition, tenfold increases in blood eosinophil and two- to three-fold increases in neutrophil and monocyte levels were observed. The intraperitoneal injections also resulted in 6- to 15-fold increases in peritoneal phagocytes with an increase in macrophage phagocytic activity.

These experiments clearly demonstrate that murine IL-3 influences the replication and growth potential of primitive hemopoietic progenitors, and strongly suggest that whatever effects such hormones have on blood counts are related to their influences on progenitor function rather than to their effects on peripheral blood cell kinetics. They also suggest that the function of mature cells can be altered in vivo, an effect that would be expected to decrease rather than increase numbers of circulating phagocytes.

Similarly, the first indications that the human hemopoietic growth factor, granulocyte-macrophage colony-stimulating factor (GM-CSF), could broadly stimulate hematopoiesis in vivo resulted from studies of the infusion of COS cell produced GM-CSF into cynomolgous macaques (18). Recombinant (r) human (h) GM-CSF acts on simian progenitors. The disappearance curve of intravenously injected metabolically labeled factor is complex and suggests a multicompartment turnover model, but the overall

Table 14-1. Hematopoietic Growth Factors with Clinical Potential or Proven Usefulness

Class	Factor	Biologic Activity		Major Clinical Uses
		Progenitors	Mature Cells*	
Stem Cell/ synergistic	SF	Synergistic; IL-3, GM-CSF, G-CSF, EPO		Mobilization of progenitor cells; gene transfer
	Flt3L	Synergistic		Same as above
	IL-11	Synergistic; IL-3		Platelet reconstitution
	IL-6	Synergistic		Gene transfer
Multilineage	IL-3	All CFC	eo, b	Gene transfer
	GM-CSF	All CFC	n, mo, eo	Mobilization; postchemotherapy or transplantation
Lineage-restricted	G-CSF	CFU-G and other CFC	n	Mobilization; postchemotherapy or transplantation; selected neutropenias
	M-CSF	CFU-M	mo	
	EPO	BFU-E, CFU-E		Renal failure
	TPO	CEU-Meg and other CFC	Platelet	Platelet reconstitution

* eo, eosinophil; b, basophil; n, polymorphonuclear neutrophil; mo, monocyte.

initial half-time of 15 to 20 minutes clearly demonstrated that infusion of the hormone at a concentration sufficient to maintain a functional blood level could be achieved (18). The effects of such infusions into normal *Macaca fascicularis* were striking. Large increments in all classes of leukocytes, including eosinophils and lymphocytes as well as reticulocytes, were observed during the hormone infusion. When the hormone treatment was terminated, the blood counts rapidly fell toward normal.

Human granulocyte colony-stimulating factor (G-CSF) also underwent simian preclinical trials. Cynomolgous monkeys treated with two daily subcutaneous injections of purified G-CSF for 14 to 28 days showed a dosage-related increase in polymorphonuclear neutrophils, the plateau being reached after 1 week (19). At the intermediate dosage of 10 μg/kg/day, total white blood cell counts of 40,000–50,000/μL were observed. Neutrophil function was also enhanced. Encouraging results were also achieved in two cyclophosphamide-treated animals that received G-CSF either from 6 days before until 21 days after the cyclophosphamide treatment, or for 14 days from day 3 after cyclophosphamide. In both monkeys, the neutrophil count increased dramatically by day 6 to 7 after cyclophosphamide, reaching levels of 50,000/μL by the tenth day. The control animal remained pancytopenic for 3 to 4 weeks after treatment.

More recently, identification of the protooncogene c-mpl (20), based on its homology to the oncogene transduced by the murine myeloproliferative leukemia virus (21,22), revealed an orphan HGF receptor important for megakaryocytopoiesis (23), and eventually led to the cloning of thrombopoietin (TPO) (24–26). Recombinant human TPO or its polyethylene glycol–derivatized 163 residue aminoterminus megakaryocyte growth and differentiation factor (PEG-MGDF) stimulates megakaryocyte proliferation and endoreduplication in vitro and is a potent inducer of megakaryocytopoiesis and platelet production in vivo in mice and nonhuman primates (24–28). Steel factor (SF), also known as kit ligand or stem cell factor (29), and Flt3 ligand (30,31) both interact with a variety of hematopoietic progenitor cells, perhaps most importantly with very early stem cell populations.

Indications

Several recombinant HGFs have been evaluated in a variety of clinical settings. Largely because of availability, initial studies focused on GM-CSF and G-CSF in both transient and long-standing bone marrow failure syndromes, and erythropoietin (EPO) in the anemia of chronic renal failure. More recently, other HGFs, such as monocyte colony-stimulating factor (M-CSF), SF, IL-1, IL-11, and TPO, have been evaluated. The availability of recombinant growth factors that stimulate myeloid progenitors raised several possibilities. First, they might shorten or prevent the hypoplasia that follows chemotherapy and make more

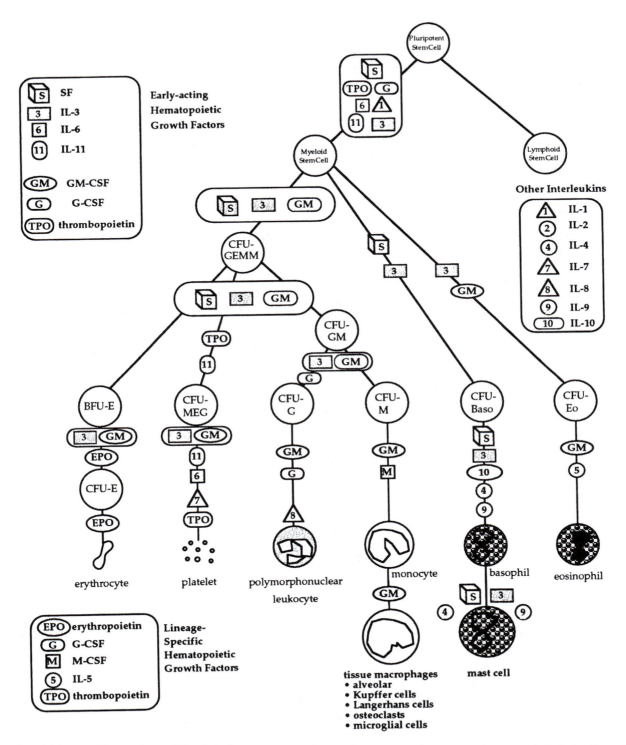

Figure 14-1. Major cytokine actions. Cells of the bone marrow microenvironment such as macrophages, endothelial cells, and reticular fibroblastoid cells produce M-CSF, GM-CSF, G-CSF, IL-6, and probably Steel factor (SF: cellular sources not yet precisely determined) after induction with endotoxin or IL-1/TNF. T cells produce IL-3, GM-CSF, and IL-5 in response to antigenic and IL-1 stimulation. These cytokines have overlapping actions during hematopoietic differentiation, as indicated, and for all lineages optimal development requires a combination of early- and late-acting factors.

intensive myeloablative chemotherapy regimes possible. However, because receptors for HGFs are expressed by several nonhematopoietic cell types, malignancies of these cell lineages might also respond to growth factor therapy. Second, they might improve hematopoiesis in conditions in which bone marrow function is more permanently impaired.

Transient Bone Marrow Failure

Malignant Disease and the Prevention of Chemotherapy-Induced Neutropenia

G-CSF. In the first phase I/II clinical studies in patients with malignant disease, administration of G-CSF by bolus or continuous intravenous infusion for 5 to 6 days before chemotherapy led to a dosage-related increase in polymorphonuclear neutrophils (32,33). Rapid increases in neutrophil counts were observed, with maximal counts of $80–100 \times 10^9$/L at dosages of 10–30 µg/kg/d. A transient depression in neutrophil counts was noted to precede this increase in one study (34). In another study, rhG-CSF was given for 14 days after alternate cycles of intensive chemotherapy (35). The period of neutropenia was reduced by a median of 80% (52% to 100%) in the chemotherapy/G-CSF cycles, with

a return to normal neutrophil counts within 2 weeks after chemotherapy. Infective episodes were observed during the cycles with chemotherapy that did not include G-CSF, while no infective episodes occurred in those that did. G-CSF treatment after chemotherapy results in a significant reduction in the number of days per patient in which the neutrophil count is less than 1.0×10^9/L (32). Antibiotic use to treat fever and neutropenia is also reduced, and all the patients could receive their next course of chemotherapy on schedule (vs. 29% of patients who did not receive G-CSF). The mature neutrophils produced in response to G-CSF have normal mobility and bactericidal capacity (36). More recently, in a double-blind, randomized, placebo-controlled U.S. multicenter trial, patients with lung carcinoma who received up to six cycles of cyclophosphamide, doxorubicin, and etoposide were given G-CSF or placebo from day 4 to day 17 of each cycle. The results showed a reduction in the median duration of severe neutropenia ($<0.5 \times 10^9$/L) from 6 to 3 days in the G-CSF arm and a 50% reduction of febrile neutropenia, hospitalizations, confirmed infections, and antibiotic use with G-CSF (Fig. 14-2) (37). This study and other reports (38,39) have led the American Society of Clinical Oncology (ASCO) to recommend the primary use of G-CSF in patients with an expected rate of neutropenia that exceeds 40% (40). The use of G-CSF has allowed dosage intensification in lung carcinoma patients, with

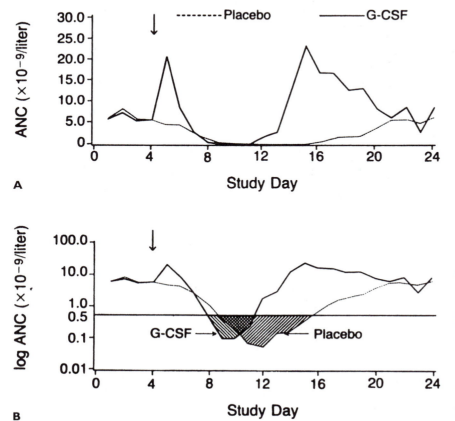

Figure 14-2. Median ANCs in the placebo and G-CSF groups represented on linear (*A*) and log (*B*) scales. Arrow represents the start of placebo or G-CSF. Hatching demonstrates the degree and duration of neutropenia. Reproduced with permission from Crawford J, Ozer H, Stoller R, et al. Reduction by granulocyte colony-stimulating factor of fever and neutropenia induced by chemotherapy in patients with small-cell lung cancer. N Engl J Med 1991;325:164–170. Copyright©1991 Massachusetts Medical Society. All rights reserved.

the suggestion that overall survival may be improved (41,42). However, larger randomized clinical trials will be needed to answer this question more conclusively. Patients in the placebo arm of the U.S. multicenter trial (37) who developed fever in the first treatment cycle were subsequently treated with G-CSF, and this reduced the duration of severe neutropenia from 6 to 3 days and neutropenic fever from 100% in cycle 1 to 23% in cycle 2. Thus, the prophylactic use of G-CSF in chemotherapy-induced neutropenia is supported. However, the literature does not support the use of G-CSF or GM-CSF once afebrile (43) or febrile neutropenia has developed (44,45), with the exception of one study (46). While the duration of neutropenia may be shortened, it has been difficult to show an effect on clinically significant endpoints such as shortened duration of hospitalization, which was reported in only one of the studies (45).

GM-CSF. Recombinant human GM-CSF (rhGM-CSF) was first administered in phase I/II studies to several groups of adult patients with advanced malignancy, both before and after chemotherapy (47–49). Glycosylated GM-CSF, produced in either mammalian (Chinese hamster ovary, or CHO) cells or yeast, and *E. coli*–derived nonglycosylated GM-CSF have been evaluated with comparable results, Rapid, dosage-related increases in polymorphonuclear neutrophils, monocytes, and eosinophils are observed in patients treated before chemotherapy. Neutrophils peak at around $20–30 \times 10^9$/L at dosages of 4–32 mg/kg/d, and are well tolerated at dosages up to this level. A capillary leak syndrome and venous thrombi are observed at higher dosages (64 mg/kg/d) (47). More recent phase III randomized trials in patients with lymphoma or breast cancer have confirmed that GM-CSF given after chemotherapy is associated with shorter periods of neutropenia and higher leukocyte nadirs (50–52). However, one of these studies included only the patients able to tolerate treatment and was not significant on an intention-to-treat basis. Furthermore, another study of GM-CSF after chemotherapy showed decreased neutropenia after the first treatment cycle only (53), while two other studies showed no improvement in neutrophil counts (54,55). In one of these studies (54), patients with small cell lung cancer were given chemotherapy and radiation; compared with the placebo control, patients in the GM-CSF arm suffered more infections, toxic deaths, and longer hospital stays, and therefore the ASCO panel has cautioned against the use of CSFs in combined chemotherapy/radiation regimens (40,56).

Similarly encouraging results have been obtained in children with solid tumors undergoing intensive chemotherapy (57–59). Significantly shorter durations of severe neutropenia and thrombocytopenia were observed in a study of 25 children in whom yeast-derived GM-CSF was given at 60–1500 µg/m²/d for 14 days after chemotherapy (57).

IL-3. A phase I/II study of the effect of rhIL-3 in patients with nonhematopoietic malignancies with normal marrow function, as well as lymphomas and bone marrow failure, was reported (60). Doses that ranged from 30–500 mg/m² were given for 15 days by daily subcutaneous injection. In the patients with normal hematopoiesis, a dosage-dependent (1.4- to 3.0-fold) increase in

neutrophils was observed, with the major increase during the second week. This contrasts with the rapid neutrophil response that has been the experience with GM-CSF or G-CSF. Platelets and eosinophils also increased in a dosage-dependent fashion up to a dosage of 250 mg/m²/d (1.3- to 1.9-fold), and increases in basophil and lymphocytes were noted. Increases in reticulocytes that did not appear to be dosage-related were also observed in 70% of the patients. Similar results were observed in the patients with bone marrow failure, but stimulation of malignant B cells was seen in two patients with lymphoma. Examination of the bone marrow showed increases in cycling of granulocyte erythroid monocyte megakaryocyte colony-forming units (CFU-GEMM), erythroid burst-forming units (BFU-E), and granulocyte monocyte colony-forming units (CFU-GM), with increased bone marrow cellularity (61). There was also an increase in blood CFU-GEMM and CFU-GM, but a reduction in BFU-E.

In conclusion, results from this initial human IL-3 study indicate that IL-3 can induce a multilineage hematopoietic response, but that increases in eosinophils and basophils may not be desirable.

TPO. Because of TPO's potent in vitro activity and its role as the factor essential for terminal megakaryocytic differentiation, analogous to EPO for the erythroid lineage, clinical studies designed to assess its effect on platelet production have recently been performed. Both rhTPO and PEG-MGDF are safe and show no organ toxicity, and in normal volunteers a single bolus of 3 µg/kg/day PEG-MGDF doubles the blood platelet concentration by day 12 with a return to baseline by day 28 [reviewed in (28)]. A stimulatory effect on platelet production was observed when TPO or PEG-MGDF was administered after chemotherapy to more than 100 cancer patients, resulting in a decrease in the time for platelet counts to return to normal and elevated platelet nadirs (62–64).

Other HGFs. IL-11 has been shown to ameliorate the thrombocytopenia associated with chemotherapy for breast cancer (65,66), and has been approved by the Food and Drug Administration for secondary prophylaxis of thrombocytopenia following chemotherapy. Partially purified urinary M-CSF has been evaluated in patients with different malignancies who received myelotoxic chemotherapy. After treatment, patients received M-CSF for 5 days, and a modest increase in neutrophils was observed. Monocytes and other hematopoietic lineages were unaffected (67). IL-1, given at 0.03, 0.1, or 0.3 µg/kg/d for 5 days, was used in 43 adults with advanced neoplasms, before or after carboplatin chemotherapy (68). A third of the patients (5/15) given one of the higher two doses after chemotherapy had minimal thrombocytopenia (platelets > 90,000/µL vs. median of 19,000/µL without IL-1).

Bone Marrow Transplantation
GM-CSF, G-CSF, and M-CSF have been evaluated in clinical autotransplantation trials.

GM-CSF. Patients with nonhematopoietic malignancies were treated with high-dosage combination chemotherapy, autologous bone marrow transplantation, and rhGM-CSF given by continuous intravenous infusion for 14 days beginning 3 hours after bone marrow infusion. There was a dosage-related increase in the neutrophil count at day 14 (1411 per μL at 2–8 mg/kg/day, 2575 per μL at 16 mg/kg/day, and 3120 per μL at 32 mg/kg/day, compared with 863 per μL in 24 historical controls) (69). Although not statistically significant, there was an improved neutrophil response in patients who had not received previous chemotherapy compared with those who had (1832 vs. 833 per μL). Lower morbidity and mortality were also noted among the patients who received the GM-CSF; bacteremia occurred in 16% of treated patients compared with 35% of evaluable controls. Comparable results were reported in a study of patients with lymphoid malignancies who received rhGM-CSF as a 2-hour infusion daily for 14 days following chemotherapy, radiotherapy, and autologous bone marrow transplantation (70). Neutrophil and platelet counts recovered more rapidly, there were fewer days with fever, and the extent of hospitalization was reduced in comparison with a historical control group. In a pediatric study, nine patients received 5–10 μg/kg/d GM-CSF after BMT. Neutrophil recovery was accelerated, although there was no difference in fever, infection, or length of hospitalization when compared with historical controls (71).

The response to GM-CSF after myelosuppression may be dependent on the infusion of sufficient progenitor cells. In an autotransplantation study of patients with acute lymphoblastic leukemia, bone marrows were purged with 4-hydroperoxycyclophosphamide and anti-T or -B cell lineage specific antibodies before transplantation (72). Thirty percent of the patients who received more than 64 μg/m^2/d achieved an absolute neutrophil count of more than 1000/μL by day 21, whereas none of the nonresponders reached this level by day 27 post transplant. The responders required only one-third as many platelet transfusions, and there were trends toward fewer red cell transfusions, higher M:E ratio, and earlier day of discharge in the responder group as well. Although bone marrow cell dosage did not differ between the two groups, the number of CFU-GM progenitors infused per kilogram was significantly higher in the responders than in the nonresponders [17.5 (12–27) × 10^3/kg vs. 2 (0–7.2) × 10^3/kg]. Although it is possible that this accounts for the more rapid recovery rather than the rhGM-CSF infusion, the responders all showed a rapid decrease in ANC within 48 to 72 hours of discontinuing GM-CSF; this is consistent with a stimulatory effect on bone marrow. One can conclude that GM-CSF is effective in this context provided that sufficient progenitor cells are present.

G-CSF. Recombinant human G-CSF was evaluated in patients with hematopoietic and nonhematopoietic malignancies after intensive chemotherapy and reinfusion of cryopreserved autologous bone marrow (73). The rhG-CSF was given by continuous IV infusion from 24 hours after marrow infusion for a maximum of 28 days, beginning at 20 μg/kg/day and reducing the dosage after the neutrophil count persistently exceeded 1×10^9/L. The

mean time to neutrophil recovery ($>0.5 \times 10^9$/L) occurred by day 11, 9 days earlier than in historical controls. This led to significantly fewer days of parental antibiotic therapy, but there was no effect on red cell or platelet recovery. Although the rate of recovery from neutropenia was faster than that reported for rhGM-CSF, the later studies were phase I dosage-escalation evaluation, and many patients did not receive an optimal dosage of GM-CSF. One study compared G-CSF with GM-CSF in exactly the same analogous bone marrow transplant protocol (74). The G-CSF group contained more patients with breast carcinoma who had received previous chemotherapy, and this group did not show a dosage-related increase in neutrophil count after a 14-day continuous IV infusion at dosages of 16, 32, and 64 μg/kg/day. Overall, however, total leukocyte recovery was slightly more rapid in the G-CSF group in comparison with the GM-CSF group. G-CSF administration resulted in two leukocyte peaks. The first, at day 10, comprised lymphocytes, while the second, at day 14, comprised mostly granulocytes; in contrast, GM-CSF produced a single peak at the end of the period of infusion. A major difference was observed with respect to neutrophil migration to an inflammatory site during CSF infusion after hematopoietic reconstitution (74). Neutrophils did not migrate to skin chambers filled with autologous serum during GM-CSF treatment, a defect not encountered during the administration of G-CSF. There were, however, similar reductions in the incidence of bacteremia with both GM-CSF and G-CSF (18% and 19%, respectively) in comparison with the historical controls (35%).

In conclusion, if neutrophil recovery is the goal following bone marrow transplantation, then G-CSF appears to be the factor of choice. It preserves neutrophil function and is well tolerated.

TPO. PEG-MGDF was evaluated in a controlled trial of 50 breast cancer patients who received chemotherapy with autologous bone marrow; the time during which the number of platelets remained below 20,000/μL was reduced ($p < 0.6$), and the time to recovery of normal platelets was significantly shortened. However, when mobilized blood progenitor support was given rather than bone marrow, the more rapid recovery made it difficult to demonstrate an effect of PEG-MGDF on duration of thrombocytopenia or platelet transfusion requirements [for a review, see (28)].

M-CSF. Human urinary M-CSF was evaluated in a phase II study of patients with different malignancies who received cyclophosphamide, total body irradiation, and either allogeneic or autologous bone marrow (75). Human urinary CSF was given for 14 days by 2-hour IV infusion daily starting at day 1, day 4, or day 14. In patients who received CSF early, there was a significant reduction in the time to a neutrophil count above 1×10^9/L when compared with a control group (16.7 vs. 25.4 days). However, the time to recovery of the control group was somewhat delayed in comparison with other reports (17 to 21 days).

Myelodysplasia

GM-CSF. Despite the theoretical risks of treating patients with myeloid stem cell clonal diseases with the CSFs, the factors have been evaluated in patients with refractory anemia (RA), RA with an excess of blasts (RAEB), RAEB in transformation (RAEBIT), and chronic myelomonocytic leukemia (76–78). In an early study, GM-CSF was given by continuous infusion for 14 days, which was repeated after a 2-week rest period (76). Five of the eight patients had received chemotherapy for up to 4 weeks before the study. Doses of 30–500 µg/m² were used. Blood leukocytes rose 5- to 70-fold and neutrophils 5- to 373-fold, and absolute increases in monocytes, eosinophils, and lymphocytes were also observed. Three of the eight patients also had 2- to 10-fold increases in platelet count and improvement in erythropoiesis, and two of the three became transfusion independent. Marrow cellularity increased and there was a reduction in the proportion of blasts, although there was a transient and dosage-related increase in the absolute number of circulating blasts. No patient developed overt leukemia during the period of follow-up (up to 32 weeks). There was no cytogenetic evidence for a reduction in abnormal clones, and it is likely that the stimulatory effect on hematopoiesis affected both normal and abnormal cells. Dosage-related increases in neutrophils, monocytes, eosinophils, and lymphocytes were also noted in a study of 11 patients with myelodysplasia. However, four patients who presented with 14% blasts in the bone marrow showed an increase in blasts after therapy, while an additional three patients showed an increase in blasts in the blood; five patients progressed to acute leukemia either during, or within 4 weeks after, treatment (78). Unlike the earlier report, none of these patients had received previous chemotherapy.

G-CSF. Patients have also been treated with G-CSF (79,80). Neutrophil responses were seen in five patients with myelodysplasia who received 50–1600 µg/m²/d by intravenous infusion daily for 6 days. At the higher dosages (400 µg/m²/d) the increase was sustained and associated with an increase in bone marrow cellularity. No reticulocyte or platelet increases were observed, and no patient progressed to an acute phase. Similar results were reported in a study of 12 patients given G-CSF by daily subcutaneous injection, with dosage escalation from 0.1 to 3 µg/kg/day over an 8-week period (80). While 10 of the 12 patients showed elevations in neutrophils (5- to 40-fold), increases in reticulocytes occurred in five patients and reductions in transfusion requirement in two. There was no response in other cell lineages and no conversion to acute leukemia.

Other HGFs and HGF Combinations. Approximately 20% of patients show increases in platelet count during treatment with IL-3 (81,82), and a similar proportion show increases in hematocrit or reduced transfusion requirements with EPO (83). This erythroid response can be increased to about 40% if EPO is combined with either G-CSF (84,85) or GM-CSF (86).

Chronic Bone Marrow Failure

Aplastic Anemia

GM-CSF. Establishing a role for the HGFs in aplastic anemia (AA) will challenge investigators. Severe AA is a heterogeneous disease that may result from either absent or defective stem cells, from microenvironmental defects, or from immunologically mediated suppression. Mortality is high and therapeutic options are limited to bone marrow transplantation if an appropriate donor is available, or to immunosuppression (see Chapter 6). While BMT can be curative, treatment with antithymocyte globulin (ATG) is sometimes effective but generally not curative. Other modalities such as cyclosporin A and androgens may be partially effective in some patients. For these reasons, rhGM-CSF has been evaluated in a number of phase I/II studies. Administration of rhGM-CSF by bolus or continuous IV infusion for 7 or 14 days resulted in increased granulocytes, monocytes, and reticulocytes in six of eight cases (77). In another small study, rhGM-CSF was given to cohorts of patients in escalating dosages from 4 to 64 µg/kg/day by continuous IV infusion for 14 days. While no dosage-related effect was observed, 10 of 11 evaluable patients had partial or complete responses in neutrophils, monocytes, and eosinophils, with increases in bone marrow cellularity. Importantly, the greatest increments occurred in patients with higher pretreatment neutrophil counts and more cellular marrows. Only 10% to 20% of patients show increases in hemoglobin concentration and platelet count, and in all cases counts return to baseline after cessation of treatment (87,88). In the first report of rhGM-CSF treatment in childhood, three-quarters of the evaluable patients responded with significant rises in neutrophil count during the 28-day induction period (89). While neutrophil counts returned to baseline after cessation of treatment in all the responders with severe AA, one patient with moderate aplasia maintained a trilineage response off therapy for more than 1 year. One cannot extrapolate from such a small experience, but the data underscore the point that responses are more likely in less severely affected cases.

Thus, in summary, it appears as though rhGM-CSF is palliative in AA, with greater neutrophil responses evident in less severely affected patients. The most severely affected patients respond poorly (90). No infections were observed during the study period in several reports, while infections were observed in others. Longer-term prospective comparative studies will be necessary to investigate morbidity.

G-CSF. Neutrophil responses have also been reported in a study of 20 children given 400 µg/m²/d G-CSF for 14 days (91). Twelve patients responded by doubling their neutrophil counts, but other lineages were unaffected. In another pediatric study, high dosages of G-CSF (400–2000 µg/m²/d) induced neutrophil responses in six of 10 patients with very severe AA (92). Long-term treatment may be associated with multilineage responses when G-CSF is given alone (93) or in combination with cyclosporine (94).

IL-3, IL-6, and EPO. Hematopoietic responses have been reported in a small phase I study of nine AA patients given IL-3 at 250–500 µg/m². Five of nine doubled their neutrophil counts; four of nine showed increases in reticulocyte counts but no reductions in transfusion requirement; and one exhibited an increased platelet count, from 1–31 × 10^9/L (60). An increase in platelet count was reported in one of six patients entered in a phase I study of IL-6, although dosage-related decreases in neutrophils, monocytes, and lymphocytes were observed, and a proportion (ca. 1/3) of patients given EPO showed reduced transfusion requirements and/or increases in Hb [reviewed by Kojima (95)]. Other promising preliminary results, including trilineage responses, have been reported in a small number of refractory AA patients treated with low-dosage GM-CSF plus EPO (96) or G-CSF plus EPO (97). The effects of EPO are unexpected since endogenous levels are very high in AA.

Human Immunodeficiency Virus (HIV) Infection

GM-CSF. HIV infection is associated with several hematologic abnormalities including neutropenia, anemia, and thrombocytopenia. Anemia and neutropenia can be exacerbated by treatment with azidothymidine, and rhGM-CSF has been evaluated in an effort to enhance immunologic and hematopoietic function and improve tolerance to therapeutic agents. In the first report of the use of rhGM-CSF in humans, cohorts of AIDS patients were treated with increasing dosages of factor given by 14-day continuous IV infusion (98). This resulted in rapid, dosage-related increases in neutrophils, bands, and eosinophils, with a slight increase in monocytes. A follow-up study with subcutaneous administration showed that these effects could be sustained for up to 6 months without evidence of tachyphylaxis (99).

A concern with the use of GM-CSF in AIDS is possible enhancement of HIV replication. In one study of azidothymidine given on an alternate-week schedule with GM-CSF, some patients showed increased viral p24 levels during therapy with GM-CSF. There is evidence, however, that GM-CSF may in fact augment azidothymidine levels in monocytes, which suggests that the combination of azidothymidine and GM-CSF might be advantageous (100). This is not the case with newer nucleoside analogues such as dideoxycytidine and dideoxyinosine [reviewed by Mueller (101)]. Two clinical studies have documented an increase in HIV p24 antigen while on GM-CSF (102,103), and therefore GM-CSF has been replaced by G-CSF for the treatment of neutropenia.

G-CSF. In a pilot study at the National Institutes of Health, G-CSF was evaluated in 19 pediatric AIDS patients who developed neutropenia while receiving azidothymidine. The neutrophil count increased from a median of 1 × 10^9/L to 2.9 × 10^9/L at dosages from 1–20 µg/kg/d, and in 17 of the 19 patients continued azidothymidine was well tolerated (104). Of note was the development of thrombocytopenia in some patients; two patients developed G-CSF dependent disseminated intravascular coagulation, and one patient developed an increase in myeloblasts that disappeared after stopping the G-CSF (101).

EPO. EPO has been used in 12 anemic pediatric patients to determine if tolerance to azidothymidine could be improved (101). EPO was well tolerated, and at dosages of 150–400 U/kg subcutaneously or intravenously three times per week, all patients could be maintained on azidothymidine with marked (four patients) or moderate (four patients) reduction in transfusion requirement.

TPO. Polyethylene glycol (PEG)–derivatized megakaryocyte growth and development factor (PEG-MGDF) has been evaluated in six HIV-infected thrombocytopenic patients in a randomized placebo-controlled study (105). Platelet counts increased 10-fold within 14 days and were sustained for the 16 weeks of the study, returning to previous levels within 2 weeks of cessation of treatment. There was no evidence of increased viral load or anti-PEG-MGDF antibodies. Megakaryocytic apoptosis, which was abnormal prior to treatment, was shifted into the normal range by TPO treatment, suggesting that the mechanism of action involves increased effectiveness of the platelets that are produced.

Bone Marrow Failure Syndromes

The use of HGFs in the treatment of inherited bone marrow failure syndromes has been reviewed in detail (106).

Fanconi Anemia (FA). GM-CSF has been studied in seven patients with FA (107), and more recently, trials of IL-3 and G-CSF have been evaluated (106). Results show that all three HGFs can improve the neutrophil counts in most pancytopenic patients, but platelet and hemoglobin levels are unaffected. On a more encouraging note, Rackoff et al treated 12 neutropenic FA patients with G-CSF for 40 weeks (108). All patients showed increases in absolute neutrophil count (ANC), and eight maintained ANC levels above 1500/mm³ on G-CSF given on alternate days; four untransfused patients exhibited increases in hemoglobin of at least 2.0 g/dL; and four showed increases in platelet count that were not maintained when the G-CSF dosage was reduced.

Diamond-Blackfan Anemia (DBA). Although there is no evidence that DBA results from deficiency of EPO (109), IL-3, or GM-CSF (110), or an abnormality of c-kit or its ligand SF (111,112), it is possible that pharmacologic dosages of these factors might stimulate erythropoiesis. Niemeyer et al (113) observed no reticulocyte or hemoglobin responses in nine patients treated with rhEPO dosages as high as 2000 U/kg/d. In contrast, three of six patients treated with IL-3 (60–125 µg/m²/d subcutaneously for 4 to 6 weeks) exhibited reticulocyte increases, and two of the responders remained transfusion independent for 1.5 to 2 years off therapy (114). Another IL-3 study (115) showed four responders out of 18 patients treated with 0.5–10 µg/kg subcutaneously. Two responders developed deep vein thromboses necessitating discontinuation of treatment, while the other two patients sustained their responses, one on maintenance IL-3 for 31 months and one off treatment for 12 months after 30 months of therapy. In another study of 13 patients, no responses were observed (116). Thus, six patients have had significant erythroid responses to IL-3 out of a total of 37 (16%), a rate similar to that reported by the European working group for DBA (3/25) (117).

Amegakaryocytic Thrombocytopenia (AMT).   AMT is a rare disease that presents in infancy or early childhood with thrombocytopenia, frequent anemia, and progression to pancytopenia. Bone marrow (BM) megakaryocytes are absent or extremely scarce. A phase I/II IL-3 dosage-escalation study without or with sequential GM-CSF in five children with AMT showed that IL-3 (but not IL-3/GM-CSF) induced platelet responses in two patients and improvements in bruising, bleeding, and transfusion requirement in the other three (118). The two platelet responders became unresponsive after several months of IL-3 maintenance ($125-250\,\mu g/m^2/d$), while another patient became platelet transfusion independent after 4 months of IL-3 and had a trilineage response sustained for almost 2 years. Five patients have been treated with PIXY321 (IL-3/GM-CSF fusion protein) and in two the platelet count increased (106). Trilineage responses were observed in three of 14 patients with AMT and other BM failure syndromes, and PIXY321 was well tolerated and may be considered as potential therapy (119). However, antibodies to the fusion protein have been reported.

Kostmann Disease.   Severe congenital neutropenia or Kostmann disease (KD) is a disorder of myelopoiesis characterized by impaired neutrophil differentiation and absolute neutrophil counts less than $200/\mu L$. In contrast, monocytes and eosinophils are normal or increased. The bone marrow shows maturation arrest at the promyelocyte stage, and these cells are often atypical, with abnormal nuclei and vacuolated cytoplasm. The pathophysiology is uncertain. Serum from these patients contains normal or elevated levels of G-CSF, as determined by Western blot and bioassay (120). A progenitor defect is more likely, since in vitro cultures show normal CFU-M and CFU-Eo but impaired differentiation of CFU-G in the presence of either GM-CSF or G-CSF. G-CSF receptors show normal number and affinity in other KD patients (121), and single-strand conformational polymorphism analysis of the cytoplasmic domain of the receptor showed no evidence for structural abnormality in six patients (122). Furthermore, JAK2, a nonreceptor tyrosine kinase involved in G-CSF signaling, shows increased phosphorylation in response to G-CSF in neutrophils from KS patients in comparison with normal (123). It is still possible, however, that a defect in the G-CSF signal transduction pathway will be identified.

The responses of these patients to exogenous G-CSF and GM-CSF are therefore of great interest. One study has compared the effects of GM-CSF and G-CSF in a small number of patients, and G-CSF alone was evaluated in other studies (124–126). In these investigations, *G-CSF produced a remarkable increase in neutrophils in all patients.* The dosage necessary to maintain a neutrophil count above $1000/\mu L$ varied, and ranged from $3-15\,\mu g/kg/day$. The monocyte count was also increased. In contrast, rhGM-CSF produced an increase in neutrophils in only one

patient, while the others showed increases in both eosinophils and monocytes. Although the period of study was short, no new episodes of severe bacterial infection occurred during either GM-CSF or G-CSF treatment; this contrasts with the recurrent bacterial and fungal infections that occurred before treatment. A multicenter phase III study of G-CSF in 120 patients with severe chronic neutropenic disorders including KD, Shwachman-Diamond syndrome, and myelokathexis showed complete responses in 108 patients (ANC $> 1.5 \times 10^9/L$), partial responses in four patients, and failure to respond in eight patients (127).

Somatic mutations of a single allele of the G-CSFR that result in loss of the c-terminal "differentiation" domain of the receptor were described in several KS patients, and were shown to act as a dominant negative in transduced cells (128,129). These patients may go on to develop myelodysplastic syndrome (MDS) and/or acute myeloblastic leukemia (AML) (130). Data from the SCN International Registry (131) on 506 patients with severe congenital neutropenia, cyclic neutropenia, and idiopathic neutropenia who were treated in phase I–III clinical G-CSF trials showed that 23 of 249 KS/Shwachman-Diamond (neutropenia and pancreatic insufficiency) patients developed MDS/AML, in comparison with none of the 97 cyclic or 160 idiopathic neutropenia patients. The observation that KS but not cyclic or idiopathic neutropenia patients on G-CSF develop MDS/AML is consistent with reports of AML in KS before the introduction of G-CSF treatment (132,133), and show that KS is a preleukemic disease. Additional cytogenetic changes (translocations and monosomy 7) and oncogene (ras) mutations are common in the patients that go on to develop MDS/AML (134). The G-CSFR mutation is present in myeloid cells only and was not present in first-degree relatives of affected patients, including a sibling with KS (135), demonstrating that the mutation is acquired.

In summary, although the genetic abnormality that causes KS has not yet been identified, treatment with recombinant G-CSF has had a major positive impact on the lives of the majority of these patients. This continued treatment has increased the risk of emergence of leukemic clones in this preleukemic disease, and patients need to be monitored regularly for their acquisition.

Cyclic Neutropenia.   Cyclic neutropenia is a rare hematopoietic stem cell disease characterized by regular 21-day cyclic fluctuations in numbers of neutrophils, monocytes, eosinophils, lymphocytes, platelets, and reticulocytes. Patients typically have recurrent episodes of fever, malaise, mucosal ulceration, and occasionally life-threatening infection during periods of neutropenia. Six patients were treated with intravenous or subcutaneous rhG-CSF for 3 to 15 months at dosages ranging from 3–$10\,\mu g/kg/day$ (136). The median neutrophil count increased from $0.7 \times 10^9/L$ to $9.8 \times 10^9/L$. In five of the patients, cycling of blood counts continued, but the length of the cycles decreased from 21 to 14 days. The number of days of severe neutropenia ($<200/\mu L$) was reduced from a mean of 12.7 per month to less than 1 per month and, importantly, the nadir counts increased; neutrophil turnover increased almost 4-fold; and migration to a skin window was normal. Average counts of other cells did not increase. One patient with disease of adult onset had a qualitatively different response with an increase in neutrophils and disappearance of the cyclic fluctuations in count. Therapy reduced the frequency of oropharyngeal inflammation, fever, and infections, demonstrating that treatment with rhG-CSF is effective management for such patients. These results have been confirmed, and rhG-CSF has been well tolerated, in other studies (137–139). GM-CSF was not effective in two patients but eliminated severe neutropenia when given in a low dosage (0.3 µg/kg/d) (140–142).

Chronic Idiopathic Neutropenia. This disorder of myelopoiesis is characterized by maturation arrest of neutrophil precursors in the bone marrow, neutrophil counts of less than 1.5×10^9/L, and normal other cell lineages. Patients have mucosal ulcers, periodontal disease, and recurrent infections. The pathophysiology is uncertain; in vitro bone marrow cultures show normal numbers of myeloid progenitors, and antineutrophil antibodies are absent. A single patient who received 1–3 µg/kg/day rhG-CSF by subcutaneous injection showed normalization of the absolute neutrophil count with healing of chronic oral ulceration, reduction of episodes of recurrent infection, and minimal side effects (143). Cycling of neutrophils, monocytes, and platelets was induced with a 40-day periodicity; this contrasts with the normal 21-day cycle and out-of-phase fluctuation of neutrophils and monocytes seen in cyclic neutropenia.

Anemia of Chronic Renal Failure (CRF)

Erythropoietin. Anemia is a major complication of end-stage renal failure, and is due primarily to a reduction in EPO production. Other mechanisms that may be involved are shortened red cell survival, iron deficiency, hypersplenism, possible circulating inhibitors of erythropoiesis, and aluminum-induced microcytosis. Several phase I, II, and III studies have documented that rhEPO can induce a dosage-dependent increase in effective erythropoiesis (144–146).

In a phase III study, patients received 150 or 300 U rhEPO three times per week following hemodialysis, and reached a target hematocrit of 35% by 8 to 12 weeks (145,146). The majority of patients required 50–125 U/kg IV three times per week following dialysis to maintain a hematocrit of approximately 35%. The increase in erythropoiesis required to normalize the hemoglobin requires mobilization of a considerable amount of iron; patients who improve, and particularly those who improve rapidly, can develop absolute or relative iron deficiency. If iron is not given, the response to rhEPO becomes blunted; the standard corrective measure is IV administration of iron dextran or oral iron supplementation. Regular measurements of ferritin and transferrin saturation are necessary to ensure that iron stores are adequate.

Erythropoietin has been well tolerated, has resulted in elimination of transfusion dependency, and has not led to antibody formation. *Hypertension*, occasionally with *encephalopathy*, has been observed, particularly with rapid rises in hematocrit that lead to an increase in peripheral vascular resistance; induction with doses not greater than 150 U/kg is recommended to produce a gradual increase in hemoglobin level. Some patients require

either the initiation of antihypertensive medication or an adjustment of dosage.

The effect of rhEPO in most studies appears to be restricted to the erythroid lineage. However, data from a phase III study of 303 patients show a significant increase in mean platelet count (224×10^9/L to 241×10^9/L at 6 months), which is not biologically meaningful. There is also a slight increase in blood urea nitrogen, creatinine, and serum potassium levels. The bone marrow progenitors from patients with end-stage renal failure were studied before and 2 weeks after rhEPO treatment. The concentrations of BFU-E, CFU-E, and CFU-Meg increased after therapy. Surprisingly, an increment in CFU-GM also occurred, and the number of progenitors of all classes in cell cycle almost doubled (147).

Subjective improvements in appetite, energy, sleep pattern, and libido are also noted. A Canadian double-blind placebo-controlled study of rhEPO treatment has provided objective evidence of benefit.

Extending this treatment to patients who do not yet require dialysis has met with similar success (148). An issue that has yet to be resolved is financial; rhEPO is not inexpensive, and the National Kidney Foundation in the USA has issued guidelines for the use of rhEPO in which all patients with a hematocrit of <30% will be eligible. rhEPO is more effective when administered by the subcutaneous route, and this will be more convenient for patients and also will allow a dosage reduction (149,150). In predialysis patients, 100 U/kg given subcutaneously provided a response similar to that of 150 U/kg given intravenously (149). There is evidence that the bioavailability of subcutaneous EPO is 7 times greater than that of intravenously administered drug, and a recent large controlled study showed that the mean EPO dosage to maintain a stable hematocrit was 32% lower by the subcutaneous than the intravenous route (151).

Similar results have been obtained in several rhEPO studies in children [reviewed by Müller-Wiefel and Amon (152)]. Anemia was corrected within 3 to 4 months in 24 children with preterminal CRF treated with rhEPO and iron treatment, which was adjusted by careful monitoring of iron status. Hypertension is the most common side effect (153–156). Interestingly, while the growth failure of children with terminal CRF is unaffected by rhEPO treatment, mean growth velocity in 22 children with preterminal CRF increased from −2.29 to −0.56 within the first 6 months of treatment (152). Other reported benefits include delay in progression of renal dysfunction in children with preterminal CRF and improvement in cognitive function.

Other Indications for Recombinant Erythropoietin Therapy

Several small clinical trials have evaluated the use of rhEPO in the anemia of prematurity (157–163). These studies have been reviewed by Mentzer and Shannon (164), and although study differences in patient population, transfusion criteria, rhEPO dosage, and iron therapy make comparisons difficult, rhEPO treatment is safe and stimulates a reticulocyte response. An effect on hematocrit was observed only in the studies in which dosages greater than 500 U/kg/week were used (157,159,161,162), and there appears to be a modest effect on transfusion requirement. Increasing the dosage from 750 U/kg/week to 1500 U/kg/week was not supported by a large European study of 184 very-low-birth-weight infants (165).

Preliminary data suggest that rhEPO may be useful in the treatment of patients with the anemia of chronic disease associated with rheumatoid arthritis (166) and the anemia that complicates azidothymidine treatment in patients with AIDS (discussed above).

In simian studies, hemoglobin F levels can be increased by administration of EPO (167). If similar changes occur in humans, EPO may have a role in the management of sickle cell disease and thalassemia. Several small studies in sickle cell disease have shown that an F reticulocytosis can occur in some patients, while other patients show an increase in hemoglobin without a sustained F reticulocyte response, a finding that is of some concern since blood viscosity might be increased (168). There are also data to suggest that hydroxyurea in combination with EPO can augment the F reticulocyte response, although the contribution of EPO is still uncertain (169,170). In patients with transfusion-dependent or untransfused thalassemia, variable responses to EPO alone have also been reported (171–174), with some patients showing increases in hemoglobin and F cells. The only report to show a consistent increase in fetal hemoglobin was a study of 10 untransfused thalassemic patients who received rhEPO (400–800 U/kg three times weekly) as well as iron and hydroxyurea 4 days per week. Hemoglobin increased significantly in eight of the 10 patients, with concomitant increases in fetal hemoglobin 5% to 20% above baseline (174).

Finally, EPO can be used to increase the number of units of blood that can be obtained preoperatively in the context of autologous blood donation (175).

Osteopetrosis

An interesting series of studies showed that osteopetrotic op/op mice do not produce M-CSF (176,177), that the op locus maps to the same region of chromosome 3 as the M-CSF gene, and that fibroblasts from the mice have a single base insertional mutation in the M-CSF gene that results in a premature stop codon (178). Based on the observations that osteopetrosis in op/op mice can be corrected by M-CSF treatment (179–181) a phase I/II study was designed to evaluate escalating dosages of M-CSF in children with severe infantile osteopetrosis (182). Preliminary results in one patient showed a partial response; in particular, growth velocity was maintained, and relatively normal bone trabecular formation was observed on biopsy after 2 months of treatment. However, biochemical evidence of bone resorption was not seen.

Osteoclastic superoxide production and bone resorption can be stimulated by IFN-γ in osteopetrotic mi/mi mice (183), and this cytokine has been evaluated in a phase I/II study in 14 patients with osteopetrosis (184). An increase in leukocyte superoxide production, a decrease in trabecular bone volume, and an increase in hemoglobin and platelet counts after 6 months of treatment were measured.

Stem and Progenitor Cell Mobilization

The effect of G-CSF on progenitor cells is interesting. After melphalan and G-CSF, the absolute numbers of *circulating* progenitor cells of the granulocyte-macrophage, erythroid, mixed, and megakaryocyte lineages show dosage-related increases up to 100-fold after 4 days of treatment with rhG-CSF (185), confirming earlier animal studies (186,187). The relative proportions of the early and late granulocyte progenitors and of early progenitors of different lineages remain unchanged; however, CFU-E, normally undetectable in blood, is markedly increased. The mechanism for the increase in all progenitors in the blood is unclear; G-CSF has been shown to affect immature blast colony-forming cells, and it is possible that stem cells are stimulated in vivo to produce increased progenitors of all classes. Alternatively, G-CSF may indirectly stimulate progenitors by induction of HGF production, or by release into the circulation of bone marrow progenitor cells. Like G-CSF, GM-CSF also produced an increase in blood progenitor cells of both erythroid and myeloid lineages. Before chemotherapy, an 18-fold increase in blood CFU-GM and an 8-fold increase in BFU-E were noted; after chemotherapy, GM-CSF produced a much greater increase of progenitors (60-fold) when given during the recovery period (188).

These early studies set the stage for attempts at high-dosage chemotherapy followed by mobilized blood progenitor cell rescue in a number of chemosensitive tumors such as lymphoma, breast cancer, and multiple myeloma. Time to engraftment is critically related to the number of CD34+ cells infused, and several studies indicate that a dosage of no less than 5×10^6 CD34+ cells/kg results in prompt neutrophil and platelet engraftment (189–192). G-CSF is the usual HGF used to mobilize progenitors, and four or more apheresis procedures are commonly required to achieve this dosage of CD34+ cells. Strategies to increase the yield and thereby reduce the number of apheresis procedures include the combination of G-CSF with chemotherapy, SF (192–195), TPO (196,197), a high-affinity IL-3 receptor agonist (198), and FL in animal studies (199–203). Two studies suggest that SF in combination with G-CSF can decrease the number of required apheresis procedures (192,204), which might be expected to have several advantages, including reduction of apheresis-associated morbidity, less delay in administration of chemotherapy, and decreased cost.

Ex Vivo Expansion of Stem and Progenitor Cells

The recognition that HGFs play a major role in the proliferation and differentiation of immature cells has led to intense interest in ex vivo expansion of stem and progenitor cells for clinical use. Since the rapidity, degree, and longevity of engraftment are dependent on the number and quality of transplanted stem cells, the ability to expand these critical cells might have great clinical potential in graft engineering, tumor purging, and gene therapy. Current efforts to achieve the goal of ex vivo culture and amplification of hematopoietic stem cells (HSCs) have mainly involved the use of different cytokine combinations. However, there is little evidence to support the notion that the true long-term repopulating HSC (LTR-HSC) can be induced to divide and self-renew in such conditions, raising the concern that even if cell division is induced, the dividing cells may differentiate and eventually die. Several factors, such as SF, FL, TPO IL-3, IL-6, IL-11, G-CSF, and GM-CSF, appear to act on very primitive hematopoietic cells, including stem cells. Despite intensive investigation, only murine studies have demonstrated that cytokines can indeed increase self-renewal among the most immature HSCs capable of self-renewal and long-term hematopoietic reconstitution (205,206). In human studies, the lack of a suitable stem cell assay has made it difficult to investigate the regulatory mechanisms of HSC self-renewal. Very high concentrations of a combination of SF, FL, and IL-3 can lead to significant expansion of primitive human hematopoietic long-term culture-initiating cells (LTC-ICs) (207), but the relationship of this cell to LTR-HSC is uncertain. Recent data using a xenogeneic assay in which human cells are injected into immunodeficient nonobese diabetic/severe combined immu-nodeficient (NOD/SCID) mice suggest that the SCID repopu-lating cell (SRC) assay detects a cell more primitive than the LTC-IC (208–211). Recent reports suggest that it may be possi-ble to maintain or increase SRC numbers in serum-free cultures supplemented with a cytokine combination that comprises SF, FL, IL-3, IL-6, and G-CSF (212,213). However, our data (214) show that incubation of cord blood CD34$^+$ cells in a similar com-bination of cytokines (SF, FL, IL-3) results in rapid loss of SRC activity over 3 days. These data emphasize the need for new approaches to investigate and induce HSC self-renewal and for caution in the clinical use of these ex vivo expanded cells.

Ex vivo expanded progenitors were first used clinically by Brugger et al (215), who cultured CD34$^+$ mobilized blood prog-enitors in the combination of SF, IL-1, IL-3, IL-6, and EPO and showed rapid short-term engraftment of autografts given to breast cancer patients after high-dosage chemotherapy. However, it was not possible to assess the contribution of these unmarked cells to long-term reconstitution. When expanded progenitors were used in a similar protocol in myeloablated patients with hematopoietic malignancies, short-term but not long-term engraftment was observed, with failure to achieve sustained neu-trophil engraftment and no evidence of platelet reconstitution (216).

In addition to attempts to expand the stem cell population and perhaps partly because this aim has been rather difficult to achieve, there is considerable interest in amplifying "post-progenitor" cells—that is, myeloid and platelet precursors—for therapeutic use. Although a number of different HGF combina-tions can generate impressive amplification, clinically effective use of these cells has yet to be achieved [reviewed by Scheding et al (217)].

Gene Transfer into Hematopoietic Stem Cells

Retrovirus-mediated gene transfer into long-lived pluripotent HSCs could provide permanent correction of hematopoietic gene dysfunction in a variety of genetic diseases. However, the results of clinical gene therapy trials have been disappointing, owing to the low efficiency of gene transfer into HSCs and/or poor expres-sion in the differentiated progeny of these cells (218–221). Major problems regarding human retrovirus–mediated gene transfer include poor HSC expression of amphotropic receptors for the retroviral envelope gene (222,223) and the quiescent state of the majority of HSCs, which does not favor the integration of retro-viral vectors, since cell division is thought to be required (224). Difficulties in assaying human HSCs have compounded these problems, and protocols for clinical trials based on results from in vitro clonogenic assays of human progenitors, in particular the long-term culture-initiating cell (LTC-IC) assay, have not corre-lated with clinical outcomes.

One approach to the amphotropic receptor problem has been the development of new vectors such as Moloney murine leukemia virus–based retrovirus pseudotyped with the vesicular stomatitis virus G protein (VSV-G) (225). VSV-G pseudotyped retroviruses, like conventional retroviruses, can stably integrate into the host genome, but have a much broader host range than conventional retroviruses and are more stable, thus permitting concentration by ultracentrifugation to more than 10^9 infectious particles per milliliter (226,227). These vectors can efficiently infect mammalian and nonmammalian cells that are resistant to infection by conventional Moloney-based retroviruses.

The problem of stem cell quiescence is usually approached by using HGFs ex vivo to stimulate murine (228) or human (229–231) stem and progenitor cells into cycle, and this paradigm has driven much research in animal models and clinical trials. The human studies are based on investigations showing that stimula-tion with combinations of HGFs such as IL-3, IL-6, and SF can increase the efficiency of gene transfer into LTC-ICs in clinically applicable supernatant infection procedures in the absence of stroma (232,233). While stromal support has been shown to increase the efficiency of gene transfer, and may be necessary for optimal stem cell survival (233–235), stromal-based gene transfer methods are impractical. Despite these laboratory advances, HSC gene transfer efficiency in primate (236,237) and human (218–221) clinical studies has been disappointingly low. Although strategies using combinations of HGFs have increased the effi-ciency of gene transfer into in vitro clonogenic progenitors, there is little evidence that cytokines increase the frequency of gene transfer into long-term repopulating stem cells as measured in blood cells obtained from patients. Indeed, it is possible that stimulation with HGFs may irreversibly alter HSC proper-ties, and there is now strong evidence that sustained HSC self-renewal may not be possible (238–240). Instead, the potential of HSCs to self-renew is finite, determined by replicative history (241,242).

Ex Vivo Response of SRC to Hematopoietic Growth Factors

In a system that is modeled closely on human bone marrow trans-plantation and the long-term repopulation assay in mice, Kamel-Reid and Dick injected 10^7 human bone marrow cells into irradiated bg/nu/xid mice. By molecular analysis, low levels (0.1% to 1%) of DNA from bone marrow and spleen were positive with a human probe, and these organs also contained human progenitor cells (208). Improved results with this technique have come from increasing the cell dosage, regular intraperitoneal injections of SF, IL-3/GM-CSF fusion protein (PIXY-321), and EPO (243), and use of the NOD/SCID strain, which in addition to the T- and B-cell defects present in SCID mice has defects of innate immunity in NK cells, macrophages, and complement (244–246). Cell fractionation and gene marking studies provide some evidence that the NOD/SCID repopulating cell (SRC) is more primitive than the LTC-IC (211,247). Although SRC may still be a heterogeneous population of cells that includes long-term repopulating HSC, this assay provides a better measure of stem cell properties than the LTC-IC assay, especially with regard to the multipotent (i.e., myeloid and lymphoid) and self-renewal properties of HSCs. Recent reports suggest that it may be possible to maintain or increase SRC numbers in serum-free cultures supplemented with a cytokine combination comprising SF, FL, IL-3, IL-6, and G-CSF (212,213). These findings appear to conflict with our data that SRC number and quality decline rapidly in culture (214). However, Conneally et al (212) report that after culture the numbers of CFCs and LTC-ICs generated per SRC are lower than before culture, despite correction for the observed twofold increase in the number of SRCs. Data from Bhatia et al (213) suggest a decline in the quality of SRCs as well. They calculate a fourfold increase in SRCs after 4 days in culture; however, despite this increase, the level of engraftment of 500 CD34$^+$CD38$^-$ cells was low (<1%), similar to the level obtained with fourfold fewer day 0 cells (247). This is consistent with their further observation that by day 9 no SRC activity was detectable at all. Thus, in summary, it is still uncertain whether human HSCs can be maintained, expanded, or induced to cycle ex vivo, and these obstacles still present major challenges to successful gene therapy.

Toxicity of CSF Treatment

The CSFs tested in all these clinical trials have in general been well tolerated. Both GM-CSF and G-CSF induce a *transient leukopenia* in the first 30 minutes after administration by intravenous bolus injection. GM-CSF rapidly induces surface expression of the leukocyte adhesion protein CD11b (MO1) in vitro, and this is accompanied by an increase in neutrophil aggregation (248). CD11a (LFA-1) and CD11c (gp 150, 95), two other members of this family of cell surface adhesion glycoproteins that have distinct α-chains but share a common β-chain (CD18) with CD11b, are unaffected by GM-CSF. These results have been corroborated by in vivo studies of sarcoma patients who received 32 or 64 µg/kg/day GM-CSF. A marked increase of CD11b was noted that was evident by 30 minutes and persisted for 12 to 24 hours after treatment (188). Radionuclide-labeled leukocytes are sequestered in the lungs after GM-CSF treatment (34), probably owing to the aggregability and adhesiveness induced by increased CD11b expression. Breathlessness and hypoxia have been observed in some patients, particular after short-duration IV administration. CD11b is not modulated by G-CSF, and the reason for the transient leukopenia following treatment with G-CSF is at present unclear.

Both GM-CSF and G-CSF have been associated with *bone pain* coincident with or shortly after administration. Occasional increases in leukocyte alkaline phosphatase and/or lactate dehydrogenase have been noted. In contrast, GM-CSF has also induced *flu-like symptoms*, including fever, flushing malaise, myalgia, arthralgia, anorexia, and headache. Mild elevations of *transaminase levels* and *rash* are also reported. These effects are usually mild, are alleviated by antipyretics, and disappear with continued administration. More serious GM-CSF toxicity has been observed at higher dosage levels (>32 µg/kg/day IV or >15 µg/kg/day SC). These include a *capillary leak syndrome* with weight gain due to fluid retention, manifested as pericardial or pleural effusions, ascites, and/or edema (47,69). *Phlebitis* was noted in initial studies when the GM-CSF was infused into small veins; large-vessel thrombosis has occurred with infusion of high doses into central veins (47). Subcutaneously administered SF frequently causes injection-site reactions (204) and has also been associated with severe systemic allergic reactions that are thought to be mast cell–related (249).

Antibodies to Recombinant Factors

rhGM-CSF that is produced in mammalian cells [Chinese hamster ovary (CHO) cells] is variably glycosylated on both O-linked and N-linked sites. Production in *E. coli* results in nonglycosylated GM-CSF, and the yeast product is glycosylated on N-linked sites. All three products appear to be equally efficacious, but antibodies have been reported in four of 13 patients given the yeast-derived product in phase I/II studies (250). The IgG antibodies developed by 7 days after the start of the infusion in all four patients, three of whom had received bolus test doses; the antibodies were non-neutralizing as judged by bone marrow colony-forming assay, and they were directed at sites on the protein backbone of the GM-CSF molecule that are normally protected by O-linked glycosylation but that are exposed in the yeast-derived and *E. coli*–derived products. Antibodies to TPO have been reported in one cancer patient (251) and in volunteers given PEG-MGDF, and further clinical development of this TPO formulation has been stopped, since transient decreases in platelet count were noted (28,252). No dosage-limiting toxicity has been observed with G-CSF. However, one case of pathogenic *neutrophil infiltration* (*acute febrile neutrophilic dermatosis* or *Sweet's syndrome*) has been reported (253). One patient with Kostmann disease (KD) developed *cutaneous necrotizing vasculitis* (*leukoclastic vasculitis*) while on G-CSF treatment (120,125). As noted above, there is also concern that G-CSF will induce or accelerate the development of *acute myeloblastic leukemia or myelodysplasia with monosomy 7* in aplastic anemia and KD, perhaps more likely in those patients with G-CSF receptor mutations that can transduce a proliferative but not a differentiation signal.

Fever is the most frequent side effect associated with administration of human urinary M-CSF (67,75). Malaise, headache, and slight depression of blood pressure have also been observed.

Future Directions

It is interesting that of all the HGFs, two lineage-specific factors, G-CSF and EPO, have proven to be most useful clinically as stimulators of granulocytic and erythroid progenitors and precursors for both transient and selected chronic bone marrow failure states. Combinations of these late-acting factors with those that act synergistically on stem cells will certainly find roles in mobilization strategies to harvest stem and progenitor cells. However, a better understanding of the molecular mechanisms that control stem cell trafficking would potentially allow specific manipulation of these events. Papayannopoulou and colleagues (254–256) have demonstrated the importance of VLA-4, expressed on progenitor cells, and its receptor VCAM-1, expressed by stromal cells, in the localization of stem cells to the marrow. Antibodies to these molecules show that they play a role in the homing of stem cells to the marrow and in the mobilization of stem/progenitor cells from bone marrow to blood, an active mechanism that appears to require signaling through the SF receptor c-kit (257).

Whether a combination of factors will allow expansion of stem cells is perhaps more doubtful, and one may have to move toward more novel methods of manipulating self-renewal as understanding of this key event in hematopoiesis is increased. As an example, murine bone marrow cells engineered to overexpress HOXB4 by retrovirus-mediated gene transfer show a dramatic up-regulation in stem cell activity both in vitro and in vivo (258). Serial transplantation studies have shown a greatly enhanced ability of HOXB4-transduced bone marrow cells to regenerate the most primitive hematopoietic stem cell compartment, resulting in 50-fold higher numbers of transplantable totipotent hematopoietic stem cells in primary and secondary recipients, compared with serially passaged control (neotransduced) cells. It is possible that overexpression of other transcription factors that drive hematopoietic development might allow stem cell decisions to be manipulated.

Another area that holds great promise for future manipulation of the hematopoietic system is the development of small molecules or peptides that bind to specific receptors, with the objective of finding high-affinity second-generation drugs that may be developed into oral agents. Remarkable progress has been made in the identification of a 13 amino acid EPO mimetic peptide (259–261) whose activity can be markedly increased by the construction of covalent dimers of the peptide (262–264). A second example is the high-affinity IL-3 receptor agonist that shows promise in preclinical large animal studies (265–267).

Conclusion

Advances in molecular and cell biology have led to an unraveling of some of the most challenging and confusing aspects of the study of hematopoiesis. Therapeutic benefits are rapidly emerging from these discoveries. The field of hematopoiesis, once a jumble of unknown factors and activities, has come of age and is providing direct benefits to countless patients.

References

1. Bradley TR, Metcalf D. The growth of mouse bone marrow cells in vitro. Aust J Exp Biol Med Sci 1966;44:287–293.
2. Pluznik DH, Sachs L. The cloning of normal "mast" cells in tissue cultures. J Cell Comp Physiol 1965;66:319–324.
3. Metcalf D. The molecular control of blood cells. Cambridge: Harvard University Press, 1988.
4. Metcalf D. Hemopoietic regulators and leukemia development: a personal retrospective. Adv Cancer Res 1994;63:41–91.
5. Clark SC, Kamen R. The human hematopoietic colony-stimulating factors. Science 1987;236:1229–1237.
6. Metcalf D. The colony stimulating factors. Cancer 1990;65:2185–2195.
7. Moore MAS. Haemopoietic growth factor interactions: in vitro and in vivo preclinical evaluation. Cancer Surv 1990;9:7–80.
8. Wong GG, Clark SC. Multiple actions of interleukin-6 within a cytokine network. Immunol Today 1988;9:137–139.
9. Bazan JF. Neuropoietic cytokines in the hematopoietic fold. Neuron 1991;7:197–208.
10. Bazan JF. Emerging families of cytokines and receptors. Curr Biol 1993;3:603.
11. Pestka S, Langer JA, Zoon KC, Samuel CE. Interferons and their actions. Annu Rev Biochem 1987;56:727–777.
12. Strober W, James SP. The interleukins. Ped Res 1988;24:549–557.
13. Shalaby MR, Pennica D, Palladino MA Jr. An overview of the history and biologic properties of tumor necrosis factors. Springer Semin Immunopathol 1986;9:33–37.
14. Fung MC, Hapel AJ, Yuner S, et al. Molecular cloning for cDNA for murine interleukin-3. Nature 1984;307:233–237.
15. Yokota T, Lee T, Rennick D, et al. Isolation and characterization of a mouse cDNA clone that expresses mast-cell growth factor activity in monkey cells. Proc Natl Acad Sci USA 1984;81:1070–1074.
16. Kindler J, Thorens B, De Kossodo S, et al. Stimulation of hematopoiesis in vivo by recombinant bacterial murine interleukin 3. Proc Natl Acad Sci USA 1986;83:1001–1005.
17. Metcalf D, Begley CG, Johnson GR, et al. Effects of purified bacterially synthesized murine multi-CSF (IL-3) on hematopoiesis in normal adult mice. Blood 1986;68:46–57.
18. Donahue RE, Wang EA, Stone DK, et al. Stimulation of hematopoiesis in primates by continuous infusion of recombinant human GM-CSF. Nature 1986;321:872–875.
19. Welte K, Bonilla MA, Gillio AP, et al. Recombinant human granulocyte-colony-stimulating factor: effects on hematopoiesis in normal and cyclophosphamide treated primates. J Exp Med 1987;165:941–948.
20. Wendling F, Maraskovsky E, Debili N, et al. c-Mpl ligand is a humoral regulator of megakaryocytopoiesis. Nature 1994;369:571–574.
21. Wendling F, Varlet P, Charon M, et al. A retrovirus complex including an acute myeloproliferative leukemia virus immortalizes hematopoietic progenitors. Virology 1986;149:242.
22. Souyri M, Vigon I, Penciolelli JF, et al. A putative truncated cytokine receptor gene transduced by the myeloproliferative leukemia virus immortalizes hematopoietic progenitors. Cell 1990;63:1137–1147.

23. Methia N, Louache F, Vainchenker W, Wendling F. Oligodeoxynucleotides antisense to the protooncogene c-mpl specifically inhibit in vitro megakaryocytopoiesis. Blood 1993;82:1395–1401.
24. de Sauvage FJ, Hass PE, Spencer SD, et al. Stimulation of megakaryocytopoiesis and thrombopoiesis by the c-Mpl ligand. Nature 1994;369:533–538.
25. Bartley TD, Bogenberger J, Hunt P, et al. Identification and cloning of a megakaryocyte growth and development factor that is a ligand for the cytokine receptor Mpl. Cell 1994;77: 1117–1124.
26. Lok S, Kaushansky K, Holly RD, et al. Cloning and expression of murine thrombopoietin cDNA and stimulation of platelet production in vivo. Nature 1994;369:565.
27. Harker LA, Marzec UM, Hunt P, et al. Dose-response effects of pegylated human megakaryocyte growth and development factor on platelet production and function in nonhuman primates. Blood 1996;88:511–521.
28. Harker LA. Physiology and clinical applications of platelet growth factors [In Process Citation]. Curr Opin Hematol 1999;6:127–134.
29. Galli SJ, Zsebo KM, Geissler EN. The kit ligand, stem cell factor. Adv Immunol 1994;55:1–95.
30. Hannum C, Culpepper J, Campbell D, et al. Ligand for FLT3/FLK2 receptor tyrosine kinase regulates growth of haematopoietic stem cells and is encoded by variant RNAs. Nature 1994;368:643–648.
31. Lyman SD, James L, Johnson L, et al. Cloning of the human homologue of the murine flt3 ligand: a growth factor for early hematopoietic progenitor cells. Blood 1994;83:2795–2801.
32. Gabrilove J, Jakubowski A, Scher H, et al. Effect of granulocyte colony-stimulating factor on neutropenia and associated morbidity due to chemotherapy for transitional-cell carcinoma of the urothelium. N Engl J Med 1988;318:1414–1422.
33. Morstyn G, Campbell L, Souza LM, et al. Effect of granulocyte colony stimulating factor on neutropenia induced by cytotoxic chemotherapy. Lancet 1988;I:667–672.
34. Devereaux S, Linch DC, Campos-Costa D, et al. Transient leucopenia induced by granulocyte-macrophage colony-stimulating factor. Lancet 1987;2:1523.
35. Bronchud MH, Scarffe JH, Thatcher N, et al. Phase I/II study of recombinant human granulocyte colony-stimulating factor in patients receiving intensive chemotherapy for small cell lung cancer. Br J Cancer 1987;56:809–813.
36. Kodo H, Tajika K, Takahashi S, et al. Acceleration of neutrophilic granulocyte recovery after bone-marrow transplantation by the administration of recombinant human granulocyte colony-stimulating factor. Lancet 1988;2:38–39.
37. Crawford J, Ozer H, Stoller R, et al. Reduction by granulocyte colony-stimulating factor of fever and neutropenia induced by chemotherapy in patients with small-cell lung cancer. N Engl J Med 1991;325:164–170.
38. Pettengell R, Gurney H, Radford JA, et al. Granulocyte colony-stimulating factor to prevent dose-limiting neutropenia in non-Hodgkin's lymphoma: a randomized controlled trial. Blood 1992;80:1430–1436.
39. Zinzani PL, Pavone E, Storti S, et al. Randomized trial with or without granulocyte colony-stimulating factor as adjunct to induction VNCOP-B treatment of elderly high-grade non-Hodgkin's lymphoma. Blood 1997;89:3974–3979.
40. American Society of Clinical Oncology. Update of recommendations for the use of hematopoietic colony-stimulating factors: evidence-based clinical practice guidelines. J Clin Oncol 1996;14:1957–1960.
41. Negoro S, Masuda N, Furuse K, et al. Dose-intensive chemotherapy in extensive-stage small-cell lung cancer. Cancer Chemother Pharmacol 1997;40(suppl):S70–S73.
42. Woll PJ, Hodgetts J, Lomax L, et al. Can cytotoxic dose-intensity be increased by using granulocyte colony-stimulating factor? A randomized controlled trial of lenograstim in small-cell lung cancer. J Clin Oncol 1995;13: 652–659.
43. Hartmann LC, Tschetter LK, Habermann TM, et al. Granulocyte colony-stimulating factor in severe chemotherapy-induced afebrile neutropenia [see comments]. N Engl J Med 1997;336:1776–1780.
44. Maher DW, Lieschke GJ, Green M, et al. Filgrastim in patients with chemotherapy-induced febrile neutropenia. A double-blind, placebo-controlled trial [see comments]. Ann Intern Med 1994;121:492–501.
45. Mayordomo JI, Rivera F, Diaz-Puente MT, et al. Improving treatment of chemotherapy-induced neutropenic fever by administration of colony-stimulating factors [see comments]. J Natl Cancer Inst 1995;87:803–808.
46. Aviles A, Guzman R, Garcia EL, et al. Resutls of a randomized trial of granulocyte colony-stimulating factor in patients with infection and severe granulocytopenia. Anticancer Drugs 1996;7:392–397.
47. Antman KS, Griffin JD, Elias A, et al. Effect of recombinant human granulocyte-macrophage colony-stimulating factor on chemotherapy-induced myelosuppression. N Engl J Med 1988;319:593–598.
48. Herrmann F, Schulz G, Lindemann A, et al. Hematopoietic responses in patients with advanced malignancy treated with recombinant human granulocyte-macrophage colony-stimulating factor. J Clin Oncol 1989;7:159–167.
49. Steward WP, Scarffe JH, Austin R, et al. Recombinant human granulocyte macrophage colony stimulating factor (rhGM-CSF) given as daily short infusions—a phase I dose-toxicity study. Br J Cancer 1989;59:142–145.
50. Kaplan LD, Kahn JO, Crowe S, et al. Clinical and virologic effects of recombinant human granulocyte-macrophage colony-stimulating factor in patients receiving chemotherapy for human immunodeficiency virus-associated non-Hodgkin's lymphoma: results of a randomized trial. J Clin Oncol 1991;9:929–940.
51. Jones SE, Schottstaedt MW, Duncan LA, et al. Randomized double-blind prospective trial to evaluate the effects of sargramostim versus placebo in a moderate-dose fluorouracil, doxorubicin, and cyclophosphamide adjuvant chemotherapy program for stage II and III breast cancer. J Clin Oncol 1996;14:2976–2983.
52. Gerhartz HH, Engelhard M, Meusers P, et al. Randomized, double-blind, placebo-controlled, phase III study of recombinant human granulocyte-macrophage colony-stimulating factor as adjunct to induction treatment of high-grade malignant non-Hodgkin's lymphomas [see comments]. Blood 1993;82:2329–2339.
53. Yau JC, Neidhart JA, Triozzi P, et al. Randomized placebo-

controlled trial of granulocyte-macrophage colony-stimulating-factor support for dose-intensive cyclophosphamide, etoposide, and cisplatin. Am J Hematol 1996;51: 289–295.

54. Bunn PA Jr, Crowley J, Kelly K, et al. Chemoradiotherapy with or without granulocyte-macrophage colony-stimulating factor in the treatment of limited-stage small-cell lung cancer: a prospective phase III randomized study of the Southwest Oncology Group [published erratum appears in J Clin Oncol 1995 Nov;13(11):2860]. J Clin Oncol 1995;13:1632–1641.

55. Bajorin DF, Nichols CR, Schmoll HJ, et al. Recombinant human granulocyte-macrophage colony-stimulating factor as an adjunct to conventional-dose ifosfamide-based chemotherapy for patients with advanced or relapsed germ cell tumors: a randomized trial. J Clin Oncol 1995;13:79–86.

56. American Society of Clinical Oncology. Recommendations for the use of hematopoietic colony-stimulating factors: evidence-based, clinical practice guidelines. J Clin Oncol 1994;12:2471–2508.

57. Furman WL. Cytokine support following cytotoxic chemotherapy in children. Int J Ped Hem/Onc 1995;2:163–171.

58. Saarinen UM, Hovi L, Riikonen P, et al. Recombinant human granulocyte-macrophage colony-stimulating factor in children with chemotherapy-induced neutropenia. Med Ped Onc 1992;20:489–496.

59. Burdach S. Molecular regulation of hematopoietic cytokines: implications and indications for clinical use in pediatric oncology. [Review]. Med Ped Onc 1992;2(suppl): 10–17.

60. Ganser A, Lindemann A, Seipelt G, et al. Effects of recombinant human interleukin-3 in patients with normal hematopoiesis and in patients with bone marrow failure. Blood 1990;76:666–676.

61. Ottmann OG, Ganser A, Seipelt G, et al. Effects of recombinant human interleukin-3 on human hematopoietic progenitor and precursor cells in vivo. Blood 1990;76:1494–1502.

62. O'Malley CJ, Rasko JE, Basser RL, et al. Administration of pegylated recombinant human megakaryocyte growth and development factor to humans stimulates the production of functional platelets that show no evidence of in vivo activation. Blood 1996;88:3288–3298.

63. Vadhan-Raj S, Murray LJ, Bueso-Ramos C, et al. Stimulation of megakaryocyte and platelet production by a single dose of recombinant human thrombopoietin in patients with cancer [see comments]. Ann Intern Med 1997; 126:673–681.

64. Fanucchi M, Glaspy J, Crawford J, et al. Effects of polyethylene glycol-conjugated recombinant human megakaryocyte growth and development factor on platelet counts after chemotherapy for lung cancer [see comments]. N Engl J Med 1997;336:404–409.

65. Gordon MS, Battiato L, Hoffman R, et al. Subcutaneously (SC) administered recombinant human interleukin-11 (neumega rhIL-11 growth factor; rhIL-11) prevents thrombocytopenia following chemotherapy (CT) with cyclophosphamide (C) and doxorubicin (A) in women with breast cancer. Blood 1993;82:318a.

66. Tepler I, Elias L, Smith JWII, et al. A randomized placebo-controlled trial of recombinant human interleukin-11 in cancer patients with severe thrombocytopenia due to chemotherapy. Blood 1996;87:3607–3614.

67. Motoyoshi K, Takaku F, Maekawa T, et al. Protective effect of partially purified human urinary colony-stimulating factor on granulocytopenia after antitumor chemotherapy. Exp Hematol 1986;14:1069–1075.

68. Smith JW, Longo DL, Alvord WG, et al. The effects of treatment with interleukin-1 alpha in platelet recovery after high-dose carboplatin. N Engl J Med 1993;328:756–761.

69. Brandt SJ, Peters WP, Atwater SK, et al. Effect of recombinant human granulocyte-macrophage colony-stimulating factor of hematopoietic reconsitution after high-dose chemotherapy and autologous bone marrow transplantation. N Engl J Med 1988;318:869–876.

70. Nemunaitis J, Singer JW, Buckner CD, et al. Use of recombinant human granulocyte-macrophage colony-stimulating factor in graft failure after bone marrow transplantation. Blood 1990;76:345–353.

71. Tapp H, Vowels M. Prophylactic use of GM-CSF in pediatric marrow transplantation. Transplant Proc 1992;24:2267–2268.

72. Blazar BR, Kersey JH, McGlave PB, et al. In vivo administration of recombinant human granulocyte/macrophage colony-stimulating factor in acute lymphoblastic leukemia patients receiving purged autografts. Blood 1989;73:849–857.

73. Sheridan WP, Morstyn G, Wolf M, et al. Granulocyte colony-stimulating factor and neutrophil recovery after high-dose chemotherapy and autologous bone marrow transplantation. Lancet 1989;2:891–895.

74. Peters WP, Stuart A, Affronti ML, et al. Neutrophil migration is defective during recombinant human granulocyte-macrophage colony-stimulating factor infusion after autologous bone marrow transplantation in humans. Blood 1988;72:1310–1315.

75. Masaoka T, Motoyoshi K, Takaku F, et al. Administration of human urinary colony stimulating factor after bone marrow transplantation. Bone Marrow Transplant 1988;3:121–127.

76. Vadhan-Raj S, Keating M, LeMaistre A, et al. Effects of recombinant human granulocyte-macrophage colony-stimulating factor in patients with myelodysplastic syndromes. N Engl J Med 1987;317:1545–1552.

77. Antin JH, Smith BR, Holmes W, Rosenthal DS. Phase I/II study of recombinant human granulocyte-macrophage colony-stimulating factor in aplastic anemia and myelodysplastic syndrome. Blood 1988;72:705–713.

78. Ganser A, Volkers B, Greher J, et al. Recombinant human granulocyte-macrophage colony-stimulating factor in patients with myelodysplastic syndromes—a phase I/II trial. Blood 1989;73:31–37.

79. Kobayashi Y, Okabe T, Ozawa K, et al. Treatment of myelodysplastic syndromes with recombinant human granulocyte colony-stimulating factor: a preliminary report. Am J Med 1989;86:178–182.

80. Negrin RS, Haeuber D, Nagler A, et al. Treatment of myelodysplastic syndromes with recombinant human granulocyte colony-stimulating factor: a phase I/II trial. Ann Intern Med 1989;110:976–984.

81. Ganser A, Ottmann OG, Seipelt G, et al. Effect of long-term treatment with recombinant human interleukin-3 in patients with myelodysplastic syndromes. Leukemia 1993;7: 696–701.

82. Nimer SD, Paquette RL, Ireland P, et al. A phase I/II study of interleukin-3 in patients with aplastic anemia and myelodysplasia. Exp Hematol 1994;22:875–880.

83. Hellstrom-Lindberg E. Efficacy of erythropoietin in the myelodysplastic syndromes: a meta-analysis of 205 patients from 17 studies [see comments]. Br J Haematol 1995;89: 67–71.

84. Hellstrom-Lindberg E, Negrin R, Stein R, et al. Erythroid response to treatment with G-CSF plus erythropoietin for the anaemia of patients with myelodysplastic syndromes: proposal for a predictive model. Br J Haematol 1997; 99:344–351.

85. Hellstrom-Lindberg E, Ahlgren T, Beguin Y, et al. Treatment of anemia in myelodysplastic syndromes with granulocyte colony-stimulating factor plus erythropoietin: results from a randomized phase II study and long-term follow-up of 71 patients. Blood 1998;92:68–75.

86. Economopoulos T, Mellou S, Papageorgiou E, et al. Treatment of anemia in low risk myelodysplastic syndromes with granulocyte-macrophage colony-stimulating factor plus recombinant human erythropoietin. Leukemia 1999;13: 1009–1012.

87. Champlin RE, Nimer SD, Ireland P, et al. Treatment of refractory aplastic anemia with recombinant human granulocyte-macrophage-colony-stimulating factor. Blood 1989;73:694–699.

88. Vadhan-Raj S, Buescher S, Broxmeyer HE, et al. Stimulation of myelopoiesis in patients with aplastic anemia by recombinant human granulocyte-macrophage colony-stimulating factor. N Engl J Med 1988;319:1628–1634.

89. Guinan EC, Sieff CA, Oette DH, Nathan DG. A phase I/II trial of recombinant granulocyte-macrophage colony-stimulating factor for children with aplastic anemia. Blood 1990;76:1077–1082.

90. Nissen C, Tichelli A, Gratwohl A, et al. Failure of recombinant human granulocyte-macrophage colony-stimulating factor therapy in aplastic anemia patients with very severe neutropenia. Blood 1988;72:2045–2047.

91. Kojima S, Fukuda M, Miyajima Y, Horibe K. Treatment of aplastic anemia in children with recombinant human granulocyte colony-stimulating factor. Blood 1991;77:937–941.

92. Kojima S, Matsuyama T. Stimulation of granulopoiesis by high-dose recombinant human granulocyte colony-stimulating factor in children with aplastic anemia and very severe neutropenia. Blood 1994;83:1474–1478.

93. Sonoda Y, Yashige H, Fujii H, et al. Bilineage response in refractory aplastic anemia patients following long-term administration of recombinant human granulocyte colony-stimulating factor. Eur J Haematol 1992;48:41–48.

94. Gluckman E, Esperou-Bourdeau H. Recent treatments of aplastic anemia. The international group on SAA. Nou Rev Fran d Hematol 1991;33:507–510.

95. Kojima S. Cytokine treatment of aplastic anemia. Int J Ped Hem/Onc 1995;2:135–141.

96. Kurzrock R, Talpaz M, Gutterman JU. Very low doses of GM-CSF administered alone with erythropoietin in aplastic anemia. Am J Med 1992;93:41–48.

97. Hirashima K, Bessho M, Jinnai I, Murohashi I. Successful treatment of aplastic anemia and refractory anemia by combination therapy with recombinant human granulocyte colony-stimulating factor and erythropoietin. Exp Hematol 1993;21:1080a.

98. Groopman JE, Mitsuyasu RT, DeLeo MJ, et al. Effects of recombinant human granulocyte-macrophage colony-stimulating factor on myelopoiesis in the acquired immunodeficiency syndrome. N Engl J Med 1987;317:593–598.

99. Groopman JE, Molina J-M, Scadden DT. Hematopoietic growth factors: biology and clinical applications. N Engl J Med 1989;321:1449–1459.

100. Perno CF, Yarchoan R, Conney DA, et al. Replication of human immunodeficiency virus in monocytes: granulocyte/macrophage colony-stimulating factor (GM-CSF) potentiates viral production yet enhances the antiviral effect mediated by 3'-azido-2'3'-dideoxythymidine (AZT) and other dideoxynucleoside congeners of thymidine. J Exp Med 1989;169:933–951.

101. Mueller BU. Role of cytokines in children with HIV infection. Int J Ped Hem/Onc 1995;2:151–161.

102. Pluda JM, Yarchoan R, Smith PD, et al. Subcutaneous recombinant granulocyte-macrophage colony-stimulating factor used as a single agent and in an alternating regimen with azidothymidine in leukopenic patients with severe human immunodeficiency virus infection. Blood 1990;76:463–472.

103. Kaplan LD, Kahn JO, Crowe S, et al. Clinical and virologic effects of recombinant human granulocyte-macrophage colony-stimulating factor in patients receiving chemotherapy for human immunodeficiency virus–associated non-Hodgkin's lymphoma: results of a randomized trial. J Clin Oncol 1991;9:929–940.

104. Mueller BU, Jacobsen F, Butler KM, et al. Combination treatment with azidothymidine and granulocyte colony-stimulating factor in children with human immunodeficiency virus infection. J Pediatr 1992;121:797–802.

105. Cole JL, Marzec UM, Gunthel CJ, et al. Ineffective platelet production in thrombocytopenic human immunodeficiency virus–infected patients. Blood 1998;91:3239–3246.

106. Gillio AP, Guinan EC. Cytokine treatment of inherited bone marrow failure syndromes. Int J Ped Hem/Onc 1992;2: 123–133.

107. Guinan EC, Lopez KD, Huhn RD, et al. Evaluation of granulocyte-macrophage colony-stimulating factor for treatment of pancytopenia in children with Fanconi anemia. J Pediatr 1994;124:144–150.

108. Rackoff WR, Orazi A, Robinson CA, et al. Prolonged administration of granulocyte colony-stimulating factor (filgrastim) to patients with Fanconi anemia: a pilot study. Blood 1996;88:1588–1593.

109. Hammond D, Keighley G. The erythrocyte-stimulating factor in serum and urine in congenital hypoplastic anemia. Am J Dis Child 1960;100:466–468.

110. Bagnara GP, Zauli G, Vitale L, et al. In vitro growth and regulation of bone marrow enriched $CD34^+$ hematopoietic progenitors in Diamond-Blackfan anemia. Blood 1991;78: 2203–2210.

111. Abkowitz JL, Broudy VC, Bennett LG, et al. Absence of abnormalities of *c-kit* or its ligand in two patients with Diamond-Blackfan anemia. Blood 1992;79:25–28.

112. Sieff CA, Yokoyama CT, Zsebo KM, et al. The production of Steel factor mRNA in Diamond-Blackfan anaemia long-term cultures and interactions of Steel factor with erythropoietin and interleukin-3. Br J Haematol 1992;82:640–647.

113. Niemeyer CM, Baumgarten E, Holldack J, et al. Treatment trial with recombinant human erythropoietin in children with congenital hypoplastic anemia. Contrib Nephrol 1991;88:276–280. Discussion.

114. Dunbar CE, Smith DA, Kimball J, et al. Treatment of Diamond-Blackfan anaemia with haematopoietic growth factors, granulocyte-macrophage colony stimulating factor and interleukin 3: sustained remissions following IL-3. Br J Haematol 1991;79:316–321.

115. Gillio AP, Faulkner LB, Alter BP, et al. Treatment of Diamond-Blackfan anemia with recombinant human interleukin-3. Blood 1993;82:744–751.

116. Olivieri NF, Feig SA, Valentino L, et al. Failure of recombinant human interleukin-3 therapy to induce erythropoiesis in patients with refractory Diamond-Blackfan anemia. Blood 1994;83:2444–2450.

117. Bastion Y, Bordigoni P, Debre M, et al. Sustained response after recombinant interleukin-3 in patients with bone marrow failure. Blood 1994;83:617.

118. Guinan EC, Lee YS, Lopez KD, et al. Effects of interleukin-3 and granulocyte-macrophage colony-stimulating factor on thrombopoiesis in congenital amegakaryocytic thrombocytopenia. Blood 1993;81:1691–1698.

119. Taylor DS, Lee Y, Sieff CA, et al. Phase I/II trial of PIXY321 (granulocyte-macrophage colony stimulating factor/interleukin-3 fusion protein) for treatment of inherited and acquired marrow failure syndromes. Br J Haematol 1998;103:304–307.

120. Pietsch T, Buhrer C, Mempel K, et al. Blood mononuclear cells from patients with severe congenital neutropenia are capable of producing granulocyte colony-stimulating factor. Blood 1991;77:1234–1237.

121. Kyas U, Pietsch T, Welte K. Expression of receptors for granulocyte colony-stimulating factor on neutrophils from patients with severe congenital neutropenia and cyclic neutropenia. Blood 1992;79:1144–1147.

122. Guba SC, Sartor CA, Hutchinson R, et al. Granulocyte colony-stimulating factor (G-CSF) production and G-CSF receptor structure in patients with congenital neutropenia. Blood 1994;83:1486–1492.

123. Rauprich P, Kasper B, Tidow N, Welte K. The protein tyrosine kinase JAK2 is activated in neutrophils from patients with severe congenital neutropenia. Blood 1995;86:4500–4505.

124. Bonilla MA, Gillio AP, Ruggiero M, et al. Effects of recombinant human granulocyte colony-stimulating factor on neutropenia in patients with congenital agranulocytosis. N Engl J Med 1989;320:1574–1580.

125. Welte K, Zeidler C, Reiter A, et al. Differential effects of granulocyte-macrophage colony-stimulating factor and granulocyte-stimulating factor in children with severe congenital neutropenia. Blood 1990;75:1056–1063.

126. Boxer LA, Hutchinson R, Emerson S. Recombinant human granulocyte-colony-stimulating factor in the treatment of patients with neutropenia. Clin Immunol Immunopathol 1992;62:539.

127. Dale DC, Bonilla MA, Davis MW, et al. A randomized controlled phase III trial of recombinant human granulocyte colony-stimulating factor (filgrastim) for treatment of severe chronic neutropenia. Blood 1993;81:2496–2502.

128. Dong F, van Buitenen C, Pouwels K, et al. Distinct cytoplasmic regions of the human G-CSF receptor involved in induction of proliferation and maturation. Mol Cell Biol 1993;13:7774–7781.

129. Dong F, Hoefsloot LH, Schelen AM, et al. Identification of a nonsense mutation in the granulocyte-colony-stimulating factor receptor in severe congenital neutropenia. Proc Natl Acad Sci USA 1994;91:4480–4484.

130. Dong F, Brynes RK, Tidow N, et al. Mutations in the gene for the granulocyte colony-stimulating-factor receptor in patients with acute myeloid leukemia preceded by severe congenital neutropenia. N Engl J Med 1995;333:487–493.

131. Welte K, Boxer LA. Severe chronic neutropenia: pathophysiology and therapy. Semin Hematol 1997;34:267–278.

132. Gilman PA, Jackson DP, Guild HG. Congenital agranulocytosis: prolonged survival and terminal acute leukemia. Blood 1970;36:576–585.

133. Rosen RB, Kang SJ. Congenital agranulocytosis terminating in acute myelomonocytic leukemia. J Pediatr 1979;94:406–408.

134. Kalra R, Dale D, Freedman M, et al. Monosomy 7 and activating RAS mutations accompany malignant transformation in patients with congenital neutropenia. Blood 1995;86:4579–4586.

135. Tidow N, Pilz C, Teichmann B, et al. Clinical relevance of point mutations in the cytoplasmic domain of the granulocyte colony-stimulating factor receptor gene in patients with severe congenital neutropenia [see comments]. Blood 1997;89:2369–2375.

136. Hammond WP IV, Price TH, Souza LM, Dale DC. Treatment of cyclic neutropenia with granulocyte colony-stimulating factor. N Engl J Med 1989;320:1306–1311.

137. Sugimoto K, Togawal A, Miyazono K. Treatment of childhood-onset cyclic neutropenia with recombinant human granulocyte colony stimulating factor. Eur J Haematol 1990;45:110–111.

138. Hanada T, Ono I, Nagasawa T. Childhood cyclic neutropenia treated with granulocyte colony-stimulating factor. Br J Haematol 1990;75:135–137.

139. Dale D, Bolyard A, Hammond W. Cyclic neutropenia: natural history and effects of long-term treatment with recombinant human granulocyte colony-stimulating factor. Cancer Invest 1993;11:219–223.

140. Wright D, Oette D, Malech H. Treatment of cyclic neutropenia with recombinant human granulocyte-macrophage colony-stimulating factor (rhGM-CSF). Blood 1989;74:231a.

141. Freund M, Luft S, Schober C, et al. Differential effect of GM-CSF and G-CSF in cyclic neutropenia. Lancet 1990;336:313.

142. Kurzrock R, Talpaz M, Gutterman J. Treatment of cyclic neutropenia with very low doses of GM-CSF. Am J Med 1991;91:317–318.

143. Jakubowski AA, Souza L, Kelly F, et al. Effects of human granulocyte colony-stimulating factor in a patient with idiopathic neutropenia. N Engl J Med 1989;320:38–42.

144. Winearls CG, Oliver DO, Pippard MJ, et al. Effect of human erythropoietin derived from recombinant DNA on the anemia of patients maintained by chronic haemodialysis. Lancet 1986;11:1175–1178.

145. Eschbach JW, Abdulhadi MH, Browne JK, et al. Recombinant human erythropoietin in anemic patients with end-stage renal disease. Ann Intern Med 1989;111:992–1000.

146. Adamson JW. The promise of recombinant human erythropoietin. Semin Hematol 1989;26(suppl 2):5–8.
147. Dessypris EN, Graber SE, Krantz SB, Stone WJ. Effects of recombinant erythropoietin on the concentration and cycling status of human marrow hematopoietic progenitor cells in vivo. Blood 1988;72:2060–2062.
148. Laupacis A. Changes in quality of life and functional capacity in hemodialysis patients treated with recombinant human erythropoietin. Semin Nephrol 1990;10(suppl 1):11–19.
149. Eschbach JW, Kelly MR, Haley NR, et al. Treatment of the anemia of progressive renal failure with recombinant human erythropoietin. N Engl J Med 1989;321:158–163.
150. Bommer J, Ritz E, Weinrich T, et al. Subcutaneous erythropoietin. Lancet 1988;2:406.
151. Kaufman JS, Reda DJ, Fye CL, et al. Subcutaneous compared with intravenous epoetin in patients receiving hemodialysis. Department of Veterans Affairs Cooperative Study Group on Erythropoietin in Hemodialysis Patients [see comments]. N Engl J Med 1998;339:578–583.
152. Müller-Wiefel DE, Amon O. Erythropoietin treatment of anemia associated with chronic renal failure in children. Int J Ped Hem/Onc 1995;2:87–95.
153. Offner G, Hoyer PF, Latta K, et al. One year's experience with recombinant erythropoietin in children undergoing continuous ambulatory or cycling peritoneal dialysis. Ped Nephrol 1990;4:498–500.
154. Scigalla P, Bonzel KE, Bulla M, et al. Therapy of renal anemia with recombinant human erythropoietin in children with end-stage renal disease. Contrib Nephrol 1989;76:227–240. Discussion.
155. Scharer K, Klare B, Braun A, et al. Treatment of renal anemia by subcutaneous erythropoietin in children with preterminal chronic renal failure. Acta Pediatr 1993;82:953–958.
156. Onkingco JRC, Ruley EJ, Turner ME. Use of low-dose subcutaneous recombinant human erythropoietin in end-stage renal disease: experience with children receiving continuous cycling peritoneal dialysis. Am J Kidney Dis 1991;18:446–450.
157. Ohls R, Christensen R. Recombinant erythropoietin compared with erythrocyte transfusion in the treatment of anemia of prematurity. J Pediatr 1991;119:781–788.
158. Soubasi V, Kremenopoulos G, Diamandi E, et al. In which neonates does early recombinant human erythropoietin treatment prevent anemia of prematurity? Results of a randomized, controlled study. Ped Res 1993;34:675–679.
159. Messer J, Haddad J, Donato L, et al. Early treatment of premature infants with recombinant human erythropoietin [see comments]. Pediatrics 1993;92:519–523.
160. Bechensteen AG, Haga P, Halvorsen S, et al. Erythropoietin, protein, and iron supplementation and the prevention of anaemia of prematurity. Arch Dis Childhood 1993;69:19–23.
161. Shannon KM, Mentzer WC, Abels RI, et al. Enhancement of erythropoiesis by recombinant human erythorpoietin in low birth weight infants: a pilot study. J Pediatr 1992;120:586–592.
162. Carnielli V, Montini G, Da Riol R, et al. Effect of high doses of human recombinant erythropoietin on the need for blood transfusions in preterm infants [see comments]. J Pediatr 1992;121:98–102.
163. Halperin D, Felix M, Wacker P, et al. Recombinant human erythropoietin in the treatment of infants with anemia of prematurity. Eur J Pediatr 1992;151:661–667.
164. Mentzer WC, Shannon KM. The use of recombinant human erythropoietin in preterm infants. Int J Ped Hem/Onc 1995;2:97–103.
165. Maier RF, Obladen M, Kattner E, et al. High- versus low-dose erythropoietin in extremely low birth weight infants. The European Multicenter rhEPO Study Group. J Pediatr 1998;132:866–870.
166. Means RT, Olsen NJ, Krantz SB, et al. Treatment of the anemia of rheumatoid arthritis with recombinant human erythropoietin: clinical and in vitro studies. Arth Rheum 1989;32:638–642.
167. Umemura T, al-Khatti A, Donahue RE, et al. Effects of interleukin-3 and erythorpoietin on *in vitro* erythropoiesis and F cell formation in primates. Blood 1989;74:1561–1576.
168. al-Khatti A, Umemura T, Clow J, et al. Erythropoietin stimulates F-reticulocyte formation in sickle cell anemia. Trans Assoc Amer Phys 1988;101:54–61.
169. Goldberg MA, Brugnara C, Dover GJ, et al. Treatment of sickle cell anemia with hydroxyurea and erythropoietin. N Engl J Med 1990;323:366–372.
170. Rodgers GP, Dover GJ, Uyesaka N, et al. Augmentation by erythropoietin of the fetal-hemoglobin response to hydroxyurea in sickle cell disease [see comments]. N Engl J Med 1993;328:73–80.
171. Rachmilewitz EA, Goldfarb A, Dover G. Administration of erythropoietin to patients with β-thalassemia intermedia: a preliminary trial. Blood 1991;78:1145–1147.
172. Olivieri NF, Freedman MH, Perrine SP, et al. Trial of recombinant human erythropoietin: three patients with thalassemia intermedia [letter]. Blood 1992;80:3258–3260.
173. Aker M, Dover G, Schrier S, et al. Sustained increase in the hemoglobin, hematocrit and RBC following long term administration of recombinant human erythropoietin to patients with beta thalassemia intermedia. Blood 1993;82:358a. Abstract.
174. Loukopoulos D, Voskaridou E, Cozma C, et al. Effective stimulation of erythropoiesis in thalassemia intermedia with recombinant human erythropoietin and hydroxyurea. Blood 1993;82:357a.
175. Goodnough LT, Rudnick S, Price TH, et al. Increased preoperative collection of autologous blood with recombinant human erythropoietin therapy. N Engl J Med 1989;321:1163–1168.
176. Felix R, Cecchini MG, Hofstetter W, et al. Impairment of macrophage colony-stimulating factor production and lack of resident bone marrow macrophages in the osteopetrotic op/op mouse. J Bone Mineral Res 1990;5:781–789.
177. Wiktor-Jedrzejczak W, Bartocci A, Ferrante AW Jr, et al. Total absence of colony-stimulating factor 1 in the macrophage-deficient osteopetrotic (op/op) mouse [published erratum appears in Proc Natl Acad Sci USA 1991 Jul 1;88(13):5937]. Proc Natl Acad Sci USA 1990;87:4828–4832.
178. Yoshida H, Hayashi S-I, Kunisada T, et al. The murine mutation osteopetrosis is in the coding region of the macrophage colony stimulating factor gene. Nature 1990;345:442–444.
179. Felix R, Cecchini MG, Fleisch H. Macrophage colony stim-

ulating factor restores in vivo bone resorption in the op/op osteopetrotic mouse. Endocrinology 1990;127:2592–2594.

180. Wiktor-Jedrzejczak W, Urbanowska E, Aukerman SL, et al. Correction by CSF-1 of defects in the osteopetrotic op/op mouse suggests local, developmental, and humoral requirements for this growth factor. Exp Hematol 1991;19:1049–1054.

181. Kodama H, Yamasaki A, Nose M, et al. Congenital osteoclast deficiency in osteopetrotic (op/op) mice is cured by injections of macrophage colony-stimulating factor. J Exp Med 1991;173:269–272.

182. Key LL Jr, Rodriguiz RM, Wang WC. Cytokines and bone resorption in osteopetrosis. Int J Ped Hem/Onc 1995;2:143–149.

183. Rodriguiz RM, Key LL Jr, Ries WL. Combination macrophage-colony stimulating factor and interferon-gamma administration ameliorates the osteopetrotic condition in microphthalmic (mi/mi) mice. Ped Res 1993;33:384–389.

184. Key LL, Ries WL, Rodriguiz RM, Hatcher HC. Recombinant human interferon gamma therapy of osteopetrosis. J Pediatr 1992;121:119–124.

185. Duhrsen U, Villeval J-L, Boyd J, et al. Effects of recombinant human granulocyte colony-stimulating factor on hematopoietic progenitor cells in cancer patients. Blood 1988;72:2074–2081.

186. Tamura M, Hattori K, Nomura H, et al. Induction of neutrophilic granulocytes in mice by administration of purified human native granulocyte colony-stimulating factor (G-CSF). Biochem Biophys Res Comm 1987;142:454.

187. Shimamura M, Kobayashi Y, Yuo A, et al. Effect of human recombinant granulocyte colony-stimulating factor on hematopoietic injury in mice induced by 5-fluorouracil. Blood 1987;69:353.

188. Socinski MA, Cannistra SA, Elias A, et al. Granulocyte-macrophage colony stimulating factor expands the circulating haemopoietic progenitor cell compartment in man. Lancet 1988;1:1194–1198.

189. Bensinger W, Appelbaum F, Rowley S, et al. Factors that influence collection and engraftment of autologous peripheral-blood stem cells. J Clin Oncol 1995;13:2547–2555.

190. Weaver CH, Hazelton B, Birch R, et al. An analysis of engraftment kinetics as a function of the CD34 content of peripheral blood progenitor cell collections in 692 patients after the administration of myeloablative chemotherapy. Blood 1995;86:3961–3969.

191. Pecora AL, Preti RA, Gleim GW, et al. CD34+CD33– cells influence days to engraftment and transfusion requirements in autologous blood stem-cell recipients. J Clin Oncol 1998;16:2093–2104.

192. Glaspy JA, Shpall EJ, LeMaistre CF, et al. Peripheral blood progenitor cell mobilization using stem cell factor in combination with filgrastim in breast cancer patients. Blood 1997;90:2939–2951.

193. Moskowitz CH, Stiff P, Gordon MS, et al. Recombinant methionyl human stem cell factor and filgrastim for peripheral blood progenitor cell mobilization and transplantation in non-Hodgkin's lymphoma patients—results of a phase I/II trial. Blood 1997;89:3136–3147.

194. Weaver A, Ryder D, Crowther D, et al. Increased numbers of long-term culture-initiating cells in the apheresis product

of patients randomized to receive increasing doses of stem cell factor administered in combination with chemotherapy and a standard dose of granulocyte colony-stimulating factor. Blood 1996;88:3323–3328.

195. Begley CG, Basser R, Mansfield R, et al. Enhanced levels and enhanced clonogenic capacity of blood progenitor cells following administration of stem cell factor plus granulocyte colony-stimulating factor to humans. Blood 1997;90:3378–3389.

196. Basser RL, Rasko JE, Clarke K, et al. Randomized, blinded, placebo-controlled phase I trial of pegylated recombinant human megakaryocyte growth and development factor with filgrastim after dose-intensive chemotherapy in patients with advanced cancer [published erratum appears in Blood 1997 Sep 15;90(6):2513]. Blood 1997;89:3118–3128.

197. Rasko JE, Basser RL, Boyd J, et al. Multilineage mobilization of peripheral blood progenitor cells in humans following administration of PEG-rHuMGDF. Br J Haematol 1997;97:871–880.

198. Tricot G, Jagannath S, Vesole D, et al. Peripheral blood stem cell transplants for multiple myeloma: identification of favorable variables for rapid engraftment in 225 patients. Blood 1995;85:588–596.

199. Pless M, Wodnar-Filipowicz A, John L, et al. Synergy of growth factors during mobilization of peripheral blood precursor cells with recombinant human Flt3-ligand and granulocyte colony-stimulating factor in rabbits. Exp Hematol 1999;27:155–161.

200. Brasel K, McKenna HJ, Charrier K, et al. Flt3 ligand synergizes with granulocyte-macrophage colony-stimulating factor or granulocyte colony-stimulating factor to mobilize hematopoietic progenitor cells into the peripheral blood of mice. Blood 1997;90:3781–3788.

201. Papayannopoulou T, Nakamoto B, Andrews RG, et al. In vivo effects of Flt3/Flk2 ligand on mobilization of hematopoietic progenitors in primates and potent synergistic enhancement with granulocyte colony-stimulating factor. Blood 1997;90:620–629.

202. Molineux G, McCrea C, Yan XQ, et al. Flt-3 ligand synergizes with granulocyte colony-stimulating factor to increase neutrophil numbers and to mobilize peripheral blood stem cells with long-term repopulating potential. Blood 1997;89:3998–4004.

203. Sudo Y, Shimazaki C, Ashihara E, et al. Synergistic effect of FLT-3 ligand on the granulocyte colony-stimulating factor-induced mobilization of hematopoietic stem cells and progenitor cells into blood in mice. Blood 1997;89:3186–3191.

204. Shpall EJ. The utilization of cytokines in stem cell mobilization strategies. Bone Marrow Transplant 1999;23(suppl 2):S13–S19.

205. Bodine DM, Seidel NE, Orlic D. Bone marrow collected 14 days after in vivo administration of granulocyte colony-stimulating factor and stem cell factor to mice has 10-fold more repopulating ability than untreated marrow. Blood 1996;88:89–97.

206. Miller CL, Eaves CJ. Expansion in vitro of adult murine hematopoietic stem cells with transplantable lympho-myeloid reconstituting ability. Proc Natl Acad Sci USA 1997;94:13648–13653.

207. Zandstra PW, Conneally E, Petzer AL, et al. Cytokine

manipulation of primitive human hematopoietic cell self-renewal. Proc Natl Acad Sci USA 1997;94:4698–4703.

208. Kamel-Reid S, Dick JE. Engraftment of immune-deficient mice with human hematopoietic stem cells. Science 1988;242:1706–1709.

209. Vormoor J, Lapidot T, Pflumio F, et al. Immature human cord blood progenitors engraft and proliferate to high levels in severe combined immunodeficient mice. Blood 1994;83: 2489–2497.

210. Gan OI, Murdoch B, Larochelle A, Dick JE. Differential maintenance of primitive human SCID-repopulating cells, clonogenic progenitors, and long-term culture-initiating cells after incubation on human bone marrow stromal cells. Blood 1997;90:641–650.

211. Larochelle A, Vormoor J, Hanenberg H, et al. Identification of primitive human hematopoietic cells capable of repopulating NOD/SCID mouse bone marrow: implications for gene therapy. Nat Medicine 1996;2:1329–1337.

212. Conneally E, Cashman J, Petzer A, Eaves C. Expansion in vitro of transplantable human cord blood stem cells demonstrated using a quantitative assay of their lympho-myeloid repopulating activity in nonobese diabetic-scid/scid mice. Proc Natl Acad Sci USA 1997;94:9836–9841.

213. Bhatia M, Bonnet D, Kapp U, et al. Quantitative analysis reveals expansion of human hematopoietic repopulating cells after short-term ex vivo culture. J Exp Med 1997;186: 619–624.

214. Rebel VI, Tanaka M, Lee JS, et al. One-day ex vivo culture allows effective gene transfer into human nonobese diabetic/severe combined immune-deficient repopulating cells using high-titer vesicular stomatitis virus G protein pseudotyped retrovirus. Blood 1999;93:2217–2224.

215. Brugger W, Heimfeld S, Berenson RJ, et al. Reconstitution of hematopoiesis after high-dose chemotherapy by autologous progenitor cells generated ex vivo. N Engl J Med 1995;333:283–287.

216. Holyoake TL, Alcorn MJ, Richmond L, et al. CD34 positive PBPC expanded ex vivo may not provide durable engraftment following myeloablative chemoradiotherapy regimens. Bone Marrow Transplant 1997;19:1095–1101.

217. Scheding S, Kratz-Albers K, Meister B, et al. Ex vivo expansion of hematopoietic progenitor cells for clinical use. Semin Hematol 1998;35:232–240.

218. Dunbar CE, Cottler-Fox M, O'Shaughnessy JA, et al. Retrovirally marked CD34-enriched peripheral blood and bone marrow cells contribute to long-term engraftment after autologous transplantation. Blood 1995;85:3048–3057.

219. Bordignon C, Notarangelo LD, Nobili N, et al. Gene therapy in peripheral blood lymphocytes and bone marrow for ADA immunodeficient patients. Science 1995;270:470–475.

220. Blaese RM, Culver KW, Miller AD, et al. T lymphocyte-directed gene therapy for ADA-SCID: initial trial results after 4 years. Science 1995;270:475–480.

221. Kohn DB, Weinberg KI, Nolta JA, et al. Engraftment of gene-modified umbilical cord blood cells in neonates with adenosine deaminase deficiency. Nat Medicine 1995;1:1017–1023.

222. Kavanaugh MP, Miller DG, Zhang W, et al. Cell-surface receptors for gibbon ape leukemia virus and amphotropic murine retrovirus are inducible sodium-dependent

phosphate symporters. Proc Natl Acad Sci USA 1994;91: 7071–7075.

223. Orlic D, Girard LJ, Jordan CT, et al. The level of mRNA encoding the amphotropic retrovirus receptor in mouse and human hematopoietic stem cells is low and correlates with the efficiency of retrovirus transduction. Proc Natl Acad Sci USA 1996;93:11097–11102.

224. Miller DG, Adam MA, Miller AD. Gene transfer by retrovirus vectors occurs only in cells that are actively replicating at the time of infection [published erratum appears in Mol Cell Biol 1992 Jan;12(1):433]. Mol Cell Biol 1990;10: 4239–4242.

225. Emi N, Friedmann T, Yee JK. Pseudotype formation of murine leukemia virus with the G protein of vesicular stomatitis virus. J Virol 1991;65:1202–1207.

226. Burns JC, Friedmann T, Driever W, et al. Vesicular stomatitis virus G glycoprotein pseudotyped retroviral vectors: concentration to very high titer and efficient gene transfer into mammalian and nonmammalian cells. Proc Natl Acad Sci USA 1993;90:8033–8037.

227. Friedmann T, Yee JK. Pseudotyped retroviral vectors for studies of human gene therapy. [Review]. Nat Medicine 1995;1:275–277.

228. Bodine DM, Karlsson S, Nienhuis AW. Combination of interleukins 3 and 6 preserves stem cell function in culture and enhances retrovirus-mediated gene transfer into hematopoietic stem cells. Proc Natl Acad Sci USA 1989;86:8897–8901.

229. Laneuville P, Chang W, Kamel-Reid S, et al. High-efficiency gene transfer and expression in normal human hematopoietic cells with retrovirus vectors. Blood 1988;71:811–814.

230. Dick JE, Kamel-Reid S, Murdoch B, Doedens M. Gene transfer into normal human hematopoietic cells using in vitro and in vivo assays. Blood 1991;78:624–634.

231. Hughes PF, Eaves CJ, Hogge DE, Humphries RK. High-efficiency gene transfer to human hematopoietic cells maintained in long-term marrow culture. Blood 1989;74:1915–1922.

232. Hughes PFD, Thacker JD, Hogge D, et al. Retroviral gene transfer to primitive normal and leukemic hematopoietic cells using clinically applicable procedures. J Clin Invest 1992;89:1817–1824.

233. Xu LC, Kluepfel-Stahl S, Blanco M, et al. Growth factors and stromal support generate very efficient retroviral transduction of peripheral blood CD34+ cells from Gaucher patients. Blood 1995;86:141–146.

234. Moore KA, Deisseroth AB, Reading CL, et al. Stromal support enhances cell-free retroviral vector transduction of human bone marrow long-term culture-initiating cells. Blood 1992;79:1393–1399.

235. Nolta JA, Smogorzewska EM, Kohn DB. Analysis of optimal conditions for retroviral-mediated transduction of primitive human hematopoietic cells. Blood 1995;86:101–110.

236. van Beusechem VW, Kukler A, Heidt PJ, Valerio D. Long-term expression of human adenosine deaminase in rhesus monkeys transplanted with retrovirus-infected bone-marrow cells. Proc Natl Acad Sci USA 1992;89:7640–7644.

237. Bodine DM, Moritz T, Donahue RE, et al. Long-term in vivo expression of a murine adenosine deaminase gene in rhesus monkey hematopoietic cells of multiple lineages after retro-

viral mediated gene transfer into CD34$^+$ bone marrow cells. Blood 1993;82:1975–1980.

238. Harrison DE, Stone M, Astle CM. Effects of transplantation on the primitive immunohematopoietic stem cell. J Exp Med 1990;172:431–437.

239. Spangrude GJ, Brooks DM, Tumas DB. Long-term repopulation of irradiated mice with limiting numbers of purified hematopoietic stem cells: in vivo expansion of stem cell phenotype but not function. Blood 1995;85:1006–1016.

240. Van Zant G, de Haan G, Rich IN. Alternatives to stem cell renewal from a developmental viewpoint. Exp Hematol 1997;25:187–192.

241. Morrison SJ, Wandycz AM, Akashi K, et al. The aging of hematopoietic stem cells. Nat Medicine 1996;2:1011–1016.

242. Van Zant G, Holland BP, Eldridge PW, Chen JJ. Genotype-restricted growth and aging patterns in hematopoietic stem cell populations of allophenic mice. J Exp Med 1990;171:1547–1565.

243. Lapidot T, Pflumio F, Doedens M, et al. Cytokine stimulation of multilineage hematopoiesis from immature human cells engrafted in SCID mice. Science 1992;255:1137–1141.

244. Hesselton RM, Greiner DL, Mordes JP, et al. High levels of human peripheral blood mononuclear cell engraftment and enhanced susceptibility to human immunodeficiency virus type 1 infection in NOD/LtSz-scid/scid mice. J Infect Dis 1995;172:974–982.

245. Greiner DL, Shultz LD, Yates J, et al. Improved engraftment of human spleen cells in NOD/LtSz-scid/scid mice as compared with C.B-17-scid/scid mice. Am J Pathol 1995;146:888–902.

246. Shultz LD, Schweitzer PA, Christianson SW, et al. Multiple defects in innate and adaptive immunologic function in NOD/LtSz-scid mice. J Immunol 1995;154:180–191.

247. Bhatia M, Wang JCY, Kapp U, et al. Purification of primitive human hematopoietic cells capable of repopulating immune-deficient mice. Proc Natl Acad Sci USA 1997;94:5320–5325.

248. Arnaout MA, Wang EA, Clark SC, Sieff CA. Human recombinant granulocyte macrophage colony-stimulating factor increases cell to cell adhesion and surface expression of adhesion promoting surface glycoproteins on mature granulocytes. J Clin Invest 1986;78:597–601.

249. Costa JJ, Demetri GD, Harrist TJ, et al. Recombinant human stem cell factor (kit ligand) promotes human mast cell and melanocyte hyperplasia and functional activation in vivo. J Exp Med 1996;183:2681–2686.

250. Gribben JG, Devereux S, Thomas NSB, et al. Development of antibodies to unprotected glycosylation sites on recombinant human GM-CSF. Lancet 1990;335:434–437.

251. Vadhan-Raj S, Murray LJ, Bueso-Ramos C, et al. Stimulation of megakaryocyte and platelet production by a single dose of recombinant human thrombopoietin in patients with cancer [see comments]. Ann Intern Med 1997;126:673–681.

252. Goodnough LT, Dipersio J, Mccullough J, et al. Pegylated recombinant human megakaryocyte growth and development factor (PEG-rHuMGDF) increases platelet count and

apheresis yields of normal platelet donors: initial results. Transfusion 1997;37(suppl 9S):67S. Abstract.

253. Glaspy JA, Baldwin GC, Robertson PA, et al. Therapy for neutropenia in hairy cell leukemia with recombinant human granulocyte colony-stimulating factor. Ann Intern Med 1988;109:789–795.

254. Papayannopoulou T, Nakamoto B. Peripheralization of hemopoietic progenitors in primates treated with anti-VLA4 integrin. Proc Natl Acad Sci USA 1993;90:9374–9378.

255. Papayannopoulou T, Craddock C, Nakamoto B, et al. The VLA4/VCAM-1 adhesion pathway defines contrasting mechanisms of lodgement of transplanted murine hemopoietic progenitors between bone marrow and spleen. Proc Natl Acad Sci USA 1995;92:9647–9651.

256. Craddock CF, Nakamoto B, Andrews RG, et al. Antibodies to VLA4 integrin mobilize long-term repopulating cells and augment cytokine-induced mobilization in primates and mice. Blood 1997;90:4779–4788.

257. Papayannopoulou T, Priestley GV, Nakamoto B. Anti-VLA4/VCAM-1-induced mobilization requires cooperative signaling through the kit/mkit ligand pathway. Blood 1998;91:2231–2239.

258. Sauvageau G, Thorsteinsdottir U, Eaves CJ, et al. Overexpression of HOXB4 in hematopoietic cells causes the selective expansion of more primitive populations in vitro and in vivo. Genes Devel 1995;9:1753–1765.

259. Livnah O, Stura EA, Johnson DL, et al. Functional mimicry of a protein hormone by a peptide agonist: the EPO receptor complex at 2.8 A. Science 1996;273:464–471.

260. Wrighton NC, Farrell FX, Chang R, et al. Small peptides as potent mimetics of the protein hormone erythropoietin. Science 1996;273:458–464.

261. Johnson DL, Farrell FX, Barbone FP, et al. Identification of a 13 amino acid peptide mimetic of erythropoietin and description of amino acids critical for the mimetic activity of EMP1. Biochemistry 1998;37:3699–3710.

262. Barbone FP, Johnson DL, Farrell FX, et al. New epoetin molecules and novel therapeutic approaches. Nephrol Dial Transplant 1999;14(suppl 2):80–84.

263. Livnah O, Stura EA, Middleton SA, et al. Crystallographic evidence for preformed dimers of erythropoietin receptor before ligand activation. Science 1999;283:987–990.

264. Johnson DL, Farrell FX, Barbone FP, et al. Amino-terminal dimerization of an erythropoietin mimetic peptide results in increased erythropoietic activity. Chem Biol 1997;4:939–950.

265. Fleming WH, Lankford-Turner P, Turner CW, et al. Administration of daniplestim and granulocyte colony-stimulating factor for the mobilization of hematopoietic progenitor cells in nonhuman primates. Biol Blood Marrow Transplant 1999;5:8–14.

266. MacVittie TJ, Farese AM, Herodin F, et al. Combination therapy for radiation-induced bone marrow aplasia in nonhuman primates using synthokine SC-55494 and recombinant human granulocyte colony-stimulating factor. Blood 1996;87:4129–4135.

267. Farese AM, Herodin F, McKearn JP, et al. Acceleration of hematopoietic reconstitution with a synthetic cytokine (SC-55494) after radiation-induced bone marrow aplasia. Blood 1996;87:581–591.

Chapter 15

Cytokines Regulating Immune Inflammation: Interleukin-4, Interleukin-10, and Interleukin-12

Richard N. Mitchell
Abul K. Abbas

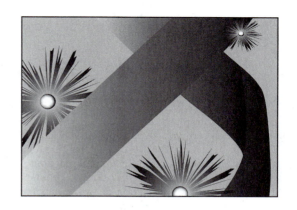

Immune and inflammatory reactions are an integral part of host defense, serving to protect the host by neutralizing or eliminating a variety of infectious agents. They also have a role in the surveillance and destruction of tumors. However, exuberant inflammatory responses have the potential to cause local tissue injury (e.g., abscesses or granulomas), systemic pathology (e.g., autoimmune disease or anaphylaxis), and allograft rejection.

The host response to microbes is comprised of antigen-non-specific cells and serum components (*innate immunity*) as well as antigen-specific T and B cells and antibodies (*specific immunity*). The components of innate immunity are activated prior to the development of specific immunity, and are also secondarily recruited in the effector phase of specific immune reactions. Neutrophils, macrophages, natural killer cells, mast cells, and complement constitute the principal mediators of innate immunity. Depending on the nature of the initial inciting antigen and the types of antigen-specific cells that are activated, the components of innate immunity will be differentially elicited, and the resulting reactions will have different morphologic appearances. Finally, depending on the circumstances, the components of specific immunity have the capacity to either enhance or moderate innate immunity.

This chapter describes the biology of three *cytokines* that are important effectors of immunologic inflammation, and discusses potential therapies aimed at modulating their activities. Cytokines are protein hormones that regulate the growth and differentiation of lymphocytes (e.g., in T-cell activation), or regulate the activation of other inflammatory cells (e.g., effector macrophages or eosinophils). Although many cytokines can also affect the proliferation or activation of other cell types (e.g., vascular wall endothelium and smooth muscle), we will concentrate here on the effects of cytokines on inflammatory cells. A critical concept in this discussion is that cytokines not only regulate inflammatory cell activation, but also interact through feedback pathways to regulate the expression of each other.

As we will discuss, *interleukin-4* plays a central role in allergic and parasitic disorders; moderating or augmenting its activity may allow the treatment of a variety of conditions ranging from asthma to helminth infestation. *Interleukin-10* is an anti-inflammatory cytokine; regulating its expression may be important in treating a variety of clinically important inflammatory states, including ulcerative colitis, rheumatoid arthritis, and allograft rejection. Finally, *interleukin-12* tends to be strongly proinflammatory; modulation of its activity may provide a handle on improving host responses to certain infectious agents and tumors.

Overview of T-Lymphocyte Function and Cytokines

T lymphocytes initiate and regulate all specific immune responses to protein antigens. These cells classically fall into two major categories: CD4+ T-helper (Th) cells and CD8+ T-cytotoxic (Tc) cells. The CD4 and CD8 molecules on T cells recognize nonpolymorphic regions of class II or class I major histocompatibility complex (MHC) molecules, respectively, and function as coreceptors for antigen recognition. T-cell antigen recognition is followed in short order by T-cell activation and subsequent generation of effector functions.

Antigen-stimulated CD4+ Th cells are sources of cytokines that provide "help" for the proliferation and activation of a variety of cells, including B cells, macrophages, and other T lymphocytes. Some of these cytokines, such as interleukin-2 (IL-2), interleukin-4 (IL-4), and transforming growth factor-β (TGF-β), act in autocrine fashion, regulating the activity (e.g., proliferation and/or differentiation) of the same cells that secrete them. These cytokines may also act in a paracrine manner, influencing the behavior of other cells including neighboring T and B cells. Other T cell–derived cytokines, such as interleukin-5, interleukin-13, and interferon-γ (IFN-γ), act primarily on nonlymphoid cells such as eosinophils, macrophages, and endothelium. In general, each differentiated Th cell makes only a discrete subset of cytokines. Th cells in culture or in chronic immune reactions appear to undergo differentiation from functionally inactive precursors into one of two predominant Th cell types, called Th1 and Th2, that make defined cytokine profiles (1,2). A third "Th3" population, which suppresses the responses of both Th1 and Th2 populations, has also been recently described (3). Although the differentiation into distinct Th subsets has been best documented in mice, it also clearly occurs in humans (4,5).

Th1 cells make cytokines (e.g., IL-2 and IFN-γ) which heighten macrophage-dependent host defense mechanisms such as delayed-type hypersensitivity (Fig. 15-1). Conversely, Th2 cells make cytokines (e.g., IL-4 and IL-5) that preferentially amplify IgE- and eosinophil-mediated reactions (Fig. 15-2). Both subsets will augment antibody production, although Th1 cells favor the production of Ig isotypes (such as IgG2a in mice) that promote opsonization and complement fixation, while Th2 cells induce Ig isotypes that activate mast cells and basophils (IgE). Both subsets can also drive the maturation of Tc cells.

Activated CD8⁺ Tc cells are cytolytic effector cells that kill their targets. In recent years, however, cytotoxic activity by a subset of CD4⁺ cells and cytokine production by CD8⁺ cells have been increasingly documented (6,7). Thus, although we will focus here on cytokines produced by Th cells, the contribution of analogous Tc populations may also be important (8).

Finally, some cytokines are produced primarily by the cells of innate immunity (e.g., macrophages) and also play a role in stimulating or inhibiting inflammatory responses. In this category

fall interleukin-1 (IL-1) and tumor necrosis factor-α (TNF-α), both of which have proinflammatory effects, including endothelial activation that promotes inflammatory cell adhesion and a thrombotic diathesis. Interleukin-12 (IL-12) is another cytokine made predominantly by macrophages; among its functions are the activation of natural killer cell and Tc cell activity. Importantly, IL-12 also induces the differentiation of naïve CD4⁺ T cells into Th1 cells, thereby serving as a crucial link between innate and specific immunity. A large family of "chemotactic cytokines," or *chemokines*, is also important in recruiting the appropriate effector cells to the sites of inflammation. All chemokines contain two internal disulfide loops, and are subtyped on the basis of whether the amino terminal cysteines that participate in the disulfide bonds are adjacent (*C-C chemokines*) or separated by one amino acid (*C-X-C chemokines*). The C-X-C chemokines are produced by activated macrophages, as well as endothelium and fibroblasts, and serve primarily to recruit neutrophils; interleukin-8 (IL-8) is the best characterized of this group. The C-C chemokines are produced largely by activated T cells, and act predominantly on T cells, monocytes, eosinophils, and basophils. They each show some degree of specificity; consequently, the chemokine *eotaxin* preferentially recruits eosinophils, while another chemokine, *RANTES*, has a predilection for memory CD4⁺ T cells (9).

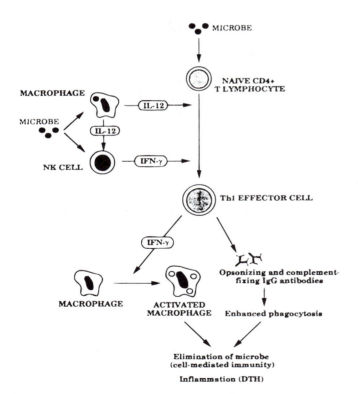

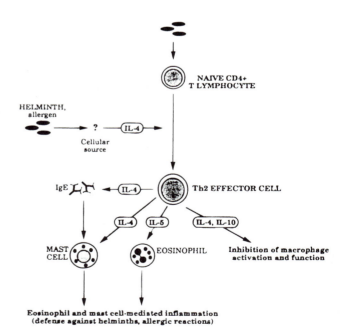

Figure 15-1. Development and functions of Th1 effector cells. Naive CD4+ T lymphocytes recognize an antigen (microbe) in the context of IL-12 and IFN-γ, cytokines that induce the differentiation of the naive cells to Th1 effectors. Th1 cells produce IFN-γ, which stimulates phagocyte-mediated defense mechanisms and inflammation (DTH). Note that IL-12 and IFN-γ provide an amplification mechanism for T cell–macrophage interactions.

Figure 15-2. Development and functions of Th2 effector cells. Naive CD4+ T lymphocytes recognize an antigen (helminth, or allergen) in the context of IL-4, which stimulates the differentiation of the naive cells to Th2 effectors. Th2 cells produce cytokines that stimulate mast cell and eosinophil-mediated defense reactions and inflammation (IL-4 and IL-5), and that suppress macrophage activation (IL-4 ad IL-10).

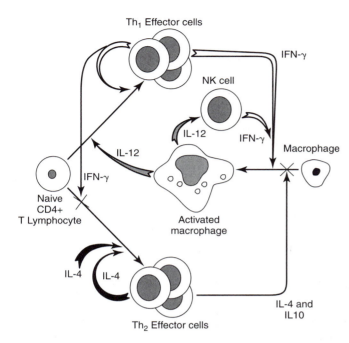

Figure 15-3. Interaction and counter-regulation of Th1 and Th2 cells. Differentiated Th1 cells secrete cytokines (principally IFN-γ) that feed back and inhibit the development of Th2 cells. Differentiated Th2 cells secrete cytokines (principally IL-4 and IL-10) that inhibit the activation of macrophages. This, in turn, results in less IL-12 production, and thus reduced Th1 cell development.

The cytokines produced by Th1 or Th2 cells tend to sustain their own development, and are frequently antagonistic to one another (Fig. 15-3). Thus, IFN-γ produced by Th1 cells blocks the expansion and differentiation of Th2 cells. IFN-γ also activates macrophages to produce more IL-12, which leads to further expansion of Th1 cells and inhibition of Th2 cells. Conversely, IL-4 produced by Th2 cells antagonizes Th1-cell effector functions. Locally elevated IL-4 drives the selective differentiation of activated T cells toward a Th2 phenotype. Interleukin-10 (IL-10) is a cytokine produced by Th2 cells (hence, its frequent classification as a "Th2 cytokine"), as well as some Th1 populations, activated macrophages, and perhaps B cells. It is an important cytokine in antagonizing the inflammatory response; by inhibiting macrophage activation, it indirectly causes decreased IL-12 production and thus a diminished drive to develop a Th1 phenotype. By depressing MHC, costimulator, and adhesion molecule expression, IL-10 can also directly modulate a variety of immune and inflammatory reactions (10–12).

Types of Immune-Mediated Inflammation

There are two distinct types of inflammation elicited by specific immune responses. These inflammatory reactions are character-

ized by their histologic features, mechanisms of induction, physiologic functions, and pathologic effects (Table 15-1). Delayed type hypersensitivity (DTH) reactions (see also Chapter 1) are characterized by the presence of activated macrophages and lymphocytes, as well as variable numbers of neutrophils and other granulocytes. Such reactions classically occur in response to chronic infections by organisms that resist phagocytic elimination—e.g., mycobacteria. Activated macrophages are required to destroy such microbes, and the generation of such cells is the protective function of DTH reactions. Granulomatous inflammation is a prototypical example of a protective DTH response to *Mycobacterium tuberculosis*. At the same time, activated macrophages and other leukocytes can have pathologic consequences, resulting in nonspecific tissue injury with subsequent scarring (as occurs often in granulomatous inflammation).

The second type of immune-mediated inflammation is characterized by the accumulation and activation of eosinophils and mast cells. This reaction is typically seen in allergic reactions, and probably plays a protective role against parasitic infections—e.g., trichinosis and schistosomiasis. As described in greater detail below, DTH and eosinophil-mediated inflammatory responses are driven by the secreted cytokines of the Th1 and Th2 subpopulations of T lymphocytes, respectively. Predictably, if multiple cytokines are produced during an immune response, the accompanying inflammatory reaction may exhibit features of both DTH and eosinophilic inflammation.

Role of T Cells and Cytokines in DTH

DTH reactions are usually triggered by antigen-mediated stimulation of the Th1 effector subset of CD4+ helper T cells producing IL-2, IFN-γ, and tumor necrosis factor-β (TNF-β or lymphotoxin) (1,13). In the DTH response, antigen stimulates secretion of the relevant cytokines from Th1 cells that have been activated and differentiated in response to previous exposure to that antigen (see Fig. 15-1). TNF-β from Th1 cells and TNF-α from activated macrophages stimulate endothelial cells at the site of antigen challenge to express ligands for leukocyte integrins (14). Monocytes, neutrophils, and activated T lymphocytes expressing high levels of the integrins bind to the activated endothelium and—driven by local chemokine production—migrate to the extravascular site where antigen is present. T cells that specifically recognize the antigen are preferentially retained at this site, and continue to produce cytokines. IL-2 promotes expansion of the antigen-responsive lymphocyte clones. IFN-γ activates macrophages to increase their phagocytic and degradative functions, improving antigen elimination. IFN-γ also stimulates the production of IgG antibody subclasses that promote phagocytosis of opsonized microbes. Activated macrophages, in turn, secrete IL-12 that stimulates greater T-cell IFN-γ production in an amplification loop. Thus, IL-2, IFN-γ, and TNF are the principal effector cytokines in DTH reactions, and IL-12 is important for local augmentation of the process. This form of inflammation is critical in protecting against a variety of infectious

Table 15-1. Types of Immune Inflammation

Feature	Delayed-Type Hypersensitivity (DTH)	Eosinophil/Mast Cell–Mediated Inflammation
Histologic appearance	Activated macrophages, lymphocytes, neutrophils, endothelial activation	Eosinophils, mast cells, vascular reaction (edema)
Type of T cells involved	Typically Th1 cells; sometimes CD8$^+$ T cells	Typically Th2 cells
Roles of cytokines:		
Induction	IFN-γ, TNF, IL-12	IL-4, IL-5
Inhibition	IL-10, IL-4	IFN-γ
Physiologic function	Elimination of intracellular microbes	Defense against helminths; regulation of Th1 responses
Pathologic effects	Tissue necrosis, scarring; typically chronic granulomatous inflammation	Allergic reactions, acute inflammation

organisms, and may also play a role in immune surveillance of tumors. Conversely, exuberant or unregulated DTH responses are responsible for much of the pathology that occurs in a variety of autoimmune diseases.

Role of T Cells and Cytokines in Eosinophil- and Mast Cell–Mediated Inflammation

Inflammatory reactions characterized by eosinophil and mast cell accumulation and activation are triggered by stimulation of the Th2 effector subset of helper T cells producing IL-4, IL-5, IL-10, and IL-13 (1,13) (see Fig. 15-2). IL-4 and IL-13 promote expansion of the antigen-responsive Th2 clones, and stimulate production of IgE antibody, which in turn sensitizes mast cells for subsequent degranulation in response to antigen binding. IL-4 also promotes eosinophil recruitment by inducing the expression of appropriate endothelial adhesion molecules (vascular cell adhesion molecule-1) and chemokines such as eotaxin (15,16); TNF can potentiate this process (16). IL-5 produced by Th2 cells is a potent eosinophil-activating cytokine, promoting eosinophil binding and killing of IgE-opsonized targets. Moreover, tissue mast cells and recruited eosinophils are potential sources of Th2 cytokines, and so tend to maintain a local environment rich in Th2-differentiated lymphocytes (17–20). Th2-driven inflammatory responses play important roles in protection against a host of extracellular parasitic infections. However, dysregulated eosinophil- and mast cell–mediated inflammation also underlies the pathology associated with allergic states.

Th2 cells not only induce eosinophil- and mast cell–mediated inflammation, but also serve a crucial role as inhibitors of Th1-induced DTH reactions. Thus, IL-10 inhibits macrophage activation, and IL-4 antagonizes the actions of IFN-γ. Therefore, besides providing protection against parasites, inhibitory Th2 cytokines may also have a physiologic role in modulating Th1 responses and thereby limiting tissue injury in DTH reactions (see Fig. 15-3).

Development and Functions of Helper T-Cell Subsets

It is apparent that the nature of any immune response to a given antigen is influenced by the types of T cells that are stimulated. Following antigen recognition, naive CD4$^+$ T cells may be induced to differentiate into polarized Th1 or Th2 cells, or into some mixture of the two. The major determinants of the patterns of T-cell differentiation are the cytokines produced at the site of antigen exposure (see Figs. 15-1 and 15-2). If naive T cells are stimulated by antigen in the presence of IL-12 or IFN-γ, the T cells differentiate to become Th1 effectors. By contrast, antigenic stimulation in the presence of IL-4 or IL-10 promotes the development of Th2 effectors. Thus, the cytokines that function in the effector phases of T cell–mediated immune responses are also key participants in the activation phases of T-cell responses. The initial stimulus for Th1-cell differentiation appears to be IL-12 secreted by cells of innate immunity—e.g., nonspecifically activated macrophages (21) or dendritic cells (22). The initial driving force for Th2 differentiation is much less clear; workers have variously suggested IL-4 derived from mast cells (20), basophils (23), eosinophils (18,19), low-level production by T cells (22), or a major output from minor T-cell subsets (24).

The dual function of cytokines provides a powerful amplification system. Thus, macrophages infected with intracellular microbes such as mycobacteria will secrete IL-12 (21), which stimulates production of IFN-γ by NK cells and T lymphocytes, and induces T cells to develop into IFN-γ–producing Th1 effectors (25). The IFN-γ in turn activates macrophages to destroy the intracellular microbes (see Fig. 15-1). Similarly, helminths can induce production of IL-4 from basophils (23), and perhaps from eosinophils (18,19). In turn, IL-4 promotes the development of Th2 effectors, and the reactions triggered by Th2 cells—to make IgE and to recruit and activate eosinophils—serve to eliminate helminths.

Finally, it has been observed that the initial immune response to many protein antigens consists mainly of Th1 cells, and chronic antigenic stimulation leads to a progressive increase in Th2 populations (1). This sequence of events supports the conceptual framework that Th1 cells are the subpopulation initially elicited to eliminate most microbes and bear the primary responsibility for phagocyte-mediated host defense and antigen elimination. In this paradigm, Th2 cells develop secondarily and serve an important role in limiting the tissue injury that accompanies macrophage activation.

Figure 15-3 schematically demonstrates how Th1 and Th2 effector cells and cytokines are interrelated, and how they can cross-modulate each other. Thus, Th1 responses may be augmented either by increasing local IFN-γ or IL-12 production, or by inhibiting IL-4 and IL-10 output. Conversely, Th1 responses can be dampened by directly blocking IFN-γ or IL-12, or by locally enhancing IL-4 and IL-10. Th2 populations may be similarly regulated by appropriate manipulation of either Th1 or Th2 cytokines.

In practical terms, a number of approaches have been used to alter Th1/Th2 cell ratios or, more specifically, the in vivo cytokine milieu, all with certain advantages and drawbacks (Table 15-2).

In experimental models, the adoptive transfer of purified Th1 or Th2 cells specific for a particular antigen has been used to shift the in vivo response toward a particular phenotype (26,27). The recognition of a cell-surface molecule apparently uniquely expressed on Th2 cells in mice [ST2L (28,29)] permits the selective antibody-mediated depletion of these cells with a resultant augmented Th1 response (29). Antibodies to adhesion molecules and integrins that prolong cardiac allograft survival have also been reported to shift the immune response toward a Th2 predominance (30). Immunotherapy with selected allergen extracts to reduce allergies may achieve clinical benefit by reducing Th2 responses and augmenting Th1 responses to the specific antigen (31,32). Similar benefits of enhanced Th1 responses have been reported in animal tumor vaccine models (33). These approaches all suffer from the potential shortcoming that entire panels of Th1 or Th2 cytokines may be altered rather than a single selected molecule.

Pharmacologic inhibition of selected cytokines has also been reported; thus, pentoxifylline inhibits IL-12 production (34), lysofylline inhibits IL-12 receptor signaling (35), and monomethylfumarate augments the production of IL-4 and IL-5 (36). In addition, pharmacologic inhibition of intracellular mitogen-activated protein (MAP) kinase or calcineurin signaling pathways results in differential modulation of cytokine expression (37). Nevertheless, most experimental work has used direct administration of cytokines (38), or blocking antibodies directed against the cytokines *or their receptors*, to achieve specific

cytokine blockade. The expanding availability of recombinant cytokines and monoclonal humanized antibodies has made these approaches increasingly attractive.

From this brief summary it is clear that regulating the activities of the cytokines that are involved in the differentiation and effector functions of CD4⁺ (and likely CD8⁺) T cells can be of therapeutic importance in a variety of disease states. In the remainder of this chapter we will discuss three cytokines that play important roles in immune-mediated inflammation: IL-4, IL-10, and IL-12. A fourth, IFN-γ, is described in Chapter 16.

Interleukin-4 (IL-4)

The potential clinical importance of IL-4 stems from its central role in the development of IgE-mediated allergic reactions, and its ability to suppress cell-mediated immunity and DTH. IL-4 antagonism is clearly desirable in the treatment of allergic diseases (39–41). On the other hand, specific IL-4 agonists may be helpful in ameliorating autoimmunity (42) or transplant rejection (43,44). Although one might anticipate that IL-4 agonists would be efficacious for enhancing the elimination of certain extracellular parasites via IgE- and eosinophil-mediated pathways, a beneficial outcome has been only rarely reported (45). In fact, it is much more commonly observed that IL-4 antagonism either accelerates clearance of the microorganisms or prevents infection-related disease (46,47).

History

IL-4 was discovered in 1982 as a T cell–derived factor (originally called B-cell stimulatory factor or BSF-1) that enhanced the proliferation of B lymphocytes induced to undergo polyclonal proliferation by culture with anti-immunoglobulin antibodies (48). In 1986, the murine IL-4 gene was identified by expression cloning, using induction of antibody synthesis as the bioassay (49). Cloning of the human IL-4 gene, and of mouse and human IL-4 receptors, followed in short order.

IL-4, IL-4 Receptor, and Mechanisms of IL-4 Action

IL-4 is a 20-kD glycoprotein (129 amino acids) containing six cysteine residues that are involved in the formation of disulfide bonds essential for its activity. IL-4 forms a four α-helical structure characteristic of cytokines that stimulate lymphoid and hematopoietic cells, including IL-2, IL-3, IL-5, IL-7, and GM-CSF (so-called "type I cytokines") (50). Both mouse and human IL-4 are species specific, although their sequences diverge only at residues 91–128. The IL-4 molecule has one structural domain that mediates high-affinity binding to the IL-4 receptor [$K_d = 150$ pM (51)], and a separate domain that induces receptor signaling. Substitution of an aspartate residue for TYR_{124} in human IL-4 thus preserves binding but eliminates IL-4-dependent T-cell proliferation, and results in a potent IL-4 antagonist (52).

Table 15-2. Approaches to Modulation of Cytokine Profiles

Agent	Effect	Advantage	Disadvantage
Pharmacologic agents:		• Potential oral agents	• ? Specificity
Pentoxifylline	Inhibits IL-12 production		
Lysofylline	Inhibits IL-12 receptor signaling		
Monomethylfumarate	Augments IL-4 and IL-5 production		
Cytokines:		• Potent	• Usually short half-life (min-hr)
IL-4	Induces Th2 response and inhibits macrophage cytokine production		• Peptides requiring injection
IL-10	Blocks IL-12 production and reduces macrophage costimulation		• Systemic toxicity (e.g., IL-4, IL-12)
IL-12	Induces Th1 response and increased IFN-γ production		
Cytokines delivered by viral vectors	Same as cytokines directly	• Longer, sustained delivery • Less systemic toxicity	• Vectors themselves may modulate the immune response
Anticytokine antibodies:		• Selective depletion of one effector cytokine	• Short half-life (days)
Anti-IL-4	Blocks Th2 responses (e.g., allergy, anaphylaxis)		• Requires systemic injection
Anti-IL-10	Augments Th1 response		• Difficult to sustain blockade at local level
Anti-IL-12	Augments Th2 response and inhibits Th1 response		
Cytokine antagonists (e.g., mutant IL-4)	Effects similar to cytokine blocking antibodies	• No immune response to the antagonists (as opposed to antibodies that may elicit responses to foreign proteins)	• Short half-life (days) • Require systemic injection • Difficult to sustain blockade at local level
Anticytockine receptor antibodies	Effects similar to cytokine blocking antibodies	• May block only activated cells with expressed receptor	• Short half-life (days) • Require systemic injection
Adoptive transfer of differentiated antigen-specific cells:		• Well-characterized, antigen-specific cells	• Difficult to target to lesional tissue
Th1 cells	Augmented Th1 response, blunted or absent Th2 response		• Impractical except for research purposes
Th2 cells	Augmented Th2 response, blunted Th1 response		• Global modification of Th1 or Th2 cytokine milieu
Anti-ST2L (anti-Th2)	Augmented Th1 response	• Selective Th2 subpopulation depletion with intact cell-mediated immunity	• Global Th2 depletion (i.e., not antigen-specific)
Anti-ICA-1/anti-LFA-1 (adhesion molecules)	Augmented Th2 response	• May preferentially target activated cells	• Global Th1/Th2 modulation • Affects other inflammatory responses (e.g., neutrophil recruitment)

The IL-4 receptor (also called CD124) is expressed at densities of 100 to 5000 copies per cell. Like other type I cytokine receptors, it is a heterodimer, composed of a 130-kD α-chain that confers ligand binding specificity, and a signal-transducing 150-kD γ_c chain that is shared with the IL-2, IL-7, IL-9, and IL-15 receptors. The ligand-binding α-chain has a conserved domain defined by two cysteine residues and a trytophan-serine-X (any residue)–trytophan–serine (WSXWS) peptide motif characteristic of type I cytokine receptors. Signal transduction may also be achieved by α-chain association with the signaling subunit of the

IL-13 receptor. The various complexes act through different JAK kinases, but in inducing Th2 differentiation events, ultimately act by means of phosphorylation of the same STAT-6 transcription factor (STAT stands for signal transducer and activator of transcription) (53,54).

The IL-4 receptor is expressed on a wide variety of hematopoietic cells, including lymphocytes, macrophages, and mast cells. Soluble IL-4 receptors have been detected in mice and humans, generated by proteolytic cleavage of the membrane-bound receptors or direct translation of mRNAs encoding the soluble form of the molecule (55). Recombinant soluble IL-4 receptors can theoretically act as competitive inhibitors of IL-4. However, soluble receptors form long-lived IL-4 complexes and will release IL-4 even after prolonged incubation; thus, they can have both antagonistic and agonistic activities, depending on the relative concentrations of IL-4 (56).

IL-4-induced cell *proliferation* occurs by means of IL-4 receptor γ_c-chain–mediated tyr_{497} phosphorylation of the IL-4 receptor α-chain, involving JAK kinases. This is followed by binding and phosphorylation of insulin-responsive substrate-1 or -2; IRS-2 is active in hematopoietic cells, while IRS-1 is active in nonhematopoietic cells. The signaling cascade downstream of IRS phosphorylation is not well defined. IL-4–mediated *differentiation* events are mediated by phosphorylation of more distal sites on the IL-4 receptor α-chain, including a series of STAT-6 binding sites. Phosphorylated STAT-6 ultimately translocates to the nucleus and binds to target sequences in the promoters of IL-4–responsive genes, including the immunoglobulin C_ε and $C_{\gamma 1}$ genes and the IL-4 gene itself (24).

Cellular Sources and Actions

In all species, IL-4 is produced by CD4$^+$ helper T cells of the Th2 subset; indeed, IL-4 production is used as the criterion for classifying Th cells in this subset. Activated mast cells, basophils, and some CD8$^+$ T cells and perhaps eosinophils can also produce IL-4. In T lymphocytes, IL-4 production is elicited by specific antigen recognition and is regulated at the level of transcription. Cells of the basophil/mast cell lineage secrete IL-4 as a result of cross-linking of Fc receptor-bound IgE by antigen (57). In several parasitic infections and model immune responses to protein antigens in mice, these non-T cells produce at least as much IL-4 as do helper T lymphocytes (58).

The biologic effects of IL-4 are exerted on several cell types.

B Lymphocytes

IL-4 is required for isotype switching of antigen-stimulated B cells to the production of IgE antibodies, and inhibits switching to isotypes augmented by interferon-γ (e.g., IgG2a in mice) (59). IL-4 also promotes switching to the IgG1 heavy chain isotype in mice (IgG4 isotype in humans). Since these isotypes do not fix complement or bind to Fc receptors on phagocytes, they do not participate in phagocyte-dependent defense. In addition to antibody production, IL-4 is a growth factor for B lymphocytes. It also promotes MHC class II expression on B cells, thus augmenting helper T cell–B cell interactions.

T Lymphocytes

IL-4 is required for the differentiation of naive CD4$^+$ T lymphocytes to the Th2 effector subset. IL-4 is also an autocrine growth factor for Th2 cells, and may function as a growth and differentiation factor for some CD8$^+$ cells.

Macrophages

IL-4 inhibits IFN-γ–induced production of proinflammatory cytokines (TNF-α, IL-1), nitric oxide, and prostaglandins by macrophages (60,61). Because of these activities, IL-4 suppresses cell-mediated immunity and DTH.

Mast Cells

IL-4 is a growth factor for mast cell lines, and synergizes with IL-3 to stimulate mast cell proliferation (59).

Other Cells

IL-4 stimulates the expression of VCAM-1 on vascular endothelium, promoting the binding and transmigration of lymphocytes, monocytes, and especially eosinophils. IL-4–treated endothelial cells also secrete chemokines such as monocyte chemotactic protein-1 (MCP-1) (62), and IL-4–treated fibroblasts and epithelial cells secrete eotaxin (63), potentially responsible for selectively inducing monocyte- and eosinophil-rich inflammatory reactions.

IL-13 is structurally distinct from IL-4 but shares many of the same biologic activities. However, IL-13 can only activate the IL-13 receptor, while IL-4 can bind and activate both the IL-4 and IL-13 receptors. Since T lymphocytes predominantly express the IL-4 receptor, and the IL-13 receptor is found on B cells and nonlymphoid cells (e.g., macrophages and endothelium), IL-13 mimics many IL-4 effects but does not function as a growth or differentiation factor for T cells. Interestingly, IL-13 does stimulate isotype switching to IgE and IgG1 (64).

Role in Disease

Overproduction of IL-4 and the other Th2 cytokines relative to Th1 cytokines plays an important part in the pathogenesis of three categories of diseases. First, as mentioned above, allergic reactions are mediated by IL-4 and IL-5. Severely atopic individuals may generate larger numbers of allergen-specific Th2 cells than normal individuals, and the Th2 cells of atopic patients often secrete abnormally high levels of IL-4 per cell (4,65).

Second, imbalanced Th2 activation suppresses cell-mediated immunity and leads to severe, disseminated infections—especially with intracellular microbes. Disseminated leishmaniasis and lepromatous leprosy are two examples of such infections (1,66). It has also been suggested that evolution of a predominant Th2 response (67) may augment the progression of AIDS by increasing susceptibility to opportunistic infections (68,69). This theory is extremely controversial, and there is abundant evidence against generalized Th1 or Th2 predominance in HIV-infected individuals (70), even with falling CD4$^+$ T cell counts and clinical symptoms (71). Nevertheless, it is intriguing that, owing to the intrinsic variability of HIV strains, different responses may occur. Thus, macrophage-tropic HIV replicates more efficiently in Th1-type cultures, while T cell-tropic strains preferentially infect Th2-type cells (72). In addition, IL-4 down-modulates the expression of the C-C chemokine receptor 5 (CCR5) "HIV coreceptor" on macrophages and inhibits HIV replication in macrophages (73), while increasing the C-X-C chemokine receptor 4 (CXCR4) "HIV coreceptor" expression on T cells and stimulating their HIV expression (74). Although the vast majority of sexually transmitted HIV uses the CCR5 coreceptor, the transition from clinical latency to full-blown AIDS is marked by an apparent conversion of the virus to the use of the CXCR4 coreceptor (75). However, whether this transition in HIV tropism is cause or effect of the clinical disease is not clear; it is noteworthy that no clinical trial involving Th1/Th2 modulation in AIDS has yet been performed.

Third, because of the negative feedback loops involving Th2 cytokines, administration of IL-4 (and IL-10) is being increasingly evaluated in the treatment of a variety of autoimmune diseases (42) and for modulating transplant rejection (76,77). IL-4 released from tumor-associated Th2 cells has also been implicated in aggravating the severity of metastatic disease (78), so that therapy directed against IL-4 may result in a more potent antitumor cellular immune response.

Therapeutic Potential of IL-4 and IL-4 Antagonists

The main therapeutic possibilities for IL-4 antagonists are for the disorders in which excessive production of this cytokine is implicated in disease pathogenesis. Thus, IL-4 antagonists may be useful for treating allergies, for inhibiting IgE production, and for blocking local eosinophil- and mast cell–mediated inflammatory reactions. In support of this, and as mentioned above, immunotherapy to ameliorate allergies may achieve clinical benefit in humans by reducing Th2 responses and augmenting Th1 responses to the specific antigen (31,32), although this is not a uniform finding (79). Anti–IL-4 monoclonal antibodies have also been demonstrated to prevent fatal anaphylaxis in an animal model (80).

Moreover, IL-4 antagonists may be useful adjuncts for treating infectious diseases associated with depressed cell-mediated immunity, including disseminated leishmaniasis and lepromatous leprosy (47). As described above, possible IL-4 antagonists for clinical use include neutralizing monoclonal antibodies and recombinant soluble receptors, as well as specifically engineered IL-4 mutant proteins that block all IL-4 signaling (81). While being extensively applied in several animal models, none of these antagonists has yet found use in human clinical trials.

Administration of IL-4 directly may also be useful for counteracting exuberant Th1-type responses. For example, IL-4 has shown efficacy as antigen-specific therapy for inducing immune deviation to a presumptively less inflammatory Th2 phenotype in several autoimmune disease models (42). Thus, IL-4—with or without IL-10—suppresses collagen-induced arthritis (82,83), autoimmune diabetes (84), experimental autoimmune

encephalomyelitis (a model for multiple sclerosis) (85), and inflammatory bowel disease (86). Although there is a strong theoretical basis for its efficacy, the utility of IL-4 administration or Th2 cell deviation in moderating rejection in animal models of transplantation is much less clear; results thus far have been contradictory (76,77). IL-4 has also been tested for the treatment of metastatic cancers, based on the demonstration that IL-4–transfected tumor cells elicit local inflammation and are rejected rapidly, and may also stimulate systemic T cell–dependent immunity to the parent tumor (87,88).

Systemic administration of cytokines such as IL-4 is fraught with difficulties related to therapeutic availability and potential toxicities. However, the extremely short half-life of IL-4 in vivo (minutes) can be modulated by binding to soluble IL-4 receptors (56) or by using IL-4–immunoglobulin fusion proteins (89). Moreover, half-life and toxicity issues related to systemic administration of IL-4 may be bypassed by targeted delivery of IL-4 genes using viral vector strategies (85,86,90). The utility of these compounds and approaches in human disease has not yet been demonstrated.

Interleukin-10 (IL-10)

IL-10 and TGF-β are the major known physiologic inhibitors of inflammation. TGF-β acts mainly on neutrophils, and knockout mice lacking the TGF-β cytokine develop fatal widespread, acute inflammation (91). Conversely, the anti-inflammatory action of IL-10 is directed mainly against macrophages, and its physiologic function appears to be control of Th1-mediated inflammation. Thus, the principal potential therapeutic utility of this cytokine is for disorders caused by excessive T cell– and macrophage-mediated inflammatory reactions (92), including autoimmune diseases (93) and transplant rejection (94). IL-10 blockade may also have efficacy in augmenting the immune response to a variety of infectious organisms (95,96).

History

The discovery of IL-10 is a remarkable example of the successful search for a cytokine whose existence was predicted largely on a theoretical basis. Following identification of Th1 and Th2 subsets among mouse CD4$^+$ T cells, Mosmann and his colleagues postulated that each subset should produce cytokines that cross-regulated—i.e., inhibited—the development and/or effector functions of the other subset. It had already been demonstrated that IFN-γ inhibited Th2 proliferation in vitro. The search for a cytokine acting in the reverse direction led to the identification of a Th2-cell product that inhibited IFN-γ production by Th1 clones; the cytokine was called IL-10 (97). It is now clear that the inhibitory effects on IFN-γ production are indirect and largely attributable to blockade of IL-12 synthesis by IL-10. IL-10 also inhibits the synthesis of other cytokines, including TNF-α and -β, IL-1, and IL-6. Although the actions of IL-10 can be conceptualized primarily as anti-inflammatory, IL-10 is also a potent CD8$^+$ T-cell chemoattractant and cytotoxic T-cell differentiation factor, and in vitro is an important B-cell stimulator and differentiation factor (98,99).

IL-10, IL-10 Receptor, and Mechanisms of IL-10 Action

IL-10 is an 18-kD homodimeric polypeptide composed of two noncovalently associated 160 amino acid subunits (99); its tertiary structure is remarkably similar to that of IFN-γ (100). Interestingly, the Epstein-Barr virus expresses a structurally homologous protein (84% homology at the protein level) called BCRF-1 (Bam HI C fragment rightward reading frame; also called viral IL-10 or vIL-10) that exhibits many of the biologic activities of the natural cytokine (101). It is postulated that the Epstein-Barr virus incorporated the cellular IL-10 gene as a mechanism for inhibiting antiviral defense and promoting its own survival.

The IL-10 receptor is a heavily glycosylated 110-kD transmembrane glycoprotein protein with sequence homologies to the IFN receptors (102,103), and with a high affinity for the IL-10 ligand ($K_d = 70–250 \, pM$). The structural similarity of IL-10 and IFN-γ and their receptors is intriguing in light of the fact that IL-10 inhibits many of the macrophage functions activated by IFN-γ. Thus, both receptors may interact with the same downstream signaling pathways, but with different consequences. The IL-10 receptor is expressed on a variety of hematopoietic cell lineages in bone marrow, spleen, and thymus, and to a lesser extent on nonhematopoietic cells; 5000 to 10,000 receptors are present on B cells (103). Engagement of the receptor by IL-10 results in JAK1 and tyk2 kinase phosphorylation, and subsequent activation of STAT-1 and STAT-3 (104).

Cellular Sources and Actions

Although IL-10 was first identified as a product of mouse Th2 cells, it is not strictly a Th2-specific cytokine. Indeed, monocytes/macrophages, CD4+ T cells of both Th1 and Th2 subsets, and some B cells and CD8+ T cells can all produce IL-10 on appropriate stimulation; keratinocyte production has also been documented. In humans, the monocyte/macrophage lineage is the major source of endogenous IL-10 (105). IL-10 synthesis is transcriptionally regulated with NFκB and cAMP response elements in the upstream promoter sequence (99,105); its synthesis is negatively regulated by IL-1, IL-4, and IFN-γ (106).

The principal action of IL-10 is inhibition of the proinflammatory response (98,107). Thus, although IL-1, IL-12, and TNF-α are all rapidly elevated following endotoxin challenge (30 minutes), IL-10 production peaks 6 to 8 hours later, suggesting a role in reducing cytokine-induced inflammation (108,109).

Macrophages
Much of the anti-inflammatory effect of IL-10 is attributable to inhibition of macrophage activation and accessory function (107,110). IL-10 blocks the expression of costimulators and IFN-γ–induced class II MHC molecules on macrophages, and directly inhibits production of TNF-α, IL-1, IL-12, and reactive oxygen species (111,112). The inhibition of IFN-γ production, the first

activity attributed to IL-10, results primarily from decreased production of IL-12 and diminished costimulator expression on macrophages (11,107). Owing to its ability to inhibit IL-12 production by macrophages, IL-10 inhibits the development of Th1 effector cells from naive CD4+ T lymphocytes and induces a Th2-dominant population (111,113).

B Lymphocytes
IL-10 is a B-cell proliferation and differentiation factor in vitro, contributing to clonal expansion and plasma cell maturation (114). IL-10 also participates in immunoglobulin class switching to IgG1 and IgG3 (115), the isotypes that most avidly bind to Fc receptors and fix complement. Coincidentally, IL-10 augments Fc-γ receptor expression on a variety of cell types (99), so that the net effect of IL-10 will be an augmented antibody synthesis and enhanced effector function of humoral immunity.

T Lymphocytes
In addition to the indirect effects on cytokine synthesis in T cells, IL-10 has chemotactic activity for CD8+ T cells (116) and induces CD8+ cytotoxic T-cell differentiation (117).

Mast Cells
Although IL-10 is reported to stimulate mast cell proliferation in mice (99), it inhibits cytokine generation by these cells (118).

Other Cells
IL-10 augments IL-2–induced natural killer (NK) cell proliferation and activates NK-cell cytolytic activity while suppressing IFN-γ and TNF cytokine synthesis by these cells (99,105).

Role in Disease

A relative deficiency of IL-10 production has been implicated in diseases associated with excessive macrophage-mediated inflammation. For example, mice with their IL-10 genes disrupted by homologous recombination ("IL-10 knock-outs") develop uncontrolled inflammation in response to minor trauma and a severe, uniformly fatal inflammatory bowel disease (119). Similar colonic inflammation occurs in SCID (severe combined immunodeficiency) mice given IFN-γ–producing Th1 cells, presumably owing to a relative predominance of IFN-γ over IL-10 (120). The "spontaneous" inflammatory lesions are typically most severe in the lower GI tract because it naturally harbors a wealth of pathogenic microbes and thus has an active immune response presumably requiring tight regulation.

Deficient IL-10 is also implicated in several human diseases with a presumed autoimmune basis, including Wegener's granulomatosis (121), psoriasis (122), and rheumatoid arthritis (123). On the other hand, elevated IL-10 is readily measured in the peripheral blood of patients in whom immune modulation would be important, including in the recovery phase of meningococcal septic shock (124), where IL-10 is presumably inducing monocyte deactivation. IL-10 is systemically elevated following major surgery or injury, potentially to create a post-traumatic immune refractory state (92,125). It is also increased systemically in infections and inflammatory disease syndromes (126), where it may play a role in limiting cell-mediated immune injury.

Relevant to therapy, protective anti-inflammatory effects of IL-10 have been demonstrated in animal models of autoimmune uveoretinitis (127), autoimmune encephalomyelitis (128), and collagen-induced arthritis (129). Evidence has also accrued that generation of T-cell anergy to selected antigens in both mice and humans (e.g., in specific immunotherapy for allergies) may occur through generation of IL-10–producing regulatory T cells (130–133).

In a variety of infectious disease models, the importance of IL-10 varies with the nature of the infectious challenge. Thus, in IL-10–deficient mice, *Toxoplasmosis gondii* infection was uniformly fatal owing to IL-12, IFN-γ, and TNF-α overproduction (134), whereas lack of IL-10 was protective to the host animal in the setting of a *Listeria monocytogenes* infection (96). Thus, as recombinant IL-10 is used more extensively for clinical immune modulation, the associated risks relating to infectious disease will become increasingly important (126), although not necessarily predictable.

Therapeutic Potential of IL-10

In animal experiments, recombinant IL-10 has proved to be extremely well tolerated at therapeutically effective dosages, and human clinical trials for several disease entities are under way (126,135). Healthy human volunteers receiving IL-10 exhibited marked reductions in IL-2-induced T-cell proliferation and monocyte IL-1 and TNF-α synthesis; high dosages resulted in only mild flulike symptoms (136,137).

A principal therapeutic use of IL-10 may be for modulation of acute inflammation in endotoxin shock (108). Thus, pretreatment with IL-10 before a low-dosage endotoxin challenge in volunteers resulted in attenuation of proinflammatory cytokine production, neutrophil degranulation, and coagulation activation (138,139). Clinical trials with IL-10 in clinical septic shock have yet to be reported, although titration of IL-10 to ameliorate the effects of excessive inflammation without causing potentially lethal immunosuppression may prove challenging (126).

IL-10 also shows great promise for treating chronic inflammatory disorders such as ulcerative colitis and Crohn's disease, rheumatoid arthritis, psoriasis, and multiple sclerosis (126,135). Clinical trials are ongoing for each, with those for inflammatory bowel disease currently in phase 3 (126).

With regards to other applications, IL-10 may have efficacy in limiting the extent of inflammatory damage following ischemia and reperfusion—i.e., in lung (140), gastrointestinal tract (141), or brain (e.g., following stroke) (142). Although IL-10 has been promoted as a potential immunosuppressive agent for transplantation (94), results thus far have been contradictory. Thus, retroviral transfer of viral IL-10 significantly prolonged survival in a nonvascularized murine heart transplant model, although it did not prevent eventual graft failure (143). Conversely, in a vascularized murine heart transplant model, IL-10 accelerated allograft rejection, and anti–IL-10 prolonged allograft survival,

particularly in presensitized hosts in which alloantibody responses would have been expected to be important (144). Based on animal experiments in SCID mice reconstituted with human hematopoietic cells, IL-10 also appears to reduce the HIV burden by inhibiting transcription activation in infected cells and/or by altering the proliferative cytokine milieu (145); a phase 1 trial in HIV infection is underway (126). IL-10 has also been reported to induce apoptosis in malignant B cells, and therefore may have utility in the treatment of certain leukemias (146).

The use of IL-10 antagonists could potentially be beneficial in pathologic conditions where cell-mediated immunity is defective, perhaps as a result of excessive Th2 activation (e.g., lepromatous leprosy and generalized tuberculosis). Like IL-4 antagonists, agents that interfere with the actions of IL-10 (e.g., monoclonal blocking antibodies) would reduce Th2-mediated suppression and enhance protective cellular immunity. Few studies examining these points have been reported.

Interleukin-12 (IL-12)

Since the molecular cloning of IL-12 in 1991, an astonishing amount of information has accumulated. The major physiologic importance of IL-12 is its central role in macrophage–T cell interactions and in eliciting protective cell-mediated immunity against intracellular microbes. It is in this context that IL-12–modulating agents are likely to be of greatest therapeutic benefit (147,148). IL-12 augmentation may also be efficacious in antitumor immunity (149,150). On the flip side, pharmacologic damping of IL-12 activity may have utility in treating chronic inflammatory diseases (151) or transplant rejection (152).

History

As outlined at the beginning of this chapter, phagocytic cells and NK cells are important effectors of innate resistance, representing early lines of defense against infectious pathogens. During the early host response to microorganisms, these cells produce cytokines that amplify their own effector functions. Thus, IFN-γ secreted by NK cells is a powerful activator of macrophages and important in driving Th1-cell differentiation (see Fig. 15-1). Activation of NK cells—as well as CD8⁺ cytotoxic T lymphocytes (CTL)—in turn is accomplished by means of cytokines produced by macrophages and Th cells. IL-12, produced by infected phagocytic and dendritic cells, is a critical cytokine in this process. It stimulates IFN-γ production by NK cells and CTL, and enhances the cytotoxic activity of both CTL and NK cells, hence its original name of natural killer stimulatory factor (NKSF) (153,154). Consequently, IL-12 functions as a key initiator of cell-mediated immunity.

IL-12, IL-12 Receptor, and Mechanisms of IL-12 Action

IL-12 is a glycosylated, covalently linked heterodimer of 70 kD (p70) composed of two nonhomologous subunits of approximately 40kD (p40, 306 amino acids) and 35kD (p35, 197 amino acids) coded by differentially regulated and distinct genes on different chromosomes (155,156). Since antibodies to the p40 component effectively block IL-12 association with its receptors, this subunit putatively expresses the relevant binding site; the free p40 subunit also antagonizes the effects of the IL-12 heterodimer (157). The individual chains have no biologic activity, and cotransfection of cDNA from both genes is required for production of functional IL-12 (156). However, biologically active single-chain fusion constructs of IL-12 have been engineered (158,159).

The IL-12 receptor is a heterodimeric transmembrane protein composed of β1 and β2 subunits; each subunit alone has very low IL-12 binding affinity (K_d = 2–5nM), whereas the combined molecule exhibits high-affinity (K_d = 50pM) and low-affinity (K_d = 5nM) binding sites (160). Since IL-12 mediates many of its biologic functions at picomolar concentrations (153), the highest-affinity receptors are probably responsible for the biologic effects of IL-12. IL-12 p40 interacts predominantly with the β1 chain, while p35 binds to the β2 molecule. The IL-12 receptor heterodimer is highly expressed on activated CD4$^+$ and CD8$^+$ T cells, as well as on activated NK cells. It is not present—or is present at very low levels—on resting T and NK cells, and is not expressed on B lymphocytes (161), although the latter do synthesize β1 subunit mRNA (162).

Both subunits have cytoplasmic domains with motifs characteristic of several other cytokine receptors. However, the β1 chain lacks cytoplasmic tyrosines, while the β2 protein has three and is probably therefore the chain responsible for signal transduction. Binding of IL-12 to the heterodimeric receptor induces tyrosine phosphorylation of JAK2 and tyk2 kinases, with subsequent phosphorylation and nuclear translocation of the STAT-3 and STAT-4 transcription factors; IL-12 is the only known inducer of STAT-4 (163,164). IL-12 induces production of IFN-γ and expression of other cellular proteins mostly by enhancing gene transcription. However, its effect in the context of other inducers is often attributable to a combination of transcriptional and post-transcriptional modifications. For instance, IL-12 induces IFN-γ transcription and IL-2 stabilizes the transcripts, accounting for the synergistic action of these two cytokines (165).

Cellular Sources and Actions

Multiple cell types synthesize the p35 subunit of IL-12, but production of the p40 subunit to generate fully active IL-12 is largely restricted to mononuclear phagocytic cells and dendritic cells. Cells that synthesize active IL-12 tend to secrete a large excess (up to 1000-fold) of free p40 chain (166), which may play a local regulatory role by forming p40 homodimers that bind (but do not activate) the IL-12 receptor (167). Although IL-12 was originally described as a product of B-cell lines (153,154), it is unlikely that B cells are a physiologically relevant source of the cytokine. Rather, phagocytic cells (particularly monocytes and macrophages) and dendritic cells are the major producers of IL-12 (166).

IL-12 synthesis is increased in these cells in response to bacteria, bacterial products such as lipopolysaccharide (LPS), or intracellular parasites (166); neutrophils also respond to LPS by secreting IL-12 (168). In addition to monocytes/macrophages, other cell types with potent antigen-presenting cell (APC) functions (e.g., dendritic cells and epidermal Langerhans cells) can produce IL-12. Besides infectious agents, IL-12 synthesis by macrophages and dendritic cells can be stimulated via CD40 on these APCs interacting with CD40 ligand on activated T cells (169,170). IFN-γ also enhances the production of IL-12 by phagocytes (168,171), an important aspect in feedback amplification of the T cell–APC interaction (see below).

IL-12 acts primarily on T lymphocytes and NK cells, resulting in four major biological effects.

Cytokine Production

IL-12 induces T lymphocytes and NK cells to produce several cytokines (e.g., GM-CSF and TNF), and it is particularly efficient in inducing production of IFN-γ (172,173). IL-12 not only potently induces IFN-γ production but also synergizes with many other stimuli to facilitate this activity (165,173).

Th1-Cell Development

IL-12 is required for Th1-cell development during the response to pathogens; the ratio between IL-4 and IL-12 production early after infection affects the ultimate balance of Th1 and Th2 cells (174–176). Mechanisms by which IL-12 induces T-cell differentiation toward the Th1 subset include: 1) priming T cells for high IFN-γ production in response to antigenic stimulation (177); 2) a preferential proliferative effect on Th1 cells (178); and 3) suppressing the development of IL-4–producing cells (174). Once a Th1 response is generated, IL-12 is generally not necessary to maintain the phenotype (179); however, Th1-differentiated T cells retain IL-12 responsiveness, and IL-12 produced by APC may be significant for generating autoamplification loops in autoimmune diseases (180).

Lymphocyte Proliferation

IL-12 does not directly induce resting T lymphocytes or NK cells to proliferate, although it does potentiate T-cell proliferation induced by other means (153,181). IL-12 can directly induce activated T and NK cells to proliferate in response to activation-induced conformational changes in the IL-12 receptors that transduce proliferative signals (182,183). Costimulation through the T-cell CD28 receptor (via B7 ligands on APCs) strongly synergizes with IL-12 to induce even greater T-cell proliferation (173,184).

Lymphocyte Cytotoxicity

IL-12 enhances the generation of cytotoxic lymphocytes (CTLs) and lymphokine-activated killer (LAK) cells, and potentiates the cytotoxic activity of CTLs and NK cells (153,185,186). IL-12 mediates these effects mainly by enhancing the expression of cytotoxic cell granule associated proteins (e.g., perforin) (187), as well as increasing the expression of adhesion molecules involved in target cell binding (188).

Role in Disease

Because it is the primary inducer of Th1-cell development, IL-12 is required for infections by intracellular microbes for which Th1 responses are protective. Within hours of contact with bacteria or other intracellular pathogens, infected macrophages produce IL-12, which in turn induces NK-cell and T-lymphocyte production of IFN-γ. This IFN-γ then activates phagocytic cells and enhances their microbicidal activity. Effective host responses to *Leishmania major* (189), *Mycobacterium tuberculosis* and *M. leprae* (190), *Candida albicans* (191), and *Toxoplasma gondii* (192) all require initial IL-12 production.

In experimental models of infection, treatment with neutralizing anti–IL-12 antibodies abrogates host resistance, whereas IL-12 treatment enhances it (193–195). Thus, IL-12 may represent a clinically useful adjuvant in the treatment of a variety of bacterial and intracellular parasite infections (147,196).

In comparison to its efficacy with bacteria, IL-12 plays a relatively minor role in viral infections, which tend to trigger IL-12–independent mechanisms of IFN-γ production (197). Nevertheless, use of IL-12 has been advocated for treatment of persistent hepatitis (198), and IL-12 has demonstrated efficacy in reducing the expression of the BM5def retrovirus responsible for murine acquired immunodeficiency syndrome, as well as inhibiting progression of the disease (199).

In contrast to this protective role, IL-12 also induces harmful and frequently lethal responses in endotoxin (septic) shock, resulting in exaggerated production of TNF-α, IL-1, and IL-12, and followed a few hours later by IFN-γ secretion. The fatal outcome of endotoxin shock is prevented by anti-IL-12 antibody blockade (147,200,201) although this has not been used in any human trials.

Therapeutic Potential of IL-12

A unique feature of recombinant IL-12 supporting its potential clinical utility is its long in vivo half-life (3 hours in rodents and 17 hours in rhesus monkeys). Moreover, in several animal models, low-dosage IL-12 is reasonably well tolerated. High-dosage IL-12 therapy (0.1–1 µg/day in mice), however, leads to acute toxicity attributable to IFN-γ production and primarily involving the hematopoietic, hepatic, and gastrointestinal systems (202). Chronic IL-12 administration in animals also induced a severe pulmonary macrophage infiltrate that invariably led to lethal pulmonary edema, even in the absence of IFN-γ (202). In humans, acute IL-12 toxicity involving the same organ systems occurred at much lower dosages than expected based on the animal data. Indeed, in an early phase II oncology trial, two therapy-related deaths and severe toxicity frequently requiring hospitalization were reported (203). Subsequent work demonstrated that protection from the adverse effects of daily IL-12 administration may be achieved by a single high dose of IL-12 delivered 1 to 2 weeks earlier, perhaps by modulating subsequent IFN-γ production (203).

Because IL-12 is a powerful inducer of cell-mediated immunity, it may be useful in treating disseminated infections by intracellular pathogens. In proof of concept, systemic administration of IL-12 cures mice of *Leishmania major* infection, even in strains that develop fatal disseminated leishmaniasis (204,205). However, it is significant that IL-12 therapy to generate a Th1 response needs to be initiated early in the course of infection; once a Th2 environment is developed, it is extremely difficult to reverse it by IL-12 treatment alone (205). This is a crucial point; most studies examining the efficacy of IL-12 demonstrate that coadministration of IL-12 at the time of inoculation with infectious agent (or tumor) leads to resistance. However, with the exception of vaccinations (see below), most clinical situations involve IL-12 being given only after the pathologic state is established. Antigen load (i.e., number of microbes) can influence the ability to reverse the cytokine environment, so that adjunctive IL-12 therapy in concert with microbicidal agents may represent a therapeutic option even late in the course of disease (206).

Another promising application of IL-12 is its use as an adjuvant in vaccination against those infectious diseases in which a Th1-dependent cell-mediated immune response is protective. Although IL-12 potentially acts as an adjuvant for both Th1 and Th2 cells (207), it usually promotes a strong Th1 outcome, even in strains more typically prone to Th2-type responses (176). Thus, immunization of certain mouse strains with a soluble *Leishmania major* extract results in induction of a Th2 response that is not protective; vaccination that includes IL-12 with the antigenic extract induces a memory Th1 response that completely protects the mice from subsequent infection (208). Similarly, in an animal model of *Schistosoma mansoni* infection, vaccines that included IL-12 prevented the Th2 response responsible for pathologic granuloma formation (209). IL-12 has also been shown to be an effective adjuvant in vaccines against *Listeria monocytogenes* (210) and *Bordetella pertussis* (211). IL-12 is an effective adjuvant when given subcutaneously with antigen, or when administered systemically separate from the antigen (212). To date, no clinical trials of this vaccination approach have been reported.

IL-12 has been shown in vitro partially to correct the depressed NK-cell activity observed in advanced AIDS patients and to induce production of IFN-γ from lymphocytes of HIV-positive patients (185). Furthermore, IL-12 can correct the defective in vitro proliferative responses of T cells from HIV-positive patients to HIV peptides, alloantigens, and recall antigens—e.g., influenza virus (213,214). This corrective effect of IL-12 may be attributable to the fact that peripheral blood mononuclear cells of HIV-positive patients produce 5- to 20-fold less IL-12 than do cells from healthy donors (215). The potential efficacy of IL-12 in AIDS to augment cellular immunity against opportunistic pathogens, and possibly against HIV itself, has prompted the initiation of phase I clinical trials.

In addition to infectious diseases, IL-12 is already undergoing several clinical trials as an antitumor agent. IL-12 stimulates tumoricidal NK cells (216), tumor-specific CTLs (216), and a novel population of CD18+ and CD8+ T cells with high IFN-γ production and enhanced non-MHC-restricted cytolytic activity (217); IL-12–induced IFN-γ is also directly tumoricidal (218). IL-12 may also have antitumor effects by inducing a potent Th1-driven antitumor response wherein macrophages kill tumor cells using nitric oxide (219). To optimize the efficacy of IL-12 tumoricidal activity and minimize the toxic side effects, strategies for targeted or local delivery—including gene therapy—have been advocated (196). IL-12 and B7 costimulation (with B7-transfected tumor cells) also yields an augmented antitumor response (173).

As mentioned above, neutralizing antibodies to IL-12 are effective in preventing mortality associated with endotoxin shock in animal models (147,200,201). However, the utility of this approach in human septic shock may be limited because IL-12 is produced within 2 to 3 hours of LPS administration and only pretreatment with antibodies is effective. Moreover, a pivotal role for IL-12 or IFN-γ in human septic shock is less clear than in rodents (220). IL-12 antagonists may also be useful in treating autoimmune diseases (151) or for preventing allograft rejection or graft-versus-host disease in bone marrow transplantation (152).

References

1. Abbas A, Murphy K, Sher A. Functional diversity of helper T lymphocytes. Nature 1996;383:787–793.
2. Mosmann T, Sad S. The expanding universe of T cell subsets: Th1, Th2 and more. Immunol Today 1996;17:138–146.
3. Hafler D, Kent S, Pietrusewicz M, et al. Oral administration of myelin induces antigen-specific TGF-beta 1 secreting T cells in patients with multiple sclerosis. Ann NY Acad Sci 1997;835:120–131.
4. Romagnani S. Lymphokine production by human T cells in disease states. Annu Rev Immunol 1994;12:227–257.
5. DelPrete G. The concept of type-1 and type-2 helper T cells and their cytokines in humans. Int Rev Immunol 1998;16:427–455.
6. Hahn S, Gehri R, Erb P. Mechanism and biological significance of CD4-mediated cytotoxicity. Immunol Rev 1995;146:57–79.
7. Mosmann T, Li L, Hengartner H, et al. Differentiation and function of T cell subsets. Ciba Found Symp 1997;204:148–154.
8. Cerwenka A, Carter L, Reome J, et al. In vivo persistence of CD8 polarized T cell subsets producing type 1 or type 2 cytokines. J Immunol 1998;161:97–105.
9. Baggiolini M, Dewald B, Moser B. Human chemokines: an update. Annu Rev Immunol 1997;15:675–705.
10. deWaal-Malefyt R, Haanen R, Spits H, et al. Interleukin 10 (IL-10) and viral IL-10 strongly reduce antigen-specific human T cell proliferation by diminishing antigen-presenting capacity of monocytes via down-regulation of class II major histocompatibility complex expression. J Exp Med 1991;174:915–924.
11. Ding L, Linsley P, Huang L, et al. IL-10 inhibits macrophage costimulatory activity by selectively inhibiting up-regulation of B7 expression. J Immunol 1993;151:1224–1234.
12. Chang C, Furue M, Tamaki K. Selective regulation of ICAM-1 and major histocompatibility complex class I and II expression on epidermal Langerhans cells by some of the cytokines released by keratinocytes and T cells. Eur J Immunol 1994;24:2889–2895.
13. Mosmann T, Coffman R. TH1 and TH2 cells: different patterns of lymphokine secretion lead to different functional properties. Annu Rev Immunol 1989;7:145–173.
14. Bevilacqua M. Endothelial leukocyte adhesion molecules. Annu Rev Immunol 1993;11:767–804.
15. Li L, Xia Y, Nguyen A, et al. Effects of Th2 cytokines on chemokine expression in the lung: IL-13 potently induces eotaxin expression by airway epithelial cells. J Immunol 1999;162:2477–2487.
16. Teran L, Mochizuki M, Bartels J, et al. Th1- and Th2-type cytokines regulate the expression and production of eotaxin and RANTES by human lung fibroblasts. Am J Respir Cell Mol Biol 1999;20:777–786.
17. Bradding P, Feather I, Wilson S, et al. Immunolocalization of cytokines in the nasal muscosa of normal and perennial rhinitic subjects. The mast cell as a source of IL-4, IL-5, and IL-6 in human allergic mucosal inflammation. J Immunol 1993;151:3853–3865.
18. Bjerke T, Gaustadnes M, Nielsen S, et al. Human blood eosinophils produce and secrete interleukin 4. Respir Med 1996;90:271–277.
19. Rumbley C, Sugaya H, Zekavat S, et al. Activated eosinophils are the major source of Th2-associated cytokines in the schistosome granuloma. J Immunol 1999;162:1003–1009.
20. Wang M, Saxon A, Diaz-Sanchez D. Early IL-4 production driving Th2 differentiation in a human in vivo allergic model is mast cell derived. Clin Immunol 1999;90:47–54.
21. Wang J, Wakeham J, Harkness R, Xing Z. Macrophages are a significant source of type 1 cytokines during mycobacterial infection. J Clin Invest 1999;103:1023–1029.
22. Ohshima Y, Delespesse G. T cell-derived IL-4 and dendritic cell-derived IL-12 regulate the lymphokine-producing phenotype of alloantigen-primed naive human CD4 T cells. J Immunol 1997;158:629–636.
23. Dahinden C, Rihs S, Ochsensberger B. Regulation of cytokine expression by human blood basophils. Int Arch Allergy Immunol 1997;113:134–137.
24. Paul W. Interleukin 4: signalling mechanisms and control of T cell differentiation. Ciba Found Symp 1997;204:208–216.
25. Trinchieri G. Immunobiology of interleukin-12. Immunol Res 1998;17:269–278.
26. Ohta A, Sato N, Yahata T, et al. Manipulation of Th1/Th2 balance in vivo by adoptive transfer of antigen-specific Th1 or Th2 cells. J Immunol Method 1997;209:85–92.
27. Li X, Schofield B, Wang Q, et al. Induction of pulmonary allergic responses by antigen-specific Th2 cells. J Immunol 1998;160:1378–1384.
28. Lohning M, Coyle AS, Grogan J, et al. T1/ST2 is preferentially expressed on murine Th2 cells, independent of interleukin 4, interleukin 5, and interleukin 10, and important for Th2 effector function. Proc Natl Acad Sci USA 1998;95:6930–6935.
29. Xu D, Chan W, Leung B, et al. Selective expression of a stable cell surface molecule on type 2 but not type 1 helper T cells. J Exp Med 1998;187:787–794.
30. Isobe M, Suzuki J, Yamazaki S, et al. Regulation by differential development of Th1 and Th2 cells in peripheral tolerance to cardiac allograft induced by blocking ICAM-1/LFA-1 adhesion. Circulation 1997;96:2247–2253.
31. Ebner C, Siemann U, Bohle B, et al. Immunological changes during specific immunotherapy of grass pollen allergy: reduced lymphoproliferative responses to allergen and shift from a Th2 to Th1 in T-cell clones specific for Phl p 1, a major grass pollen allergen. Clin Exp Allergy 1997;27:1007–1015.

32. Durham S, Till S. Immunologic changes associated with allergen immunotherapy. J Allergy Clin Immunol 1998;102: 157–164.

33. Hu H, Urba W, Fox B. Gene-modified tumor vaccine with therapeutic potential shifts tumor-specific T cell response from a type 2 to a type 1 cytokine profile. J Immunol 1998; 161:3033–3041.

34. Moller D, Wysocka M, Greenlee B, et al. Inhibition of human interleukin-12 production by pentoxyifylline. Immunology 1997;91:197–203.

35. Bright J, Du C, Coon M, et al. Prevention of experimental allergic encephalomyelitis via inhibition of IL-12 signaling and IL-12-mediated Th1 differentiation: an effect of the novel anti-inflammatory drug lysofylline. J Immunol 1998;161:7015–7022.

36. deJong R, Bezemer A, Zomerdijk T, et al. Selective stimulation of T helper 2 cytokine responses by the antipsoriasis agent monomethylfumarate. Eur J Immunol 1996;26:2067–2074.

37. Dumont F, Staruch M, Fischer P, et al. Inhibition of T cell activation by phramacologic disruption of the MEK1/ERK MAP kinase or calcineurin signaling pathways results in differential modulation of cytokine production. J Immunol 1998;160:2579–2589.

38. Rempel J, Wang M, HayGlass K. In vivo IL-12 administration induces profound but transient commitment to T helper cell type 1-associated patterns of cytokine and antibody production. J Immunol 1997;159:1490–1496.

39. Daser A, Meissner N, Herz U, Renz H. Role and modulation of T-cell cytokines in allergy. Curr Opin Immunol 1995;7:762–770.

40. Hogan S, Foster P. Cytokines as targets for the inhibition of eosinophilic inflammation. Pharmacol Ther 1997;74:259–283.

41. Rolland J, O'Hehir R. Immunotherapy of allergy: anergy, deletion, and immune deviation. Curr Opin Immunol 1998; 10:640–645.

42. Rocken M, Racke M, Shevach E. IL-4-induced immune deviation as antigen-specific therapy for inflammatory autoimmune disease. Curr Opin Immunol 1996;17:225–231.

43. Takeuchi T, Ueki T, Sunaga S, et al. Murine interleukin 4 transgenic heart allograft survival prolonged with down-regulation of the Th1 cytokine mRNA in grafts. Transplantation 1997;64:152–157.

44. He X, Chen J, Verma N, et al. Treatment with interleukin-4 prolongs allogeneic neonatal heart graft survival by inducing T helper 2 responses. Transplantation 1998;65:1145–1152.

45. Carter K, Gallagher G, Baillie A, Alexander J. The induction of protective immunity to Leishmania major in the BALB/c mouse by interleukin 4 treatment. Eur J Immunol 1989;19:779–782.

46. Pearlman E, Lass J, Bardenstein D, et al. Interleukin 4 and T helper type 2 cells are required for the development of experimental onchocercal keratitis (river blindness). J Exp Med 1995;182:931–940.

47. Wakil A, Wang Z, Locksley R. Leishmania major: targeting IL-4 in successful immunomodulation of murine infection. Exp Parasitol 1996;84:214–222.

48. Howard M, Farrar J, Hilfiker M, et al. Identification of a T cell-derived B cell growth factor distinct from interleukin 2. J Exp Med 1982;155:914–923.

49. Noma Y, Sideras T, Naito T, et al. Cloning of cDNA encoding the murine IgG induction factor by a novel strategy using SP6 promoter. Nature 1986;319:640–646.

50. Boulay J-L, Paul W. Hematopoietin sub-families: classification based on size, gene organization, and secondary structure. Curr Biol 1993;3:573–581.

51. Wang Y, Shen B, Sebald W. A mixed-charge pair in human interleukin 4 dominates high-affinity interaction with the receptor alpha chain. Proc Natl Acad Sci USA 1997;94: 1657–1662.

52. Kruse N, Tony H, Sebald W. Conversion of human interleukin-4 into a high affinity antagonist by a single amino acid replacement. EMBO J 1992;11:3237–3244.

53. He Y, Malek T. The structure and function of gamma c-dependent cytokines and receptors: regulation of T lymphocyte development and homeostasis. Crit Rev Immunol 1998;18:503–524.

54. Nelms K, Huang H, Ryan J, et al. Interleukin-4 receptor signalling mechanisms and their biological significance. Adv Exp Med Biol 1998;452:37–43.

55. Fernandez-Botran R, Chilton P, Ma Y, et al. Control of the production of soluble interleukin-4 receptors: implications in immunoregulation. J Leukoc Biol 1996;59:499–504.

56. Jung T, Wagner K, Neumann C, Heusser C. Enhancement of human IL-4 activity by soluble IL-4 receptors in vitro. Eur J Immunol 1999;29:864–871.

57. Brown M, Hural J. Functions of IL-4 and control of its expression. Crit Rev Immunol 1997;17:1–32.

58. Paul W, Seder R, Plaut M. Lymphokine and cytokine production by FcERI+ cells. Adv Immunol 1993;53:1–29.

59. Paul W. Interleukin-4: a prototypic immunoregulatory lymphokine. Blood 1991;77:1859–1870.

60. Essner R, Rhoades K, Bride WM, et al. IL-4 down-regulates IL-1 and TNF gene expression in human monocytes. J Immunol 1989;142:3857–3861.

61. Gautam S, Tebo J, Hamilton T. IL-4 suppresses cytokine gene expression induced by IFN-gamma and/or IL-2 in murine peritoneal macrophages. J Immunol 1992;148: 1725–1730.

62. Colotta F, Sironi M, Borre A, et al. Interleukin 4 amplifies monocyte chemotactic protein and interleukin 6 production by endothelial cells. Cytokine 1992;4:24–28.

63. Mochizuki M, Bartels J, Mallet A, et al. IL-4 induces eotaxin: a possible mechanism of selective eosinophil recruitment in helminth infection and atopy. J Immunol 1998;160:60–68.

64. Chomarat P, Banchereau J. Interleukin-4 and interleukin-13: their similarities and discrepancies. Int Rev Immunol 1998;17:1–52.

65. Romagnani S. Regulation and dysregulation of human IgE synthesis. Immunol Today 1990;11:316–321.

66. Sher A, Coffman R. Regulation of immunity to parasites by T cells and T cell-derived cytokines. Annu Rev Immunol 1992;10:385–409.

67. Sousa A, Chaves A, Doroana M, et al. Kinetics of the changes of lymphocyte subsets defined by cytokine production at single cell level during highly active antiretroviral therapy for HIV-1 infection. J Immunol 1999;162:3718–3726.

68. Clerici M, Shearer G. A TH1→TH2 switch is a critical step in the etiology of HIV infection. Immunol Today 1993;14: 107–111.
69. Clerici M, Fusi M, Ruzzante S, et al. Type 1 and type 2 cytokines in HIV infection—a possible role in apoptosis and disease progression. Ann Med 1997;29:185–188.
70. Graziosi C, Pantaleo G, Gantt KR, et al. Lack of evidence for the dichotomy of TH1 and TH2 predominance in HIV-infected individuals. Science 1994;265:248–252.
71. Canaris A, Caruso A, Licenziati S, et al. Lack of polarized type 1 or type 2 cytokine profile in asymptomatic HIV-1-infected patients during a two-year bimonthly follow-up. Scand J Immunol 1998;47:146–151.
72. Suzuki Y, Koyanagi Y, Tanaka Y, et al. Determinant in human immunodeficiency virus type 1 for efficient replication under cytokine-induced CD4(+) T-helper 1 (Th1)- and Th2-type conditions. J Virol 1999;73:316–324.
73. Wang J, Roderiquez G, Oravecz T, Norcross M. Cytokine regulation of human immunodeficiency virus type 1 entry and replication in human monocytes/macrophages through modulation of CCR5 expression. J Virol 1998;72:7642–7647.
74. Valentin A, Lu W, Rosati M, et al. Dual effect of interleukin 4 on HIV-1 expression: implications for viral phenotypic switch and disease progression. Proc Natl Acad Sci USA 1998;21:8886–8891.
75. Littman D. Chemokine receptors: keys to AIDS pathogenesis? Cell 1998;93:677–680.
76. Piccotti J, Chan S, VanBuskirk A, et al. Are Th2 helper T lymphocytes beneficial, deleterious, or irrelevant in promoting allograft survival? Transplantation 1997;63:619–624.
77. Nickerson P, Steiger J, Zheng X, et al. Manipulation of cytokine networks in transplantation: false hope or realistic opportunity for tolerance? Transplantation 1997;63:489–494.
78. Kobayashi M, Kobayashi H, Pollard R, Suzuki F. A pathogenic role of Th2 cells and their cytokine products on the pulmonary metastasis of murine B16 melanoma. J Immunol 1998;160:5869–5873.
79. Muller U, Akdis C, Fricker M, et al. Successful immunotherapy with T-cell epitope peptides of bee venom phospholipase A2 induces specific T-cell anergy in patients allergic to bee venom. J Allergy Clin Immunol 1998;101:747–754.
80. Park J, Choi I, Lee D, et al. Anti-IL-4 monoclonal antibody prevents antibiotics-induced active fatal anaphylaxis. J Immunol 1997;158:5002–5006.
81. Grunewald S, Kunzmann S, Schnarr B, et al. A murine interleukin-4 antagonistic mutant protein completely inhibits interleukin-4-induced cell proliferation, differentiation, and signal transduction. J Biol Chem 1997;272:1480–1483.
82. Joosten L, Lubberts E, Durez P, et al. Role of interleukin-4 and interleukin-10 in murine collagen-induced arthritis. Protective effect of interleukin-4 and interleukin-10 treatment on cartilage destruction. Arthritis Rheum 1997;40:249–260.
83. Horsfall A, Butler D, Marinova L, et al. Suppression of collagen-induced arthritis by continuous administration of IL-4. J Immunol 1997;159:5687–5696.
84. Rabinovitch A, Suarez-Pinzon W, Sorensen O, et al. Combined therapy with interleukin-4 and interleukin-10 inhibits autoimmune diabetes recurrence in syngeneic islet-transplanted nonobese diabetic mice. Analysis of cytokine mRNA expression in the graft. Transplantation 1995;60: 368–374.
85. Shaw M, Lorens J, Dhawan A, et al. Local delivery of interleukin 4 by retrovirus-transduced T lymphocytes ameliorates experimental autoimmune encephalomyelitis. J Exp Med 1997;185:1711–1714.
86. Hogaboam C, Vallance B, Kumar A, et al. Therapeutic effects of interleukin-4 gene transfer in experimental inflammatory bowel disease. J Clin Invest 1997;100:2766–2776.
87. Tepper R, Pattengale P, Leder P. Murine interleukin-4 displays potent anti-tumor activity in vivo. Cell 1989;57:503–512.
88. Golumbek P, Lazenby A, Levitsky H, et al. Treatment of established renal cancer by tumor cell engineered to secrete interleukin-4. Science 1991;254:713–716.
89. Nickerson P, Zheng X, Steiger J, et al. Prolonged islet allograft acceptance in the absence of interleukin 4 expression. Transplant Immunol 1996;4:81–85.
90. Bennedetti S, Bruzzone M, Pollo B, et al. Eradication of rat malignant gliomas by retroviral-mediated, in vivo delivery of the interleukin 4 gene. Cancer Res 1999;59:645–652.
91. Kulkarni A, Huh C, Becker D, et al. Transforming growth factor beta 1 null mutation in mice causes excessive inflammatory response and early death. Proc Natl Acad Sci USA 1993;90:770–774.
92. Selzman C, Shames B, Miller S, et al. Therapeutic implications of interleukin-10 in surgical disease. Shock 1998;10: 309–318.
93. Weckman A, Alcocer-Varela J. Cytokine inhibitors in autoimmune disease. Semin Arthritis Rheum 1996;26:539–557.
94. Bromberg J. IL-10 immunosuppression in transplantation. Curr Opin Immunol 1995;7:639–643.
95. Kobayashi F, Morii T, Matsui T, et al. Production of interleukin 10 during malaria caused by lethal and nonlethal variants of Plasmodium yoelii yoelii. Parasitol Res 1996;82: 385–391.
96. Dai W, Kohler G, Brombacher F. Both innate and acquired immunity to Listeria monocytogenes infection are increased in IL-10-deficient mice. J Immunol 1997;158:2259–2267.
97. Fiorentino D, Band M, Mosmann T. Two types of mouse helper T cell. IV. Th2 clones secrete a factor that inhibits cytokine production by Th1 clones. J Exp Med 1989;170: 2081–2095.
98. deWaal-Malefyt R, Yssel H, Roncarolo M, et al. Interleukin-10. Curr Opin Immunol 1992;4:314–320.
99. Moore K, O'Garra A, deWaal-Malefyt R, et al. Interleukin-10. Annu Rev Immunol 1993;11:165–190.
100. Zdanov A, Schalk-Hihi C, Wlodawer A. Crystal structure of human interleukin-10 at 1.6A and a model of a complex with its soluble receptor. Protein Sci 1996;5:1955–1962.
101. Moore K, Vieira P, Fiorentino D, et al. Homology of cytokine synthesis inhibitory factor (IL-10) to the Epstein Barr virus gene BCRF1. Science 1990;248:1230–1234.
102. Suk-Yue-Ho A, Liu Y, Khan T, et al. A receptor for interleukin 10 is related to interferon receptors. Proc Natl Acad Sci USA 1993;90:11267–11271.
103. Liu Y, Wei S, Ho A, et al. Expression cloning and characterization of a human IL-10 receptor. J Immunol 1994;152: 1821–1829.

104. Finbloom D, Weinstock K. Interleukin-10 induces the tyrosine phosphorylation of tyk2 and jak1 in the differential assembly of STAT1 and STAT3 complexes in human T cells and monocytes. J Immunol 1995;155:1079–1090.

105. deVries J. Immunosuppressive and anti-inflammatory properties of interleukin-10. Ann Med 1995;27:537–541.

106. Chomarat P, Rissoan N, Banchereau J, Miossec P. Interferon gamma inhibits interleukin-10 production by monocytes. J Exp Med 1993;177:523–527.

107. Fiorentino D, Zlotnik A, Vieira P, et al. IL-10 acts on the antigen-presenting cell to inhibit cytokine production by Th1 cells. J Immunol 1991;146:3444–3451.

108. Howard M, Muchamuel T, Andrade S, Menon S. Interleukin 10 protects mice from lethal endotoxemia. J Exp Med 1993;177:1205–1208.

109. vanderPoll T, Jensen P, Montegut WJ, et al. Effects of interleukin-10 on systemic inflammatory responses during sublethal primate endotoxemia. J Immunol 1997;158:1971–1975.

110. Bogdan C, Vodovotz Y, Nathan C. Macrophage deactivation by interleukin-10. J Exp Med 1991;174:1549–1555.

111. D'Andrea A, Aste-Amezaga M, Valiante N, et al. Interleukin-10 (IL-10) inhibits human lymphocyte interferon gamma production by suppressing natural killer cell stimulatory factor/IL-12 synthesis in accessory cells. J Exp Med 1993;178:1041–1048.

112. Marchant A, Bruyns C, vanDenabeele P, et al. Interleukin-10 controls interferon gamma and tumor necrosis factor production during experimental endotoxemia. Eur J Immunol 1994;24:1167–1171.

113. Hsieh C, Heimberger A, Gold J., et al. Differential regulation of T helper phenotype development by interleukins 4 and 10 in an alpha beta T cell receptor transgenic system. Proc Natl Acad Sci USA 1992;89:6065–6069.

114. Rousset F, Garcia E, DeFrance T, et al. Interleukin-10 as a potent growth and differentiation factor for activated human B lymphocytes. Proc Natl Acad Sci USA 1992;85:1890–1898.

115. Fujieda S, Saxon A, Zhang K. Direct evidence that gamma-1 and gamma-3 switching in human B cells is IL-10 dependent. Mol Immunol 1996;33:1335–1343.

116. Jinquan T, Larsen C, Gresser B, et al. Human IL-10 is a chemoattractant for CD8+ lymphocytes and an inhibitor of IL-8-induced CD4+ T lymphocyte migration. J Immunol 1993;151:4545–4551.

117. Chen W, Zlotnick A. IL-10: a novel cytotoxic T cell differentiation factor. J Immunol 1991;147:528–534.

118. Arock M, Zuany-Amorim C, Singer M, et al. Interleukin-10 inhibits cytokine generation from mast cells. Eur J Immunol 1996;26:166–170.

119. Kuhn R, Lohler J, Rennick D, et al. Interleukin-10-deficient mice develop chronic enterocolitis. Cell 1993;75:263–274.

120. Powrie F, Leach M, Mauze S, et al. Phenotypically distinct subsets of CD4+ T cells induce or protect from chronic intestinal inflammation in C.B-17 scid mice. Int Immunol 1993;5:1461–1471.

121. Ludviksson B, Sneller M, Chua K, et al. Active Wegener's granulomatosis is associated with HLA-DR+ CD4+ T cells exhibiting an unbalanced Th1-type T cell cytokine pattern: reversal with IL-10. J Immunol 1998;160:3602–3609.

122. Asadullah K, Sterry W, Stephanek K, et al. IL-10 is a key cytokine in psoriasis. Proof of principle by IL-10 therapy: a new therapeutic approach. J Clin Invest 1998;101:783–794.

123. Keystone E, Wherry J, Grint P. IL-10 as a therapeutic strategy in the treatment of rheumatoid arthritis. Rheum Dis Clin North Am 1998;24:629–639.

124. vanDeuren M, vanderVenJongekrijg J, Demacker P, et al. Differential expression of pro-inflammatory cytokines and their inhibitors during the course of meningococcal infection. J Infect Dis 1994;169:157–161.

125. Klava A, Windsor A, Farmery S, et al. Interleukin-10: a role in the development of post-operative immunosuppression. Arch Surg 1997;132:425–429.

126. Opal S, Wherry J, Grint P. Interleukin-10: potential benefits and possible risks in clinical infectious diseases. Clin Infect Dis 1998;27:1497–1507.

127. Rizzo L, Xu H, Chan C, et al. IL-10 has a protective role in experimental autoimmune uveoretinitis. Int Immunol 1998;10:807–814.

128. Bettelli E, Das M, Howard E, et al. IL-10 is critical in the regulation of autoimmune encephalomyelitis as demonstrated by studies of IL-10- and IL-4-deficient and transgenic mice. J Immunol 1998;161:3299–3306.

129. Ma Y, Thornton S, Duwel L, et al. Inhibition of collagen-induced arthritis in mice by viral IL-10 gene transfer. J Immunol 1998;161:1516–1524.

130. Groux H, O'Garra A, Bigler M, et al. A CD4+ T-cell subset inhibits antigen-specific T-cell responses and prevents colitis. Nature 1997;389:737–742.

131. Akdis C, Blesken T, Akdis M, et al. Role of interleukin 10 in specific immunotherapy. J Clin Invest 1998;102:98–106.

132. Buer J, Lanoue A, Franzke A, et al. Interleukin 10 secretion and impaired effector function of major histocompatibility complex class II-restricted T cells anergized in vivo. J Exp Med 1998;187:177–183.

133. Akdis C, Blaser K. IL-10-induced anergy in peripheral T cell and reactivation by microenvironmental cytokines: two key steps in specific immunotherapy. FASEB J 1999;13:603–609.

134. Gazzinelli R, Wysocka M, Hieny S, et al. In the absence of endogenous IL-10, mice acutely infected with Toxoplasma gondii succumb to a lethal immune response dependent on CD4+ T cells and accompanied by over-production of IL-12, IFN-gamma and TNF-alpha. J Immunol 1996;157:798–805.

135. Geissler K. Current status of clinical development of interleukin-10. Curr Opin Hematol 1996;3:203–208.

136. Chernoff A, Granowitz E, Shapiro L, et al. A randomized-controlled trial of interleukin-10 in humans: inhibition of inflammatory cytokine production and immune responses. J Immunol 1995;154:5492–5499.

137. Huhn R, Rodwanski E, O'Connell S, et al. Pharmacokinetics and immunomodulatory properties of intravenously administered recombinant human interleukin-10 in health volunteers. Blood 1996;87:699–705.

138. Pajkart D, Camoglio L, Tiel-vanBuul M, et al. Attenuation of proinflammatory response by recombinant human IL-10 in human endotoxemia: the effect of timing of rhIL-10 administration. J Immunol 1997;158:3971–3977.

139. Pajkart D, vanderPoll T, Levi M, et al. Interleukin-10 inhibits activation of coagulation and fibrinolysis during human endotoxemia. Blood 1997;89:2701–2705.

140. Eppinger M, Ward P, Bolling S, Deeb G. Regulatory effects

of interleukin-10 in lung ischemia reperfusion injury. J Thorac Cardiovasc Surg 1996;112:1301–1305.

141. Lane J, Todd K, Lewis M, et al. Interleukin-10 reduces systemic inflammatory response syndrome in a murine model of intestinal ischemia reperfusion. Surgery 1997;122:288–294.

142. Spera P, Ellison J, Feuerstein G, Barone F. IL-10 reduces rat brain injury following focal stroke. Neurosci Lett 1998;251: 189–192.

143. Qin L, Chavin K, Ding Y, et al. Retrovirus-mediated transfer of viral IL-10 gene prolongs murine cardiac allograft survival. J Immunol 1996;156:2316–2323.

144. Li W, Fu F, Lu L, et al. Systemic administration of anti-interleukin-10 antibody prolongs organ allograft survival in normal and presensitized recipients. Transplantation 1998; 66:1587–1596.

145. Kollman T, Pettoello-Mantavani M, Katopodis N, et al. Inhibition of acute in vivo human immunodeficiency virus infection in SCID mice implanted with human fetal thymus and liver. Proc Natl Acad Sci USA 1996;93:3126–3131.

146. Fluckiger A, Durand I, Banchereau J. Interleukin-10 induces apoptotic death of B-chronic lymphocytic leukemia cells. J Exp Med 1994;179:91–99.

147. Gazzinelli R. Molecular and cellular basis of interleukin 12 activity in prophylaxis and therapy against infectious diseases. Mol Med Today 1996;2:258–267.

148. Romani L, Puccetti P, Bistoni F. Interleukin-12 in infectious diseases. Clin Microbiol Rev 1997;10:611–636.

149. Kumagai K, Takeda K, Hashimoto W, et al. Interleukin-12 as an inducer of cytotoxic effectors in anti-tumor immunity. Int Rev Immunol 1997;14:229–256.

150. Hiscox S, Jiang W. Interleukin-12, an emerging anti-tumour cytokine. In Vivo 1997;11:125–132.

151. Caspi R. IL-12 in autoimmunity. Clin Immunol Immunopathol 1998;88:4–13.

152. Orr D, Bolton E, Bradley J. Neutralising IL-12 activity as a strategy for prolonging allograft survival and preventing graft-versus-host disease. Scott Med J 1998;43:109–111.

153. Kobayashi M, Fitz L, Ryan M, et al. Identification and purification of natural killer cell stimulatory factor (NKSF), a cytokine with multiple biologic effects on human lymphocytes. J Exp Med 1989;170:827–846.

154. Stern A, Podlaski F, Hulmes J, et al. Purification to homogeneity and partial characterization of cytotoxic lymphocyte maturation factor from human B-lymphoblastoid cells. Proc Natl Acad Sci USA 1990;87:6808–6812.

155. Wolf S, Temple P, Kobayashi M, et al. Cloning of cDNA for natural killer cell stimulatory factor, a heterodimeric cytokine with multiple biologic effects on T and natural killer cells. J Immunol 1991;146:3074–3081.

156. Gubler U, Chua A, Schoenhaut D, et al. Coexpression of two distinct genes is required to generate secreted bioactive cytotoxic lymphocyte maturation factor. Proc Natl Acad Sci USA 1991;88:4143–4147.

157. Chizzonite R, Truitt T, Podlaski F, et al. IL-12: monoclonal antibodies specific for the 40-kDa subunit block receptor binding and biologic activity on activated human lymphoblasts. J Immunol 1991;147:1548–1556.

158. Lieschke G, Rao P, Gately M, Mulligan R. Bioactive murine and human interleukin-12 fusion proteins which retain anti-tumor activity in vivo. Nat Biotechnol 1997;15:35–40.

159. Anderson R, Macdonald I, Corbett T, et al. Construction and biological characterization of an interleukin-12 fusion protein (Flexi-12): delivery to acute myeloid leukemic blasts using adeno-associated virus. Hum Gene Ther 1997;8: 1125–1135.

160. Presky D, Yang H, Minetti J, et al. A functional interleukin 12 receptor complex is composed of two beta-type cytokine receptor subunits. Proc Natl Acad Sci USA 1996;93:14002–14007.

161. Desai B, Quinn P, Wolitzky A, et al. The IL-12 receptor: II. Distribution and regulation of receptor expression. J Immunol 1992;148:3125–3132.

162. Benjamin D, Sharma V, Kubin M, et al. IL-12 expression in AIDS-related lymphoma B cell lines. J Immunol 1996;156: 1626–1637.

163. Bacon C, McVicar D, Ortaldo J, et al. Interleukin 12 (IL-12) induces tyrosine phosphorylation of JAK2 and TYK2: differential use of janus family tyrosine kinases by IL-2 and IL-12. J Exp Med 1995;181:399–404.

164. Jacobson N, Szabo S, Weber-Nordt R, et al. Interleukin 12 signaling in T helper 1 (Th1) cells involves tyrosine phosphorylation of signal transducer and activator of transcription (Stat) 3 and Stat4. J Exp Med 1995;181:1755–1762.

165. Chan S, Kobayashi M, Santoli D, et al. Mechanisms of IFN-g induction by natural killer cell stimulatory factor (NKSF/IL-12): role of transcription and mRNA stability in the synergistic interaction between NKSF and IL-2. J Immunol 1992;148:92–98.

166. D'Andrea A, Rengaraju M, Valiante N, et al. Production of natural killer cell stimulatory factor (NKSF/IL-12) by peripheral blood mononuclear cells. J Exp Med 1992;176: 1387–1398.

167. Gillessen S, Carvajal D, Ling P, et al. Mouse interleukin-12 (IL-12) p40 homodimer: a potent IL-12 antagonist. Eur J Immunol 1995;25:200–206.

168. Cassatella M, Meda L, Gasperini S, et al. Interleukin-12 production by human polymorphonuclear leukocytes. Eur J Immunol 1995;25:1–5.

169. Shu U, Kiniwa M, Wu C, et al. Activated T cells induce interleukin-12 production by monocytes via CD40-CD40 ligand interaction. Eur J Immunol 1995;25:1125–1128.

170. Cella M, Scheidegger D, Plamer-Lehmann K, et al. Ligation of CD40 on dendritic cells triggers production of high levels of interleukin-12 and enhances T cell stimulatory capacity: T-T help via APC activation. J Exp Med 1996;184:747–752.

171. Ma X, Chow J, Gri G, et al. The interleukin-12 p40 gene promoter is primed by interferon-g in monocytic cells. J Exp Med 1996;183:147–157.

172. Chan S, Perussia B, Gupta J, et al. Induction of IFN-g production by NK cell stimulatory factor (NKSF): characterization of the responder cells and synergy with other inducers. J Exp Med 1991;173:869–879.

173. Kubin M, Kamoun M, Trinchieri G. Interleukin-12 synergizes with B7/CD28 interaction in inducing efficient proliferation and cytokine production of human T cells. J Exp Med 1994;180:211–222.

174. Manetti R, Parronchi P, Giudizi M, et al. Natural killer cell stimulatory factor (NKSF/IL-12) induces Th1-type specific immune responses and inhibits the development of IL-4 producing Th cells. J Exp Med 1993;177:1199–1204.

175. Hsieh C, Macatonia S, Tripp C, et al. Listeria-induced Th1

development in ab-TCR transgenic CD4+ T cells occurs through macrophage production of IL-12. Science 1993;260: 547–549.

176. McKnight A, Zimmer G, Fogelman I, et al. Effects of IL-12 on helper T cell-dependent immune responses in vivo. J Immunol 1994;152:2172–2179.

177. Manetti R, Gerosa F, Giudizi M, et al. Interleukin-12 induces stable priming for interferon-g (IFN-g) production during differentiation of human T helper (Th) cells and transient IFN-g production in established Th2 cell clones. J Exp Med 1994;179:1273–1283.

178. Germann T, Gately M, Schoenhaut D, et al. Interleukin-12/T cell stimulating factor, a cytokine with multiple effects on T helper type 1 (Th1) but not on Th2 cells. Eur J Immunol 1993;23:1762–1770.

179. Gazzinelli R, Wysocka M, Hayashi S, et al. Parasite induced IL-12 stimulates early IFN-g synthesis and resistance during acute infection with Toxoplasma gondii. J Immunol 1994;153:2533–2543.

180. Seder R, Kelsall B, Jankovic D. Differential roles for IL-12 in the maintenance of immune responses in infectious versus autoimmune disease. J Immunol 1996;157:2745–2748.

181. Perussia B, Chan S, D'Andrea A, et al. Natural killer cell stimulatory factor or IL-12 has differential effects on the proliferation of TCRab+, TCRgd+ T lymphocytes and NK cells. J Immunol 1992;149:3495–3502.

182. Chizzonite R, Truitt T, Desai B, et al. IL-12 receptor: I. Characterization of the receptor on PHA-activated human lymphoblasts. J Immunol 1992;148:3117–3124.

183. Gately M, Desai B, Wolitzky A, et al. Regulation of human lymphocyte proliferation by a heterodimeric cytokine, IL-12 (cytotoxic lymphocyte maturation factor). J Immunol 1991;147:874–882.

184. Murphy E, Terres G, Macatonia S, et al. B7 and IL-12 cooperate for proliferation and IFN-g production by mouse T helper clones that are unresponsive to B7 costimulation. J Exp Med 1994;180:223–231.

185. Chehimi J, Starr S, Frank I, et al. Natural killer cell stimulatory factor (NKSF) increases the cytotoxic activity of NK cells from both healthy donors and HIV-infected patients. J Exp Med 1992;175:789–796.

186. Chehimi J, Valiante N, D'Andrea A, et al. Enhancing effect of natural killer cell stimulatory factor (NKSF/IL-12) on cell-mediated cytotoxicity against tumor-derived and virus-infected cells. Eur J Immunol 1993;23:1826–1830.

187. Salcedo T, Azzoni L, Wolf S, Perussia B. Modulation of perforin and granzyme messenger RNA expression in human natural killer cells. J Immunol 1993;151:2511–2520.

188. Rabinowich H, Herberman R, Whiteside T. Differential effects of IL-12 and IL-2 on expression and function of cellular adhesion molecules on purified human natural killer cells. Cell Immunol 1993;152:481–498.

189. Vieira L, Hondowicz B, Afonso L, et al. Infection with Leishmania major induces interleukin-12 production in vivo. Immunol Lett 1994;40:157–161.

190. Zhang M, Gately M, Wang E, et al. Interleukin 12 at the site of disease in tuberculosis. J Clin Invest 1994;93:1733–1739.

191. Romani L, Mencacci A, Tonnetti L, et al. Interleukin-12 but not interferon-g production correlates with induction of T helper type-1 phenotype in murine candidiasis. Eur J Immunol 1994;24:909–915.

192. Gazzinelli R, Amichay D, Sharton-Kersten T, et al. Role of macrophage-derived cytokines in the induction and regulation of cell-mediated immunity to Toxoplasma gondii. Curr Top Microbiol Immunol 1996;219:127–139.

193. Tripp C, Wolf S, Unanue E, et al. Interleukin 12 and tumor necrosis factor alpha are costimulators of interferon gamma production by natural killer cells in severe combined immunodeficiency mice with listeriosis, and interleukin 10 is a physiologic antagonist. Proc Natl Acad Sci USA 1993;90: 3725–3729.

194. Tripp C, Gately M, Hakimi J, et al. Neutralization of IL-12 decreases resistance to Listeria in SCID and CB-17 mice. J Immunol 1994;152:1883–1887.

195. Gazzinelli R, Hieny S, Wynn T, et al. Interleukin-12 is required for the T-lymphocyte independent induction of interferon-g by an intracellular parasite and induces resistance in T-deficient hosts. Proc Natl Acad Sci USA 1993;90: 6115–6119.

196. Trinchieri G, Scott P. Interleukin-12: basic principles and clinical applications. Curr Top Microbiol Immunol 1999;238: 57–78.

197. Biron C, Gazzinelli R. Effects of IL-12 on immune responses to microbial infections: a key mediator in regulating disease outcome. Curr Opin Immunol 1995;7:485–496.

198. Carreno V, Quiroga J. Biological properties of interleukin-12 and its therapeutic use in persistent hepatitis B virus and hepatitis C virus infection. J Viral Hepat 1997;4(suppl 2):83–86.

199. Gazzinelli R, Giese N, Morse H. In vivo treatment with interleukin 12 protects mice from immune abnormalities observed during murine acquired immunodeficiency syndrome (MAIDS). J Exp Med 1994;180:2199–2208.

200. Trinchieri G, Wysocka M, D'Andrea A, et al. Natural killer cell stimulatory factor (NKSF) or interleukin-12 is a key regulator of immune response and inflammation. Prog Growth Factor Res 1992;4:355–368.

201. Ozmen L, Pericin M, Hakimi J, et al. IL-12, IFN-g and TNF-a are the key cytokines of the generalized Shwartzman reaction. J Exp Med 1994;180:907–915.

202. Car B, Eng V, Schnyder B, et al. Role of interferon-g in IL-12 induced pathology in mice. Am J Pathol 1995;147:1693–1707.

203. Leonard J, Sherman M, Fisher G, et al. Effects of a single-dose interleukin-12 exposure on interleukin-12-associated toxicity and interferon-gamma production. Blood 1997;90: 2541–2548.

204. Heinzel F, Schoenhaut D, Rerko R, et al. Recombinant interleukin 12 cures mice infected with Leishmania major. J Exp Med 1993;177:1505–1509.

205. Sypek J, Chung C, Mayor S, et al. Resolution of cutaneus leishmaniasis: interleukin-12 initiates a protective T helper type 1 immune response. J Exp Med 1993;177:1797–1802.

206. Nabors G, Afonso L, Farrell J, Scott P. Switch from a type 2 to a type 1 T helper response and cure of established Leishmania major infection in mice is induced by combined therapy with interleukin 12 and Pentostam. Proc Natl Acad Sci USA 1995;92:3142–3146.

207. Bliss J, VanCleave V, Murray K, et al. IL-12 as an adjuvant, promotes a T helper 1 cell, but does not suppress a T helper 2 cell recall response. J Immunol 1996;156:887–894.

208. Afonso L, Scharton T, Vieira L, et al. IL-12 functions as an

effective adjuvant in a vaccine against Leishmania major by directing the development of leishmanial specific CD4+ Th1 cells. Science 1994;263:235–237.

209. Wynn T, Eltoum I, Oswald I, et al. Endogenous interleukin 12 (IL-12) regulates granuloma formation induced by eggs of Schistosoma mansoni and exogenous IL-12 both inhibits and prophylactically immunizes against egg pathology. J Exp Med 1994;179:1551–1561.

210. Miller M, Skeen M, Ziegler H. Nonviable bacterial antigens administered with IL-12 generate antigen-specific T cell responses and protective immunity against Listeria mono-cytogenes. J Immunol 1995;155:4817–4828.

211. Mahon B, Ryan M, Griffin F, Mills K. Interleukin-12 is produced by macrophages in response to live or killed Borde-tella pertussis and enhances the efficacy of an acellular pertussis vaccine by promoting induction of Th1 cells. Infect Immun 1996;64:5295–5301.

212. Bliss J, Maylor R, Stokes K, et al. Interleukin-12 as vaccine adjuvant: characteristics of primary, recall, and long-term resistance. Ann NY Acad Sci 1996;795:26–35.

213. Clerici M, Lucey D, Berzofsky J, et al. Restoration of HIV-specific cell-mediated immune responses by interleukin-12 in vitro. Science 1993;262:1721–1724.

214. Nagy-Agren S, Cooney E. Interleukin-12 enhancement of antigen-specific lymphocyte proliferation correlates with stage of human immunodeficiency virus infection. J Infect Dis 1999;179:493–496.

215. Chehimi J, Starr S, Frank I, et al. Impaired interleukin-12 production in human immunodeficiency virus-infected patients. J Exp Med 1994;179:1361–1366.

216. Brunda M, Luistro L, Warrier R, et al. Antitumor and antimetastatic activity of interleukin 12 against murine tumors. J Exp Med 1993;178:1223–1230.

217. Gollob J, Schnipper C, Orsini E, et al. Characterization of a novel subset of CD8(+) T cells that expands in patients receiving interleukin-12. J Clin Invest 1998;102:561–575.

218. Nastala C, Edington H, McKinney T, et al. Recombinant IL-12 administration induces tumor regression in association with IFN-g production. J Immunol 1994;153:1697–1706.

219. Tsung K, Meko J, Peplinski G, et al. IL-12 induces T helper 1-directed antitumor response. J Immunol 1997;158:3359–3365.

220. Calandra T, Baumgartner J, Grau G, et al. Prognostic values of tumor necrosis factor/cachectin, interleukin-1, interferon-alpha, and interferon-gamma in the serum of patients with septic shock. J Infect Dis 1990;161:982–987.

Chapter 16

The Interferons: Basic Biology and Therapeutic Potential

Vijay Shankaran
Robert D. Schreiber

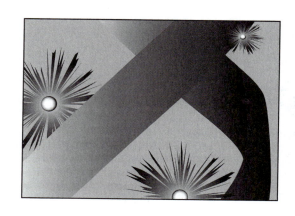

Much progress has been made in our understanding of interferon (IFN) biology since the initial description in 1957 by Isaacs and Lindenmann of an activity present in the supernatants of virally infected cells that interfered with the ability of a wide variety of viruses to infect other cells (1). Progress has been especially rapid in the last 20 years, during which time the genes encoding the IFNs and their receptors have been cloned and expressed. The production of large amounts of recombinant IFN and soluble IFN receptors and the generation of specific monoclonal antibodies to these proteins have facilitated their molecular definition and yielded insights into their in vivo function. Structure-function studies of these proteins have identified the key regions required for their biologic activity, and these insights have been supported by the solving of the crystal structures of IFN-γ and the IFN-γ–IFN-γ receptor complex. Recently, mice lacking expression of IFN family members, IFN receptors, or IFN signaling components have been generated, and have confirmed and extended the results from previous studies utilizing anti-IFN neutralizing antibodies concerning the physiologic roles of these proteins. In addition, our understanding of the role of IFNs in preventing human disease has recently been advanced by the identification of human patients with IFN-γ production or signaling deficiencies and the demonstration that IFN-γ plays a critical role in eliminating primary tumors in immunocompetent hosts. Therefore, we now have a relatively clear view of the biochemistry and biology of the IFN system in both mice and humans. In this chapter, we will review key aspects of the IFN system, paying special attention to IFN-γ because of its central role in modulating immune system activity and its ability to coordinate host defense to both microbial pathogens and tumors.

Structure of Interferon Genes and Proteins

The interferons were originally described as antiviral agents produced by virally infected cells or mitogen-stimulated leukocytes (1,2). We now know that this antiviral activity results from the actions of a family of proteins that have been divided into two classes on the basis of structural and functional criteria as well as the stimuli that induce their expression. The first class of proteins, termed type I IFNs, are primarily induced in response to viral infection of cells and have been further subdivided into two groups (IFN-α and IFN-β) based on their cellular origins (3). The IFN-α family consists of more than 22 structurally related polypeptides encoded by distinct genes and produced largely by leukocytes (4,5). IFN-β is the product of a single distinct gene and is produced by fibroblasts (3). The second class of IFNs, termed type II IFN, immune IFN, or IFN-γ, are the products of a single gene and are produced by T lymphocytes and natural killer (NK) cells following activation with immune and inflammatory stimuli rather than viral infection (6,7).

IFN-α and IFN-β Genes and Proteins

A total of 26 IFN-α genes have been identified to date, although at least five of these are pseudogenes (4). These genes lack introns, are organized in an identical manner, and reside together in a gene cluster on human chromosome 9 and mouse chromosome 4 (8). It is currently thought that this gene family evolved from a single ancestral gene. However, the individual roles of the multiple IFN-α gene products remain undefined. IFN-α proteins are single-chain polypeptides that contain 165 to 167 amino acids in their mature forms. At least 25 distinct forms of mature human IFN-α protein have been identified with Mr values that range from 16 to 27.5 kD in part as a result of differential glycosylation (5). Most of the IFN-α polypeptides are heat and pH stable. The different human IFN-α proteins display 68% sequence identity with one another and approximately 40% homology with their murine IFN-α counterparts. Some of the IFN-α gene products display species specificity in their ability to bind cell surface receptors and activate cellular responses, while others do not.

IFN-β is encoded by a single gene located next to the IFN-α gene cluster in both the human and mouse genomes. Both human and murine IFN-β proteins are glycosylated, consist of 166 and 161 amino acids, respectively, and display Mr values of 20 kD and 28 to 35 kD, respectively. Despite the overall similarity in the organization of the IFN-α and IFN-β genes, the proteins they encode share only 15% to 30% identity at the amino acid level. However, sufficient similarity exists between the key functional domains of these proteins that they bind to the same cell surface receptor. In this manner, they induce a highly overlapping array of biologic responses (9).

IFN-γ Genes and Proteins

IFN-γ is unrelated to either IFN-α or IFN-β at both the genetic and protein levels, and is encoded by a single 6-kb gene that resides on human chromosome 12 and murine chromosome 10 (10,11). The gene is organized in an identical manner in humans and mice and contains four exons and three introns. The human IFN-γ gene encodes a 1.2-kb mRNA that is translated into a 166 amino acid polypeptide. After removal of its 23 amino acid signal sequence, the mature human IFN-γ polypeptide consists of 143 amino acids. Differential glycosylation at two N-linked glycosylation sites gives rise to mature human IFN-γ polypeptides with Mr values of 17, 20, and 25 kD (12). The murine IFN-γ gene encodes a 1.2-kb mRNA that gives rise to a 134 amino acid mature polypeptide that, depending on its glycosylation state, displays an Mr value of 15.4, 20, or 25 kD. In both species, the fully glycosylated IFN-γ polypeptide predominates. Human and murine IFN-γ coding sequences display 60% identity, while the polypeptides share only 40% identity. This primary amino acid sequence diversity is the basis for the strict species specificity that human and murine IFN-γ display in binding to and inducing responses in human and murine cells, respectively (6). Under physiologic conditions, two IFN-γ polypeptides self-associate to form a noncovalent homodimer with a molecular mass of 50 kD (13,14). The IFN-γ homodimer is a labile molecule that can be denatured by extremes of temperature (>65°C) or pH (pH <4 or >9). Importantly, only the homodimeric form of IFN-γ is fully capable of binding to the IFN-γ receptor on cells and inducing biologic responses. The crystal structure of the IFN-γ dimer has been solved and indicates that two IFN-γ monomers associate in an antiparallel fashion to form a symmetric dimer (15). Subsequent crystallographic studies of the complex of IFN-γ bound to the ligand-binding chain of the IFN-γ receptor indicate that the IFN-γ homodimer contains two identical receptor binding sites and interacts with two receptor molecules (16).

Interferon Biosynthesis

IFN-α/β Biosynthesis

Most cells are capable of producing at least one form of type I IFN following exposure to the appropriate inducing stimuli (17–20). Viral infection is the most important physiologic inducer of type I IFNs. Other stimuli, including double-stranded RNA, inflammatory stimuli such as bacterial endotoxin, interleukin-1 (IL-1), and tumor necrosis factor (TNF), and even IFN itself, can also stimulate IFN-α/β production. The promoters of the type I interferon genes contain binding sites for the transcription factors NF-κB and interferon regulatory factor-1, which are activated by the known IFN inducers. The induction of IFN-α/β is rapid and can be detected in the extracellular environment within 6 hours after cellular stimulation.

IFN-γ Biosynthesis

In contrast to IFN-α/β production, IFN-γ production is restricted to appropriately stimulated T lymphocytes and NK cells (6,7). CD8+ T cells and the Th0 and Th1 CD4+ T helper (Th) subsets secrete IFN-γ and other T cell–derived cytokines in response to antigen presented in the context of the proper major histocompatibility complex (MHC) protein and costimulation. Agents that mimic T-cell activation, such as antibodies that cross-link the T-cell receptor (TCR), mitogens, or pharmacologic agents (such as the combination of phorbol myristate acetate and calcium ionophore), can also stimulate IFN-γ production in these cells. Neither IFN-γ message nor protein can be detected in resting T cells. However, IFN-γ transcripts can be detected within 6 to 8 hours of T-cell activation, reach maximum levels by 12 to 24 hours, and then subsequently decline to baseline values. The IFN-γ protein is secreted immediately after synthesis and reaches maximal extracellular levels 18 to 24 hours after T-cell stimulation (6). A second, TCR-independent pathway has been shown to induce robust IFN-γ production by T cells. This pathway involves the cytokines interleukin-12 (IL-12) and interleukin-18 (IL-18), which synergize to induce IFN-γ production through mechanisms involving the transcription factors STAT4 and NF-κB (21–27). However, activation of these transcription factors is not sufficient to induce IFN-γ transcription in T cells, because additional protein synthesis is required (27). Further work is needed to define the other proteins that regulate IFN-γ production.

Activated NK cells comprise the other cellular source of IFN-γ. Unlike T cells, NK cells produce IFN-γ solely in an MHC-unrestricted manner. Analysis of lymphocyte-deficient SCID mice infected with the gram-positive bacteria *Listeria moncytogenes* identified a cytokine amplification loop that leads to the production of large amounts of IFN-γ by NK cells (28,29). On interaction with bacterial products, tissue macrophages produce small amounts of tumor necrosis factor α (TNF-α) and IL-12, which together stimulate NK cells to secrete low levels of IFN-γ. This NK cell–derived IFN-γ in turn stimulates the macrophages to increase their production of TNF-α and IL-12, which subsequently leads to enhanced production of IFN-γ by NK cells. This reciprocal stimulation forms a positive amplification loop that results in the rapid production of substantial quantities of IFN-γ early in the course of infection and facilitates the generation of large numbers of activated macrophages with antimicrobial activity. Therefore, the interdependent synergistic effects of IFN-γ, IL-12, and TNF-α on macrophages and NK cells provide the host with an innate mechanism for IFN-γ production and macrophage activation that facilitates early control of infection (30).

Interleukin-10 (IL-10) is a cytokine produced late in the course of infection that, through indirect mechanisms, down-regulates the production of IFN-γ by both NK and T cells (26,29,31). IL-10 functions by preventing macrophage secretion of TNF-α and IL-12, although its mechanism of action remains undefined.

The IFN Receptors

The IFN-α/β Receptor

All type I interferons bind to a single high-affinity cell surface IFN-α/β receptor (9,32). Functionally active IFN-α/β receptors are comprised of two distinct subunits: a 110-kD IFNAR1 polypeptide (also known as IFN-αR1) and a 102-kD IFNAR2 polypeptide (also called IFN-αR2). The IFNAR1 and IFNAR2 subunits are members of the class 2 cytokine receptor family, which also includes one of the subunits of the IFN-γ receptor, both IL-10 receptor subunits, and tissue factor (33). The genes encoding IFNAR1 and IFNAR2 are located in a gene cluster on human chromosome 21 and murine chromosome 16, which also contains the genes for some of the other class 2 cytokine receptor family members—i.e., the α subunit of the IFN-γ receptor and the β subunit of the IL-10 receptor (34,35).

The human IFNAR1 gene encodes a 557 amino acid polypeptide that contains a 27 amino acid signal sequence (9). The mature 530 amino acid IFNAR1 polypeptide consists of a 409 amino acid extracellular domain, a 21 amino acid transmembrane domain, and a 100 amino acid cytoplasmic domain. The human IFNAR2 gene encodes a mature polypeptide of 489 amino acids and consists of a 217 amino acid extracellular domain, a 21 amino acid transmembrane domain, and a 251 amino acid intracellular domain. Although expression of human IFNAR1 is sufficient to confer on cells the ability to bind and respond to one IFN-α family member (IFN-α8), binding of all type I IFN family members requires the coexpression of both IFN-α/β receptor subunits (9,36).

The IFN-γ Receptor

IFN-γ interacts with a distinct high-affinity ($Ka = 10^{10}$–$10^{11}\,M^{-1}$) receptor that is expressed on nearly all cell surfaces (16,37). IFN-γ receptors consist of two species-matched polypeptides. The first is a 90-kD protein known as the IFN-γ receptor α chain, IFNGR1, IFN-γR1, or CDw119, and is encoded by a gene on human chromosome 6 and murine chromosome 10. The IFNGR1 subunit is responsible for ligand binding and ligand trafficking through the cell, and is required but not sufficient for signal transduction. The second is a 62-kD protein termed the IFN-γ receptor β chain, IFNGR2, IFN-γR2, or accessory factor-1 and is encoded by a gene on human chromosome 21 and murine chromosome 16. The IFNGR2 subunit plays only a minor role in ligand binding but is required for IFN-γ signaling.

The two IFN-γ receptor subunits differ significantly in terms of their cell surface expression. IFNGR1 is expressed constitutively at moderate levels on the surfaces of nearly all cells (200 to 25,000 sites per cell), and its expression does not appear to be modulated by external stimuli. In contrast, IFNGR2 is expressed on cells at very low levels, and its expression is regulated in certain cell types (such as T lymphocytes) by external stimuli (38,39). In some cells, expression of the IFNGR2 gene is a critical factor in determining IFN-γ responsiveness.

The human IFNGR1 gene encodes a 489 amino acid precursor that contains a 17 amino acid signal sequence (40), while the murine IFNGR1 gene encodes a 477 amino acid polypeptide containing a 26 amino acid signal peptide (41–45). The human and murine proteins are organized in a similar manner: both contain a 228 amino acid extracellular domain and a 23 amino acid transmembrane domain and relatively large, serine- and threonine-rich intracellular domains that also contain several tyrosine residues. Despite this organizational similarity, the two polypeptides exhibit only 52.5% overall sequence identity, which applies to both extracellular and intracellular domains. The Mr values of mature human IFNGR1 proteins from different cells range from 80 to 95 kD due to cell-specific differences in glycosylation (46–48).

Human and murine IFNGR2 subunits are also structurally similar to one another. Human IFNGR2 is a 337 amino acid type I transmembrane polypeptide that contains a 21 amino acid signal sequence, an extracellular domain of 226 amino acids, a single 24 amino acid transmembrane domain, and a relatively short intracellular domain of only 66 amino acids (49). Murine IFNGR2 consists of an 18 amino acid signal sequence, a 224 amino acid extracellular domain, a 24 amino acid transmembrane domain, and a 64 amino acid intracellular domain (50). Although human and murine IFNGR2 polypeptides exhibit only 58% overall identity, their cytoplasmic domains display 73% identity. The human and murine cDNAs encode polypeptides of 38 kD. However, mature forms of both human IFNGR2 and murine IFNGR2 display an Mr value of 62 kD (39). This difference is most likely explained by postsynthetic glycosylation of the polypeptides, although the composition and location of IFNGR2-associated carbohydrates have not yet been established.

Signal Transduction through the IFN Receptors

JAKs and STATs

Work performed in many laboratories over the past 9 years has demonstrated that both the IFN-α/β and IFN-γ receptors as well as many other cytokine and growth factor receptors function as a result of the ligand-induced coupling of the cognate cell surface receptor to a signal transduction pathway named the JAK-STAT pathway (16,32,51–54). The JAK-STAT pathway rapidly transfers signals directly from the cell surface to the nucleus. To do so, the pathway utilizes two families of molecules. The first is a family of related protein tyrosine kinases known as Janus kinases, or JAKs (Table 16-1). The second is a family of latent cytosolic transcription factors termed signal transducers and activators of transcription, or STATs (see Table 16-1).

The Janus kinase family currently consists of four molecules: JAK1, JAK2, JAK3, and Tyk2 (51,54,55). The JAK family members are structurally distinguished from other protein tyrosine kinases in that they contain dual kinase domains at their carboxy-terminus, although only the most extreme C-terminal

Table 16-1. Phenotypes of Mice Lacking JAK-STAT Pathway Proteins

Gene Deleted	KO Mouse Phenotype	Cytokine Receptors Affected	Reference(s)
JAK1	Perinatal lethality, T- and B-cell deficits, no innate immunity, neuronal survival deficit	IFN-α/β, IFN-γ, IL-10, γ_c family, gp130 family	(56)
JAK2	Early embryonic lethality, no blood formation, lack of IFN-γ signaling	IFN-γ, Epo	(57,58)
JAK3	T- and B-cell deficits	γ_c family	(174–176)
Tyk2	N.D.	N.D.	–
STAT1	Innate immunity defect, poor Th1 response	IFN-α/β, IFN-γ	(60,61)
STAT2	Enhanced viral susceptibility	IFN-α/β	(177)
STAT3	Early embryonic lethality, dysregulated macrophage production of inflammatory cytokines	IL-10, gp130 family	(178–180)
STAT4	Th1 defect	IL-12	(181,182)
STAT5A	Lactation defect	Prolactin	(183,184)
STAT5B	Dwarfism	GH	(184,185)
STAT5A × B	T-cell defect	Il-2	(184)
STAT6	Th2 defect	Il-4	(186,187)

kinase domain has documented kinase activity. The JAKs associate with cytokine receptor subunits in a specific and constitutive manner and, on ligand addition, are able to phosphorylate both activated cytokine receptors and STAT proteins (56–59).

The STAT protein family currently consists of seven distinct polypeptides: STAT1, STAT2, STAT3, STAT4, STAT5A, STAT5B, and STAT6 (52,54). This family of transcription factors is unusual in that its members have src homology 2 (SH2) domains capable of binding to phosphotyrosine-containing sequences. Studies utilizing cells and mice engineered to lack particular STAT proteins have demonstrated that the STATs play a major role in determining cytokine receptor signaling specificity (51,60,61). This property derives from sequence differences within the SH2 domains of the STAT proteins, which enables the selective recruitment of distinct STATs to different activated, tyrosine phosphorylated cytokine receptor subunits, and allows for the subsequent specific pairing that occurs between two tyrosine phosphorylated STAT proteins that form the functionally active transcription factor complex. Recently, the crystal structure of an activated STAT1 homodimer has been solved (62).

IFN-γ Receptor Signaling

Detailed structure/function analyses performed on the IFN-γ receptor and its signaling proteins has defined the proximal IFN-γ signal transduction events and facilitated the construction of a model of IFN-γ signal transduction that currently serves as a paradigm for cytokine receptor signaling (Fig. 16-1). We now know that in unstimulated cells, the IFN-γ receptor subunits are not preassociated with one another (63) but rather associate constitutively by means of their intracellular domains with inactive forms of specific Janus kinases (63–66). JAK1 binds to a $_{266}$LPKS$_{269}$ sequence in the membrane proximal portion of the intracellular domain of the human IFNGR1 chain and JAK2 associates with a 12 amino acid sequence ($_{263}$PPSIPLQIEEYL$_{274}$) in the intracellular domain of the human IFNGR2 chain. Signal

transduction is initiated when a homodimeric IFN-γ molecule binds to two IFNGR1 subunits leading to the formation of a complex to which two IFNGR2 proteins subsequently bind. Within the ligand assembled receptor complex, the inactive subunit-associated kinases are brought into close juxtaposition with one another and are activated by mechanisms involving auto- and transphosphorylation. The activated kinases then phosphorylate a key tyrosine residue within a $_{440}$YDKPH$_{444}$ sequence near the carboxy-terminus of the human IFNGR1 chain, thereby forming the phosphorylated sequence that is specifically recognized by the SH2 domain of STAT1 (67,68). Two STAT1 molecules then bind to the paired docking sites on the activated receptor complex, are brought into close proximity with the receptor-associated, activated tyrosine kinases, and are themselves phosphorylated at a specific tyrosine residue (Y701) near their C-terminus (69,70). The two phosphorylated STAT1 proteins then dissociate from the IFNGR1 subunits, form reciprocal homodimers that have also been serine phosphorylated during the activation process, and then translocate to the nucleus. In the nucleus, the STAT1 homodimers bind to specific promoter elements (known as gamma-interferon activated sites, or GAS elements) and thereby effect transcription of IFN-γ–induced genes (16,51). Studies utilizing cells and mice with induced genetic deficiencies of different JAKs and STATs have demonstrated that most IFN-γ–induced biologic responses require JAK1, JAK2, and STAT1 (see Table 16-1) (56–58,60,61). These studies therefore unequivocally establish the physiologic relevance of this IFN-γ signaling model.

IFN-α/β Receptor Signaling

IFN-α/β receptor signaling is similar to IFN-γ receptor signaling, with some important differences. Like the chains of the IFN-γ receptor, IFN-α/β receptor subunits constitutively and specifically associate with inactive JAKs in unstimulated cells. Tyk2 binds to the membrane-proximal region of the IFNAR1 intra-

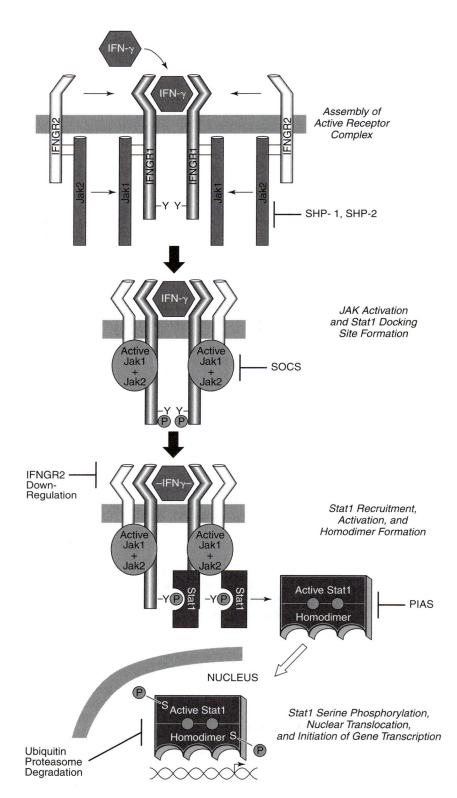

Figure 16-1. Model of IFN-γ signaling.

cellular domain (71) while JAK1 associates with a $_{274}LPKV_{277}$ sequence in the intracellular domain of IFNAR2 (72,73). However, in contrast to the IFN-γ receptor complex, latent forms of STAT1 and STAT2 are preassociated with the membrane-proximal region of the cytoplasmic domain of one of the IFN-α/β receptor subunits (IFNAR2) in unstimulated cells (74). The molecular basis for the association of STAT1 and STAT2 with IFNAR2 is not well understood but is not mediated through the interaction of phosphotyrosine-containing receptor sequences and the SH2 domains of the STATs. When type I IFN molecules encounter cells bearing IFN-α/β receptors, they bind to the IFNAR1 and IFNAR2 subunits, causing them to oligomerize, leading to JAK activation and consequent phosphorylation of a $_{466}YVFFP_{470}$ sequence in the IFNAR1 intracellular domain (75). This tyrosine phosphorylated sequence serves as a binding site for the SH2 domain of STAT2, enabling the formation of a high-affinity association between STAT2 and the activated IFN-α/β receptor (76). STAT2 is subsequently tyrosine phosphorylated by the receptor-associated JAKs, and is then bound by a STAT1 molecule, which binds by way of its own SH2 domain to the tyrosine phosphorylated STAT2 sequence. The STAT1 molecule is also tyrosine phosphorylated after binding to an IFNAR1-associated STAT2 protein. The STAT1/STAT2 complex that forms on the activated IFN-α/β receptor has two fates (32). First, some of the activated STAT1 proteins dissociate from their STAT2 tethers and form STAT1 homodimers, which translocate to the nucleus, bind to GAS elements, and effect the transcription of genes driven by GAS elements. This mechanism can to some extent explain the overlapping pattern of genes induced by IFN-α/β and IFN-γ. Second, the STAT1/STAT2 dimer (known as ISGF3α) can dissociate as an intact heterocomplex from the IFN-α/β receptor. This heterodimer cannot translocate to the nucleus or bind DNA on its own. However, it can associate with a cytosolic DNA binding protein named p48 or ISGF3γ, thus forming a trimolecular complex known as ISGF3, which can translocate to the nucleus and activate transcription. In the nucleus, ISGF3 interacts with a specific promoter element (termed the interferon-stimulated response element, or ISRE) that is distinct from the GAS element, and thus promotes the transcription of a distinct set of IFN-α/β–inducible genes (51,75).

Regulation of IFN-Dependent JAK-STAT Signaling

Role of Phosphatases

Several different mechanisms have been proposed to regulate IFN signaling. Experiments demonstrating the transient nature of IFN receptor and STAT protein tyrosine phosphorylation inspired the straightforward hypothesis that IFN signaling is directly regulated by specific protein tyrosine phosphatases. Several groups have studied this issue, and some initial data have emerged. SHP-1, an SH2 domain-containing tyrosine phosphatase, was found to bind to the IFN-α/β receptor complex in a reversible manner (77,78). In this study, SHP-1 was found to associate constitutively with the receptor complex, presumably maintaining the complex in an inactive state. Following receptor engagement, SHP-1 transiently dissociated from the complex, perhaps facilitating JAK activation and STAT recruitment. Macrophages taken from SHP-1–deficient *motheaten* mice showed increased JAK1 and STAT1 tyrosine phosphorylation in response to IFN-α stimulation compared with macrophages from normal littermate controls (78). Taken together, these results suggest that SHP-1 may play a negative regulatory role in IFN-α/β–induced signaling. Another group proposed an opposite, positive role for SHP-1 in regulating IFN-γ signaling based on their observation that overexpression of a catalytically inactive SHP-1 protein in HeLa cells led to a 30% to 50% increase in STAT1 activation in response to IFN-γ (79). Recently, another protein tyrosine phosphatase, SHP-2, was reported to interact constitutively with the IFN-α/β and IFN-γ receptors (80). Embryonic fibroblasts from SHP-2–deficient mice displayed hyperactive STAT activation after either IFN-α/β or IFN-γ stimulation, indicating that SHP-2 plays a negative role in regulating *both* IFN-α/β and IFN-γ signaling (80). However, detailed analyses of the magnitude of IFN-dependent biologic responses in the phosphatase-deficient cells need to be performed to establish the importance of tyrosine phosphatases in regulation of the IFN pathways.

Role of JAK Inhibitors

Recently, three groups independently cloned a family of proteins [termed suppressor of cytokine signaling (SOCS), JAK-binding (JAB) protein, or STAT-induced STAT inhibitor (SSI)] whose production is induced by many different cytokines, and that appear to function by binding via their SH2 domain to activated JAKs and inhibiting their catalytic activity (81–83). One member of this family, cytokine-inducible SH2 (CIS) protein, appears to function in a different manner because it binds directly to activated receptors that contain phosphorylated STAT5 recruitment sequences (such as the receptors for erythropoietin and IL-3) and thereby blocks STAT5 recruitment and activation at the receptor (84). The SOCS proteins contain an N-terminal region that is variable in length and sequence, a central SH2 domain, and a 40 amino acid region at the C-terminus termed the SOCS box. The formal SOCS family includes eight proteins: SOCS-1 through SOCS-7 and CIS. Twelve additional proteins have been identified that contain the SOCS box (85). However, the function of these related proteins remains unknown. The induction of SOCS gene transcription by cytokines appears to be mediated by STAT transcription factors. The time course of induction of many of the SOCS family genes is rapid and transient (transcript appears within 20 minutes of cytokine stimulation and disappears 2 to 4 hours later), but for some (such as SOCS-5 and CIS) the time course of induction is delayed or prolonged (86). Because many of the functional analyses of the SOCS proteins have relied on overexpression approaches in intact cells and cell-free systems, and because many of the SOCS family members are promiscuously induced by many different cytokines, the in vivo role of the SOCS proteins remains unclear. However, an initial view of the physiologic role of these proteins has come from the work of two different groups that generated mice that were devoid of SOCS-1/SSI-1 (87,88). SOCS-1/SSI-1 gene targeted mice display retarded growth and die within 3 weeks of birth. These mice exhibit fatty degeneration of the liver and accelerated apoptosis of lymphocytes with aging, which correlates with an up-regulation of Bax in the thymus and spleen. Further work, including the generation of mice lacking expression of other SOCS family members, needs to be done to place the role of these proteins in a proper perspective. Key questions that need to be addressed are whether the different SOCS proteins specifically regulate distinct cytokine signaling responses and whether they function as a generalized mechanism to effect the return of activated cytokine signaling pathways to their homeostatic baselines.

Role of STAT Inhibitors

A third family of novel inhibitory proteins termed proteins that inhibit activated STATs (PIAS) has been recently identified, and appears to function downstream of the activated receptor complex. The first of these proteins to be described (PIAS-1) was cloned using a yeast 2-hybrid screen for STAT1 interacting proteins, and another four PIAS family members were subsequently cloned on the basis of homology to PIAS-1 (89,90). The PIAS proteins, which contain a putative zinc-binding motif, are expressed constitutively, and are thought to associate specifically with activated STAT molecules after cytokine stimulation of cells. The PIAS proteins show a high degree of specificity for particular activated STAT complexes. Of the two family members that have been characterized thus far, PIAS-1 binds selectively to activated STAT1 molecules while PIAS-3 binds selectively to activated STAT3 molecules. More work needs to be done to determine whether the other PIAS proteins display specificity for other activated STAT molecules and to determine the mechanism of action of the PIAS proteins.

Role of the Ubiquitin-Proteasome Pathway

A fourth mechanism proposed to control the amount of activated STAT after IFN stimulation is degradation by the ubiquitin-proteasome pathway. One group showed that an inhibitor of the proteasome (MG132) stabilized STAT1 phosphorylation following IFN-γ treatment of HeLa cells. Phosphorylated STAT1 was ubiquitinated in vivo, implying that at some time after activation, STAT1 is targeted for degradation by the proteasome (91). However, these data do not exclude the possibility that signaling intermediates upstream of the STATs are also targeted for proteasome degradation. In fact, another group, using ^{35}S labeling to study the distribution of total STAT1 and activated STAT1 after IFN-γ treatment of cells, showed that STAT1 molecules translocate into the nucleus as tyrosine phosphorylated molecules but later return quantitatively to the cytoplasm as nonphosphorylated molecules (92). This result indicates that phosphorylated STAT1 molecules are not the main targets of proteasome degradation. Interestingly, a third group recently reported that the SOCS box of SOCS family proteins mediates interactions with

elongins B and C, which may target SOCS-bound proteins (i.e., Janus kinases or cytokine receptor chains) to the proteasomal degradation pathway (93).

Role of Receptor Down-regulation

Finally, IFN signaling can be regulated by a mechanism involving inhibition of expression of particular receptor subunits. IFNGR2 has been shown to be down-regulated (probably at the transcriptional level) in T cells as they differentiate to the Th1 CD4$^+$ subset (38,39). In newly developing T-cell clones, exposure of the cells to IFN-γ leads to a loss of IFNGR2 message and protein. In long-term Th1 clones, IFNGR2 expression is permanently suppressed. The generality and molecular basis of the mechanism underlying this unusual type of homologous desensitization remains poorly understood.

IFN-Inducible Genes

The rapid signaling of the JAK-STAT pathway makes it an ideal system for regulating the activation of immediate early genes that provide the host with a rapid mechanism for responding to an infectious agent. In fact, over the years it has been possible to identify a large number of interferon-stimulated genes (or ISGs) that are induced rapidly (i.e., within 15 to 30 minutes) after IFN treatment of cells, and whose transcription does not depend on new protein synthesis (94,95). The promoter regions of these ISGs contain two types of conserved nucleotide sequences that direct their rapid transcriptional activation (51,52). One is the interferon-stimulated response element (ISRE). The ISRE is a 12- to 15-nucleotide sequence that displays a consensus motif of AGTTTCNNTTTCNC/T and is responsible for driving expression of IFN-α/β–inducible genes. This site is recognized by the trimolecular ISGF3 signaling complex induced by IFN-α/β. The other is the GAS element, which functions to promote transcription of IFN-γ–inducible genes. The GAS site is a nine-nucleotide sequence with a consensus motif of TTNCNNNAA, and is specifically bound by STAT1 homodimers.

Examples of IFN-γ–induced immediate early genes include interferon regulatory factor-1 (IRF-1), guanylate binding protein-1 (GBP-1), and the type I Fcγ receptor (FcγRI), which encode proteins that participate in inflammatory and immune responses. Several IFN-γ–regulated intermediate genes have also been identified. These genes are induced within 6 to 8 hours of stimulation and require additional protein synthesis for transcriptional activation to occur. Examples of these genes include those that encode class I and class II MHC proteins, which play a central role in determining adaptive immune responses. Studies utilizing STAT1-, JAK1-, or JAK2-deficient mice have shown that these proteins play an obligate role in activating most IFN-γ– and IFN-α/β–inducible genes (57,58,60,61). More than 100 IFN-regulated genes have been identified. This subject has been recently reviewed elsewhere, and the reader is referred to several excellent reviews on the subject (7,94,96).

IFN Biologic Activities

Antiviral and Antiproliferative Activities

Both type I and type II interferons can protect cells from viral infection and have profound antiproliferative actions on normal and neoplastic cells. The molecular basis of the antiviral effects of the interferons has been extensively studied over the last 15 years. The IFNs promote antiviral responses that are either intrinsic to the infected cell itself or extrinsic in that they effect recognition and destruction of infected cells by components of either the innate or specific limbs of the host immune response.

Interferons induce several proteins in cells that promote intrinsic mechanisms of resistance to viral infection (97). Three distinct mechanisms have thus far been identified. The first relies on the actions of a family of enzymes known as $2'–5'$ oligoadenylate synthetases, which are induced by both type I and type II IFNs and activated by double-stranded RNA (98). The activated enzymes polymerize ATP into $2'–5'$ linked oligomers that in turn activate RNAse L, a latent constitutively expressed endoribonuclease. Activated RNAse L degrades single-stranded RNA and thereby inhibits protein synthesis in cells. The second antiviral mechanism is dependent on the protein PKR (also known as double-stranded RNA-dependent kinase, P1 kinase, p68 kinase, or eIF-2 kinase), which is a serine/threonine kinase that is also induced by IFN and activated by double-stranded RNA (99,100). PKR phosphorylates and inactivates the eukaryotic protein synthesis initiation factor (eIF-2), thereby blocking protein synthesis in cells. Thus, these two mechanisms produce their antiviral effects by inhibiting cellular protein synthesis. The third mechanism depends on the Mx protein, which is induced only by type I and not by type II interferons, and is directed primarily at inhibiting replication of orthomyxoviruses such as influenza virus (101). The human MxA protein belongs to the dynamin superfamily of high-molecular-weight GTPases, and has been shown to bind to influenza nucleocapsids in the cytoplasm and block their movement into the nucleus, thereby preventing the nuclear replication of the viral genome (102).

Extrinsic antiviral mechanisms induced by the IFNs are largely those that direct the development of innate and specific immune responses. Type I interferons are known to induce enhanced cytolytic activity in NK cells and thereby promote the capacity of these cells to lyse virally infected target cells. Both type I and type II interferons promote antigen processing and presentation and thereby play a key role in the induction of antiviral cellular and humoral immune responses. These actions will be discussed in more detail later in this chapter.

Both classes of IFNs have been shown to manifest antiproliferative effects on cells. However, although these biologic effects are well documented, their molecular bases are not yet well defined. Recent work has revealed that at least some of the antiproliferative actions of the IFNs are attributable to the induction of proteins that inhibit the enzymes involved in cell cycle progression. For example, IFN has been shown to induce, by way of the JAK-STAT pathway, expression of the protein p21$^{WAF1/CIP1/CAP1}$, which is an inhibitor of CDK2 (103,104). However, this process occurs in a relatively cell-specific manner, and it is presently unclear whether other cell cycle inhibitors may also be involved in the process. Nevertheless, this negative biologic response can still be attributed to a positive induction of a particular gene product.

Macrophage Activation and Innate Immunity

Of the interferon family members, IFN-γ is clearly distinct in its ability to function as the major macrophage-activating factor (MAF) (105–107). As such, it plays a critical role in promoting nonspecific host defense mechanisms against a number of pathogens. Data supporting this concept come from both in vitro and in vivo studies that have demonstrated that IFN-γ can induce in macrophages the capacity to kill nonspecifically a variety of intracellular and extracellular parasites as well as neoplastic cells (6,108). In addition, IFN-γ reduces the susceptibility of macrophages to microbial infection and enhances recognition of targets during the early innate phase of immunity through regulation of macrophage cell surface proteins that are to date undefined (109). The physiologic significance of the role of IFN-γ in macrophage activation and host defense against microbial pathogens has been clearly established by several in vivo murine infection models. Mice pretreated with neutralizing antibodies to IFN-γ lose the ability to resist sublethal challenges of a variety of microbial pathogens such as *Listeria monocytogenes* (28,106), *Toxoplasma gondii* (110), and *Leishmania major* (111). In addition, mice with disrupted genes for IFN-γ, the IFNGR1 chain, or the IFN signaling protein STAT1 die when challenged with sublethal doses of microbial pathogens such as *Mycobacterium bovis*, *Listeria monocytogenes*, and *Leishmania major* (60,112,113).

Activated macrophages kill microbial targets using a variety of toxic substances such as reactive oxygen and nitrogen intermediates that are induced by IFN-γ. Much of the antimicrobial function of IFN-γ–activated macrophages can be attributed to the actions of nitric oxide (NO) and/or reactive oxygen intermediates (ROIs) (114,115). NO is produced in activated macrophages by the inducible form of nitric oxide synthase (iNOS or NOS2). The gene encoding iNOS is transcriptionally activated following treatment of cells with IFN-γ plus a variety of second signals that activate the transcription factor NF-κB, such as TNF-α, IL-1, or bacterial endotoxin. The enzyme catalyzes the conversion of L-arginine to L-citrulline, giving rise to large amounts of NO. NO is thought to kill target cells by one of two mechanisms. First, it can form an iron-nitrosyl complex with Fe-S groups of aconitase and complex I and complex II, thereby causing the inactivation of the mitochondrial electron transport chain. Alternatively, NO may react with superoxide anion (a reactive oxygen intermediate formed by the IFN-γ–induced enzyme NADPH oxidase) to form peroxynitrite, which decays rapidly once protonated to form the highly toxic compound hydroxyl radical. Evidence that NO is responsible for macrophage killing of intracellular parasites comes from several studies with *Listeria* and *Leishmania*. Mice pretreated with the L-arginine analogue N-monomethyl-L-arginine (NMMA), which is an iNOS inhibitor, were unable to resolve footpad infection with *Leishmania* parasites. Similarly, mice treated with another iNOS inhibitor (aminoguanidine) succumbed to sublethal *Listeria* infection (116). Furthermore, mice lacking the iNOS gene are highly susceptible to infection with microbial pathogens (114,115,117).

Antigen Processing and Presentation

One of the major immunoregulatory roles of the interferons is their ability to promote the inductive phase of immune responses. These cytokines significantly influence the generation and presentation of antigenic peptides on cell surfaces (6,7). Among the IFN family members, IFN-γ is uniquely capable of regulating the expression of MHC class II proteins, thereby promoting enhanced CD4$^+$ T-cell responses (7,118). IFN-γ induces MHC class II protein expression on many cells, such as mononuclear phagocytes, endothelial cells, and epithelial cells. Interestingly, IFN-γ inhibits IL-4–dependent class II expression on B cells (119), although the molecular basis for this apparently discordant effect is unknown. Type I IFN cannot induce MHC class II proteins on cells by itself. However, it can either inhibit or enhance the ability of IFN-γ to induce MHC class II. In the case of mononuclear phagocytes, pre-exposure of cells to type I IFNs induces a state of unresponsiveness to IFN-γ. In contrast, treatment of cells with IFN-α/β, either together with or after IFN-γ treatment, leads to enhanced class II expression. A similar type of modulation of the MHC class II–inducing activity of IFN-γ is also observed with other stimuli such as TNF, bacterial endotoxin, and immune complexes. Thus, a cell's ability to express MHC class II in response to IFN-γ is influenced by the composition of the microenvironment (6).

One function that all IFN family members share is their ability to regulate the expression of molecules involved in the MHC class I antigen processing and presentation pathway (7). Some of these effects are at the level of regulating cell surface molecules. Both type I IFN and IFN-γ enhance the expression of MHC class I proteins and beta-2-microglobulin in a wide variety of cell types. The proteins also enhance the expression of several cell surface components such as ICAM-1 and B7, which are responsible for increasing target cell–T cell contact and T-cell costimulation, respectively (120,121).

The IFNs also promote antigen processing by regulating expression of many intracellular proteins required for antigenic peptide generation (7,121). IFN-γ has been shown to play a key role in modifying the activity of the proteasome, a multisubunit enzyme complex that is responsible for generating the peptides that bind to MHC class I proteins. It does so in part by modulating the expression of the enzymatic proteasome subunits. IFN-γ increases expression of the inducible subunits—namely, LMP2, LMP7, and MECL1—while at the same time decreasing expression of the constitutive subunits x, y, and z, thereby altering proteasome composition and specificity (121–123). In addition, IFN-γ enhances the production of nonenzymatic proteasome components, such as the α and β subunits of PA28 (also known as the 11S regulator of the proteasome), that function to regulate pro-

teasome enzymatic activity (124). Purified 20S and 26S proteasomes from IFN-γ–treated cells show an increased capacity to cleave peptides after hydrophobic and basic residues, revealing that IFN-γ alters the proteasome in a way that changes the types of antigenic peptides that it produces (122).

IFN-γ additionally increases expression of the peptide transporters TAP1 and TAP2, which transfer peptides that have been generated in the cytoplasm by the proteasome into the endoplasmic reticulum where they can bind to nascently produced MHC class I proteins (120,121). Moreover, IFN-γ increases expression of the heat shock protein gp96, which may play a role in transferring peptide both within the cell, from the TAPs to MHC class I, and between cells, from nonprofessional antigen-presenting cells to a subset of macrophages (125). Taken together, these data strongly suggest that IFN-γ plays an important role in enhancing immunogenicity by increasing both the quantity and the repertoire of peptides displayed on MHC class I.

Helper T-Cell Phenotype Development

Human and murine CD4$^+$ T cells can be divided into two subsets based on their patterns of cytokine secretion after stimulation (26,126). T helper 1 (Th1) cells promote cell-mediated immunity and delayed type hypersensitivity (DTH) responses through their production of IFN-γ, lymphotoxin (LT), and IL-2. In contrast, T helper 2 (Th2) cells predominantly produce IL-4, -5, and -10 and thereby provide help for humoral immune responses. IFN-γ plays an important role in Th1 development. In vitro, antibody neutralization of IFN-γ greatly reduces the development of Th1 cells and augments the development of Th2 cells. Importantly, administration of exogenous IFN-γ either in vitro or in vivo does not drive a Th1 response. Thus, IFN-γ is necessary, but is not sufficient, for Th1 development.

Both in vitro and in vivo studies have demonstrated that IL-12 is the single most important cytokine that drives T cells to the Th1 pole (127,128). Bacterial products promote Th1 cell development by inducing IL-12 production from antigen-presenting cells such as macrophages. In addition, mice deficient in either the gene for IL-12 or the IL-12 signaling protein STAT4 are unable to generate Th1 cells and display reduced DTH responses. The role of IFN-γ in Th development has recently been shown to be attributable to its effects at the levels of both the macrophage and the CD4$^+$ T cell. The effects of IFN-γ on macrophages were elucidated in studies that used transgenic mice lacking IFN-γ sensitivity specifically in the macrophage compartment. IFN-γ–insensitive macrophages were unable to support efficient Th1 development owing to a severely reduced capacity to produce IL-12 (129). More recently, IFN-γ has been shown to have direct effects on the developing Th cells themselves. IFN-γ maintains expression of the β2 subunit of the IL-12 receptor on developing T cells, thereby preserving sensitivity of these cells to IL-12 and promoting their development into a Th1 phenotype (130). IFN-γ also blocks development of Th2 phenotype through two mechanisms. First, it inhibits synthesis of IL-4 from undifferentiated, antigen-stimulated T cells, thereby inhibiting production of the cytokine that is required for Th2 development (131). Second, it inhibits Th2 cell expansion by directly inhibiting proliferation of Th2 cells (132). The antiproliferative effects of IFN-γ are not observed on Th1 cells because these cells do not express the IFNGR2 subunit (38,39). Thus, IFN-γ simultaneously promotes cell-mediated immunity (through facilitation of Th1 cell formation) and inhibits development of humoral immunity (through blockading of Th2 cell expansion).

Humoral Immunity

The interferons play complex and conflicting roles in regulation humoral immunity. Up until now, most studies have been focused on defining the actions of IFN-γ in modulating humoral responses, although more recent observations suggest that type I interferons may also cause many of the same biologic effects. The interferons exert their effects either indirectly by regulating the development of specific T helper cell subsets (as described above) or directly at the level of the B cell. In the latter case, the IFNs are predominantly responsible for regulating three specialized B-cell functions: 1) B-cell development and proliferation, 2) Ig secretion, and 3) Ig heavy chain switching.

IFN-γ has been shown to regulate B-cell differentiation negatively by inhibiting IL-4–dependent induction of MHC class II protein expression and proliferation of murine B cells stimulated with anti-Ig and IL-4. In contrast, IFN-γ enhances proliferative responses in human B cells activated with anti-Ig. IFN-γ can also enhance or inhibit Ig secretion by either murine or human B cells. However, in this process the effects of IFN-γ are dependent on the differentiation state of the B cell, the timing of IFN-γ stimulation, and the nature of the activating stimulus.

The best-characterized B-cell–directed effect of the interferons is their ability to influence Ig heavy chain switching. Immunoglobulin class switching is significant because the different Ig isotypes promote distinct effector functions in the host. IgE is the only isotype that can bind to Fcε receptors on mast cells and basophils and thereby promotes immediate type hypersensitivity and allergic reactions. IgG2a fixes complement and can also, in monomeric form, bind to FcγRI on murine macrophages, a high-affinity Fc receptor that is up-regulated during IFN-γ–induced macrophage activation. Activated macrophages can efficiently use antibodies of the IgG2a isotype to mediate antibody-dependent cellular cytotoxicity (ADCC). IgG3 is an isotype that can self-aggregate, a process that may enhance its opsonic activity. Along with IgG2a, IgG3 can also bind to the NK cell IgG receptor CD16 and effect NK-mediated ADCC. Interferons, by favoring the production of IgG2a and IgG3 and inhibiting the production of IgE isotypes, can facilitate the interaction between the humoral and cellular effector limbs of the immune response and enhance host defense against certain bacteria and viruses.

In vitro IFN-γ is able to direct immunoglobulin class switching from IgM to the IgG2a subtype in LPS-stimulated murine B cells and to IgG2a and IgG3 in murine B cells that have been stimulated with activated T cells (133,134). Moreover, IFN-γ blocks IL-4–induced Ig class switching in murine B cells to IgG1 or IgE (135). The validity of these observations has been strin-

gently tested in experiments in which Ig subclass production was monitored in mice that were injected with IgD-specific antiserum to achieve polyclonal activation of B cells. Mice treated in this manner produced large quantities of IgG1 and IgE. However, when IFN-γ was administered to the mice prior to anti-IgD treatment, they produced high levels of IgG2a and decreased levels of IgG1. Thus, IFN-γ is clearly an important regulator of Ig class switching in vivo (136).

Recently, a role for the type I IFNs in this process has also been identified (137). Mice deficient in the receptors for either IFN-γ, IFN-α/β, or both IFN-γ and IFN-α/β were infected with live lymphocytic choriomeningitis virus (LCMV), and the profile of the LCMV-specific antibodies generated was determined. Comparable levels of LCMV-specific IgG2a antibodies were observed in the sera of normal mice and of mice that were unresponsive to *either* IFN-γ or IFN-α/β. In contrast, IgG2a anti-bodies were not produced in mice with combined unresponsiveness to *both* types of IFN. These results demonstrate that if induced during the immune response, type I IFNs can indeed function in the same way IFN-γ functions in effecting Ig class switching.

Tumor Immunity

An accumulating body of evidence suggests that IFN family members play important roles in promoting host defense to tumors. The IFNs can exert profound antiproliferative effects on a variety of tumor cells. IFN-α/β is, in general, more active in promoting this response than IFN-γ. The IFNs have also been proposed to inhibit tumor generation by directly increasing expression of several tumor suppressor genes such as IRF-1 and PKR.

However, there are several antitumor activities that are unique to IFN-γ. In vitro, IFN-γ is able to activate macrophages to nonspecifically lyse certain tumor cells, through mechanisms involving the generation of reactive oxygen and nitrogen intermediates and the production of cytotoxic ligands of the tumor necrosis family, such as TNF, Fas ligand (FasL), and TNF-related apoptosis-inducing ligand (TRAIL) (108,138,139). In addition, IFN-γ is required for robust IL-12 secretion by macrophages. IL-12 has been shown in several studies to exhibit potent antitumor effects even in mice with pre-established tumors (128). Injection of recombinant IL-12 into tumor-bearing mice reduces the rate of metastasis, slows tumor growth, and in some cases effects complete tumor regression. IFN-γ is required for IL-12–mediated antitumor effects. This conclusion is based on the observation that neutralizing IFN-γ–specific mAbs ablate the effects of IL-12 on tumors in vivo (140,141).

Many experiments indicate that the major mechanism of the antitumor effects of IFN-γ involves its ability to promote the generation of specific immune responses to tumors. As discussed earlier, IFN-γ up-regulates MHC class I and class II molecules on a wide variety of cells, and increases the magnitude and changes the nature of MHC class I antigen processing. In vitro experiments showed that IFN-γ treatment of a wide variety of nonantigenic tumors made them highly antigenic, and correlated with an increase in expression levels of IFN-γ–inducible genes that regulate MHC class I processing and presentation, including LMP2, LMP7, Tap1, and Tap2 (142,143). Another study showed that the ability of lymphocytes harvested from draining lymph nodes of mice harboring the fibrosarcoma MCA 105 to effect adoptive transfer of immunity to MCA 105 was abrogated by in vivo administration of neutralizing IFN-γ antibodies to the recipient mice (144). Together, these studies suggest that a major effect of IFN-γ is to increase the antigenicity of tumors and augment tumor immunity.

A clear demonstration of a role for IFN-γ in immune-mediated tumor rejection comes from a series of studies using chemically induced fibrosarcomas such as the Meth A tumor cell line (145). Meth A is a methylcholanthrene (MCA)-induced fibrosarcoma of BALB/c mice that grows progressively when transplanted intradermally in syngeneic mice. Although the tumor is highly aggressive and eventually kills the host, a tumor-bearing mouse can be induced to reject the tumor by administration of LPS. Using neutralizing mAb specific for murine IFN-γ, it was determined that IFN-γ is obligatorily required for LPS-induced tumor rejection. In addition, Meth A tumors grew significantly more rapidly in anti-IFN-γ–treated syngeneic mice.

Although these results established the importance of IFN-γ in Meth A growth regulation, they did not identify the cellular target of the actions of IFN-γ. By introducing a mutant nonfunctional IFNGR1 protein into Meth A tumor cells, it was possible specifically to ablate tumor cell responsiveness to the cytokine and demonstrate that the tumor itself was a major target of the actions of IFN-γ. IFN-γ–insensitive Meth A grew more rapidly in naive syngeneic mice than did control tumors and was not rejected when the tumor-bearing mice were treated with LPS. In addition, the IFN-γ–insensitive tumors neither primed naive mice for induction of Meth A immunity nor were rejected in mice with pre-established immunity to the wild type tumor cell. This effect was not attributable to the antiproliferative actions of IFN-γ. Similar studies using different murine fibrosarcomas have yielded similar results. Thus, the ability of the immune system to recognize and reject certain tumors is critically dependent on the tumor's ability to respond to IFN-γ (145).

A subsequent study suggests that IFN-γ may also exert its antitumor effects in tumor transplant models through a mechanism involving the inhibition of blood vessel recruitment by tumors (146). Overexpression of a mutant nonfunctional IFNGR1 chain in tumor cells rendered them relatively insensitive to IFN-γ, highly tumorigenic, and relatively unresponsive to IL-12 therapy in vivo. IL-12 was found to induce ischemic damage only in IFN-γ–responsive tumors. In vivo Matrigel assays showed that while both IFN-γ–sensitive and -insensitive tumors recruited blood vessels equally well, IL-12 therapy only inhibited angiogenesis in the IFN-γ–responsive tumors. IFN-γ induces the expression of several angiostatic molecules in target cells, including the chemokines IP-10 and Mig, which may mediate its antiangiogenic activity.

Although the tumor transplantation studies described above identified a critical role for IFN-γ in promoting rejection of transplantable tumors, they did not address the question of whether IFN-γ participates in the elimination of primary developing tumor cells (147). To examine this question, IFN-γR−/− mice, STAT1−/− mice, and wild type mice, all of which were derived on a pure inbred 129/Sv/Ev background, were treated with different dosages of the chemical carcinogen methylcholanthrene (MCA) and tumor development followed through 165 days. At every MCA dosage examined, IFN-γ–insensitive mice developed tumors significantly more rapidly and with greater frequency compared with wild type mice (Fig. 16-2). IFN-γ–insensitive mice also displayed enhanced tumor development in a model of spontaneous tumor formation. Mice lacking the p53 tumor suppressor gene were bred onto a wild type 129/Sv/Ev, IFN-γR−/−, or STAT1−/− background, and tumor development in the single or double knockout offspring was assessed. IFN-γ–insensitive p53−/− mice developed spontaneous tumors significantly earlier than did their IFN-γ–sensitive counterparts (Fig. 16-3). Furthermore, the two groups of mice displayed differences in the types of tumors that formed. While all of the IFN-γ–sensitive p53−/− mice developed lymphoid tumors, 35% of the IFN-γR−/− × p53−/− mice and 38% of the STAT1−/− × p53−/− mice formed nonlymphoid tumors without concomitant lymphoid tumors.

Two sets of experiments indicate that the increased tumor incidence in IFN-γ–unresponsive hosts is due to IFN-γ unresponsiveness at the level of the transformed cell itself. First, tumor cells derived from MCA-treated IFN-γ–insensitive mice grew progressively with identical kinetics when transplanted into either wild type mice or the corresponding IFN-γ–insensitive mouse strain. Second, introduction of the missing IFN-γ signaling protein into these cells by gene transfer reconstituted their capacity to respond to IFN-γ and converted them into immunogenic tumors that were rejected in wild type 129/Sv/Ev mice but not in Rag2−/− mice, which are devoid of lymphocytes. Together, these results thus demonstrate that the interplay between IFN-γ and the specific immune system forms the basis of an effective tumor surveillance system in the normal host. In addition, these observations indicate that a major target of the antitumor functions of IFN-γ is the tumor cell itself. A critical role for lymphocytes in this process has recently been confirmed by studies showing that lymphocyte-deficient Rag2−/− mice are highly susceptible to tumor induction by MCA, and that tumors that develop in the absence of lymphocytes are strongly immunogenic.

The existence of an IFN-γ–dependent antitumor system is further supported by the identification of tumor cells that have developed spontaneous and specific insensitivity to IFN-γ (147). A screen of human tumor cell banks revealed that lung adenocarcinomas show a tendency to develop permanent IFN-γ unresponsiveness spontaneously. Four out of 17 lines tested failed to initiate IFN-γ–dependent signaling (as measured using an electrophoretic mobility shift assay) and failed to develop biologic responses to human IFN-γ as determined by monitoring of enhanced MHC class I expression. Using immunochemical and molecular genetic approaches, the IFN-γ unresponsiveness in each cell line was determined to be the result of a discrete lesion in a proximal IFN-γ signaling component. One tumor cell line lacked the IFNGR1 chain, two others produced abnormal forms of JAK2, and the fourth lacked JAK1. Recently, a subset of *primary* MCA-induced murine tumors have been identified that develop quantitative insensitivity to IFN-γ. These IFN-γ–insensitive tumors grow in a highly aggressive manner when transplanted into syngeneic immunocompetent mice.

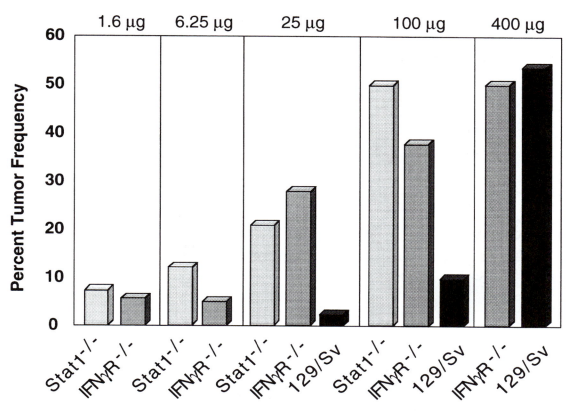

Figure 16-2. IFN-γ–insensitive mice demonstrate an increased susceptibility to development of chemically induced tumors. Groups of wild type, IFN-γR$^{-/-}$, and STAT1$^{-/-}$ mice were injected with one of a range of dosages of MCA and tumor development monitored for 165 days. Values represent the composite of four independent experiments.

In Vivo Dysfunction of IFN-γ Signaling

Mice with Targeted Disruption of Genes Involved in IFN-γ Signaling

The physiologic consequences of global in vivo inactivation of the IFN-γ signaling pathway in mice were originally uncovered using neutralizing monoclonal antibodies specific for IFN-γ. However, the physiologic role of IFN-γ has been more fully elucidated using mice with engineered disruptions in either the IFN-γ structural gene (112), the genes encoding the two IFN-γ receptor subunits (IFNGR1 and IFNGR2) (113,148,149), or the genes encoding any of the three signaling proteins required by IFN-γ for biologic response induction—i.e., STAT1 (60,61), JAK1 (56), or JAK2 (57,58). As a group, these mice display a greatly impaired ability to resist infection by a variety of microbial pathogens including *L. monocytogenes, L. major,* and several mycobacterial species, including *M. bovis* and *M. avium.* Importantly, mice lacking either IFNGR1 or IFNGR2 are able to mount curative responses to many viruses, while mice lacking the IFN-α/β receptor or STAT1, and cells from mice deficient in JAK1, are not. These results thus demonstrate that under physiologic conditions the majority of

the antiviral effects of the IFN system are largely mediated via type I interferons (150).

Identification of Human Patients with Defects in IFN-γ Signaling or Production

Results obtained from IFNGR1-deficient mice suggest that individuals with inactivating mutations in the human IFN-γ receptor genes might suffer from recurrent microbial but not viral infections. In 1996, two research groups identified children from three unrelated families with such mutations who manifested a severe susceptibility to weakly pathogenic mycobacterial species (151,152). Genetic analysis of these patients' families revealed that susceptibility to atypical mycobacterial infection was inherited in an autosomal recessive manner. Sequence analysis of the patients' IFNGR1 alleles identified missense mutations in genetic regions coding for the extracellular domain of the IFNGR1 polypeptide, leading to the production of truncated receptor proteins that were not able to be retained at the cell surface. The clinical syndromes of these patients were similar. In one study, a group of related Maltese children showed extreme susceptibility to infection with *M. fortuitum, M. avium,* and *M. chelonei* (151).

A

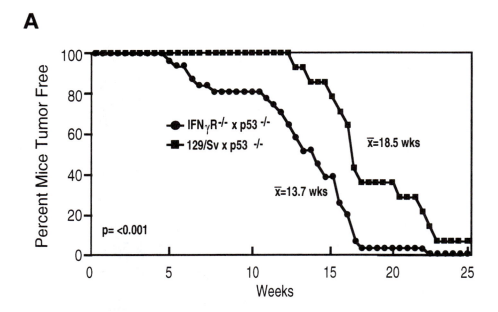

B

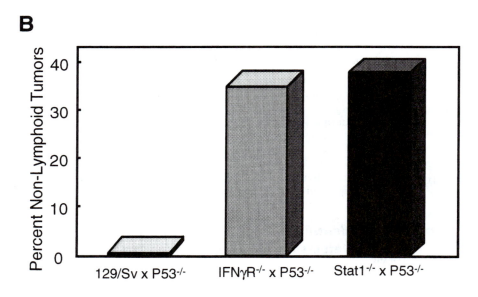

Figure 16-3. IFN-γ–insensitive mice demonstrate an increased susceptibility to development of spontaneous tumors. Panel A: spontaneous tumor development in IFN-γR$^{-/-}$ × p53$^{-/-}$ and 129/Sv/Ev × p53$^{-/-}$ mice. The difference in average tumor development times between 129/Sv/Ev × p53$^{-/-}$ (18.5 weeks) and IFN-γR$^{-/-}$ × p53$^{-/-}$ (13.7 weeks) is statistically significant by the Wilcoxon rank sum test ($P < 0.001$). Panel B: percent 129/Sv/Ev × p53$^{-/-}$, IFN-γR$^{-/-}$ × p53$^{-/-}$, and STAT1$^{-/-}$ × p53$^{-/-}$ mice developing nonlymphoid tumors without concomitant lymphoid tumors.

In another study, a Tunisian child was identified with disseminated *M. bovis* infection following Bacillus Calmette-Guérin (BCG) vaccination (152). A third study identified a child of distinct ancestry who had a similar immunocompromised phenotype (153). Biopsies from these patients revealed the presence of multibacillary, poorly defined granulomas, which contained scattered macrophages but lacked epithelioid and giant cells and surrounding lymphocytes. Importantly, these patients showed enhanced susceptibility to mycobacteria and occasionally to salmonella but not to other typical bacteria or other common microbial pathogens or fungi. Moreover, in all three kindred, the

patients were able to mount antibody and/or curative responses to several different viruses.

Subsequently, several patients were identified who developed less severe mycobacterial disease than the children described above. These patients were successfully treated with IFN-γ and antibiotics. On analysis of their IFN-γ receptor genes, some of the patients were found to display distinct mutations in the IFNGR1 gene, leading to reduced but not ablated receptor function (154). A Portuguese family was identified in which one child developed disseminated BCG infection and a sibling who had not been BCG vaccinated developed clinical tuberculosis.

Both patients were homozygous for a point mutation in the extracellular domain-encoding region of the IFNGR1 gene that produced an isoleucine-to-threonine amino acid substitution. The mutant receptors were found to require 100- to 1000-fold higher concentrations of IFN-γ than normal receptors in order to activate STAT1 (154).

Another set of 19 patients from 12 unrelated families were found to have inherited partial IFN-γ insensitivity in an autosomal-dominant manner (155). All of these patients were found to be heterozygous for a wild type IFNGR1 allele and an IFNGR1 allele with a frameshift mutation that produced an IFNGR1 protein that lacked most of the intracellular domain including the JAK1 and STAT1 binding sites. Interestingly, in this group of patients, there were 12 independent mutation events at a single site, defining a small deletion hotspot in the IFNGR1 gene. The truncated receptor chain accumulated on cell surfaces and was shown to act in a dominant negative manner to inhibit IFN-γ responses in cells. The definition of the molecular basis for this defect was facilitated by the observation that the IFN-γ–response phenotype of these patients resembled that of IFN-γ–insensitive cells or transgenic mice generated earlier that overexpressed a genetically engineered truncated IFNGR1 subunit (145,156). In all of these patients, defects in IFN-γ responsiveness were partial, and cells from the patients retained some degree of sensitivity to IFN-γ. This correlates with the milder infections in these patients, and their positive responses to exogenous IFN-γ therapy.

Recently, a case of a child with severe, disseminated infections attributed to *M. fortuitum* and *M. avium* who lacked mutations in the IFNGR1 gene was described (157). This child was found to be homozygous for mutations in the gene encoding the IFNGR2 chain protein. The mutation resulted in a premature stop codon in the extracellular domain-encoding region, and led to the production of IFNGR2 proteins that could not be expressed at the cell surface. The clinical and histopathologic phenotype of this patient closely resembled that of patients lacking expression of the IFNGR1 chain.

An interesting additional group of patients were identified whose clinical syndromes resembled partial IFN-γR deficiency, but on analysis were found to express normal IFN-γ receptor polypeptides. Seven of these patients lacked functional IL-12 receptor complexes as a result of null mutations in the IL-12Rβ1 gene (158,159). Lymphocytes from these patients were deficient in producing IFN-γ. This defect could not be corrected by addition of recombinant IL-12. One case of an individual with a homozygous frameshift deletion encompassing two exons of the IL-12 p40 gene was also reported (160). This patient's lymphocytes had a reduced capacity to secrete IFN-γ, which could be complemented by exogenous IL-12. All of these patients with functional defects in IFN-γ production developed atypical mycobacterial infections that could be cured by exogenous IFN-γ therapy. As a group, the patients with defects in either IFN-γ signaling or IL-12–induced IFN-γ production have taught us that IFN-γ plays a critical role in host defense to mycobacterial infections in humans. It will be important in the future to determine why IFN-γ receptor defects in humans lead almost exclusively to enhanced susceptibility to mycobacterial infection.

Clinical Applications of the Interferons

Soon after their discovery, the possibility of using the interferons to treat a wide variety of human diseases, including infectious diseases and malignancies, captured the imagination of both the discoverers of the interferons and the general public. The interferons have turned out to be highly effective in the clinics for a limited number of disorders, and have been approved by regulatory agencies for the treatment of at least 13 viral and malignant diseases (161). However, the clinical utility of these proteins has not fulfilled the great expectations that were predicted on their discovery more than four decades ago.

The IFNs are currently being used clinically to treat several different infectious diseases. IFN-α has become the treatment of choice for individuals with chronic hepatitis B virus (HBV) and hepatitis C virus (HCV) infections. In response to treatment with this cytokine, 40% of HBV-infected patients and 10% to 25% of HCV-infected individuals show a decrease in viral load and an improvement in liver function tests (117,161). IFN-α is also highly effective in the treatment of condylomata acuminata and laryngeal papilloma, which are benign epithelial tumors associated with human papilloma virus types 6 and 11 (117,161). IFN-γ administration has been shown to be a useful adjuvant to antibiotic therapy in decreasing the severity and frequency of infections in patients with chronic granulomatous disease (CGD) (162). CGD patients suffer from chronic bacterial infections as a result of defects in the phagocyte-specific NADPH oxidase system that generates superoxide radicals during the respiratory burst. IFN-γ was selected as a candidate therapeutic for CGD because it is known to increase superoxide production and the microbicidal activity of phagocytes. However, the mechanism of the therapeutic action of IFN-γ appears to be independent of these direct effects on the NADPH oxidase system, because cells from patients who responded to IFN-γ therapy did not display enhanced superoxide production or in vitro bacterial killing (162).

As both single agents and in combination therapy, the interferons (especially IFN-α) have also been found to be effective in treating certain malignancies. IFN-α2 is used widely in the treatment of two different hematologic malignancies, hairy cell leukemia (HCL) and chronic myelogenous leukemia (CML). More than 85% of patients with HCL, a rare B-cell neoplasm involving the dysregulated growth of preplasma cells, respond completely or partially to IFN-α2 treatment. After even low-dosage IFN-α2 therapy, patients experience a decrease in malignant cell infiltration of the bone marrow and a normalization of peripheral hematologic cell counts (163,164). The reason for the high sensitivity of HCL to IFN-α remains undefined. CML is a multilineage hematologic cancer whose clinical course can be separated into two major stages. The first stage, called the chronic stage, is characterized by a gradual increase in peripheral granulocyte levels and gradual splenic enlargement. The second stage, termed the acute phase, is marked by a progression to undifferentiated leukemia, with the expansion of undifferentiated myeloid or lymphoid blast cells. At dosages higher than those used to treat HCL, IFN-α has been shown to induce a sustained clinical improvement in more than 75% of patients with chronic phase CML (165–168). IFN-α is, however, relatively ineffective therapeutically in CML cases that have progressed to the acute phase. Responses to IFN-α treatment are characterized by a reduction in leukemic mass as well as the suppression of cells carrying the Philadelphia chromosome, which results in the aberrant expression of the abl oncogene (168). Some other hematologic malignancies are sensitive to IFN-α, although response rates are not as dramatic as for HCL and CML. These include multiple myeloma, chronic lymphocytic leukemia, and several different lymphomas (169,170).

As a group, nonhematologic solid tumors are relatively refractory to IFN therapy. IFNs have been tested in clinical trials against a variety of solid tumors, and response rates are generally less than 30%. However, IFN-α has been found to be especially efficacious against one tumor (hemangioma of infancy), effecting complete hemangioma regression in more than 80% of children bearing this life-threatening tumor (171). The dramatic regression of this particular tumor, which is a cancer of endothelial cells, highlights the potent angiostatic effects of the IFNs.

One of the IFN family members, IFN-β, has been shown to be highly effective in treating multiple sclerosis (MS), an inflammatory disease that is pathologically characterized by demyelination of neurons of the brain and spinal cord. The mechanism of the therapeutic actions of IFN-β is unclear (172). However, the ability of IFN-β to decrease attack frequency starkly contrasts with the tendency of IFN-γ to increase attack frequency, which led to the halting of a trial of IFN-γ in MS (173).

Taken together, the clinical trials of the IFNs demonstrate that this group of cytokines can be a highly effective therapeutic for certain human diseases. Interestingly, type I IFNs have more clinical efficacy than IFN-γ. This is somewhat surprising because of the more potent immunomodulatory activity of IFN-γ versus IFN-α/β. These results thus suggest that more research is needed before these cytokines can be used most effectively in a clinical setting.

Acknowledgments

Vijay Shankaran is supported by a predoctoral training award from the Cancer Research Institute. Work from Robert D. Schreiber's lab quoted in this chapter was supported by grants from the National Institutes of Health (CA43039 and CA76464), Genentech, Inc, and the Cancer Research Institute.

References

1. Isaacs A, Lindenmann J. Virus interference. I. The interferon. Proc R Soc London Ser 1957;147:258.
2. Wheelock EF. Interferon-like virus-inhibitor induced in human leukocytes by phytohemagglutinin. Science 1965;149:310–311.
3. Pestka S, Langer JA, Zoon KC, Samuel CE. Interferons and their actions. Annu Rev Biochem 1987;56:727–777.
4. Henco K, Brosius J, Fujisawa A, et al. Structural relationships of human interferon alpha genes and pseudogenes. J Mol Biol 1985;185:227–260.
5. Zoon KC, Miller D, Bekisz J, et al. Purification and characterization of multiple components of human lymphoblastoid interferon alpha. J Biol Chem 1992;267:15210–15216.
6. Farrar MA, Schreiber RD. The molecular cell biology of interferon-γ and its receptor. Annu Rev Immunol 1993;11:571–611.
7. Boehm U, Klamp T, Groot M, Howard JC. Cellular responses to interferon-γ. Annu Rev Immunol 1997;15:749–795.
8. Trent JM, Olson S, Lawn RM. Chromosomal localization of human leukocyte, fibroblast, and immune interferon genes by means of in situ hybridization. Proc Natl Acad Sci USA 1982;79:7809–7813.
9. Uzé G, Lutfalla G, Mogensen KE. Alpha and beta interferon and their receptor and their friends and relations. J Interferon Res 1995;15:3–26.
10. Naylor SL, Sakaguchi AY, Shows TB, et al. Human immune interferon gene is located on chromosome 12. J Exp Med 1983;157:1020–1027.
11. Naylor SL, Gray PW, Lalley PA. Mouse immune interferon (IFNγ) gene is on human chromosome 10. Somat Cell Mol Genet 1984;10:531–534.
12. Kelker HC, Le J, Rubin BY, et al. Three molecular weight forms of natural human interferon-gamma revealed by immunoprecipitation with monoclonal antibody. J Biol Chem 1984;259:4301–4304.
13. Scahill SJ, Devos R, Van der Heyden J, Fiers W. Expression and characterization of the product of a human immune interferon cDNA gene in Chinese hamster ovary cells. Proc Natl Acad Sci USA 1983;80:4654–4658.
14. Chang TW, McKinney S, Liu V, et al. Use of monoclonal antibodies as sensitive and specific probes for biologically active human gamma-interferon. Proc Natl Acad Sci USA 1984;81:5219–5222.
15. Ealick SE, Cook WJ, Vijay-Kumar S, et al. Three-dimensional structure of recombinant human interferon-γ. Science 1991;252:698–702.
16. Bach EA, Aguet M, Schreiber RD. The IFNγ receptor: a paradigm for cytokine receptor signaling. Annu Rev Immunol 1997;15:563–591.
17. Maniatis T. Mechanisms of human β-interferon gene regulation. Harvey Lectures 1988;82:71–104.
18. Taniguchi T. Regulation of interferon-β gene: structure and function of cis-elements and trans-acting factors. J Interferon Res 1989;9:633–640.
19. Pitha PM, Au W-C. Induction of interferon alpha genes expression. Virology 1995;6:151–159.
20. Tanaka N, Taniguchi T. Cytokine gene regulation: regulatory cis-elements and DNA binding factors involved in the interferon system. Adv Immunol 1992;52:263–281.
21. Wolf SF, Temple PA, Kobayashi M, et al. Cloning of cDNA for natural killer cell stimulatory factor, a heterodimeric cytokine with multiple biologic effects on T and natural killer cells. J Immunol 1991;146:3074–3080.
22. Stern AS, Podlaski FJ, Hulmes JD, et al. Purification to homogeneity and partial characterization of cytotoxic lymphocyte maturation factor from human B-lymphoblastoid cells. Proc Natl Acad Sci USA 1990;87:6808–6812.
23. Jacobson NG, Szabo SJ, Weber-Nordt RM, et al. Interleukin 12 signaling in T helper type 1 (Th1) cells involves tyrosine phosphorylation of signal transducer and activator of transcription (Stat)3 and Stat4. J Exp Med 1995;181:1755–1762.

24. Okamura H, Tsutsul H, Komatsu T, et al. Cloning of a new cytokine that induces IFN-γ production by T cells. Nature 1995;378:88–91.

25. Robinson D, Shibuya K, Mui A, et al. IGIG does not drive Th1 development, but synergizes with IL-12 for IFN-γ production, and activates IRAK and NF-kB. Immunity 1997; 7:571–581.

26. O'Garra A. Cytokines induce the development of functionally heterogeneous T helper cell subsets. Immunity 1998;8: 275–283.

27. Yang J, Murphy TL, Ouyang W, Murphy KM. Induction of interferon-gamma production in Th1 CD4+ T cells: evidence for two distinct pathways for promoter activation. Eur J Immunol 1999;29:548–555.

28. Bancroft GJ, Schreiber RD, Unanue ER. Natural immunity, a T-cell-independent pathway of macrophage activation, defined in the scid mouse. Immunol Rev 1991;124:5–24.

29. Tripp CS, Wolf SF, Unanue ER. Interleukin-12 and tumor necrosis factor alpha are costimulators of interferon-gamma production by natural killer cells in severe combined immunodeficiency mice with listeriosis, and interleukin-10 is a physiologic antagonist. Proc Natl Acad Sci USA 1993;90: 3725–3729.

30. Unanue ER. Interrelationship among macrophages, NK cells and neutrophils in early stages of Listeria resistance. Curr Opin Immunol 1997;9:35–43.

31. Fiorentino DF, Zlotnik A, Mosmann TR, et al. IL-10 inhibits cytokine production by activated macrophages. J Immunol 1991;147:3815–3822.

32. Stark GR, Kerr IM, Williams BRG, et al. How cells respond to interferons. Annu Rev Biochem 1998;67:227–264.

33. Bazan JF. Structural design and molecular evolution of a cytokine receptor superfamily. Proc Natl Acad Sci USA 1990;87:6934–6938.

34. Cook JR, Emanuel SL, Donnelly RJ, et al. Sublocalization of the human interferon-gamma receptor accessory factor gene and characterization of accessory factor activity by yeast artificial chromosomal fragmentation. J Biol Chem 1994;269:7013–7018.

35. Spencer SD, Di Marco F, Hooley J, et al. The orphan receptor CRF2-4 is an essential subunit of the interleukin 10 receptor. J Exp Med 1998;187:571–578.

36. Uzé G, Lutfalla G, Gresser I. Genetic transfer of a functional human interferon alpha receptor into mouse cells: cloning and expression of its cDNA. Cell 1990;60:225–234.

37. Pestka S, Kotenko SV, Muthukumaran G, et al. The interferon gamma (IFN-γ) receptor: a paradigm for the multichain cytokine receptor. Cytokine Growth Fac Rev 1997; 8:189–206.

38. Pernis A, Gupta S, Gollob KJ, et al. Lack of interferon-γ receptor β chain and the prevention of interferon-γ signaling in T$_H$1 cells. Science 1995;269:245–247.

39. Bach EA, Szabo SJ, Dighe AS, et al. Ligand-induced autoregulation of IFN-γ receptor β chain expression in T helper cell subsets. Science 1995;270:1215–1218.

40. Aguet M, Dembic Z, Merlin G. Molecular cloning and expression of the human interferon-γ receptor. Cell 1988;55: 273–280.

41. Gray PW, Leong S, Fennie EH, et al. Cloning and expression of the cDNA for the murine interferon gamma receptor. Proc Natl Acad Sci USA 1989;86:8497–8501.

42. Kumar CS, Muthukumaran G, Frost LJ, et al. Molecular characterization of the murine interferon-γ receptor cDNA. J Biol Chem 1989;264:17939–17946.

43. Munro S, Maniatis T. Expression and cloning of the murine interferon-γ receptor cDNA. Proc Natl Acad Sci USA 1989; 86:9248–9252.

44. Hemmi S, Peghini P, Metzler M, et al. Cloning of murine interferon gamma receptor cDNA: expression in human cells mediates high-affinity binding but is not sufficient to confer sensitivity to murine interferon gamma. Proc Natl Acad Sci USA 1989;86:9901–9905.

45. Cofano F, Moore SK, Tanaka S, et al. Affinity purification, peptide analysis, and cDNA sequence of the mouse interferon-γ receptor. J Biol Chem 1990;265:4064–4071.

46. Hershey GK, Schreiber RD. Biosynthetic analysis of the human interferon-gamma receptor. Identification of N-linked glycosylation intermediates. J Biol Chem 1989;264: 11981–11988.

47. Mao C, Aguet M, Merlin G. Molecular characterization of the human interferon-gamma receptor: analysis of polymorphism and glycosylation. J Interferon Res 1989;9:659–669.

48. Fischer T, Thoma B, Scheurich P, Pfizenmaier K. Glycosylation of the human interferon-gamma receptor. N-linked carbohydrates contribute to structural heterogeneity and are required for ligand binding. J Biol Chem 1990;265:1710–1717.

49. Soh J, Donnelly RO, Kotenko S, et al. Identification and sequence of an accessory factor required for activation of the human interferon-γ receptor. Cell 1994;76:793–802.

50. Hemmi S, Bohni R, Stark G, et al. A novel member of the interferon receptor family complements functionality of the murine interferon γ receptor in human cells. Cell 1994;76: 803–810.

51. Darnell JE Jr, Kerr IM, Stark GR. Jak-STAT pathways and transcriptional activation in response to IFNs and other extracellular signaling proteins. Science 1994;264:1415–1421.

52. Schindler C, Darnell JE Jr. Transcriptional responses to polypeptide ligands: the JAK-STAT pathway. Annu Rev Biochem 1995;64:621–651.

53. Darnell JE Jr. STATs and gene regulation. Science 1997;277: 1630–1635.

54. O'Shea JJ. Jaks, STATs, cytokine signal transduction, and immunoregulation: are we there yet? Immunity 1997;7(1): 1–11.

55. Ihle JN, Witthuhn BA, Quelle FW, et al. Signaling through the hematopoietic cytokine receptors. Annu Rev Immunol 1995;13:369–398.

56. Rodig SJ, Meraz MA, White JM, et al. Disruption of the Jak1 gene demonstrates obligatory and nonredundant roles of the Jaks in cytokine-induced biologic responses. Cell 1998; 93:373–383.

57. Paraganas E, Wang D, Stravopodis D, et al. Jak2 is essential for signaling through a variety of cytokine receptors. Cell 1998;93:385–395.

58. Neubauer H, Cumano A, Muller M, et al. Jak2 deficiency defines an essential developmental checkpoint in definitive hematopoiesis. Cell 1998;93:397–409.

59. Kotenko SV, Izotova LS, Pollack BP, et al. Other kinases can substitute for Jak2 in signal transduction by interferon-γ. J Biol Chem 1996;271:17174–17182.

60. Meraz MA, White JM, Sheehan KCF, et al. Targeted disruption of the STAT1 gene in mice reveals unexpected physiologic specificity in the JAK-STAT signaling pathway. Cell 1996;84:431–442.

61. Durbin JE, Hackenmiller R, Simon MC, Levy DE. Targeted disruption of the mouse Stat1 gene results in compromised innate immunity to viral infection. Cell 1996;84:443–450.

62. Chen X, Vinkemeier U, Zhao Y, et al. Crystal structure of a tyrosine phosphorylated STAT-1 dimer bound to DNA. Cell 1998;93:827–839.

63. Bach EA, Tanner JW, Marsters, SA, et al. Ligand-induced assembly and activation of the gamma interferon receptor in intact cells. Mol Cell Biol 1996;16:3214–3221.

64. Kaplan DH, Greenlund AC, Tanner JW, et al. Identification of an interferon-γ receptor α chain sequence required for JAK-1 binding. J Biol Chem 1996;271:9–12.

65. Kotenko S, Izotova L, Pollack B, et al. Interaction between the components of the interferon gamma receptor complex. J Biol Chem 1995;270:20915–20921.

66. Sakatsume M, Igarashi K, Winestock KD, et al. The Jak kinases differentially associate with the α and β (accessory factor) chains of the interferon-γ receptor to form a functional receptor unit capable of activating STAT transcription factors. J Biol Chem 1995;270:17528–17534.

67. Greenlund AC, Farrar MA, Viviano BL, Schreiber RD. Ligand induced IFNγ receptor phosphorylation couples the receptor to its signal transduction system (p91). EMBO J 1994;13:1591–1600.

68. Greenlund AC, Morales MO, Viviano BL, et al. STAT recruitment by tyrosine-phosphorylated cytokine receptors: an ordered reversible affinity-driven process. Immunity 1995;2:677–687.

69. Schindler C, Shuai K, Prezioso VR, Darnell JE Jr. Interferon-dependent tyrosine phosphorylation of a latent cytoplasmic transcription factor. Science 1992;257:809–813.

70. Shuai K, Stark GR, Kerr IM, Darnell JE Jr. A single phosphotyrosine residue of stat 91 required for gene activation by interferon-γ. Science 1993;261:1744–1746.

71. Colamonici O, Yan H, Domanski P, et al. Direct binding to and tyrosine phosphorylation of a subunit of the type 1 interferon receptor by p135tyk2 tyrosine kinase. Mol Cell Biol 1994;14:8133–8142.

72. Gauzzi MC, Velazquez L, McKendry R, et al. Interferon-α-dependent activation of Tyk2 requires phosphorylation of positive regulatory tyrosines by another kinase. J Biol Chem 1996;271:20494–20500.

73. Novick D, Cohen B, Rubinstein M. The human interferon α/β receptor: characterization and molecular cloning. Cell 1994;77:391–400.

74. Li X, Leung S, Kerr IM, Stark GR. Functional subdomains of STAT2 required for preassociation with the α interferon receptor and for signaling. Mol Cell Biol 1997;17:2048–2056.

75. Yan H, Krishnan K, Greenlund AC, et al. Phosphorylated interferon-α receptor 1 subunit (IFNαR1) acts as a docking site for the latent form of the 113kDa STAT2 protein. EMBO J 1996;15:1064–1074.

76. Leung S, Qureshi SA, Kerr IM, et al. Role of STAT2 in alpha interferon signaling pathway. Mol Cell Biol 1995;15:1312–1317.

77. David M, Zhou G, Pine R, et al. The SH2 domain-containing tyrosine phosphatase PTP1D is required for interferon α/β-induced gene expression. J Biol Chem 1996;271:15862–15865.

78. David M, Chen HE, Goelz S, et al. Differential regulation of the alpha/beta interferon-stimulated JAK/STAT pathway by the SH2 domain-containing tyrosine phosphatase SHPTP1. Mol Cell Biol 1995;15:7050–7058.

79. You M, Zhao Z. Positive effects of SH2 domain-containing tyrosine phosphatase SHP-1 on epidermal growth factor- and interferon-gamma-stimulated activation of STAT transcription factors in HeLa cells. J Biol Chem 1997;272: 23376–23381.

80. You M, Yu D, Feng G. SHP-2 tyrosine phosphatase functions as a negative regulator of the interferon-stimulated JAK/STAT pathway. Mol Cell Biol 1999;19:2416–2424.

81. Starr R, Wilson TA, Viney EM, et al. A family of cytokine-inducible inhibitors of signaling. Nature 1997;387:917–920.

82. Endo TA, Masuhara M, Yokouchi M, et al. A new protein containing an SH2 domain that inhibits JAK kinases. Nature 1997;387:921–924.

83. Naka T, Narazaki M, Hirata M, et al. Structure and function of a new STAT-induced STAT inhibitor. Nature 1997;387: 924–928.

84. Matsumoto A, Masuhara M, Mitsui K, et al. CIS, a cytokine inducible SH2 protein, is a target of the JAK-STAT5 pathway and modulates STAT5 activation. Blood 1997;89: 3148–3154.

85. Hilton DJ, Richardson RT, Alexander WS, et al. Twenty proteins containing a C-terminal SOCS box form five structural classes. Proc Natl Acad Sci USA 1998;95:114–119.

86. Starr R, Hilton DJ. Negative regulation of the JAK/STAT pathway. BioEssays 1999;21:47–52.

87. Starr R, Metcalf D, Elefanty AG, et al. Liver degeneration and lymphoid deficiencies in mice lacking suppressor of cytokine signaling-1. Proc Natl Acad Sci USA 1998;95: 14395–14399.

88. Naka T, Matsumoto T, Narazaki M, et al. Accelerated apoptosis of lymphocytes by augmented induction of Bax in SSI-1 (STAT-induced STAT inhibitor-1) deficient mice. Proc Natl Acad Sci USA 1998;95:15577–15582.

89. Chung CD, Liao JY, Liu B, et al. Specific inhibition of Stat3 signal transduction by PIAS3. Science 1997;278:1803–1805.

90. Liu B, Liao J, Rao X, et al. Inhibition of Stat1-mediated gene activation by PIAS1. Proc Natl Acad Sci USA 1998;95: 10626–10631.

91. Kim TK, Maniatis T. Regulation of interferon-gamma-activated Stat1 by the ubiquitin-proteasome pathway. Science 1996;273:1717–1719.

92. Haspel RL, Salditt-Georgieff M, Darnell JE. The rapid inactivation of nuclear tyrosine phospnhorylated Stat1 depends upon a protein tyrosine phosphatase. EMBO J 1996;15: 6262–6268.

93. Zhang J, Farley A, Nicholson SE, et al. The conserved SOCS box motif in suppressors of cytokine signaling binds to elongins B and C and may couple bound proteins to proteasomal degradation. Proc Natl Acad Sci USA 1999;96: 2071–2076.

94. Kerr IM, Stark GR. The control of interferon-inducible gene expression. FEBS Lett 1991;285:194–198.

95. Lewin AR, Reid LE, McMahon M, et al. Molecular analysis of a human interferon-inducible gene family. Eur J Biochem 1991;199:417–423.

96. Der SD, Zhou A, Williams BR, Silverman RH. Identification of genes differentially regulated by interferon alpha, beta, or gamma using oligonucleotide arrays. Proc Natl Acad Sci USA 1998;95:15623–15628.

97. Vilcek J, Sen GC. Interferons and other cytokines. In: Fields BN, Knipe DM, Howley PM, eds. Fields virology. 3rd ed. Philadelphia: Lippincott-Raven, 1996:375.

98. Silverman RH, Cirino NM. RNA decay by the interferon-regulated 2-5 A system as a host defense against viruses. In: Morris DR, Harford JB, eds. mRNA metabolism and post-transcriptional gene regulation. New York: John Wiley & Sons, 1997:295.

99. Meurs E, Chong K, Galabru J, et al. Molecular cloning and characterization of the human double-stranded RNA-activated protein kinase induced by interferon. Cell 1990;62:379–390.

100. McMillan NAJ, Williams BRG. Structure and function of the interferon-induced protein kinase, PKR, and related enzymes. In: Clemens MJ, ed. Protein phosphorylation in cell growth regulation. London: Harwood Academic, 1996:225.

101. Arnheiter H, Frese M, Kambadur R, et al. Mx transgenic mice—animal models of health. Curr Top Microbiol Immunol 1996;206:119–147.

102. Kochs G, Haller O. Interferon-induced human MxA GTPase blocks nuclear import of Thogoto virus nucleocapsids. Proc Natl Acad Sci USA 1999;96:2082–2086.

103. Chin YE, Kitagawa M, Su WS, et al. Cell growth arrest and induction of cyclin-dependent kinase inhibitor p21 mediated by Stat1. Science 1996;272:719–722.

104. Bromberg JF, Horvath CM, Wen Z, et al. Transcriptionally active Stat1 is required for the antiproliferative effects of both interferon alpha and interferon gamma. Proc Natl Acad Sci USA 1996;93:7673–7678.

105. Schreiber RD, Pace JL, Russell SW, et al. Macrophage-activating factor produced by a T cell hybridoma: physiochemical and biosynthetic resemblance to gamma-interferon. J Immunol 1983;131:826–832.

106. Buchmeier NA, Schreiber RD. Requirement of endogenous interferon-gamma production for resolution of Listeria monocytogenes infection. Proc Natl Acad Sci USA 1985;82:7404–7408.

107. Nathan CF, Murray HW, Wiebe ME, Rubin BY. Identification of interferon-gamma as the lymphokine that activates human macrophage oxidative metabolism and antimicrobial activity. J Exp Med 1983;158:670–689.

108. Schreiber RD, Celada A. Molecular characterization of interferon gamma as a macrophage activating factor. Lymphokines 1985;11:87–118.

109. Belosevic M, Davis CE, Meltzer MS, Nacy CA. Regulation of activated macrophage antimicrobial activities. Identification of lymphokines that cooperate with IFN-gamma for induction of resistance to infection. J Immunol 1988;141:890–896.

110. Suzuki Y, Orellana MA, Schreiber RD, Remington JS. Interferon-gamma: the major mediator of resistance against Toxoplasma gondii. Science 1988;240:516–518.

111. Nacy CA, Fortier AH, Meltzer MS, et al. Macrophage activation to kill Leishmania major: activation of macrophages for intracellular destruction of amastigotes can be induced by both recombinant interferon-gamma and non-interferon lymphokines. J Immunol 1985;135:3505–3511.

112. Dalton DK, Pitts-Meek S, Keshav S, et al. Multiple defects of immune function in mice with disrupted interferon-γ genes. Science 1993;259:1739–1742.

113. Huang S, Hendriks W, Althage A, et al. Immune response in mice that lack the interferon-γ receptor. Science 1993;259:1742–1745.

114. Nathan C. Natural resistance and nitric oxide. Cell 1995;82:873–876.

115. MacMicking J, Xie Q-W, Nathan C. Nitric oxide and macrophage function. Annu Rev Immunol 1997;15:323–350.

116. Beckerman KP, Rogers HW, Corbett JA, et al. Release of nitric oxide during the T cell-independent pathway of macrophage activation. Its role in resistance to Listeria monocytogenes. J Immunol 1993;150:888–895.

117. Shiloh MU, MacMicking JD, Nicholson S, et al. Phenotype of mice and macrophages deficient in both phagocyte oxidase and inducible nitric oxide synthase. Immunity 1999;10:29–38.

118. Mach B, Steimle V, Martinez-Soria E, Reith W. Regulation of MHC class II genes: lessons from a disease. Annu Rev Immunol 1996;14:301–331.

119. Mond JJ, Carman J, Sarma C, et al. Interferon-gamma suppresses B cell stimulation factor (BSF-1) induction of class II MHC determinants on B cells. J Immunol 1986;137:3534–3537.

120. Germain RN. Antigen processing and presentation. In: Paul WE, ed. Fundamental immunology. 3rd ed. New York: Raven Press, 1993:629.

121. Pamer E, Cresswell P. Mechanisms of MHC class I restricted antigen processing. Annu Rev Immunol 1998;16:323–358.

122. Gaczynska M, Rock KL, Spies T, Goldberg AL. Peptidase activities of proteasomes are differentially regulated by the major histocompatability complex-encoded genes for LMP2 and LMP7. Proc Natl Acad Sci USA 1994;91:9213–9217.

123. York IA, Rock KL. Antigen processing and presentation by the class I major histocompatibility complex. Annu Rev Immunol 1996;14:369–396.

124. Groettrup M, Soza A, Eggers M, et al. A role for the proteasome regulator PA28α in antigen presentation. Nature 1996;381:166–168.

125. Suto R, Srivastava PK. A mechanism for the specific immunogenicity of heat shock proteins-chaperoned peptides. Science 1995;269:1585–1588.

126. Abbas AK, Murphy KM, Sher A. Functional diversity of helper T lymphocytes. Nature 1997;383:787–793.

127. Hsieh C-S, Macatonia S, Tripp CS, et al. Development of Th1 CD4+ T cells through IL-12 produced by Listeria-induced macrophages. Science 1993;260:547–549.

128. Gately MK, Renzetti LM, Magram J, et al. Interleukin-12/Interleukin-12-receptor system: role in normal and pathologic immune responses. Annu Rev Immunol 1998;16:495–521.

129. Dighe AS, Campbell D, Hsieh C-S, et al. Tissue specific targeting of cytokine unresponsiveness in transgenic mice. Immunity 1995;3:657–666.

130. Szabo SJ, Dighe AS, Gubler U, Murphy KM. Regulation of the interleukin (IL)-12R β2 subunit expression in developing T helper 1 (Th1) and Th2 cells. J Exp Med 1997;185:817–824.

131. Szabo SJ, Jacobson NG, Dighe AS, et al. Developmental commitment to the Th2 lineage by extinction of IL-12 signaling. Immunity 1995;2:665–675.

132. Gajewski TF, Fitch FW. Anti-proliferative effect of IFN-gamma in immune regulation. IV. Murine CTL clones produce IL-3 and GM-CSF, the activity of which is masked by the inhibitory action of secreted IFN-gamma. J Immunol 1990;144:548–556.

133. Snapper CM, Peschel C, Paul WE. IFN-gamma stimulates IgG2a secretion by murine B cells stimulated with bacterial lipopolysaccharide. J Immunol 1988;140:2121–2127.

134. Snapper CM, McIntyre TM, Mandler R, et al. Induction of IgG3 secretion by interferon gamma: a model for T cell-independent class switching in response to T cell-independent type 2 antigens. J Exp Med 1992;175:1367–1371.

135. Snapper CM, Paul WE. Interferon-gamma and B cell stimulatory factor-1 reciprocally regulate Ig isotype production. Science 1987;236:944–947.

136. Snapper CM. Interferon-gamma. In: Snapper CM, ed. Cytokine regulation of humoral immunity. West Sussex, England: John Wiley & Sons, 1996:325.

137. van den Broek MF, Muller U, Huang S, et al. Antiviral defense in mice lacking both alpha/beta and gamma interferon receptors. J Virol 1995;69:4792–4796.

138. Adams DO, Hamilton TA. The cell biology of macrophage activation. Annu Rev Immunol 1984;2:283–318.

139. Griffith TS, Wiley SR, Kubin MZ, et al. Monocyte-mediated tumoricidal activity via the tumor necrosis factor-related cytokine, TRAIL. J Exp Med 1999;189:1343–1354.

140. Nastala CL, Edington HD, McKinney TG, et al. Recombinant IL-12 administration induces tumor regression in association with IFN-γ production. J Immunol 1994;153:1697–1706.

141. Brunda MJ. Interleukin-12. J Leukoc Biol 1994;55:280–288.

142. Restifo NP, Esquivel F, Asher AL, et al. Defective presentation of endogenous antigens by a murine sarcoma. J Immunol 1991;147:1543–1549.

143. Restifo NP, Esquivel F, Kawakami Y, et al. Identification of human cancers deficient in antigen processing. J Exp Med 1993;177:265–272.

144. Tuttle TM, McCrady CW, Inge TH, et al. Gamma interferon plays a key role in T-cell-induced tumor regression. Cancer Res 1993;53:833–839.

145. Dighe AS, Richards E, Old LJ, Schreiber RD. Enhanced in vivo growth and resistance to rejection of tumor cells expressing dominant negative IFNγ receptors. Immunity 1994;1:447–456.

146. Coughlin CM, Salhany KE, Gee MS, et al. Tumor cell responses to IFNγ affect tumorigenicity and response to IL-12 therapy and antiangiogenesis. Immunity 1998;9:25–34.

147. Kaplan DH, Shankaran V, Dighe AS, et al. Demonstration of an IFNγ dependent tumor surveillance system in immunocompetent mice. Proc Natl Acad Sci USA 1998;95:7556–7561.

148. Kamijo R, Le J, Shapiro D, et al. Mice that lack the interferon-γ receptor have profoundly altered responses to infection with Bacillus Calmette-Guérin and subsequent challenge with lipopolysaccharide. J Exp Med 1993;178:1435–1440.

149. Lu B, Ebensperger C, Dembic Z, et al. Targeted disruption of the interferon-gamma receptor 2 gene results in severe immune defects in mice. Proc Natl Acad Sci USA 1998;95:8233–8238.

150. Müller U, Steinhoff U, Reis LFL, et al. Functional role of type I and type II interferons in antiviral defense. Science 1994;264:1918–1921.

151. Newport MJ, Huxley CM, Huston S, et al. A mutation in the interferon-γ-receptor gene and susceptibility to mycobacterial infection. N Engl J Med 1996;335:1941–1949.

152. Jouanguy E, Altare F, Lamhamedi S, et al. Interferon-γ-receptor deficiency in an infant with fatal bacille Calmette-Guerin infection. N Engl J Med 1996;335:1956–1961.

153. Pierre-Audigier C, Jouanguy E, Lamhamedi S, et al. Fatal disseminated Mycobacterium smegmatis infection in a child with inherited interferon γ receptor deficiency. Clin Infect Dis 1997;24:982–984.

154. Jouanguy E, Lamhamedi-Cherradi S, Altare F, et al. Partial interferon-gamma receptor 1 deficiency in a child with tuberculoid bacillus Calmette-Guerin infection and a sibling with clinical tuberculosis. J Clin Invest 1997;100:2658–2664.

155. Jouanguy E, Lamhamedi-Cherradi S, Lammas D, et al. A human IFNGR1 small deletion hotspot associated with dominant susceptibility to mycobacterial infection. Nat Genet 1999;21:370–378.

156. Dighe AS, Farrar MA, Schreiber RD. Inhibition of cellular responsiveness to interferon-γ (IFNγ) induced by overexpression of inactive forms of the IFNγ receptor. J Biol Chem 1993;268:10645–10653.

157. Dorman SE, Holland SM. Mutation in the signal-transducing chain of the interferon-gamma receptor and susceptibility to mycobacterial infection. J Clin Invest 1998;101:2364–2369.

158. Altare F, Durandy A, Lammas D, et al. Impairment of mycobacterial immunity in human interleukin-12 receptor deficiency. Science 1998;280:1432–1435.

159. de Jong R, Altare F, Haagen I, et al. Severe myocbacterial and salmonella infections in interleukin-12 receptor-deficient patients. Science 1998;280:1435–1438.

160. Altare F, Lammas D, Revy P, et al. Inherited interleukin-12 deficiency in a child with bacille Calmette-Guerin and Salmonella enteritidis disseminated infection. J Clin Invest 1998;102:2035–2040.

161. Gutterman JU. Cytokine therapeutics: lessons from interferon alpha. Proc Natl Acad Sci USA 1994;91:1198–1205.

162. Dinauer MC, Orkin SH. Chronic granulomatous disease. Annu Rev Med 1992;43:117–124.

163. Quesada JR, Hersh EM, Manning J, et al. Treatment of hairy cell leukemia with recombinant alpha interferon. Blood 1986;68:493–497.

164. Foon KA, Maluish AE, Abrams PG, et al. Recombinant leukocyte A interferon therapy for advanced hairy cell leukemia. Therapeutic and immunologic results. Am J Med 1986;80:351–356.

165. Talpaz M, Kantarijian HM, McCredie K, et al. Hematologic remission and cytogenetic improvement induced by recombinant human interferon alpha A in chronic myelogenous leukemia. N Engl J Med 1986;314:1065–1069.

166. Talpaz M, Kantarajian H, Kurzrock R, et al. Interferon-alpha produces sustained cytogenetic responses in chronic myelogenous leukemia in Philadelphia chromosome-positive patients. Ann Intern Med 1991;114:532–538.

167. Al Alimna G, Morra E, Lazzarino M, et al. Interferon alpha-2b as therapy for Ph′-positive chronic myelogenous leukemia: a study of 82 patients treated with intermittent or daily administration. Blood 1988;72:642–647.
168. Kantarjian HM, Deisseroth A, Kurzrock R, et al. Chronic myelogenous leukemia: a concise update. Blood 1993;82: 691–703.
169. Borden EC. Innovative treatment strategies for non-Hodgkin's lymphoma and multiple myeloma. Semin Oncol 1994;21(6 suppl 14):14–22.
170. O'Connell MJ, Colgan JP, Oken MM, et al. Clinical trial of recombinant leukocyte A interferon as initial therapy for favorable histology non-Hodgkin's lymphomas and chronic lymphocytic leukemia. An Eastern Cooperative Oncology Group pilot study. J Clin Oncol 1986;4:128–136.
171. Ezekowitz RAB, Mulliken JB, Folkman J. Interferon alpha-2a therapy for life-threatening hemangiomas of infancy. N Engl J Med 1992;326:1456–1463.
172. Arnason BGW. Immunologic therapy of multiple sclerosis. Annu Rev Med 1999;50:291–302.
173. Panitch HS, Haley AS, Hirsch RL, Johnson KP. Exacerbations of multiple sclerosis in patients treated with gamma interferon. Lancet 1987:893–895.
174. Nosaka T, van Deursen JMA, Tripp RA, et al. Defective lymphoid development in mice lacking Jak3. Science 1995;270:800–802.
175. Thomis DC, Gurniak CB, Tivol E, et al. Defects in B lymphocyte maturation and T lymphocyte activation in mice lacking Jak3. Science 1995;270:794–797.
176. Park SY, Saijo K, Takahashi T, et al. Developmental defects of lymphoid cells in Jak3 kinase-deficient mice. Immunity 1995;3:771–782.
177. Schindler C. Personal communication.
178. Takeda K, Noguchi K, Shi W, et al. Targeted disruption of the mouse Stat3 gene leads to early embryonic lethality. Proc Natl Acad Sci USA 1997;94:3801–3804.
179. Takeda K, Kaisho T, Yoshida N, et al. Stat3 activation is responsible for IL-6-dependent T cell proliferation through preventing apoptosis: generation and characterization of T cell-specific Stat3-deficient mice. J Immunol 1998;161:4652–4660.
180. Takeda K, Clausen BE, Kaisho T, et al. Enhanced Th1 activity and development of chronic enterocolitis in mice devoid of Stat3 in macrophages and neutrophils. Immunity 1999;10: 39–49.
181. Thierfelder WE, van Deursen JM, Yamamoto K, et al. Requirement for Stat4 in interleukin-12-mediated responses of natural killer and T cells. Nature 1996;382:171–174.
182. Kaplan MH, Sun Y-L, Hoey T, Grusby MJ. Impaired IL-12 responses and enhanced development of Th2 cells in Stat4-deficient mice. Nature 1996;382:174–177.
183. Feldman GM, Rosenthal LA, Liu X, et al. STAT5A-deficient mice demonstrate a defect in granulocyte-macrophage colony-stimulating factor-induced proliferation and gene expression. Blood 1997;90:1768–1776.
184. Teglund S, McKay C, Schuetz E, et al. Stat5a and Stat5b proteins have essential and nonessential, or redundant, roles in cytokine responses. Cell 1998;93:841–850.
185. Udy GB, Towers RP, Snell RG, et al. Requirement of STAT5b for sexual dimorphism of body growth rates and liver gene expression. Proc Natl Acad Sci USA 1997;94: 7239–7244.
186. Shimoda K, van Deursen J, Sangster MY, et al. Lack of IL-4-induced Th2 response and IgE class switching in mice with disrupted Stat6 gene. Nature 1996;380:630–633.
187. Kaplan MH, Schindler U, Smiley ST, Grusby MJ. Stat6 is required for mediating responses to IL-4 and for the development of Th2 cells. Immunity 1996;4:313–319.

Chapter 17

Interleukin-2 Immunostimulation

Kendall A. Smith

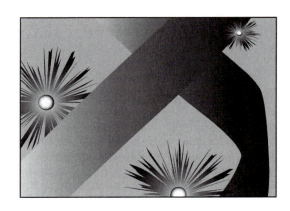

In the history of medicine, the stimulation of host defenses has been an elusive goal that has become attainable only within the past decade. By comparison, immunosuppression has been a part of the therapeutic armamentarium for the latter half of this century. Immunostimulation has lagged so far behind immunosuppression as a result of two fundamental difficulties. First, there was inadequate knowledge concerning the cellular composition of the immune system and how the system is regulated by immunologic molecules. Second, as a consequence of this lack of knowledge, there have been no suitable therapeutic agents that could be used to make the system function better. As a result, early attempts at immunostimulation yielded severe toxicity. A century ago, living bacteria and then bacterial extracts were used in attempts to promote inflammation for the treatment of cancer. However, the treatments were so toxic that the therapy was often worse than the disease, and such attempts were largely abandoned with the advent of radiotherapy in the 1920s and then chemotherapy in the 1940s. However, we have come a long way since the use of bacterial toxins, and nontoxic immunostimulation is finally within our grasp. This chapter is devoted to a detailed examination of the therapeutic use of the first hormone of the immune system, interleukin-2 (IL-2).

Historic Considerations

The Humoral and Cellular Schools

To understand why immunostimulatory therapy lagged so far behind immunosuppressive therapy, and to understand why immunostimulatory therapy can be so toxic, it is necessary to study the history of immunology in the past century. At the turn of the 20th century the science of immunology was just beginning, and two schools of thought developed. With the discovery of antibodies by Von Behring and Kitasato in 1890 (1), the humoralist school developed at the Robert Koch Institute in Berlin, and the notion of using serotherapy to treat infectious diseases evolved. At the time, great excitement was generated, as the transfer of sera from immunized animals to infected humans could be efficacious. However, the phenomenon of "serum sickness," a systemic inflammation resulting from the immune response to the heterologous serum components, limited the use of serotherapy. Therefore, when chemotherapeutics and antibiotics were developed in the 1930s and 1940s, serotherapy gradually became forgotten.

The second immunologic school in the early part of the 20th century formed around Eli Metchnikoff, a Russian biologist who first described phagocytosis. Metchnikoff recognized that the host defenses must have a cellular basis, and as Chef de Service at the Pasteur Institute, Metchnikoff's studies forwarded the concept that the cellular immune response was primary and responsible for the humoral immune response. Unfortunately, Metchnikoff was several generations ahead of his time. Although he recognized the phenomenon of phagocytosis and identified two distinct phagocytic cells, namely, macrophages and microphages (polymorphonuclear leukocytes), the composition and cellular origin of antibodies still remained unknown. Metchnikoff postulated that the phagocytes themselves were responsible for elaborating the "fixatives" detectable within plasma (2). The role of lymphocytes in the immune system had not yet been recognized. Moreover, the promise of attenuated microorganisms introduced by Pasteur for use as vaccines was not realized (3,4). It proved difficult, if not impossible, to weaken the virulence of most pathogens. Accordingly, during the first half of the 20th century the science of immunology became preoccupied with studies focused on the identification and characterization of the structures and functions of antibodies, and the science of microbiology focused on studies of the characteristics of individual microbes. Any thoughts regarding the cellular origin of the antibodies, serotherapy, vaccines, and immunotherapy were largely abandoned.

The Antibody Puzzle

By the 1950s, as the structures of antibody molecules gradually became determined (5,6), immunologists started to ponder how the tremendous diversity of antigen recognition could be created. Niels Jerne proposed that the diversity of recognition was inherent in the system and that, on introduction of antigen, antibodies were selected naturally, as in a Darwinian sense, from the population that already existed (7). However, the underlying cellular basis for such diversity remained problematic until Burnet proposed the clonal selection hypothesis, which held that a single cell was responsible for the production of only one specific antibody (8).

Proceeding beyond theory proved difficult, as the cells responsible for the formation of antibodies remained obscure. Like Metchnikoff 50 years earlier, Jerne postulated that phagocytosis of antigen-antibody complexes by the antibody-forming cells was the stimulus for the production of additional antibodies (7). Various theories were proposed to account for this phenomenon, but there appeared to be no way of testing the hypotheses. Sir McFarland Burnet succinctly stated the problem confronting immunology in 1959 (9): "Until such methods of handling pure clones of cells in vitro are available, a choice between the clonal selection hypothesis of antibody formation and other alternatives can only be on the basis of convenience and their heuristic value in stimulating new experiments."

Cellular Immunology

Consequently, investigators focused on identifying and studying the cells comprising the immune system for the next 2 decades, thereby creating the science of cellular immunology. Nowell pioneered this new science by reporting in 1960 that lymphocytes are capable of proliferating in response to stimulation by mitogens (10), and his discovery was soon followed by the demonstration that specific antigens could also activate the proliferative expansion of antigen-selected cells. Prior to this discovery it had been thought that lymphocytes were end-stage cells, incapable of self-renewal, and they were not thought to be the source of the antibody-forming plasma cells. This understanding allowed Burnet's clonal selection hypothesis to be modified to include the proliferative expansion of the clones of antigen-specific cells after they had been selected. Then, in 1963 Jerne and Nordin introduced an assay capable of detecting individual antibody-forming cells, and for the first time the selection of antigen-specific cells, as well as their proliferative expansion, was visualized and quantified (11).

Subsequently, in 1967 Dutton and Mishell improved on Jerne's assay for antibody-forming cells by performing the entire immune response in vitro (12). This development was critical, as it permitted a reductionist approach to both the activation phase, as well as the effector phase, of the immune response for the first time. Armed with these new cellular assays, it became recognized that there were at least three distinct types of cells comprising the immune system, namely, B cells, T cells, and macrophages. Although plasma cells were found to be the actual antibody-forming cells, it was not shown that B cells are the precursors of plasma cells until 1970 when B cells were found to express immunoglobulin molecules on the cell surface (13,14). However, by 1970 it was realized that antibody formation by B cells/plasma cells depended on help derived from T cells and macrophages, although the mechanisms responsible for this help remained obscure (15).

The interdependence of the cells in generating an antibody response was further confounded by the observations of Benacerraf and coworkers, who reported that antibody production was genetically determined and that the cellular immune response was somehow related to this genetic linkage (16,17). Subsequently, McDevitt and coworkers reported that the magnitude of antibody production reactive with synthetic peptide antigens depended on the genes encoded by the major histocompatability complex (MHC) (18,19). Together, Benacerraf and McDevitt demonstrated that this immune response (Ir) gene effect depended on T-cell recognition of antigen (20).

Throughout the 1970s the process by which B cells, T cells, and macrophages cooperated to generate the production of antibodies remained a mystery. However, between 1965 and 1975 many investigators noted activities in the culture medium of proliferating lymphocytes that promote in vitro immune responses. Depending on the assays used to detect the activities, these functions augment either the generation of antibody-forming cells, the so-called T-cell replacing factors (TRF) (21), or the proliferation of T cells, the so-called blastogenic factors (BF) (22,23). However, the exact chemical nature of these activities remained obscure. As well, it was unclear whether these activities were required for the generation of an immune response or whether they merely served to amplify the response. Moreover, it remained controversial whether there were many such factors or whether one or a few molecules were responsible for all of the activities detected. In addition, the cellular sources of these various activities were equally mysterious, as both T cells (24) and macrophages (25,26) were implicated.

Assays that detected the capacity of T cells to kill target cells through direct cell-cell contact were devised in 1968 by Brunner et al (27). Subsequently, Zinkernagel and Doherty reported in 1974 that cytotoxic T lymphocytes (CTL) could only recognize specific antigens if expressed by histocompatible target cells (28), a phenomenon that came to be known as MHC restriction of CTL antigen recognition. This finding and the previous observations regarding the MHC restriction of antibody production led to an explosive controversy, concerning the nature of the T-cell antigen receptor (TCR) and how it recognized both antigen and MHC-encoded molecules, that continued unabated for the next decade.

In 1975 Rolf Keissling, Eva Klein, and Hans Wigzell and, independently, Ronald Herberman's group discovered a different type of killer cell that did not appear to recognize specific antigens or to be restricted by the MHC. This cell became known as the natural killer (NK) cell, which was thought to be analogous to the natural antibodies that were found in individuals in the absence of specific immunization. The origin of NK cells remained controversial for more than 2 decades; however, with additional methods for identifying B cells and T cells, it became known that NK cells represent a distinct lineage of lymphocytes.

Also in 1975 Kohler and Milstein made the surprising discovery that somatic-cell hybrids between immunized splenic B cells and murine plasmacytoma cell lines could make continuous quantities of monoclonal antibodies (MoAbs) (29). Thus, Burnet's clonal selection hypothesis was finally proved correct, and his prediction that the proof would rest with the ability to manipulate and study the clonal progeny of a single cell was borne out. The discovery of hybridomas and MoAbs revived the idea of using antibodies as therapeutic "magic bullets." However, the technology to make human monoclonal antibodies proved difficult, and the human antimouse antibody (HAMA) response, which is really a form of serum sickness, effectively precluded the widespread use of mouse MoAbs as therapeutic agents.

In 1976 Morgan and Ruscetti working in Robert Gallo's laboratory reported that culture medium conditioned by proliferating lymphocytes promoted the long-term growth of T cells (30). Subsequently, using conditioned medium containing the T-cell growth factor (TCGF) activity, we reported the creation of the first, antigen-specific T-cell clones in 1979, 20 years after Burnet first forwarded his clonal selection hypothesis (31). Having reduced the tremendous diversity of antigen recognition by the cell population to the progeny of a single cell, it was then possible to prove that antigen recognition by T cells, like B cells, was also clonal. At the time, we predicted that monoclonal T cells would be just as important for future studies directed at determining the function of T cells as monoclonal antibody-producing cells were for understanding the function of B cells. Thus, we felt that "the growth of large numbers of monoclonal antigen-specific T cells would lead to the identification and molecular characterization of the TCR, the mechanisms responsible for T cell cytolysis, and the identification of T cell differentiation markers" (31).

Monoclonal antibodies reactive with distinct, human T-cell subsets were generated at the same time that we had generated T-cell clones (32), and in a series of reports Reinherz et al demonstrated that these antibodies were useful in defining helper (CD4+) and cytotoxic (CD8+) T cells (33). Subsequently, they discovered that an antibody that recognized a molecule expressed on all peripheral T cells (CD3) blocked T-cell proliferation in response to mitogens, while this same MoAb was mitogenic itself (34).

Molecular Immunology

While the 1960s and 1970s were devoted to identifying and isolating the cells responsible for the immune response, the 1980s and 1990s were devoted to discovering and characterizing the molecules involved in promoting the proliferation and differentiation of the various cells, particularly the T cells. With TCGF-dependent T-cell clones available, we created a quantitative assay for the TCGF activity (35), which we then used together with standard biochemical methods to identify, characterize, and purify the molecule responsible for the activity (36). Subsequently, we generated monoclonal antibodies reactive with the purified molecule, and then used these antibodies to purify the molecule to homogeneity (37). These findings were also the first to show that a lymphokine or cytokine *activity* could be ascribed to a single molecule and not several molecules, as had been proposed by others. Moreover, these findings directed us to a series of experiments that eventually identified the first cytokine receptor (38) and to the conclusion that cytokines function in exactly the same way as classic hormones, that is, by binding with high affinity to specific cell-surface receptors.

Anticipating the discovery of additional cytokines, in 1979 this new class of molecules was named interleukins, to designate that they functioned to signal *between leukocytes*. At that time, an activity derived from macrophages had been identified that we had shown functioned to augment TCGF production by T cells (39,40). Therefore, the macrophage product, which

had been termed lymphocyte-activating factor, was renamed interleukin-1 (IL-1), and the TCGF molecule was renamed interleukin-2 (IL-2).

The decade of the 1980s produced an exponential increase in the amount of information available regarding the molecules of the immune system and in our understanding of how those molecules function to initiate and regulate the immune reaction, all of which set the stage for immunostimulatory therapy. Using antigen-specific T-cell clones and hybridomas and clone-specific monoclonal antibodies, the T-cell antigen receptor (TCR) was identified and characterized biochemically by Meuer et al (41,42) and by Haskins et al (43). Soon thereafter, Hedrick et al isolated the first cDNA encoding one of the four chains of the receptor (44). This information placed the TCR into the immunoglobulin superfamily and revealed that the basic structures of the TCR and immunoglobulins are quite similar. Subsequent studies focused on TCR signaling and gene activation revealed that TCR triggering is obligatory for the transcriptional activation of the IL-2 gene (45–47), as well as of the genes encoding the IL-2 receptor (IL-2R) (48–50). Subsequently, the same TCR triggering was found to be responsible for the expression of additional cytokines as they came to be discovered.

Dendritic cells were discovered and found to present antigen to T cells with marked efficiency (51). Moreover, B cells were also shown to present antigen effectively to T cells (52). Also, macrophages were found to process protein antigens and present peptides as antigens to the TCR, revealing that T cells recognized fundamentally different antigenic molecules as compared with antibodies (53). Ultimately, the structure of MHC-encoded molecules was determined, and for the first time it was realized how antigenic peptides are bound to the MHC molecules and presented to T cells, thereby solving the controversy of MHC restriction of TCR antigen recognition (54). The TCR recognizes a complex of peptide antigen and MHC-encoded molecules. This revelation explained the MHC restriction of immune responses, which is that CD4+ helper T cells recognize antigens bound to MHC class II–encoded molecules and that CD8+ CTL recognizes antigens bound to MHC class I–encoded molecules.

During the 1980s and 90s, almost two dozen new interleukins were discovered, most of them with homologies to IL-2. Some of these interleukins such as IL-4 (55), IL-6 (56), and IL-10 (57) were found to be important in the production of antibodies. Therefore, the T-cell replacing factor activity described in the early 1970s was explained in part by the discovery and characterization of these cytokines. Direct cell-cell contact between helper T cells and B cells, mediated by T-cell–derived CD40 ligand and B-cell CD40, was also demonstrated to be necessary for optimal T-cell help in antibody formation (58). Other cytokines, in particular IFN-γ (59) and IL-12 (60), were found to be crucial to the generation of classic, cell-mediated, immune responses such as the delayed type hypersensitivity (DTH) reaction. IL-2 was found to be important for the production and action of both the so-called TH-1 cytokines (i.e., DTH cytokines) and the TH-2 cytokines (i.e., antibody-related cytokines) (61,62). IL-2 became the first interleukin to be resolved at the genetic level by Taniguchi et al (63), and recombinant DNA technology become the method of choice to identify and characterize the new interleukins.

Two other cytokine families were found to differ structurally and functionally from the interleukins, the interferons (IFN) (64,65) and the tumor necrosis factor (TNF) family (66). Although closely related to the interleukins, the IFNs are distinct, both structurally and functionally, in that the IFNs have direct antiviral activity (hence their name as substances that *interfered* with viral replication). As the name connotes, TNF is capable of causing the necrosis of tumors (67). However, in addition, subsequent to its identification at the molecular level, TNF was discovered to be one of the primary mediators of inflammation and to be responsible for much of the toxicity associated with severe infection, including the systemic inflammatory response syndrome (SIRS), or septic shock (66). Bacterial toxins such as endotoxin from coliforms and exotoxins from pyogenic organisms are potent stimuli for the production of TNF-α. One of the major functions of TNF-α is to increase vascular permeability, which promotes the extravasation of cells and plasma at the site of inflammation. Thus, the classic signs of inflammation (i.e., rubor, dolor, calor, and tumor) in large part can be ascribed to the effects of TNF-α and the other proinflammatory cytokines. When localized, this inflammatory response is beneficial to the host, as the immune effector cells and serum components can readily access the site. However, if TNF-α is released in large quantities systemically, there is a generalized extravasation of cells and plasma that results in hypotension. Thus, proinflammatory cytokines were responsible for the toxicities observed when bacteria and bacterial extracts were administered in attempts to treat malignancies at the turn of the last century. This understanding solved a long-standing controversy regarding the origin of the toxicities of bacteria and other microbes. The signs and symptoms of inflammation result from the microbial toxin–induced production of "endogenous pyrogens" (cytokines) and not from the direct effects of the microbes or microbial toxins themselves.

The cellular origins of the various cytokines were identified as these molecules became purified and cloned. Thus, in addition to T cells, NK cells and macrophages became known as major sources of cytokines during an immune/inflammatory reaction. Only three of these cytokines were found to be restricted to T cells—IL-2, IL-4, and IL-5. By comparison, IFN-γ is produced by both T cells and NK cells, while TNF-α is produced by T cells, NK cells, and macrophages. Macrophages are also the source of such proinflammatory cytokines as IL-1 and IL-6. In retrospect, the original lymphocyte activating factor was most probably a mixture of these macrophage-derived, proinflammatory cytokines. The cells that participate in the immune/inflammatory reactions are connected with one another by these cytokines, which is of major importance when cytokines are administered therapeutically.

The mechanisms involved in the interaction of the cytokines with their respective target cells were found to reside in the expression of high-affinity, ligand-specific receptors expressed on the cell surface (38,68,69). The IL-2R is comprised of three chains that cooperate to form a very high affinity receptor (Kd = 10 pM). These high-affinity heterotrimeric receptors are expressed tran-

siently only on antigen-selected T cells, thereby conserving the specificity of the immune response. By comparison, NK cells differ from T cells by expressing IL-2Rs constitutively. However, unlike T cells, approximately 90% of NK cells lack the α chain of the IL-2R (70,71). This results in IL-2Rs comprised of only the β and γ chains, which have a 100-fold lower affinity for IL-2 compared with heterotrimeric IL-2Rs. This difference between T-cell and NK-cell IL-2R expression eventually became important when IL-2 was administered as a therapeutic (72).

Also, in the 1990s, immunoglobulin Fc receptors (FcR) were characterized at the molecular level and were shown to be the major molecular connections between the humoral immune response and the cellular immune system of phagocytes, as proposed originally by Metchnikoff (73). In addition, B cells and NK cells were found to express FcRs, and these special FcRs are now known to be important in the regulation of the production of antibodies, as well as in the function of cytolytic cells, through a phenomenon termed antibody-dependent cellular cytotoxicity (ADCC).

History of the Use of IL-2 in the Clinic: High-Dose, Intermittent Therapy for Cancer

In the early 1980s before IL-2 was available in pure form and in large enough quantities for therapeutic use, Steven Rosenberg attempted to use a lymphocyte-conditioned medium containing TCGF (IL-2) activity to generate large quantities of tumor-specific lymphocytes in vitro. He intended to then reinfuse these cells as adoptive immunotherapy for the treatment of cancers that were refractory to conventional radiotherapy and chemotherapy. Unfortunately, it was difficult to generate tumor-specific CTL reactive to autologous tumor cells; therefore, Rosenberg simply cultured PBMCs from his patients for several days in the lymphocyte-conditioned medium and then reinfused the in vitro cultured cells, which he termed lymphokine-activated killer (LAK) cells. Concomitantly, the lymphocyte-conditioned medium was also administered. The identity of the LAK cells, whether T cell, NK cell, or monocyte, remained obscure.

As purified, natural IL-2 became available, soon followed by purified recombinant IL-2, Rosenberg et al began using IL-2 as a continuous infusion, together with the cultivated LAK cells, as immunotherapy (74). Based on experimental tumor models in mice, they used the principles of cytotoxic chemotherapy of dose intensification to toxicity to establish their IL-2 dosing regimens (75). Thus, doses of 150 million units of IL-2 per day, or approximately 10 mg of recombinant IL-2 protein, became standard. This total dose is administered as an intravenous bolus in three divided doses daily every 8 hours for 3 to 5 days and is still in use today, having been approved by the FDA for the treatment of renal cell carcinoma and malignant melanoma. The initial 25 patients treated with high doses of IL-2 together with LAK cells were reported to undergo either a partial or complete remission rate of approximately 40%, an unprecedented response rate (74). Subsequent studies by many investigators revealed that the LAK cells added no benefit to the IL-2 therapy, and the LAK infusions were abandoned. Now, 15 years later, several hundred patients have received this treatment, and the overall results reveal that 9% of patients enjoy a long-term (i.e., >5 years), disease-free remission, while 10% achieved a partial remission, with a greater than 50% decrease in measurable tumor mass (76).

The mechanisms responsible for the antitumor effects of high-dose IL-2 therapy remain obscure to this day. Rosenberg has maintained that the severe, clinical, grade III–IV toxicity is necessary for the antitumor response (76). However, 100% of the patients experience the toxicity, while only 19% achieve an objective diminution of tumor mass. The toxicities experienced are remarkably similar to those symptoms described for the SIRS, or septic shock. Thus, patients experience high fevers, 104 to 105°F, with severe rigors, followed by hypotension and hypoxemia. Accordingly, this therapy is administered in the hospital, usually in an intensive care unit, and most patients require assisted ventilation and blood pressure support in the form of IV fluids and vasopressors. Most patients who undergo high-dose IL-2 therapy gain approximately 20 kg of body weight as a consequence of fluid retention.

Biologic Effects of IL-2

IL-2 is a potent growth factor for T cells in vivo and also serves as a growth factor for NK cells (77,78). In addition, IL-2 promotes the differentiation of T cells (both TH and CTL) and NK cells, serving to promote the differentiated function of these cell types. Accordingly, IL-2 triggers the expansion of mature, antigen-selected T cells and NK cells. Moreover, the differentiated functions of these cells, that is, the secretion of cytokines and the capacity to effect cytolysis, are promoted by IL-2. Because these effects of IL-2 set in play a cascade of additional cytokines and cytolytic effector molecules, IL-2 has the potential of eventually leading to a severe inflammatory reaction. In essence, the IL-2 produced by antigen-stimulated T cells acts to further expand the number and function of these cells. Moreover, by activating NK cells, IL-2 communicates between the antigen-specific, acquired immune response and the nonspecific, innate host defenses mediated by NK cells and macrophages. On IL-2 activation, NK cells produce a restricted subset of cytokines that include granulocyte-macrophage colony-stimulating factor (GM-CSF), IFN-γ, and TNF-α. These cytokines, in turn, are potent stimuli for monocytes and macrophages. Accordingly, the stimulation of macrophages that occurs indirectly through the IL-2–activation of NK cells eventually results in the production of cytokines by macrophages, in particular the proinflammatory cytokines TNF-α, IL-1, and IL-6 (79). Moreover, the macrophage production of IL-2 then feeds back to further enhance the function of the NK cells, thereby creating a circuit that can promote itself to create the inflammatory response. The NK cell–derived monocytotropic cytokines also enhance macrophage antigen processing and presentation by MHC molecules, as well as antigen clearance by potentiation of Fc receptor expression.

IL-2 also imparts survival signals to its target cells, mediated by the activation of the expression of a set of genes that encode molecules such as Bcl2 and related family members that are anti-apoptotic (80). However, if IL-2 is withdrawn from IL-2R+ cells, the expression of these genes is extinguished, and subsequently the cells undergo programmed cell death. This "cytokine withdrawal apoptosis" is a major phenomenon regulating the size of the expanded pool of antigen-selected cells, particularly after antigen is cleared and no longer promotes the production of IL-2 (81).

When antigen persists, even though the immune system has been activated, activation-induced cell death (AICD) ensues, which also leads to apoptosis (82). This form of programmed cell death can be mediated by the activation of the FasL/Fas pathway (83), as well as the TNF-α/TNF-αR pathway (84), and depends on both TCR triggering and IL-2R activation. At present the physiologic significance of this phenomenon remains obscure, but some have proposed that it underlies the mechanisms responsible for peripheral tolerance, as well as the phenomenon of "high zone tolerance" (85).

IL-2 Pharmacodynamics and the Therapeutic Index

When Rosenberg and Lotze first used high-dose IL-2 therapy in the mid 1980s, it was not immediately obvious why so much toxicity was generated. Theoretically, low IL-2 concentrations should fully saturate the high-affinity IL-2Rs expressed by antigen-activated T cells, and higher doses should have no further effect. However, it was not appreciated that most NK cells expressed a different type of IL-2R compared with antigen-activated T cells. Also, it was not appreciated that there are approximately 1 billion (10^9) circulating NK cells. Understanding the effects of IL-2 therapy has required a detailed determination of IL-2 pharmacodynamics, as well as pharmacokinetics. Moreover, the determination of the interaction between IL-2 target cells and other cells responsible for the generation of the inflammatory response was necessary to fully comprehend why high doses of IL-2 are toxic and therefore how to effectively use IL-2 in the clinic.

IL-2 only directly affects target cells that express IL-2Rs (i.e., T cells and NK cells). However, because these target cells produce bioactive cytokines that can have wide-ranging effects on many tissues, it is important to understand the pharmacodynamics of IL-2, which depend on the type and distribution of the IL-2Rs. As described, the only cells that express IL-2Rs are NK cells and antigen-activated T cells. The T cells express high-affinity (Kd = 10 pM) heterotrimeric IL-2Rs, which bind and respond to IL-2 in the 1- to 100-pM concentration range (15 pg/mL to 1.5 ng/mL) (68,69). It is convenient to express the plasma IL-2 concentrations in molar concentrations because the equilibrium dissociation constants of the receptors are expressed in these units of measure. However, as doses of drugs are usually expressed in protein weights, or units of biologic activity, it can be confusing when trying to understand the pharmacodynamics and pharmacokinetics. In this regard, it is helpful to make the calculation of molar concentration into molecules/mL, using Avogadro's number (6.02×10^{23} molecules/mole). Thus, $1\,pM = 10^{-12}$ moles/L = 600 million molecules/mL. Therefore, the effective range of concentration of IL-2 for T cells in molecules/mL is 600 million molecules/mL to 60 billion molecules/mL.

By comparison, the equilibrium dissociation constant of the intermediate-affinity IL-2R expressed by approximately 90% of NK cells is 100-fold lower than the high-affinity IL-2R (i.e., Kd = 1 nM). Accordingly, the IL-2 concentration range that binds to this class of IL-2Rs varies from 100 pM to 10 nM, which in molecular terms is 60 billion molecules/mL to 6 trillion molecules/mL. The difference between the high-affinity and intermediate-affinity IL-2R resides in the absence of the α chain (86). Thus, the intermediate-affinity IL-2R is comprised of only the β and γ chains, and thus these receptors lack the fast association rate imparted by the α chain.

The therapeutic index is influenced by these two distinct receptor classes, as 100-fold higher doses of IL-2 are required to generate IL-2 concentrations high enough to bind to the intermediate-affinity IL-2Rs expressed by the majority of NK cells. Since there are approximately 10^9 circulating NK cells, most of the systemic toxicity can be avoided if the doses of IL-2 are kept low, resulting in IL-2 concentrations <100 pM. This results in the activation of less than 10% of the intermediate-affinity IL-2Rs expressed by NK cells, while saturating the high-affinity IL-2Rs expressed by antigen-activated T cells (87,88). Whether systemic toxicity is produced at any IL-2 concentration depends on how many cells express IL-2Rs, because the absolute number of cells that produce secondary proinflammatory cytokines such as TNF-α, IFN-γ, and GM-CSF essentially determines how great the symptoms of the SIRS will be. Accordingly, if there is a systemic, persistent infection, as occurs in untreated HIV infection, one would expect greater numbers of antigen-activated T cells to be present. Therefore, it is more likely that lower doses of IL-2 may produce toxicity in this setting than in a situation when the number of IL-2R+ cells is lower.

IL-2 Pharmacokinetics

IL-2 is a small (15-kDa) globular glycoprotein. Therefore, when injected intravenously, IL-2 rapidly passes between capillary endothelial cells and distributes into total extracellular space, which in a normal adult is approximately 14 liters (89). When injected either subcutaneously or intramuscularly, IL-2 is rapidly taken up by the lymphatics and distributed by the circulatory system to total extracellular space. Subsequently, IL-2 is filtered by the glomeruli, then reabsorbed by the tubular epithelial cells, and metabolized. Consequently, it is cleared fairly rapidly.

The half-time for distribution after an intravenous injection is approximately 10 minutes. Therefore, within 40 minutes more than 94% of the injected IL-2 is distributed into the 14 liters of extracellular space. This explains why, in the initial experiments from Rosenberg's group, the intravenous bolus doses of IL-2 disappeared from the circulation so rapidly and why they attempted to counteract this phenomenon by injecting higher and higher

doses. Once distributed into the extracellular space, the renal clearance of IL-2 proceeds with a t½ of 2½ hours. Therefore, more than 94% of the intravenously administered IL-2 is cleared within 10 to 11 hours.

After a subcutaneous injection, IL-2 is absorbed into the lymphatics and appears in the blood with a t½ of approximately 50 minutes, and peak plasma IL-2 concentrations are attained by 2 to 3 hours (89). Thereafter, the same rate of renal clearance ensues as found after intravenous administration, and by 12 to 14 hours only very low levels are detectable. Accordingly, to achieve a constant IL-2 concentration within the extracellular space, the administration of IL-2 every 12 hours would be ideal. In practice, we find that daily subcutaneous administration of $1.2\,mU/m^2$ BSA is sufficient to achieve an ongoing IL-2 response. This dose of IL-2 results in a peak plasma IL-2 concentration of 20 to 30 pM, which is high enough to saturate approximately 70% of the high-affinity IL-2Rs on antigen-activated T cells, but will only bind to approximately 2% to 3% of the intermediate-affinity IL-2Rs expressed by the majority of NK cells.

IL-2 Treatment Regimens: Intermittent versus Continuous Therapy

At present, there are two schools of practice regarding dosing regimens. The initial dosing, as used by the oncologists, employed intermittent, ultra-high doses of IL-2, and this regimen has been maintained and has been approved by the FDA for use in the treatment of renal cell carcinoma and malignant melanoma. The daily dose amounts to 150 million U (10 mg), given in three divided bolus intravenous injections. This regimen is administered for 3 to 5 days and is repeated within 6 to 8 weeks if there is an objective response but not a complete disappearance of detectable tumor.

For the treatment of HIV infection, Kovacs et al (90) and Davey et al (91) have also used intermittent administration, but the dose has been reduced approximately 10-fold from that used in cancer therapy to 15 million U/day (1 mg/d). This dose is divided into twice-daily dosing and is either given as a subcutaneous injection or as a continuous intravenous infusion. An intermediate dose of 9 to 10 million U/day (~600 μg) has recently been described for the treatment of HIV infection, given in two daily doses subcutaneosly.

When these high, intermittent dosing schedules are used, during the treatment interval a marked lymphopenia is observed, and all circulating mononuclear cells decrease to very low levels. Simultaneously, a capillary leak syndrome occurs, and hypotension can result. After the cessation of IL-2 injections, a rebound lymphocytosis occurs, with all circulating mononuclear cells increasing to concentrations 10 times the pretreatment values. Over the ensuing weeks the lymphocyte and monocyte concentrations gradually return toward the pretreatment values. Thus, high-dose, intermittent IL-2 administration results in marked cellular and fluid shifts, and it is difficult to determine whether there is actually a net gain or loss of lymphocytes with this regimen.

We developed the low-dose, continuous dosing regimen in an attempt to arrive at a dose and schedule that was nontoxic; it also would provide fairly continuous exposure of the cells to IL-2 (88,92). Continuous IL-2 exposure, rather than intermittent dosing, was considered preferable to maximize the IL-2 cellular signaling. The rationale is based on a series of experiments where we found that the T-cell proliferative response was proportional to the IL-2 concentration, the IL-2R density, and the duration of the IL-2/IL-2R interaction (45,48). Accordingly, if antigen-activated T cells expressing optimal levels of IL-2Rs are exposed to an IL-2R saturating concentration (i.e., ~100 pM), the magnitude of the proliferative response directly depends on the duration of the IL-2 exposure. In addition, the withdrawal of IL-2 from IL-2R+ cells results in rapid apoptosis, such that the cells are irreversibly damaged within 12 to 24 hours without IL-2. Therefore, intermittent exposure to IL-2 may well create a situation where recently antigen-activated IL-2R+ cells are actually killed by withdrawal of the survival-enhancing properties of IL-2.

Therapeutic Uses for IL-2

Intermittent IL-2 therapy at all of the high doses is used primarily to promote rapid changes within the immune system, either for the treatment of cancer or in situations where there is a need to enhance the number of circulating lymphocytes rapidly. As already mentioned, the ultra-high IL-2 dose used in cancer treatment does result in long-term, disease-free intervals for a small number of patients. In patients infected with HIV, the high and the intermediate intermittent IL-2 doses can rapidly increase the concentration of circulating CD4+ T cells, which then can remain elevated for several months after the treatment interval. However, whether these changes in the concentrations of circulating CD4+ T cells translate into a clinical benefit remains unknown. Consequently, there are currently two, large-scale, clinical trials under way that are designed to determine the answer to this question.

The problem with all high IL-2 dose protocols is toxicity. The systemic side effects generated, including fatigue, fever, rigor, and capillary leak, are remarkably similar to the symptoms and signs described a century ago, when bacteria and bacterial extracts were used in cancer treatment. Because of these toxicities, a wider range of illnesses, that is, those in which it might be beneficial to augment the function of the immune system, are precluded. It is important to realize that the toxic side effects are IL-2 dose-dependent, which accounts for the progressive decreases in dosing that have occurred since the initiation of the ultra-high dose used for cancer treatment.

Low doses of IL-2 can be given daily for prolonged intervals. We have administered low-dose IL-2 to asymptomatic HIV+ individuals for as long as 5 years without significant adverse events (89). In particular, we have not experienced the development of autoimmune phenomena, a danger that many have thought probable with continuous IL-2 therapy. We now have had experience with approximately 100 individuals treated continuously with low-dose IL-2 for at least 1 year, and we are finding that the earliest change detectable in the immune system is a 5- to 10-fold increase in eosinophils within the first 2 weeks of initiation of therapy. Thereafter, the next change that is readily detectable is a progressive increase in the concentration of circulating NK cells. The NK-cell concentration increases by a mean of approximately 200 cells/µL over 2 months and then stabilizes at this increment as long as IL-2 is administered. In asymptomatic HIV+ individuals treated with highly active antiretroviral therapy (HAART) and low-dose IL-2 for 1 year, there is an increase in the concentration of circulating CD4+ T cells at a rate of approximately 10 cells/month. This rate is about 2.5 times faster than that reported for HAART alone. A randomized, controlled trial to test the effectiveness of IL-2 for the acceleration of the recovery of the immune system is presently in progress. The preliminary data analyzed after 6 months of combined HAART + IL-2 have revealed a significant difference in the rate of increase in the concentration of naive CD4+ T cells and in the concentration of NK cells. Whether these changes in the concentration of circulating lymphocytes will translate into a clinical benefit remains to be determined.

From our earliest experiments it was clear that IL-2 is effective in promoting T-cell proliferation only after antigen activation of IL-2R expression (77). Moreover, IL-2R expression was transient. On removal of the antigen, a progressive decline in the density of IL-2Rs is detectable, such that after 14 days in culture most cells lose expression of the IL-2R and become unresponsive to IL-2 (48). However, if antigen is reintroduced, the cells rapidly reexpress IL-2Rs and once again become IL-2–responsive. Accordingly, the proliferative response to IL-2 is antigen-dependent, and antigen-nonreactive cells will not expand even though IL-2R saturating concentrations of IL-2 are present. Extrapolating these in vitro findings to clinical situations, it follows that it will be beneficial to introduce the desired antigen at the time that IL-2 is administered to expand the number of antigen-specific cells.

Recently, we have used the interruption of HAART in HIV+ individuals, combined with low-dose, daily IL-2 therapy (93). We have found that plasma virus becomes detectable within 19 ± 3 days on cessation of HAART. Thereafter, there is a rapid increase in viral concentration (doubling time 1.6 ± 0.1 days) to a peak concentration after a mean of 17 days. Subsequently, there is a progressive decline of detectable plasma virus with a $t\frac{1}{2}$ of 3.5 ± 0.7 days, with a trough concentration that is approximately 10-fold lower than the peak reached in 18 ± 3 days. Coincident with the viral relapse, there is a CD8+ lymphocytosis, which peaks at about twice the baseline concentration just after the peak of viremia. Subsequently, the CD8+ T-cell concentration remains elevated as the virus progressively decreases. Moreover, the rate and magnitude of viral decline correlate with the magnitude of the CD8+ lymphocytosis.

These data are consistent with the interpretation that the viral relapse activates the CD8+ memory T cells to become IL-2R+, and the administered IL-2 then promotes their expansion. However, we need to do additional experiments to support this hypothesis. In particular, experiments are indicated to identify and quantify the number of HIV-specific T cells and also to evaluate whether the increase in the concentration of CD8+ T cells is the result of their proliferative expansion. However, these data support the notion that antigen plus IL-2 will be more effective in stimulating an antigen-specific immune response than either antigen or IL-2 alone, and that the next step will be to combine IL-2 therapy with a therapeutic immunization schedule.

The principles that we have used to develop low-dose, nontoxic, daily IL-2 administration now permit the extension of this therapeutic dosing and regimen to other infectious diseases and to cancer. Accordingly, we are developing protocols to test the efficacy of the addition of low-dose, daily IL-2 therapy to the standard therapy for the treatment of hepatitis C virus (HCV) infection, which consists of IFN-α and ribavirin. In addition, these same principles can now be applied to the use of IL-2 as an adjuvant given in combination with vaccines. Most adjuvants in use today are focused on enhancing antigen processing and presentation by antigen-presenting cells. However, if IL-2 production is limited or compromised in any way, the resultant proliferative expansion of antigen-selected cells will necessarily be abbreviated. Accordingly, IL-2 adjuvant use may well markedly improve the immunogenicity of weak vaccines.

Combination Antibody–IL-2 Therapy

As discussed in the introduction, the use of mouse MoAbs as therapeutics has been hampered by the human antimouse antibody response (HAMA). However, over the past 20 years genetic engineering approaches have succeeded in "humanizing" the mouse MoAbs (94). Thus, the mouse variable regions are retained, while the rest of the antibody (i.e., the constant regions) are replaced with human sequences. Furthermore, the antigen-binding complementarity determining region 3 (CDR3) of the mouse antibody is the only part that is not of human sequences. These approaches have demonstrated the "proof of principle" that it is possible to markedly diminish the HAMA so that MoAbs are once again feasible to consider as therapeutics.

More recently, transgenic mice have been created that express only human genetic sequences (95–97). These mice are remarkable because they contain almost the entire genomic DNA encoding both heavy and light chains, but they are tolerant to the human gene products because they have been exposed to the human antibodies during embryogenesis. Thus, their entire antibody production is from human sequences, yet they can recognize all human molecules as foreign. Consequently, it is now possible to create human MoAbs reactive with all foreign molecules and all human molecules as well. Accordingly, the prospects for future therapeutics using human MoAbs now appear limitless.

Anticipating the future, the combination of human MoAbs with cytokines such as IL-2 should enhance the efficacy of the MoAbs. IL-2 will function to augment the capacity of the reticuloendothelial system to recognize antigen-antibody complexes by its effects on NK cells and macrophages. Thus, by stimulating NK cells to release IFN-γ, GM-CSF, and TNF-α, these cytokines will increase the cell-surface density of Fc receptors, as well as the phagocytic capacities of the cells. Therefore, both the humoral and cellular effector arms can be artificially enhanced for the first time. The net effect will be to improve the efficiency of MoAb therapy, so that a maximal response may be obtained with lower doses of MoAbs. Also, the frequency of MoAb administration may be influenced by the use of immunomodulating cytokines such as IL-2.

Conclusions

At this juncture, we stand on a new therapeutic threshold. The separation of the immune response into a humoral and cellular school resulted in a century of reductionist science that has finally given us a fairly complete picture of the cells involved in the system and of the molecules that direct their activities. Armed with cytokines, the hormones of the immune system, and the knowledge that they mediate their effects by interacting with high-affinity stereospecific cellular receptors, it is now possible for the first time to design rational, therapeutic strategies to improve the function of the system without generating undue toxicities. Moreover, the principles of therapeutic cytokine administration can now be applied together with vaccines to maximize immune responses after immunization. In addition, with the availability of human MoAbs, it will be possible to harness the power of the specificity and diversity of the immune response and direct therapy at specific molecules and cells. These advances should transform medicine as we presently know it.

References
1. Behring EAS, Kitasato K. Ueber das Zustandekommen der Diphtherie-Immunaitat und der Tetanus-Immunitat bei Thieren. Ttsch Med Wochenschr Leipzig 1890;16:113.
2. Metchnikoff E. Immunity in infective diseases. Cambridge, UK: Cambridge University Press, 1905:576.
3. Pasteur L, Joubert, Chamberland. La theorie des germes et ses applications a la medicine et a la chirurgie. Comptes Rendus Hebdomadaires des Seances de l'Academie des Sciences 1878;86:1037.
4. Pasteur L. Sur les maladies virulentes, et en particulier sur la maladie appelee vulgairement cholera des poules. Comptes Rendus Hebdomadaires des Seances de l'Academie des Sciences 1880;90:249.
5. Porter RR. The hydrolysis of rabbit gamma globulin and antibodies with crystalline papain. Biochem J 1959;73:119.
6. Edelman GM. Dissociation of gamma globulin. J Am Chem Soc 1959;81:3155.
7. Jerne NK. The natural selection theory of antibody formation. Proc Natl Acad Sci USA 1955;41:849.
8. Burnet FM. A modification of Jerne's theory of antibody production using the concept of clonal selection. Aust J Sci 1957; 20:67.
9. Burnet FM. Clonal selection theory of acquired immunity. Cambridge, England: Cambridge and Vanderbilt University Presses, 1959.

10. Nowell PC. Phytohemagglutinin: an initiator of mitosis in cultures of normal human leukocytes. Cancer Res 1960;20: 462.

11. Jerne NK, Nordin AA. Antibody formation in agar by single antibody-producing cells. Science 1963;140:405.

12. Dutton RW, Mishell RI. Cell populations and cell proliferation in the in vitro response of normal mouse spleen to heterologous erythrocytes. Analysis by the hot pulse technique. J Exp Med 1967;126:443.

13. Raff M, Sternberg M, Taylor RB. Immunoglobulin determinants on the surface of mouse lymphoid cells. Nature 1970; 225:553.

14. Pernis B, Forni L, Amante L. Immunoglobulin spots on the surface of rabbit lymphocytes. J Exp Med 1970;132:1001.

15. Dutton RW, McCarthy MM, Mishell RI, Raidt DJ. Cell components in the immune response. IV. Relationships and possible interactions. Cell Immunol 1970;1:196.

16. Kantor FS, Ojeda A, Benacerraf B. Studies on artificial antigens. I. Antigenicity of DNP-polylysine and DNP copolymer of lysine and glutamic acid in guinea pigs. J Exp Med 1963; 117:55.

17. Green I, Paul WE, Benacerraf B. The behavior of hapten-poly-L-lysine conjugates as complete antigens in genetic responder and as haptens in non-responder guinea pigs. J Exp Med 1966;123:859.

18. McDevitt HO, Tyan ML. Genetic control of the antibody response in inbred mice: transfer of response by spleen cells and linkage to the major histocompatability (H2) locus. J Exp Med 1968;128:1.

19. McDevitt HO, Chinitz A. Genetic control of the antibody response: relationship between immune response and histocompatability (H-2) type. Science 1969;163:273.

20. Benacerraf B, McDevitt HO. Histocompatability-linked immune response genes. Science 1972;175:273.

21. Dutton RW, Folkoff R, Hirst JA, et al. Is there evidence for a non–antigen specific diffusable chemical mediator from the thymus-derived cell in the initiation of the immune response? Prog Immunol 1971;1:355.

22. Kasakura S, Lowenstein L. A factor stimulating DNA synthesis derived from the medium of leukocyte cultures. Nature 1965;208:794.

23. Gordon J, MacLean LD. A lymphocyte-stimulating factor produced in vitro. Nature 1965;208:795.

24. Janis M, Bach FH. Potentiation of in vitro lymphocyte reactivity. Nature 1970;225:238.

25. Hoffman M, Dutton RW. Immune response restoration with macrophage supernatants. Science 1971;172:1047.

26. Gery I, Waksman BH. Potentiation of the T-lymphocyte response to mitogens: the cellular source of potentiating mediators. J Exp Med 1972;136:143.

27. Brunner KT, Mauel J, Cerottini J-C, Chapius B. Quantitative assay of the lytic action of lymphoid cells on 51-Cr labelled allogeneic target cells in vitro. Inhibition by isoantibody and drugs. Immunology 1968;14:181.

28. Zinkernagel RM, Doherty PC. Immunological surveillance against altered self components by sensitized T lymphocytes in lymphocytic choriomeningitis. Nature 1974;251:547.

29. Kohler G, Milstein C. Continuous culture of fused cells secreting antibody of predefined specificity. Nature 1975;256: 495.

30. Morgan DA, Ruscetti FW, Gallo R. Selective in vitro growth of T lymphocytes from normal human bone marrows. Science 1976;193:1007.

31. Baker PE, Gillis S, Smith KA. Monoclonal cytolytic T-cell lines. J Exp Med 1979;149:273.

32. Kung P, Goldstein G, Reinherz EL, Schlossman SF. Monoclonal antibodies defining distinctive human T-cell surface antigens. Science 1979;206:347.

33. Reinherz EL, Kung PC, Goldstein G, Schlossman SF. Separation of functional subsets of human T cells by a monoclonal antibody. Proc Natl Acad Sci USA 1979;76:4061.

34. Reinherz EL, Hussey RE, Schlossman SF. A monoclonal antibody blocking human T-cell function. Eur J Immunol 1980; 10:758.

35. Gillis S, Ferm MM, Ou W, Smith KA. T-cell growth factor: paramenters of production and a quantitative microassay for activity. J Immunol 1978;120:2027.

36. Robb RJ, Smith KA. Heterogeneity of human T-cell growth factor(s) due to variable glycosylation. Mol Immunol 1981; 18:1087.

37. Smith KA, Favata MF, Oroszlan S. Production and characterization of monoclonal antibodies to human interleukin-2: strategy and tactics. J Immunol 1983;131:1808.

38. Robb RJ, Munck A, Smith KA. T-cell growth factor receptors. Quantitation, specificity, and biological relevance. J Exp Med 1981;154:1455.

39. Smith KA, Gilbride KJ, Favata MF. Lymphocyte activating factor promotes T-cell growth factor production by cloned murine lymphoma cells. Nature 1980;287:853.

40. Smith KA, Lachman LB, Oppenheim JJ, Favata MF. The functional relationship of the interleukins. J Exp Med 1980;151: 1551.

41. Meuer SC, Fitzgerald KA, Hussey RE, et al. Clonotypic structures involved in antigen-specific human T-cell function. Relationship to the T3 molecular complex. J Exp Med 1983; 157:705.

42. Meuer SC, Hodgdon JC, Hussey RE, et al. Antigen-like effects of monoclonal antibodies directed at receptors on human T-cell clones. J Exp Med 1983;158:988.

43. Haskins K, Kubo R, Pigeon M, et al. The major histocompatability complex–restricted antigen receptor in T cells. I. Isolation with a monoclonal antibody. J Exp Med 1983;157: 1149.

44. Hedrick S, Cohen D, Nielson E, Davis MM. Isolation of cDNA clones encoding T-cell–specific membrane-associated proteins. Nature 1984;308:149.

45. Cantrell DA, Smith KA. The interleukin-2 T-cell system: a new cell growth model. Science 1984;224:1312.

46. Meuer SC, Hussey RE, Cantrell DA, et al. Triggering the T3-Ti antigen-receptor complex results in clonal T-cell proliferation through an interleukin-2–dependent autocrine pathway. Proc Natl Acad Sci USA 1984;81:1509.

47. Shaw JP, Utz PJ, Durand DB, et al. Identification of a putative regulator of early T-cell activation. Science 1988;241: 202.

48. Cantrell DA, Smith KA. Transient expression of interleukin-2 receptors. Consequences for T-cell growth. J Exp Med 1983;158:1895.

49. Leonard WJ, Depper JM, Crabtree GR, et al. Molecular cloning and expression of cDNAs for the human interleukin-2 receptor. Nature 1984;311:626.

50. Nikaido T, Shimizu A, Ishida N, et al. Molecular cloning of

cDNA encoding human interleukin-2 receptor. Nature 1984; 311:631.

51. Steinman R, Kaplan G, Whitmer MD, Cohn ZA. Identification of a novel cell type in peripheral lymphoid organs of mice. J Exp Med 1979;149:1.
52. Chestnut RW, Grey HM. Studies on the capacity of B cells to serve as antigen-presenting cells. J Immunol 1981;126:1075.
53. Zeigler HK, Unanue ER. Decrease in macrophage antigen catabolism caused by ammonia and chloroquin is associated with inhibition of antigen presentation to T cells. Proc Natl Acad Sci USA 1982;79:175.
54. Bjorkman PJ, Saper MA, Samaoui B, et al. Structure of the human class I histocompatability antigen, HLA-A2. Nature 1987;329:506.
55. Howard M, Farrar J, Hilfiker M, et al. Identification of a T-cell–derived B-cell growth factor distinct from interleukin-2. J Exp Med 1982;155:914.
56. Muraguchi A, Nishimoto H, Karamura N, et al. B-cell–derived BCGF functions as an autocrine growth factor(s) in normal and transformed B lymphocytes. J Immunol 1986; 137:179.
57. Vieira P, de Waal-Malefyt R, Dang MN, et al. Isolation and expression of human cytokine synthesis inhibitory factor cDNA clones: homology to Epstein-Barr virus open-reading frame. Proc Natl Acad Sci USA 1991;88:1172.
58. Lederman S, Yellin MJ, Inghirami G, et al. Molecular interactions mediating T-B lymphocyte collaboration in human lymphoid follicles. Roles of T cell-B cell activating molecules (5c8 antigen) and CD40 in contact-dependent help. J Immunol 1992;149:3817.
59. Nathan C, Pendergast TJ, Wiebe ME, et al. Activation of human macrophages. Comparison of other cytokines with interferon gamma. J Exp Med 1984;160:600.
60. Gately MK, Wilson DE, Wong HL. Synergy between recombinant interleukin-2 (rIL-2) and IL-2–depleted lymphokine-containing supernatants in facilitating allogeneic human cytolytic T-lymphocyte responses in vitro. J Immunol 1986;136:1274.
61. Le Gros G, Ben-Sasson SZ, Seder R, et al. Generation of interleukin-4 (IL-4)–producing cells in vivo and in vitro: IL-2 and IL-4 are required for in vitro generation of IL-4–producing cells. J Exp Med 1990;172:921.
62. Swain SL. Generation and in vivo persistence of polarized Th1 and Th2 memory cells. Immunity 1994;1:543.
63. Taniguchi T, Matsui H, Fujita T, et al. Structure and expression of a cloned cDNA for human interleukin-2. Nature 1983;302:305.
64. Isaacs A, Lindeman J. Virus interference. I. The interferon. Proc R Soc Lond [Biol] 1957;147:258.
65. Issacs A, Lindeman J, Valentine RC. Virus interference. II. Some properties of interferon. Proc R Soc Lond [Biol] 1957;147:268.
66. Tracey KJ, Cerami A. TNF and other cytokines in disease. Annu Rev Cell Biol 1993;9:317.
67. Green S, Dobrjansky A, Carswell E, et al. Partial purification of a serum factor that causes necrosis of tumors. Proc Natl Acad Sci USA 1976;73:381.
68. Smith KA. The interleukin-2 receptor. Annu Rev Cell Biol 1989;5:397.
69. Smith KA. Cell growth signal transduction is quantal. Ann NY Acad Sci 1995;766:263.
70. Caligiuri MA, Zmuidzinas A, Manley TJ, et al. Functional consequences of interleukin-2 receptor expression on resting human lymphocytes. Identification of a novel natural killer cell subset with high affinity receptors. J Exp Med 1990;171: 1509.
71. Nakarai T, Robertson MJ, Streuli M, et al. Interleukin-2 receptor gamma chain expression on resting and activated lymphoid cells. J Exp Med 1994;180:241.
72. Smith KA. Rational interleukin-2 therapy. Cancer J 1997;3: S137.
73. Ravetch JV, Clynes RA. Divergent role for Fc receptors and complement in vivo. Annu Rev Immunol 1998;16:1657.
74. Rosenberg SA, Lotze MT, Muul LM, et al. Observations on the systemic administration of autologous lymphokine-activated killer cells and recombinant interleukin-2 to patients with metastatic cancer. N Engl J Med 1985;313: 1485.
75. Lotze MT, Matory YL, Ettinghausen SE, et al. In vivo administration of purified human interleukin-2. II. Half-life, immunologic effects, and expansion of peripheral lymphoid cells in vivo with recombinant IL-2. J Immunol 1985;135: 2865.
76. Rosenberg SA. Perspectives on the use of interleukin-2 in cancer treatment. Cancer J 1997;3(suppl 1):S2.
77. Smith KA. T-cell growth factor. Immunol Rev 1980;51:337.
78. Smith KA. Interleukin-2: inception, impact, and implications. Science 1988;240:1169.
79. Mier JW, Vachino G, Klempner MS, et al. Inhibition of interleukin-2–induced tumor necrosis factor release by dexamethasone: prevention of an acquired neutrophil chemotaxis defect and differential suppression of interleukin-2–associated side effects [see comments]. Blood 1990; 76:1933.
80. Smith K, Beadling C, Jacobson E. Interleukin-2. In: Gallin J, Snyderman R, eds. Inflammation: basic principles and clinical correlates. Philadelphia: Lippincott Williams & Wilkins, 1999:463.
81. Kuroda K, Yagi J, Imanishi K, et al. Implantation of IL-2–containing osmotic pump prolongs the survival of superantigen-reactive T cells expanded in mice injected with bacterial superantigen. J Immunol 1996;157:1422.
82. Lenardo MJ. Interleukin-2 programs mouse alpha beta T lymphocytes for apoptosis. Nature 1991;353:858.
83. Van Parijs L, Ibraghimov A, Abbas AK. The roles of costimulation and Fas in T-cell apoptosis and peripheral tolerance. Immunity 1996;4:321.
84. Zheng L, Fisher G, Miller RE, et al. Induction of apoptosis in mature T cells by tumour necrosis factor. Nature 1995; 377:348.
85. Zheng L, Boehme SA, Critchfield JM, et al. Immunological tolerance by antigen-induced apoptosis of mature T lymphocytes. Adv Exp Med Biol 1994;365:81.
86. Wang HM, Smith KA. The interleukin-2 receptor. Functional consequences of its bimolecular structure. J Exp Med 1987; 166:1055.
87. Smith KA. Lowest dose interleukin-2 immunotherapy [see comments]. Blood 1993;81:1414.
88. Jacobson EL, Pilaro F, Smith KA. Rational interleukin-2 therapy for HIV-positive individuals: daily low doses enhance immune function without toxicity. Proc Natl Acad Sci USA 1996;93:10405.

89. Smith KA, Jacobson EL, Emert R, et al. Restoration of immunity with interleukin-2 therapy. Aids Reader 1999;9: 563.

90. Kovacs JA, Vogel S, Albert JM, et al. Controlled trial of interleukin-2 infusions in patients infected with the human immunodeficiency virus [see comments]. N Engl J Med 1996; 335:1350.

91. Davey RT Jr, Chaitt DG, Albert JM, et al. A randomized trial of high- versus low-dose subcutaneous interleukin-2 outpatient therapy for early human immunodeficiency virus type 1 infection. J Infect Dis 1999;179:849.

92. Caligiuri MA, Murray C, Soiffer RJ, et al. Extended continuous infusion low-dose recombinant interleukin-2 in advanced cancer: prolonged immunomodulation without significant toxicity. J Clin Oncol 1991;9:2110.

93. Smith KA, Jacobson EL, Sohn T, et al. HIV and lymphocyte dynamics after interruption of antiviral therapy but continuation of interleukin-2 therapy. Submitted for publication, 2000.

94. Casadevall A. Passive antibody therapies: progress and continuing challenges. Clin Immunol 1999;93:5.

95. Jakobovits A, Moore AL, Green LL, et al. Germ-line transmission of a human-derived yeast artificial chromosome. Nature 1993;362:255.

96. Green LL, Hardy MC, Maynard-Currie CE, et al. Antigen-specific human monoclonal antibodies from mice engineered with human Ig heavy and light chain YACS. Nat Genet 1994;7:13.

97. Yang X-D, Jia X-C, Corvalan JRF, et al. Eradication of established tumors by a fully human monoclonal antibody to the epidermal growth factor receptor without concomitant chemotherapy. Cancer Res 1999;59:1236.

Chapter 18

A Soluble TNF Receptor–Fc Fusion Protein (Etanercept) in the Treatment of Inflammatory Diseases

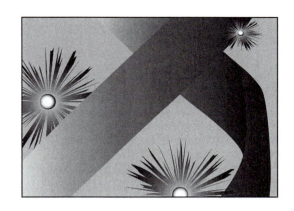

Michael B. Widmer
Leslie Garrison
Kendall M. Mohler

The processes of immunity and inflammation are orchestrated in large part by cytokines, which serve as a means of communication among the cellular components of the immune system. In addition to performing their normal immunoregulatory functions, cytokines have been implicated in the pathogenesis of several autoimmune and inflammatory diseases. As a result, considerable interest has developed in exploring the therapeutic potential of agents that can interfere with cytokine synthesis or biologic activity. One approach to cytokine antagonism that has proven to be therapeutically useful involves soluble cytokine receptors. These molecules consist of the extracellular, ligand-binding portions of cell surface cytokine receptors and act as competitive inhibitors of cytokine binding. An antagonist of the proinflammatory cytokine TNF (tumor necrosis factor), in the form of a soluble p75 TNF receptor–Fc fusion protein (TNFR:Fc, Enbrel, generic name of etanercept), was recently approved by the FDA for the treatment of rheumatoid arthritis. This chapter contains a description of the preclinical rationale and experimentation leading to the development of etanercept, clinical trial results obtained in rheumatoid arthritis studies, and a discussion of potential additional therapeutic indications for etanercept.

Rationale

Soluble Cytokine Receptors

The precise function of the naturally occurring soluble cytokine receptors is not clear; presumably, they constitute a means of regulating biologic activities of the corresponding cytokines (1–3). Whatever their natural function may be, soluble cytokine receptors exhibit several characteristics that make them attractive candidates as pharmacologic agents for inhibiting the biologic activity of cytokines and the disease processes in which they are involved. Their properties include the following: 1) They are specific. Because each cytokine mediates its biologic activity by binding to one or a restricted set of cell surface receptors, the use of soluble receptors represents a specific means by which to modulate the activity of particular cytokines. This property may

confer a therapeutic and safety advantage over other, more broadly acting substances conventionally used for immunosuppression. 2) They occur naturally (4–7). In some cases (e.g., soluble murine IL-4R), alternative splicing of the RNA encoding the full-length receptor results in RNA species encoding only the extracellular, ligand-binding portion of the protein (8). In other cases (e.g., soluble TNFRs), no unique transcript for the extracellular domain has been identified, and the soluble receptor proteins are produced by proteolytic cleavage of the cell surface receptor (9). Recombinant cytokine receptors used clinically are based on naturally occurring human molecules, and thus have the potential to be more weakly immunogenic than other specific cytokine antagonists such as monoclonal antibodies generated in a heterologous species. 3) A compelling evolutionary argument for the potential utility of soluble cytokine receptors stems from the fact that certain members of the pox virus family have captured genetic information for the extracellular portions of some proinflammatory cytokine receptors (TNFR, IL-1R, and IFN-γR) and appear to use the proteins encoded by those sequences as a means of diverting the inflammatory, antiviral response (10–13). 4) They exhibit no intrinsic biologic activity. Soluble cytokine receptors act as a cytokine "sponge" and may be anticipated to be relatively free of some of the untoward effects of agents that stimulate biologic responses. 5) They exhibit beneficial effects in preclinical disease models and clinical settings.

TNF and TNFR: Structure-Function Relationship

TNF exists in both membrane-bound and soluble (primarily homotrimeric) forms (14–16), and its biologic activity is dependent on cross-linking of cell surface TNF receptors (17,18).

There are two distinct cell surface receptors for TNF: the 55-kD (p55) and the 75-kD (p75) TNF receptors (19,20). The affinity of TNF for these receptors is virtually identical, on the order of $10^{10} M^{-1}$ (19,20). The p55 TNFR is thought to be the primary signaling receptor for inflammatory responses. The p75 TNFR can signal in some cell types (e.g., T cells). The p75 receptor may also function as a natural antagonist of inflammatory responses (18,21). Both p55 and p75 receptors exist in cell-bound and soluble forms (17).

Another proinflammatory cytokine, lymphotoxin α (LTα), also binds to cell surface TNF receptors when LTα is expressed as a soluble homotrimer. A second form of lymphotoxin, composed of a heterotrimeric mixture of LTα and LTβ is a cell surface molecule that binds to a receptor distinct from either the p55 or p75 TNF receptors [the so-called LTβ receptor (22,23)]. The heterotrimeric molecule is thought to be important in lymph node development, because LTα, LTβ, and LTβR knockout mice fail to develop normal lymph nodes (24–26).

Etanercept Structure and Mechanism of Action

Recombinant human TNFR:Fc is a fusion protein consisting of the extracellular, ligand-binding domain of the human p75 TNF receptor linked to the Fc portion of human IgG1 (Fig. 18-1). The Fc element consists of the hinge region and the CH$_2$ and CH$_3$ domains but not the CH$_1$ domain of IgG1. This soluble TNF receptor–Fc fusion construct is produced in a mammalian expression system [Chinese hamster ovary (CHO) cells] for use as a therapeutic inhibitor of the proinflammatory cytokine TNF. It acts as a competitive inhibitor of TNF binding to cell surface TNF receptors and thereby functions as an inhibitor of the biologic activity of TNF (Fig. 18-2).

TNFR:Fc binds to both TNF and LTα_3 homotrimers but not to LTα/β heterotrimers (Fig. 18-3). Thus, the biologic effects of TNFR:Fc may be attributable to its ability to inhibit the biologic activity of TNF and/or LTα.

Divalent soluble receptors have a higher affinity for TNF than do monovalent soluble receptors and are considerably more potent competitive inhibitors of TNF binding (27,28). In addition, the use of an immunoglobulin Fc region as a fusion element in the construction of a dimeric receptor imparts a longer serum half-life. The elimination half-lives of radiolabeled forms of

TNFR:Fc and monovalent soluble p75 TNFR after intravenous administration in mice are approximately 19 hours and 4 hours, respectively.

The affinity of TNF for the TNFR:Fc construct is $10^{10}\,\text{M}^{-1}$, which is approximately the same affinity as TNF exhibits for its cell surface receptors (19,20). In contrast, the affinity of TNF for a soluble recombinant human monomeric p75 TNFR is $10^8\,\text{M}^{-1}$. The difference in TNF binding properties of TNFR:Fc and monomeric TNFR is readily apparent when the two molecules are tested for inhibition of TNF biologic activity. In an assay involving TNF-mediated cytolysis of the murine L929 cell line, TNFR:Fc was approximately 100 times more potent than

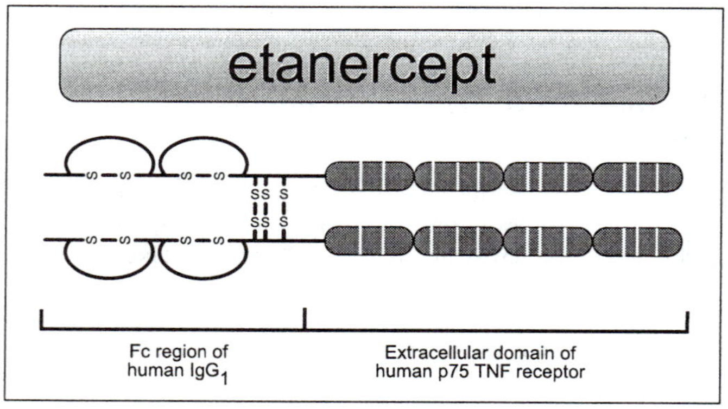

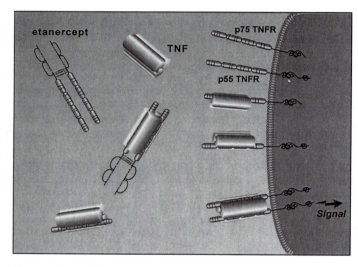

Figure 18-2. TNF binding to cell surface receptors and inhibition by naturally occurring monomeric soluble TNF receptor and etanercept.

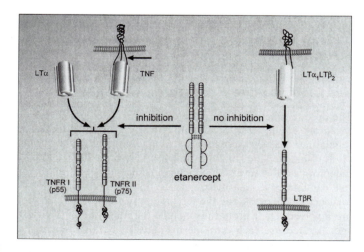

Figure 18-1. Diagrammatic depiction of etanercept, consisting of the extracellular portion of the p75 TNF receptor linked to the Fc region of human IgG1.

Figure 18-3. Etanercept binds to TNF and LTα_3 but not to LTα/β complex.

monomeric p75 TNFR as an inhibitor of rhu TNF (28). The biologic activities of recombinant murine TNF and native murine TNF in this assay were also inhibited to a greater extent by TNFR:Fc than by monomeric p75 TNFR.

Because TNFR:Fc is a fusion protein consisting, in part, of the CH_2 and CH_3 domains of the Fc region of human IgG1, it has also been tested for activities normally ascribed to the Fc region—namely, the ability to bind to Fc receptors and to fix complement. The molecule does indeed bind to Fc receptors on the cell surface, but this binding is inhibited by concentrations of human immunoglobulin far lower than those present in human plasma; Fc receptor binding is therefore considered to have little impact on the biologic activity of the construct. In a direct complement fixation assay with human serum as a source of complement, TNFR:Fc was found to be inactive. In addition, TNFR:Fc did not induce complement-mediated cytolysis of cells expressing TNF on the cell surface (29). Taken together with the fact that TNFR:Fc acts as a competitive inhibitor of TNF binding to its cell surface receptors, the data indicate that the major biologic effects of TNFR:Fc in preclinical and clinical studies can be ascribed primarily to the ligand-binding, soluble receptor portion of the molecule, as opposed to the Fc portion.

TNFR:Fc has exhibited efficacy preclinically in several disease models. In two of these model systems, experiments were conducted to determine the effect of TNFR:Fc administration on the concentration of endogenous TNF in biologic fluids. The first model involves inflammation of the lung that occurs in response to intranasal administration of the actinomycete *Micropolyspora faeni*. The inflammatory response in this model, as measured by influx of neutrophils to the lung, was markedly inhibited by administration of TNFR:Fc at the time of antigen administration. Bronchoalveolar lavage (BAL) fluids from mice challenged with *M. faeni* were examined for the presence of bioactive TNF as assessed by cytolysis of the murine cell line, L929. TNF biologic activity was nearly absent in the BAL of TNFR:Fc-treated mice in comparison with control mice treated with human IgG, which had significant levels of bioactive TNF. However, when an antihuman p75 TNFR monoclonal antibody that displaces bound TNF from TNFR:Fc was included in the bioassay mixture, TNF bioactivity was readily detectable in BAL fluids of mice that had been treated with TNFR:Fc (K. Mohler, unpublished observation).

Similar observations were made in a second model dependent on production of endogenous TNF, an endotoxin challenge model in mice. In this model, the lethal effects of endotoxin are inhibited by administration of TNFR:Fc. Analysis of serum samples from mice given TNFR:Fc revealed almost no biologically active TNF in the serum in comparison with the high TNF levels observed in IgG-treated controls. However, when the serum samples were examined for TNF in the presence of the antihuman p75 TNFR antibody, TNF was readily detectable and was found to be present in higher concentrations and for longer periods of time in mice treated with TNFR:Fc than in control mice treated with human IgG (28).

TNFR:Fc had a similar effect on serum TNF concentration in humans, as demonstrated by analysis of serum samples from solid organ transplant recipients treated with anti-CD3 antibody (OKT3) for graft rejection crisis (30). While serum concentrations of antigenic TNF as determined by ELISA were higher in patients treated with TNFR:Fc than in placebo controls, TNF bioactivity was significantly reduced.

Taken together, the results obtained in these preclinical models (*M. faeni* and endotoxin challenge) and the clinical trial (OKT3 in organ transplantation) indicate that administration of TNFR:Fc does not lead to accelerated clearance of TNF from biologic fluids, but renders the TNF that is present biologically unavailable. These observations have led to the concept that TNFR:Fc can act as both a cytokine "carrier," in the sense of prolonging the existence of inactive TNF in biologic fluids, and as an effective TNF antagonist at the same time.

TNF in Rheumatoid Arthritis

TNF was originally described as a molecule that could induce the hemorrhagic necrosis of tumors (31) and wasting (cachexia) (32) when induced in or administered to experimental animals. Numerous subsequent studies revealed a central role for TNF in the induction and propagation of inflammatory processes (reviewed in 33–36). As a proinflammatory cytokine, TNF has been implicated in the pathogenesis of several inflammatory diseases, including rheumatoid arthritis (37–39).

There are several properties of TNF that may contribute to the disease process in rheumatoid arthritis (Fig. 18-4). 1) TNF has been observed to be expressed at the cartilage-pannus junction, in synovial fluids, and in cultures of synoviocytes from rheumatoid arthritis patients (40,41). 2) The concentrations of soluble p55 and p75 TNF receptors are elevated in biologic fluids obtained from patients with inflammatory conditions, including rheumatoid arthritis (42). 3) TNF induces the production of tissue degradative enzymes, or matrix metalloproteases (MMPs) (37). These enzymes are thought to contribute to joint destruction in

Role of TNF in the Pathophysiology of RA

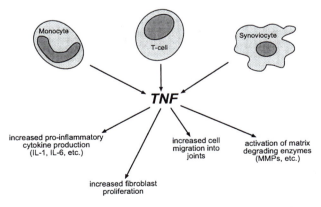

Figure 18-4. Some biological activities of TNF pertinent to rheumatoid arthritis.

rheumatoid arthritis. 4) TNF stimulates production of other proinflammatory cytokines such as IL-1 and IL-6. Furthermore, the addition of TNF blocking antibodies to synovial cultures inhibits the production of IL-1 (43). 5) TNF induces the expression of adhesion molecules on vascular endothelial cells, an effect that may facilitate the migration of inflammatory cells into the rheumatoid joint (44). 6) When TNF is expressed as a transgene in mice under the control of its endogenous promoter, the resulting phenotype is a polyarticular inflammation reminiscent of rheumatoid arthritis (45). 7) TNF antagonists are beneficial in animal models of experimentally induced arthritis (46–50).

Collectively, these considerations have led to the notion that TNF is a major driver of inflammation in rheumatoid arthritis, and have led some to propose that TNF may occupy a position at or near the top of an inflammatory cascade in rheumatoid arthritis (39). The results of clinical trials with etanercept (51–53) and with a monoclonal antibody to TNF (54–56) provide direct evidence for the involvement of TNF in this disease.

Effects in Models of Rheumatoid Arthritis

The model most extensively employed to examine clinical potential of TNFR:Fc in arthritis is the collagen-induced arthritis (CIA) model, in which mice develop joint inflammation and tissue degradation in response to the administration of heterologous collagen.

In a bovine CIA model, mice were given TNFR:Fc according to either of two protocols: a preventative protocol or a therapeutic protocol. Daily IP administration of TNFR:Fc (50 µg/mouse) starting on day 21 and ending on day 28 relative to collagen administration (a time during which the disease is developing) reduced the incidence of disease to 28%, in comparison to the 86% disease incidence in saline-treated controls. When treatment initiation was delayed until disease symptoms had already occurred, mice given TNFR:Fc (50 µg/mouse) by daily IP injection for two weeks developed a less severe arthritis than mice given human serum albumin as a control. Thus, TNFR:Fc was effective in both prophylactic and therapeutic settings (49).

Dosage-response effects of TNFR:Fc were examined in a separate series of CIA experiments. In these experiments, mice were immunized with collagen, then challenged 21 days later. Dosages of TNFR:Fc as low as 0.1 µg per day for 10 days or 1 µg per day for 14 days after collagen challenge led to a significant reduction in clinical arthritis score. Administration of 10 µg or 50 µg per mouse per day produced reductions in arthritis score greater than those in the 0.1-µg group and similar to those in the 1-µg group.

In addition to its beneficial effects on clinical symptoms in the CIA model, TNFR:Fc administration resulted in reduced joint damage as assessed histopathologically. In a double-blind study, daily administration of TNFR:Fc for 10 days beginning on the day of collagen challenge resulted in a lower clinical arthritis score, less joint destruction as assessed by microscopic examination of joint sections, and less cartilage depletion in

comparison with controls (K. Mohler and J. Schuh, unpublished observations).

Effects in Other Preclinical Models

TNFR:Fc has been tested as a TNF antagonist in several preclinical models in addition to the arthritis models summarized in the previous section. These secondary pharmacology studies are summarized here.

One of the earliest described biologic activities of TNF is the induction of wasting, or cachexia (32). TNFR:Fc prevented cachexia in two murine models. In mice bearing a TNF-secreting tumor, weight loss was prevented and reversed by TNFR:Fc (57). In addition, TNF transgenic mice, which normally runt and die early as a result of constitutive TNF production, grew to normal size and reproduced when treated continuously with TNFR:Fc (57).

TNFR:Fc has been tested in several preclinical models of lung inflammation. As discussed previously, intranasal administration of TNFR:Fc concomitantly with *M. faeni* antigen decreased cellular infiltration to the lung in a model of hypersensitivity pneumonitis. In other models of lung inflammation, systemic administration of TNFR:Fc also resulted in beneficial effects. Mice injected with TNFR:Fc IP prior to administration of lipopolysaccharide (LPS) and formyl-norleucyl-leucyl-phenylalanine (FNLP) in a model of respiratory distress syndrome exhibited a reduction in lung vascular permeability, neutrophil influx, and tissue damage (58). As observed in the *M. faeni* model, TNF concentration was increased in the lungs of mice treated with TNFR:Fc, but the TNF was not biologically active. Inflammatory granuloma formation in the lung in response to systemic administration of *Schistosoma mansoni* eggs was also reduced by IP administration of TNFR:Fc (59). The effect of TNFR:Fc was associated with decreased expression of RNA for intercellular adhesion molecule 1 (ICAM-1) in the lung and with a reduced splenocyte response to soluble *S. mansoni* egg antigen in vitro.

The role of TNF in inflammation may also contribute to the processes involved in allograft rejection and the response to vascular injury. In a model of heterotopic cardiac transplantation in rabbits, neointimal thickening of donor coronary arteries was significantly less pronounced in comparison with controls following daily subcutaneous (SC) TNFR:Fc administration beginning on the day of transplantation (60). Expression of the vascular endothelial adhesion molecule, VCAM-1, was reduced in murine heterotopic cardiac allografts following TNFR:Fc administration, although the graft rejection rate was not affected in this model (61). TNFR:Fc administration prolonged graft survival in nonhuman primate recipients of kidney allografts, and the effect was enhanced by combining TNFR:Fc with subtherapeutic doses of cyclosporin A (62). Administration of TNFR:Fc for 15 days following transfer of allogeneic spleen cells to irradiated SCID mice reduced the death rate due to acute graft-versus-host disease (GVHD) by approximately 50%; mice surviving past 15 days exhibited a chronic form of GVHD for a 6-month follow-up period (63). In another model of allogeneic bone marrow transplantation to irradiated mice, administration of TNFR:Fc for 2 days prior to and on the day of transplantation, then every other day for 2 weeks, increased the recipient 50-day survival incidence from 22% to 70% (64). Engraftment of both syngeneic and allogeneic islets of Langerhans in diabetic mice was promoted by TNFR:Fc administration, although graft rejection was not prevented (65). These tissue and organ transplantation models involve inflammation at local sites and, in the case of GVHD, systemic inflammation. It is likely that the beneficial effects of TNFR:Fc in these models are related to its ability to modulate the multiple components of inflammation associated with the immune response to the allograft.

TNF has been implicated in the pathogenesis of cardiovascular disease and is a mediator of hemodynamic dysfunction during systemic inflammation. Studies of isolated feline cardiac myocytes in vitro demonstrated a negative inotropic effect of TNF, and a reversal of that effect by TNFR:Fc (66). In an in vivo model of burn shock in guinea pigs, administration of TNFR:Fc prevented myocardial dysfunction (67).

Pathology of Rheumatoid Arthritis in Humans

Rheumatoid arthritis (RA) is a chronic articular disorder estimated to occur in 1% of the U.S. population. Its signs and symptoms include joint pain, swelling, stiffness, and deformity that result in significant morbidity and increased mortality. Affected individuals have functional impairment, avocational and occupational disability, and a consequential decrease in their quality of life (QOL). More than 50% of RA patients experience substantial functional loss within 5 years of diagnosis.

There is no cure for RA. Current therapies are directed at controlling the disease through a variety of pathways, including inhibitors of prostaglandin synthesis (nonsteroidal anti-inflammatory drugs), immunosuppressive agents (azathioprine and cyclosporine A), antimetabolites (methotrexate), and other drugs that control disease symptoms through mechanisms that are unknown (gold salts, antimalarials, and corticosteroids). Of these, only methotrexate has been proven to slow joint erosions, the most devastating of the long-term sequelae (68), and is therefore considered to be the "gold standard" of therapy. However, all of these treatments, including methotrexate, are limited by lack or loss of efficacy over time, as well as by side effects ranging from those with serious health consequences, such as pneumonitis, to those of only nuisance value, such as nausea or hair loss. As a result, only a small percentage of RA patients continue many of the available drug therapies for an extended period of time.

The primary pathology of RA is a chronic, symmetric, and erosive inflammation of the synovium of the peripheral joints, resulting ultimately in joint destruction. The swelling and inflammation result from the marked increase in cellularity in the synovial membrane, which becomes infiltrated by leukocytes under the influence of TNF-driven cytokines. The cellular infiltrate causes a thickening of the lining layer of the joint, and produc-

tion of a pannus. This structure is formed by the junction of the thickened synovium lining the joint capsule with the cartilage and bone. The cells of the pannus migrate over the underlying cartilage into the subchondral bone, causing destruction of the cartilage, destruction of the margins of the joints, and erosion of the periarticular bone. As the disease progresses, the joint capsule is distended or ruptured. The massive tumor-like expansion of the new stromal connective tissue cells forming the pannus is supported by neoangiogenesis. This network of new blood vessels is essential for the massive hyperplasia of the synovium because it provides the vascular support for this tissue.

The central role of TNF in the inflammatory process of RA has been confirmed recently by the therapeutic efficacy of etanercept. On the basis of extensive data from the etanercept clinical trials, this agent became the first biologic response modifier approved by the FDA for use in patients with RA or juvenile rheumatoid arthritis (JRA) who have not responded to treatment with at least one other disease-modifying drug. Recently, a clinical trial investigating the efficacy of etanercept as initial therapy for newly diagnosed RA, and as an agent for slowing of joint destruction, was completed (69).

Studies of Etanercept in Patients with RA

Etanercept Therapy in Adults with RA

The potential clinical utility of etanercept in adults with RA was assessed in three placebo-controlled, double-blind, randomized clinical trials involving more than 500 patients. In the first placebo-controlled etanercept trial, a phase II trial involving 180 patients who had failed therapy with from one to four disease-modifying antirheumatic drugs (DMARDs), patients received SC injections of placebo or etanercept (0.25, 2, or 16 mg per square meter of body-surface area) twice weekly for 3 months. Etanercept produced a significantly greater improvement in disease activity than did placebo as assessed by all measures (51). On the basis of the favorable results from the phase II study, a placebo-controlled phase III study was conducted using a simplified etanercept dosing schema and a duration of therapy extended to 6 months (52). In this trial, 234 patients with refractory RA (inadequate response to one to four prior DMARDs) were randomized to receive placebo, etanercept 10 mg, or etanercept 25 mg SC (total dose per patient, as a bolus injection) twice weekly. All patients were required to have at least 12 tender and 10 swollen joints, and at least one of the following: erythrocyte sedimentation rate (ESR) $\geq$28 mm, C-reactive protein (CRP) >2.0 mg/dL, or morning stiffness for at least 45 minutes. The endpoints were 20% and 50% improvement in disease activity at 3 and 6 months, as defined in the American College of Rheumatology (ACR) response criteria (70), and other parameters measuring disease activity.

In the phase II study, the mean reduction from baseline in total swollen and tender joint count was 61% with etanercept 16 mg/m^2, and 25% with placebo (Fig. 18-5). The difference

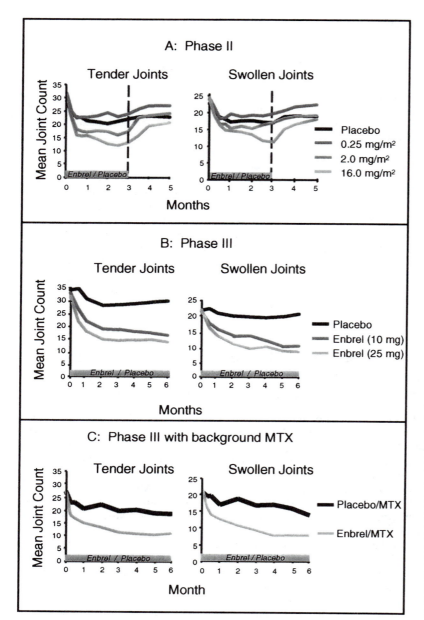

Figure 18-5. Mean joint count change with time in three randomized double-blind placebo controlled studies. In all cases, etanercept was administered SC biweekly. *A*, Phase II study in which RA patients who had not responded adequately to one to four DMARDs were randomized to receive placebo or to receive one of three doses of etanercept, the lowest of which was a "no effect" dose. Etanercept treatment was stopped at month 3, and patients were followed for 2 more months. *B*, Phase III study in which RA patients who had not responded adequately to DMARDs were randomized to receive placebo or to receive one of two doses of etanercept. Treatment was continued for 6 months. *C*, Phase III study in which RA patients who were receiving MTX, but still had persistently active disease, were randomized to two groups, one with placebo added to the MTX therapy and the other with etanercept added to the MTX therapy. Treatment was continued for 6 months.

between the two groups was apparent as early as 2 weeks after initiation of treatment. At the end of the 3-month treatment period, a significantly larger percentage of patients in the etanercept 16 mg/m² group (75%) than in the placebo group (14%) had at least a 20% improvement in ACR response. Similarly, significantly more patients (57%) receiving etanercept 16 mg/m² experienced a 50% improvement in symptoms, compared with only 7% of the placebo group. After the drug was withdrawn at 3 months, patients were followed for an additional 2 months, and disease activity returned within 1 to 2 months toward baseline (but did not fully reach baseline levels).

Results of the first phase III study (see Fig. 18-5) were similar. At 6 months, 59% of patients in the etanercept 25 mg group, 51% of patients in the etanercept 10 mg group, and 11% of patients in the placebo group achieved a 20% ACR response ($p < 0.001$ for each etanercept group compared with the placebo group). The percentages of patients achieving 50% and 70% ACR responses were also superior in patients receiving etanercept ($p \leq 0.001$ for etanercept 25 mg vs. placebo) (52).

In both studies, a dosage-response relationship was observed between etanercept dosage and the efficacy endpoints, with the greatest response observed with 16 mg/m², or 25 mg biweekly.

Figure 18-6. Response of JRA patients receiving etanercept or placebo. Patients with polyarticular-course JRA enrolled in a two-part study. In the first part, all patients received etanercept 0.4 mg/kg biweekly. In the second part, patients who had responded in the first part were randomized to receive either etanercept at the same dosage, or placebo for 4 months, or until disease flare. At the end of this period, all patients entered the open-label long-term study in which they were given etanercept 0.4 mg/kg biweekly. Response was assessed on the basis of a 30% or greater improvement in 3/6 JRA core set variables (number of active joints, LOM, MD and patient global assessment, childhood HAQ and ESR).

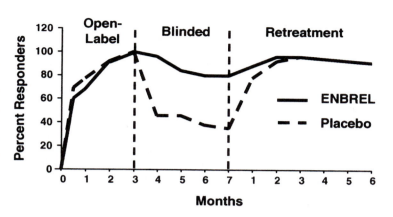

The combination of methotrexate and etanercept was compared with methotrexate plus placebo in a phase III randomized, double-blind trial in adult RA (53). In this study, 89 patients with persistently active RA despite methotrexate treatment received SC injections of either placebo or etanercept 25 mg twice weekly in addition to continuing methotrexate (12.5 to 25 mg per week). There was a significant decrease in the joint count in patients treated with etanercept plus methotrexate in comparison with patients treated with placebo plus methotrexate (see Fig. 18-5). The combination of etanercept and methotrexate resulted in 71% of patients achieving a 20% ACR response, compared with only 27% of patients who received methotrexate plus placebo. The percentages of patients achieving 50% and 70% ACR responses were also significantly greater for patients receiving etanercept. Responses were rapid and durable.

Etanercept Therapy in Juvenile RA

A placebo-controlled trial of etanercept in pediatric patients between the ages of 4 and 17 with active, polyarticular-course juvenile RA (JRA) has been completed (71,72). The two-part design was unusual, in that the first part was an open-label trial, and all patients initially received etanercept 0.4 mg/kg SC twice weekly for up to 3 months. The 0.4-mg/kg dose is roughly equivalent to the 25-mg dose used in adults. The maximum allowed was 25 mg per dose. Patients who met the JRA definition of improvement (73) at the end of 3 months were then randomized into the second part of the study, which was placebo controlled. They continued on etanercept or placebo for 4 months or until disease flare occurred. Sixty-nine patients enrolled in the trial, and 51 (74%) met the criteria for improvement at 3 months and entered the placebo-controlled part of the study. More than 80% of patients who continued on etanercept maintained their response, as compared with less than 40% of the patients who received placebo. The response was regained when patients on the placebo arm were again given etanercept (Fig. 18-6).

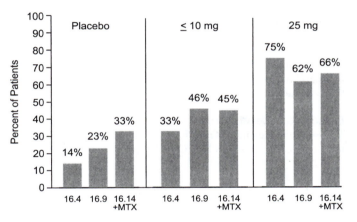

Figure 18-7. Dose-response in randomized studies. Percent of patients achieving 20% ACR response at the end of the study in randomized blinded controlled phase II and phase III studies.

Overview of the Three Placebo-Controlled Clinical Trials

Efficacy

In all three studies of adult subjects, disease activity in the patients in the placebo group was either relatively unchanged from, or worse than, baseline disease. In the first study, response in the lowest dose group, 0.25 mg/m^2, was comparable to that in the placebo group. In contrast, patients receiving higher doses in all three studies of adult subjects (16 mg/m^2, 10 mg, and 25 mg) exhibited significantly improved responses throughout each study. Mean tender and swollen joint count values, and mean percent changes from baseline to 3 and 6 months, are summarized in Figure 18-5. ACR$_{20}$ responses are shown in Figure 18-7. In general, ACR responses in all studies demonstrated a dose-response effect. In almost all cases, the higher doses of etanercept produced significantly ($p < 0.05$) more 20% and 50% ACR responses compared with lower doses.

Major clinical responses, here defined as an ACR 70% response, were observed in approximately 15% to 20% of etanercept-treated patients in the three placebo-controlled, randomized, double-blind studies. These responses were sustained over 24 months.

The clinical responses to etanercept treatment generally occurred rapidly and were more rapid at the 25-mg dose than at lower doses. ACR responses were observed as quickly as 1 week after the first dose in many patients. By 2 weeks of treatment, significantly higher percentages of patients treated in the higher-dose groups (10 mg, 25 mg, and 16 mg/m²) achieved a 20% ACR response compared with patients in the placebo groups, and by 1 month there was also a statistically significant difference in the number of ACR 50% and ACR 70% responses between the etanercept groups and the placebo groups.

Laboratory Values

High CRP and ESR values are commonly associated with RA. Patients in the higher-dose groups in all three controlled studies had complete normalization of CRP and ESR values, as compared with patients in the placebo-treated group, which did not. Platelet counts and albumin levels, which are commonly low in RA patients, were normalized in the first two studies but not in the last study, in which all patients were receiving methotrexate.

Quality of Life Measurements

The Health Assessment Questionnaire (HAQ) is a standard used to calculate the quality of life (QOL) in patients with RA. Its spe-

cific categories are: disability index (or physical function), general health status, arthritis-specific health status, mental health, and vitality. The first category, the disability index, assesses eight activities (dressing and grooming, arising, eating, walking, hygiene, reach, grip, and general activities). Patients are also queried about requirements for aids or devices, or help from another person. The general health area is measured with a "feeling thermometer," on a scale of 1 to 10. The mental health domains include questions such as "feel calm and peaceful" and "feel downhearted and blue." The vitality measures include questions such as "feel full of pep" and "have enough energy to do the things you want to do."

Only the first category, disability, was measured in the phase II randomized study, and at month 3 there was a significant improvement in the treated groups (data not shown). The full HAQ was performed in the two phase III studies (Table 18-1). Treatment with etanercept significantly improved patients' functional ability, especially at the highest dose. At 6 months after the start of therapy, etanercept-treated patients had 39% to 44% improvement in physical function (disability). The average patient in these studies had a baseline disability index of 1.3 to 1.7, and the disability index dropped by 0.5 unit or greater in more than 53% of etanercept-treated patients.

Health-related QOL also improved significantly as assessed by the other parameters. Improvements ranged from 33% to 51% in general health status, 44% to 47% in arthritis-specific health status, 34% to 35% in mental health, and 25% to 30% in vitality.

Table 18-1. HAQ: Disability/QOL (Mean % Improvement from Baseline)

Parameter	Placebo N = 80	Phase III Etanercept 10 mg N = 76	Phase III Etanercept 25 mg N = 78	p-value	Placebo N = 30	Phase III with background MTX Etanercept 25 mg N = 59	p-value
Disability							
Week 2	4	16	17	0.012	19	21	0.52
Month 3	8	30	36	<0.001	14	37	0.006
Month 6	2	34	39	<0.001	12	44	<0.001
General Health Status							
Week 2	6	23	19	0.095	−8	21	0.006
Month 3	−6	35	30	0.001	−5	45	0.002
Month 6	−12	34	33	0.001	1	51	<0.001
Arthritis–Specific Health Status							
Week 2	−11	11	15	0.079	−11	26	0.001
Month 3	−19	38	42	<0.001	−4	48	<0.001
Month 6	−22	31	44	<0.001	0	47	0.011
Mental Health							
Week 2	−2	1	11	0.555	9	20	0.213
Month 3	4	11	29	0.008	13	31	0.200
Month 6	3	17	35	0.001	0	34	<0.001
Vitality							
Week 2	3	8	12	0.001	5	17	0.061
Month 3	5	19	26	<0.001	11	26	0.052
Month 6	2	22	25	<0.001	8	30	0.007

In almost all of these categories, improvement over placebo was significantly different at $p < 0.001$.

Improvements in physical function and health-related QOL have been sustained for as long as etanercept has been administered. The patients treated in the randomized, placebo-controlled, double-blind trials have been enrolled in an open-label safety trial without interruption of etanercept. Patients have demonstrated consistent improvements in physical function and health-related QOL for more than 24 months.

Long-Term Safety and Efficacy

All patients treated in the three studies of adult RA patients and in the study of children with JRA were eligible to enter a long-term, open-label study. Safety analysis included all 782 patients (713 adults and 69 children) who participated in the four placebo-controlled studies and who were eligible to enter the open-label study (74). Six hundred and thirty-eight patients entered the open-label study and were analyzed for efficacy. The 144 patients who did not enter either were lost to follow-up or elected not to enroll.

The mean age of the overall population of 782 patients was 51 years. The demographics of the population were 77% female and 89% Caucasian, with a 12-year mean duration of RA. Almost all of the patients (513) have now been followed for at least 12 months, for 891.6 patient years. The only side effect that was increased in frequency in treated patients over placebo-treated patients in the controlled trials was mild to moderate injection site reactions. These reactions, which were reported in 43% of etanercept-treated patients in the long-term study, occurred with approximately one to two injections, and were usually seen during the first 4 weeks of therapy. No other side effect was clearly associated with etanercept treatment. Furthermore, no increase in frequency of adverse events has been observed with increasing time on etanercept.

With any drug that is an immunomodulator, infections and cancer (especially lymphoproliferative) are theoretical concerns. Table 18-2 lists the incidence of infections in the first three (placebo-controlled) trials, and the incidence in the patients from those three trials who entered the long-term follow-up. The overall incidence of infections and serious infections were similar in the etanercept and placebo groups in the controlled clinical trials. Furthermore, the overall incidence of infections in the long-term follow-up were comparable to the incidence in the controlled trials of the placebo and etanercept groups. This was also the case in the serious infection category (defined as those requiring hospitalization or IV antibiotics). However, etanercept should be used with caution in patients with serious infections, and these patients should be closely monitored.

In these trials, there were nine cancers (892 patient years) in the etanercept treated group, of which one was Hodgkin's disease and one was non-Hodgkin's lymphoma. This is the same incidence as that expected in the age-matched population (9.2 cases/892 patient years).

The efficacy observed with etanercept therapy is maintained with continued treatment, as shown in Figures 18-8 and 18-9. Not only is the ACR composite score maintained (Fig. 18-8), but, importantly, as shown in Figure 18-9, joint scores remained improved with time.

The experience obtained to date in clinical trials leaves little doubt about the efficacy of etanercept in controlling symptoms in these patients with longstanding disease. In a recent trial (69) of patients with early RA (less than 3 years since diagnosis and no prior methotrexate therapy), patients were randomized to

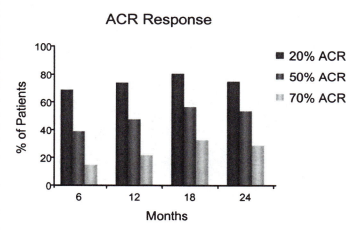

Figure 18-8. Percent of patients who participated in the open-label, long-term study who achieved an ACR 20%, 50%, or 70% response at 6, 12, 18, or 24 months.

Table 18-2. Rate of Infections in All Patients Treated with Etanercept (Reported as Event/Patient Year)

| | **Controlled Trials** | | **Long-Term Data** |
	Placebo	**Etanercept**	**(up to 33 months)**
All Infections	1.86	1.82	1.64
Upper Respiratory	0.68	0.82	0.54
Sinusitis	0.42	0.31	0.18
Skin Infection	0.31	0.16	0.14
Serious*	0.059	0.045	0.053

*Associated with hospitalization or IV antibiotics.

Longterm Treatment Trial - Joint Counts

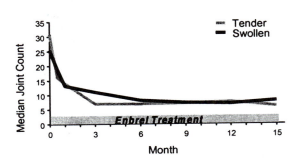

Figure 18-9. Median tender or swollen joint count in patients who participated in the open-label, long-term study.

receive etanercept 10 mg, etanercept 25 mg, or optimal doses of methotrexate for 12 months. Patients were evaluated clinically, as in previous trials, and radiographically, to determine the extent of progression of bony erosions. The results of this trial are likely to have a major impact on the ultimate place of etanercept in the treatment of RA. In addition, as more experience with etanercept is gained, effects on corticosteroid, NSAID, and DMARD requirements will likely become available, as well as information about long-term health impacts such as effects on disability and requirements for joint replacements.

New Indications

As TNF has been implicated in a variety of diseases, there is a wide range of potential applications for etanercept. Ongoing clinical trials include psoriatic arthritis and vasculitis. A clinical trial for Crohn's disease is under development, and large trials in chronic heart failure are underway.

Psoriatic arthritis is similar to RA except that these patients also have psoriasis. This skin disease is characterized by scaling and by erythematous, indurated skin. Approximately 10% to 15% of these patients also have arthritis. Although there are some differences in terms of which joints are involved and in the pathology, it is still very similar to RA in terms of joint destruction. Methotrexate is the drug of choice for psoriatic arthritis. A 60-patient, 3-month, double-blind, placebo-controlled study of etanercept has been completed (75). As expected, there was the same dramatic response in the joints as has been seen in the studies of RA. In addition, there was significant improvement in the psoriasis.

Many of the autoimmune diseases involve vasculitis—inflammation of the small or large vessels of the body. Vasculitis may be the main manifestation of disease, or it may be a feature of another autoimmune disease such as systemic lupus erythematosis. Most of the vasculitides affect vessels in a specific anatomic location. One example is Wegener's granulomatosis. The lesions consist of granulomas that form primarily around the small vessels of the upper and lower respiratory tracts and kidneys. The lesions are necrotizing, and result in acute or chronic inflammation of the sinus, nasopharyngeal tract, or trachea. The lung infiltrates are typically multiple, nodular, cavitating lesions, and renal involvement presents as focal necrotizing glomerulonephritis. Nearly 70% of patients have some form of joint involvement during the course of the disease, either a nondeforming arthritis of ankles and knees or a symmetric polyarticular arthralgia. Eye involvement is also common. The only treatment is a combination of corticosteroids and a cytotoxic agent such as cyclophosphamide. An initial open-label, 20-patient clinical trial of etanercept in this disease has just been completed (76).

Crohn's disease is an autoimmune disease that affects the entire intestinal tract, especially the distal ileum, colon, and anorectal region. This is a chronic inflammatory process, which also consists of granulomatous lesions. These lesions are transmural as opposed to superficial, and extend through the mucosa of the gut. The usual victim is a young person in the second or third decade who presents with episodic abdominal pain with mild diarrhea. With time, the pain localizes to the right lower quadrant, and the symptoms often include weight loss. A major problem with Crohn's disease is the development of perirectal or perianal fistulas with pain, mass, purulent drainage and fever, and deep penetrating ulceration. It can be accompanied by extraintestinal manifestations such as arthritis. Crohn's disease has been shown to respond to anti-TNF therapy (77), and clinical trials examining the efficacy of etanercept in this disease are ongoing.

Perhaps the most novel potential indication for etanercept is congestive heart failure (CHF). Serum TNF concentrations are elevated in patients with heart failure, and these elevated concentrations have been linked with left ventricular dysfunction (78–82). Preclinical studies have shown that soluble TNF receptors can reverse the negative inotropic effects of TNF (66). A 30-patient clinical trial demonstrated some activity of etanercept in heart failure (83). On the basis of these data, two 900-patient, double-blind, randomized, placebo-controlled studies of etanercept in class II-IV CHF patients are in progress.

Conclusion

In conclusion, TNF has been implicated in a variety of inflammatory diseases. TNF antagonists have already been approved in the treatment of RA (etanercept and infliximab) and Crohn's disease (infliximab). In theory, virtually any disease with an inflammatory or autoimmune component could be a candidate for etanercept treatment. It will be of great interest to determine the spectrum of additional diseases in which TNF inhibitors exhibit efficacy.

Acknowledgments
We thank Dr. Vera Byers for helping to compose the clinical results section of this chapter and Linda Robbins and Susan Moon for help in preparation of the manuscript.

References

1. Aderka D, Engelmann H, Maor Y, et al. Stabilization of the bioactivity of tumor necrosis factor by its soluble receptors. J Exp Med 1992;175:323–329.
2. Girardin E, Roux-Lombard P, Grau GE, et al. Imbalance between tumour necrosis factor-alpha and soluble TNF receptor concentrations in severe meningococcaemia. The J5 Study Group. Immunology 1992;76:20–23.
3. Fernandez-Botran R, Chilton PM, Ma Y. Soluble cytokine receptors: their roles in immunoregulation, disease, and therapy. Adv Immunol 1996;63:269–336.
4. Novick D, Engelmann H, Wallach D, Rubinstein M. Soluble cytokine receptors are present in normal human urine. J Exp Med 1989;170:1409–1414.
5. Seckinger P, Isaaz S, Dayer JM. Purification and biologic characterization of a specific tumor necrosis factor alpha inhibitor. J Biol Chem 1989;264:11966–11973.
6. Fernandez-Botran R, Vitetta ES. A soluble, high-affinity, interleukin-4-binding protein is present in the biological fluids of mice. Proc Natl Acad Sci USA 1990;87:4202–4206.
7. Fanslow WC, Clifford K, VandenBos T, et al. A soluble form of the interleukin 4 receptor in biological fluids. Cytokine 1990;2:398–401.
8. Mosley B, Beckmann MP, March CJ, et al. The murine interleukin-4 receptor: molecular cloning and characterization of secreted and membrane bound forms. Cell 1989;59:335–348.
9. Peschon JJ, Slack JL, Reddy P, et al. An essential role for ectodomain shedding in mammalian development [see comments]. Science 1998;282:1281–1284.
10. Smith CA, Davis T, Wignall JM, et al. T2 open reading frame from the Shope fibroma virus encodes a soluble form of the TNF receptor. Biochem Biophys Res Commun 1991;176:335–342.
11. Upton C, Macen JL, Schreiber M, and McFadden G. Myxoma virus expresses a secreted protein with homology to the tumor necrosis factor receptor gene family that contributes to viral virulence. Virology 1991;184:370–382.
12. Spriggs MK, Hruby DE, Maliszewski CR, et al. Vaccinia and cowpox viruses encode a novel secreted interleukin-1-binding protein. Cell 1992;71:145–152.
13. Alcami A, Smith GL. A soluble receptor for interleukin-1 beta encoded by vaccinia virus: a novel mechanism of virus modulation of the host response to infection. Cell 1992;71:153–167.
14. Kriegler M, Perez C, DeFay K, et al. A novel form of TNF/cachectin is a cell surface cytotoxic transmembrane protein: ramifications for the complex physiology of TNF. Cell 1988;53:45–53.
15. Eck MJ, Sprang SR. The structure of tumor necrosis factor-alpha at 2.6 A resolution. Implications for receptor binding. J Biol Chem 1989;264:17595–17605.
16. Jones EY, Stuart DI, Walker NP. Structure of tumour necrosis factor. Nature 1989;338:225–228.
17. Engelmann H, Novick D, Wallach D. Two tumor necrosis factor-binding proteins purified from human urine. Evidence for immunological cross-reactivity with cell surface tumor necrosis factor receptors. J Biol Chem 1990;265:1531–1536.
18. Tartaglia LA, Goeddel DV, Reynolds C, et al. Stimulation of human T-cell proliferation by specific activation of the 75-kDa tumor necrosis factor receptor. J Immunol 1993;151:4637–4641.
19. Loetscher H, Pan YC, Lahm HW, et al. Molecular cloning and expression of the human 55kd tumor necrosis factor receptor. Cell 1990;61:351–359.
20. Smith CA, Davis T, Anderson D, et al. A receptor for tumor necrosis factor defines an unusual family of cellular and viral proteins. Science 1990;248:1019–1023.
21. Peschon JJ, Torrance DS, Stocking KL, et al. TFN receptor-deficient mice reveal divergent roles for p55 and p75 in several models of inflammation. J Immunol 1998;160:943–952.
22. Browning JL, Ngam-ek A, Lawton P, et al. Lymphotoxin beta, a novel member of the TNF family that forms a heteromeric complex with lymphotoxin on the cell surface. Cell 1993;72:847–856.
23. Crowe PD, VanArsdale TL, Walter BN, et al. A lymphotoxin-beta-specific receptor [see comments]. Science 1994;264:707–710.
24. De Togni P, Goellner J, Ruddle NH, et al. Abnormal development of peripheral lymphoid organs in mice deficient in lymphotoxin [see comments]. Science 1994;264:703–707.
25. Futterer A, Mink K, Luz A, et al. The lymphotoxin beta receptor controls organogenesis and affinity maturation in peripheral lymphoid tissues. Immunity 1998;9:59–70.
26. Koni PA, Sacca R, Lawton P, et al. Distinct roles in lymphoid organogenesis for lymphotoxins alpha and beta revealed in lymphotoxin beta-deficient mice. Immunity 1997;6:491–500.
27. Peppel K, Crawford D, Beutler B. A tumor necrosis factor (TNF) receptor-IgG heavy chain chimeric protein as a bivalent antagonist of TNF activity. J Exp Med 1991;174:1483–1489.
28. Mohler KM, Torrance DS, Smith CA, et al. Soluble tumor necrosis factor (TNF) receptors are effective therapeutic agents in lethal endotoxemia and function simultaneously as both TNF carriers and TNF antagonists. J Immunol 1993;151:1548–1561.
29. Barone D, Krantz C, Lambert D, et al. Comparative analysis of the ability of etanercept and infliximab to lyse TNF-expressing cells in a complement dependent fashion. American College of Rheumatology 63rd Annual Scientific Meeting, Boston, 1999;S90. Abstract 116.
30. Wee S, Pascual M, Eason JD, et al. Biological effects and fate of a soluble, dimeric, 80-kDa tumor necrosis factor receptor in renal transplant recipients who receive OKT3 therapy. Transplantation 1997;63:570–577.
31. Old LJ. Tumor necrosis factor (TNF). Science 1985;230:630–632.
32. Beutler B, Cerami A. The biology of cachectin/TNF—a primary mediator of the host response. Annu Rev Immunol 1989;7:625–655.
33. Vassalli P. The pathophysiology of tumor necrosis factors. Annu Rev Immunol 1992;10:411–452.
34. Bazzoni F, Beutler B. The tumor necrosis factor ligand and receptor families. N Engl J Med 1996;334:1717–1725.
35. Ruddle NH. Tumor necrosis factor (TNF-alpha) and lymphotoxin (TNF-beta). Curr Opin Immunol 1992;4:327–332.
36. Zhang M, Tracey KJ. Tumor necrosis factor. In: Thomson A, ed. The cytokine handbook. 3rd ed. San Diego: Academic Press, 1998:517–548.

37. Dayer JM, Beutler B, Cerami A. Cachectin/tumor necrosis factor stimulates collagenase and prostaglandin E2 production by human synovial cells and dermal fibroblasts. J Exp Med 1985;162:2163–2168.

38. Saklatvala J. Tumour necrosis factor alpha stimulates resorption and inhibits synthesis of proteoglycan in cartilage. Nature 1986;322:547–549.

39. Feldmann M, Brennan FM, Maini RN. Role of cytokines in rheumatoid arthritis. Annu Rev Immunol 1996;14:397–440.

40. Saxne T, Palladino MA Jr, Heinegard D, et al. Detection of tumor necrosis factor alpha but not tumor necrosis factor beta in rheumatoid arthritis synovial fluid and serum. Arthritis Rheum 1998;31:1041–1045.

41. Chu CQ, Field M, Feldmann M, Maini RN. Localization of tumor necrosis factor alpha in synovial tissues and at the cartilage-pannus junction in patients with rheumatoid arthritis. Arthritis Rheum 1991;34:1125–1132.

42. Cope AP, Aderka D, Doherty M, et al. Increased levels of soluble tumor necrosis factor receptors in the sera and synovial fluid of patients with rheumatic diseases. Arthritis Rheum 1992;35:1160–1169.

43. Brennan FM, Chantry D, Jackson A, et al. Inhibitory effect of TNF alpha antibodies on synovial cell interleukin-1 production in rheumatoid arthritis. Lancet 1989;2:244–247.

44. Moser R, Schleiffenbaum B, Groscurth P, Fehr J. Interleukin 1 and tumor necrosis factor stimulate human vascular endothelial cells to promote transendothelial neutrophil passage. J Clin Invest 1989;83:444–455.

45. Keffer J, Probert L, Cazlaris H, et al. Transgenic mice expressing human tumour necrosis factor: a predictive genetic model of arthritis. Embo J 1991;10:4025–4031.

46. Thorbecke GJ, Shah R, Leu CH, et al. Involvement of endogenous tumor necrosis factor alpha and transforming growth factor beta during induction of collagen type II arthritis in mice. Proc Natl Acad Sci USA 1992;89:7375–7379.

47. Piguet PF, Grau GE, Vesin C, et al. Evolution of collagen arthritis in mice is arrested by treatment with anti-tumour necrosis factor (TNF) antibody or a recombinant soluble TNF receptor. Immunology 1992;77:510–514.

48. Williams RO, Feldmann M, Maini RN. Anti-tumor necrosis factor ameliorates joint disease in murine collagen-induced arthritis. Proc Natl Acad Sci USA 1992;89:9784–9788.

49. Wooley PH, Dutcher J, Widmer MB, Gillis S. Influence of a recombinant human soluble tumor necrosis factor receptor FC fusion protein on type II collagen-induced arthritis in mice. J Immunol 1993;151:6602–6607.

50. Williams RO, Ghrayeb J, Feldmann M, Maini RN. Successful therapy of collagen-induced arthritis with TNF receptor-IgG fusion protein and combination with anti-CD4. Immunology 1995;84:433–439.

51. Moreland LW, Baumgartner SW, Schiff MH, et al. Treatment of rheumatoid arthritis with a recombinant human tumor necrosis factor receptor (p75)-Fc fusion protein [see comments]. N Engl J Med 1997;337:141–147.

52. Moreland LW, Schiff MH, Baumgartner SW, et al. Etanercept therapy in rheumatoid arthritis. A randomized, controlled trial. Ann Intern Med 1999;130:478–486.

53. Weinblatt ME, Kremer JM, Bankhurst AD, et al. A trial of etanercept, a recombinant tumor necrosis factor receptor: Fc fusion protein, in patients with rheumatoid arthritis receiving methotrexate [see comments]. N Engl J Med 1999;340:253–259.

54. Elliott MJ, Maini RN, Feldmann M, et al. Treatment of rheumatoid arthritis with chimeric monoclonal antibodies to tumor necrosis factor alpha. Arthritis Rheum 1993;36:1681–1690.

55. Elliott MJ, Maini RN, Feldmann M, et al. Randomised double-blind comparison of chimeric monoclonal antibody to tumour necrosis factor alpha (cA2) versus placebo in rheumatoid arthritis. Lancet 1994;344:1105–1110.

56. Elliott MJ, Maini RN, Feldmann M, et al. Repeated therapy with monoclonal antibody to tumour necrosis factor alpha (cA2) in patients with rheumatoid arthritis. Lancet 1994;344:1125–1127.

57. Teng MN, Turksen K, Jacobs CA, et al. Prevention of runting and cachexia by a chimeric TNF receptor-Fc protein. Clin Immunol Immunopathol 1993;69:215–222.

58. Denis M, Guojian L, Widmer M, Cantin A. A mouse model of lung injury induced by microbial products: implication of tumor necrosis factor. Am J Respir Cell Molec Biol 1994;10:658–664.

59. Lukacs NW, Chensue SW, Strieter RM, et al. Inflammatory granuloma formation is mediated by TNF-alpha-inducible intercellular adhesion molecule-1. J Immunol 1994;152:5883–5889.

60. Clausell N, Molossi S, Sett S, Rabinovitch M. In vivo blockade of tumor necrosis factor-alpha in cholesterol-fed rabbits after cardiac transplant inhibits acute coronary artery neointimal formation. Circulation 1994;89:2768–2779.

61. Bergese SD, Huang EH, Pelletier RP, et al. Regulation of endothelial VCAM-1 expression in murine cardiac grafts. Expression of allograft endothelial VCAM-1 can be manipulated with antagonist of IFN-alpha or IL-4 and is not required for allograft rejection. Am J Pathol 1995;147:166–175.

62. Eason JD, Wee S, Kawai T, et al. Inhibition of the effects of TNF in renal allograft recipients using recombinant human dimeric tumor necrosis factor receptors. Transplantation 1995;59:300–305.

63. Xun CQ, Thompson JS, Jennings CD, et al. Effect of total body irradiation, busulfan-cyclophosphamide, or cyclophosphamide conditioning on inflammatory cytokine release and development of acute and chronic graft-versus-host disease in H-2-incompatible transplanted SCID mice. Blood 1994;83:2360–2367.

64. Hill GR, Crawford JM, Cooke KR, et al. Total body irradiation and acute graft-versus-host disease: the role of gastrointestinal damage and inflammatory cytokines. Blood 1997;90:3204–3213.

65. Farney AC, Xenos E, Sutherland DE, et al. Inhibition of pancreatic islet beta cell function by tumor necrosis factor is blocked by a soluble tumor necrosis factor receptor. Transplant Proc 1993;25:865–866.

66. Kapadia S, Torre-Amione G, Yokoyama T, Mann DL. Soluble TNF binding proteins modulate the negative inotropic properties of TNF-alpha in vitro. Am J Physiol 1995;268:H517–H525.

67. Giroir BP, Horton JW, White DJ, et al. Inhibition of tumor necrosis factor prevents myocardial dysfunction during burn shock. Am J Physiol 1994;267:H118–H124.

68. Rau R, Herborn G, Karger T, Werdier D. Retardation of radiologic progression in rheumatoid arthritis with methotrexate therapy. A controlled study [see comments]. Arthritis Rheum 1991;34:1236–1244.

69. Finck B, Martin R, Fleischmann R, et al. A phase III trial of etanercept vs. methotrexate (MTX) in early rheumatoid arthritis (Enbrel ERA trial). American College of Rheumatology 63rd Annual Scientific Meeting, Boston, 1999. Abstract.

70. Felson DT, Anderson JJ, Boers M, et al. American College of Rheumatology. Preliminary definition of improvement in rheumatoid arthritis [see comments]. Arthritis Rheum 1995; 38:727–735.

71. Lovell DJ, Gianni EH, Whitmore JB, et al. Safety and efficacy of tumor necrosis factor receptor p75 Fc fusion protein (TNFR:Fc; ENBREL™) in polyarticular course juvenile rheumatoid arthritis. American College of Rheumatology 62nd National Meeting, San Diego, 1998:S130. Abstract 584.

72. Lovell DJ, Giannini EH, Lange M, et al. Safety and efficacy of Enbrel (etanercept) in the extended treatment of polyarticular course JRA. American College of Rheumatology Annual Scientific Meeting, Boston, 1999. Abstract.

73. Giannini EH, Ruperto N, Ravelli A, et al. Preliminary definition of improvement in juvenile arthritis [see comments]. Arthritis Rheum 1997;40:1202–1209.

74. Moreland LW, Baumgartner SW, Tindall EA, et al. Long-term safety and efficacy of etanercept (ENBREL) in DMARD refractory rheumatoid arthritis (RA). European League against Rheumatism, 1999.

75. Mease P, Goffe B, Metz J, Vanderstoep A. Enbrel (etanercept) in patients with psoriatric arthritis and psoriasis. Arthritis Rheum 1999;42:1835. Abstract.

76. Stone JH, Hellmann DB, Uhlfelder ML, et al. Etanercept in Wegener's granulomatosis (WG): results of an open-label trial. Arthritis Rheum 1999;42:1467. Abstract.

77. Present DH, Rutgeerts P, Targan S, et al. Infliximab for the treatment of fistulas in patients with Crohn's disease. N Engl J Med 1999;340:1398–1405.

78. Levine B, Kalman J, Mayer L, et al. Elevated circulating levels of tumor necrosis factor in severe chronic heart failure. N Engl J Med 1990;323:236–241.

79. McMurray J, Abdullah I, Dargie HJ, Shapiro D. Increased concentrations of tumour necrosis factor in "cachectic" patients with severe chronic heart failure. Br Heart J 1991;66: 356–358.

80. Matsumori A, Yamada T, Suzuki H, et al. Increased circulating cytokines in patients with myocarditis and cardiomyopathy. Br Heart J 1994;72:561–566.

81. Katz SD, Rao R, Berman JW, et al. Pathophysiological correlates of increased serum tumor necrosis factor in patients with congestive heart failure. Relation to nitric oxide-dependent vasodilation in the forearm circulation. Circulation 1994;90:12–16.

82. Torre-Amione G, Kapadia S, Benedict C, et al. Proinflammatory cytokine levels in patients with depressed left ventricular ejection fraction: a report from the Studies of Left Ventricular Dysfunction (SOLVD). J Am Coll Cardiol 1996;27:1201–1206.

83. Bozkurt B, Torre-Amione G, Soran OZ, et al. Results of a multidose phase I trial with tumor necrosis factor receptor (p75) fusion protein (etanercept) in patients with heart failure. J Am Coll Cardiol 1999;33(suppl A):184A–185A. Abstract.

Chapter 19

Intravenous Immunoglobulin Therapy

Francisco A. Bonilla
Raif S. Geha

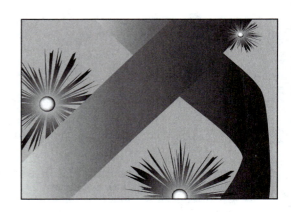

The use of antibodies in the prophylaxis and treatment of infections began in 1890 when von Behring and Kitasato in Germany demonstrated the effects of immune serum in the prevention of tetanus and diphtheria. In fact, the first Nobel Prize in Medicine and Physiology was awarded to von Behring for this work. Within a short time, antisera against snake venoms were produced. Crude attempts to purify antibodies to measles were made by McKhann and Chu, who fractionated globulins from placenta with ammonium sulfate. The historic observations of Tiselius and Kabat, in 1939, that the antibodies of the plasma were in the gamma globulin fraction, prepared the way for Edwin J. Cohn's massive effort during World War II to fractionate plasma on a vast scale. Cohn's fraction II is almost pure immunoglobulin G (IgG), and is still used today as the starting material for the manufacture of gamma globulin. Early attempts to administer this material by the intravenous route led to several fatalities at the Peter Bent Brigham Hospital in Boston. It became clear that these early preparations of gamma globulin could be administered safely only by intramuscular injection (intramuscular immunoglobulin, or IMIG). Barandun, Hassig, and Isliker at the Swiss Red Cross demonstrated that the untoward effects of intravenous administration of gamma globulin could be circumvented by removing aggregates of gamma globulin from the preparation. Over the following decade, many attempts were made to render gamma globulin aggregate free by treatment with acid (pH 4), or by the use of proteolytic enzymes. Several methods have now been established for the preparation of immunoglobulin for intravenous administration (IVIG), and a variety of these products have been approved by the Food and Drug Administration (FDA) for clinical use in the United States (Table 19-1), and several more are in use worldwide.

Characteristics of Immunoglobulin Preparations

Immunoglobulin can be administered by intramuscular, subcutaneous, or intravenous routes, and has also been given orally. Preparations intended solely for intramuscular or subcutaneous injection must not be given intravenously, although IVIG may be administered subcutaneously. IMIG has been available for more than 40 years. IMIG preparations do not transmit viral infections, such as hepatitis B, hepatitis C, or human immunodeficiency virus

(HIV). However, the injections are painful, it is difficult to increase serum IgG levels by more than 200 mg/dL, and the risk of a severe adverse reaction is significant (1). The introduction of IVIG has overcome these problems. Such preparations are well tolerated and effective in most patients, and adverse reactions are so infrequent that administration of IVIG at home is a safe and acceptable form of therapy. Subcutaneous administration of IMIG and IVIG is safe (2,3), and is gaining acceptance in Europe because of reduced cost and convenience, although the total dose infused is smaller in comparison with intravenous administration, and doses must be more frequent to achieve similar blood levels.

Intravenous Immunoglobulin Preparations

Intravenous infusion is the preferred route of administration of immunoglobulin for patients. Several different preparations of IVIG have been approved for use in the United States (see Table 19-1). All are well tolerated and effective but show individual differences in immunoglobulin subclass distribution and antibody content (4,5). All IVIG preparations are isolated initially from normal plasma by the Cohn alcohol fractionation method or a modification of it. The World Health Organization has established the following production criteria: each lot of IVIG should be derived from plasma pooled from at least 1000 donors; it should contain at least 90% intact IgG, with the subclasses present in normal ratios; its IgG molecules should maintain biologic activity, such as complement fixation; it should be free of prekallikrein activator, kinins, plasmin, and preservatives; and it should be free of infectious agents (6). All plasma donations are now screened for hepatitis B surface antigen (HBsAg) and for antibodies to human immunodeficiency virus (HIV) and hepatitis C virus (HCV). FDA approval of an IVIG product in the United States requires minimum titers against diphtheria, hepatitis B (HBV), measles, and polio viruses.

Mechanisms of Action of IVIG

IVIG exerts two major modes of action: antigen-specific activity and immunomodulation. The proposed mechanisms of the therapeutic effects of IVIG administration are listed in Table 19-2. It is highly probable that several of these mechanisms are operating in concert in any given clinical situation.

Table 19-1. IVIG Preparations Approved for Use in the United States

Name	Preparation[a]	Form	Stabilizer
Gamimune-N, 5%	Diafiltration, pH 4.0, solvent/detergent	Liquid, 5%	Maltose
Gaminune-N, 10%	Diafiltration, pH 4.0, solvent/detergent	Liquid, 10%	Glycine
Gammagard-S/D	Ultrafiltration, ion-exchange chromatography, solvent/detergent	Lyophilized, 5%, 10%	Albumin, glycine, glucose, PEG[b]
Gammar-P I.V.	Pasteurization	Lyophilized, 5%	Albumin, sucrose
IVEEGAM	Trypsin digestion, PEG[b], precipitation	Lyophilized, 5%	Glucose
Panglobulin	Ultrafiltration	Lyophilized, 3%, 6%, 9%, 12%	Sucrose
Polygam S/D	Ultrafiltration, ion-exchange chromatography, solvent/detergent	Lyophilized, 5%, 10%	Albumin, glycine, glucose, PEG[b]
Sandoglobulin	pH 4, pepsin digestion	Lyophilized, 3%, 6%, 9%, 12%	Sucrose
Venoglobulin-S, 5%, 10%	Ion-exchange chromatography, PEG[b] precipitation, solvent/detergent	Lyophilized, 5%, 10%	Sorbitol

[a] All preparations begin with cold ethanol fractionation.
[b] Polyethylene glycol.
SOURCE: *Physicians' Desk Reference* (209).

Table 19-2. Proposed Mechanisms of the Therapeutic Effects of IVIG

Antigen-specific Effects

Neutralization of toxins
Neutralization of viruses
Opsonization of bacteria

Immunomodulatory Effects

Alterations in the populations of lymphocytes in the circulation and in lymphoid tissues
Inhibition of lymphocyte (and other leukocyte) activation as determined by proliferation, cytokine production, or expression of activation markers (e.g., adhesion molecules), mediated by:
　IVIG interaction with cell surface proteins
　IVIG binding to cytokines
FcγR blockade
Interaction with the complement pathways
Idiotype network regulation

Antigen-Specific Activity of IVIG

IVIG is prepared from plasma pools collected from thousands of donors. It is estimated that it contains ten million antibody specificities. IVIG has been shown to contain measurable antibody titers against a variety of bacteria and viruses (Table 19-3), as well as against bacterial toxins including exotoxins and endotoxins. As mentioned above, minimum titers against diphtheria toxin, measles, HBV, and polio are required for product approval in the United States. The levels of antibodies binding to other viruses and bacteria show great variability from one product to another, and even between lots from the same manufacturer. This presumably results from the uniqueness of a particular donor pool at one point in time that constitutes each lot of IVIG.

Antibodies in IVIG may opsonize infectious organisms, and the resulting immune complexes fix complement and are readily phagocytosed following binding to IgG Fc receptors (FcγR) and complement receptors on phagocytic cells. In addition, antibodies in IVIG neutralize viruses and toxins, preventing their attachment to cellular receptors. These properties underlie the therapeutic value of IVIG in primary and secondary antibody deficiency syndromes, in neonatal sepsis, and possibly in Kawasaki disease (see below).

Immunomodulatory Activity of IVIG

The beneficial effects of IVIG in several autoimmune and inflammatory diseases have spurred a flurry of investigation into the potential immunomodulatory activity of IVIG. The information available to date suggests multiple actions of IVIG on the immune system.

Alterations in Circulating Lymphocytes and Inhibition of T- and B-Cell Activation

Changes in the relative proportions of lymphocyte subsets during IVIG therapy have been reported. One study found a mean 30% reduction in total lymphocytes, predominantly T cells, in patients receiving high-dose infusions (2 g/kg) (7). Counts slowly returned to baseline values over 30 days. Others have observed a reduction in the CD4/CD8 T cell ratio owing to an increase in the number of CD8 cells (8). Lymphocytes in the circulation constitute only about 2% of the total in the body. Although it has not been studied, it is possible, or even likely, that IVIG may induce significant changes in patterns of lymphocyte recirculation and in the makeup of various secondary lymphoid tissues.

IVIG may inhibit T-cell proliferation and interleukin-2 (IL-2) receptor (IL-2R) expression in response to mitogens, anti-CD3 antibody, superantigens and antigens, and agents that bypass surface receptor signaling such as phorbol ester (PMA) with a

Table 19-3. Antibody Activities in IVIG

Bacteria	Viruses
Corynebacterium diphtheriae toxin	Cytomegalovirus (CMV)
Clostridium tetani toxin	Epstein-Barr virus (EBV)
Escherichia coli	Hepatitis A virus (HAV)
Hemophilus influenzae type B (HIB)	Hepatitis B virus (HBV)
Pseudomonas aeruginosa	Measles virus
Salmonella minnesota	Parainfluenza virus
Staphylococcus epidermidis	Polio virus
Streptococcus pneumoniae	Respiratory syncytial virus (RSV)
Group B streptococcus	Rubella virus
	Varicella/Zoster virus (VZV)

This list includes specificities detected with varying degrees of consistency among different preparations and lots of IVIG. Many more specificities may be found in IVIG; their detectability depends on the degree to which they are generally represented in the plasma donor pool. See text for additional discussion.

calcium ionophore (ionomycin) (9). More strikingly, IVIG inhibits immunoglobulin production by B cells in vitro. This has been shown to depend on FcγR binding and to correlate with inhibition of IL-6 production (10).

One group has reported that T cells expressing TCR Vβ regions characteristically stimulated by the superantigen staphylococcal enterotoxin B (SEB) are selectively expanded in cultures after the addition of IVIG (11). As shown in other studies, IVIG caused a general inhibition of proliferation. However, the relative proportions of Vβ3$^+$ and Vβ17$^+$ cells increased threefold. This finding might appear to argue against a role for IVIG in inhibiting the activity of superantigen exotoxins, as has been suggested for Kawasaki disease (12) (see below). However, the functional state of the Vβ3$^+$ and Vβ17$^+$ cells was not addressed.

Some have reported that ingredients acting as stabilizers in IVIG preparations may, in fact, have therapeutically important immunomodulatory effects (13). For example, sucrose and maltose were found to provide partial (20% to 30%) inhibition of in vitro proliferative responses of PBMC to mitogenic stimuli (lectins, anti-CD3 antibody, PMA plus ionomycin). The concentrations used were similar to those occurring in blood after IVIG administration.

Antibodies to Cytokines

Antibodies to IL-1 and to tumor necrosis factor (TNF) are found in pooled IgG. However, it is unlikely that the levels of these antibodies achieved following even large doses of IVIG play a significant role in the immunomodulatory effect of IVIG (14). IVIG also contains antibodies that bind interferon-γ (IFN-γ) and can inhibit proliferation in mixed lymphocyte culture in vitro (15). This inhibition is abrogated by the addition of exogenous IFN-γ. Again, the relevance of this finding with respect to the in vivo action of IVIG is not known.

Alteration of Cytokine Production and Expression of Adhesion Molecules

In vitro, IVIG inhibits IL-2, IL-3, IL-4, and IL-5 production by T cells stimulated by PMA and ionomycin, or via the T-cell receptor (TCR) (16). In a similar study using exclusively accessory cell-independent stimuli (immobilized anti-CD3 antibody, or PMA plus ionomycin), IVIG was found to cause inhibition of T-cell cytokine secretion only in the presence of accessory cells (17). This suggests that IVIG in some way enables or facilitates an inhibitory interaction of accessory cells with T cells.

Indeed, several studies have shown alterations in cytokine release from monocytes and macrophages exposed to IVIG. For example, IVIG inhibits production of IL-1 TNF and macrophages stimulated by lipopolysaccharide (17a). This inhibition has been shown to depend on FcγR binding. In contrast, IL-8 production is increased by IVIG in vitro (16). Furthermore, IVIG induces release of IL-1 receptor antagonist (IL-1Ra) from macrophages (14). However, the in vivo significance of IL-1Ra release is in question, because the levels of serum IL-1Ra are barely measurable and are below baseline levels already present in the sera of patients with inflammatory and autoimmune diseases treated with IVIG.

Cultured endothelial cells exposed to TNF or IL-1β proliferate and express adhesion molecules and produce cytokines and chemokines. The addition of IVIG to this system inhibits the generation of mRNA for intercellular adhesion molecule-1 (ICAM-1), vascular cell adhesion molecule-1 (VCAM-1), macrophage CSF (M-CSF), monocyte chemoattractant protein-1 (MCP-1), and IL-6 (19).

Perhaps more clinically relevant than the above mentioned in vitro effects, administration of IVIG to patients with Kawasaki disease results in reduction of circulating levels of IL-1, TNF, and IFN-γ (20). Similarly, M-CSF and IL-6 levels are reduced in a subset of patients having elevated levels and receiving high-dose IVIG for the treatment of immune thrombocytopenic purpura (ITP) (21). Changes in markers of monocyte/macrophage activity have also been observed in vivo. Increases in serum neopterin levels are closely correlated with in vitro suppression of peripheral blood mononuclear cell (PBMC) responses to mitogens and with decreases in phagocytic cell respiratory burst induced by zymosan (8).

Antibodies to Cell Surface Antigens

Antibodies present in IVIG may react with a variety of surface antigens on B and T cells and on other cell types. Antibodies binding the T-cell receptor (TCR) may inhibit T-cell (and, indirectly, B-cell) activation in vitro (22,23). Inhibition of T-cell proliferation in mixed lymphocyte culture has been ascribed to antibodies interacting with uncharacterized membrane glycoproteins (24). Antibodies interacting with human leukocyte antigen (HLA) class I molecules have been implicated in the suppression of specific T-cell cytotoxicity (25). IVIG induces apoptosis via the CD95 (Fas, APO-1) pathway in vitro in human leukemic lymphoid and monocytic cell lines, as well as in activated tonsillar B cells (26). This study found direct Fas-binding activity in IVIG, as did a group reporting the benefit of IVIG in toxic epidermal necrolysis (see below).

FcγR Blockade

FcγRs are expressed on a variety of cell types. High-affinity FcγRI (CD64) is expressed on monocytes and macrophages; intermediate-affinity FcγRII (CD32) is expressed on monocytes, macrophages, and B cells; and low-affinity FcγRIII (CD16) is expressed on granulocytes and NK cells. There is strong evidence to suggest that in vivo administration of IVIG inhibits the binding of antibody-coated platelets to phagocytic cells by means of FcγR blockade. Indeed, IVIG increases the survival of anti-Rh (D) antibody-coated red cells (27), and an anti-FcγR antibody has been shown to be effective in ITP (28) (see below).

Increased Rate of IgG Catabolism

Evidence is growing that IgG is catabolized mainly (if not exclusively) by vascular endothelial cells (ECs), which take it up from the circulation by pinocytosis (29). Within the phagosome of the EC, IgG binds to a receptor called the "neonatal" FcR, or FcRn, because this same receptor mediates transfer of IgG from the gut lumen of the newborn into the circulation. Within the EC phagosome, FcRn protects IgG from degradation and mediates its recycling to the cell surface, where it is re-released into the circulation. Unbound IgG remains within the EC and is digested by proteases. As the level of IgG in serum rises, this receptor system becomes increasingly saturated, and the fractional catabolic rate of IgG increases accordingly. Stated in another way, the serum half-life of IgG falls as its concentration in serum rises.

Depending on the dose and frequency, IVIG infusions can greatly increase the total amount of IgG in the body. For example, 0.4 gm/kg daily for five days will roughly triple the body's total content of IgG, and the rate of catabolism will also triple (30). The infused IVIG now dilutes any pathogenic antibody and increases its rate of destruction. Assuming continued production of a pathogenic antibody at the same rate, its level in the circulation will be reduced by about 40% after 2 weeks, and by about 50% after 4 weeks. Soon thereafter, the balance will begin to shift, and the fraction of endogenous IgG will rise again without further addition of exogenous IVIG.

Some have proposed that this mass effect of dilution and increased catabolism of endogenous Ig is an important component of the therapeutic effect of IVIG (30,31). As others have

pointed out (30), this mechanism certainly cannot account for the sometimes rapid decreases of two to three orders of magnitude that have been observed for some autoantibodies after IVIG administration (32), as well as for persistent decreases in autoantibody production lasting months after a course of IVIG therapy. It is possible that some threshold effects for tissue damage by pathogenic autoantibodies could be significantly altered by changes of the magnitudes described above. Only further study will clarify the role of increased IgG catabolism in the benefit of IVIG.

Interaction with Complement Pathways

Several investigators have reported that IVIG can activate complement, and that it may also interact with activated complement components. One group reported that the complement-activating property resided predominantly in the monomeric fraction of IVIG, with less activity in multimers and dimers (33). These authors found that IVIG protected against complement-mediated red blood cell (RBC) lysis by shifting complement activation from the surface to the fluid phase, and that administration of IVIG resulted in increases in circulating markers of complement activation (C3bc, Bb, and C5a) in vivo (34).

Several studies have shown that IVIG can prevent complement binding to tissues. A single dose of IVIG can prevent shock and death in guinea pigs injected with Forssman antiserum, even though serum complement levels are unchanged (35). IVIG blocks complement deposition leading to hyperacute rejection of porcine hearts transplanted into baboons (36). IVIG has also been shown to inhibit deposition of complement on endomysial capillaries in patients with dermatomyositis (37). Some have shown that IVIG can inhibit C3 binding to sensitized human erythrocytes and protect them from phagocytosis (38). However, not all studies uniformly show RBC-protective complement-related effects of IVIG. One group reported that dimeric and multimeric fractions of IVIG bound complement and could interact with RBC CR1, leading to erythrophagocytosis in vitro; monomeric IgG was inactive (39).

Idiotype–Anti-Idiotype Interactions

Deletion of autoreactive T cells occurs in the thymus, and failure of this deletion step may lead to the appearance in the periphery of mature autoreactive T-cell clones with potential to cause disease. "Backup" mechanisms of anergy and suppression may be called into play in order to prevent the activation and expansion of autoreactive T cells. Among the mechanisms that may regulate autoreactivity is the ability of lymphocytes and antibodies to interact with V regions on the antigen receptors of other lymphocytes and thereby influence humoral and cell-mediated immune responses. This V region– (idiotype-) determined network prevents autoantibody production (or antiself cellular responses) by suppressing activation and expansion of autoreactive clones. Autoantibodies are one of the hallmarks of autoimmune diseases, and their titers generally correlate well with disease activity. They may arise from disruption of network regulation, and its restoration may lead to decreased autoantibody levels and improvement in disease symptoms.

Because 1 g of IVIG contains 4×10^{18} IgG molecules capable of recognizing more than 10 million antigenic determinants, it is likely that there are many anti-idiotypes with the potential to regulate autoantibody production. The finding that pooled IgG contains up to 40% dimers in which the antigen-binding sites are in contact (40) supports the notion that anti-idiotypes are present and may play a role in the beneficial effects of IgG in autoimmune disorders. In this regard, the presence in IVIG of anti-idiotypic antibodies to factor VIII inhibitors, anti-neutrophil cytoplasmic antibodies (ANCA), anti-Smith (anti-Sm) antigen, and other autoantibodies has been demonstrated (41–44).

Adverse Effects of Intravenous Immunoglobulin

Generalized Reactions

Nonspecific Generalized Reactions
Systemic reactions occurring independently of specific hypersensitivity to a component of an IVIG preparation may arise by several mechanisms. It is likely that characteristics of the recipient, such as the underlying disease, the presence and type of intercurrent infectious illness, and the properties of specific IVIG preparations, may all interact in the pathogenesis of these adverse reactions.

IVIG contains varying amounts of aggregated immunoglobulin molecules and these may cause complement activation (see above). Infused IVIG may interact with (infectious) antigens in the recipient, leading to immune complex–mediated phenomena. Unknown serum-derived vaso- or hemodynamically active molecules may exist as contaminants in IVIG, and may be responsible for some adverse effects. Ingredients added during the manufacturing process may also contribute. One recent study found elevated blood levels of IL-6 and thromboxane in adults experiencing generalized symptoms during rapid infusion (0.08 mL/kg/min, or 4 mg/kg/min) of IVIG (45). Others have reported that at therapeutically relevant concentrations in vitro, IVIG induces FcγRII-dependent degranulation of neutrophils (46).

The incidence of generalized reactions occurring during and/or after the administration of IVIG is reported to be in the range of 1% to 15% (usually less than 5%), and may be mild, moderate, or severe (47). Mild reactions usually begin within 30 minutes of the start of the infusion and are characterized by back pain, flushing, chills, and myalgia. Mild reactions rarely require the infusion to be discontinued, but the rate of administration should be slowed until symptoms have subsided. Pretreatment prophylaxis with aspirin, or nonsteroidal anti-inflammatory drugs (NSAIDs) and antihistamines, is often sufficient. If necessary, a dose of hydrocortisone or other glucocorticoid may be added to the regimen.

Moderate reactions, such as bronchospasm, wheezing, vomiting, and progressive "mild" symptoms unresponsive to slowing of the infusion, require that the infusion be stopped and that appropriate emergency treatment be instituted. Nonanaphylactic reactions to IVIG are usually rate-related, and are observed most often in newly treated patients or in those with active infections. The frequency of reactions falls once infections have been treated with antibiotics and IVIG replacement. Some patients have delayed symptoms, particularly fatigue and headaches, within 24 hours following an infusion. These symptoms are usually mild, but can last for several hours or sometimes for several days.

Hypersensitivity and Anaphylactic Reactions
True anaphylactic reactions to IVIG are rare (48). Signs and symptoms begin seconds to minutes after infusion is begun and typically consist of flushing, facial swelling, dyspnea, and hypotension. Such reactions are most commonly attributable to antibodies to IgA in patients with severe IgA deficiency (49). These antibodies are usually of the IgG class (50), although IgM and IgE anti-IgA antibodies have also been reported (49). In these patients, IVIG preparations low in IgA may be administered safely (51).

Organ-Specific Adverse Effects

Hemolytic Anemia
Cases of acute Coombs-positive hemolytic anemia mediated by antibodies to blood group antigens have been reported during IVIG treatment (52,53). In these instances, hemolysis by IVIG could be demonstrated. Decreased haptoglobin levels and mild reticulocytosis have been observed in normal volunteers receiving IVIG, but without a change in hemoglobin level, suggesting that clinically insignificant, well-compensated hemolysis occurs during IVIG treatment (54). One study of 42 patients identified 12 who had developed passive sensitization to RBC antigens, and 11 who had hemolysis sufficient to lower hemoglobin by 1 g/dL (55). The reason for this finding of such a high rate of significant hemolysis in this study is unclear.

Neurological Complications
Headache is not uncommonly reported by patients receiving IVIG; this symptom is effectively treated by analgesics and/or antihistamines. Acute aseptic meningitis has been reported as a rare cause of recurrent severe IVIG-associated headaches (56–58). The mechanism of this reaction remains unknown. Cases of recurrent migraine after IVIG therapy have also been described. These patients have presented with typical migraine symptoms, and have been treated successfully with prophylactic propranolol (59) or with sumatriptan or dihydroergotamine mesylate (60).

Renal Complications
A recent analysis of 22 reports involving 52 patients experiencing renal failure following administration of IVIG showed that 58% had known preexisting renal insufficiency (61). In the four fatalities resulting from complications of kidney dysfunction, various forms of renal injury were observed. These included osmotic injury, tubular vacuolization, tubulointerstitial infiltrates,

and cryoglobulin deposition. Renal functional status should be determined wherever the potential for compromise exists. Reduced doses of IVIG and slow infusions should be used initially in patients with renal impairment, with monitoring of function after infusion.

Cardiovascular Compromise

Seriously ill patients with compromised cardiac function, and fluid-restricted patients, may be at increased risk of cardiac complications manifested by elevated blood pressure and/or cardiac failure. The kallikrein activity of some IVIG preparations has been incriminated in these adverse vasomotor reactions. Dysrhythmias have also been observed in two children treated for ITP with IVIG (62). Both children had previous histories of rhythm disturbances (supraventricular tachycardia, and long QT syndrome). Children or adults with preexisting electrophysiologic abnormalities may be at increased risk of cardiac complications of IVIG administration, but further study is required.

Thrombotic/Veno-Occlusive Events

Four cases of fatal stroke in elderly patients (62 to 83 years old) all receiving IVIG for ITP have been reported (63,64). The rise in platelet count during IVIG treatment could have played a role in these thrombotic events. However, few severe thrombotic episodes have been observed with IVIG therapy overall, and the link between the treatment and these otherwise frequent events in old and severely ill patients is not clear.

A hyperviscosity syndrome with CNS symptoms was observed in an HIV-infected child with very high serum IgG levels (65). This syndrome responded to slowing of the infusion rate. Hyperviscosity with central retinal vein occlusion has also been observed with IVIG administration (66). The rise in viscosity that may occur in some patients after IVIG therapy could impair blood flow and might be sufficient to cause myocardial or cerebral ischemia or infarction in predisposed patients, especially the elderly.

Miscellaneous Side Effects

Sporadic case reports of many side effects of IVIG are in the literature. Alopecia (67), hypothermia (68), arthritis (69), and other symptoms have been observed after infusion of IVIG. The link between IVIG administration and the specific complication is often unclear, and no pathogenetic explanation can be given. These complications may represent idiosyncratic responses.

Disease Transmission by IVIG

Several mechanisms operate in concert to make IVIG one of the safest human blood-derived products with respect to the transmission of infectious disease. First, potential plasma donors are screened for risk factors for infection with blood-borne pathogens such as intravenous drug use, history of blood transfusions, etc. Donated plasma is then screened for the presence of antibodies to HIV-1 and -2, HCV, and HBsAg. The same testing is applied to pooled plasma prior to processing. During IgG

purification, many viruses segregate preferentially in waste fractions. The product itself is then subjected to conditions that inactivate many different viruses. Finally, antibodies in IVIG may neutralize viruses present in the final product.

The cold-ethanol fractionation process developed by Cohn substantially reduces the amount of HBV present in plasma products, and inactivates HIV. Experiments in which donor plasma was spiked with HIV-1 showed that the Cohn process reduced the level of virus to 10^{-15} of the initial dose (70). There have been no reports of HIV transmission through IVIG, even though batches of IVIG were unintentionally prepared from plasma of HIV-infected donors in the early 1980s.

Prior to screening for HBsAg, there were several cases of HBV transmission, probably resulting from suboptimal fractionation procedures using plasma from infected donors. HBsAg has not been found in the Cohn fraction of plasma used to make IVIG, and no cases of hepatitis B have occurred with the use of IVIG in the United States. However, batches of IVIG have been associated with outbreaks of severe hepatitis C (71,72). In a recent outbreak of hepatitis C (approximately 115 cases) associated with particular lots of a single IVIG preparation, HCV transmission may have occurred because hepatitis C antibody–positive donors were *excluded* by a very sensitive assay. As a result, there were no longer hepatitis C–neutralizing antibodies present in the final preparation (73–75). This allowed HCV that entered the plasma pool from antibody-negative donors to persist in the final product in an infective form.

Additional steps in the production of IVIG have been incorporated for the purpose of viral inactivation. These procedures include adjustment to pH 4, the use of propionic acid, enzymatic treatment, pasteurization, and treatment with solvent/detergent. These measures, particularly solvent/detergent treatment, inactivate lipid-enveloped viruses including HCV, and greatly enhance the safety of IVIG with respect to viral transmission. All IVIG preparations currently approved for use in the United States have demonstrated inactivation of HCV. The possibility that nonenveloped viruses, such as parvovirus, may escape inactivation must be kept in mind. To date, there is no evidence that these agents are transmitted. The presence of high antibody titers in IVIG against such viruses may be critical in preventing infection.

In the United Kingdom, and elsewhere, there has recently arisen great concern regarding the potential for transmission of prion agents in human blood products. These fears have been spurred by the finding that some people who had eaten beef from cows that later developed bovine spongiform encephalopathy (BSE) developed "new variant" Creutzfeldt-Jakob disease (nvCJD) (76). These diseases are caused by the same agent (77,78). Some of these individuals, as well as individuals with "sporadic" CJD (spCJD), had been regular blood donors. At present, there is no method capable of detecting small amounts of potentially infectious prion agents in blood.

There are only two unconfirmed case reports of suspected transmission of CJD by a blood product (albumin) in the medical literature. In one case, the diagnosis in the donor was established on clinical grounds only, without biopsy or genetic analysis of prion protein (PrP^CJD) (79). In the second case, the occurrence of CJD in the recipient could not be definitively linked to that in the donor (80). It is interesting to note that in the few animal studies of the infectivity of various blood products with respect to prion agents, Cohn fraction V (albumin) has the least (81). To date, there are no established cases of human transmission of prion agents by whole blood, blood cells, plasma, or any plasma-derived product.

Clinical Uses of Intravenous Immunoglobulin

IVIG for Primary Antibody Deficiency

The clearest indication for immunoglobulin replacement therapy is primary antibody deficiency (82). Antibody deficiencies range from virtually complete absence of all major immunoglobulin classes to more selective decreases. Not all require treatment with gamma globulin, since they vary in their clinical severity. The more classic forms of primary antibody deficiency are X-linked agammaglobulinemia (XLA), common variable immunodeficiency (CVID), and the hyper-IgM syndrome. These conditions uniformly require replacement therapy. Transient hypogammaglobulinemia of infancy (THI) is relatively common, and patients with specific antibody defects with or without associated IgG subclass deficiency are increasingly recognized. These two conditions, particularly THI, have a high likelihood of benefiting from prophylactic antibiotics, but a sizable proportion of patients with antibody defects require replacement therapy. Indeed, recurrent infection associated with impaired antibody production, following test immunization if necessary, and not merely a low level of an immunoglobulin isotype, is the key indication for replacement therapy. Because almost all antigen-specific antibody responses are T cell dependent, patients with primary T-cell immunodeficiency diseases, such as severe combined immunodeficiency, Wiskott-Aldrich syndrome, and ataxia-telangiectasia, also require immunoglobulin replacement.

The availability of immunoglobulin has greatly reduced the morbidity due to bacterial infections in patients with severe antibody deficiency (83,84). The efficacy of IVIG in IgG subclass deficiencies is more debatable. For significant IgG1 and/or IgG2 deficiency, coupled with distinct antibody deficits, the use of IVIG is justified. For IgG3 and IgG4 deficiency, the data are less clear because no placebo-controlled trials have been published. One open trial of IVIG in 12 patients with IgG3 subclass deficiency who failed to respond to antibiotic prophylaxis found significant reductions in the frequency of acute sinusitis and otitis media (85).

Dosage

Studies in patients with agammaglobulinemia (serum IgG <100 mg/mL) have clearly established that IVIG is superior to IMIG when given at the same dosage of 100 mg/kg/month (84). The efficacy of high-dose (600 mg/kg) versus low-dose

(200 mg/kg) replacement regimens was also clear in a study comparing subjective criteria such as chest x-rays, pulmonary function, and rates of major and minor infections (86). Furthermore, maintenance of a trough serum IgG level greater than 500 mg/dL appeared to be of clinical benefit. The dose of IVIG needed to keep a patient symptom free depends on the severity of the antibody defect and the catabolic rate of the infused IVIG. Postinfusion serum IgG levels increase by about 225 mg/dL for each 100 mg/kg infused. About half the IgG is redistributed to the extravascular compartment during the first 3 to 5 days after intravenous infusion. Elimination of IgG depends on the serum concentration. In normal individuals, the half-life of IgG is 18 to 23 days. The half-life of serum IgG is variable in patients with antibody deficiency, but most IVIG preparations show half-lives of 30 to 40 days. Most practitioners aim to maintain trough IgG levels above 500 mg/dL. This is achieved in most patients by the administration of about 400–500 mg/kg, usually at intervals of 2 to 4 weeks (48). Adjustment of both the dose and the infusion interval is empirical.

Adverse Reactions

Adverse reactions are not uncommon in antibody-deficient patients during the first few infusions. These infusions should be given slowly and under medical supervision (48). The starting rates are 0.01–0.02 mL/kg/min, with progressive increases of up to 0.1 mL/kg/min. This results in a maximal rate of 150–300 mg/kg/h. Selected patients can tolerate even higher infusion rates (87). Newer IVIG preparations are tolerated much better than first-generation preparations.

Monitoring of IVIG Therapy

The benefits of IVIG therapy can take up to 4 months to become apparent. Serum IgG should be checked at regular intervals prior to infusion to ensure that target levels of trough serum IgG (about 500–600 mg/dL) are maintained or exceeded. In children, it is important to ensure that the dose is adjusted as they grow. Liver function, especially serum transaminase levels, should be measured at about 3-month intervals to exclude subclinical, passively transmitted hepatitis (48). The lot numbers of preparations infused must be recorded. Patients should be evaluated by their physicians about every 6 months.

Personal symptom diaries are recommended to record the number, duration, site, and severity of infections, antibiotic usage, symptoms possibly related to IVIG infusion, and other relevant clinical information. Chronic lung disease is the most common, serious, and potentially fatal complication of primary antibody deficiency. Regular measurement of pulmonary function and structure is important in determining the efficacy of IVIG therapy.

Home Therapy

Infusion of IVIG in the patient's home is an increasingly accepted alternative to hospitalization, because IVIG replacement is often a life-long requirement. Selection of patients is important. They must have good venous access, have received at least one infusion in a hospital or clinic setting without a significant reaction, and be well motivated. The wide availability of providers of home intravenous infusion therapy is a boon to these patients, who are thus able to receive IVIG with the greatest convenience and at lower cost.

IVIG for Secondary Antibody Deficiency

Chronic Lymphocytic Leukemia (CLL)
The most common complication of chronic lymphocytic leukemia (CLL) is infection. It is the cause of death in up to 57% of patients (88). Hypogammaglobulinemia is more frequent in long-term survivors, in patients with diffuse bone marrow infiltration, and in the higher clinical stage groups (stages III and IV of the Rai staging system). Higher values of serum β2-microglobulin at the time of diagnosis correlate with a rapid development of hypogammaglobulinemia. The efficacy of IVIG in the prevention of infection in CLL was shown in two randomized, controlled, double-blind clinical trials over 1 year in patients with B-CLL and hypogammaglobulinemia, or a history of one or more serious infections (89). In one study the patients in the IVIG-treated group had significantly fewer bacterial infections than those in the placebo group and remained free of serious bacterial infections for longer periods after entering the study. No difference was noted between IVIG doses of 250 mg/kg and 500 mg/kg with respect to the incidence of viral or fungal infections. IgG levels were helpful for predicting infections, because they tended to occur when the serum IgG level was below 640 mg/dL, although there were patients with low levels who did not get infections. Therefore, other factors may be of importance as indicators of infection risk, such as neutrophil count, functional ability, and number of NK cells (90). Furthermore, as is the case for primary antibody deficiency, the absence of specific antibodies is likely to be a more precise indication for benefit from IVIG therapy (89). A recent crossover study involving 30 patients found low-dosage of IVIG (300 mg/kg every 4 weeks) to be adequate for infection prophylaxis (91). However, the treatment was judged not to be cost effective.

Multiple Myeloma
Patients with multiple myeloma suffer from serious bacterial infections throughout the course of the disease. This is probably associated with reduced polyclonal immunoglobulin synthesis. Infection is the cause of death in as many as 42% of patients with myeloma (88). These infections are predominantly caused by encapsulated bacteria, and involve the respiratory and urinary tracts. There is a high incidence of septicemia. The infrequency of viral and fungal infections suggests that cell-mediated immune defects are less significant in myeloma patients.

A randomized, placebo-controlled, double-blind study of IVIG (400 mg/kg/month) in 82 selected patients with stable-phase multiple myeloma has been conducted (92). Serious infections were considerably reduced by immunoglobulin prophylaxis, and there was a striking reduction in life-threatening infections. Episodes of septicemia and pneumonia were reduced by IVIG. The incidence of adverse events was higher (12%) than that in

an age-matched population of patients with CLL (3%). The relatively high reaction rate (5%) in the placebo-treated patients may reflect the increased susceptibility of patients with myeloma to hemodynamic changes. There were transient, but nonsignificant, rises in serum creatinine. In conclusion, IVIG can be given safely to selected patients with multiple myeloma in a stable phase of the disease, and it protects them against life-threatening infections.

Allogeneic Bone Marrow Transplantation (BMT)
As BMT protocols continue to be refined, this therapy is applied to an ever broader array of hematologic abnormalities. Its success depends to a large extent on the supportive care of the transplant recipient, which is aimed at the prevention of opportunistic infections and graft-versus-host disease (GVHD). Marrow engraftment usually occurs within 2 to 4 weeks after transplantation, and neutrophil counts return to normal levels by 4 to 6 weeks post-transplant. Full immune reconstitution develops 9 to 12 months after autologous, syngeneic, or HLA-matched allogeneic transplantation (93). HLA disparity and development of GVHD delay immune reconstitution after marrow grafting (94).

GVHD. Acute GVHD is observed in 20% to 50% of recipients of HLA-identical unmodified marrow, and in more than 75% of HLA-nonidentical and unrelated donor grafts (95). Increases in opportunistic infection are seen in patients with acute GVHD in association with immune deficiency, immunosuppressive treatment, and damaged skin and gut (95–98).

Recently, IVIG was shown to reduce the incidence of acute GVHD after transplantation (97,99). The specific mechanism of this immune modulation by IVIG remains unclear. Chronic GVHD develops after day 100 post-transplant in 25% to 45% of long-term survivors of HLA-matched BMT and in 50% to 65% of HLA-mismatched or unrelated donor transplants. It is similar in clinical presentation to several naturally occurring autoimmune disorders (95,96). The incidence of chronic GVHD increases with patient age and HLA disparity. Stable graft host tolerance eventually develops, but early institution of immunosuppressive therapy is indicated to decrease the incidence of permanent disability from chronic GVHD. Bacteremia, sinusitis, and pulmonary infections are common in this setting. Antibiotic prophylaxis with penicillin and trimethoprim sulfamethoxazole prevents overwhelming infections with encapsulated organisms and *Pneumocystis carinii*.

A meta-analysis of 379 patients studied in controlled trials of IVIG to reduce GVHD revealed a decrease of 30% or more in acute GVHD as well as a 25% reduction in mortality in patients receiving IVIG (0.5–1.0 g/kg weekly during days 90–120 post-transplant) (101). However, in the absence of hypogammaglobulinemia, there was no benefit of IVIG with respect to chronic GVHD or late complications.

Cytomegalovirus (CMV) Infection. CMV infection has been a major cause of morbidity and mortality following allogeneic BMT (98). Although CMV infections are now less frequently observed, CMV interstitial pneumonia continues to have a mortality rate of approximately 50%, despite ganciclovir and IVIG (102). For CMV-seronegative patients, the use of CMV negative blood products has proven effective in preventing transfusion-associated CMV disease (103). Several studies have evaluated the use of prophylactic IVIG in preventing major complications of BMT in both CMV-seronegative and CMV-seropositive patients (97,99,104,105). Winston et al (97) and Kapoor et al (105) reported a reduction in symptomatic CMV infection and prevention of interstitial pneumonia in recipients of CMV-immune plasma compared with untreated controls, who also had a 21-fold increased risk of developing septicemia. Recipients who were more than 20 years of age also had reduced rates of interstitial pneumonia and non-relapse-related mortality. An analysis of 12 randomized, controlled trials of IVIG prophylaxis in BMT revealed a significant reduction in post-transplant complications in patients receiving IVIG prophylaxis (106). Reductions in fatal CMV infection, CMV pneumonia, non-CMV interstitial pneumonia, and transplant-related mortality were confirmed. Because serum IgG half-life in BMT recipients may be very short (3 to 10 days), weekly dosing may be advantageous for maintaining adequate levels for protection from CMV pneumonia.

One recent study compared IVIG having a high titer to CMV (CMV-IVIG, 100 mg/kg weekly) with "regular" IVIG (400 mg/kg weekly) for prophylaxis of CMV infection after BMT (107). Both groups had similar rates of CMV antigenemia (61% CMV-IgG, 71% IVIG, not significant). There were no differences in the course of CMV infection, GVHD, or other transplant-related complications. IVIG cost approximately 50% more than CMV-IgG.

Solid Organ Transplantation

Rejection. In 52 pediatric recipients of renal grafts who were treated with IVIG for CMV prophylaxis, graft survival ranged from 88% to 95% over the first 3 years, versus 79% to 88% in the group who did not receive IVIG (108). Ten patients receiving cardiac and renal transplants had episodes of acute rejection with anti-HLA antibodies treated with IVIG (109). All episodes were reversed, and in nine patients there was no recurrence after (in some cases) 5 years of follow-up. Reversal of rejection was associated with a rapid fall in the titer of anti-HLA antibodies. Another study of 41 HLA-sensitized recipients of second cadaveric renal transplants showed an increase in 5-year survival from 50% to 68% with IVIG treatment (0.4 g/kg daily for the first 5 days after transplantation) (110).

CMV Infection. A prospective study of pediatric renal transplant recipients receiving IVIG, using retrospective controls, showed a reduction from 71% to 17% in the incidence of CMV infection among CMV-seronegative recipients of grafts from seropositive donors (111). The infections that occurred in IVIG recipients were later and less severe than those in controls. There was no difference in graft rejection or survival. Another recent study showed a somewhat higher overall incidence of CMV infection (55%) in 33 CMV-seronegative children who were treated

with CMV-IVIG after receiving kidneys from CMV-seropositive donors (112).

HIV Infection and the Acquired Immunodeficiency Syndrome (AIDS)

The main immunologic abnormality in HIV-infected patients, with or without AIDS, is a deficiency in cellular immunity. However, children infected with HIV also display laboratory evidence of a deficiency in humoral immunity, with depressed specific antibody responses to keyhole limpet hemocyanin, pneumococcal polysaccharides (113,114), tetanus toxoid, and bacteriophage ΦX174 (115). Infections with *Streptococcus pneumoniae* and other gram-positive encapsulated bacteria, which are normally cleared by opsonizing antibody, are relatively common in HIV-infected patients (particularly children), and may occur before and after the development of AIDS.

The definitive study of IVIG therapy in HIV-infected children to date was undertaken by The National Institute of Child Health and Human Development Intravenous Immunoglobulin Study Group, which demonstrated convincing evidence of benefit in a double-blind, placebo-controlled trial (116). Three hundred and seventy-two children with HIV disease categorized as CDC P2 (symptomatic) or P1.B (asymptomatic but with abnormal immune function) were randomly allocated to receive either IVIG (400 mg/kg) or placebo every 28 days. Children with CD4$^+$ lymphocyte counts greater than 200/mm^3 showed a significant increase in the time free from infection and a reduction in the number of serious bacterial infections and admissions for acute care. These benefits were not observed in the group with CD4$^+$ lymphocyte counts less than 200/mm^3. Subsequent analyses revealed that IVIG therapy was associated with a slowing of the decline in the CD4$^+$ lymphocyte count and a reduction in the rate of viral infections and minor bacterial infections (117,118). There was no apparent difference in the rate of opportunistic infections between the IVIG and placebo arms of the trial. It can be concluded that IVIG therapy should be instituted for HIV-infected children with recurrent viral or bacterial infections. The role of IVIG therapy in delaying the progression of HIV-related disease and in children with CD4$^+$ lymphocyte counts less than 200/mm^3 remains to be evaluated.

A randomized placebo-controlled trial of 200 mg/kg IVIG monthly for 1 year was recently conducted in HIV-infected infants during the first year of life (119). Reductions in bacterial infections of the respiratory, urinary, and gastrointestinal systems, as well as increases in weight and length, were observed in the treated infants, compared with those who received placebo.

The value of IVIG therapy in HIV-infected adults is more difficult to assess. Clinical trials to date have not shown conclusive benefit. Demonstration of efficacy in a double-blind, placebo-controlled trial of IVIG therapy in patients with AIDS or with HIV infection using mortality and severe infections as endpoints is required before IVIG therapy can be recommended for such patients routinely. IVIG should also be assessed in a subset of adult HIV-infected patients with recurrent bacterial infections and/or septicemia. Finally, there is no evidence that IVIG therapy has any role to play in asymptomatic HIV-infected patients. In particular, there is no conclusive evidence that it delays progression of HIV-related disease.

Thrombocytopenia occurs with relatively high frequency in HIV-infected patients; the incidence may be as much as 40-fold greater than in the HIV-negative population (120). Standard regimens for ITP have been used with some success in thrombocytopenic patients with HIV (121). One recent study used a very low dosage (40 mg/kg weekly for five weeks) (122). The authors observed responses in 10 of 13 patients; the responses were prolonged (3 months) in four patients. There was significant cost savings with the low-dosage regimen.

Prophylaxis and Therapy of Infections in Immunocompetent Hosts

Sepsis in Adults

Infections remain the leading cause of death among patients admitted to surgical intensive care units (ICUs). The mortality rate related to gram-negative sepsis varies from 20% to 40% (123), and with the development of gram-negative septic shock it reaches 50% to 75% (124,125). Thus, novel therapies are needed to prevent and to treat infections in critically ill patients. Two studies suggested that hyperimmune serum or plasma from healthy volunteers who had been vaccinated with heat-killed *E. coli* J5 strain might be effective in the prevention or treatment of gram-negative septic shock (125,126), whereas two other studies were negative (127,128). The favorable outcomes in the two successful studies could not be significantly correlated with the levels of antibody to *E. coli* J5 administered to patients. The reduction of nosocomial pneumonia recorded in both trials, and the shortening of the stay in the ICU, resulted in savings in hospital costs. In two other studies where IVIG preparations were given prophylactically to high-risk patients, there was no difference in the incidence of sepsis, in the overall mortality, or in mortality attributed to infections (127,128). However, the incidence of pneumonia was significantly reduced.

A double-blind, randomized, three-arm study compared the prophylactic efficacies of hyperimmune IVIG (400 mg/kg) obtained from blood donors with naturally high levels of antibody directed to the core of LPS, standard IVIG (400 mg/kg), and placebo in preventing infections in high-risk surgical patients (129). Infections were significantly lower in the group receiving standard IVIG than in the placebo group, as was the incidence of pneumonia. The administration of standard IVIG prevented mainly infections of late onset—i.e., infections not already incubating at the time of randomization. The number of days spent in the ICU was significantly lower in the standard IVIG group than in the placebo group. In contrast, the hyperimmune IVIG preparation had no detectable prophylactic effect on infection. The prophylactic efficacy of standard IVIG might be related to a larger repertoire of specific antibodies, because 10,000 to 30,000 donors were used for the preparation of the standard IVIG compared with 300 for the preparation of the hyperimmune IVIG. Neither standard IVIG nor hyperimmune IVIG prevented systemic infectious episodes or septic shock.

The efficacy of IVIG given therapeutically to critically ill adult patients with established infections has also been studied. In two unblinded, randomized, controlled trials with 104 surgical intensive care patients, administration of IVIG over 2 days, in conjunction with antibiotics, had no effect on mortality attributed to infections, or on overall mortality (130,131). In another multicenter, randomized, double-blind, therapeutic study, Calandra et al compared the efficacy of IVIG collected from volunteers immunized with *E. coli* J5 with that of standard IVIG in the treatment of gram-negative septic shock (124). No difference in a high mortality rate (50%) was observed between the two groups. Because of the lack of demonstrable benefit, the prevention and treatment of adult sepsis is not considered an indication for IVIG therapy. New antibody- and immunoglobulin-based modalities are under investigation, including the use of monoclonal antibodies specific for bacterial antigens, and IgM-enriched preparations (132).

Infection with toxin-producing strains of *Staphylococcus aureus* leading to toxic shock syndrome may be one form of sepsis for which IVIG is beneficial. Several authors have reported sometimes dramatic clinical improvement when IVIG was added to conventional antimicrobial therapy (133–135). No controlled trials have been performed.

Neonatal Sepsis

Bacterial infections remain a major cause of morbidity and mortality in neonates, particularly premature infants. Many of these infections are caused by encapsulated organisms such as group B streptococcus (GBS); *E. coli* is another common pathogen in this setting. Neonates may be antibody deficient if the mother does not have antibody to the specific neonatal pathogens, or if the child is born prematurely, because most of the maternal-derived antibody passes across the placenta in the last 4 to 6 weeks of pregnancy. IVIG enhances immunity to neonatal bacterial pathogens by facilitating opsonization and phagocytosis.

IVIG prophylaxis has not consistently provided protection from late-onset sepsis (136–138). IVIG preparations contain variable levels of antibody to *Staphylococcus epidermidis*, a major cause of late-onset sepsis, with many lots having nearly undetectable titers. The lack of consistent levels of antibody to staphylococci may explain why IVIG prophylaxis of neonatal sepsis has not been uniformly effective.

In early-onset neonatal sepsis, IVIG has generally improved survival when used therapeutically in combination with antibiotics (139). However, individual IVIG lots may not contain sufficient pathogen-specific antibody to provide effective therapy, and this has been shown in some studies to correlate with lack of efficacy.

A recent meta-analysis of the use of IVIG in the prophylaxis and treatment of neonatal sepsis has been performed (140). The authors reported that IVIG provides a small but statistically significant benefit for the prevention of sepsis. On the other hand, adjunctive use of IVIG in the therapy of established sepsis results in a sixfold reduction in mortality.

Kawasaki Disease

Kawasaki disease (KD) is an acute vasculitis of childhood that involves mainly the medium and large arteries, particularly the coronary arteries. Its clinical features include fever, skin rash, mucocutaneous inflammation, conjunctivitis, peripheral edema, desquamation, and cervical lymphadenopathy (141). The etiology of KD is unknown. Based on both epidemiologic and clinical findings, it is widely agreed that KD represents an infectious disease. Indirect evidence, in the form of expansion of T cells utilizing Vβ2, has been used to suggest that a superantigen is responsible for many of the manifestations of KD (18). Leung et al reported finding superantigen toxin-producing staphylococci and streptococci from various anatomic sites in 13 of 16 patients with KD, and in only one of 15 controls (12). These authors speculated that KD may be the result of widespread T-cell activation due to superantigen toxins, and that the efficacy of IVIG may be related to toxin-binding activity. These findings need to be confirmed in additional studies.

The mechanism of action of IVIG in KD could be neutralization of an infectious agent or toxin. Alternatively, IVIG may act as an immunomodulator to decrease the inflammation in KD, which is associated with evidence of immune activation. Circulating T cells bear activation antigens, B cells spontaneously produce immunoglobulins (142), and there is evidence of autoantibodies to antigens expressed by endothelial cells following activation with IL-1 and TNF (143,144). High levels of circulating cytokines (TNF, IFN-γ, and IL-1) have been detected in KD patients, and these levels decrease after IVIG therapy (20). Furthermore, IVIG inhibits the expression of endothelial cell activation markers such as endothelial leukocyte adhesion molecule-1 (ELAM-1) and ICAM-1 in KD patients through inhibition of IL-1 (143–145).

Untreated KD is generally a self-limited illness. Coronary artery involvement (aneurysm formation) occurs in 20% to 25% of patients who do not receive therapy within 10 days of the onset of fever. Studies in Japan and the United States have shown that treatment with IVIG plus aspirin given within the first 10 days of onset reduces the prevalence of coronary artery disease to 5%. Early studies evaluated IVIG at a dosage of 400 mg/kg/day for 4 consecutive days (146). A subsequent multicenter study demonstrated that a single dose of IVIG 2 g/kg with aspirin was even more protective against coronary artery aneurysm formation (147). In addition to reducing coronary artery disease, IVIG therapy results in a more rapid normalization of laboratory values as well as faster resolution of clinical symptoms. It was noted that a lower peak IgG level is associated with prolonged duration of acute symptoms and with a worse clinical outcome.

A recent survey of data from 378 patients with KD treated at nine North American centers showed that 48 hours after the initial infusion of gamma globulin, only 13.2% of patients remained febrile (148). Although not well-studied, it has become common to administer a second dose of gamma globulin to persistently febrile patients, and 58% of such patients in the survey were treated a second time. Only 1.4% of patients who defer-vesced with a single dose of gamma globulin developed coronary artery abnormalities; this occurred in 12.2% of patients who were febrile after the first IVIG dose.

Bronchiolitis Secondary to Respiratory Syncytial Virus (RSV)

IVIG prepared from donors with high titer antibodies to respiratory syncytial virus constitutes RSV-IVIG. A recent large (510 patients) randomized, double-blind, placebo-controlled trial demonstrated that premature infants, and infants with bronchopulmonary dysplasia, who received monthly injections of 750 mg/kg during the RSV season (October/December through March/May, depending on the region) had a 41% reduction in hospitalization due to RSV, a 53% reduction in hospital days, and a 60% reduction in days requiring supplemental oxygen (149). In addition, recipients of RSV-IVIG had a 38% reduction in hospitalization for respiratory disease of any cause and a 46% reduction in total hospital days for respiratory illness per 100 children. An earlier and smaller (102 children) randomized, blinded, placebo-controlled trial did not show a benefit for a prophylactic regimen consisting of a single infusion of 1500 mg/kg RSV-IVIG (150).

Palivizumab is a humanized monoclonal antibody that recognizes a conserved antigenic determinant of the F glycoprotein of RSV. This drug is administered by IM injection 15 mg/kg monthly during the RSV season. A double-blind, placebo-controlled, randomized study comprised of 1502 infants with prematurity and/or chronic lung disease showed a 55% reduction in RSV-related hospitalization. There were similar reductions in RSV-related outcome measures as described above for RSV-IVIG. Palivizumab does not yield any reduction in non-RSV-related morbidity (151).

Current guidelines for the use of RSV-IVIG or palivizumab include 1) children under 2 years of age with chronic lung disease requiring medical therapy within 6 months of the beginning of the RSV season; 2) infants born between 29 and 32 weeks of gestation without chronic lung disease up to 6 months of age; and 3) infants born at 28 weeks or earlier up to 12 months of age (152). Additional patients who may be considered for therapy are those with primary or secondary immune deficiency. RSV-IVIG (but not palivizumab) is contraindicated in infants with cyanotic congenital heart disease (153).

In general, palivizumab is preferred on the basis of considerations of ease of use, safety, and equal effectiveness in comparison with RSV-IVIG. In some cases, the anticipated benefits of the non-RSV-specific antibodies in RSV-IVIG are desirable. Studies of cost effectiveness of RSV-IVIG have yielded conflicting results. No formal studies of the cost effectiveness of palivizumab have been conducted.

Additional Anti-Infective Uses of IVIG

Gastroenteritis Secondary to Rotavirus. In a double-blind, placebo-controlled trial of oral IVIG in 71 children with gastroenteritis caused by rotavirus, a single oral dose of 300 mg/kg resulted in statistically significant reductions in the duration of diarrhea (−42%) and virus excretion (−37%) (154). No adverse effects were noted. Neutralizing titers ranging from 1:800 to 1:3200 were found for four rotavirus serotypes in the single preparation tested.

Toxic Epidermal Necrolysis (TEN). In TEN, a severe (30% mortality rate) form of drug hypersensitivity with widespread skin sloughing, keratinocytes die by apoptosis initiated by surface CD95 (Fas) and CD95L (Fas ligand) interaction. In an open study of 10 patients with TEN, administration of IVIG 0.2–0.75 mg/kg daily for 5 days halted the progression of skin detachment, and promoted healing in all patients (155). There were no deaths. These authors provide evidence that IVIG contains antibodies that bind to human Fas, and suggest that the effectiveness of IVIG in TEN may result from blocking of the CD95-CD95L interaction.

Clostridium Difficile Colitis. Salcedo et al found neutralizing activity against *C. difficile* toxins A and B in several IVIG products. They treated two patients with refractory pseudomembranous colitis and achieved rapid resolution of symptoms (156). Leung et al induced remission of chronic relapsing *C. difficile* colitis in five children by administration of IVIG 400 mg/kg every 3 weeks (157).

IVIG in Autoimmune and Inflammatory Diseases

IVIG has been shown to be an effective therapy for the treatment of several autoimmune diseases, and continues to be investigated in experimental protocols for an increasing number of autoimmune and inflammatory disorders. A list of the autoimmune conditions in which IVIG has been reported to be effective is shown in Table 19-4.

The capacity of IVIG to down-regulate dysfunctional immune responses has been attributed to several mechanisms (see above). These include interference with FcγR binding of endogenous ligands, down-regulation of antibody production through ligating FcγR on B cells, alterations in T-cell subsets and T-cell function, inhibition of cytokine and other inflammatory mediator release, inhibition of complement-mediated cytolysis, solubilization of immune complexes, and the reestablishment of normal idiotypic regulation of pathogenic autoantibody responses by passive transfer of anti-idiotypic antibodies. IVIG contains antibodies reactive against the idiotypic regions of several pathogenic autoantibodies, including anti–factor VIII (41), anti-thyroglobulin (43), anti–neutrophil cytoplasmic antibody (ANCA) (42), anti–endothelial cell (158), anti–acetylcholine receptor (159), and anti-Sm (44). Since the half-life of infused IVIG is approximately 3 weeks, one would expect the pathogenic autoantibody responses to return rapidly. However, this is usually not the case. In many instances, IVIG infusions

Table 19-4. Autoimmune Diseases or Diseases with an Autoimmune Component in Which IVIG Therapy Has Been Studied

Hematologic Disorders	**Neurologic Disorders**
Thrombocytopenia	Amyotrophic lateral sclerosis
Neutropenia	Chronic inflammatory demyelinating
Anemia	polyneuropathy
Coagulopathy	Intractable childhood epilepsy
Von Willebrand's disease	Guillain-Barré syndrome
	Lambert-Eaton myasthenic syndrome
Arthritides	Multiple sclerosis
	Myasthenia gravis
Rheumatoid arthritis	
Juvenile rheumatoid	**Systemic Autoimmune Diseases/Vasculitides**
arthritis	
	Systemic lupus erythematosus
Skin Diseases	ANCA-associated vasculitis
	Henoch-Schönlein purpura
Pemphigus vulgaris	Churg-Strauss syndrome
Bullous pemphigoid	Essential mixed cryoglobulinemia
Epidermolysis bullosa	
acquisita	
Other Diseases	
Dermatomyositis/polymyositis	
Graves' disease	
Inflammatory bowel disease	
Recurrent spontaneous abortion	
Uveitis	

have resulted in a long-lasting modulation of autoreactivity, suggesting that IVIG actively induces a down-regulation of autoantibody responses resulting in the amelioration of disease.

It is possible that a large donor pool is necessary for the effectiveness of IVIG as an immunomodulator, because pooled IgG, but not IgG obtained from a limited number of donors, has been shown to contain as much as 40% dimers that contact each other in the antigen-binding site, suggesting that they consist of idiotype–anti-idiotype complexes (40). Alternatively, IVIG derived from selected individuals who have recovered from autoimmune diseases, or who for some reason have exceptionally high titers of anti-idiotypic antibodies, would determine the effectiveness of IVIG in autoimmune disorders. The latter would explain the lot-to-lot variations in the efficacy of IVIG in the control of various autoimmune and inflammatory diseases (23,158).

Space does not permit discussion of all of the autoimmune disorders listed in Table 19-4. Presented below is a large selection of some of the more well-studied diseases in which IVIG has been shown to be, or suggested to be, of benefit.

Immune Thrombocytopenic Purpura (ITP)

In ITP, antibodies are often directed against the platelet surface glycoprotein IIb/IIIa complex (integrin αIIb/β3; CD41/CD61). The rapid destruction of platelets is attributable to autoantibodies that bind, by means of the interaction of their combining sites, to the antigenic site, or to immune complexes that bind via FcγR on the platelets. Opsonized platelets are rapidly removed by cells of the mononuclear phagocyte system, especially in the spleen. There is a significant correlation among platelet autoantibody level, the patient's age at the time of diagnosis, and prognosis. Younger children with moderate autoantibody levels may have a greater chance of spontaneous remission or of compensated disease. The course of adolescents with high autoantibody levels seems similar to that of adults, in whom spontaneous remission or compensation is unusual.

The key observation of the value of IVIG treatment in ITP was made in a 12-year-old boy who was unresponsive to conventional treatment and developed secondary hypogammaglobulinemia (160). Within the first 24 hours after the initial dose of 400 mg/kg IVIG, his platelet count increased dramatically. Subsequent multicenter randomized double-blind studies established the efficacy of IVIG in ITP (161,162). Table 19-5 summarizes the recommendations for IVIG treatment in ITP. There are three categories of treatment:

1. In patients with severe bleeding or at risk of bleeding (i.e., before surgery), 800 mg/kg IVIG should be given initially. The subsequent treatment depends on the initial response (platelet increase within 72 hours, duration of effect). For life-threatening situations, a combination of IVIG, high-dosage corticosteroids (8–12 mg/kg body weight/day), and platelet transfusion is indicated.
2. In patients with long-term bleeding problems, and particularly in children, 400 mg/kg IVIG given at intervals of 2 to 8 weeks is recommended, depending on hemorrhagic symptoms.
3. In patients with no, or only occasional, bleeding, no routine treatment is required. However, patients participating in special activities (e.g., sports) may need individualized treatment.

ITP during pregnancy poses a risk for both the third-trimester fetus and the newborn, because maternal antibodies cross the placenta. Platelets are eliminated before and within the first few weeks after delivery. The incidence of severe ITP ($<50 \times 10^3$/mm^3 platelets) is about 20%. Fetal platelet counts should be determined by percutaneous umbilical vessel sampling or by scalp vein sampling during delivery. If the platelet count is below 50×10^3/mm^3, cesarean section should be performed (163). If the platelet count is higher than this level, the newborn should be treated with IVIG prophylactically, because the platelet count often continues to decrease within the first few days after birth (164). The dosage of IVIG and the rate of response are the same as in children with acute ITP.

Table 19-5. The Treatment of ITP with IVIG

Initial Treatment

Day 1:   IVIG 0.8 g/kg body weight
Day 3:   If platelet count is $>30 \times 10^9$/L, no further treatment
         If platelet count is $<30 \times 10^9$/L, repeat IVIG as on day 1
         If platelet count is $<10 \times 10^9$/L, bone marrow analysis for exclusion of production disorders of platelets, leukemia, etc.

Emergency Treatment (Severe Bleeding, Presurgery)

IVIG 1–2 g/kg body weight until platelet counts are at least 30×10^9/L or there is no more bleeding; eventually, combination with high-dose methylprednisolone (8–12 mg/kg body weight, intravenously or orally) and/or with platelet transfusion

Preventive Treatment and Treatment in Chronic ITP (Platelet Count $<10–30 \times 10^9$/L)

IVIG 0.4–0.8 g/kg body weight, once

Recently, anti-D (Rh) immunoglobulin has emerged as a potentially more cost-effective treatment of immune thrombocytopenia in Rh-positive individuals. This therapy is useful only in patients who are Rh-positive and have not had splenectomy. In one retrospective study of 33 children, those who received anti-D exhibited clinical responses that were comparable to responses of children receiving IVIG with respect to kinetics of platelet recovery and days in hospital (165). Not surprisingly, recipients of anti-D had greater hemolysis than those who used IVIG, but the difference was not statistically significant, and no patients required therapy for hemolysis. One open prospective study of 15 adult patients with chronic immune thrombocytopenia administered home IM injections of anti-D (166). The treatment was effective and safe, and no clinically significant hemolysis was observed. Some have estimated through retrospective analysis that anti-D therapy may yield a 36% reduction in cost per treated episode (120).

Mechanism of Action of IVIG in ITP. The immediate effect of IVIG in ITP may be attributable to inhibition of FcγR-mediated phagocytosis resulting in reduced platelet destruction. There is an association between the increase in platelet counts induced by IVIG and the prolonged survival of anti-D–coated erythrocytes (27). Furthermore, a monoclonal antibody directed against the FcγR has been successfully used in the treatment of refractory ITP (27,28). The possibility that IVIG may modify complexes on the platelet surface, including those consisting of viral products and antibodies directed against them, remains to be examined.

Modulation of immune responsiveness with decreased autoantibody production may be responsible for the long-term effects of IVIG in ITP. Such a mechanism could result from the presence of anti-idiotype antibodies in IVIG, or inhibition of B-cell responses by engagement of FcγR, or other B- and T-cell molecules by IVIG.

Systemic Lupus Erythematosus (SLE)

SLE is an autoimmune disease in which autoantibodies are produced against multiple autoantigens. This results in immune complex formation and immune complex–mediated tissue injury through complement activation. There are ample experimental data to suggest a role for IVIG in the treatment of the immune abnormalities encountered in SLE. IVIG could inhibit autoantibody production through anti-idiotypic networks (see above). For example, anti-idiotypic antibodies binding to the 4B4 idiotype of anti-Sm autoantibodies have been detected in IVIG (44). IVIG binds activated complement, preventing its binding to target cells, with subsequent inhibition of tissue injury and destruction. IVIG might also act to solubilize immune complexes, reducing their size and their ability to activate complement and cause tissue injury. IVIG may also inhibit the induction of cytokine release mediated by immune complexes.

No blinded, placebo-controlled studies of IVIG in SLE have been published. One open trial of IVIG 400 mg/kg for 5 consecutive days monthly for 6 to 24 months in patients with SLE

refractory to standard immunosuppressive therapy reported improvement in 11 of 12 treated patients with respect to clinical status, as well as to hemoglobin and complement levels, renal function, decreases in sedimentation rate, and antinuclear antibodies (167). In addition, there are numerous isolated case reports of various clinical manifestations of SLE (encephalitis, cytopenias, polyradiculopathy, etc.) responding to IVIG (168). On the other hand, several authors have reported a worsening of proteinuria in SLE patients treated with IVIG (22,169,170). A blinded, controlled trial of IVIG therapy in active SLE is needed before its routine use in these patients can be recommended.

Anti-Neutrophil Cytoplasmic Antibody (ANCA)–Associated Vasculitis

In contrast to SLE, systemic vasculitic disorders, especially those associated with ANCA positivity, have shown rather impressive responses to IVIG therapy. ANCA appears to play a significant pathogenic role in the development of systemic vasculitis (42). ANCA has been detected in the sera of normal individuals at very low levels, and in pooled human immunoglobulin preparations. IVIG preparations also contain anti-ANCA antibodies and inhibit ANCA-mediated neutrophil activation in vitro (42,171). This may be critical for their beneficial effect, because a most important determinant predicting remission from ANCA-positive vasculitis has been the detection of anti-ANCA anti-idiotypic antibodies in patients' sera (42).

IVIG is beneficial in Wegener's granulomatosis, even in some cases refractory to prednisone and cytoxan. The only instances in which IVIG has failed to show a benefit have been in patients with terminal lung hemorrhage and patients with fulminant renal failure. The largest study of IVIG in the treatment of systemic vasculitis was reported by Jayne et al, who found clinical benefit in 15 of 16 patients, with sustained remissions in eight (42). The ability of IVIG to produce a lasting remission was associated with a fall in ANCA titers and with stimulation of endogenous IgM anti-ANCA production. The improvement of severe ANCA-associated vasculitis by IVIG and the subsequent downregulation of ANCA titers point to IVIG as an immunomodulatory agent with the potential to control vasculitic disorders without predisposition to infectious complications. Controlled clinical trials are necessary to establish the efficacy of IVIG for these indications.

Guillain-Barré Syndrome

Guillain-Barré syndrome (GBS) is an acute, immune-mediated polyneuropathy with a severe clinical course. This disease usually leads to severe quadriparesis, and artificial ventilation is often needed. Although functional recovery is the rule, 15% of patients show a residual deficit. For these reasons, more specific therapy has been sought in addition to supportive care. Plasma exchange (PE) was the first proven effective treatment ameliorating morbidity and outcome (172). However, it is not always readily available, and contraindications and complications frequently occur.

IVIG can be administered easily, quickly, and without specialized equipment. In a recently published randomized trial of 150 patients that compared IVIG with PE, 34% of the patients in the PE group improved by one or more functional grades after 4 weeks, compared with 53% in the IVIG group ($P = 0.024$) (173). The median time to improve at least one grade on the functional scale and the median time to regain the ability of independent ambulation were less in the IVIG group than in the PE group. Pneumonia, atelectasis, thrombosis, and hemodynamic difficulties all occurred more often in the PE group, and fewer patients in the IVIG group required artificial ventilation. IVIG treatment has the additional advantage that other medications may be given simultaneously. In PE, comedication is removed together with the disease-causing factors. Recent data suggest that the combination of IVIG and high-dose methylprednisolone might be synergistic in the treatment of GBS.

A randomized study of 379 adults comparing PE, IVIG, and sequential treatment (PE followed by IVIG) in GBS showed equal efficacy of all three regimens. IVIG was administered at a dosage of 0.4 g/kg daily for 5 days (174). Similar regimens in smaller studies of patients of varying ages (50 patients) (175), and in seven pediatric patients (176), have yielded similar conclusions. The latter studies have found generally lower rates of complications in the IVIG-treated groups. This fact, combined with the relative ease of use of IVIG, has led to the suggestion that it be used as first-line therapy in this disorder.

One recent report of 67 patients with chronic inflammatory demyelinating polyneuropathy (CIDP) described equal response rates (roughly 40%) to prednisone, PE, and IVIG, although symptom scores showed the greatest improvement with PE (177). As with GBS, the efficacy, safety, and ease of use of IVIG have led some to recommend it as first-line therapy in this disorder as well (178).

Multiple Sclerosis

One double-blind, placebo-controlled trial involving 148 patients has shown a benefit of relatively low dosages of IVIG (0.1–0.2 g/kg monthly for 2 years) in improving disability in multiple sclerosis (MS) (179). A smaller study using a much higher dosage (1 g/kg daily for 2 days each month for 6 months) has shown similar benefit (180). Other studies have failed to demonstrate significant benefit (181). At present, IVIG is not recommended routinely for therapy of MS (182).

Myasthenia Gravis

Myasthenia gravis (MG) is an autoimmune disease characterized by a deficit in neuromuscular transmission. Acetylcholine receptor (AchR) antibodies, present in 80% to 90% of patients, are specific for this illness. These antibodies are deposited with complement on the postsynaptic membrane, and play a crucial role in the impairment of neuromuscular transmission by accelerating the degradation of the receptors and the membrane, and/or by blocking AchR (183). Injection of IgG from myasthenics into mice reproduces the disease, suggesting that the anti-AchR IgG is pathogenic (183).

The neuromuscular deficit in MG varies in intensity throughout the day and from one day to another. Studies evaluating treatment modalities have been difficult to carry out because of the unpredictable short- and long-term evolution of MG, the rarity of the illness, and difficulties in objectively measuring the deficit. Anticholinesterase compounds are used as first-line treatment in all patients. Thymectomy is proposed for patients with generalized disease presenting before the age of 40 years. Generalized forms with significant impairment are treated with corticosteroids and immunosuppressants. These therapies lead to a significant improvement in 80% to 90% of cases (184). PE is used for acute exacerbations of the illness and is thought to be effective despite the lack of controlled trials.

Several studies, excluding one that used a low dosage of IVIG, have reported beneficial effects of adding IVIG to the standard regimens for MG. However, the durations of the improvements obtained have been poorly documented. In two series, reductions in anti-AChR Ab were noted (159,185), while in two others (100,186), no changes occurred. No complications have been reported.

The effectiveness of IVIG in comparison with placebo has not been demonstrated definitively. It is difficult from an ethical point of view to propose a study with IVIG versus placebo. One randomized trial involving 87 patients compared PE with 3 to 5 days of IVIG (0.4 g/kg daily). This group reported equal efficacy of both treatments, with a lower rate of complications with IVIG (187). A smaller study of 16 exacerbations in 11 patients treated with a 5-day regimen reported a similar benefit (188). In general, IVIG appears to have a relatively delayed onset of effect (a few days) in comparison with PE, but its ease of use and better tolerability make it a valid therapeutic alternative (189).

Epilepsy

An analysis of 29 separate, largely uncontrolled studies involving a total of 374 patients with intractable childhood epilepsy found consistent response rates of 30% to 50% to therapy with IVIG (190).

Additional Autoimmune Disorders Treated with IVIG

Arthritis. In one double-blind, placebo-controlled study of 31 children with systemic juvenile rheumatoid arthritis (JRA) who exhibited inadequate responses to standard therapy, the treated group received IVIG 1.5 g/kg biweekly for 2 months, then monthly for 4 more months (191). The response rate with respect to physicians' assessments of disease activity in the IVIG group was 50%, compared with 27% for placebo, but the results did not reach statistical significance. Similarly, joint counts and several laboratory measures of inflammation were not significantly different in the two groups. IVIG was judged to be of limited benefit. Another blinded, placebo-controlled phase I/II study in polyarticular JRA found that a regimen essentially identical to the one described above yielded improvements in approximately 75% of patients receiving IVIG (192). Improvement was more likely in patients with disease of less than 3 years' duration. At this time, IVIG is not considered standard therapy for autoimmune arthritides.

Diabetes Mellitus. Several studies have examined the utility of IVIG in the treatment of diabetes mellitus (DM) (193,194). Regimens have varied from 0.4gm/kg daily for brief periods to 2g/kg over 2 days monthly for extended (2-year) periods. A subgroup of patients has responded with increased duration of remissions, but the overall results do not support routine use of IVIG for new-onset autoimmune insulin-dependent DM.

Urticaria. A subgroup of patients (as many as 30% of the total) with chronic urticaria have been found to produce autoantibodies which bind autologous IgE or the high-affinity IgE receptor (FcεRI) (195). Patients' sera are capable of causing wheal and flare reactions when injected intradermally and of stimulating histamine release from basophils in vitro. One study of IVIG in 10 of these patients, using a regimen of 0.4g/kg daily for 5 days, reported remissions of 3 years' duration in three patients, two temporary remissions, and clinical improvement in four of the five remaining patients (196).

Coagulopathies. In several case reports, IVIG has been found to be beneficial in the treatment of patients with bleeding diatheses resulting from autoantibody coagulation inhibitors. These reports include cases of factor VIII (197) and factor V (198) inhibitors.

Additional Disorders Treated with IVIG

Recurrent Spontaneous Abortion (RSA)

From the point of view of the mother, a fetus can be regarded as an allograft. Local immunosuppression is thought to play an important role in the survival of the trophoblast and fetus. Both T cells and non-T cells, and soluble placental suppressor factors, contribute to local immunosuppression. Habitual abortion or RSA is defined as a series of three or more pregnancies ending in miscarriage. Most early gestation miscarriages are caused by chromosomal aberrations; in some, endocrinologic or anatomic problems may be the cause. In approximately 40% of these spontaneous abortions, no causative factor can be determined. In this group of patients, an immunologic rejection reaction is suspected.

It is postulated that patients with RSA lack "blocking" antibodies or factors to protect the fetus against immunologic rejection. The beneficial but unexplained effect of pretransplantation blood transfusions in kidney allografts has led to the use of allogeneic leukocyte therapy in patients with RSA, under the assumption that this therapy will elicit blocking antibodies that inhibit fetal rejection (199). Reported success rates vary from 58% to 100% for this form of therapy (200). It has been reasoned that IVIG should contain preformed antibodies of similar specificity and might be effective as passive immunization in patients with RSA (201,202). Moreover, experiments in mice have

demonstrated an antiresorptive effect (i.e., an increase in number of viable neonates) after intraperitoneal treatment with pooled normal mouse immunoglobulin preparations (203).

The advantages of IVIG treatment in RSA would be the avoidance of immunization against HLA antigens, a lesser risk of viral transmission, and the fact that IVIG treatment does not have to begin until pregnancy has been confirmed. Several clinical trials in RSA using 500–600mg/kg IVIG every 3–4 weeks administered as soon as possible after pregnancy was diagnosed, and lasting through week 22–24 of gestation, showed a success rate of approximately 75%. However, one has to bear in mind that the probability of carrying out a successful pregnancy for a woman with a history of three spontaneous abortions is about 60% without any treatment. In a recently conducted double-blind, placebo-controlled study, differences between pregnancy success rates of women treated with IVIG and those treated with placebo did not achieve statistical significance (204). Furthermore, these rates were in the range of results reported for allogeneic leukocyte treatment, casting doubt on the efficacy of the latter treatment as well.

In another study, administration of 200–250mg/kg IVIG every 3 weeks for the first 8 months of pregnancy resulted in live births in 28 (85%) of 33 women who had had three or more prior miscarriages (205). Twenty-three of these patients had one or more autoimmune abnormalities, including thyroid autoantibodies and/or Hashimoto's disease, circulating immune complexes, anticardiolipin antibodies, ITP, and Crohn's disease. A decrease in autoantibody levels occurred in all women having successful pregnancies.

Asthma

IVIG has been shown to be therapeutically useful in the management of severe steroid-dependent asthma. In a double-blind, randomized, placebo-controlled study, Salmun et al found a significant reduction in steroid use among a subgroup of patients with high systemic steroid requirements in the year prior to the study (206). This group administered IVIG 2g/kg for the first dose, followed by 400mg/kg every 3 weeks for 9 months. In another open study of 11 adult and adolescent patients, a regimen of 2g/kg every 4 weeks for 14 months led to significant improvement in pulmonary function and symptom scores, together with a reduction in steroid doses (207). Airway hyperreactivity as measured by methacholine challenge was unchanged. Another prospective, controlled, randomized study of 31 children, adolescents, and young adults did not show a statistically significant benefit of IVIG with respect to symptom scores, bronchial hyperreactivity, or variability in the measurement of peak airway flow (208). However, this group used a much smaller total dosage of IVIG: 1g/kg given each day for the first 2 days followed by only two more doses at 4-week intervals.

Conclusion

Gamma globulin was rendered safe for intravenous administration 15 years ago. This enabled the administration of large doses of gamma globulin to patients with humoral immunodeficiency diseases, particularly those with XLA and CVID who had been inadequately treated prior to that time. It has proved to be very effective prophylaxis, and has improved the quality of life of these patients. Intravenous gamma globulin has proved to be effective therapy for KD, in which the cardiac morbidity has been decreased sevenfold after the administration of a single large dose of gamma globulin. IVIG has also found utility in a variety of situations for the prophylaxis of infection associated with secondary antibody deficiency, such as malignancy, and immune suppression occurring during solid organ of bone marrow transplantation. IVIG also shows great promise for the treatment of some autoimmune diseases. As our knowledge of both the actions of IVIG in vivo and the pathophysiology of autoimmune diseases continues to grow, more effective applications in these disorders may be possible. In addition to its neutralizing effect on viruses, bacteria, and toxins, gamma globulin appears to have an immunomodulatory effect on inflammatory responses. More work is needed for better elucidation of its role in this regard.

References

1. Hill L, Mollison P. Hypogammaglobulinaemia in the United Kingdom. 13 Conclusions. Medical Research Council Special Report Series (London) 1971;310:124–127.
2. Stiehm ER, Casillas AM, Finkelstein JZ, et al. Slow subcutaneous human intravenous immunoglobulin in the treatment of antibody immunodeficiency: use of an old method with a new product. J Allergy Clin Immunol 1998;101(6 Pt 1):848–849.
3. Gaspar J, Gerritsen B, Jones A. Immunoglobulin replacement treatment by rapid subcutaneous infusion. Arch Dis Child 1998;79(1)48–51.
4. Romer J, Morgenthaler J-J, Scherz R, Skvaril F. Characterization of various immunoglobulin preparations for intravenous application. I. Protein composition and antibody content. Vox Sang 1982;42:62–73.
5. Lundblad J, Londeree N, Mitra G. Characterisation of various intravenous immunoglobulin preparations. J Infect 1987;15(suppl 1):3–12.
6. Appropriate uses of human immunoglobulin in clinical practice: memorandum from an IUIS/WHO meeting. Bull World Health Organ 1982;60:43–47.
7. Koffman BM, Dalakas MC. Effect of high-dose intravenous immunoglobulin on serum chemistry, hematology, and lymphocyte subpopulations; assessments based on controlled treatment trials in patients with neurological diseases. Muscle Nerve 1997;20(9):1102–1107.
8. Aukrust P, Muller F, Nordoy I, et al. Modulation of lymphocyte and monocyte activity after intravenous immunoglobulin administration in vivo. Clin Exp Immunol 1997;107(1):50–56.
9. Andersson U, Bjork L, Skansen-Saphir U, Andersson J. Pooled human IgG modulates cytokine production in lymphocytes and monocytes. Immunol Rev 1994;139:21–42.
10. Toyoda M, Jordan S. Intravenous immunoglobulin inhibits immunoglobulin production and cytokine mRNA production in human PBMCs. Proceedings of the Fourth International Symposium on Kawasaki Disease (American Heart Foundation) 1993;4:423–430.
11. Baudet V, Hurez V, Lapeyre C, et al. Intravenous immunoglobulin (IVIg) modulates the expansion of V beta 3$^+$ and V beta 17$^+$ T cells induced by staphylococcal enterotoxin B superantigen in vitro. Scand J Immunol 1996;43(3):277–282.
12. Leung DY, Meissner HC, Fulton DR, et al. Toxic shock syndrome toxin-secreting Staphylococcus aureus in Kawasaki syndrome. Lancet 1993;342(8884):1385–1388.
13. Alder LB, Morgan LA, Spickett GP. Contribution of stabilizing agents present in intravenous immunoglobulin preparations to modulation of mononuclear cell proliferation in vitro. Scand J Immunol 1996;44(6):585–591.
14. Dinarello C. Is there a role for interleukin-1 blockade in intravenous immunoglobulin therapy? Immunol Rev 1994;139:173–188.
15. Toungouz M, Denys C, Dupont E. Blockade of proliferation and tumor necrosis factor-alpha production occurring during mixed lymphocyte reaction by interferon-gamma-specific natural antibodies contained in intravenous immunoglobulins. Transplantation 1996;62(9):1292–1296.
16. Andersson J, Skansen-Saphir U, Sparrelid E, Andersson U. Intravenous immune globulin affects cytokine production in T lymphocytes and monocytes/macrophages. Clin Exp Immunol 1996;104(suppl 1):10–20.
17. Skansen-Saphir U, Andersson J, Bjork L, et al. Down-regulation of lymphokine synthesis by intravenous gammaglobulin is dependent upon accessory cells. Scand J Immunol 1998;47(3):229–235.
17a. Shimozato T, Iwata M, Kawada H, T'amura N. Human immunoglobulin preparation for intravenous use induces elevation of cellular cyclic adenosine 3′:5′-monophosphate levels, resulting in suppression of tumour necrosis factor alpha and interleukin-1 production. Immunol 1991;72:497–501.
18. Abe J, Kotzin B, Jujo K, et al. Selective expansion of T cells expressing T-cell receptor variable regions Vβ2 and Vβ8 in Kawasaki disease. Proc Natl Acad Sci USA 1992;89:4066.
19. Xu C, Poirier B, Van Huyen JP, et al. Modulation of endothelial cell function by normal polyspecific human intravenous immunoglobulins: a possible mechanism of action in vascular diseases. Am J Pathol 1998;153(4):1257–1266.
20. Furukawa S, Matsubara T, Jujoh K, et al. Peripheral blood monocyte/macrophage and serum tumor necrosis factor in Kawasaki disease. Clin Exp Immunol 1988;48:247–251.
21. Nomura S, Yasunaga K, Fujimura K, et al. High-dose intravenous gamma globulin reduces macrophage colony-stimulating factor levels in idiopathic thrombocytopenic purpura. Int J Hematol 1996;63(3):227–234.
22. Jordan S. Intravenous gammaglobulin therapy in systemic lupus erythematosus and immune complex disease. Clin Immunol Immunopathol 1989;53:S164–S169.
23. Jordan S, Toyoda M. Treatment of autoimmune diseases and systemic vasculitis with pooled human intravenous immune globulin. Clin Exp Immunol 1994;97(suppl 1):31–38.
24. Vuist WM, Van Schaik IN, Van Lint M, Brand A. The growth arresting effect of human immunoglobulin for intravenous use is mediated by antibodies recognizing membrane glycolipids. J Clin Immunol 1997;17(4):301–310.

25. Kaveri S, Vassilev T, Hurez V, et al. Antibodies to a conserved region of HLA class I molecules, capable of modulating CD8 T cell-mediated function, are present in pooled normal immunoglobulin for therapeutic use. J Clin Invest 1996;97(3):865–869.
26. Prasad NK, Papoff G, Zeuner A, et al. Therapeutic preparations of normal polyspecific IgG (IVIg) induce apoptosis in human lymphocytes and monocytes: a novel mechanism of action of IVIg involving the Fas apoptotic pathway. J Immunol 1998;161(7):3781–3790.
27. Fehr J, Hofmann V, Kappeler U. Transient reversal of thrombocytopenia in idiopathic thrombocytopenic purpura by high dose intravenous gammaglobulin. N Engl J Med 1982;306:1254–1258.
28. Clarkson S, Bussel J, Kimberly R, et al. Treatment of refractory immune thrombocytopenic purpura with an anti Fc receptor antibody. N Engl J Med 1986;314:1236–1239.
29. Ghetie V, Ward ES. FcRn: the MHC class I-related receptor that is more than an IgG transporter. Immunol Today 1997;18(12):592–598.
30. Masson PL. Elimination of infectious antigens and increase of IgG catabolism as possible modes of action of IVIg. J Autoimmun 1993;6(6):683–689.
31. Yu Z, Lennon VA. Mechanism of intravenous immune globulin therapy in antibody-mediated autoimmune diseases. N Engl J Med 1999;340(3):227–228.
32. Kaveri SV, Dietrich G, Hurez V, Kazatchkine MD. Intravenous immunoglobulins (IVIg) in the treatment of autoimmune diseases. Clin Exp Immunol 1991;86(2):192–198.
33. Mollnes TE, Andreassen IH, Hogasen K, et al. Effect of whole and fractionated intravenous immunoglobulin on complement in vitro. Mol Immunol 1997;34(10):719–729.
34. Mollnes TE, Hogasen K, De Carolis C, et al. High-dose intravenous immunoglobulin treatment activates complement in vivo. Scand J Immunol 1998;48(3):312–317.
35. Basta M, Kirshbom P, Frank MM, Fries LF. Mechanism of therapeutic effect of high-dose intravenous immunoglobulin. Attenuation of acute, complement-dependent immune damage in a guinea pig model. J Clin Invest 1989;84(6):1974–1981.
36. Magee JC, Collins BH, Harland RC, et al. Immunoglobulin prevents complement-mediated hyperacute rejection in swine-to-primate xenotransplantation. J Clin Invest 1995;96(5):2404–2412.
37. Basta M, Dalakas MC. High-dose intravenous immunoglobulin exerts its beneficial effect in patients with dermatomyositis by blocking endomysial deposition of activated complement fragments. J Clin Invest 1994;94(5):1729–1735.
38. Wagner E, Platt JL, Frank MM. High dose intravenous immunoglobulin does not affect complement-bacteria interactions. J Immunol 1998;160(4):1936–1943.
39. Shoham-Kessary H, Naot Y, Gershon H. Immune complex-like moieties in immunoglobulin for intravenous use (i.v.Ig) bind complement and enhance phagocytosis of human erythrocytes. Clin Exp Immunol 1998;113(1):77–84.
40. Tankersley D. Dimer formation in immunoglobulin preparations and speculations on the mechanism of action of intravenous immune globulin in autoimmune diseases. Immunol Rev 1994;139:159–172.
41. Blanchette V, Kirby M, Turner C. Role of immunoglobulin G in autoimmune hematologic disorders. Semin Hematol 1992;29:72–82.
42. Jayne D, Esnault V, Lockwood C. ANCA anti-idiotype antibodies and the treatment of systemic vasculitis with intravenous immunoglobulin. J Autoimmun 1993;6:207–219.
43. Dietrich G, Kazatchkine M. Normal immunoglobulin G (IgG) for therapeutic use (intravenous IgG)) contains anti-idiotypic specificities against an immunodominant, disease-associated, cross-reactive idiotype of human anti-thyroglobulin autoantibodies. J Clin Invest 1990;85:620–625.
44. DeKeyser F, DeKeyser H, Kazatchkine MD, et al. Pooled human immunoglobulins contain anti-idiotypes with reactivity against the SLE-associated 4B4 cross-reactive idiotype. Clin Exp Rheumatol 1996;14(6):587–591.
45. Bagdasarian A, Tonetta S, Harel W, et al. IVIG adverse reactions: potential role of cytokines and vasoactive substances. Vox Sang 1998;74(2):74–82.
46. Teeling JL, De Groot ER, Eerenberg AJ, et al. Human intravenous immunoglobulin (IVIG) preparations degranulate human neutrophils in vitro. Clin Exp Immunol 1998;114(2):264–270.
47. Misbah S, Chapel H. Adverse effects of immunoglobulin therapy. Drug Safety 1993;4:254–262.
48. Chapel H. Consensus Panel for the Diagnosis and Management of Primary Antibody Deficiencies. Consensus on diagnosis and management of primary antibody deficiencies. Br Med J 1994;308:581–585.
49. Burks A, Sampson H, Buckley R. Anaphylactic reactions following gammaglobulin administration in patients with hypogammaglobulinaemia: detection of IgE antibodies to IgA. N Engl J Med 1986;314:560–564.
50. Bjorkander J, Hammarstrom L, Smith C, et al. Immunoglobulin prophylaxis in patients with antibody deficiency syndromes and anti-IgA antibodies. J Clin Immunol 1987;7:8–15.
51. Cunningham-Rundles C, Zhou Z, Mankarious S, Courter S. Long-term use of IgA-depleted intravenous immunoglobulin in immunodeficient subjects with anti-IgA antibodies. J Clin Immunol 1993;13(4):272–278.
52. Brox A, Cournoyer D, Sternbach M, Spurll G. Hemolytic anemia following intravenous gammaglobulin administration. Am J Med 1987;82:633–635.
53. Comenzo R, Malachowski M, Meissner H, et al. Immune hemolysis, disseminated intravascular coagulation and serum sickness after large dose of immune globulin given intravenously for Kawasaki disease. J Pediatr 1992;120:926–928.
54. Salama A, Mueller-Eckhardt C, Kieffel V. Effect of intravenous immunoglobulin in immune thrombocytopenia. Lancet 1983;ii:193–195.
55. Wilson JR, Bhoopalam H, Fisher M. Hemolytic anemia associated with intravenous immunoglobulin. Muscle Nerve 1997;20(9):1142–1145.
56. Kato E, Shindo S, Eto Y, et al. Administration of immune globulin associated with aseptic meningitis. JAMA 1988;22:3269–3270.
57. Watson J, Gibson J, Joshua D, Kronenberg H. Aseptic meningitis associated with high-dose intravenous immunoglobulin therapy. J Neurol Neurosurg Psychiatr 1991;54:275–276.

58. Vera-Ramirez M, Charlet M, Parry G. Recurrent aseptic meningitis complicating intravenous immunoglobulin therapy for chronic inflammatory demyelinating polyradiculoneuropathy. Neurology 1992;43:1636–1637.

59. Constantinescu C, Chang A, McCluskey L. Recurrent migraine and intravenous immune globulin therapy. N Engl J Med 1993;229:583–584.

60. Finkel AG, Howard JF Jr, Mann JD. Successful treatment of headache related to intravenous immunoglobulin with antimigraine medications. Headache 1998;38(4):317–321.

61. Ahsan N. Intravenous immunoglobulin induced-nephropathy: a complication of IVIG therapy. J Nephrol 1998;11(3):157–161.

62. Savasan S, Tuzcu V, Warrier I, Karpawich P. Cardiac rhythm abnormalities during intravenous immunoglobulin G infusion for treatment of thrombocytopenia. J Pediatr Hematol Oncol 1997;19(3):254–257.

63. Woodruff R, Griff A, Firkin F, Smith I. Fatal thrombic events during treatment of autoimmune thrombocytopenia with intravenous immunoglobulins in elderly patients. Lancet 1986;ii:217–218.

64. Frame W, Crawford R. Thrombotic events after intravenous immunoglobulin. Lancet 1986;ii:468.

65. Hague R, Eden O, Yap P, et al. Hyperviscosity in HIV infected children—a potential hazard during intravenous immunoglobulin therapy. Blut 1990;61:66–67.

66. Oh KT, Boldt HC, Danis RP. Iatrogenic central retinal vein occlusion and hyperviscosity associated with high-dose intravenous immunoglobulin administration. Am J Ophthalmol 1997;124(3):416–418.

67. Chan-Lam D, Fitzsimons EJ, Douglas WS. Alopecia after immunoglobulin infusion [letter]. Lancet 1987;i:1436.

68. Duhem C, Ries F, Dicato M. Intravenous immune globulins and hypothermia [letter]. Am J Hematol 1996;51(2):172–173.

69. Lisak RP. Arthritis associated with circulating immune complexes following administration of intravenous immunoglobulin therapy in a patient with chronic inflammatory demyelinating polyneuropathy. J Neurol Sci 1996;135(1):85–88.

70. Stiehm E. Human gamma globulins as therapeutic agents. Adv Pediatr 1988;35:1–72.

71. Lever A, Webster A, Brown D, Thomas H. Non-A, non-B hepatitis occurring in agammaglobulinaemic patients after intravenous immunoglobulin. Lancet 1984;ii:1062–1064.

72. Bjorkander J, Cunningham-Rundles C, Lundin P, et al. Intravenous immunoglobulin prophylaxis causing liver damage in 16 of 77 patients with hypogammaglobulinaemia or IgG subclass deficiency. Am J Med 1988;84:107–111.

73. Schneider LC, Jonas MM, Baron MJ, et al. Intravenous immunoglobulin and hepatitis C virus: the Boston episode. Clin Ther 1996;18:108–109.

74. Flora K, Schiele M, Benner K, et al. An outbreak of acute hepatitis C among recipients of intravenous immunoglobulin. Ann Allergy Asthma Immunol 1996;76(2):160–162.

75. Bresee JS, Mast EE, Coleman PJ, et al. Hepatitis C virus infection associated with administration of intravenous immune globulin. A cohort study. JAMA 1996;276(19):1563–1567.

76. Will RG, Ironside JW, Zeidler M, et al. A new variant of Creutzfeldt-Jakob disease in the UK. Lancet 1996;347(9006):921–925.

77. Bruce ME, Will RG, Ironside JW, et al. Transmissions to mice indicate that "new variant" CJD is caused by the BSE agent. Nature 1997;389(6650):498–501.

78. Hill AF, Desbruslais M, Joiner S, et al. The same prion strain causes vCJD and BSE [letter]. Nature 1997;389(6650):448–450, 526.

79. Creange A, Gray F, Cesaro P, et al. Creutzfeldt-Jakob disease after liver transplantation. Ann Neurol 1995;38(2):269–272.

80. Patry D, Curry B, Easton D, et al. Creutzfeldt-Jakob disease (CJD) after blood product transfusion from a donor with CJD. Neurology 1998;50(6):1872–1873.

81. Brown P, Rohwer RG, Dunstan BC, et al. The distribution of infectivity in blood components and plasma derivatives in experimental models of transmissible spongiform encephalopathy. Transfusion 1998;38(9):810–816.

82. Primary immunodeficiency diseases. Report of a WHO scientific group. Clin Exp Immunol 1997;109(suppl 1):1–28.

83. Hermaszewski R, Webster A. Primary hypogammaglobulinaemia: a survey of clinical manifestations and complications. Quart J Med 1993;86:31–42.

84. Roifman C, Lederman H, Lavis S, et al. Benefit of intravenous IgG replacement in hypogammaglobulinemic patients with chronic sinopulmonary disease. Am J Med 1985;79:171–174.

85. Barlan IB, Geha RS, Schneider LC. Therapy for patients with recurrent infections and low serum IgG3 levels. J Allergy Clin Immunol 1993;92(2):353–355.

86. Roifman C, Levison H, Gelfand E. High-dose versus low-dose intravenous immunoglobulin in hypogammaglobulinaemia and chronic lung disease. Lancet 1987;i:1075–1077.

87. Schiff R, Sedlak D, Buckley R. Rapid infusion of Sandoglobulin in patients with primary disorders of humoral immunity. J Allergy Clin Immunol 1991;88:61–67.

88. Salonen J, Nikoskelainen J. Lethal infections in patients with hematological malignancies. Eur J Haematol 1993;51(2):102–108.

89. Besa E. Recent advances in the treatment of chronic lymphocytic leukemia: defining the role of intravenous immunoglobulin. Semin Hematol 1992;29:14–23.

90. Molica S. Infections in chronic lymphocytic leukemia: risk factors, and impact on survival, and treatment. Leuk Lymphoma 1994;13(3–4):203–214.

91. Molica S, Musto P, Chiurazzi F, et al. Prophylaxis against infections with low-dose intravenous immunoglobulins (IVIG) in chronic lymphocytic leukemia. Results of a crossover study. Haematologica 1996;81(2):121–126.

92. Chapel HM, Lee M, Hargreaves R, et al. Randomised trial of intravenous immunoglobulin as prophylaxis against infection in plateau-phase multiple myeloma. The UK Group for Immunoglobulin Replacement Therapy in Multiple Myeloma. Lancet 1994;343(8905):1059–1063.

93. Lum L. A review: the kinetics of immune reconstitution after human marrow transplantation. Blood 1987;69:369–380.

94. Atkinson K, Farewell V, Storb R, et al. Analysis of late infections after human bone marrow transplantation: role of genotypic nonidentity between marrow donor and recipient

and of nonspecific suppressor cells in patients with chronic graft-versus-host disease. Blood 1982;60:714–720.

95. Sullivan K. Acute and chronic graft-versus-host disease in man. Int J Cell Cloning 1986;4:49–93.

96. Sullivan K, Agura E, Anasetti C, et al. Chronic graft-versus-host disease and other late complications of bone marrow transplantation. Semin Hematol 1991;28:250–259.

97. Winston D, Ho W, Lin C-H, et al. Intravenous immune globulin for prevention of cytomegalovirus infection and interstitial pneumonia after bone marrow transplantation. Ann Intern Med 1987;106:12–18.

98. Winston D, Ho W, Champlin R. Cytomegalovirus infections after allogenic bone marrow transplantation. Rev Infect Dis 1990;12(suppl 7):S776–S792.

99. Sullivan K, Kopecky K, Jocom J, et al. Immunomodulatory and antimicrobial efficacy of intravenous immunoglobulin in bone marrow transplantation. N Engl J Med 1990;323:705–712.

100. Arsura E, Bick A, Brunner N, et al. High dose intravenous immunoglobulin in the management of myasthenia gravis. Arch Int Med 1986;146:1365–1368.

101. Sullivan KM, Storek J, Kopecky KJ, et al. A controlled trial of long-term administration of intravenous immunoglobulin to prevent late infection and chronic graft-vs.-host disease after marrow transplantation: clinical outcome and effect on subsequent immune recovery. Biol Blood Marrow Transplant 1996;2(1):44–53.

102. Schmidt G, Kovacs A, Zaia J, et al. Ganciclovir/immunoglobulin combination therapy for the treatment of human cytomegalovirus-associated interstitial pneumonia in bone marrow allograft recipients. Transplantation 1988;46:905–907.

103. Bowden R, Sayers M, Flournoy N, et al. Cytomegalovirus immune globulin and seronegative blood products to prevent primary cytomegalovirus infection after marrow transplantation. N Engl J Med 1986;314:1006–1010.

104. Meyers J, Leszczynski J, Zaia J, et al. Prevention of cytomegalovirus infection by cytomegalovirus immune globulin after marrow transplantation. Ann Intern Med 1983;98:442–446.

105. Kapoor N, Copelan E, Tutschka P. Cytomegalovirus infection in bone marrow transplant recipients: use of intravenous gamma globulin as a prophylactic and therapeutic agent. Transplant Proc 1989;21:3095–3096.

106. Bass E, Powe N, Goodman S, et al. Efficacy of immune globulin in preventing complications of bone marrow transplantation: a meta analysis. Bone Marrow Transplant 1993;12:273–282.

107. Zikos P, Van Lint MT, Lamparelli T, et al. A randomized trial of high dose polyvalent intravenous immunoglobulin (HDIgG) vs. cytomegalovirus (CMV) hyperimmune IgG in allogeneic hemopoietic stem cell transplants (HSCT). Haematologica 1998;83(2):132–137.

108. Bunchman TE, Parekh RS, Kershaw DB, et al. Beneficial effect of Sandoglobulin upon allograft survival in the pediatric renal transplant recipient. Clin Transplant 1997;11(6):604–607.

109. Jordan SC, Quartel AW, Czer LS, et al. Posttransplant therapy using high-dose human immunoglobulin (intravenous gammaglobulin) to control acute humoral rejection in renal and cardiac allograft recipients and poten-

110. Peraldi MN, Akposso K, Haymann JP, et al. Long-term benefit of intravenous immunoglobulins in cadaveric kidney retransplantation. Transplantation 1996;62(11):1670–1673.

111. Flynn JT, Kaiser BA, Long SS, et al. Intravenous immunoglobulin prophylaxis of cytomegalovirus infection in pediatric renal transplant recipients. Am J Nephrol 1997;17(2):146–152.

112. Ginevri F, Losurdo G, Fontana I, et al. Acyclovir plus CMV immunoglobulin prophylaxis and early therapy with ganciclovir are effective and safe in CMV high-risk renal transplant pediatric recipients. Transpl Int 1998;11(suppl 1):S130–S134.

113. Ammann A, Ashman R, Buckley R, et al. Use of intravenous gamma-globulin in antibody immunodeficiency: results of a multicenter controlled trial. Clin Immunol Immunopathol 1982;22:60–67.

114. Ammann A, Schiffman G, Abrams D, et al. B-cell immunodeficiency is acquired immune deficiency syndrome. JAMA 1984;251:1447–1449.

115. Bernstein L, Ochs H, Wedgwood R, Rubinstein A. Defective humoral immunity in pediatric acquired immune deficiency syndrome. J Pediatr 1985;107:352–357.

116. The National Institute of Child Health and Human Development Intravenous Immunoglobulin Study Group. Intravenous immune globulin for the prevention of bacterial infections in children with symptomatic human immunodeficiency virus infection. N Engl J Med 1991;325:78–80.

117. Mofenson L, Moye J, Bethe J, et al. Prophylactic intravenous immunoglobulin in HIV-infected children with CD4+ counts of 0.20×10^9/l or more. Effect on viral, opportunistic and bacterial infections. JAMA 1992;268:483–488.

118. Mofenson L, Bethel J, Moye J, et al. Effect of intravenous immunoglobulin (IVIG) on CD4+ lymphocyte decline in HIV-infected children in a clinical trial of IVIG infection prophylaxis. J Acq Immune Def Syndr 1993;6:1103–1113.

119. Olopoenia L, Young M, White D, et al. Intravenous immunoglobulin in symptomatic and asymptomatic children with perinatal HIV infection. J Natl Med Assoc 1997;89(8):543–547.

120. Simpson KN, Coughlin CM, Eron J, Bussel JB. Idiopathic thrombocytopenic purpura: treatment patterns and an analysis of cost associated with intravenous immunoglobulin and anti-D therapy. Semin Hematol 1998;35(1 suppl 1):58–64.

121. Nydegger UE, Castelli D. Review on therapeutic options in HIV associated thrombocytopenia with emphasis on i.v. immunoglobulin treatment. Immunol Invest 1991;20(2):223–229.

122. Majluf-Cruz A, Luna-Castanos G, Huitron S, Nieto-Cisneros L. Usefulness of a low-dose intravenous immunoglobulin regimen for the treatment of thrombocytopenia associated with AIDS. Am J Hematol 1998;59(2):127–132.

123. Bryan CS, Reynolds KL, Brenner ER. Analysis of 1186 episodes of gram-negative bacteremia in non-university hospitals: the effects of antimicrobial therapy. Rev Infect Dis 1983;5:29–38.

124. Calandra T, Glauser M, Schellekens J, Verhoef J, Group TS-DJIS. Treatment of gram-negative septic shock with

human IgG antibody to *Escherichia coli* J5: a prospective, double-blind, randomized study. J Infect Dis 1988;158: 312–319.

125. Ziegler E, McCutchan J, Fierer J, et al. Treatment of gram-negative bacteremia and shock with human antiserum to a mutant Escherichia coli. N Engl J Med 1982;307:1225–1230.

126. Baumgartner J, Glauser M, McCutchan J, et al. Prevention of gram-negative shock and death in surgical patients by prophylactic antibody to endotoxin core glycolipid. Lancet 1985;ii:59–63.

127. Duswald K, Muller K, Seifert J, Ring J. Wirksamkeit von i.v. Gammaglobulin gegen backterielle Infektionen chirurgischer Patienten. Muench med Wschr 1980;122:832.

128. Glinz W, Grob J, Nydegger U, et al. Polyvalent immunoglobulins for prophylaxis of bacterial infections in patients with multiple trauma. Intensive Care Med 1985;11:288–294.

129. Prophylactic intravenous administration of standard immune globulin as compared with core-lipopolysaccharide immune globulin in patients at high risk of postsurgical infection. The Intravenous Immunoglobulin Collaborative Study Group. N Engl J Med 1992;327(4):234–240.

130. Just H, Vogel W, Metzger M, et al. Treatment of intensive care unit patients with severe nosocomial infections. In: Morel A, Nydegger UE, eds. Clinical use of intravenous immune globulins. London: Academic Press, 1986:345–352.

131. Jesdinsky J, Tenpel G, Castrup H, Seifert J. Cooperative Group of Additional Immunoglobulin Therapy in Severe Bacterial Infections: results of a multicenter randomized controlled trial in cases of diffuse fibrinopurulent peritonitis. Klin Wochenschr 1987;65:1132–1138.

132. Nydegger UE. Sepsis and polyspecific intravenous immunoglobulins. J Clin Apheresis 1997;12(2):93–99.

133. Barry W, Hudgins L, Donta ST, Pesanti EL. Intravenous immunoglobulin therapy for toxic shock syndrome. JAMA 1992;267(24):3315–3316.

134. Lamothe F, D'Amico P, Ghosn P, et al. Clinical usefulness of intravenous human immunoglobulins in invasive group A streptococcal infections: case report and review. Clin Infect Dis 1995;21(6):1469–1470.

135. Perez CM, Kubak BM, Cryer HG, et al. Adjunctive treatment of streptococcal toxic shock syndrome using intravenous immunoglobulin: case report and review. Am J Med 1997;102(1):111–113.

136. Baker C, Melish M, Hall R, et al. Intravenous immune globulin or the prevention of nosocomial infection in low-birth-weight neonates. N Engl J Med 1992;327:213–219.

137. Fanaroff A, Wright E, Korones S, et al. A controlled trial of prophylactic intravenous immunoglobulin to reduce nosocomial infections in VLBW infants. Pediatr Res 1992;31:202A. Abstract.

138. Fischer G. Use of intravenous immune globulin in newborn infants. Clin Exp Immunol 1994;97:73–77.

139. Weisman L, Cruess D, Fischer G. Standard versus hyperimmune intravenous immunoglobulin in preventing or treating neonatal bacterial infections. Clin Perinatol 1993;20: 211–224.

140. Jenson HB, Pollock BH. Meta-analyses of the effectiveness of intravenous immune globulin for prevention and treatment of neonatal sepsis. Pediatrics 1997;99(2):E2.

141. Leung D, Chu E, Wood N, et al. Immunoregulatory T cell abnormalities in mucocutaneous lymph node syndrome. J Immunol 1983;130:2002–2004.

142. Meissner H, Schlievert P, Leung D. Mechanisms of immunoglobulin action: observations on Kawasaki syndrome and RSV prophylaxis. Immunol Rev 1994;139:109–123.

143. Leung D, Geha R, Newburger J, et al. Two monokines, interleukin 1 and tumor necrosis factor, render cultured vascular endothelial cells susceptible to lysis by antibodies circulating during Kawasaki syndrome. J Exp Med 1986;164:1958–1972.

144. Leung D, Collins T, LaPierre L, et al. IgM antibodies present in the acute phase of Kawasaki syndrome lyse cultured vascular endothelial cells stimulated by gamma interferon. J Clin Invest 1986;77:1428–1435.

145. Leung D, Cotran R, Kurt-Jones E, et al. Endothelial cell activation and increased interleukin 1 secretion in the pathogenesis of acute Kawasaki disease. Lancet 1986;2: 1298–1302.

146. Newburger J, Takahashi M, Burns J, et al. The treatment of Kawasaki syndrome with intravenous gammaglobulin. N Engl J Med 1986;315:341–347.

147. Newburger JW, Takahashi M, Beiser AS, et al. A single intravenous infusion of gamma globulin as compared with four infusions in the treatment of acute Kawasaki syndrome. N Engl J Med 1991;324(23):1633–1639.

148. Burns JC, Capparelli EV, Brown JA, et al. Intravenous gammaglobulin treatment and retreatment in Kawasaki disease. US/Canadian Kawasaki Syndrome Study Group. Pediatr Infect Dis J 1998;17(12):1144–1148.

149. Reduction of respiratory syncytial virus hospitalization among premature infants and infants with bronchopulmonary dysplasia using respiratory syncytial virus immune globulin prophylaxis. The PREVENT Study Group. Pediatrics 1997;99(1):93–99.

150. Rodriguez WJ, Gruber WC, Welliver RC, et al. Respiratory syncytial virus (RSV) immune globulin intravenous therapy for RSV lower respiratory tract infection in infants and young children at high risk for severe RSV infections: Respiratory Syncytial Virus Immune Globulin Study Group. Pediatrics 1997;99(3):454–461.

151. Palivizumab, a humanized respiratory syncytial virus monoclonal antibody, reduces hospitalization from respiratory syncytial virus infection in high-risk infants. The IMpact-RSV Study Group. Pediatrics 1998;102(3 Pt 1):531–537.

152. American Academy of Pediatrics Committee on Infectious Diseases and Committee of Fetus and Newborn. Prevention of respiratory syncytial virus infections: indications for the use of palivizumab and update on the use of RSV-IGIV. Pediatrics 1998;102(5):1211–1216.

153. Meissner HC, Groothuis JR. Immunoprophylaxis and the control of RSV disease. Pediatrics 1997;100:260–262.

154. Guarino A, Canani RB, Russo S, et al. Oral immunoglobulins for treatment of acute rotaviral gastroenteritis. Pediatrics 1994;93(1):12–16.

155. Viard I, Wehrli P, Bullani R, et al. Inhibition of toxic epidermal necrolysis by blockade of CD95 with human intravenous immunoglobulin. Science 1998;282(5388):490–493.

156. Salcedo J, Keates S, Pothoulakis C, et al. Intravenous immunoglobulin therapy for severe Clostridium difficile colitis. Gut 1997;41(3):366–370.

157. Leung DY, Kelly CP, Boguniewicz M, et al. Treatment with intravenously administered gamma globulin of chronic relapsing colitis induced by Clostridium difficile toxin. J Pediatr 1991;118(4 Pt 1):633–637.

158. Ronda N, Kaveri S, Kazatchkine M. Treatment of autoimmune diseases with normal immunoglobulin through manipulation of the idiotypic network. Clin Exp Immunol 1993;93:14–15.

159. Gajdos P, Outin H, Morel E, et al. High dose intravenous gamma globulin for myasthenia gravis: an alternative to plasma exchange? Ann NY Acad Sci 1987;505:842–844.

160. Imbach P, Barandun S, d'Apuzzo V, et al. High-dose intravenous gamma-globulin for idiopathic thrombocytopenic purpura in childhood. Lancet 1981;i:1228-1231.

161. Imholz B, Imbach P, Baumgartner C, et al. Intravenous immunoglobulin (i.v. IgG) for previously treated acute or for chronic idiopathic thrombocytopenic purpura (ITP) in childhood: a prospective multicenter study. Blut 1988;56:63–68.

162. Imbach P, Wagner H, Berchtold W, et al. Intravenous immunoglobulin versus oral corticosteroids in acute immune thrombocytopenic purpura in childhood. Lancet 1985;ii:464–468.

163. Martin J, Morrison J, Files J. Autoimmune thrombocytopenic purpura: current concepts and recommended practices. Am J Obstet Gynecol 1984;150:86–96.

164. Kelton J. Management of the pregnant patient with idiopathic thrombocytopenic purpura. Ann Intern Med 1983;99:796–800.

165. Tarantino MD, Madden RM, Fennewald DL, et al. Treatment of childhood acute immune thrombocytopenic purpura with anti-D immune globulin or pooled immune globulin. J Pediatr 1999;134(1):21–26.

166. Sagripanti A, Ferretti A, Giannessi D, et al. Anti-D treatment for chronic immune thrombocytopenic purpura: clinical and laboratory aspects. Biomed Pharmacother 1998;52(7–8):293–297.

167. Francioni C, Galeazzi M, Fioravanti A, et al. Long-term i.v. Ig treatment in systemic lupus erythematosus. Clin Exp Rheumatol 1994;12(2):163–168.

168. Lesprit P, Mouloud F, Bierling P, et al. Prolonged remission of SLE-associated polyradiculoneuropathy after a single course of intravenous immunoglobulin. Scand J Rheumatol 1996;25(3):177–179.

169. Corvetta A, Della Britta R, Gabrielli A, et al. Use of high-dose intravenous immunoglobulin in systemic lupus erythematosus; report of 3 cases. Clin Exp Rheumatol 1989;7:295–299.

170. Lin R, Racis S. In vivo reduction of circulating C1q binding immune complexes by intravenous gammaglobulin administration. Int Arch Allergy Appl Immunol 1986;79:286–290.

171. Tuso P, Moudgil A, Hay J, et al. Treatment of ANCA-positive glomerulonephritis associated with Wegener's granulomatosus with pooled intravenous gammaglobulin. Am J Kidney Dis 1992;20:504–508.

172. French Cooperative Group on Plasma Exchange in Guillain-Barre Syndrome. Efficiency of plasma exchange in Guillain-Barre syndrome: role of replacement fluids. Ann Neurol 1987;22:753–761.

173. van der Meche FG, Schmitz PI. A randomized trial comparing intravenous immune globulin and plasma exchange in Guillain-Barre syndrome. Dutch Guillain-Barre Study Group. N Engl J Med 1992;326(17):1123–1129.

174. Randomised trial of plasma exchange, intravenous immunoglobulin, and combined treatments in Guillain-Barre syndrome. Plasma Exchange/Sandoglobulin Guillain-Barre Syndrome Trial Group. Lancet 1997;349(9047):225–230.

175. Bril V, Ilse WK, Pearce R, et al. Pilot trial of immunoglobulin versus plasma exchange in patients with Guillain-Barre syndrome. Neurology 1996;46(1):100–103.

176. Abd-Allah SA, Jansen PW, Ashwal S, Perkin RM. Intravenous immunoglobulin as therapy for pediatric Guillain-Barre syndrome. J Child Neurol 1997;12(6):376–380.

177. Gorson KC, Allam G, Ropper AH. Chronic inflammatory demyelinating polyneuropathy: clinical features and response to treatment in 67 consecutive patients with and without a monoclonal gammopathy. Neurology 1997;48(2):321–328.

178. Hahn AF. Treatment of chronic inflammatory demyelinating polyneuropathy with intravenous immunoglobulin. Neurology 1998;51(6 suppl 5):S16–S21.

179. Fazekas F, Deisenhammer F, Strasser-Fuchs S, et al. Randomised placebo-controlled trial of monthly intravenous immunoglobulin therapy in relapsing-remitting multiple sclerosis. Austrian Immunoglobulin in Multiple Sclerosis Study Group. Lancet 1997;349(9052):589–593.

180. Sorensen PS, Wanscher B, Schreiber K, et al. A double-blind, cross-over trial of intravenous immunoglobulin G in multiple sclerosis: preliminary results. Mult Scler 1997;3(2):145–148.

181. Francis GS, Freedman MS, Antel JP. Failure of intravenous immunoglobulin to arrest progression of multiple sclerosis: a clinical and MRI based study. Mult Scler 1997;3(6):370–376.

182. Lisak RP. Intravenous immunoglobulins in multiple sclerosis. Neurology 1998;51(6 suppl 5):S25–S29.

183. Engel A. Myasthenia gravis and myasthenic syndromes. Ann Neurol 1984;16:519–534.

184. Rowland L. Controversies about the treatment of myasthenia gravis. Neurol Neurosurg Psych 1980;43:644–659.

185. Besinger U, Fateh-Moghadam A, Knorr-Held S, et al. Immunomodulation in myasthenia gravis by high dose intravenous 7-S immunoglobulin. Ann NY Acad Sci 1987;505:828–831.

186. Cosi V, Lombardi M, Piccolo G, Erbetta A. Treatment of myasthenia gravis with high dose intravenous immunoglobulin. Acta Neurol Scand 1991;84:81–84.

187. Gajdos P, Chevret S, Clair B, et al. Clinical trial of plasma exchange and high-dose intravenous immunoglobulin in myasthenia gravis. Myasthenia Gravis Clinical Study Group. Ann Neurol 1997;41(6):789–796.

188. Jongen JL, van Doorn PA, van der Meche FG. High-dose intravenous immunoglobulin therapy for myasthenia gravis. J Neurol 1998;245(1):26–31.

189. Howard JF Jr. Intravenous immunoglobulin for the treatment of acquired myasthenia gravis. Neurology 1998;51(6 suppl 5):S30–S36.

190. Duse M, Notarangelo LD, Tiberti S, et al. Intravenous immune globulin in the treatment of intractable childhood epilepsy. Clin Exp Immunol 1996;104(suppl 1):71–76.

191. Silverman ED, Cawkwell GD, Lovell DJ, et al. Intravenous immunoglobulin in the treatment of systemic juvenile rheumatoid arthritis: a randomized placebo controlled trial. Pediatric Rheumatology Collaborative Study Group. J Rheumatol 1994;21(12):2353–2358.

192. Giannini EH, Lovell DJ, Silverman ED, et al. Intravenous immunoglobulin in the treatment of polyarticular juvenile rheumatoid arthritis: a phase I/II study. Pediatric Rheumatology Collaborative Study Group. J Rheumatol 1996;23(5): 919–924.

193. Colagiuri S, Leong GM, Thayer Z, et al. Intravenous immunoglobulin therapy for autoimmune diabetes mellitus. Clin Exp Rheumatol 1996;14(suppl 15):S93–S97.

194. Heinze E. Immunoglobulins in children with autoimmune diabetes mellitus. Clin Exp Rheumatol 1996;14(suppl 15):S99–S102.

195. Hide M, Francis DM, Grattan CE, et al. Autoantibodies against the high-affinity IgE receptor as a cause of histamine release in chronic urticaria. N Engl J Med 1993;328(22): 1599–1604.

196. O'Donnell BF, Barr RM, Black AK, et al. Intravenous immunoglobulin in autoimmune chronic urticaria. Br J Dermatol 1998;138(1):101–106.

197. Lafferty TE, Smith JB, Schuster SJ, DeHoratius RJ. Treatment of acquired factor VIII inhibitor using intravenous immunoglobulin in two patients with systemic lupus erythematosus. Arthritis Rheum 1997;40(4):775–778.

198. Tarantino MD, Ross MP, Daniels TM, Nichols WL. Modulation of an acquired coagulation factor V inhibitor with intravenous immune globulin. J Pediatr Hematol Oncol 1997;19(3):226–231.

199. Taylor C, Faulk W. Prevention of recurrent abortion with leucocyte transfusions. Lancet 1981;ii:68–70.

200. Unander AM. The role of immunization treatment in preventing recurrent abortion. Transf Med Rev 1992;6:1–16.

201. Mueller-Eckhardt G, Heine O, Neppert J, et al. Prevention of recurrent spontaneous abortion by intravenous immunoglobulin. Vox Sang 1989;51:122–126.

202. Mueller-Eckhardt G, Heine O, Polten B. IVIG to prevent recurrent spontaneous abortion. Lancet 1991;337:424–425.

203. Heine O, Mueller-Eckhardt G, Stitz L, Pabst W. Influence of treatment with mouse immunoglobulin on the rate of viable neonates in the CBA/JxDBA/2J model. Res Exp Med 1992;192:49–52.

204. Heine O, Mueller-Eckhardt G. Intravenous immune globulin in recurrent abortion. Clin Exp Immunol 1994;97:39–42.

205. Kiprov DD, Nachtigall RD, Weaver RC, et al. The use of intravenous immunoglobulin in recurrent pregnancy loss associated with combined alloimmune and autoimmune abnormalities. Am J Reprod Immunol 1996;36(4):228–234.

206. Salmun LM, Barlan I, Wolf HM, et al. Effect of intravenous immunoglobulin on steroid consumption in patients with severe asthma: a double-blind, placebo-controlled, randomized trial. J All Clin Immunol 1999;103:810–815.

207. Landwehr LP, Jeppson JD, Katlan MG, et al. Benefits of high-dose i.v. immunoglobulin in patients with severe steroid-dependent asthma. Chest 1998;114(5):1349–1356.

208. Niggemann B, Leupold W, Schuster A, et al. Prospective, double-blind, placebo-controlled, multicentre study on the effect of high-dose, intravenous immunoglobulin in children and adolescents with severe bronchial asthma. Clin Exp Allergy 1998;28(2):205–210.

209. Physicians' desk reference. Montvale, NJ: Medical Economics Company, 1999.

Chapter 20

Therapeutic Inhibition of Complement Activation with Emphasis on Drugs in Clinical Trials

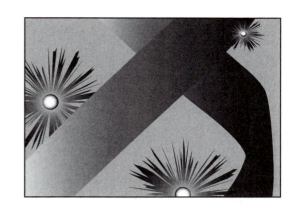

Lloyd B. Klickstein
Francis D. Moore, Jr.
John P. Atkinson

The complement system was discovered over 100 years ago as a "complement" to antibody in the lysis of microorganisms. Within 2 years of its description as a powerful lytic substance, it was recognized that a rare form of hemolytic anemia (paroxysmal cold hemoglobinuria) was caused by this same duo of autoantibody and complement. Thus, like other elements of the immune system, complement is a double-edged sword. Without it, the host is susceptible to both infectious diseases and the development of autoimmunity. At the same time, complement activation can mediate undesirable cellular and tissue injury. To turn off the complement system in clinical situations where complement-mediated injury outweighs benefits is the goal of the investigations to be discussed in this chapter. To provide a coherent discussion, emphasis is placed on the two complement inhibitors currently in clinical trials in the United States.

Complement Activation

The complement system evolved to protect the host from microorganisms. It is an ancient system of defense against pathogens that preceded antibody development and is an important part of both innate and adaptive immunity. Microorganisms do not (usually) bear complement inhibitors; thus, the alternative pathway activates on their surface to deposit opsonic fragments and to generate from precursors in the fluid phase the membrane attack complex, which disrupts the integrity of a microbial surface and leads to membrane perturbation and in many cases to lysis of the targeted organism. To recruit cellular elements of an inflammatory response, C3a and C5a anaphylatoxins are released during complement activation; these anaphylatoxins recruit leukocytes and activate a wide variety of cell types by binding to their G-protein–coupled receptors. The recruited leukocytes bear complement receptors with which they recognize and respond to the opsonized microorganisms by phagocytosis, enzyme release, and oxygen radical production. Thus, complement and leukocytes together yield an innate immune response that is effective even for pathogens that are new to the individual. Complement-opsonized antigens eventually are efficiently presented to lymphocytes to recruit adaptive immunity.

The classical pathway (Fig. 20-1) is activated primarily by immune complexes and other substances that fix C1. Once C1 binds to an activator, the C1r enzymatic component autoactivates and cleaves C1s to form activated C1s within the C1 complex. C4 binds to C1 and is cleaved by activated C1s to C4b, releasing a soluble C4a fragment. The C1 complex also binds C2, and C2 is cleaved by C1s to yield soluble C2b and generate the C4b2a complex, the classical pathway C3 convertase. The enzymatic component of this complex, C2a, cleaves C3 to form C3a and activated C3b. Activated C3b may opsonize a surface by binding covalently via the reactive internal thiolester to nearby amine or hydroxyl groups; it may be inactivated by water hydrolysis of the thiolester; or it may bind covalently (1) to a specific region of the C4b component of the C3 convertase to form the classical pathway C5 convertase, C4b3b2a.

The lectin pathway (see Fig. 20-1) shares many of the same components of the classical pathway. The initial step is binding of mannan-binding lectin (MBL) to an activating surface, for example, yeast cell walls. There are two serine esterases associated with MBL, termed MBL-associated serine protease-1 and -2 (MASP-1 and MASP-2). Each element of the MBL/MASP complex is structurally and functionally homologous to the corresponding elements of C1. The MASP-2 in the bound complex cleaves C4 to form C4a and C4b and C2 to form C2a and C2b. The C4b2a formed is the same C3 convertase as that generated in the classical pathway.

The alternative pathway (see Fig. 20-1) was the second complement activation pathway discovered (hence the name), but it is phylogenetically the most ancient. The alternative pathway is continuously active at a low level under normal circumstances, which accounts for most of the basal C3 turnover observed. With the assumptions of a glomerular filtration efficiency of 50%, normal creatinine clearance, and no other significant clearance mechanisms, the steady-state C3a desArg level of 100 ng/mL (2) yields a plasma C3 half-life of 1.8 days, which corresponds closely to the experimentally observed C3 turnover of 1% to 2% per hour (3). Soluble factors H, I, and host cell surface regulators

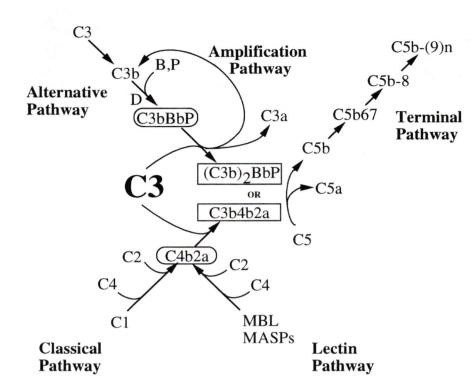

Figure 20-1. Schematic diagram of complement activation pathways, organized to illustrate the central roles of C3 and the C5 convertases. Pathways are indicated in bold. C4b2a and C3bBbP are the classical/lectin and alternative C3 convertases, respectively, and are circled. Similarly, C3b4b2a and (C3b)$_2$BbP are the classical/lectin and alternative C5 convertases, respectively, and are boxed. The C5-convertase designations reflect the covalent associations of C3b with C4b in the classical/lectin convertase and the covalent C3b dimer in the alternative convertase. At least one C5 convertase is required to generate C5a and C5b and activate the terminal pathway. MBL, mannan-binding lectin; MASPs, MBL-associated serine proteases.

limit the activation (Table 20-1); thus, under normal circumstances the alternative pathway is continuously idling, analogous to the engine of a car waiting at a traffic light. If C3b deposits on an activating surface such as that of most microbes, factor H is less effective, and since (most) microbial surfaces do not bear regulators of complement activation, the balance tilts towards activation. Factor B, which is structurally and functionally homologous to C2, binds to the deposited C3b and is cleaved by the constitutively active factor D to Bb and Ba. The C3bBb is the alternative pathway C3 convertase, which is stabilized by binding properdin (P). The serine protease Bb component of C3bBbP then cleaves C3, which may further opsonize the activating surface and in turn bind additional B to form more C3 convertases. This process is termed the amplification pathway, which may be recruited by any of the activation pathways as a positive-feedback step. The C3b may alternatively bind covalently to the C3b element of the C3 convertase to form (C3b)$_2$Bb, which is stabilized by the binding of P to form (C3b)$_2$BbP, the C5 convertase of the alternative pathway.

The terminal pathway (see Fig. 20-1) begins with the cleavage of C5 by either the classical/lectin C5 convertase or the alternative C5 convertase. The C5a generated from the cleavage is a potent chemotaxin and activator of leukocytes. The C5b binds C6, which in turn binds C7 to yield fluid phase C5b67. This complex can bind to lipid membranes and recruit C8. The C5b678 forms an initial pore in the membrane, and recruitment of multiple molecules of C9 yields C5b6789n, the membrane attack complex (MAC). The role of the fully developed MAC in adult immunology is unclear, as nearly 0.1% of 145,640 blood donors from

Osaka, Japan, were substantially deficient in C9 without an obvious phenotype (4). However, C9 may be more important for neonates and young children, who are at risk of losing transplacentally provided humoral immunity before acquisition of their own specific immunoglobulin (5,6). For more complete discussions of the complement pathways, the reader is referred to textbooks of general immunology that have excellent chapters on this subject (7–9) and to available books and monographs (10–16) that authoritatively address aspects of the complement system.

Physiologic Regulation of Complement Activation

The complement system has evolved to allow unimpeded activation on a microbe, but this activation is strictly limited in time and space. The reaction must be finite in time to avoid excessive consumption of components in any one reaction and finite in space to minimize damage to host tissue. Thus, a typical complement reaction on a microbial target occurs within a few minutes, and during this process self-tissue is protected by plasma and membrane regulators. These inhibitors function at the critical steps of initiation, convertase assembly, and membrane attack. The physiologic regulators of complement activation are listed in Table 20-1. A separate chapter is devoted to the C1 inhibitor, which will not be discussed further here. A brief discussion of the endogenous complement inhibitors follows, to clarify the mechanisms of

Table 20-1. Human Complement Regulatory Proteins

Endogenous Complement Inhibitors	Location	Pathway/Product(s) Affected	Mechanism of Action
C1 inhibitor	Plasma	Classical and lectin/C1r, C1s, MASPs	Covalently binds and inactivates C1r, C1s, and MASPs
Factor I	Plasma	All 3 activation pathways/C3b, C4b	Highly specific serine protease that cleaves and inactivates C3b and C4b; has an absolute requirement for a cofactor (see below)
Factor H	Plasma	All 3 activation pathways/C3b	Cofactor for factor I–mediated cleavage of C3b >> C4b to iC3b, primarily active in fluid phase
C4 binding protein (C4bp)	Plasma	Classical and lectin/C4b	Cofactor for factor I–mediated cleavage of C4b >> C3b to C4c + C4d, primarily active in fluid phase
Carboxypeptidase N	Plasma	Anaphylatoxins/C3a, C5a	Inactivates anaphylatoxins C3a and C5a by removal of C-terminal arginine
Vitronectin	Plasma	Terminal pathway	Binds activated C5b67 and prevents membrane insertion; binds C9 and prevents polymerization
Decay-accelerating factor (DAF, CD55)	Cell surfaces (nearly all)	All 3 activation pathways/all convertases	Binds intrinsic (located on the same surface) C3 and C5 convertases and accelerates convertase inactivation
Membrane cofactor protein (MCP, CD46)	Cell surfaces (nearly all)	All 3 activation pathways/C3b, C4b	Binds intrinsic C3 and C5 convertases and serves as cofactor for factor I cleavage of C4b and C3b
Protectin (MIRL, CD59, other names)	Cell surfaces (nearly all)	Terminal pathway/MAC	Binds C5b-8, C5b-9, and prevents pore formation
Complement receptor type 1 (CR1, CD35)	Cell surfaces (limited)	All 3 activation pathways/all convertases	Combined activities of factor H, C4bp, MCP, and DAF; not a major regulator ordinarily, due to limited expression

action of the therapeutic agents currently in clinical trials in humans.

Many of the physiologic inhibitors of complement affect the activation sequences. A major limiting factor that controls complement activation is the inherent instability of the amplification convertases. For example, the alternative pathway C3 convertase has a biologic half-life of 3 to 5 minutes, which may be extended to as long as 20 to 40 minutes in the presence of P (17). Factor H in the fluid phase catalytically accelerates the irreversible dissociation of Bb from the alternative pathway convertases. Similarly, C4bp accelerates the decay of the fluid-phase classical/lectin pathway convertases, and decay-accelerating factor (DAF, CD55) serves the same function on cell surfaces. The convertase-specific protease, factor I, requires a cofactor, which may be factor H or C4bp in the fluid phase or membrane cofactor protein (MCP, CD46) on cell surfaces. Transfection experiments (18) have suggested that MCP preferentially acts on the alternative pathway and DAF acts on the classical pathway. Complement receptor type 1 (CR1, CD35) has the combined complement inhibitory activities of factor H, C4bp, MCP, and DAF; but its expression is limited to erythrocytes, granulocytes, some lymphocytes, dendritic cells, glomerular podocytes, and possibly endothelial cells under conditions of hypoxia and reoxygenation. This limited expression and the low levels of soluble CR1 present under normal circumstances (0.2% to 1% of H and C4bp) suggest that CR1 is unlikely to serve as a physiologic complement inhibitor.

Of the cell surface regulators of complement activation, all exhibit some activity as recombinant soluble(s) molecules (19). In the single, comparative, in vitro study available, sCR1 was approximately 200-fold more potent than sDAF or sMCP as an inhibitor of the classical pathway (19). In an unusual alternative pathway assay of antibody-sensitized CHO cell lysis using serum with Mg2+/EGTA, sCR1 and sMCP were equipotent and far superior to sDAF (19).

Inhibition of the terminal pathway is accomplished at three distinct steps. The fluid-phase C5b67 is formed by action of one of the C5 convertases to cleave C5, followed by binding of C6 and C7. Nascent C5b67 bears exposed hydrophobic sites for membrane insertion and is unstable, with a half-life of only a second or so (20). If the C5b67 does not insert into a lipid membrane, it undergoes a spontaneous and irreversible conformational change to yield hemolytically inactive C5b67 (iC5b67). The plasma protein vitronectin (complement S-protein) binds to C5b67 or iC5b67, which exposes the heparin-binding site of vitronectin (21,22). Given the very short half-life of C5b67, it is unclear whether vitronectin binding to C5b67 has a physiologic role as a complement inhibitor or whether it serves a clearance, adhesion, or signaling function through cellular receptors. All normal cells express CD59 on the surface, a 20-kD membrane protein that binds to C5b-8 and C5b-9 on the same surface and prevents pore formation. Patients with homozygous deficiency of CD59 have the same phenotype as those with paroxysmal nocturnal hemoglobinuria (PNH), in which there is an acquired deficiency of DAF, CD59, and other glycosylphosphatidylinositol-(GPI) anchored proteins in hematopoietic cells, which indicates an important role for this molecule in vivo (23). The lack of a phenotype in adults with C9 deficiency, as noted in the previous section, suggests the important ligand for CD59 is C5b-8. Vitronectin also binds C9 and may limit C9 polymerization (24).

Preclinical and Clinical Trials of Complement Inhibitors

Two specific inhibitors of complement activation are currently in clinical trials in the United States, and several others are under development (Table 20-2). sCR1 inhibits the C3 and C5 convertases from all the activation pathways by two distinct mechanisms. sCR1 alone accelerates the otherwise spontaneous and irreversible decay of the convertases. sCR1 also serves as a cofactor for factor I–mediated cleavage of C3b and C4b, which results in proteolytic, irreversible inactivation of the convertases. In each of these mechanisms, sCR1 acts catalytically, that is, one molecule of sCR1 can inactivate multiple convertases. The anti-C5 mAb, h5G1.1, either as the humanized mAb or a single-chain Fv, binds stoichiometrically to C5 with a K_D in the high picomolar range and prevents all C5 convertase activity. Thus, both complement inhibitors block C5 convertase activity, both act on all three activation pathways, and both must be administered parenterally.

sCR1 in addition blocks the C3 convertases. The subsequent discussion focuses on these two agents, both of which have a reasonable chance of becoming FDA-approved pharmaceuticals.

Soluble Complement Receptor Type 1 (sCR1)

Initially, CR1 was not considered to be a practical molecule for development as a therapeutic complement inhibitor. The monomeric equilibrium dissociation constant (K_D) for C3b binding to CR1 was known to be approximately $1\,\mu M$ (25); consequently, the quantities of CR1 protein required for in vivo inhibition of convertases containing C3b would be very large and prohibitively expensive. It was also known that the K_D of CR1 for C3b dimers was in the low nanomolar range; however, the dimers were assumed to bind to two CR1 molecules on the cells studied. Several findings in the mid to late 1980s led to a reevaluation of CR1 as a potential therapeutic agent. First, CR1 was found to be a significantly better cofactor for factor I when both C3b and C4b were deposited on the surface via the classical pathway than when equivalent numbers of C3b or C4b were deposited separately (26). Second, the C3b and C4b of the classical C5 convertase were found to be covalently associated (1), as were the two C3b molecules in the C5 convertase of the alternative pathway (27). Third, expression and analysis of recombinant deletion mutants of human CR1 led to the recognition that CR1 is multivalent (28). CR1 contains two sites that preferentially bind C3b over C4b and an amino-terminal site that preferentially binds C4b over C3b; thus, the sites are arranged in an

Table 20-2. Selected Complement Activation Inhibitors Under Development

Product	Description	Actions	Company
TP10, TP20	Soluble recombinant CR1 (sCR1) without (TP10) or with sLe^x (TP20) on N-linked carbohydrate	Both degrade C3b/C4b (CA) and decay C3 and C5 convertases (DAA); in addition, TP20 blocks selectin binding	Avant Immunotherapeutics, (Needham, MA)
h5G1.1	Humanized, high-affinity anti-C5 mAb, as single-chain Fv or intact mAb	Blocks cleavage of C5 to C5a and C5b by C5 convertases, prevents C5a and C5b-9 formation	Alexion Pharmaceuticals (New Haven, CT)
APT070	Amino-terminal 3 SCR of CR1 myristoylated at the carboxyl terminus	Inserts in cell membranes and provides intrinsic protection via CR1-like mechanisms	AdProTech (Royston, Herts., UK)
CAB-2	Soluble recombinant chimera of MCP and DAF	Degrades C3b/C4b (CA) and decays C3 and C5 convertases (DAA)	Millenium Pharmaceuticals (Cambridge, MA)
C1q RNA aptamers	Small molecule inhibitors of C1q	Block C1q	NeXstar Pharmaceuticals (Boulder, CO)
C1q analogs	Low-molecular-weight inhibitor of the beta-amyloid–induced activation of C1q	Block C1q	Gliatech (Cleveland, OH)
Serine protease inhibitor analogs	Low-molecular-weight inhibitors of factor D	Inhibit AP activation	BioCryst Pharmaceuticals (Hoover, AL)

DAA, decay-accelerating activity; CA, cofactor activity; SCR, short consensus repeat, the basic structural unit of CR1, MCP, DAF, and related proteins; MAC, membrane attack complex; MCP, membrane cofactor protein; DAF, decay-accelerating factor; CR1, complement receptor type 1; AP, alternative pathway.
Adapted in part from (124,125).

order such that a single molecule of CR1 could interact with both C3b and C4b in the classical C5 convertase or with both C3b molecules in the alternative C5 convertase (28). Each of these binding sites is contained in a separate, long, homologous repeat unit of the molecule. All these observations taken together suggested that a single molecule of recombinant soluble CR1 (sCR1) would be expected to have high affinity for the C3bC4b and (C3b)$_2$ dimers in the classical/lectin and alternative C5 convertases, respectively. More recently, CR1 has been found to bind C1q and MBL via its fourth, long, homologous repeat (29). Coimmobilized C1q and C4b support binding of CR1-bearing erythrocytes in an additive fashion (30). Consequently, CR1 may also interact bivalently with the classical and lectin intermediates that cleave C2; however, whether this contributes to the complement inhibitory activity of sCR1 is currently unknown.

The initial description of sCR1 activity in vivo (31) demonstrated that the recombinant, soluble molecule retained its desirable functional properties. First, it bound the anticipated ligands, C3b and C4b. Next, at nanomolar concentrations it fully inhibited both classical and alternative pathway activation. Third, human sCR1 also blocked complement activation in rats and selected other experimental animals. Last, sCR1 was shown to inhibit an inflammatory reaction in the rat, myocardial ischemia and reperfusion. The reduced infarct size as a result of sCR1 administration was caused by complement inhibition, because

there was reduced immunostaining for C5b-9 neoantigen in treated tissues. By inference, this in vivo experiment established penetration of this large inhibitory molecule into the extravascular space.

As of this writing, more than 70 peer-reviewed publications report utilization of sCR1 to inhibit complement activation in a variety of disease models in animals. Selected models will be discussed as introductions to human trials. Of the two forms of sCR1 currently under investigation, TP10 is the recombinant soluble form of the F (also called A or CR1*1) CR1 allotype that has been used in most studies. This protein was produced by truncation of the cDNA after the sequence encoding the first alanine in the transmembrane domain, residue 1931, as numbered from the glutamine presumed to be the first amino acid of the mature protein (28,31). The recombinant protein was expressed in CHO cells and purified from conditioned medium. A newer version is TP20 in which the same sCR1 protein is expressed in a CHO cell variant (CHO LEC11) that decorates the N-linked carbohydrate with sialyl Lewis^x (sLe^x) and forms a ligand for selectins. This strategy was conceived to target the sCR1 to activated endothelium expressing E-selectin and P-selectin, to block selectin interactions, and to address in part the relatively short half-life of sCR1. Initial studies have validated this idea (32). Various models of human disease for which sCR1 has proved an effective therapy are summarized in Table 20-3.

Table 20-3. Animal Models of Disease in Which Complement Inhibition with sCR1 or h5G1.1 Anti-C5 has Shown Efficacy in Vivo

Animal Model	Human Disease	Drug tested	References
Ischemia/reperfusion			
Cerebral artery ligation/release	Stroke	sCR1	71
Mesenteric artery ligation/release	Mesenteric ischemia	sCR1	74–77
Coronary artery ligation +/– release	Myocardial infarction	sCR1	31–39
Cardiopulmonary bypass	Cardiopulmonary bypass	Anti-C5	102,123
Organ allotransplantation			
Lung allograft	Lung transplantation	sCR1	83
Cardiac allograft	Heart transplantation	sCR1	79
Renal allograft	Kidney transplantation	sCR1	81
Liver allograft	Liver transplantation	sCR1	82
Direct complement activation			
Pulmonary acid instillation	Aspiration pneumonitis	sCR1	54–56
Burn injury	Burn injury	sCR1	121,122
Endotoxin treatment/bacterial infection	Septic shock	Anti-C5	51,52
Remote lung injury			
Lung injury after mesenteric or hindlimb ischemia	Adult respiratory distress syndrome	sCR1	57,58
Autoimmunity			
Antigen-/collagen-induced arthritis	Rheumatoid arthritis	sCR1	60,61
Pulmonary IgA immune complexes	IgA-associated pneumonitis	sCR1	59
Glomerulonephritis	Glomerulonephritis	sCR1	65
Glomerulonephritis	Lupus	Anti-C5	99
Experimental autoimmune neuritis	Guillain-Barré syndrome	sCR1	69,70
Passive antiacetylcholine receptor	Myasthenia gravis	sCR1	72
Experimental allergic encephalitis	Multiple sclerosis	sCR1	73

Reperfusion Injury

From the earliest in vivo studies of sCR1 as a drug (31), efforts have focused on the critical role of complement in ischemia and reperfusion. Experimental reperfusion systems in which sCR1 has demonstrated significant benefit have included several animal models of myocardial ischemia (31,33–39). These studies were primarily models of coronary bypass and myocardial infarction. For example, in one recent study, 20 pigs were subjected to occlusion of the second and third diagonal coronary arteries for 90 minutes, followed by 45 minutes of cardioplegic arrest, and then 3 hours of reperfusion, to model emergent surgical revascularization of acutely ischemic myocardium (38). Half of the pigs were given 10 mg/kg of sCR1 before coronary occlusion. Pigs that received sCR1 had infarcts that were 40% smaller than those pigs that did not receive sCR1, and these pigs had correspondingly improved wall motion scores. Both outcomes were highly significant ($P < .0001$). sCR1 was efficacious in all the other studies, too.

An important issue that needs further attention is whether sCR1 would be efficacious when administered after the initiation of ischemia. In the models of allotransplantation, the sCR1 is given before transplantation; that is, after ischemia but before reperfusion. Thus, there is some support for initiation of the complement-mediated injury on reperfusion. However, the donor organs are washed free of blood, and presumably the organs are washed free of most complement components too. In ischemia/reperfusion where blood is present, it is likely that complement activation occurs during the time of ischemia. Two of the newer trials have addressed timing of complement inhibitor therapy, in particular a recent study in a model of ischemic stroke, discussed below.

Direct Alternative Pathway Activation

Thermal Injury.   Burns have long been known to cause complement activation (40,41), presumably the result of a direct alternative pathway activation by heat-denatured proteins (42). The complement activation may further injure the host, as demonstrated by the improved early survival rate of experimental animals with large burns that had been complement depleted before the burn compared with untreated, burned animals (43). The degree of burn wound edema can be attenuated by prior decomplementation (44). A study of eight patients (45) documented systemic complement activation with elevated C3a desArg levels and also showed a selective decrease in the patients' neutrophil chemotaxis to C5a. This was accompanied by a loss of C5a receptors and was interpreted as demonstrating that the burns had caused systemic complement activation, which generated C5a; C5a then caused systemic neutrophil activation with resulting loss of subsequent chemotaxis to C5a. This finding could possibly explain the well-known propensity of burned patients to experience invasive infections. In another study of seven patients (46), systemic neutrophil activation was directly documented and correlated highly with the loss of chemotaxis to C5a. In this study small burns demonstrated as much neutrophil activation as large burns, indicating that the complement response becomes systemic with even minor injuries. Serum concentrations of C4a desArg and C3a desArg were elevated, suggesting a role for the classical pathway as well (47). Complement inhibition with sCR1 may reduce both the degree of burn injury acutely and reduce the propensity for infection subsequently.

Sepsis and Septic Shock.   Septic shock is associated with direct activation of the alternative complement pathway (48). In a study of 48 critically ill patients, concentrations of C3a desArg were increased in those with septic shock (49). In another study of 27 septic patients, C3a desArg levels were increased and in those patients in whom levels did not normalize, acute respiratory distress syndrome (ARDS) and multisystem organ failure ensued; these findings suggested that ongoing complement activation predicts an adverse outcome (50). In vivo experimental evidence supports a pathogenic role for complement in septic shock. In rodent (51) and primate (52) models of septic shock, endotoxin infusions caused increased concentrations of C3a desArg, and the adverse cardiovascular effects of endotoxin were mimicked by C5a infusions. Furthermore, the adverse cardiovascular effects of endotoxin were improved with an anti-C5a antibody infusion. Whether the administration of sCR1 could improve survival in some forms of septic shock is uncertain, as erythrocyte CR1 is required for intravascular particle clearance, including bacterial particles (53). sCR1 conceivably could block this clearance mechanism; however, this possibility has not been evaluated experimentally.

Aspiration.   Aspiration of gastric contents is a serious illness that causes pneumonitis, which results from both the acidity of the aspirated material and the presence of oral flora. A study was undertaken to clarify further the mechanism of injury in a model of aspiration using C3, C4, or E- or P-selectin knockout mice and sCR1 treatment of wild-type mice (54). To cause an acid injury, 0.1 N HCl was instilled into the large airways. C3 deficiency and sCR1 treatment of wild-type mice each ameliorated the lung injury, as assessed by quantitative measures of pulmonary edema, while deficiencies in E-selectin, P-selectin, and C4 had no effect. Neutrophil depletion, in addition to sCR1 treatment, had an additive effect. The authors concluded that neutrophils and alternative pathway activation, but not endothelial selectins or the classical/lectin pathways, were required for acid-induced, acute lung injury. In a model of aspiration in rats, 0.2 mL of 0.1 N HCl was introduced into the trachea, and intravenous pretreatment of the rats with sCR1 (10 mg/kg) was as effective as cobra venom factor–depletion of complement (55). Pulmonary edema, leakage of protein into bronchoalveolar lavage fluid, and tissue oxygenation were all significantly improved in both treatment groups compared with the untreated group. In contrast, in a similar model in which the same dose of sCR1 was used and 0.1 mL of 0.1 N HCl was introduced into just one lung, there was no effect on edema and protein leakage in the acid-treated lung but a significant improvement in the remote injury effect on the contralateral lung and the intestine at 4 hours. There was an approximately 80% decrease in circulating tumor necrosis factor α (TNF-α) levels in the sCR1-pretreated rats, compared with the levels in the control group (56). Another study found a similar protective effect of sCR1 for the remote lung injury after 60 minutes of mesenteric arterial occlusion followed by 180 minutes of reperfusion (57). Pretreatment with sCR1 (approximately 20 to 30 mg/kg) resulted in decreased lung permeability to ^{125}I-labeled bovine serum albumin (BSA) and a decreased intestinal mucosal injury score. As in the previous study, there was no change in pulmonary myeloperoxidase level. These findings suggested that neutrophils were still sequestered in the lung but not activated. There was also a trend toward decreased mortality in the sCR1-treated animals. Significant effects were generally not seen with a lower dose of sCR1. In a similar model of remote lung injury after bilateral hindlimb ischemia in the rat, sCR1 attenuated the increase in pulmonary vascular permeability without an effect on pulmonary myeloperoxidase levels (58).

Autoimmune Diseases

In vivo models of autoimmune disease support a role for complement activation in selected circumstances. One early and dramatic example was IgA immune complex–mediated pulmonary injury in rats (59). In this model, a critical role for complement was shown by highly significant inhibition of lung injury in rats pretreated with sCR1. Blocking mAb to CD18 also attenuated the injury, but neutrophils apparently had no role. Thus, the authors suggested that the lung injury in this model is caused by complement-mediated activation of local macrophages.

Two in vivo rat studies that used sCR1 supported a role for complement in models of rheumatoid arthritis. In one study (60), periarticular injection of TNF-α and passive immunization with a low dose of anticollagen type II antibody led to florid arthritis in the hindpaw, near the site of TNF-α injection. Neither treatment alone led to clinically evident arthritis. Pretreatment of rats with sCR1 before induction of TNF-α–dependent, anticollagen antibody–induced arthritis significantly attenuated the inflammation, although not as much as prior leukocyte depletion with an antigranulocyte antibody. In the second study, rats that were immunized with methylated BSA were given an intraarticular injection of BSA and sCR1 (0.2 mg) in one knee. Control rats received sCR1 intravenously, intraperitoneal cobra venom factor, or saline. Joints that received intraarticular sCR1 demonstrated dramatically decreased swelling and much lower histologic scores, significantly better than joints from rats that had received intravenous sCR1 or even cobra venom factor, where the CH50 was zero. Relatively little effect, although still of statistical significance, was seen if sCR1 were administered after the onset of arthritis (61). These data were interpreted to indicate that locally synthesized complement is important in the development of antigen-induced arthritis. Finally, a novel derivative of CR1, APT070, contains just SCR1-3, retains activity as a complement inhibitor (62), and has been used as an intraarticular therapy in antigen-induced arthritis in rats (63). This protein is produced in bacteria, refolded in vitro after partial purification, and subsequently myristoylated. Intraarticular injection of this material

leads to insertion of the protein in cell membranes, tissue acquisition of complement inhibitory activity, and substantial therapeutic benefit in the BSA antigen-induced arthritis model (63). APT070 was also tested in a model of renal transplantation–associated ischemia/reperfusion (64). The donor kidney was perfused with the drug, held ex vivo for a 90-minute period of ischemia, and then transplanted. Histological analysis showed dramatically decreased acute tubular necrosis and neutrophil infiltrate in the treated kidneys compared with buffer-treated kidneys and with kidneys treated with a similar recombinant fragment of CR1 but without the membrane targeting modification. Immunochemically detectable APT070 remained associated with the kidney for the 3-day duration of the experiment.

In a single study that examined three experimental models of glomerulonephritis in the rat, sCR1 was given daily at high dose (60 mg/kg). The models chosen, concanavalin A, antithymocyte serum, and passive Heyman nephritis, are known to be complement-mediated, at least in part. sCR1 treatment decreased proteinuria in all cases and was associated with less severe histologic changes (65). Treatment of glomerulonephritis with sCR1 in humans might be more complex, as erythrocyte CR1 is involved in clearance of intravascular immune complexes (66), unlike rodents where immune complexes are cleared after binding to a different protein on platelets. Thus, sCR1 might be effective in glomerulonephritides where immune complexes form in situ but not in illnesses where circulating complexes are trapped by the kidney.

Neurologic Diseases

Antibody and complement have been implicated in the pathogenesis of several neurologic diseases, notably demyelinating diseases such as Guillain-Barré syndrome (GBS). Humans with these illnesses have dramatically elevated levels of SC5b-9, an average of 100 μg/mL in the plasma, which is a 100-fold increase above normal, as assessed by an antibody to a C9 neoepitope expressed on inactive, soluble MAC. Interestingly, human CSF levels of C3a and C5a (probably the desArg forms) were found to be more than 10-fold elevated above normal levels, while there was no elevation in plasma C3a and only a modest elevation of C5a (67). These findings are consistent with the primary complement activation being localized to the spinal roots, the site of the pathology in GBS. Consistent with a central role for complement in these disorders, intravenous gamma globulin and apheresis are both effective therapies. The subject of complement and neurologic disease has been reviewed recently (68). In a rat model of GBS, experimental autoimmune neuritis (EAN), animals were immunized with bovine myelin in Freund's adjuvant. Administration of daily sCR1 (30 mg/kg) begun on day 8 postimmunization dramatically suppressed the development of symptoms. None of eight sCR1-treated animals became paretic, whereas seven of nine control animals did. Furthermore, electrophysiologic and histologic studies of sciatic nerves showed highly significant prevention of nerve damage by sCR1 (69). Rats treated with a lower dose of sCR1 were not protected from experimental autoimmune neuritis to the same extent as those treated with cobra venom factor (70).

There is, to date, one published study in a murine model of stroke with the new TP20 version of sCR1 that bears approximately 10 sLe^x moieties on the N-linked carbohydrate of each protein molecule (71). One middle cerebral artery in each mouse was occluded for 45 minutes, followed by 23 hours of reperfusion. The sCR1sLe^x (0, 5, 10, or 15 mg/kg) was administered before or at the time of restoration of flow. In a dose-response fashion, the sCR1sLe^x significantly decreased infarct volume by up to 80%. There were also statistically significant decreased leukocyte and platelet accumulations in the reperfused hemisphere, a decreased clinical neurologic deficit score, decreased intracranial hemorrhage, and a modest increase in cerebral blood flow (71). There was a trend toward decreased mortality in the sCR1sLe^x-treated animals. In comparisons of sCR1 and sCR1sLe^x, the sCR1sLe^x was significantly more effective. It is unclear whether the increased efficacy represents better drug targeting, a longer drug half-life, an additional effect of blocking selectin interactions, or some combination of these factors.

Other studies have suggested efficacy of complement inhibition in models of myasthenia gravis and multiple sclerosis (72,73).

Intestinal Ischemia and Organ Allografts

It is well established that ischemia with subsequent reperfusion leads to complement activation and leukocyte-dependent tissue injury. This relationship was shown in the first in vivo study of sCR1 in ischemic rat myocardium (31) and has been confirmed subsequently in several models of disease. A stroke model of ischemia/reperfusion was discussed in the section above, where dramatic efficacy was achieved with the TP20 version of sCR1 (71).

In a murine model of intestinal ischemia, 40 minutes of jejunal ischemia was followed by 3 hours of reperfusion in mice lacking C3, C4, or Ig or in wild-type mice treated with sCR1 (74). All the knockout mice and the sCR1-treated mice had decreased permeability to ^{125}I-labeled albumin when compared with wild-type control mice. In a rat model of intestinal ischemia and reperfusion, anesthetized rats were bled until hypotensive and maintained in the hypotensive state for 1 hour. The rats were then given sCR1 (15 mg/kg) or saline and their blood reinfused with an equal volume of saline to restore central hemodynamic measurements to normal. sCR1 essentially prevented the histologic features of ischemia/reperfusion, the neutrophil influx, and the decrease in nitric oxide synthase that occurred in the saline-treated animals (75). Using the same rat model of ischemia/reperfusion and intravital videomicroscopy, the same investigators found that the arteriolar constriction appearing after ischemia/reperfusion was prevented by treatment with sCR1 (15 mg/kg) just before resuscitation (76). Finally, other investigators, using a rat model of mesenteric artery ligation and reperfusion, found sCR1 (12 mg/kg) decreased histologic injury, neutrophil influx, and leukotriene B$_4$ production in a time-dependent fashion. sCR1 administered at the time of reperfusion or 30 minutes afterward showed a protective effect, but not if given an hour after reperfusion (77). Taken together, these findings suggest that classical or lectin pathway–dependent endothelial dysfunc-

tion contributes to the ischemia/reperfusion injury in the gut. In studies of cultured human umbilical vein endothelial cells, hypoxia and reoxygenation of the cultures led to classical or lectin pathway activation but not alternative pathway activation in the presence of 30% human serum (78), as assessed by immunodepletion of the serum with anti-C2 versus anti-B antibodies. Thus, the rodent studies may indeed be relevant to the human system.

Organ transplantation is perhaps the most extreme clinical situation in which ischemia/reperfusion injury occurs. There is intense interest in complement inhibition as a step toward successful xenograft transplantation (discussed in Chapter 40). The following discussion emphasizes the effect of sCR1 on models of allograft survival and function. There are ongoing trials of sCR1 in human allograft recipients (see below). In the earliest animal study (79), Lewis rats were sensitized after rejection of three serial skin grafts from ACI rats. These sensitized rats then received heterotopic cardiac allografts from the ACI rats. Relatively low dose sCR1 (3 mg/kg) given just before allografting increased the graft survival from 3 hours to 32 hours, which suggested that the antibody-mediated, hyperacute, allograft rejection was complement-dependent. Complement-mediated, hyperacute rejection requires the late components of the terminal pathway, because C6-deficient rats, or rats treated with anti-C6 antibody, have a markedly prolonged time to rejection of guinea pig cardiac xenografts compared with that of C6-sufficient animals (80). Thus, the h5G1.1 anti-C5 antibody might be effective in these models too.

In a renal allograft model, unsensitized DA rats received a Lewis rat kidney with or without daily treatment with sCR1 (25 mg/kg). In the sCR1-treated animals, there was a delay from 5 days to 9 days in the development of histologic evidence of vascular injury and there were fewer infiltrating leukocytes and fewer activated lymphocytes (81).

In a rat model of orthotopic liver transplant, there was significantly less histologic evidence of reperfusion injury in rats that received sCR1 (20 mg/kg) than in control rats (82). This circumstance translated to an improved functional status as sCR1-treated animals had significantly improved bile production and lower serum transaminase levels than the control animals.

In models of lung allotransplantation, where the donor organ undergoes dramatic ischemia-reperfusion, treatment with sCR1 is of considerable benefit. In a pig model of lung allotransplantation (83), seven pigs were treated with 15 mg/kg sCR1 intravenously before receipt of a left lung that had been explanted, flushed to remove blood, and stored at 4°C for 30 hours. Control animals received saline. In assessments of transplanted lung function at 1 hour and again at 3 days after reperfusion, alveolar ventilation and mixed venous oxygenation were significantly improved in the sCR1-treated animals compared with the control animals. There was less edema in the transplanted lung of the sCR1-treated animals as well.

In summary, these in vivo animal studies demonstrated that complement plays a major role in the obligate reperfusion injury that accompanies organ allografting. There have been no studies in which the donor is administered sCR1 before the organ is harvested, especially the TP20 form of sCR1 bearing the N-linked sLe^x, which might provide additional therapeutic benefit. In one study, APT070 treatment of the donor kidney before transplantation showed significant efficacy, as noted previously (64).

Acute Respiratory Distress Syndrome

The hypothesis that systemic complement activation causes pulmonary dysfunction arose from studies of patients undergoing hemodialysis with complement-activating membranes, in whom hypoxemia, neutrophil aggregation, neutropenia, and pulmonary leukocyte sequestration were found (84,85). The relationship of complement to these events was inferred from the similar capacities of plasma containing C5a (activated in the absence of neutrophils) and of plasma exposed to dialysis membranes to cause neutrophil aggregation (86,87). This hypothesis was subsequently verified by study of C3a desArg levels and neutrophil activation during repeated dialyses (88) and then by the demonstration that during hemodialysis neutrophils express increased cell surface CR3, a proadhesive protein (89). The extension of this reasoning to conclude that complement activation is the seminal event leading to all cases of adult respiratory distress syndrome (ARDS) has not been accepted, primarily because of the complexity of the clinical events and the multiple other mediators present. Yet, in all reported clinical series of patients with ARDS in whom complement activation was assessed, complement activation was present. In 34 patients at risk for ARDS, the 19 who progressed to experience the syndrome had increased C3a desArg levels, decreased chemotaxis of neutrophils to C5a in vitro, and evidence of systemic neutrophil degranulation, all indicative of systemic complement activation (90). This set of findings was also noted in 44 other patients (91). Experimentally, infusion of C5a-containing plasma produces ARDS in rabbits (92). Thus, the administration of sCR1 was predicted to improve some forms of ARDS, and this prediction has been borne out in animal models.

Clinical Trials of sCR1 in Humans

On the basis of the reasoning and animal studies detailed above, recombinant soluble CR1 is currently being studied in patients undergoing lung transplantation; however, there is little published in the scientific literature so far. Two, small, phase I trials have been reported in abstract form. An open-label, dose-escalation study of 0.1 to 10 mg/kg sCR1 (TP10) was performed in 24 patients with acute lung injury. The drug was given as an infusion over 30 minutes, and the patients were followed for nearly a month. sCR1 appeared to be safe in this context as there were no adverse events attributable to it (93). There was a two-phase half-life of the drug, with the bulk of the clearance occurring relatively quickly. A similar trial in which the same dose range was studied in 24 patients with a first myocardial infarction, who received either thrombolytic therapy or revascularization by angioplasty, also found the drug safe and nonimmunogenic. In the latter study, patients were followed for 7 days, and there was a dose- and time-dependent decrease in the CH50. The rise in C3a levels that occurs in patients with myocardial infarction did not occur in the patients treated

with sCR1. In a subset analysis of the nine patients who received thrombolytic therapy, there was a trend toward lower CK-MB levels (52 versus 511) in patients who received >1 mg/kg sCR1 compared with those who received the lower doses, but this difference did not reach statistical significance, perhaps because of the very small sample size (94). It is intriguing that in a larger trial of a single-chain Fv fragment of the h5G1.1 anti-C5 monoclonal antibody in patients undergoing coronary artery bypass grafting, a decrease in CK levels also was seen that was statistically significant (95) (see below). The similar outcome in two trials with completely different inhibitors allows two tentative conclusions with respect to complement inhibition in humans with cardiac disease. First, complement may be necessary for a major element of the reperfusion injury that leads to cardiac myocyte death. Second, the component of reperfusion injury that leads to cell death and CK leak may be mediated by one or more of the C5-C9 complement components.

A single, randomized, multicenter trial of sCR1 in 59 patients undergoing lung transplantation has been reported in abstract form (96). Twenty-nine patients from five centers received a single dose of sCR1 (TP10, 10 mg/kg), and 30 patients received placebo before restoration of blood flow to the transplanted lung. Serum CH50 levels were suppressed by greater than 90% for 1 to 2 days in the patients treated with sCR1. The patients who received sCR1 were extubated significantly sooner than those who received placebo, consistent with the decreased edema and injury seen in the animal models described above. There was a trend toward a shorter time on the ventilator (4.1 +/– 7.1 versus 6.8 +/– 12.6 days) and a shorter time in the ICU (8.1 +/– 9.8 versus 9.9 +/– 14.9 days) for the patients treated with sCR1 versus those treated with placebo, respectively, but these differences did not reach statistical significance at the $P < .05$ level. In a subset analysis of the patients who required cardiopulmonary bypass during transplantation (sCR1, six patients; placebo, five patients), the time on the ventilator was significantly shorter for the patients treated with sCR1 (9.5 +/– 3.7 days versus 21.5 +/– 4.1 days). There was no difference between the groups in perioperative deaths, infections, or acute rejection. As noted previously, some of the complement activation may begin during the ischemic phase of the lung injury, before and during organ harvest. It would be worthwhile to test this possibility in animal models by pretreatment of the donor with sCR1 before organ harvest to see if the beneficial effects of complement inhibition could be augmented.

Humanized Single-Chain Monoclonal Antibody to Human C5, h5G1.1scFv

This single-chain Fv mAb recognizes an epitope near the aminoterminal of the alpha chain of C5 and blocks the cleavage of C5 by the C5 convertases (97). It binds C5 essentially irreversibly because of an extraordinarily high affinity and then takes on the half-life of the C5 protein (1% to 2% turnover/hr). Since the excess single-chain Fv mAb (not bound to C5) is rapidly metabolized, mAb infusions would be required every few days to "sop up" the newly synthesized C5. However, a humanized, four-chain mAb with the same antigenic specificity and functional capability has been prepared, and, as expected, this protein has a longer half-life. This mAb is being evaluated in illnesses where chronic complement inhibition would be useful, such as glomerulonephritis and dermatomyositis.

This antibody would not prevent C3 from depositing on a target. Therefore, the opsonizing capability of C3b and the proinflammatory effects of the C3a anaphylatoxin would still be operative. Depending on the clinical circumstances, this could be an advantage or a disadvantage. If C3b were mediating destruction of a self-target by serving as a ligand for complement receptors on phagocytic cells, then this mAb would be of no use. However, complete C3 deficiency leads to a severe illness featuring recurrent pyogenic infections (98). The possibility of infectious complications would not be nearly as much of a concern with an agent that inhibits C5 cleavage, as C5 deficiency is associated primarily with rare Neisserial infections (98). Consequently, for this mAb to be effective, the immune pathology must be mediated by C5a, an element of the terminal pathway, the MAC, or some combination thereof. In immune complex–mediated conditions, it is often not clear how much of the tissue damage is caused by the reaction cascade through C3 versus that produced by C5a or the MAC. We now have improved animal models, thanks primarily to knockout technology, to better address such issues in the mouse.

Phase I and phase II trials have demonstrated that this mAb effectively inhibits C5 activation in patients undergoing cardiopulmonary bypass for coronary artery bypass grafting (95) and in patients undergoing renal dialysis. In this cardiopulmonary bypass study, significantly less blood loss, lower total serum CK-MB postoperatively, and a dramatic decrease in "post-pump" cognitive deficits occurred in comparison with the placebo-treated patients. There were no untoward or unanticipated effects in the short-term dialysis and bypass trials. An immune response was rarely observed to this "humanized" mAb.

Although data on the clinical usefulness in the treatment of human autoimmune disease are at least one year away, this mAb has been highly efficacious in several mouse models of immune complex–mediated disease, including lupus (99). In a study in lupus-prone mice (NZB X NZW), even if treatment with the mAb were started after the appearance of anti-DNA antibodies, the glomerulonephritis that leads to renal failure and death in the F_1 female mice was curtailed, resulting in the survival of nearly 80% of the treated mice versus less than 5% of the control animals. Treatment was continued for 6 months, and the mice did not develop infections or a significant immune response to the antibody. Perhaps the most surprising aspect of this study is the conclusion that the complement cascade beyond C3 is playing a pivotal role in the tissue damage. The precise role of Fc receptors versus complement receptors in the development of experimental glomerulonephritis is a subject of ongoing investigation (100–101).

The mAb approach to inhibiting complement activation has several advantages, provided the mAb does not itself activate complement. First, there is substantial clinical experience with the use of mAbs. Second, the half-life of IgG is 2 to 3 weeks. Third, the production of large quantities of a mAb is relatively easily

accomplished. Fourth, most of the humanized mAbs have been minimally immunogenic. The major potential disadvantage is that the tissue damage must be caused by C5a or the MAC; however, both of these are likely involved in ischemia/reperfusion injury. In a porcine model of cardiac ischemia/reperfusion, an anti-C5a mAb limited the neutrophil-dependent impairment of endothelial relaxation. There was no effect on short-term myocardial contractility or left ventricular pressure (102). In studies of porcine arterial rings, complement activation and C5b-9 deposition are associated with a decrease in endothelial relaxation to several stimuli (36). In in vitro studies of human umbilical vein endothelial cells, h5G1.1scFv blocked the up-regulation of VCAM-1 induced by C5b-9, probably by limiting NF-kB translocation (103). Thus, the adverse effects on endothelial function mediated by C5a and C5b-9 are both blocked by h5G1.1 anti-C5.

Other Potential Applications of Complement Inhibitors in Human Medicine

The intravascular administration of liposomes is currently in use as a strategy to minimize the toxicity of amphotericin B (104), and several other liposome and nanoparticle applications are under investigation (105). These artificial particles may be seen as foreign by the innate immune system and fix natural antibody and/or complement (106). In vivo, this circumstance may result in pulmonary hypertension, caused in part by the release of thromboxane A_2. Complement fixation by the particles may also result in augmented particle clearance to the liver and spleen by the intravascular particle-clearance mechanism (66,107–109). In a pig model, the adverse hemodynamic consequences of complement fixation by multilamellar liposomes were blocked by sCR1 and by anti-C5 mAb (110). Particle clearance itself, however, probably does not depend on components beyond C3. For example, clearance of bacteria from the bloodstream proceeded normally in C5-deficient mice (111). Thus, considering the two drugs currently in clinical trials with respect to intravascular particulate therapeutics, the h5G1.1 anti-C5 mAb would be best to prevent C5a- and C5b-9–mediated pathology without affecting C3-mediated opsonization, while sCR1 would be best to prevent undesired particle clearance.

A minority of infertile couples have difficulty conceiving because of antisperm antibody, which fixes complement with ensuing deposition of C3 fragments and C5b-9 and loss of sperm motility (112). Complement fixation by sperm can be effectively blocked with sCR1, resulting in preserved sperm motility in vitro (113). Whether this therapy would yield improved fertility has not been tested, but more complex strategies to remove antisperm antibodies have been successful (114). Artificial insemination with sperm in sCR1-containing medium or coitus in the presence of intravaginal sCR1 might be effective, less expensive, and safer than the current, most successful strategy of drug-induced superovulation, egg harvest, and in vitro fertilization for this form of infertility (111).

CR1 has been found to bear the Knops, McCoy, and Swain-Langley blood group antigens (115), and these alloantibodies occasionally complicate the crossmatching of donors and recipients for blood transfusions. These alloantibodies from patient sera have been neutralized with sCR1 (116). It is likely that development of a sCR1-specific kit would facilitate faster, more specific, and more successful cross matching and transfusion of sensitized patients bearing these antibodies.

Erythrocyte CR1, which is critically involved in the clearance of immune complexes, is present at abnormally low levels on the erythrocytes of patients with active diseases associated with immune complexes such as lupus as a result of a consumptive process. Conceptually, augmentation of erythrocyte CR1 should improve immune complex clearance. This hypothesis has been tested in one study, where 10 anemic patients with active lupus nephritis were treated with erythropoietin (117). The therapy increased the erythrocyte count and erythrocyte immune complex binding and modestly improved renal function. Whether there will be any long-term benefit remains to be seen. An alternative strategy would be to use a CR1 molecule that can insert into cell membranes and potentially support adhesion of complexes such as the APT070 compound (63,64). This strategy, in combination with conventional therapy such as steroids and cytotoxic agents should result in more rapid improvement in renal function than conventional therapy alone.

There are many other complement inhibitors in earlier stages of development, a few of which are listed in Table 20-2. The reader is referred to the recent, comprehensive review by Makrides (118) for lists of these potential drugs.

Possible Risks and Side Effects of Complement Inhibition

No side effects have been reported with the two inhibitors of complement currently in clinical trials. However, relatively few patients have been treated, and follow-up has been limited to less than a few weeks. There is only one peer-reviewed publication available (95). It is instructive to consider the consequences of inherited complement component deficiencies in this context. Deficiencies of complement regulators are also considered, as these can be associated with complement deficiency resulting from a consumptive process (e.g., C1 INH deficiency, see Chapter 21). Complement deficiency is associated with specific syndromes, depending on which element of the various pathways is lacking, and *chronic* therapeutic complement inhibition theoretically could result in similar phenotypes. *Acute, transient* complement inhibition should be well tolerated. The deficiency of B, P, or D of the alternative pathway or one of the late components, C5, C6, C7, C8, or C9, has been reported to lead to an increased risk of neisserial infection, commonly meningitis (98). Deficiency of one of the classic pathway components, C1, C4 or C2, is strongly associated with the development of a lupus-like autoimmune syndrome. The explanation underlying this association remains obscure. There are advocates for a mechanism involving dysreg-

ulated negative selection of B cells in the bone marrow (100), and some investigators support a faulty mechanism for clearance of apoptotic cells (119); these explanations are not mutually exclusive. Deficiency of mannose-binding lectin (MBL), the first component of the lectin pathway, has a weaker association with SLE (120). Although extraordinarily rare, C3 deficiency has been reported to be associated with both an increase in infections and autoimmune disease. Thus, based on their mechanisms of action, chronic sCR1 use theoretically could be associated with infection or autoimmunity, while chronic use of h5G1.1 anti-C5 mAb theoretically could be associated with neisserial infection.

Conclusions

Basic and preclinical studies strongly support a pathogenic role for complement activation in a variety of illnesses (see Table 20-2). Two potent and specific complement inhibitors, sCR1 and the anti-C5 mAb h5G1.1, are currently under investigation in human clinical trials. On the basis of preliminary phase I/II data, both complement inhibitors appear to be safe and effective. Outcomes of subsequent trials will determine whether these new drugs reach the pharmacy.

References

1. Takata Y, Kinoshita T, Kozono H, et al. Covalent association of C3b with C4b within C5 convertase of the classical complement pathway. J Exp Med 1987;195:1494–1509.
2. Wagner JL, Hugli TE. Radioimmunoassay for anaphylatoxins: a sensitive method for detecting complement activation products in biological fluids. Anal Biochem 1984;136:75.
3. Alper C, Rosen FS. Studies of the in vivo behavior of human C'3 in normal subjects and patients. J Clin Invest 1967;46:2021.
4. Fukumori Y, Yoshimura K, Ohnoki S, et al. A high incidence of C9 deficiency among healthy blood donors in Osaka, Japan. Int Immunol 1989;1:85–89.
5. Joiner KA, Schmetz MA, Sanders ME, et al. Multimeric complement component C9 is necessary for killing of *Escherichia coli* J5 by terminal attack complex C5b-9. Proc Natl Acad Sci USA 1985;82:4808–4812.
6. Lassiter HA, Watson SW, Seifring ML, Tanner JE. Complement factor 9 deficiency in serum of human neonates. J Infect Dis 1992;166:53–57.
7. Roitt I, Brostoff J, Male D. Immunology. 4th ed., Barcelona: Mosby, 1996.
8. Abbas AK, Lichtman AH, Pober JS. Cellular and molecular immunology. 3rd ed. Philadelphia: WB Saunders, 1997.
9. Janeway Jr CA, Travers P, Hunt S, Walport M. Immunobiology: the immune system in health and disease. 3rd ed. New York: Garland, 1997.
10. Liszewski MK, Farries TC, Lublin DM, et al. Control of the complement system. Adv Immunol 1996;61:201–283.
11. Volanakis JE, Frank MM. The human complement system in health and disease. New York: Marcel Dekker, 1998.
12. Rother K, Till GO, Hansch GM. The complement system. 2nd revised ed. Berlin: Springer, 1998.

13. Lambris JD. Current topics in microbiology and immunology: the third component of complement. New York: Springer-Verlag, 1990.

14. Parker CJ. Current topics in microbiology and immunology: membrane defenses against attack by complement and perforins. New York: Springer-Verlag, 1992.

15. Whaley K, Loos M, Weiler JM. Immunology and medicine: complement in health and disease. 2nd ed. Boston: Kluwer Academic, 1993.

16. Morgan BP, Harris CL. Complement regulatory proteins. San Diego: Harcourt Brace, 1999.

17. Fearon DT, Austen KF. Properdin: binding to C3b and stabilization of the C3b-dependent C3 convertase. J Exp Med 1975;142:856.

18. Kojirna A, Iwata K, Seya T, et al. Membrane cofactor protein (CD46) protects cells predominantly from activation complement pathway–mediated C3-fragment deposition and cytolysis. J Immunol 1993;151:1519–1527.

19. Christiansen D, Milland J, Thorley BR, et al. A functional analysis of recombinant soluble CD46 in vivo and a comparison with recombinant soluble forms of CD55 and CD35 in vitro. Eur J Immunol 1996;26:578–585.

20. Gotze O, Muller-Eberhard HJ. Lysis of erythrocytes by complement in the absence of antibody. J Exp Med 1970;132:898–915.

21. Hogasen K, Mollnes TE, Harboe M. Heparin-binding properties of vitronectin are linked to complex formation as illustrated by in vitro polymerization and binding to the terminal complement complex. J Biol Chem 1992;267:23076–23082.

22. Sheehan M, Morris CA, Pussell BA, Charlesworth JA. Complement inhibition by human vitronectin involves nonheparin binding domains. Clin Exp Immunol 1995;101:136–141.

23. Yamashina M, Ueda E, Kinoshita T, et al. Inherited complete deficiency of 20-kilodalton homologous restriction factor (CD59) as a cause of paroxysmal nocturnal hemoglobinuria. N Engl J Med 1990;323:1184–1189.

24. Johnson E, Berge V, Hogasen K. Formation of the terminal complement complex on agarose beads: further evidence that vitronectin (complement S-protein) inhibits C9 polymerization. Scand J Immunol 1994;39:281–285.

25. Arnaout MA, Melamed J, Tack BF, Colten HR. Characterization of the human complement (C3b) receptor with a fluid phase C3b dimer. J Immunol 1981;127:1348–1354.

26. Medof ME, Nussenzweig V. Control of the function of substrate-bound C4b-C3b by the complement receptor CR1. J Exp Med 1984;159:1669–1685.

27. Kinoshita T, Takata Y, Kozono H, et al. C5 convertase of the alternative complement pathway: covalent linkage between two C3b molecules within the trimolecular complex enzyme. J Immunol 1988;141:3895–3903.

28. Klickstein LB, Bartow TJ, Miletic V, et al. Identification of distinct C3b and C4b recognition sites in the human C3b/C4b receptor (CR1, CD35) by deletion mutagenesis. J Exp Med 1988;168:1699–1717.

29. Klickstein LB, Barbashov SF, Liu T, et al. Complement receptor type 1 (CR1, CD35) is a receptor for C1q. Immunity 1997;7:345–355.

30. Tas SW, Klickstein LB, Nicholson-Weller A. C1q and C4b bind to independent sites on CR1 and mediate erythrocyte adhesion. J Immunol 1999;163:5056–5063.

31. Weisman HF, Bartow T, Leppo MK, et al. Soluble human complement receptor type 1: in vivo inhibitor of complement suppressing post-ischemic myocardial inflammation and necrosis. Science 1990;249:146–151.

32. Mulligan MS, Warner RL, Rittershaus CW, et al. Endothelial targeting and enhanced antiinflammatory effects of complement inhibitors possessing sialyl Lewis^x moieties. J Immunol 1999;162:4952–4959.

33. Smith EF, Griswold DE, Egan JW, et al. Reduction of myocardial reperfusion injury with human soluble complement receptor type 1 (BRL55730). Eur J Pharmacol 1993;236:477–481.

34. Shandelya SML, Kuppusamy P, Herskowitz A, et al. Soluble complement receptor type 1 inhibits the complement pathway and prevents contractile failure in the postischemic heart: evidence that complement activation is required for neutrophil-mediated reperfusion injury. Circulation 1993;88:2812–2826.

35. Gillinov AM, DeValeria PA, Winkelstein JA, et al. Complement inhibition with soluble complement receptor type 1 in cardiopulmonary bypass. Ann Thorac Surg 1993;55:619–624.

36. Stahl GL, Reenstra WR, Frendl G. Complement-mediated loss of endothelium-dependent relaxation of porcine coronary arteries. Role of the terminal membrane attack complex. Circ Res 1995;76:575–583.

37. Schaiff WT, Eisenberg PR. Direct induction of complement activation by pharmacologic activation of plasminogen. Coron Artery Dis 1997;8:9–18.

38. Lazar HL, Hamasaki T, Bao Y, et al. Soluble complement receptor type 1 limits damage during revascularization of ischemic myocardium. Ann Thoracic Surg 1998;65:973–977.

39. Homeister JW, Kuppusamy P, Herskowitz A, et al. Soluble complement receptor type 1 prevents human complement–mediated damage of the rabbit isolated heart. J Immunol 1993;150:1055–1064.

40. Fjelistrom K-E, Arturson G. Changes in the human complement system following burn injury. Acta Pathol Microbiol Scand 1963;59:257–270.

41. Daniels JC, Larson DL, Abston S, Ritzrnan SE. Serum protein profiles in thermal burns. II. Protease inhibitors, complement factors, and C-reactive protein. J Trauma 1974;14:153–162.

42. Heideman M. The effect of thermal injury on hemodynamic, respiratory, and hematologic variables in relation to complement activation. J Trauma 1979;19:239–243.

43. Gelfand JA, Donelan M, Burke JF. Alternative complement pathway activation increases mortality in a model of burn injury in mice. J Clin Invest 1982;70:1170–1176.

44. Mulligan MS, Yeh CG, Rudolph AR, Ward PA. Protective effects of soluble CR1 in complement- and neutrophil-mediated tissue injury. J Immunol 1992;148:1479–1485.

45. Solomkin JS, Nelson RD, Chenoweth DE, et al. Regulation of neutrophil migratory function in burn injury by complement activation products. Ann Surg 1984;200:742–746.

46. Moore FD Jr, Davis C, Rodrick M, et al. Neutrophil activation in thermal injury as assessed by increased expression of complement receptors. N Engl J Med 1986;314:948–953.

47. Davis CF, Moore FD Jr, Rodrick ML, et al. Neutrophil activation after burn injury: contributions of the classical complement pathway and of endotoxin. Ann Surg 1987;102:477–484.

48. Fearon DT, Ruddy S, Schur PH, McCabe WR. Activation of the properdin pathway of complement in patients with gram-negative bacteremia. N Engl J Med 1975;292:937–940.

49. Slotman GJ, Burchard KW, Williams JJ, et al. Interaction of prostaglandins, activated complement, and granulocytes in clinical sepsis and hypotension. Surgery 1986;99:744–750.

50. Bengston A, Heideman M. Anaphylatoxin formation in sepsis. Arch Surg 1988;123:645–649.

51. Smedegard G, Cui L, Hugli TE. Endotoxin-induced shock in the rat: a role for C5a. Am J Pathol 1989;135:489–497.

52. Stevens JH, O'Hanley P, Shapiro JM, et al. Effects of anti-C5a antibodies on the adult respiratory distress syndrome in septic primates. J Clin Invest 1986;77:1812–1816.

53. Toki H, Hersh EM, Gutterman JU, et al. Organ distributions and clearance studies of ^{99m}technitium-labeled *Corynebacterium parvum* in patients with leukemia. Int J Immunopharmacol 1981;3:141–145.

54. Weiser MR, Pechet TT, Williams JP, et al. Experimental murine acid aspiration injury is mediated by neutrophils and the alternative complement pathway. J Appl Physiol 1997;83:1090–1095.

55. Rabinovici R, Neville LF, Abdullah F, et al. Aspiration-induced lung injury: the role of complement. Crit Care Med 1995;23:1405–1411.

56. Nishizawa H, Yamada H, Miyazaki H, et al. Soluble complement receptor type 1 inhibited the systemic organ injury caused by acid-installation into a lung. Anesthesiology 1996;85:1120–1128.

57. Hill J, Lindsay TF, Ortiz F, et al. Soluble complement receptor type 1 ameliorates the local and remote organ injury after intestinal ischemia-reperfusion in the rat. J Immunol 1992;149:1723–1728.

58. Lindsay TF, Hill J, Ortiz F, et al. Blockade of complement activation prevents local and pulmonary albumin leak after lower torso ischemia-reperfusion. Ann Surg 1992;216:677–683.

59. Mulligan MS, Warren JS, Smith CW, et al. Lung injury after deposition of IgA immune complexes. Requirements for CD18 and L-arginine. J Immunol 1992;148:3086–3092.

60. Fava RA, Gates C, Townes AS. Critical role of peripheral blood phagocytes and the involvement of complement in tumour necrosis factor enhancement of passive collagen-arthritis. Clin Exp Immunol 1993;94:261–266.

61. Goodfellow RM, Williams AS, Levin JL, et al. Local therapy with soluble complement receptor 1 (sCR1) suppresses inflammation in rat mono-articular arthritis. Clin Exp Immunol 1997;110:45–52.

62. Mossakowska D, Dodd I, Pindar W, Smith RA. Structure-activity relationships within the N-terminal short consensus repeats (SCR) of human CR1 (C3b/C4b receptor, CD35): SCR 3 plays a critical role in inhibition of the classical and alternative pathways of complement activation. Eur J Immunol 1999;29:1955–1965.

63. Linton S, Dodd I, Smith R, Morgan BP. Therapeutic efficacy of a novel membrane-targeted complement regulator in antigen arthritis in the rat. Mol Immunol 1999;36:306. Abstract.

64. Dong J, Pram JR, Smith RAG, et al. Application of a novel membrane-targeted complement regulator to ischaemia/reperfusion injury in transplantation. Mol Immunol 1999;36:310. Abstract.

65. Couser WG, Johnson RJ, Young BA, et al. The effects of soluble recombinant complement receptor 1 on complement-mediated experimental glomerulonephritis. J Am Soc Nephrol 1995;5:1888–1894.

66. Taylor RP, Ferguson PJ, Martin EN, et al. Immune complexes bound to the primate erythrocyte complement receptor (CR1) via anti-CR1 mAbs are cleared simultaneously with loss of CR1 in a concerted reaction in a rhesus monkey model. Clin Immunol Immunopathol 1997;82:49–59.

67. Hatung H-P, Schwenke C, Bitter-Suermann D, Toyka KV. Guillain-Barre syndrome: activated complement components C3a and C5a in CSF. Neurology 1987;37:1006–1009.

68. Morgan BP, Gasque P, Singhrao S, Piddlesden SJ. The role of complement in disorders of the nervous system. Immunopharmacol 1997;38:43–50.

69. Jung S, Toyka KV, Hartung H-P. Soluble complement receptor 1 inhibits experimental autoimmune neuritis in Lewis rats. Neurosci Lett 1995;200:167–170.

70. Vriesendorp FJ, Flynn RE, Pappolla MA, Koski CL. Soluble complement receptor 1 (sCR1) is not as effective as cobra venom factor in the treatment of experimental allergic neuritis. Int J Neurosci 1997;92:287–298.

71. Huang J, Kim LJ, Mealey R, et al. Neuronal protection in stroke by an sLe^x-glycosylated complement inhibitory protein. Science 1999;285:595–599.

72. Piddlesden SJ, Jiang S, Levin JL, et al. Soluble complement receptor 1 (sCR1) protects against experimental autoimmune myasthenia gravis. J Neuroimmunol 1996;71:173–177.

73. Piddlesden SJ, Storch MK, Hibbs MJ, et al. Soluble recombinant complement receptor 1 inhibits inflammation and demyelination in antibody-mediated demyelinating experimental allergic encephalomyelitis. J Immunol 1994;152:5477–5484.

74. Williams JP, Pechet TT, Weiser MR, et al. Intestinal reperfusion injury is mediated by IgM and complement. J Appl Physiol 1999;86:938–942.

75. Spain DA, Fruchterman TM, Matheson PJ, et al. Complement activation mediates intestinal injury after resuscitation from hemorrhagic shock. J Trauma 1999;46:224–233.

76. Fruchterman TM, Spain DA, Wilson MA, et al. Complement inhibition prevents gut ischemia and endothelial cell dysfunction after hemorrhage/resuscitation. Surgery 1998;124:782–792.

77. Eror AT, Stojadinovic A, Starnes BW, et al. Antiinflammatory effects of soluble complement receptor type 1 promote rapid recovery of ischemia/reperfusion injury in rat small intestine. Clin Immunol 1999;90:266–275.

78. Collard CD, Vakeva AP, Bukusoglu C, et al. Reoxygenation of hypoxic human umbilical vein endothelial cells activated the classic complement pathway. Circulation 1997;96:326–333.

79. Pruitt SK, Bollinger RR. The effect of soluble complement receptor type 1 on hyperacute allograft rejection. J Surg Res 1991;50:350–355.

80. Brauer RB, Baldwin WM III, Wand D, et al. Functional activity of anti-C6 antibodies elicited in C6-deficient rats reconstituted by liver allografts. Ability to inhibit hyperacute rejection of discordant cardiac xenografts. Transplantation 1996;61:588–594.

81. Pratt JR, Hibbs MJ, Laver AJ, et al. Effects of complement inhibition with soluble complement receptor-1 on vascular

injury and inflammation during renal allograft rejection in the rat. Am J Pathol 1996;149:2055–2066.

82. Lehmann TG, Koeppel TA, Kirschfink M, et al. Complement inhibition by soluble complement receptor type 1 improves microcirculation after rat liver transplantation. Transplantation 1998;66:717–722.

83. Pierre AF, Xavier AM, Liu M, et al. Effect of complement inhibition with soluble complement receptor 1 on pig allotransplant lung function. Transplantation 1998;66:723–732.

84. Jacob HS, Craddock PR, Hammerschmidt S, Moldow CF. Complement-induced granulocyte aggregation: an unsuspected mechanism of disease. N Engl J Med 1980;302:789–794.

85. Craddock PR, Fehr J, Brigham KL, et al. Complement and leukocyte-mediated pulmonary dysfunction in hemodialysis. N Engl J Med 1977;296:769–774.

86. Craddock PR, Fehr J, Dalmasso AP, et al. Hemodialysis leukopenia: pulmonary vascular leukostasis resulting from complement activation by dialyzer cellophane membranes. Clin Invest 1977;59:879–888.

87. Craddock PR, Hammerschmidt D, White JG, et al. Complement (C5a)-induced granulocyte aggregation in vitro: a possible explanation of complement-mediated leukostasis and leukopenia. J Clin Invest 1977;60:260–264.

88. Lee J, Hakim RM, Fearon DT. Increased expression of the C3b receptor by neutrophils and complement activation during hemodialysis. Clin Exp Immunol 1984;56:205–214.

89. Arnaout MA, Hakim RM, Todd RF III, et al. Increased expression of an adhesion-promoting surface glycoprotein in the granutocytopenia of hemodialysis. N Engl J Med 1985;312:457–462.

90. Solomkin JS, Cotta LA, Satoh PS, et al. Complement activation and clearance in acute injury and illness: evidence for C5a as a cell-directed mediator of the adult respiratory distress syndrome in man. Surgery 1985;97:668–678.

91. Heideman M, Hugli TE. Anaphylatoxin generation in multisystem organ failure. J Trauma 1984;24:1038–1043.

92. Hohn DC, Meyers AJ, Gherini ST, et al. Production of acute pulmonary injury by leukocytes and activated complement. Surgery 1980;88:48–57.

93. Dellinger RP, Zimmerman J, Metzler MH, et al. Phase 1 trial of soluble complement receptor 1 (sCR1, TP10) in acute lung injury. Chest 1995;108(suppl).

94. Perry GJ, Eisenberg PR, Zimmerman JI, Levin J. Phase 1 safety trial of soluble complement receptor type 1 (TP10) in acute myocardial infarction. J Am Coll Cardiol 1998.

95. Fitch JCK, Rollins SA, Matis LA, et al. Pharmacology and biological efficacy of a recombinant, humanized, single-chain antibody C5 complement inhibitor in patients undergoing coronary artery bypass graft surgery utilizing cardiopulmonary bypass. Circulation 1999;100:2499–2506.

96. Keshavjee SH, Davis RD, Zamona MR, et al. Inhibition of complement in human lung transplant reperfusion injury: a multicenter clinical trial. J Heart Lung Transplant 1998.

97. Thomas TC, Rollins SA, Rother RP, et al. Inhibition of complement activity by humanized anti-C5 antibody and single-chain Fv. Mol Immunol 1996;33:1389–1401.

98. Figueroa JE, Densen P. Infectious diseases associated with complement deficiencies. Clin Microbiol Rev 1991;4:359–395.

99. Wang Y, Hu Q, Madri JA, et al. Amelioration of lupus-like autoimmune disease in NZB/W F_1 mice after treatment with a blocking monoclonal antibody specific for complement component C5. Proc Natl Acad Sci USA 1996;93:8563–8568.

100. Carroll MC. The role of complement and complement receptors in induction and regulation of immunity. Annu Rev Immunol 1998;16:545–568.

101. Ravetch JV, Clynes RA. Divergent roles for Fc receptors and complement in vivo. Annu Rev Immunol 1998;16:421–432.

102. Tofukuji M, Stahl G, Agah A, et al. Anti-C5a monoclonal antibody reduces cardiopulmonary bypass and cardioplegia-induced coronary endothelial dysfunction. J Thorac Cardiovasc Surg 1998;116:1060–1068.

103. Collard CD, Agah A, Reenstra W, et al. Endothelial nuclear factor-kB translocation and vascular cell adhesion molecule-1 induction by complement: inhibition with anti-human C5 therapy or cGMP analogues. Arterioscler Thromb Vasc Biol 1999;19:2623–2629.

104. Walsh TJ, Finberg RW, Arndt C, et al. National Institute of Allergy and Infectious Diseases Mycoses Study Group. Liposomal amphotericin B for empirical therapy in patients with persistent fever and neutropenia. N Engl J Med 1999;340:764–771.

105. Davis SS. Biomedical applications of nanotechnology: implications for drug targeting and gene therapy. Trends Biotechnol 1997;15:217–224.

106. Szebeni J, Wassef NM, Hartman KR, et al. Complement activation in vitro by the red cell substitute, liposome-encapsulated hemoglobin: mechanism of activation and inhibition by soluble complement receptor type 1. Transfusion 1997;37:150–159.

107. Kuhn SE, Nardin A, Klebba PE, et al. *Escherichia coli* bound to the primate erythrocyte complement receptor via bispecific monoclonal antibodies are transferred to and phagocytosed by human monocytes in an in vitro model. J Immunol 1998;160:5088–5097.

108. Emlen W, Burdick G, Carl V. Binding of model immune complexes to erythrocyte CR1 facilitates immune complex uptake by U937 cells. J Immunol 1989;142:4366–4371.

109. Kimberly RP, Edberg JC, Merriam LT. In vivo handling of soluble complement fixing Ab/dsDNA immune complexes in chimpanzees. J Clin Invest 1989;84:962–970.

110. Szebeni J, Fontana JL, Wassef MN, et al. Hemodynamic changes induced by liposomes and liposome-encapsulated hemoglobin in pigs: a model for pseudoallergic cardiopulmonary reactions to liposomes. Role of complement and inhibition by soluble CR1 and anti-C5a antibody. Circulation 1999;99:2302–2309.

111. Toews GB, Pierce AK. The fifth component of complement is not required for the clearance of *Staphylococcus aureus*. Am Rev Respir Dis 1984;129:597–601.

112. D'Cruz OJ, Haas GG Jr, Wang BL, et al. Activation of human complement by IgG antisperm antibody and the demonstration of C3- and C5b-9–mediated immune injury to human sperm. J Immunol 1991;146:611–620.

113. D'Cruz OJ, Toth CA, Haas GG Jr. Recombinant soluble human complement receptor type 1 inhibits antisperm antibody– and neutrophil-mediated injury to human sperm. Biol Reprod 1996;54:1217–1228.

114. Ombelet W, Vandeput H, Janssen M, et al. Treatment of male infertility due to sperm surface antibodies: IUI or IVF? Hum Reprod 1997;12:1165–1170.
115. Moulds JM, Brai M, Cohen J, et al. Reference typing report for complement receptor type 1 (CR1). Exp Clin Immunogenet 1998;15:291–294.
116. Moulds JM, Rowe KE. Neutralization of Knops system antibodies using soluble complement receptor 1. Transfusion 1996;36:517–520.
117. Kiss E, Kavai M, Csipo I, Szegedi G. Recombinant human erythropoietin modulates erythrocyte complement receptor 1 functional activity in patients with lupus nephritis. Clin Nephrol 1998;49:364–369.
118. Makrides, SC. Therapeutic inhibition of the complement system. Pharmacol Rev 1998;50:59–87.
119. Botto M, Dell' Agnola C, Bygrave AE, et al. Homozygous C1q deficiency causes glomerulonephritis associated with multiple apoptotic bodies. Nat Genet 1998;19:56–59.

120. Ip WK, Chan SY, Lau CS, Lau YL. Association of systemic lupus erythematosus with promoter polymorphisms of the mannose-binding lectin gene. Arthritis Rheum 1998;41: 1663–1668.
121. Gelfand JA, Donelan M, Burke JF. Alternative complement pathway activation increases mortality in a model of burn injury in mice. J Clin Invest 1982;70:1170–1176.
122. Mulligan MS, Yeh CG, Rudolph AR, Ward PA. Protective effects of soluble CR1 in complement- and neutrophil-mediated tissue injury. J Immunol 1992;148:1479–1485.
123. Gillinov AM, DeValeria PA, Winkelstein JA, et al. Complement inhibition with soluble complement receptor type 1 in cardiopulmonary bypass. Ann Thorac Surg 1993;55:619–624.
124. Liszewski MK, Atkinson JP. Novel complement inhibitors. Exp Opin Invest Drug 1998;7:323–332.
125. Liszewski MK, Bala Subramanian V, Atkinson JP. Complement inhibitors as therapeutic agents. Clin Immunol Newslett 1998;17:168–173.

Chapter 21

Treatment of Angioedema Resulting from C1-Inhibitor Deficiency

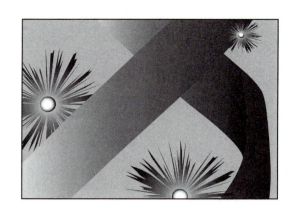

A. Thomas Waytes
Fred S. Rosen

Hereditary or acquired deficiency of the inhibitor of the first component of complement (C1-INH) results in recurrent episodes of angioedema. C1-inhibitor is one of the major serum proteinase inhibitors (serpins) and is highly homologous in structure to other serpins such as antithrombin III and alpha$_1$-antitrypsin. C1-inhibitor is the major regulator of the activation of the classic pathway of complement activation. It inhibits the trypsin-like activity of C1r and C1s by forming a covalent bond with these C1 subcomponents, which results in their dissociation from C1q. In addition, C1-INH inhibits the contact system or kallikrein as well as coagulation factors XIa, XIIa, and XIIf. It can also inhibit plasmin (1).

Hereditary angioedema (HAE) occurs in individuals who are genetically deficient in C1-INH. HAE is inherited as a mendelian autosomal-dominant trait, so that affected individuals are, in fact, heterozygous for the deficiency because they have one normal C1-INH gene from a normal parent and an abnormal C1-INH gene from an affected parent. The disease does not skip a generation (2). Acquired angioedema (AAE) occurs late in life. It is more frequently associated with monoclonal B-cell diseases, such as multiple myeloma, chronic lymphocytic leukemia, B-cell lymphoma, and Waldenström's macroglobulinemia. In these patients, a complement-fixing anti-idiotypic antibody to their own monoclonal immunoglobulin develops (3). Less frequently, AAE results from autoantibodies to C1-INH (4–6). In rare cases, the mechanism of AAE is not known (7).

HAE is characterized by recurrent attacks of localized edema of the skin or mucosa. These episodes usually begin in early childhood but are mild and may even go unnoticed. The severity and frequency of the attacks get dramatically worse around the time of pubescence. The symptoms may subside in the sixth and seventh decades of life. The attacks of edema may be induced by trauma, menses, excessive exercise, extremes of temperature, and stress. When they involve the extremities or genitalia, the swelling is benign and usually lasts no more than 48 hours. The angioedema may be accompanied by a rash that resembles erythema marginatum. Angioedema of the gut, on the other hand, is extremely painful and is accompanied by vomiting, which is usually bilious because the distal jejunum is the most common site of involvement. It may also result in profuse watery diarrhea if the colon is affected. Marked hemoconcentration occurs as a result of fluid loss into the gastrointestinal tract. When the upper airway is affected, angioedema becomes life threatening. Historically, approximately one-third of patients died of respiratory obstruction before the end of the third decade of life.

Because of the unopposed activation of C1 in patients with HAE, the fourth (C4) and second (C2) components of complement are consumed in the circulation so that serum concentration of these components is low. Because no effective C3 convertase is formed, the consumption of C3 and the late-acting components is not abnormal (8). Nor is the alternative pathway affected. Peptides that increase vascular permeability are generated from both the complement system and the contact system (9–12). The pathogenesis of angioedema is complex and may involve the generation of bradykinin and a peptide from C2, both of which can increase vascular permeability.

Because individuals with HAE are heterozygous for the deficiency, it might be expected that their serum would contain 50% of the normal level of C1-INH. This is not what is usually found. The mean C1-INH level in patients' serum is 16% of normal. This results not only from decreased synthesis of C1-INH but also from increased catabolism of the protein in affected individuals. Heterozygotes cannot maintain the equilibrium of the system with only one functional gene (13). It was found that HAE presented in two genetic forms. In type 1, the C1-INH level was very low. In type 2, the C1-INH level was normal or elevated by measurement with an antibody to C1-INH, but there is almost no normal functional C1-INH in the blood. It was subsequently found that type 2 HAE results from point mutations in the C1-INH gene, and this gives rise to nonfunctional protein (14–18). On the other hand, type 1 HAE results from nonsense mutations in the gene or deletion of exons as a result of unequal crossovers in intronic Alu sequences (19–23).

Therapy for Angioedema (C1-Inhibitor Deficiency)

A discussion of the available treatment modalities for HAE can be divided into three main areas: 1) long-term therapy to prevent or reduce the frequency or severity of attacks; 2) treatment of acute attacks; and 3) short-term prophylaxis before procedures or activities that potentially precipitate attacks. Therapy for AAE presents additional problems and is addressed separately.

Long-Term Preventive Therapy

The marked decrease in HAE-related fatalities seen in recent years is largely attributable to increased physician recognition of the disease and the availability of effective long-term preventive therapy. Two main classes of drugs have been used: antifibrinolytic agents and androgens or androgen derivatives.

The first report of an antifibrinolytic agent being beneficial in the treatment of HAE was by Nilsson et al (24), who in 1966 described a patient in whom ε-aminocaproic acid (EACA), a lysine analogue, often could decrease the severity of attacks, if taken early enough. The usefulness of this agent for long-term prophylaxis was demonstrated 2 years later in a patient with severe HAE who became attack-free during a 5-month trial (25).

Frank and coworkers (26) then conducted a double-blind study in which five patients received sequential courses of EACA (15 g/day) or placebo. Four of the five patients were free of attacks while receiving EACA, and all had multiple attacks while on placebo. No significant changes in plasma levels of C1-INH or C4 were noted in the treatment group. After this study, the same group treated 15 patients with EACA and found that only two did not respond (27). The minimal effective dosage was found to be about 8 to 10 g/day. A second double-blind study was conducted by Gwynn (28), who demonstrated a marked reduction in attack frequency over two 6-week periods in five adults (age 12 and over) and four children. Dosages as low as 6 g/day (3 g/day for children) were found to be effective in all but three patients. These three continued to have intermittent, but less severe, attacks.

A second antifibrinolytic agent, tranexamic acid, which is a cyclic derivative of EACA, has also been shown to be effective in the long-term prevention of HAE attacks. Lundh and coworkers (25) found that this agent was equivalent to EACA in their patient. A double-blind study was conducted by Sheffer et al (29) in which 12 patients received 3 g/day of tranexamic acid alternating with periods of treatment with placebo. Five patients were attack free on the drug; another six had fewer attacks than while on placebo. No differences in plasma levels of C1-INH, C2 or C4 were detected. A second double-blind study carried out in Sweden (30) demonstrated a decrease in attack frequency in two of three patients taking tranexamic acid at 3.0 to 4.5 g/day. The third patient had almost continuous severe symptoms despite treatment with this agent. Agostoni and coworkers (31) have reported tranexamic acid at dosages of 1.5 to 3.0 g/day to be effective in only seven of 27 patients studied. Effectiveness was defined as a reduction in attack frequency of greater than 80% (31).

The mechanism by which antifibrinolytic agents reduce the frequency or severity of HAE attacks is not understood. As noted, the successful use of these agents is not associated with increases in C1-INH or C4 (26,29). It has been proposed, on the basis of in vitro studies, that the action of EACA is based on the prevention of the episodic activation of C1 (32). This, however, does not explain the persistently low levels of C4 while on therapy, and the fact that some patients successfully treated with antifibrinolytic agents report having typical prodromes of attacks that do not progress (26). More likely, the activity of these agents in C1-INH deficiency is dependent on their antiplasmin activity, which results in a decreased release of vasoactive mediators (33,34). Thus, the progression of the attack is suppressed.

The use of antifibrinolytic agents in HAE may be associated with a number of minor, as well as potentially serious, adverse effects. Extensive muscle necrosis, confirmed by biopsy and associated with myoglobinuria, and a marked elevation of creatine kinase (CK) and hepatic transaminases, was described in a patient receiving EACA at a dosage of 30 g/day (35). Three of the five patients in the blind study by Frank and coworkers (26) experienced transient elevations of CK and aldolase, and there were several complaints of muscle pain, weakness, and fatigue while receiving EACA. All three female patients reported abnormally prolonged periods of slow menstrual flow, and most patients complained that EACA potentiated the sedative effects of concomitant medications or alcohol. All patients in the study by Gwynn (28) reported transient muscle pains while receiving EACA, which were particularly painful in the adults and older children. These and other complaints, including dizziness, postural hypotension, and nausea, appear to be dosage-related (27,28).

The use of tranexamic acid, which is 6 to 10 times as potent as EACA, has not been associated with muscle toxicity. Agostoni and coworkers observed 12 patients treated with tranexamic acid for periods ranging from 8 to 34 months, and found no significant changes in serum aspartate amino transferase (AST, SGOT), alanine aminotransferase (ALT, SGPT), γ-glutamyl transpeptidase, or bilirubin (36). Side effects from ingestion of this drug include nausea, diarrhea, abdominal discomfort, dysmenorrhea, and pruritis, and tend to be mild. Reports of retinal changes and oncogenicity in animals treated with large doses of tranexamic acid for prolonged periods of time, however, have raised some concerns about the safety of using this drug in HAE (27,37).

Although both of these prophylaxis agents have the potential for causing serious thrombotic events, none has yet been seen in the treatment of HAE patients. Nevertheless, this remains a concern, especially in patients who may be predisposed to the development of a deep vein thrombosis, cerebrovascular accident, or myocardial infarction.

The second main class of drugs used in the long-term preventive therapy in HAE includes the androgens or androgen derivatives. In 1960, Spaulding (38) demonstrated that methyltestosterone in dosages as low as 10 mg daily could result in a striking decrease in the frequency of HAE attacks over extended periods of time, in five of six members of the same family. The efficacy of this agent in decreasing the frequency of HAE attacks was also shown in all four adult male patients enrolled in a double-blind study by Sheffer and coworkers (39). A report that the treatment of five males for 30 to 78 months with fluoxymesterone (10 to 20 mg/day) resulted in markedly reduced HAE attack frequency came from Davis and coworkers (40). Furthermore, they achieved a successful reduction in attacks in five of six women treated for 10 to 36 months with the nonvirilizing androgen oxymetholone at dosages of 2.5 to 5.0 mg/day. The favorable response to oxymetholone was further demonstrated in a study by Sheffer and coworkers (41) in which 15 of 16 HAE patients were totally asymptomatic while receiving 5 mg/day. Lowering the dosage to 5 mg on alternate days was still efficacious, but to a lesser extent, in half of the patients.

Gelfand and coworkers (42) evaluated the efficacy of danazol, a synthetic androgen derivative with markedly attenuated virilizing side effects. In a double-blind manner, they treated five women and four men with sequential courses of danazol (200 mg) or placebo, taken three times a day. HAE attacks occurred in 44 of 47 placebo courses, but in only one of the 46 danazol courses. Mean serum levels of C1-INH increased three- to fourfold and C4 levels increased 15-fold during danazol therapy, compared with placebo, but C3 levels did not change. Several days of danazol treatment were required before these increases occurred. Elevations in C1-INH and C4 have also been demonstrated during treatment with methyltestosterone (39) and oxymetholone (41). Danazol has been found to be effective in four HAE type II patients, who have normal or elevated antigenic levels of functionless C1-INH (43). In two of these patients, the functionless C1-INH phenotype could be immunoelectrophoretically differentiated from the normal protein. Danazol therapy resulted in augmentation of the normal protein phenotype, which was associated with an overall increase in C1-INH function.

Stanozolol, another androgenic derivative with a low masculinizing activity compared with its anabolic activity, was also found to be effective in reducing the frequency of HAE attacks (44). Open, dose-ranging studies in 37 patients demonstrated that daily doses of 2 mg or less could control the frequency and severity of symptoms in many patients, and would result in increased serum concentrations of C1-INH and C4 (45,46).

As in the case with antifibrinolytics, long-term therapy with androgenic steroids can be associated with several clinically significant side effects. The 17 α-alkyl androgen derivatives such as danazol, stanozolol, and oxymetholone were selected for their low androgenic activity as well as their effectiveness in lowering the frequency of HAE attacks. Nevertheless, these agents are still associated with hirsutism and acne in a significant number of patients. The most common side effects include weight gain, menstrual irregularities and myalgias, and transient elevations of hepatocellular enzymes (46,47). One retrospective study of 36 HAE patients found that, although the long-term use of androgens was associated with relatively few side effects, 25% of the patients developed arterial hypertension (48). The development of hepatic adenomas and angiosarcomas has been reported to occur from long-term androgen therapy (49,50); however, this has not been described in the treatment of HAE patients. Microscopic hematuria was noted in nine of 69 patients treated with danazol, and subsequent cystoscopy revealed hemorrhagic cystitis in three of these patients (47). Other less common complaints include mild alopecia, decreased libido, headache, and hypertension (51). Fortunately, most adverse effects of androgens are dosage-related and can be minimized by titrating the dosage down to the lowest effective level (46,47,52).

Although impeded androgens such as danazol have been successfully used in children with HAE (53), the interfering effect of these agents on gonadal development is well established (54), and their use in children or pregnant women should be avoided except in extreme circumstances. They should also not be used in patients with hepatic disease.

Some treatment modalities that seemed to make good theoretic sense have not been found to be particularly useful in practice. Considering that many female HAE patients report a decrease in attacks during the latter months of pregnancy, and that HAE complications at the time of delivery are rare, Frank and coworkers treated three patients with medroxyprogesterone acetate (Provera) (27). Although trends toward improvement were observed with this agent (compared with placebo), no statistical differences were seen. Likewise, it has been shown that interferon-γ can induce C1-INH synthesis in cultured monocytes, leading to the speculation that use of this material in HAE patients could stimulate increased production in vivo and thus decrease the severity of disease (55). Thus far, this has not been found to be the case (56; Waytes AT, Frank MM, personal communication, 1990).

In summary, although androgens and, to a lesser extent, antifibrinolytics can successfully reduce the frequency and severity of HAE attacks, they are not benign medications, and a risk-benefit assessment must be made for each patient. Most HAE patients do not require chronic therapy with these agents. Attempting to avoid situations and activities known to precipitate attacks may be of benefit. Because plasma levels of C1-INH antigen and functional activity have been shown to be decreased in normal women taking estrogen-containing oral contraceptives (57), and the use of these agents has been shown to worsen the frequency and severity of HAE attacks (27), female patients should refrain from taking them, when possible. Also to be avoided in patients with HAE are the angiotensin-converting enzyme inhibitors, which reduce the catabolism of kinins and can potentiate the severity of HAE attacks (58,59).

The decision to institute long-term preventive therapy in an individual patient is based on the extent to which the disease is affecting his or her lifestyle. Many patients having one or more significant attacks per month or with a history of repeated laryngeal involvement would welcome the use of these agents. The goal is to reduce the frequency of symptoms to an acceptable level at the lowest effective dosage possible. Androgens are the first line of therapy, but should be avoided when possible in children and pregnant women for the reasons mentioned previously. Although the beneficial clinical effect of androgens is believed to be the result of increased hepatic synthesis of functional C1-INH, dosing should be based on clinical response and never on C1-INH or C4 determinations. Male patients can be treated with the relatively inexpensive methyltestosterone. A starting dosage of 10 mg two or three times a day can be used initially and tapered once the symptoms have been controlled. For women, daily doses of 4 mg of stanozolol or 600 mg of danazol can be started and tapered as indicated. Danazol is about four times as expensive as stanozolol, and the yearly cost of treatment at 600 mg/day can be in excess of $3000. Oxymethalone can also be used in women with a starting dosage of approximately 15 mg/day. Because of the potential of adverse reactions mentioned previously, patients receiving long-term androgen therapy should be monitored for hepatic enzyme elevations and hematuria, particularly when higher dosages are used.

The antifibrinolytic agents are second-line drugs for use in symptomatic patients who are not candidates for androgen treatment, or for those who do not respond to or cannot tolerate androgens. They, of course, should never be used in patients predisposed to thrombogenicity. Because they do not influence gonadal development, the antifibrinolytics may be more appropriate in the rare child who requires chronic therapy. Reasonable starting dosages for adults are approximately 10 g/day for EACA and 4 g/day for tranexamic acid. Monitoring for hepatic enzymes and CK is warranted, and dosages should be adjusted downward on the basis of acceptable levels of symptomatology. These agents are also expensive, with yearly costs of EACA and tranexamic acid running as high as $10,000.

Treatment of Acute Attacks

The decision whether or not to treat an acute HAE attack is based on the location as well as the severity and time course of the attack. Agents effective in treating allergic urticaria and angioedema are of limited use in HAE. Landerman (60) reported that some patients could benefit from the administration of antihistamines; however, others have found them to be of little or no benefit (2,27). The use of steroids in the treatment of acute attacks also has not been found to be beneficial (2,27,56).

Swelling attacks of the extremities are typically nonpainful and self-limiting, and therefore do not require treatment. When the frequency and severity of the attacks begin to have a significant impact on the patient's daily activities, long-term preventive therapy should be considered.

Laryngeal edema, on the other hand, can lead to asphyxiation and death, making it the most feared complication of HAE. Most attacks progress at a relatively predictable pace, usually starting as an irritating sensation in the throat, which progresses to changes in voice tone and difficulty in swallowing, before airway compromise becomes apparent. This typically takes place over a period of hours, and only rarely progresses to total airway obstruction. Thus, the patient's description of the course of an attack can have a major impact on his or her management. If a patient has reported that the throat swelling is minimal, has been present for a day or so, and is not progressing, he or she can be observed for several hours and does not require additional therapy. However, a laryngeal attack of only hours in duration that has resulted in hoarseness or difficulty in swallowing, and is continuing to progress, constitutes a medical emergency.

Because of the current lack of commercially available replacement therapy in the United States and some other countries (see later), supportive care and airway management become even more critical in these patients. An ear, nose, and throat evaluation should be requested, because intubation, if it becomes nec-

essary, should be performed electively by an experienced individual. Materials and personnel trained to perform an emergency tracheostomy should be immediately available, if needed. This procedure has saved the lives of several patients (27,60). The use of transtracheal jet ventilation through a 16-gauge cannula has been reported to reverse hypoxemia in an HAE patient with complete airway obstruction (61). Some patients have developed their own means of dealing with airway management. Donaldson and Rosen described a man who kept a scalpel in his kitchen and had his wife trained to use it in the event of severe airway compromise (2). Also, a former National Institutes of Health (NIH) patient claimed to have successfully kept his airway patent during an attack using a soup spoon. The psychological stress of a potentially fatal angioedema attack has resulted in several patients requesting and receiving permanent tracheostomies (27).

As previously mentioned, some treatments that are usually effective for reversing immunoglobulin E–mediated angioedema (e.g., antihistamines and steroids) are of limited value in HAE, and this holds true for the treatment of laryngeal attacks. Nevertheless, there have been reports that epinephrine, administered either as repeated subcutaneous injections or by a nebulized delivery system, has been found to be of modest value in some cases, and many physicians will use this agent (27). Likewise, antihistamines are often used, if for no other reason, for their sedative effects.

The primary goal in treating abdominal attacks is the relief of pain, which can be excruciating. Narcotics are often required, and have been used for more than a century (62). For whatever reason, meperidine (Demerol), at doses of 50 to 100 mg given intramuscularly, appeared to be the drug of choice for those patients treated in the NIH program. The use of narcotics, of course, brings with it the possibility of addiction (27,63). This may be a particularly difficult problem to manage, because some localized abdominal attacks may be terribly painful to the patient and yet completely void of objective clinical signs. To complicate matters further, at least one patient has informed us that abdominal discomfort resulting from a narcotic withdrawal program can simulate the pain of HAE attacks.

There can be considerable third spacing of fluids during an abdominal attack, which may result in significant discomfort and, at times, hypotension. Thus, the importance of administering intravenous fluids cannot be overemphasized. Nausea and abdominal pain often prohibit patients from attempting to drink water in spite of the presence of extreme thirst. It is also critical to remember that the diagnosis of HAE does not rule out the occurrence of abdominal pain from other causes, and the nonjudicial use of narcotics may interfere with the proper evaluation of an acute abdomen. Each abdominal attack should be evaluated carefully, with special attention given to attacks associated with pain differing in quality from previous HAE attacks or with fever, elevated sedimentation rate, or leukocytosis.

As noted earlier, available effective treatment modalities for acute attacks are limited. Androgens are of no proven value; however, antifibrinolytics, if given very early in an attack, may be of some value in limiting the progression (24,30). The kallikrein inhibitor aprotinin has been used with some success in the treatment of acute HAE attacks. Marasini and coworkers treated seven laryngeal attacks with this agent, and the mean time to the beginning of symptom regression was about 85 minutes. A single extremity attack was treated without success (64). Reports of anaphylaxis and death resulting from the use of this agent (30,65), however, have dissuaded physicians from using it for HAE treatment.

Pickering and coworkers demonstrated in 1969 that infusion of fresh frozen plasma successfully reversed acute HAE attacks in two patients (66). Others have also found this material effective in treating laryngeal and abdominal attacks (67,68). Pickering, however, raised concerns about the potential danger of supplying not only C1-INH with the fresh frozen plasma, but also complement components, kinins, and other vasoactive substances that could accelerate or increase the severity of an existing attack. These concerns have been echoed by others (31,69,70). Indeed, while infusing 2 units of fresh frozen plasma into an HAE patient for the purpose of dental prophylaxis (see later), we witnessed a dramatically accelerated swelling of the patient's foot. The patient later stated that just before the infusion she had a tingling sensation in the foot, as if an HAE attack were about to start. Had the tingling sensation been in her throat, the results could have been catastrophic. In addition, other risks, such as viral infectivity, allergic or anaphylactoid reactions, alloimmunization, and excessive intravascular volume, which may result in hypervolemia and cardiac failure, have been associated with the use of fresh frozen plasma (71).

The true breakthrough for the treatment of acute HAE attacks came about with the availability of partially purified concentrates of C1-INH made from pooled human plasma. Therapy with an experimental preparation of C1-INH concentrate manufactured by Behringwerke (Marburg, Germany) was first reported in 1973 by Brackertz and Kueppers, who used the preparation in two patients (72). The following year, Schulz described the apparent usefulness of 10 infusions of the same preparation in three patients (73). At about the same time, Vogelaar and coworkers at The Netherlands Red Cross Blood Transfusion Service in Amsterdam reported on the preparation of their own C1-INH concentrate, which they infused into five asymptomatic HAE patients in remission with no untoward effects. A 20-mL portion containing the C1-INH activity of 2 liters of fresh plasma was found to raise the functional C1-INH levels in a single patient from 0% to 75% normal (74). Also, using The Netherlands Red Cross concentrate, Marasini and coworkers treated six acute HAE attacks in five patients. All four laryngeal or facial attacks responded within 1 hour; however, resolution of arm edema took longer. Functional and antigenic levels of C1-INH were at or near maximum by 15 minutes after infusion, but increased levels of C4 were not observed until a 12-hour postinfusion measurement (64). This study was expanded to include treatment of a total of 19 attacks in 13 patients, with similar degrees of efficacy (75). The NIH group evaluated a C1-INH preparation made in cooperation with the American Red Cross (76). They found the concentrate to be effective in seven of the eight abdominal and laryngeal attacks treated. A preparation of purified C1-INH manufactured by Immuno AG (Vienna, Austria) was used by Bergamaschini

and coworkers to treat 10 acute attacks in nine patients (77). Three of these patients were children between 4 and 8 years of age. The concentrate was found to be effective in all cases. Seven attacks involving the larynx, pharynx, and abdomen all began to regress within 20 minutes of the start of the infusion. Judge and associates described four patients who were sucessfully treated for multiple HAE attacks over a 12-year period with C1-INH concentrates made by The Netherlands Red Cross and, after 1988, by Immuno. They also reported on the use of these concentrates at home by self-administration (78).

Unfortunately, the use of the early C1-INH concentrates, made from pools of plasma obtained from thousands of donors, carried with it a risk of transmission of human immunodeficiency virus (HIV) as well as transfusion hepatitis. To achieve a higher degree of viral safety, the Behringwerke preparation was stabilized with sucrose and glycine, and then heated in an aqueous solution at 60°C for 10 hours (C1-Inactivator, P. Behringwerke AG Biologicals, Marburg, Germany). The Immuno AG concentrate was subjected to a process in which the lyophylized material, in the absence of stabilizers, was subjected to vapor heating at 60°C under pressure for 10 hours [C1-Inhibitor (Human) Vapor Heated, Immuno] (Eibl J, Schwarz O, Elsinger F, et al, Method of inactivating reproducible filterable blood products as well as a method for producing blood products, U.S. patent 4,640,834). Despite the fact that C1-INH is heat labile (79), these concentrates still retain their functional activity after being exposed to the viral-inactivation procedures just mentioned. Agostoni and coworkers reported having experience with a total of 83 infusions of C1-INH concentrate, 56 of which were the vapor-heated preparation from Immuno. These concentrates have been found to be uniformly effective in reversing laryngeal and abdominal edema when given at doses of 1000 to 1500 plasma units (PU) (31). One PU is equivalent to the C1-INH activity in 1 mL of normal plasma.

The availability in the United States of Immuno's vapor-heated concentrate in the early 1990s, on an experimental basis, renewed interest in this therapeutic modality, and two double-blind, placebo-controlled studies were performed with this material. The first, a crossover study conducted at the NIH, evaluated the safety and efficacy of the concentrate when used prophylactically in six HAE patients who were unresponsive to, or could not tolerate, conventional long-term treatment with androgens or antifibrinolytics (80,81). Each patient remained at the NIH Clinical Center for two 17-day periods during which time he or she received an infusion of C1-INH (25 PU/kg body weight) every third day for 5 doses, or placebo (albumin) given at the same volume and schedule. All complaints of HAE symptoms were evaluated and objectively scored by house physicians. As a group, the patients had significantly lower symptom scores for extremity, laryngeal, abdominal, and genitourinary (GU) edema. Overall, there was a 60% reduction in the frequency and severity of objective HAE symptoms. In fact, no patient had laryngeal or GU edema while receiving C1-INH, but four had involvement in one or both of these areas while on placebo.

The second study in the United States using the vapor-heated concentrate was a double-blind evaluation of the efficacy of this material in treating acute attacks, conducted by Rosen and coworkers at Boston Children's Hospital (81). A total of 55 attacks in 11 patients were treated with the C1-INH (25 PU/kg body weight), and 28 attacks in 11 different patients were treated with an equal volume of albumin. The mean time from start of infusion to beginning of relief after C1-INH treatment was 55 minutes, compared with 799 minutes after placebo. The mean time to relief in laryngeal, abdominal, and facial attacks was 28 minutes after concentrate infusions, and 878 minutes after placebo. These are three areas in which replacement therapy would be expected to be of most benefit to the patient. Twenty-one attacks did not respond to the blind study material by 4 hours, and, at the discretion of the treating physician, the patients were successfully treated with open-label C1-INH. When the treatment code was broken, all were found to have initially been treated with placebo. Seventy-five percent of the attacks affecting the abdomen, larynx, or face responded to the C1-INH concentrate within 30 minutes, and the remainder within 4 hours. In contrast, none of the attacks involving these areas responded within 30 minutes after treatment with placebo, and only 10% responded within 4 hours. In addition to that administered in these two controlled studies, scores of infusions of open-label vapor-heated C1-INH (Hyland Immune, Baxter Healthcare) have been given in the United States on a compassionate basis.

A group of Canadian investigators used the same preparation to treat 87 HAE attacks in seven patients. Following infusions of approximately 1000 to 1700 PU of C1-INH, the mean duration of attack was reduced to 50 minutes (range, 15–150). No adverse events were reported (82).

Several important points can be made about these studies performed with a variety of different C1-INH concentrates. First, these concentrates all appear to be effective in treating attacks of HAE. Attacks of the mucosal areas such as larynx and abdomen appear, in general, to respond much earlier than extremity attacks (64,75,81). Second, in those studies in which pre- and postinfusion C1-INH and C4 levels were measured (64,74,76,80,81), maximum C1-INH activity was usually detected at 15 to 60 minutes after infusion and often fell to preinfusion levels within several days. The recovery of functional C1-INH activity following infusions was consistently about 100%, and the effective functional C1-INH half-lives for the NIH prophylaxis and Boston Children's Hospital treatment studies were estimated to be 29 and 38 hours, respectively (77,83,84). This was shorter than the 50-hour effective functional half-life seen in asymptomatic HAE patients (84a). The plasma levels attained following C1-INH concentrate infusions are several times those typically obtained after infusions of fresh frozen plasma (85). Levels of C4, however, generally did not increase until 6 to 12 hours after infusion and tended to remain elevated for longer periods of time than did C1-INH. Third, no major adverse reactions resulting from the use of these C1-INH concentrates have been reported in the literature. Although the older, untreated concentrates were believed to have had the potential for transmitting hepatitis (86), there have been no documented cases of transmission of HIV or hepatitis from the two viral-inactivated concentrates, both of which have been commercially available in Europe for years and are considered by far to be the treatments of choice for severe HAE attacks, especially those involving the larynx and abdomen. Indeed, in studies in which pre- and postinfusion samples were carefully monitored for transmission of HIV, HBV, HCV, and/or the newly described virus HGV, there was no evidence of transmission of these viruses (81,83,87).

The suspected development of an antibody to C1-inhibitor has been reported in a patient with both HAE and systemic lupus erythematosus (SLE) who was treated with multiple infusions of C1-INH concentrate (88). None of 19 patients enrolled in controlled studies and monitored for the development of anti–C1-INH antibodies did develop them, however, and the authors are not aware of any other reports concerning the development of such antibodies following treatment with C1-INH concentrates (81).

In summary, where available, the first-line treatment for significant laryngeal, facial, and abdominal attacks is the use of a purified C1-INH concentrate, given at doses of up to 25 PU/kg body weight. In those areas where these products are not available, the treater must depend primarily on providing supportive care, using intubation or tracheostomy, if necessary, to maintain an open airway. Narcotics or intravenous fluids may be of value for abdominal attacks, and extremity attacks normally do not require any therapeutic intervention.

Short-Term (Preoperative) Prophylaxis

The third major HAE treatment situation to be discussed is short-term prophylaxis before surgical procedures that are likely to precipitate acute attacks. Especially important are dental procedures. Before any dental manipulation, the patient should be evaluated by his or her physician to ensure that HAE activity has been under reasonable control. If the patient is receiving long-term preventive therapy with androgens or antifibrinolytics, these agents should be continued. Prophylactic suppressive therapy is recommended for any procedure in which local or general anesthesia is indicated, but it need not be provided for such procedures as examinations, gentle prophylaxis, or even very minor restorations (89). Short-term prophylaxis should also be provided for diagnostic procedures, such as endoscopy, which may involve manipulation of the upper airway, and for all major surgical procedures, especially those that require intubation.

The short-term use of androgens or antifibrinolytic agents has met with some success. The effective prophylaxis of a single patient treated for 6 days with 16 to 20 g/day of EACA (90), as well as several patients treated for 2 to 3 days with this agent (27), has been reported. Sheffer and coworkers described a study in which 14 patients undergoing 10 dental and four general surgical procedures received 1 g of tranexamic acid every 6 hours starting 48 hours before surgery and continuing until 48 hours postoperatively. No complications were observed (91). The use of androgens such as danazol (600 mg/day) and stanozolol (16 mg/day) for 5 to 10 days before surgery has also been described (37). When such regimens are used, however, caution must be exercised. As discussed earlier, antifibrinolytics are not totally effective in suppressing attacks. In addition, the administration of androgens is not always associated with significant increases in C1-INH (92), and treatment failures have been reported (89,93,94).

The effective use of fresh frozen plasma has been well documented at the NIH (85,89,93). The standard regimen of 2 units given the day before dental or other surgical procedures was found to be effective in the vast majority of the reported 45 patients having a total of 97 dental treatments and 30 patients undergoing other surgical procedures. Three patients had minor HAE attacks following dental treatments, and two following other surgical procedures. Interestingly, in three of these instances, the patient was also receiving either an androgen or EACA. An episode of airway obstruction requiring intubation following a single tooth extraction has been described in a patient who had received preoperative administration of both fresh frozen plasma and danazol (95).

The use of purified C1-INH concentrates given at doses of 1000 to 2000 PU within 2 hours before surgery has been reported to be effective in several anecdotal cases (92,96,97). This appears to be a reasonable alternative to fresh frozen plasma when short-term prophylaxis is required. In addition, the successful long-term prophylactic use of C1-INH concentrate, given once or twice weekly to 21 patients, has been reported (98).

Pregnancy and Cardiac Surgery

Two situations that demand separate consideration are preventive treatment modalities in HAE patients who 1) are pregnant or 2) are about to undergo cardiac surgery. Although pregnancy often results in a decrease in HAE activity (27), attacks may still occur. The use of androgens is contraindicated because of the potential virilization of a female fetus, which has been reported (52,99). The episodic use of EACA had been found to be beneficial in decreasing the severity and length of attacks throughout three pregnancies; however, rapid effective treatment was achieved in three attacks by using a purified C1-INH concentrate (100). Similar results have been reported using a C1-INH preparation to treat attacks occuring during pregnancy and 2 days postpartum (101,102). Prophylactic replacement therapy is generally not required for uncomplicated vaginal deliveries, but C1-INH concentrates have been successfully given before cesarean sections (73,103). The long-term biweekly prophylactic use of fresh frozen plasma during pregnancy has also been reported (104). One frequently cited report of a fatal HAE attack after an uneventful vaginal delivery may have, in fact, been the result of septic shock (105).

Cardiac surgery, which involves the use of cardiopulmonary bypass equipment having the potential for activating complement, may be expected to be particularly problematic for patients with C1-INH deficiency. The literature concerning this area is limited. One HAE patient received a fourfold increase in his usual 2-mg/day dosage of stanozolol for 5 days before surgery.

His C1-INH level dropped from 11 to 6 mg/dL during surgery, but he had no complications (106). An asymptomatic 7-year-old girl with a diagnosis of HAE has also been reported to have undergone uneventful open-heart surgery (107) after pretreatment with danazol and 3 units of fresh frozen plasma. One HAE patient received prophylactic C1-INH concentrate just before cardiac surgery and had no operative or postoperative complications. This patient, however, also received aprotinin, which may have further reduced the likelihood of an HAE attack (Baker J, personal communication, 1994). A patient with acquired C1-INH deficiency who had been maintained on danazol (200 mg/day) was found to have a functional C1-INH level of 28% of normal, as well as markedly decreased levels of C4, C2, C3, C1q, and factor B before open-heart surgery. Intraoperatively, bleeding started from all suture lines and needle holes. Hemostasis could not be secured despite infusions of fresh frozen plasma, coagulation factors, protamine, and EACA, and the patient died (108). The successful use of a C1-INH concentrate immediately following cardiopulmonary bypass in a patient with acquired C1-inhibitor deficiency has recently been reported (109). Although the experience in this area is scant, the prophylactic use of replacement therapy with fresh frozen plasma or, when available, C1-INH concentrates before cardiac pulmonary bypass surgery warrants serious consideration.

Treatment of Acquired Angioedema

Patients with acquired angioedema (AAE) often have swelling attacks that are indistinguishable from those resulting from HAE. Because the decrease in C1-INH in these patients results from either accelerated consumption by immune complexes or other complement-activating factors, or from inactivation by autoantibodies against this protein, the response to conventional HAE therapy may be suboptimal.

In some patients in whom a process such as a solid tumor or lymphoproliferative disease is causing the consumption of C1-INH, the surgical or chemotherapeutic treatment of the underlying disorder has resulted in reduced clinical symptoms, at times being associated with increased complement levels (110–113). The successful use of danazol in raising C1-INH levels and decreasing angioedema episodes in these patients has also been reported (114,115).

Androgen therapy has been described as being relatively ineffective in preventing angioedema in patients with autoantibodies against C1-INH; however, prophylaxis with antifibrinolytic agents was found to be effective in six of seven of these patients (116). Five of these patients received infusions of a purified C1-INH concentrate for the treatment of acute laryngeal attacks. Two responded well, and the three others had no or slow clinical responses that required progressively higher doses (up to 4000 PU). This probably reflected differences in the catabolism of the infused C1-INH by the autoantibodies (116,117). A similar disparity in response to C1-INH concentrate therapy in two patients had previously been described (4). The prophylactic use of C1-INH concentrates for longer than 1 year has been described for a patient with autoantibody-mediated angioedema, as well as a patient with HAE (118).

A sustained remission from angioedema attacks in a patient with C1-INH autoantibodies who was unresponsive to androgen therapy was obtained through a series of plasmapheresis and pulse cyclophosphamide therapy (119). A similar patient who underwent immunoadsorption using staphylococcal protein PROSORBA (IMRE Corp., Seattle, WA) columns, however, had a disastrous adverse reaction to this treatment, and its use was abandoned (120).

Summary

Long-term prevention of HAE attacks, when indicated, can usually be accomplished by daily administration of androgens or antifibrinolytic agents. To minimize side effects, the lowest doses needed to achieve acceptable clinical responses are used. Short-term prophylaxis prior to dental or other surgery can often be obtained with increased doses of these agents, with fresh frozen plasma or, where available, purified C1-INH preparations. These concentrates are also the treatments of choice for severe HAE attacks, which are otherwise managed with supportive care and pain medications or fluids, when needed. Acquired angioedema is typically more resistant to therapy than is HAE.

References

1. Davis AE III. Hereditary and acquired deficiencies of C1 inhibitor. Immunodefic Rev 1989;1:207–226.
2. Donaldson VH, Rosen FS. Hereditary angioneurotic edema: a clinical survey. Pediatrics 1966;37(6):1017–1027.
3. Geha RS, Quinti I, Austen KF, et al. Acquired C1-inhibitor deficiency associated with anti-idiotypic antibody to monoclonal immunoglobulins. N Engl J Med 1985;312:534–540.
4. Alsenz J, Bork K, Loos M. Autoantibody mediated acquired deficiency of C1 inhibitor. N Engl J Med 1987;316:1360–1366.
5. Jackson J, Sim RB, Whelan A, Feighry C. An IgG autoantibody that inactivates C1-inhibitor. Nature 1986;323:722–724.
6. Mandle R, Baron C, Roux WE, et al. Acquired C1 inhibitor deficiency as a result of an autoantibody to the reactive center region of C1 inhibitor. J Immunol 1994;152:4680–4685.
7. Cicardi M, Frangi D, Bergamaschini L, et al. Acquired C1 inhibitor deficiency with angioedema symptoms in a patient infected with Echinococcus granulosus. Complement 1985;2:133–139.
8. Donaldson VH, Rosen FS. Action of complement in hereditary angioneurotic edema: the role of C1-esterase. J Clin Invest 1964;43:2204–2213.
9. Strang CJ, Auerbach HS, Rosen FS. C1s-induced vascular permeability in C2 deficient guinea pigs. J Immunol 1986;137:631–635.
10. Strang CJ, Cholin S, Spragg J, et al. Angioedema induced by a peptide derived from complement component C2. J Exp Med 1988;168:1685–1698.
11. Schapira M, Silver LD, Scott CF, et al. Prekallikrein activation and high-molecular-weight kininogen consumption in hereditary angioedema. N Engl J Med 1983;308:1050–1053.
12. Schapira M, Scott CF, Colman RW. Protection of human plasma kallikrein from inactivation by C1-inhibitor and other protease inhibitors: the role of high molecular weight kininogen. Biochemistry 1981;20:2738–2743.
13. Quastel M, Harrison R, Cicardi M, et al. Behavior in vivo of normal and dysfunctional C1 inhibitor in normal subjects and patient with hereditary angioneurotic edema. J Clin Invest 1983;71:1041–1046.
14. Aulak KS, Pemberton PA, Rosen FS, et al. Dysfunctional C1-inhibitor (At), isolated from a type II hereditary angio-oedema plasma, contains a P1 "reactive centre" (Arg444/His) mutation. Biochem J 1988;253:615–618.
15. Levy NJ, Ramesh N, Cicardi M, et al. Type II hereditary angioneurotic edema that may result from a single nucleotide change in the codon for alanine-436 in the C1 inhibitor gene. Proc Natl Acad Sci USA 1990;87:265–268.
16. Parad RB, Kramer J, Strunk RC, et al. Dysfunctional C1 inhibitor Ta: deletion of Lys-251 results in acquisition of N-glycosylation site. Proc Natl Acad Sci USA 1990;87:6786–6790.
17. Skriver K, Wikoff WR, Patston PA, et al. Substrate properties of C1 inhibitor Ma (A434E): genetic and structural evidence suggesting that the "P12-region" contains critical determinants of serpin inhibitor/substrate status. J Biol Chem 1991;266:9216–9221.
18. Skriver K, Radziejewska E, Silberman JA, et al. Mutations in a CpG dinucleotide change reactive site arginine-444 to cysteine in dysfunctional C1 inhibitor Da and histidine in dysfunctional C1 inhibitor Ri. J Biol Chem 1989;264:3066–3071.
19. Cicardi M, Igarashi T, Rosen FS, Davis AE III. Molecular basis for the deficiency of complement 1 inhibitor in type I hereditary angioneurotic edema. J Clin Invest 1987;79:698–702.
20. Kramer K, Katz Y, Rosen FS, et al. Synthesis of C1 inhibitor in fibroblasts from patients with type I and type II hereditary angioneurotic edema. J Clin Invest 1991;87:1614–1620.
21. Stoppa-Lyonnet D, Carter PE, Meo T, Tosi M. Clusters of intragenic Alu repeats predispose the human C1 inhibitor locus to deleterious rearrangements. Proc Natl Acad Sci USA 1990;87:1551–1555.
22. Ariga T, Carter PE, Davis AE III. Recombinations between Alu repeat sequences that result in partial deletions within the C1 inhibitor gene. Genomics 1990;8:607–613.
23. Frangi D, Cicardi M, Sica A, et al. Nonsense mutations affect C1 inhibitor messenger RNA levels in patients with type I hereditary angioneurotic edema. J Clin Invest 1991;8:755–759.
24. Nilsson IM, Anderson L, Björkman SE. Epsilon-aminocaproic acid (E-ACA) as a therapeutic agent. Based on 5 years' clinical experience. Acta Med Scand 1966;448(suppl):5–46.
25. Lundh B, Laurell A, Wetterqvist H, et al. A case of hereditary angioneurotic oedema, successfully treated with ε-aminocaproic acid. Studies on C1 esterase inhibitor, C1 activation, plasminogen level and antihistamine metabolism. Clin Exp Immunol 1968;3:733–745.

26. Frank MM, Sergent JS, Kane MA, Alling DW. Epsilon aminocaproic acid therapy of hereditary angioneurotic edema: a double-blind study. N Engl J Med 1972;286(15):808–812.

27. Frank MM, Gelfand JA, Atkinson JP. Hereditary angioedema: the clinical syndrome and its management. Ann Intern Med 1966;84:580–593.

28. Gwynn CM. Therapy in hereditary angioneurotic oedema. Arch Dis Child 1974;49:636–640.

29. Sheffer AL, Austen KF, Rosen FS. Tranexamic acid therapy in hereditary angioneurotic edema. N Engl J Med 1972;287(9):452–454.

30. Blohmé G. Treatment of hereditary angioneurotic oedema with tranexamic acid. A random double-blind cross-over study. Acta Med Scand 1972;192:293–298.

31. Agostoni A, Cicardi M. Hereditary and acquired C1-inhibitor deficiency: biological and clinical characteristics in 235 patients. Medicine 1992;71(4):206–215.

32. Soter NA, Austen GF, Gigli I. Inhibition by ε-aminocaproic acid of the activation of the first component of the complement system. J Immunol 1975;114(3):928–932.

33. Cugno M, Hack CE, DeBoer JP, et al. Generation of plasmin during acute attacks of hereditary angioedema. J Lab Clin Med 1993;121(1):38–43.

34. Cugno M, Cicardi M, Agostoni A. Activation of the contact system and fibrinolysis in autoimmune acquired angioedema: a rationale for prophylactic use of tranexamic acid. J Allergy Clin Immunol 1994;93(5):870–876.

35. Korsan-Bengsten K, Ysander G, Blohmé G, Tibblin E. Extensive muscle necrosis after long-term treatment with aminocaproic acid (EACA) in a case of hereditary periodic edema. Acta Med Scand 1969;185:341–346.

36. Agostoni A, Marasini B, Cicardi M, et al. Hepatic function and fibrinolysis in patients with hereditary angioedema undergoing long-term treatment with tranexamic acid. Allergy 1978;33:216–221.

37. Sim T, Grant JA. Hereditary angioedema: its diagnostic and management perspectives. Am J Med 1990;88:656–664.

38. Spaulding WB. Methyltestosterone therapy for hereditary episodic edema (hereditary angioneurotic edema). Ann Intern Med 1960;53(4):739–745.

39. Sheffer AL, Fearon DT, Austen KF. Methyltestosterone therapy in hereditary angioedema. Ann Intern Med 1977;86:306–308.

40. Davis PJ, Davis FB, Charache P. Long-term therapy of hereditary angioedema (HAE): preventive management with fluoxymesterone and oxymetholone in severely affected males and females. Hopkins Med J 1974;135:391–398.

41. Sheffer AL, Fearon DT, Austen KF. Clinical and biochemical effects of impeded androgen (oxymetholone) therapy of hereditary angioedema. J Allergy Clin Immunol 1979;64(4):275–280.

42. Gelfand JA, Sherins RJ, Alling DW, Frank MM. Treatment of hereditary angioedema with danazol. Reversal of clinical and biochemical abnormalities. N Engl J Med 1976;295:1444–1448.

43. Gadek JE, Hosea SW, Gelfand JA, Frank MM. Response of variant hereditary angioedema phenotypes to danazol therapy. Genetic implications. J Clin Invest 1979;64:280–286.

44. Agostoni A, Cicardi M, Martignoni GC, et al. Danazol and stanozolol in long-term prophylactic treatment of hereditary angioedema. J Allergy Clin Immunol 1980;65(1):75–79.

45. Sheffer AL, Fearon DT, Austen KF. Clinical and biochemical effects of stanozolol therapy for hereditary angioedema. J Allergy Clin Immunol 1981;68(3):181–187.

46. Sheffer AL, Fearon DT, Austen KF. Hereditary angioedema: a decade of management with stanozolol. J Allergy Clin Immunol 1987;80(6):855–860.

47. Hosea SW, Santaella ML, Brown EJ, et al. Long-term therapy of hereditary angioedema with danazol. Ann Intern Med 1980;93(6):809–812.

48. Cicardi M, Castelli R, Zingale LC, Agostoni A. Side effects of long-term prophylaxis with attenuated androgens in hereditary angioedema: comparison of treated and untreated patients. J Allergy Clin Immunol 1997;99(2):194–196.

49. Westaby D, Ogle SJ, Paradinas FJ, et al. Liver damage from long-term methyltestosterone. Lancet 1977;2:261–263.

50. Falk H, Thomas LB, Popper H, Ishak KG. Hepatic angiosarcoma associated with androgenic-anabolic steroids. Lancet 1979;2:1120–1122.

51. Zurlo JJ, Frank MM. The long-term safety of danazol in women with hereditary angioedema. Fertil Steril 1990;54:64–72.

52. Cicardi M, Bergamaschini L, Cugno M, et al. Long-term treatment of hereditary angioedema with attenuated androgens. A survey of a 13-year experience. J Allergy Clin Immunol 1991;87(4):768–773.

53. Barakat AJ, Castaldo AJ. Hereditary angioedema: danazol therapy in a 5-year-old child. Am J Dis Child 1993;147:931–932.

54. Lee PA, Thompson RG, Migeon CJ, Blizzard RM. The effect of danazol in sexual precocity. Hopkins Med J 1975;137:265–269.

55. Lotz M, Zuraw BL. Interferon-γ is a major regulator of C1-inhibitor synthesis by human blood monocytes. J Immunol 1987;139(10):3382–3387.

56. Gluszko P, Undas A, Amenta S, et al. Administration of gamma interferon in human subjects decreases plasminogen activation and fibrinolysis without influencing C1 inhibitor. J Lab Clin Med 1994;123(2):232–240.

57. Gordon EM, Ratnoff OD, Saito H, et al. Rapid fibrinolysis, augmented Hageman factor (factor XII) titers, and decreased C1 esterase inhibitor titers in women taking oral contraceptives. J Lab Clin Med 1980;96(5):762–769.

58. Shepherd GM. Possible contraindication of angiotensin converting enzyme inhibitors in patients with hereditary angioedema. Am J Med 1990;88:446.

59. Agostoni A, Cicard M. Contraindications to the use of ace inhibitors in patients with C1 esterase inhibitor deficiency. Am J Med 1991;90(2):278.

60. Landerman NS. Hereditary angioneurotic edema. J Allergy 1962;33(4):316–329.

61. Baraka A, Sibai AN, Azar IA, Zaytoun G. Transtracheal jet ventilation in an adult patient with severe hereditary angioneurotic edema. Middle East J Anesthesiology 1993;12(2):171–175.

62. Osler W. Hereditary angioneurotic oedema. Am J Med Sci 1888;95:362–367.

63. Biering A. Abdominal pains in angioneurotic edema. Acta Med Scand 1956;153:373–382.

64. Marasini B, Cicardi M, Martignoni GC, Agostoni A. Treatment of hereditary angioedema. Klin Wschr 1978;56:819–823.

65. Proud G, Chamberlain J. Anaphylactic reaction to aprotinin. Lancet 1976;July 3:48–49.

66. Pickering RJ, Kelly JR, Good RA, Gewurz H. Replacement therapy in hereditary angioedema. Successful treatment of two patients with fresh frozen plasma. Lancet 1969;Feb 15:326–330.

67. Cohen G, Peterson A. Treatment of hereditary angioedema with frozen plasma. Ann Allergy 1972;30:690–692.

68. Beck P, Wills D, Davies GT, et al. A family study of hereditary angioneurotic oedema. Qtrly J Med 1973;166:317–339.

69. Rosen FS, Austen KF. The "neurotic edema" (hereditary angioedema). N Engl J Med 1969;280(24):1356–1357.

70. Donaldson VH. Therapy of "the neurotic edema." N Engl J Med 1972;286(15):835–836.

71. NIH Plasma Consensus Conference. Fresh-frozen plasma. Indications and risks. JAMA 1985;253(4):551–553.

72. Brackertz D, Kueppers F. Possible therapy in hereditary angioneurotic edema (HAE). Klin Wschr 1973;51:620–622.

73. Schulz KH. Hereditäres quincke-ödem. Neuere wege der therapie. Der Hautarzt 1974;25:12–16.

74. Vogelaar EF, Brummelhuis HGJ, Krijnen H. Contributions to the optimal use of human blood: III. Large-scale preparation of human C1 esterase inhibitor concentrate for clinical use. Vox Sang 1974;26:118–127.

75. Agostoni A, Bergamaschini L, Martignoni G, et al. Treatment of acute attacks of hereditary angioedema with C1-inhibitor concentrate. Ann Allergy 1980;44:299–301.

76. Gadek JE, Hosea SW, Gelfand JA, et al. Replacement therapy in hereditary angioedema. Successful treatment of acute episodes of angioedema with partly purified C1 inhibitor. N Engl J Med 1980;302:542–546.

77. Bergamaschini L, Cicardi M, Tucci A, et al. C1 INH concentrate in the therapy of hereditary angioedema. Allergy 1983;38:81–84.

78. Judge MR, Watson KM, Greaves MW. C1 esterase inhibitor concentrate in the management of hereditary angiooedema. J Dermatol Treat 1993;4:95–97.

79. Levy LR, Lepow IH. Assay and properties of serum inhibitor of C1-esterase. Proc Soc Exp Biol Med 1959;101:608–611.

80. Waytes AT, Huber M, Litton G, et al. Use of a vapor-heated C1-inhibitor preparation in hereditary angioedema. J Allergy Clin Immunol 1992;89:247.

81. Waytes AT, Rosen FS, Frank MM. Treatment of hereditary angioedema with a vapor-heated C1 inhibitor concentrate. N Engl J Med 1996;334:1630–1634.

82. Visentin DE, Yang WH, Karsh J. C1-esterase inhibitor transfusions in patients with hereditary angioedema. Ann Allergy Asthma Immunol 1998;80:457–461.

83. Kunschak M, Engl W, Maritsch F, et al. A randomized, controlled trial to study the efficacy and safety of C1 inhibitor concentrate in treating hereditary angioedema. Transfusion 1998;38:540–548.

84. Fritsch S, Waytes AT, Kunschak M. Recovery and half-life of C1 inhibitor in prevention and treatment of attacks of hereditary angioedema. Thromb Haemostas 69:873. Abstract.

84a. Waytes, AT, Peake B, Engl W, Wappler N, Rosen FS. Pharmacokinetic evaluation of a vapor-heated C1-Inhibitor concentrate [abstract]. J Allergy Clin Immunol 2000;105:S226.

85. Jaffe CJ, Atkinson JP, Gelfand JA, Frank MM. Hereditary angioedema: the use of fresh frozen plasma for prophylaxis in patients undergoing oral surgery. J Allergy Clin Immunol 1975;55(6):387–393.

86. Cicardi M, Mannucci PM, Castelli R, et al. Reduction in transmission of hepatitis C after the introduction of a heat-treatment step in the production of C1-inhibitor concentrate. Transfusion 1995;35(3):209–212.

87. Klarmann D, Kreuz W, Joseph-Steiner J, Ehrenforth S. Hepatitis C and pasteurized C1-inhibitor concentrate. Transfusion 1996;36(1):84–85.

88. Donaldson VH, Bissler JJ, Welch TR, et al. Antibody to C1-inhibitor in a patient receiving C1-inhibitor infusions for treatment of hereditary angioneurotic edema with systemic lupus erythematosus reacts with a normal allotype of residue 458 of C1-inhibitor. J Lab Clin Med 1996;128(4):438–443.

89. Atkinson JC, Frank MM. Oral manifestations and dental management of patients with hereditary angioedema. J Oral Pathol Med 1991;20:139–142.

90. Pence HL, Evans R, Guernsey LH, Gerhard RC. Prophylactic use of epsilon aminocaproic acid for oral surgery in a patient with hereditary angioneurotic edema. J Allergy Clin Immunol 1974;53(5):298–302.

91. Sheffer AL, Fearon DT, Austen KF, Rosen FS. Tranexamic acid: preoperative prophylactic therapy for patients with hereditary angioneurotic edema. J Allergy Clin Immunol 1977;60(1):38–40.

92. Laxenaire M, Audibert G, Janot C. Use of purified C1 esterase inhibitor in patients with hereditary angioedema. Anesthesiology 1990;72:956–957.

93. Wall RT, Frank MM, Hahn M. A review of 25 patients with hereditary angioedema requiring surgery. Anesthesiology 1989;71:309–311.

94. Peled M, Ardekian L, Schnarch A, Laufer D. Preoperative prophylaxis for C1 esterase-inhibitor deficiency in patients undergoing oral surgery: a report of three cases. Quintessence International 1997;28(3):169–171.

95. Degroote DF, Smith GL, Huttula GS. Acute airway obstruction following tooth extraction in hereditary angioedema. J Oral Maxillofac Surg 1985;Jan 43(1):52–54.

96. Leimgruber A, Jaques WA, Spaeth PJ. Hereditary angioedema: uncomplicated maxillofacial surgery using short-term C1 inhibitor replacement therapy. Int Arch Allergy Immunol 1993;101:107–112.

97. Langton D, Weiner J, Fary W. C1-esterase inhibitor concentrate prevents upper airway obstruction in hereditary angio-edema. Med J Australia 1994;160:383–384.

98. Heller Ch, Martinez I, Fischer D, et al. Hereditary angioedema—efficacy and safety of prophylaxis with pasteurized C1-inhibitor concentrate. Blood 1998;92(1):49a. Abstract.

99. Duck SL, Katayama KP. Danazol may cause female pseudohermaphroditism. Fertil Steril 1981;35:230–231.

100. Logan RA, Greaves MW. Hereditary angio-oedema: treatment with C1 esterase inhibitor concentrate. J Royal Soc Med 1984;77:1046–1048.

101. Chappatte O, De Swiet M. Hereditary angioneurotic oedema and pregnancy. Case reports and review of the literature. Br J Obstet Gynecol 1988;Sep 95:938–942.

102. Cox M, Holdcroft A. Hereditary angioneurotic oedema: current management in pregnancy. Anaesthesia 1995;50:547–549.

103. Ebert A, Pritze W, Weitzel HK. C-1-esterase-inhibitor-mangel als geburtshilfliches problem: ein fallbericht. Zent bl gynäkol 1992;114:519–522.

104. Galan HL, Reedy MB, Starr J, Knight AB. Fresh frozen plasma prophylaxis for hereditary angioedema during pregnancy. J Reprod Med 1996;41(7):541–544.

105. Postnikoff IM, Pritzker KPH. Hereditary angioneurotic edema: an unusual case of maternal mortality. J Forensic Sci 1979;24:473–478.

106. Haering JM, Comunale ME. Cardiopulmonary bypass in hereditary angioedema. Anesthesiology 1993;79(6):1429–1433.

107. Umebayashi Y, Morishita Y, Arikawa K, et al. Hereditary angioneurotic edema: report of a case undergoing open heart surgery: a case report. Vasc Surg 1987;21:138–141.

108. Bonser RS, Dave J, Morgan J, et al. Complement activation during bypass in acquired C1 esterase inhibitor deficiency. Ann Thorac Surg 1991;52:541–543.

109. Castelli R, Cicardi M, Gardinali M, et al. Cardiopulmonary by-pass in a patient with acquired C1 inhibitor deficiency. Intl J Artif Organs 1997;20(3):175–177.

110. Gelfand JA, Boss GR, Conley CL, et al. Acquired C1 esterase inhibitor deficiency and angioedema: a review. Medicine 1979;58(4):321–328.

111. Hauptmann G, Petitjean F, Lang JM, Oberling F. Acquired C1 inhibitor deficiency in a case of lymphosarcoma of the spleen. Reversal of complement abnormalities after splenectomy. Clin Exp Immunol 1979;37:523–531.

112. Bain BJ, Catovsky D, Ewan PW. Acquired angioedema as the presenting feature of lymphoproliferative disorders of mature B-lymphocytes. Cancer 1993;72(11):3318–3322.

113. Carpenter GB, Waytes AT. Reversal of acquired C1 esterase inhibitor (C1 INH) deficiency with splenic irradiation. J Allergy Clin Immunol 1996;97:367. Abstract.

114. Cohen SH, Koethe SM, Kozin F, et al. Acquired angioedema associated with rectal carcinoma and its response to danazol therapy. Acquired angioedema treated with danazol. J Allergy Clin Immunol 1978;62(4):217–221.

115. Frigas E. Subspecialty clinics: allergic diseases. Angioedema with acquired deficiency of the C1 inhibitor: a constellation of syndromes. Mayo Clin Proc 1989;64:1269–1275.

116. Cicardi M, Bisiani G, Cugno M, et al. Autoimmune C1 inhibitor deficiency: report of eight patients. Am J Med 1993;95(2):169–175.

117. Agostoni A, Cicardi M. Replacement therapy in hereditary and acquired angioedema. Pharmacol Res 1992;26(suppl 2):148–149.

118. Bork K, Witzke G. Long-term prophylaxis with C1-inhibitor (C1 INH) concentrate in patients with recurrent angioedema caused by hereditary and acquired C1-inhibitor deficiency. J Allergy Clin Immunol 1989;83:677–682.

119. Donaldson VH, Bernstein DI, Wagner CJ, et al. Angioneurotic edema with acquired C1 inhibitor deficiency and autoantibody to C1 inhibitor: response to plasmapheresis and cytotoxic therapy. J Lab Clin Med 1992;119(4):397–406.

120. Boyar A, Zuraw BL, Beall G. Brief communication. Immunoadsorption in acquired angioedema: a therapeutic misadventure. Clin Immunol Immunopathol 1993;66(2):181–183.

Chapter 22

Inhibitors of Tumor Necrosis Factor

Arthur F. Kavanaugh

Peter E. Lipsky

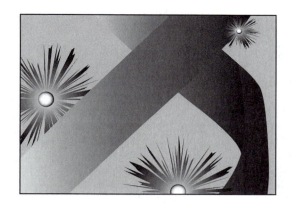

Over the past few decades, the pathogenesis of many systemic inflammatory disorders has become more clearly defined. A greater understanding of various components of the normal immune response has led to insight into the dysregulation of immunocompetent cells and their secreted products in conditions such as rheumatoid arthritis (RA), inflammatory bowel disease, psoriasis, and other diseases. Accompanying this progress, and in concert with advances in biopharmaceutical development, there has been a growing expectation that novel immunomodulatory agents might be available for the therapy of these autoimmune/inflammatory conditions. Agents that inhibit the availability of proinflammatory cytokines have shown particular promise. In this chapter, the impact of inhibitors of tumor necrosis factor-alpha (TNF-α) as therapeutic agents will be reviewed, focusing on their use in RA.

RA is a chronic, progressive disease of unknown etiology. The initiation of this aggressive systemic inflammatory disorder probably results from the exposure of a genetically susceptible host to some unidentified environmental stimulus (1–3). The propagation and sustenance of inflammation reflect an active, ongoing, immunologically driven process. Several components of the immune response are intimately involved in the pathogenesis of RA. Changes in the vasculature occur early in the disease course and facilitate its propagation. Such changes include angiogenesis and alteration of the endothelium into an activated, "high endothelial venule" phenotype. Recirculating CD4+ T lymphocytes, particularly those with a "memory" phenotype, accrue in the synovium utilizing specific adhesion molecules. These T cells, many of which have a "Th1" pattern of cytokine secretion, play a central role in the initiation and orchestration of the autoimmune response (3). Resident synovial cells such as fibroblasts, macrophages, dendritic cells, mast cells, endothelial cells, and blood-derived B cells all are crucial facets of rheumatoid inflammation (1–4). Interactions among these various cells result in the liberation of various mediators, such as cytokines, prostaglandins, and many others. These soluble mediators produce local tissue damage and cause many of the signs and symptoms of disease. In addition, some mediators, particularly cytokines, also exert prominent effects on cells. This facilitates the propagation of the chronic immunologic response that underlies rheumatoid inflammation.

Cytokines are small peptide molecules that are often released from cells on activation. By binding specific cell surface receptors, they can exert myriad biologic functions (5–7). Regarding function, cytokines may exhibit pleiotropy (i.e., one cytokine can mediate diverse functions), redundancy (i.e., several

cytokines may mediate the same activity), or antagonism (i.e., the effects of one cytokine may be inhibited by another cytokine or by soluble forms of the cytokine receptor). While cytokines can be considered individually, in vivo they function in complex networks or cascades. The overall outcome may reflect the balance between proinflammatory factors (e.g., inflammatory cytokines) and anti-inflammatory factors (e.g., soluble forms of cytokine receptors and cytokines with anti-inflammatory function) that are present in the local milieu (5–7).

In RA, there is substantial evidence that cytokines, particularly proinflammatory cytokines such as TNF-α and interleukin-1 (IL-1), subserve a crucial role in disease propagation and expression (1–7). Thus, these cytokines may be particularly appropriate therapeutic targets in RA (8–10). Several trials have attempted to modulate the availability or function of these important cytokines in autoimmune or inflammatory disease states. This review will focus on the progress using inhibitors of TNF-α in patients with RA.

Tumor Necrosis Factor (TNF)

Background

TNF, the prototype of a family of molecules involved in immune regulation and inflammation, was named for its ability to induce necrosis of tumors when injected into certain tumor-bearing animals. Although the initial observation of this effect was made in the 1890s, most knowledge of the role of TNF has been ascertained over the past two decades. Soon after it was cloned in 1984, TNF was found to be identical to another molecule that had been called "cachectin"; it was also found to be approximately 30% homologous to the molecule known as "lymphotoxin" (LT) (11). Genes encoding both TNF-α (cachectin) and the two forms of LT (formerly called TNF-β, now LT-α; and LT-β) are closely linked on chromosome 6, between loci for class I and class II molecules of the major histocompatibility complex (MHC) (12).

Although TNF-α can be synthesized and secreted by various types of cells, at inflammatory sites it is produced primarily by macrophages. It is synthesized and secreted in very large quantities by macrophages in response to various proinflammatory stimuli such as bacterial lipopolysaccharide (LPS). Production of TNF-α is closely regulated at transcriptional and post-transcriptional (i.e., mRNA stability and translational efficiency) levels. TNF-α is synthesized and expressed as a transmembrane protein and can be functional on the cell surface. However, as a result of the actions of a specific metalloproteinase (referred to as TNF-α converting enzyme, or TACE), it is cleaved and released from the cell surface. Secreted TNF-α functions as a soluble homotrimer of 17-KD subunits. LT exists in two forms: LT-α and LT-β. LT-α, which also functions as a soluble homotrimer, is produced and secreted almost exclusively by lymphocytes after antigenic or mitogenic stimulation.

Both TNF-α and LT-α bind to two specific cell surface receptors; the 55-kD (also referred to as CD120a or TNF-RI) and the 75-kD TNF receptors (also referred to as CD120b or TNF-RII) (12). These receptors, which are type I transmembrane proteins, are present on numerous cell types. It is thought that CD120a and CD120b can mediate largely overlapping activities in most tissues, although important differences in the signaling properties of the two receptors have been noted (12,13). Differences between the receptors have also been suggested in affinity for ligand and in function (14,15). Soluble forms of both CD120a and CD120b, which bind TNF-α or LT-α with high avidity and compete with cell surface receptors for binding, can be detected in blood. LT-β, which functions as a heterotrimer of one LT-α and two LT-β subunits, is a transmembrane protein present on the surfaces of T cells and some other cells. LT-β does not bind to the 55-kD or 74-kD TNF-R; rather, it binds to a distinct cell surface receptor (LT-βR).

TNF and the TNF receptors are members of families of related pairs of coreceptor molecules that include Fas-ligand (FasL)/Fas (CD95), CD40L (CD154)/CD40, CD27L (CD70)/CD27, CD30L/CD30, and others. Molecules in this family play a critical role not only in the activation of cells but also in programmed cell death (i.e., apoptosis).

Activities of TNF

TNF mediates numerous inflammatory and immunoregulatory activities; it can be involved in virtually all facets of the inflammatory cascade (Table 22-1). These diverse effects provide the basis for the important role TNF plays in the pathogenesis of RA. Moreover, deficiencies of TNF highlight its relevance to normal immunocompetence and host defense. Thus, animals that have been made deficient in TNF/TFN-R molecules exhibit defects in the development in their secondary lymphoid tissues and are susceptible to certain infections (see below) (16).

There are several activities of TNF that are of particular relevance to its role in RA and other systemic inflammatory diseases. For example, TNF exerts prominent effects on the vasculature. Indeed, the originally described ability of TNF to induce necrosis of tumors relates to the vaso-occlusive changes it causes. Exposure of endothelial cells to TNF stimulates the production of tissue factor and down-modulates thrombomodulin. This changes the normal anticoagulant function of the endothelium toward procoagulant activities, which can play a role in inflammatory responses. Perhaps of greater relevance to RA is

Table 22-1. Activities of TNF

Effects on the Vasculature

Up-regulates adhesion receptors (ICAM-1, VCAM-1, E-selection) via activation of NF-κB
Stimulates angiogenesis
Alters the normal anticoagulant function of the endothelium toward procoagulant activities (e.g., stimulates tissue factor production and down-modulates thrombomodulin)

Effects on Cells

Lymphocytes (activates lymphocytes; plays a role in lymphoid tissue development; modifies CD44 and enhances its capacity to bind ligand)
Dendritic cells (promotes maturation of dendritic cells and their migration from nonlymphoid tissue into secondary lymphoid organs)
Activates neutrophils and platelets
Induces proliferation of fibroblasts/synoviocytes

Effects on Mediators

Induces synthesis of proinflammatory cytokines (e.g., IL-1, IL-6, GM-CSF)
Induces synthesis of proinflammatory chemokines (RANTES, IL-8, MIP-1α, MCP-1)
Induces other inflammatory mediators: prostaglandins (e.g., PGE$_2$, via Cox-2 up-regulation), leukotrienes, platelet activating factor (PAF), nitric oxide, and reactive oxygen species
Induces synthesis of metalloproteinases (e.g., collagenases, gelatinases, stromolysins) that mediate bone and cartilage damage

Other Effects

Mediates pain
Mediates cachexia
Mediates fever
Mobilizes calcium from bone ("osteoclast activating factor" activity)
Modulates apoptosis

the ability of TNF to up-regulate the expression of several endothelial adhesion receptors, including E-selectin (CD62E), ICAM-1 (CD54), and VCAM-1 (CD106)—effects mediated through activation of the gene transcription factor NF-κB. TNF also alters the sulfation of the adhesion receptor CD44, increasing its binding ability (17). The effects of TNF on adhesion receptors facilitate the adhesion and subsequent transendothelial migration of circulating leukocytes into the inflamed synovium (18,19). Adhesion molecule interactions are central to the pathogenesis of RA, and treatment-induced alterations in adhesive processes may be among the most important effects of TNF inhibition in this disease. Finally, TNF plays a role in the stimulation of new blood vessel growth (angiogenesis), which is critical to the growth and propagation of the rheumatoid synovium.

Many of the notable effects of TNF in RA relate to its ability to cause signs and symptoms of inflammation. For example, TNF can directly mediate pain, fever, and cachexia (20,21). Moreover, TNF exerts substantial effects on other inflammatory mediators. For example, TNF induces the synthesis of prostaglandins (by inducing expression of cyclooxygenase 2), leukotrienes, platelet activating factor (PAF), nitric oxide (TNF stimulates the inducible form of nitric oxide synthetase), and reactive oxygen species. The effects of these mediators not only confer many of the signs and symptoms of inflammation, they also potentiate the inflammatory response.

Mediated by NF-κB activation, TNF induces the synthesis of several key proinflammatory cytokines, including IL-1, IL-6, and GM-CSF. It also stimulates production of various chemokines such as RANTES, IL-8, MCP-1, and MIP-1α (21,22). The combined effect of these mediators on cell recruitment, cell activation, and other inflammatory activities may be fundamental to the pathogenesis of RA. Because TNF induces the synthesis of so many other mediators, it serves a central role in this process and therefore is a particularly attractive target for therapy.

TNF exerts other effects that may be relevant to tissue damage in RA. It induces synthesis of metalloproteinase enzymes (e.g., collagenases, gelatinases, and stromolysins) that mediate bone and cartilage damage. Stimulation of fibroblast proliferation contributes to the formation of invasive pannus tissue. Damage to bone and surrounding structures is accentuated because TNF also decreases the de novo synthesis of matrix constituents and facilitates mobilization of calcium from bone, by contributing to the activation of osteoclasts.

Whereas the induction of inflammation mediated by TNF is important to the signs and symptoms of RA, it may also contribute to the immunologic process that drives this chronic disease. It has been suggested that productive immune responses are facilitated by cognate immune interactions that take place in the setting of an active inflammatory milieu (23,24). Thus, inflammatory cytokines released in the course of tissue injury and in response to various noxious stimuli may activate antigen-presenting dendritic cells and subsequently promote specific immunoreactivity. A correlate of this hypothesis would be that inhibition of TNF could be truly immunomodulatory. In addition, TNF exerts effects on various immunocompetent cells, particularly lymphocytes (25). TNF/TNF-R interactions can induce or regulate apoptosis. Therefore, the inhibition of TNF may well be expected to modulate the immune response.

Evidence for a Role of TNF in RA

While consideration of the above mentioned proinflammatory activities strongly suggests a potential role for TNF in RA, more direct evidence comes from two sources: analysis of RA patients and animal models. In addition to the evidence for a role of TNF in RA, there is also a growing body of data supporting the role of TNF in other inflammatory conditions, such as inflammatory bowel disease (IBD) (26).

Paralleling the progress that has been made in immunologic methods over the past decade, investigators have employed various techniques to detect cytokines in the rheumatoid synovium. These studies consistently show a relative abundance of immunoreactive TNF-α in the synovial fluid and synovial tissues of RA patients (27,28). It should be noted, however, that little if any bioactive TNF-α can be detected in synovial fluid or serum of patients with RA. The predominance of macrophage produced cytokines (i.e., TNF-α, IL-1, IL-6, and IL-8) and the relative paucity of T-cell–associated cytokines (i.e., IL-2 and IFN-γ) in the rheumatoid synovium have not only highlighted the potential utility of inhibiting proinflammatory cytokines such as TNF-α, but have also called into question the role T cells play in RA (4).

There are also increased levels of soluble forms of the TNF receptors in the serum and synovial fluid of patients with RA (29). The complete in vivo functions of these soluble receptors are not known (30). However, it is assumed that they serve primarily an inhibitory function, binding to TNF-α and LI-α and interfering with their ability to bind to cell surface receptors. While their concentrations are increased in RA, it remains uncertain whether their concentrations are sufficient to counterbalance the abundance of TNF. A similar situation has been noted regarding the balance between IL-1 and IL-1Ra in Lyme arthritis (31).

Additional evidence for a potential role of inhibiting TNF in arthritis comes from animal studies. Using susceptible strains of animals, various models, such as collagen-induced arthritis, adjuvant arthritis, and streptococcal cell wall arthritis, bear resemblance to some features of human RA. Anti–TNF-α therapy has proven efficacious in each of these models (32,33). Such therapy has been shown to attenuate inflammation and partially to reduce joint destruction. Perhaps of greatest relevance to human RA, anti-TNF therapy in animal models is effective not only when treatment is begun at the onset of disease, but also later in the disease course, when the arthritis has become established. It should be noted that blockade of IL-1 or IL-6 is also effecitve in preventing or treating many of these animal models. Moreover, it has been claimed that TNF-α may play a more critical role in mediating inflammation, whereas IL-1 may be more important in the causation of cartilage damage (10). Additional evidence of the role of TNF in arthritis comes from studies of transgenic mice. Mice that overexpress human TNF-α spontaneously develop an erosive, inflammatory arthritis (34). The arthritis can be effectively abrogated by blocking TNF-α. It is of note that in this model the inflammation can also be attenuated by blocking IL-1. This highlights the potential role of TNF-α in the induction of the inflammatory cytokine cascade (35).

In summary, these data indicate that TNF-α should be an important therapeutic target in RA.

Inhibitors of TNF in Patients with RA

Agents/Trial Designs

Several studies have evaluated inhibitors of TNF in RA (Table 22-2) (36–51). Almost all of the studies published to date have utilized one of the following agents: 1) a chimeric monoclonal anti-TNF-α antibody [infliximab (Remicade), previously designated cA2], 2) a recombinant p75TNF-R(CD120b)-Fc fusion protein [etanercept (Enbrel)], or 3) a humanized monoclonal anti-TNF-α antibody (CDP571). Several additional TNF inhibitors are in the early stages of clinical development (see below).

Infliximab is a chimeric monoclonal antibody (mAb) that consists of the variable regions of a murine anti–TNF-α mAb engrafted onto a human IgG1κ molecule. The resulting construct is approximately two-thirds human. Infliximab has a high affinity for trimeric TNF-α (K_d ~100 pmol) and has been shown to inhibit both secreted and cell-associated TNF-α effectively in numerous in vitro systems (10). Etanercept was developed by linking DNA encoding the extracellular portion of the CD120b TNF receptor (p75TNFR) with DNA encoding the Fc portion of human IgG1 (C_H2, C_H3, and hinge domains) (45,46). The resulting dimeric construct is expressed in a mammalian cell line, and binds soluble trimers of TNF-α or LT-α with higher affinity than the naturally occurring monomers of soluble TNFR. CDP571 is a humanized anti–TNF-α mAb, consisting of the complementarity determining regions (CDRs) of a murine anti–TNF-α mAb engrafted onto a human IgG4κ molecule. The resulting construct is approximately 95% human. It binds trimeric TNF-α with high affinity comparable to that of infliximab.

There are important similarities among the designs of most of the trials assessing TNF inhibitors in RA (47–52). All trials enrolled patients with established and active RA. Activity was defined as some combination of numbers of swollen joints, numbers of tender joints, elevated concentrations of acute phase reactants, and prolonged early morning stiffness. In addition, most trials enrolled groups of RA patients that might be considered somewhat refractory by virtue of long disease duration and failure to respond to several disease-modifying antirheumatic drugs (DMARDs) (see Table 22-2). During the trials, patients were typically allowed to continue stable doses of NSAIDs and prednisone (≤7.5 mg/d or ≤10 mg/d in different trials). Efficacy was often assessed on the basis of composite criteria, such as the Paulus criteria or the American College of Rheumatology (ACR) criteria (53,54). Such criteria, which require improvements in multiple variables, are more stringent than analysis of improvement in one or only selected clinical variables. For example, in order to be classified as a responder according to ACR criteria,

patients must demonstrate 1) at least 20% improvement in swollen joint count, 2) at least 20% improvement in tender joint count, and 3) at least 20% improvement in three of five other measures [patient global assessment of disease activity, physician global assessment of disease activity, patient assessment of pain, an acute phase reactant (e.g., ESR), and a measure of disability (e.g., the Health Assessment Questionnaire, or HAQ)]. The Paulus criteria and EULAR criteria are similar. As would be expected, trials progressed in phases from early, open trials through the more rigorous double-blind, placebo-controlled, randomized clinical trials. Finally, after initial studies of TNF inhibitors as monotherapy, additional trials used these agents in combination with a traditional DMARD, methotrexate (MTX).

Clinical Efficacy

As summarized in Table 22-2, a number of trials have examined the clinical efficacy of anti–TNF-α agents.

Infliximab

The initial study of infliximab, an open-label trial, demonstrated significant efficacy for this anti–TNF-α mAb (36). All patients treated with this mAb, which is administered intravenously, demonstrated clinical responses based on the composite Paulus criteria. The extent of improvement was substantial, with individual parameters, such as swollen joint count, pain score, ESR, and CRP, all improving by more than 50% for the entire group. The duration of response after this single treatment course ranged from 8 to 25 weeks. Treatment was well tolerated. Based on these promising results, a more rigorous double-blind, placebo-controlled trial was performed (37).

In the subsequent double-blind trial of 4 weeks' duration, efficacy was significantly superior in the two groups receiving single doses of infliximab compared with the placebo group (31). Using the Paulus criteria to define response, only two (8%) of 24 placebo-treated patients exhibited responses, compared with 11 (44%) of 25 patients treated with 1 mg/kg infliximab and 19 (79%) of 24 patients treated with 10 mg/kg infliximab. In addition to dose dependency of response, the duration of clinical response was also greater for patients receiving the higher dose of infliximab. As in the open trial, the extent of improvement among responding patients in the double-blind trial was quite substantial. For the infliximab-treated groups, improvements of more than 50% were noted in many individual parameters. Indeed, analysis using a modification of the Paulus criteria to require improvements of more than 50% (instead of the typical 20%) in the individual parameters resulted in 58% responders in the high-dose group and 28% of the lower-dose group at 4 weeks after therapy. The effects observed in this study appeared to be of a more profound nature than those in other clinical studies of other agents in RA.

In an open-label follow-up study, eight patients from the double-blind trial received up to four additional treatments with infliximab (38). Although all treated patients exhibited responses, there was a trend toward shorter durations of response with

Table 22-2. Trials of TNF Inhibitors in RA

Reference	Trial Design	Agent	Agent/Dosage	Concurrent DMARD	Patients	Results/Comments
36	Open	Infliximab	Infliximab: 20 mg/kg divided over 2 weeks	None	n = 20; 85% RF+; mean disease duration, 10 yr; mean DMARDs failed, 4	Substantial improvements in all variables; at week 6, all patients were responders by the composite Paulus criteria
37	DBPCRCT*	Infliximab	Infliximab: single dose of 0, 1, or 10 mg/kg	None	n = 73; 81% RF+; mean disease duration, 8 yr; mean DMARDs failed, 3.2	Significant improvements in anti-TNF groups; extent and duration of response increase with higher dose [Paulus 20% improvements at week 4: 79% (10 mg), 44% (1 mg), 8% (placebo)]
38	Open, repeated treatment (of patients in Ref. 37)	Infliximab	Infliximab: 1 dose of 20 mg/kg; up to 3 further doses of 10 mg/kg	None	n = 8 (follow-up of patients from Ref. 37 who were treated when arthritis flared)	All treated patients responded; trend toward shorter duration of response with repeated treatments; 4 of 8 patients did not receive all doses due to adverse effects
39	DBPCRCT*	Infliximab	Infliximab: single dose of 0, 5, 10, or 20 mg/kg	Methotrexate (MTX) 10 mg/week	n = 28; 82% RF+; mean disease duration, 6.2 yr; mean DMARDs failed, 2.8	81% anti-TNF-treated patients, 14% placebo responded by ACR composite criteria; extent and duration of response are dose dependent
40	Open repeated treatment (of patients in Ref. 39)	Infliximab	Infliximab: 3 doses of 10 mg/kg at 8-week intervals	MTX 10 mg/week	n = 23 (follow-up of patients from Ref. 39)	Many patients responded to repeat treatments; some responses sustained through 40-week follow-up period
41	DBPCRCT*	Infliximab	Infliximab: 0, 1, 3, or 10 mg/kg at weeks 0, 2, 6, 10, and 14	MTX 7.5 mg/week or placebo	n = 101; mean disease duration, 10 yr; mean DMARDs failed, 2.4	Concurrent MTX enhanced and prolonged clinical response to cA2; ~80% of patients receiving MTX +3 or 10 mg/kg cA2 sustained response through the 26 weeks of the trial
42	DBPCRCT* study	Infliximab	Infliximab: 0, 3, or 10 mg/kg every 4 or 8 weeks	MTX ≥12.5 mg/week	n = 428; 81% RF positive; mean disease duration, 8.4 yr; 37% had prior joint surgery	ACR 20% response: placebo, 20%; infliximab, 52% (3 and 10 mg/kg given every 4 or 8 weeks had comparable efficacy). ACR 50%: placebo, 5%; infliximab, 28%. ACR 70%: placebo, 0%; infliximab, 12%

Table 22-2. *Continued*

Reference	Trial Design	Agent	Agent/Dosage	Concurrent DMARD	Patients	Results/Comments
43	DBPCRCT*	CDP571	Single dose of 0, 0.1, 1, or 10 mg/kg	None	$n = 36$; mean disease duration, 6 yr; mean DMARDs failed, 3.5	Dose-dependent improvements in several clinical parameters
44	Repeated treatment (of patients in Ref. 43)	CDP571	1.0 or 10 mg/kg (up to 4 doses)	None	$n = 14$ (follow-up of patients from Ref. 43)	Dose-dependent responses to repeat treatments
47	DBPCRCT*	Etanercept	0, 2, 4, 8, or 16 mg/m² twice weekly for 4 weeks (after loading dose)	None	$n = 22$ (6 assessed for safety only, 16 for safety and efficacy)	Joint and pain scores decreased in 45% of treated patients compared with 22% of placebo patients
48	DBPCRCT*	Etanercept	0, 0.25, 2, or 16 mg/m² twice weekly for 12 weeks	None	$n = 180$; 77% had RA > 5 yr	ACR 20%: placebo, 14%; 0.25 mg/m², 33%; 2 mg/m², 46%; 16 mg/m², 75%. ACR 50%: placebo, 7%; 0.25 mg/m², 9%; 2 mg/m², 22%; 16 mg/m², 57%
49	DBPCRCT*	Etanercept	0, 10, or 25 mg twice weekly for 6 months	None	$n = 234$	ACR 20%: placebo, 11%; 10 mg, 51%; 25 mg, 59%. ACR 50%: placebo, 5%; 10 mg, 24%; 25 mg, 40%
50	Open follow-up	Etanercept	25 mg twice weekly	None	$n = 105$	Persistent efficacy through 2 years of follow-up
51	DBPCRCT*	Etanercept	0 or 25 mg twice weekly for 6 months	MTX 15–25 mg/week	$n = 89$; 86% RF+; mean disease duration, 13 yr; mean DMARDs failed, 2.7	ACR 20%: 27% placebo, 71% etanercept. ACR 50%: 3% placebo, 39% etanercept. ACR 70%: 0% placebo, 15% etanercept

*DBPCRCT = double-blind, placebo-controlled, randomized clinical trial.

repeated treatments. In addition, adverse effects appeared to be more frequent; four of eight patients did not receive all planned doses.

While the utility of infliximab in RA had thus been clearly established, clinical benefit was transient when the anti–TNF-α mAb was used as monotherapy. Using results from several studies, the median durations of response after single doses of infliximab were calculated to be 3 weeks for 1 mg/kg, 6 weeks for 3 mg/kg, and 8 weeks for 10 mg/kg (10). In an attempt to sustain the clinical improvements observed in trials of infliximab as monotherapy, additional studies were carried out assessing the use of this anti–TNF-α mAb in RA patients who were using a DMARD concurrently. These studies enrolled patients who had active disease despite using MTX. The hypothesis was that the clinical response achieved with the anti–TNF-α mAb might be sustained by the concurrent use of MTX. Moreover, in clinical practice patients with active RA despite concurrent therapy might represent the type of patient most likely to receive anti–TNF-α therapy in the clinic.

A randomized, double-blind, placebo-controlled study enrolled patients with active RA despite receiving concurrent MTX (treatment with MTX for 3 months or more; stable dosage of 10 mg/week for 4 weeks or more) (39). Twenty-eight patients received single doses of 0, 5, 10, or 20 mg/kg anti–TNF-α mAb and were followed for 12 weeks. Patients continued treatment with MTX at 10 mg/week throughout the trial. As assessed by the ACR composite criteria, clinical responses were achieved much more frequently among patients receiving anti–TNF-α mAb (17 of 21; 81%) as compared with placebo (1 of 7; 14%). As in the other infliximab trials, the magnitude of the clinical responses were notable. The mean number of tender joints among all infliximab-treated patients decreased from 30.1 at baseline to 13.3 at week 12, and mean CRP decreased from 3.0 at baseline to 1.1 at week 12. The duration of clinical response appeared to be dose dependent; 2 of 6 (33%) of the responding patients treated with 5 mg/kg cA2 sustained clinical responses through 12 weeks of follow-up, compared with 7 of 11 (64%) of the responding patients who received 10 or 20 mg/kg. In addition, patients were eligible to receive three further treatments of 10 mg/kg infliximab at 8-week intervals. Approximately two-thirds of patients receiving infliximab in the open trial were able to maintain clinical responses throughout the 40 weeks of this study (40).

Another double-blind, placebo-controlled trial assessed the effects of three doses of anti–TNF-α mAb (1, 3, and 10 mg/kg) and placebo in 101 patients with active RA. In addition to treatment with infliximab at weeks 0, 2, 6, 10, and 14, patients also received concurrent therapy with either MTX (7.5 mg/week) or placebo (41). The primary outcome of the study was clinical response, defined according to the 20% Paulus criterion. Overall, approximately 60% of patients receiving infliximab achieved therapeutic responses. In the infliximab treatment groups, concurrent therapy with methotrexate seemed to prolong and accentuate the clinical response. This effect was most prominent at the lowest dose; median total time of response at 1 mg/kg infliximab was greater than 16 weeks with MTX but less than 4 weeks without MTX. In the groups receiving the higher doses of

anti–TNF-α mAb (3 mg/kg or 10 mg/kg) plus MTX, approximately 80% of the patients responded, and approximately 60% sustained clinical responses throughout the 26 weeks of the trial. While the effect of MTX was less pronounced at the higher doses, synergy was observed when the Paulus 50% criterion was analyzed. Median total times of response (Paulus 50%) at 10 mg/kg infliximab were greater than 13 weeks with MTX but less than 6 weeks without MTX. Interestingly, the addition of MTX appeared to increase the blood levels of infliximab, especially those resulting from the lower dose. The addition of MTX may have altered the immune response to the chimeric anti–TNF-α mAb (see below).

Preliminary data have recently become available from a trial of 428 patients who had active RA despite receiving concurrent therapy with MTX at dosages of at least 12.5 mg/week (42). Patients received 3 or 10 mg/kg of infliximab, or placebo, at intervals of 4 to 8 weeks. Interim efficacy was assessed at 30 weeks. While only 20% of the patients receiving placebo responded according to the ACR 20% criterion, 52% of the infliximab groups responded. Interestingly, for the infliximab-treated patients, efficacy was comparable at both doses and both dosing frequencies. When more rigorous response criteria were assessed, the infliximab groups again had significant improvements as compared with placebo. Thus, using the ACR 50% criterion, approximately 28% of infliximab patients responded, compared with 5% of placebo patients. In addition, none of the placebo patients achieved a 70% ACR response, whereas approximately 12% of the infliximab patients exhibited this level of response.

CDP571 mAb

A double-blind, placebo-controlled study assessed the efficacy of the humanized anti–TNF-α mAb CDP571 in patients with active RA (43). Single intravenous doses of 0.1, 1.0, and 10 mg/kg were assessed. Responses were dose dependent. Significant improvements in tender joint count and pain score were noted for patients receiving 10 mg/kg at weeks 1 and 2 after therapy; decreases in CRP were also marked for this group at these time points. Although small patient numbers and individual trials preclude specific comparison, it appears that cA2 may achieve a somewhat greater effect than CDP571 on certain clinical variables (e.g., swollen joint count) (10).

After the single treatment in the blinded trial, some patients received additional open-label treatments with CDP571 at 8-week intervals (43,44). Clinical responses were again dose dependent, with patients receiving 10 mg/kg demonstrating greater improvements in all variables than those receiving 1 mg/kg. Mild adverse effects were noted with repeat administration.

Etanercept

The initial trial of etanercept demonstrated substantial efficacy for this soluble TNF receptor fusion protein in a small, dose-escalating, double-blind study (47). Twenty-two patients were randomized to receive etanercept or placebo subcutaneously twice weekly for 4 weeks after a single intravenous loading dose.

Doses of etanercept used were 4 mg/m^2 (load)/2 mg/m^2 (maintenance), 8 mg/m^2 (load)/4 mg/m^2 (maintenance), 16 mg/m^2 (load)/8 mg/m^2 (maintenance), and 32 mg/m^2 (load)/16 mg/m^2 (maintenance). Of the 16 patients analyzed for efficacy (six patients were analyzed for safety only), there was a 45% mean improvement in joint and pain scores among patients receiving etanercept compared with a 22% mean improvement among patients receiving placebo. The main adverse effect in the etanercept groups was injection-site reaction, which did not require study discontinuation. Based on these promising results, a more rigorous double-blind, placebo-controlled trial was performed (48).

In the subsequent trial, 180 patients with refractory RA were randomized to receive one of three doses of etanercept (0.25 mg/m^2, 2 mg/m^2, or 16 mg/m^2) or placebo, administered subcutaneously on a twice-weekly schedule for 3 months. Substantial, dose-dependent efficacy was noted (48). Utilizing the ACR 20% measure of improvement, response rates at 3 months were: placebo, 14%; 0.25 mg/m^2, 33%; 2 mg/m^2, 46%; and 16 mg/m^2, 75%. Notably using the more stringent ACR 50% measure of improvement, response rates at 3 months were: placebo, 7%; 0.25 mg/m^2, 9%; 2 mg/m^2, 22%; and 16 mg/m^2, 57%. Treatment was generally well tolerated, with injection site reactions being the most common adverse event. In all groups, efficacy achieved was transient, and measures of disease activity began to rise soon after treatment was discontinued.

In a subsequent study using a similar design, 234 patients with active RA were randomized to receive placebo or one of two doses of etanercept (10 mg or 25 mg) subcutaneously twice weekly for 6 months. As in the earlier study, significant and dose-dependent efficacy was noted (49). At 6 months, response rates using the ACR 20% measure were: placebo, 11%; 10 mg, 51%; and 25 mg, 59%. Using the ACR 50% response criterion, response rates were: placebo, 5%; 10 mg, 24%; and 25 mg, 40%. Because the efficacy dissipated after discontinuation of etanercept, a longer, open trial was conducted in order to assess the feasibility of long-term treatment. In this study, 105 patients who had participated in earlier trials were eligible to receive long-term therapy with etanercept at a twice-weekly dose of 25 mg subcutaneously (50). Notably, drop-out rates were minimal, and efficacy was maintained throughout 2 years of treatment.

The efficacy of etanercept has also been evaluated in patients with active RA despite concurrent MTX at dosages of 15–25 mg/week. In a 24-week study, 89 patients were randomized (1:2) to receive placebo or etanercept (25 mg) twice weekly (51). At 24 weeks, response rates using the ACR 20% measure were 27% in the patients receiving MTX plus placebo, compared with 71% in patients receiving MTX plus etanercept. Using the ACR 50% response criterion, response rates were 3% in the placebo group and 39% in the etanercept group. The most common adverse effect was a mild injection-site reaction, which occurred in 42% of patients receiving etanercept, compared with 7% of those receiving placebo; notably, none of these reactions required exit from the study protocol.

Etanercept also been evaluated and has shown promising results in the treatment of juvenile chronic arthritis (52).

Use of TNF Inhibitors in Diseases Other than RA

In addition to RA, anti-TNF mAbs have been utilized in a variety of other diseases, including Crohn's disease, ulcerative colitis, sepsis, and HIV infection. The greatest experience has been in Crohn's disease, an immunologically driven inflammatory bowel disease with many pathologic similarities to RA. Both infliximab and CDP571 have been shown to be efficacious in double-blind, placebo-controlled trials in this condition (55,56).

Adverse Effects

Important adverse effects that might potentially be observed with any TNF inhibitor include risk of infection, risk of malignancy, and the development of autoimmune manifestations. In addition, there may be untoward reactions that are specific to the particular agent being used, such as immunogenicity and local reactions.

Because it mediates myriad activities relevant to normal inflammation and immunity (see Table 22-1), TNF serves a central role in host defense. Therefore, increased susceptibility to specific infections (e.g., *Listeria monocytogenes*, mycobacteria, histoplasma, etc.) is a potential concern with any agent that inhibits TNF. This is perhaps illustrated most clearly by animal experiments. For example, "knockout" animals that have been genetically engineered to be deficient in the p55 or p75 TNF-receptor are highly susceptible to infection with *Listeria monocytogenes* and mycobacteria (11,57,58). Also, inhibition of TNF abrogates the protective effect of mast cell reconstitution in mast cell deficient mice challenged in peritonitis and pneumonitis models (59,60).

Complicating the analysis of any increased risk of infection that could be caused by TNF inhibitors in diseases such as RA and Crohn's disease is a high baseline prevalence of infection in these patients. In RA, infections occur more frequently and are important contributors to the accelerated morbidity of this condition (3,61). How much of this susceptibility relates to the disease itself and how much is caused instead by the effects of immunomodulatory therapies (e.g., steroids and cytotoxic drugs) is difficult to assess. Notably, the subset of RA patients with the greatest susceptibility to infection (those with severe, active disease) has also been the type of patient most commonly enrolled in trials of TNF inhibitors.

In RA trials, several infections have occurred among patients receiving TNF inhibitors (infliximab, etanercept, and CDP571), especially upper and lower respiratory infections. However, in studies with placebo arms, similar infections have also been noted among patients treated with placebo, illustrating RA patients' predilection to infection. In summary, the data presently available do not indicate that treatment with anti–TNF-α mAb results in substantially increased susceptibility to infection in patients with RA. However, because of the relatively small numbers of patients treated to date, as well as the relatively short mean duration of therapy, this remains an area of concern and deserves further study.

Immunosurveillance is also critical to the host defense against malignancy. Therefore, there is also a theoretical risk of an increase in malignancy with immunomodulatory therapies such as TNF inhibitors. As is the case for infections, patients with RA also appear to have an increased susceptibility to certain malignancies, particularly lymphoproliferative cancers (61–63). This risk must be kept in mind when evaluating results and implying causality in therapeutic trials. In trials of the various TNF inhibitors in RA patients, several cases of hematologic and other malignancies have been reported. At present, it does not appear that the incidence of cancers observed significantly exceeds the rate that would be expected in this population, although the relatively short patient exposure to these agents does not permit a definitive conclusion. This is another area that will require further study in the future.

An interesting observation in the early trials of TNF inhibitors was that approximately 10% of treated patients developed antibodies to double-stranded DNA (anti-DNA) (36–38; etanercept package insert). As for predisposition to infection and malignancy, the development of autoantibodies seems to be a common adverse effect of all agents capable of inhibiting TNF. The significance of the development of autoantibodies is uncertain, because there has been a dearth of cases involving development of symptoms suggestive of SLE (10). The mechanisms underlying the development of these autoantibodies also have not been defined. Interestingly, in some animal models of lupus, TNF-α is protective of disease progression whereas inhibition of TNF-α exacerbates it (64,65). In addition, it has been hypothesized that TNF, perhaps driven by malarial or other parasitic infection, is protective against systemic lupus erythematosus (SLE) in West African populations (66). Because molecules in the TNF/TNF-receptor family serve a critical role in mediating normal apoptosis, it is possible that inhibition of TNF modulates this in some manner, facilitating the development of autoantibodies. The significance of the development of anti-DNA antibodies with the use of TNF inhibitors requires further study.

Considerations of antigenicity are germane to any biologic therapy. The development of antibodies to a therapeutic agent could diminish its serum half-life and thereby decrease its efficacy. In addition, these antibodies could produce adverse effects by means of immune complex formation or the development of immediate hypersensitivity. Moreover, determination and quantification of antibodies to the biologic agents used in clinical studies is a complex issue. By definition, these agents are novel, and specific assays to test for antibodies to the agents have not been widely standardized. Other factors, such as the presence of rheumatoid factor, can potentially interfere with the assays. These factors make direct comparisons of the relative antigenicities of different biologic agents difficult and potentially tenuous.

Various factors affect the immunogenicity of foreign antigens. The degree of antigenic variation (or "foreignness") is an important factor. Thus, murine mAbs are more immunogenic than chimeric mAbs, which are more immunogenic than humanized mAbs. However, even completely human products (e.g., insulin, factor VIII) can be immunogenic and elicit antibody responses in certain circumstances. Other factors affecting immunogenicity include 1) dose (both high and low doses of an antigen are capable of inducing tolerance), 2) route of administration (cutaneous administration is more likely to induce antibody responses than intravenous or oral administration), 3) frequency of treatment, and 4) immunomodulatory effects of the agent or of concurrent treatment. The impact of concurrent therapy may be particularly relevant to RA. For example, concurrent use of immunosuppressive medications is known to suppress the immunogenicities of foreign antigens. In addition, some agents modulate the immune system such that they induce tolerance to themselves. These factors may be relevant in the treatment of RA.

In studies performed to date, single doses of the chimeric anti-TNF-α antibody infliximab have been associated with the formation of human antichimeric antibodies (HACAs) in 0–5% (36,56) up to 25% (10) of patients. The frequency of HACAs may vary with dose, with higher doses inducing lesser responses (41). In some studies, the persistence of the treating antibody at the time of HACA measurement may have affected the assays. With repeated administration, the prevalence of HACAs may increase to 50% or more (10,38). Although the data available to date are not extensive, the development of antibodies may have clinical relevance; in one small study, the duration of clinical response decreased with repeated administration (38). Importantly, concurrent therapy may affect immunogenicity. In one study, concurrent therapy with MTX decreased the prevalence of HACAs (41). Thus, among patients receiving cA2 as monotherapy, HACAs were seen in 53% (1 mg/kg cA2 dose), 21% (3 mg/kg), and 7% (10 mg/kg); in patients taking concurrent MTX, the corresponding frequencies of HACAs were 17%, 7%, and 0%. These data show that the development of antibodies to the treating agent varied with dose, and was affected by MTX therapy. This suggests that adjusting the treatment paradigm in terms of dosages and concurrent therapies may be a potentially useful method of decreasing immunogenicity of anti-TNF-α mAb.

For patients treated with etanercept, the most common unique adverse effect has been the development of local reactions at the site of injection. In general, these reactions have been mild and have resolved spontaneously, and only rarely have required withdrawal from the studies. Interestingly, reactions at sites of previous injections have been noted to develop after injections at other sites.

Mechanisms of Action of TNF Inhibitors

While TNF inhibitors have clearly been shown to be efficacious, there is still some speculation as to the precise mechanisms by which they exert their beneficial clinical effects. Perhaps the most straightforward mechanism of action relates to binding and inhibition of inflammatory mediators. In support of this mechanism, substantial decreases in IL-6 (36,67,68) and IL-1 (67) have been demonstrated after anti-TNF-α mAb therapy. Decreases in IL-6 provide an explanation of the pronounced improvements in acute phase reactants seen during treatment. Because IL-1 also produces numerous inflammatory effects, decreases in IL-1 would be associated with improvements in many of the signs and symptoms of inflammation. Other mediators that are triggered in vivo by TNF-α have also decreased after therapy, including IL-1Ra, sCD14, IL-8, MCP-1, nitric oxide (NO), collagenase, and stromolysin (10,67–69). The effects on matrix metalloproteinases (collagenase and stromolysin) may be important in attenuating joint damage in RA. In summary, these data highlight the central role of TNF-α in triggering the inflammatory cytokine cascade in RA and confirm its utility as a therapeutic target. Inhibition of various inflammatory mediators may also provide some explanation for the improvements noted in patients treated with TNF inhibitors.

As noted, TNF-α exerts diverse effects on the vasculature, such as activation of the endothelium and up-regulation of adhesion molecule expression. This may provide an explanation for one of the most important mechanisms of action of TNF inhibitors. In one of the placebo-controlled trials of cA2, soluble adhesion molecules were measured in the serum (70). Because they are expressed and then shed from the cell surface on activation, soluble forms of adhesion molecules provide an indirect measure of endothelial activation. Treatment with anti–TNF-α mAb resulted in dose-dependent decreases in soluble forms of ICAM-1 and E-selectin (70). In addition, increases in the numbers of circulating lymphocytes and a decrease in circulating neutrophils were noted. These changes in circulating lymphocytes are reminiscent of those achieved in another study of RA patients in which the adhesion molecule ICAM-1 was directly targeted (71). Interestingly, in the anti–TNF-α study, changes in soluble E-selectin, soluble ICAM-1, and circulating lymphocytes correlated with clinical outcome, implying mechanistic relevance. Confirmation of these effects of anti–TNF-α mAb on endothelial activation and inflammatory cell recirculation has come from additional studies, in that the decrease in serum soluble ICAM-1 has been reproduced by another group (67). More directly, histopathologic analysis of a small number of synovial biopsy specimens has shown reduction in the expression of E-selectin and VCAM-1 consequent to anti–TNF-α therapy (72). It is notable that this decrease in adhesion molecule expression was accompanied by a reduction in the infiltration of T lymphocytes into the synovium (72). Labeling studies have shown a decreased accumulation of neutrophils into joints with anti–TNF-α therapy (69). In summary, these data indicate that a crucial mechanism of action of anti–TNF-α mAb in RA patients may be the inhibition of TNF-α–dependent endothelial cell activation. This, in turn, could alter cellular recirculation and inhibit the accrual of cells into the rheumatoid synovium.

There are other potential mechanisms of TNF inhibitors. TNF/TNF-R interactions can regulate apoptosis, including that mediated by Fas/Fas-ligand interactions. Therefore, inhibition of TNF may modulate apoptosis in the rheumatoid synovium and, for example, down-regulate synovial hyperplasia (73). In diseases that are characterized by a predominant TH-1 phenotype, such as RA and Crohn's disease, it is also possible that TNF inhibitors may alter the milieu within the inflammatory site, possibly by means of an increase in IL-10 (56,74). Additional mechanisms may still be delineated as experience with TNF inhibitors as therapeutic agents expands.

Comparisons of TNF Inhibitors

There are several considerations that are relevant to the comparison of novel TNF inhibitors (Table 22-3). Important characteristics that vary among the agents include 1) avidity for ligand, 2) half-life, and 3) specificity (e.g., does the agent bind TNF-α, LT-α, or both, and does it bind cell-bound forms of the cytokines, soluble forms, or both?). The optimal characteristics for these variables remain a matter of speculation. For example, an agent with higher avidity may achieve better results but may also increase the susceptibility to infection. Likewise, an agent that has a very long half-life could be more convenient to administer, but such prolonged inhibition of TNF may have untoward effects. Agents that block both TNF-α and LT-α may exert different effects and be associated with different adverse effects than agents specific for TNF-α. Similarly, agents that interact with both soluble and cell-bound forms of the cytokines may exert immunomodulatory effects not seen with agents that bind only soluble forms (75). The optimal characteristics will need to be defined by long-term comparison studies. Another area of comparison between TNF inhibitors relates to complications. Some complications (e.g., risk of infection, malignancy, and autoimmune disease) are expected to be common to all TNF inhibitors, although factors such as avidity and half-life may affect the incidence or severity. Other complications may depend on the particular agent and may be best delineated by comparison studies. Finally, because biologic agents are expected to be more expensive than traditional drugs, cost analyses will be germane to their utility. However, TNF inhibitors such as anti–TNF-α mAb therapy have proven to have impressive efficacy for some treated patients. Therefore, optimal cost analyses in RA require balancing of the costs of the agents themselves against costs that can be alleviated (e.g., lost wages) by controlling this chronic, pernicious disease (76).

Table 22-3. Considerations Relevant to the Comparison of TNF Inhibitors

Characteristics

Specificity
Avidity
Half-life
Frequency and route of administration

Complications

Risk of infection/malignancy/autoimmune disease
Agent-specific adverse effects
   Immunogenicity
      Development of adverse effects
      Loss of efficacy
   Development of local reactions

Cost

Cost efficacy/cost utility

Future Directions

A variety of other approaches to inhibition of TNF are under development, including inhibitors of TNF-α converting enzyme (which cleaves TNF-α from the cell surface), inhibitors of phosphodiesterase IV (which regulates TNF-α production), and gene transfer to overexpress the TNF-receptor (77–79) (Fig. 22-1). Some currently available agents may also mediate their effects at least in part by inhibition of TNF. This includes thalidomide (which enhances the degradation of TNF-α mRNA) and MTX (through induction of adenosine, which down-regulates TNF-α synthesis) (80,81).

There are many avenues that should allow refinement and optimization in the use of anti–TNF-α mAbs in RA. One potentially relevant area will be the definition of subsets of patients for whom this type of therapy is most efficacious. In animal studies, it has been shown that different therapies may be more or less effective at different stages of arthritis (32). In RA, it has also been suggested that patients may be heterogeneous in their clinical presentations as well as their responses to certain therapeutics (1,3). Although anti–TNF-α mAb has been effective for the majority of treated patients, it is possible that certain patients may be particularly responsive to this type of therapy and resistant to adverse effects. The identification of such a subset will require additional research. Interestingly, genetic polymorphisms in TNF-α have been noted and have been suggested to correlate with outcome in RA (82). Research into this and other factors may allow the definition of subsets of RA for whom anti-TNF therapy would be particularly useful.

Another area in which refinement in the use of TNF inhibitors can be expected is the treatment paradigms. Early studies with these agents used them as monotherapy. More recent studies have begun to assess the effect of concurrent use of MTX as an adjunct to TNF inhibitors. This combination, which bears a resemblance to the "induction-remission" approach to cancer chemotherapy, has proven effective. In addition to prolonging and possibly potentiating the clinical response, such combination therapy also appears to decrease the immune response to the mAb. Further study of this approach to therapy is anticipated. Definition of effective combinations of a TNF inhibitor and other

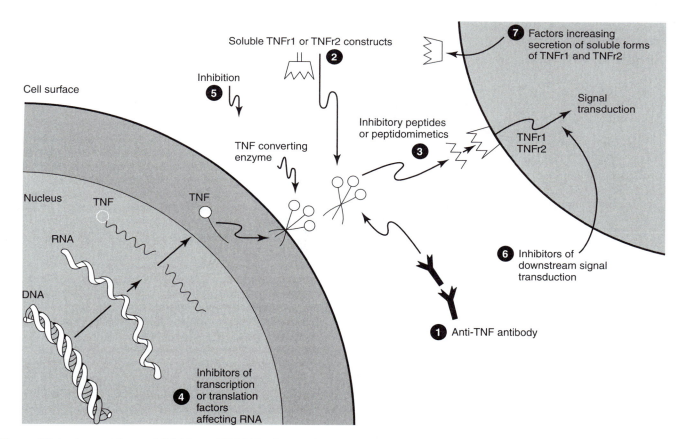

Figure 22-1. Approaches to inhibition of TNF. The interaction of TNF with its specific counter-receptors (TNF-R) can be blocked by various approaches, including: (1) antibodies specific for TNF, (2) soluble forms of the TNF-R, (3) small molecule inhibitors of TNF/TNF-R binding, (4) inhibitors of TNF synthesis, (5) inhibitors of TNF-α converting enzyme, (6) signal transduction inhibitors, and (7) factors increasing the secretion of TNF-R.

antirheumatic agents may allow lower doses of each therapy to be administered, thereby obviating toxicity. Besides MTX and other currently available antirheumatic drugs, combinations of TNF inhibitors with other immunomodulatory therapies might also prove valuable. In animal models, the combination of anti-TNF and anti-CD4 therapies have been synergistic in the therapy of arthritis (83). Preliminary studies in humans have also suggested success of this combined approach (84). Such a combined approach also has the potential to ameliorate the toxicities of both types of agents by decreasing the doses required, and also to decrease the immunogenicities of the agents. It may also be feasible to use combinations of agents that inhibit TNF-α.

Finally, another area for future research relates to minimization of adverse effects. Identifying optimal patient subsets and dosage regimens might help diminish such problems. As regards adverse effects related to antibodies to the agent, in addition to finding dosage paradigms that might diminish immunogenicity and promote tolerance, there are various methods by which biologic agents can be rendered less immunogenic. For example, polyethylene glycol treatment of mAb has the potential to engender specific immunologic tolerance. Other developments that are awaited include the development of monoclonal antibodies that are completely human.

Summary and Conclusions

Treatment of RA patients with TNF inhibitors has proven to be extremely effective. Rigorous, albeit relatively small, studies have proven the utility and acceptability of these agents. Additional studies have begun to define the optimal treatment paradigms for the use of TNF inhibitors, including combination therapy. In the near future, these powerful agents may be introduced into the therapeutic armamentarium for RA. This should afford tangible and substantial clinical benefit to some of the patients suffering from this aggressive disease. Further developments in this area can be expected to allow the clinician to refine and optimize therapy with TNF inhibitors.

References

1. Harris E. Rheumatoid arthritis; pathophysiology and implications for therapy. N Engl J Med 1990;322:1277–1289.
2. Sewell K, Trentham D. Pathogenesis of rheumatoid arthritis. Lancet 1993;341:283–286.
3. Kavanaugh A, Lipsky P. Rheumatoid arthritis. In: Rich R, ed. Clinical immunology; principles and practice. New York: Mosby, 1996:1093–1116.
4. Firestein GS, Zvaifler NJ. How important are T cells in chronic rheumatoid synovitis? Arthritis Rheum 1990;33:768–773.
5. Lipksy P, Davis L, Cush T, Oppenheimer-Marks N. The role of cytokines in the pathogenesis of rheumatoid arthritis. Springer Semin Immunopathol 1989;11:123–162.
6. Koch A, Kunkel S, Strieter R. Cytokines in rheumatoid arthritis. J Invest Med 1995;43:28–38.
7. Feldmann M, Brennan FM, Maini RN. Role of cytokines in rheumatoid arthritis. Annu Rev Immunol 1996;14:397–440.
8. Firestein G, Zvaifler N. Anticytokine therapy in rheumatoid arthritis. N Engl J Med 1997;337:195–197.
9. Arend WP, Dayer J-M. Inhibition of the production and effects of interleukin-1 and tumor necrosis factor α in rheumatoid arthritis. Arthritis Rheum 1995;38:151–160.
10. Feldmann M, Elliot M, Woody J, Maini R. Anti-tumor necrosis factor-α therapy of rheumatoid arthritis. Advances Immunol 1997;64:283–350.
11. Pennica D, Nedwin J, Hayflick P, et al. Human tumor necrosis factor: precursor structure, expression, and homology to lymphotoxin. Nature 1984;312:724–729.
12. Bazzoni F, Beutler B. The tumor necrosis factor ligand and receptor families. N Engl J Med 1996;334:1717–1725.
13. Slewik M, De Luca L, Fiers W, Pober J. Tumor necrosis factor activates human endothelial cells through the p55 tumor necrosis factor receptor but the p75 receptor contributes at low tumor necrosis factor concentration. Am J Pathol 1993;143:1724–1730.
14. Sacca R, Cuff C, Lesslauer W, Ruddle N. Differential activities of secreted lymphotoxin-α3 and membrane lymphotoxin-α1β2 in lymphotoxin-induced inflammation: critical role of TNF receptor 1 signaling. J Immunol 1998; 160:485–491.
15. Douni E, Kollias G. A critical role of the p75 tumor necrosis factor (p75TNF-R) in organ inflammation independent of TNF, lymphotoxin, or the p55TNF-R. J Exp Med 1998; 188:1343–1352.
16. Tkachuk M, Bolliger S, Ryffek B, et al. Crucial role of TNFR1 expression on nonhematopoietic cells for B cell localization within the splenic white pulp. J Exp Med 1998;187:469–477.
17. Maiti A, Maki G, Johnson P. TNF-α induction of CD44 mediated leukocyte adhesion by sulfation. Science 1998;282:941–943.
18. Fujisawa K, Aono H, Hasunuma T, et al. Activation of transcription factor NF-κB in human synovial cells in response to tumor necrosis factor α. Arthritis Rheum 1996;39:197–203.
19. Kavanaugh A. Antiadhesion therapy in rheumatoid arthritis: a review of recent progress. BioDrugs 1997;7:119–133.
20. Cunha FQ, Poole S, Lorenzetti BB, Ferreira SH. The pivotal role of tumor necrosis factor alpha in the development of inflammatory hyperalgesia. Br J Pharmacol 1992;107:660–669.
21. Dinarello C, Cannon J, Wolff S, et al. Tumor necrosis factor is an endogenous pyrogen and induces production of interleukin 1. J Exp Med 1986;163:1433–1450.
22. Brennan F, Chantry D, Turner M, et al. Inhibitory effects of TNF-α antibodies on synovial cell interleukin-1 production in rheumatoid arthritis. Lancet 1989;ii:244–247.
23. Pennisi E. Teetering on the brink of danger. Science 1996; 271:1665–1667.
24. Benoist C, Mathis D. The pathogen connection. Nature 1998; 394:227–228.
25. Cope A, Liblau R, Yang X-D, et al. Chronic tumor necrosis factor alters T cell responses by attenuating T cell receptor signaling. J Exp Med 1997;185:1573–1584.
26. van Deventer SJH. Tumour necrosis factor and Crohn's disease. Gut 1997;40:443–448.
27. Di Giovine F, Nuki G, Duff G. Tumor necrosis factor in synovial exudates. Ann Rheum Dis 1988;47:768–772.
28. Saxne T, Palladino M, Heinegard D, et al. Detection of tumor necrosis factor α but not tumor necrosis factor β in rheuma-

toid arthritis synovial fluid and serum. Arthritis Rheum 1988;31:1041–1045.

29. Cope A, Aderka D, Doherty M, et al. Increased levels of soluble tumor necrosis factor receptors in the sera and synovial fluid of patients with rheumatic diseases. Arthritis Rheum 1992;35:1160–1169.

30. Aderka D, Engelmann H, Maor Y, et al. Stabilization of the bioactivity of tumor necrosis factor by its soluble receptors. J Exp Med 1992;175:323–329.

31. Miller L, Lynch E, Isa S, et al. Balance of synovial fluid IL-1β and IL-1 receptor antagonist and recovery from Lyme arthritis. Lancet 1993;341:146–148.

32. Joosten L, Helsen M, van de Loo F, van den Berg W. Anticytokine treatment of established type II collagen-induced arthritis in DBA/1 mice; a comparative study using anti-TNFα, anti-IL-1α/β, and IL-1Ra. Arthritis Rheum 1996;39: 797–809.

33. Williams R, Feldmann M, Maini R. Anti-tumor necrosis factor ameliorates joint disease in murine collagen-induced arthritis. Proc Natl Acad Sci USA 1992;89:9784–9788.

34. Keffer J, Probert L, Cazlaris H, et al. Transgenic mice expressing human tumor necrosis factor: a predictive genetic model of arthritis. EMBO 1991;10:4025–4031.

35. Probert L, Plows D, Kontogeorgos G, Kollias G. The type 1 interleukin-1 receptor acts in series with tumor necrosis factor (TNF) to induce arthritis in TNF-transgenic mice. Eur J Immunol 1995;25:1794–1797.

36. Elliott M, Maini R, Feldmann M, et al. Treatment of rheumatoid arthritis with chimeric monoclonal antibodies to tumor necrosis factor α. Arthritis Rheum 1993;36:1681–1690.

37. Elliott M, Maini R, Feldmann M, et al. Randomized double-blind comparison of chimeric monoclonal antibody to tumor necrosis factor α (cA2) versus placebo in rheumatoid arthritis. Lancet 1994;344:1105–1110.

38. Elliott M, Maini R, Feldmann M, et al. Repeated therapy with monoclonal antibody to tumor necrosis factor α (cA2) in patients with rheumatoid arthritis. Lancet 1994;344:1125–1127.

39. Kavanaugh A, Cush J, St Clair E, et al. Anti-TNF-α monoclonal antibody treatment of rheumatoid arthritis patients with active disease on methotrexate; results of a double-blind, placebo controlled multicenter trial. Arthritis Rheum 1996;39(suppl):S123.

40. Kavanaugh A, Cush J, St Clair E, et al. Anti-TNF-α monoclonal antibody treatment of rheumatoid arthritis patients with active disease on methotrexate; results of open label, repeated dose administration following a single dose, double-blind, placebo controlled trial. Arthritis Rheum 1996; 39(suppl):S244.

41. Maini R, Breedveld F, Kalden J, et al. Therapeutic efficacy of multiple intravenous infusions of anti-tumor necrosis factor α monoclonal antibody combined with low-dose weekly methotrexate in rheumatoid arthritis. Arthritis Rheum 1998; 41:1552–1563.

42. Lipsky P, St Clair W, Kavanaugh A, et al. Long-term control of signs and symptoms of rheumatoid arthritis with chimeric monoclonal anti-TNF-α antibody (infliximab) in patients with active disease on methotrexate. Arthritis Rheum 1998; 41:S364.

43. Rankin ECC, Choy EHS, Kassimos D, et al. The therapeutic effects of an engineered human anti-tumour necrosis factor antibody (CDP571) in rheumatoid arthritis. Br J Rheumatol 1995;34:334–342.

44. Rankin E, Choy E, Sopwith M, et al. Repeated doses of 10 mg/kg of an engineered human anti-TNF-α antibody CDP571 in RA patients are safe and effective. Arthritis Rheum 1995;38(suppl):S185.

45. Peppel K, Crawford D, Beutler B. A tumor necrosis factor (TNF) receptor-IgG heavy chain chimeric protein as a bivalent antagonist of TNF activity. J Exp Med 1991;174:1483–1489.

46. Mohler KM, Torrance SD, Smith CA, et al. Soluble tumor necrosis factor (TNF) receptors are effective therapeutic agents in lethal endotoxemia and function simultaneously as both TNF carriers and TNF antagonists. J Immunol 1993; 151:1548–1561.

47. Moreland LW, Margolies G, Heck LW, et al. Recombinant soluble tumor necrosis factor receptor (p80) fusion protein: toxicity and dose finding trial in refractory rheumatoid arthritis. J Rheumatol 1996;23:1849–1855.

48. Moreland LW, Baumgartner SW, Schiff MH, et al. Treatment of rheumatoid arthritis with a recombinant human tumor necrosis factor receptor (p75)-Fc fusion protein. N Engl J Med 1997;337:141–147.

49. Weinblatt M, Moreland L, Schiff M, et al. Longterm and phase III treatment of DMARD failing rheumatoid arthritis patients with TNF receptor p75 Fc fusion protein (TNFR:Fc;Enbrel). Arthritis Rheum 1997;40:S126.

50. Moreland L, Baumgartner E, Tindall E, et al. Longterm safety and efficacy of TNF receptor (p75) Fc fusion protein (TNFR:Fc;Enbrel) in DMARD refractory rheumatoid arthritis. Arthritis Rheum 1998;41:S364.

51. Weinblatt ME, Kremer JM, Bankhurst AD, et al. A trial of etanercept, a recombinant tumor necrosis factor receptor:Fc fusion protein, in patients with rheumatoid arthritis receiving methotrexate. N Engl J Med 1999;340:253–259.

52. Lovell D, Giannini E, Whitmore J, et al. Safety and efficacy of tumor necrosis factor receptor p75 Fc fusion protein (TNFR:Fc;Enbrel) in polyarticular course juvenile rheumatoid arthritis. Arthritis Rheum 1998;41:S130.

53. Paulus H, Egger M, Ward J, Williams H. Analysis of improvement in individual rheumatoid arthritis patients treated with disease-modifying antirheumatic drugs, based on the findings in patients treated with placebo. Arthritis Rheum 1990;33: 477–484.

54. Felson D, Anderson J, Boers M, et al. The American College of Rheumatology preliminary core set of disease activity measures for rheumatoid arthritis clinical studies. Arthritis Rheum 1995;38:727–735.

55. Stack W, Mann S, Roy A, et al. Randomized controlled trial of CDP571 antibody to tumour necrosis factor-α in Crohn's disease. Lancet 1997;349:521–524.

56. Targan S, Hanauer S, Sander J, et al. A short-term study of chimeric monoclonal antibody to cA2 to tumor necrosis factor α for Crohn's disease. N Engl J Med 1997;337:109–135.

57. Rothe J, Lesslauer W, Lötscher H, et al. Mice lacking the tumour necrosis factor receptor 1 are resistant to TNF-mediated toxicity but highly susceptible to infection by *Listeria monocytogenes*. Nature 1993;364:798–802.

58. Pfeffer K, Matsuyama T, Kündig T, et al. Mice deficient for the 55 kd tumor necrosis factor receptor are resistant to

endotoxic shock, yet succumb to L. monocytogenes infection. Cell 1994;78:681–692.

59. Echtenacher B, Männel D, Hültner L. Critical protective role of mast cells in a model of acute septic peritonitis. Nature 1996;381:75–77.

60. Malaviya R, Ikeda T, Ross E, Abraham S. Mast cell modulation of neutrophil influx and bacterial clearance at sites of infection through TNF-α. Nature 1996;381:77–80.

61. Wolfe F, Mitchell D, Sibley J, et al. The mortality of rheumatoid arthritis. Arthritis Rheum 1994;37:481–494.

62. Cibere J, Sibley J, Haga M. Rheumatoid arthritis and the risk of malignancy. Arthritis Rheum 1997;40:1580–1586.

63. Gridley G, McLaughlin J, Ekbom A, et al. Incidence of cancer among patients with rheumatoid arthritis. J Natl Cancer Inst 1993;85:307–311.

64. Jacob C. Tumor necrosis factor α in autoimmunity: pretty girl or old witch? Immunol Today 1992;13:122–125.

65. Jacob C, McDevitt H. Tumour necrosis factor-α in murine autoimmune "lupus" nephritis. Nature 1988;331:356–358.

66. Adebajo A. Does tumor necrosis factor protect against lupus in West Africans? Arthritis Rheum 1992;35:839.

67. Lorenz H-M, Antoni C, Valerius T, et al. In vivo blockade of TNF-α by intravenous infusion of a chimeric monoclonal TNF-α antibody in patients with rheumatoid arthritis: short term cellular and molecular effects. J Immunol 1996;156: 1646–1653.

68. Choy E, Kassimos D, Kingsley G, et al. The effect of an engineered human anti-tumour necrosis factor antibody on interleukin-6 and bone markers in rheumatoid arthritis patients. Arthritis Rheum 1995;38(suppl):S185.

69. Taylor P, Chapman P, Elliot M, et al. Reduced granulocyte traffic and chemotactic gradients in rheumatoid joints following anti-TNFα therapy. Arthritis Rheum 1997;40(suppl): S80.

70. Paleolog E, Hunt M, Elliott M, et al. Deactivation of vascular endothelium by monoclonal anti-tumor necrosis factor α antibody in rheumatoid arthritis. Arthritis Rheum 1996;39: 1082–1091.

71. Kavanaugh A, Davis L, Nichols L, et al. Treatment of refractory rheumatoid arthritis with a monoclonal antibody to intercellular adhesion molecule-1. Arthritis Rheum 1994;37: 992–999.

72. Tak PP, Taylor PC, Breedveld FC, et al. Decrease in cellularity and expression of adhesion molecules by anti-tumor necrosis factor α monoclonal antibody treatment in patients with rheumatoid arthritis. Arthritis Rheum 1996;39:1077–1081.

73. Ohshima S, Saeki Y, Mima T, et al. Tumor necrosis factor α interferes with FAS mediated apoptotic cell death on RA synovial cells: possible mechanism for synovial hyperplasia and clinical benefit of anti-TNFα therapy in rheumatoid arthritis. Arthritis Rheum 1997;40(suppl):S79.

74. Ohshima S, Saeki Y, Mima T, et al. Possible mechanism for the long-term efficacy of anti-TNFα antibody (cA2) therapy in RA. Arthritis Rheum 1996;39(suppl):S242.

75. Scallon B, Moore M, Trinh H, et al. Chimeric anti-TNF-alpha monoclonal antibody cA2 binds recombinant transmembrane TNF-alpha and activates immune effector functions. Cytokine 1995;7:251–259.

76. Kavanaugh A, Heudebert G, Cush J, Jain R. Cost evaluation of novel therapeutics in rheumatoid arthritis (CENTRA): a decision analysis model. Seminar Arthritis Rheum 1996; 25:297–307.

77. Black R, Rauch C, Kozlosky C, et al. A metalloproteinase disintegrin that releases tumour necrosis factor-α from cells. Nature 1997;385:729–736.

78. Semmler J, Wachtel H, Endres S. The specific type IV phosphodiesterase inhibitor rolipram suppresses tumor necrosis factor-α production by human mononuclear cells. Int J Immunopharmacol 1993;15:409–413.

79. Le C, Nicolson A, Morales A, Sewell K. Suppression of collagen-induced arthritis through adenovirus-mediated transfer of a modified tumor necrosis factor α receptor gene. Arthritis Rheum 1997;40:1662–1669.

80. Moreira A, Sampaio E, Zmuidzinas A, et al. Thalidomide exerts its inhibitory action on tumor necrosis factor α by enhancing mRNA degradation. J Exp Med 1993;177:1675–1680.

81. Sajjadi F, Takabayashi K, Foster A, et al. Inhibition of TNF-α expression by adenosine: role of A3 adenosine receptors. J Immunol 1996;156:3435–3442.

82. Hajeer A, Worthington J, Silman A, Ollier W. Association of tumor necrosis factor microsatellite polymorphisms with HLA-DRB1*04-bearing haplotypes in rheumatoid arthritis patients. Arthritis Rheum 1996;39:1109–1114.

83. Williams R, Mason L, Feldmann M, Maini R. Synergy between anti-CD4 and anti-tumour necrosis factor in the amelioration of established collagen-induced arthritis. Proc Natl Acad Sci USA 1994;91:2762–2766.

84. Morgan A, Hale G, Rebello P, et al. Combination therapy with a TNF antagonist and a CD4 monoclonal antibody in rheumatoid arthritis. A pilot study. Arthritis Rheum 1997; 40(suppl):S81.

Chapter 23

Targeting the IL-2 Receptor with Antibodies or Chimeric Toxins

Terry B. Strom

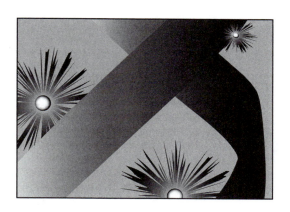

Although various mouse antirat and rat antimouse monoclonal antibodies (mAbs) produce profound immunosuppressive effects, the experience with rodent antihuman mAb has been somewhat disappointing. The impetus for creating chimeric or humanized mAbs or fusion proteins to be used as immunosuppressive agents in allograft recipients stems directly from the clinical experience with rodent antihuman mAbs. With the exception of antibodies directed against proteins of the TCR/CD3 complex, murine mAbs directed against cell surface proteins have failed to deliver on their many potential advantages for treating autoimmune diseases or preventing rejection. The favorable attributes of chimeric or humanized mAbs include 1) high specificity and affinity, 2) long circulating half-lives, and 3) a variety of mechanisms by which they can mediate an immunosuppressive effect. Cytolytic immune effector mechanisms of the host, antibody-directed cell-mediated cytotoxicity (ADCC), and complement-directed cytotoxicity (CDC) can theoretically be recruited directly against antibody-coated target cells. Moreover, mAbs can interrupt signaling at the cell surface by blocking key receptor sites.

The discrepancy between the high promise and poor delivery of therapeutic benefit through use of rodent mAbs in the clinic is explained at least in part by 1) the limiting effect of the ubiquitous human antixenoantibody response and 2) failure of most murine mAbs to activate human complement or Fc-receptor–positive cytolytic cells and thereby trigger target cell lysis. In the case of murine mAbs, this host-antibody response is denoted as the human antimurine antibody (HAMA) response (1–3). The HAMA response entails both anti-idiotypic and isotypic antibody responses, often within the first 14 to 20 days following initiation of treatment. Anti-idiotypic antibodies block the capacity of the mAb to bind antigen and are therefore neutralizing. Anti-isotypic antibodies, although not neutralizing, adversely affect the circulating half-life and volume of distribution (1). The circulating half-lives of murine mAbs in humans are considerably shorter (about 20 hours) than those of human antibodies of the same class (about 20 days), and the development of HAMA acts further to hasten clearance.

Chimeric and Humanized Monoclonal Antibodies

The majority of xenoantibodies are, at best, only poorly able to recruit ADCC or CDC human immune effector mechanisms. This means that the majority of conventional rodent antihuman cell surface protein mAbs are restricted to noncytolytic mechanisms of immunosuppression (e.g., OKT3). In order to improve the clinical utility of rodent antihuman mAbs, human sequences are introduced.

Chimeric antibodies are produced through a gene fusion strategy in which codons for the entire antigen-binding Fv region (VL + VH) from an existing murine mAb are joined to codons for human constant region sequences (Figs. 23-1 and 23-2) (see the review in 4). This simple approach has been extended and refined to create hyperchimeric, humanized antibodies (4,5). This strategy incorporates the basic concept that led to production of chimeric antibodies in which the antigen-binding portions of a rodent mAb are genetically fused to human Fc sequences but an additional step is added (see Fig. 23-2). This scheme, which seeks to introduce as little of the xenogeneic rodent V-region sequences as possible while retaining antigen specificity and affinity of a rodent mAb, is accomplished by splicing the appropriately spaced codons for the six murine antigen-binding complementarity-determining regions (CDRs) of a rodent mAb into a human V-region framework and Fc region cDNA. In practice, this approach creates a totally synthesized V-region cDNA to achieve CDR plus framework grafting. Amino acid residues outside of the CDRs, but in spatial proximity or "contact" with them, are also often grafted because they may be necessary to retain proper conformation of the antigen-binding CDR (see Fig. 23-2). The goals of these engineering efforts are to reduce immunogenicity and to gain human ADCC and CDC effector functions.

The IL-2 Receptor as a Therapeutic Target

Only certain leukemic or lymphoma cells, or recently activated immune cells, especially T cells, bear the trimolecular high-affinity interleukin-2 receptor (IL-2R). The high-affinity IL-2R is absent from the surface of resting T cells and nonlymphoid tissues (6). The de novo acquisition of high-affinity IL-2Rs is a critical event in the course of T-cell activation (6–9). The IL-2R can be expressed as high-, intermediate-, or low-affinity binding sites. The high-affinity site is a multimeric complex containing at least three peptides: the 55-kD α-chain and the 70-kD β- and 64-kD γ-chains that participate in signal transduction. The β- and γ-chains, but not the α-chain, are sparsely expressed on resting T cells and NK cells. With T-cell activation, marked amplification of expression of the β- and γ-chains and de novo expression of the

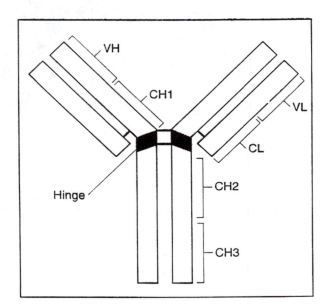

Figure 23-1. IgG structure.

α-chain ensue (6–9). The IL-2R β/γ heterodimer exhibits intermediate binding affinity, whereas the isolated 55-kD α-chain (CD25) is a low-affinity binding site (6–11).

Because the high-affinity receptor is only transiently expressed during the brief antigen-triggered proliferative burst of lymphocytes, we wondered whether administration of anti–IL-2R mAbs—e.g., anti-CD25 or chimeric IL-2 toxins—would provide a utilitarian approach to achieving selective immunosuppression aimed directly at activated lymphocytes (see the review in 12). In theory, agents directed against the IL-2R can be used in every situation of unwanted T-cell–dependent immunity to achieve selective immunosuppression.

Based on extensive and highly successful experimentation in rodent transplantation and autoimmune models (12,13), several murine antihuman-CD25 mAbs have been tested in human renal transplant recipients as an adjunct to traditional therapy. Modest beneficial effects were obtained (14–20). Nonetheless, the number of early rejection episodes were reduced and/or delayed (14–20). The HAMA response severely limited effectiveness. The modest beneficial effects produced by the conventional mAbs spurred efforts to develop refined mAbs-bearing human sequences to increase potency (21,22).

Because the HAMA response was an obvious barrier to successful employment of anti-CD25 mAbs, both the chimeric basiliximab (Simulect) (21) and the hyperchimeric daclizumab (Zenapax) (22) have been produced and tested for therapeutic efficacy as an adjunct to conventional treatment in human renal allograft recipients (23–25). Daclizumab and basiliximab are first administered in the immediate peritransplant period. Only one additional dose of basiliximab is given 4 to 5 days later (21), while five additional doses of daclizumab are given at 2-week intervals (25). The individual doses of basiliximab are greater than those

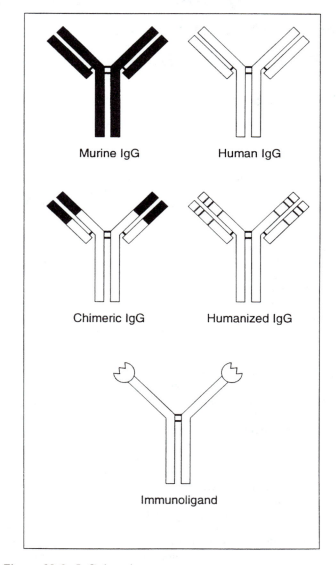

Figure 23-2. IgG domains.

used for daclizumab. Structural differences in antibodies are considerable. While daclizumab is a humanized mAb and should be less inherently immunogenic, basiliximab exerts a superior affinity for the IL-2 receptor. Thus it is difficult to assess the relative values of these mAbs using either clinical trial results or perceived superior biologic attributes.

Although intuition would suggest clear therapeutic superiority for the humanized mAb, it is not certain that this will prove to be true. Direct comparison of basiliximab and daclizumab through therapeutic trials has not been conducted. The treatment protocols are quite different in terms of the number of injections and the dose per injection.

Both the chimeric mouse-human basiliximab and hyperchimeric ("humanized") daclizumab anti-CD25 mAbs are approved by the FDA for use in renal allograft recipients. As anticipated, a single injection of mAb leads to sustained blood levels. Treatment with either mAb diminishes the incidence of acute rejection episodes by 33% to 50%. In treated patients, the rejection episodes that occur are delayed and less virulent than those observed in control patients. The incidence of neutralizing HAMA responses formed in patients treated with either mAb is very low. The overall incidence of adverse events, including lymphoma, other malignancies, and opportunistic infections, was very low and similar to the incidence noted with placebo adjustive treatment. Studies of liver and cardiac allograft recipients show a similar benefit in reducing early rejection episodes without incurring serious side effects.

Thus, it is difficult to assess the relative values of these mAbs. Because of the extreme safety and relative effectiveness of the anti-CD25, many units now use these antibodies as adjuncts to conventional immunosuppressive agents. The anti-CD25 mAbs compete with polyclonal antilymphocyte for this application. There is little question that anti-CD25 mAbs are safer than polyclonal antilymphocyte antibodies in terms of the selective targeting of activated lymphocytes, freedom from anaphylactoid reactions, and low risk for opportunistic infection. At this early date in the clinical application of anti-CD25 mAbs, it is uncertain whether the polyclonal antibodies or anti-CD25 mAbs exert similar potency in the patient populations at high risk for immunologic graft failure.

IL-2 Toxin Fusion Protein

The great German scientist Paul Ehrlich first suggested that *Zauberkugelm* (i.e., "magic bullet") hybrid molecules, consisting of cell-specific antibodies linked to a toxin (immunotoxin), be constructed for various therapeutic purposes. He envisioned the use of immunotoxins as "magic bullets" to destroy a highly selective population of target cells. By genetically linking cytokines to select portions of toxins, we and others have pursued a strategy closely related to that proposed by Ehrlich many years ago (Figs. 23-3 and 23-4). Naturally occurring bacterial and plant toxins exhibit domain-specific structure-function activity; therefore, structure can be manipulated to create biologic agents that specifically target and kill disease-causing cells (26–28).

Functional Domains of Diphtheria Toxin and Pseudomonas Exotoxin

The holotoxins used in construction of hybrid toxins have three functionally specialized domains that bind to specific target cell surface receptors, translocate the toxin into the appropriate subcellular compartment, and enzymatically intoxicate the target cell (26–28). The three functional domains of diphtheria toxin (DT) are segregated into three separate structural domains (26). In both DT and *Pseudomonas* exotoxin A (PEA) (27; see Fig. 23-4), the enzymatically active core is an ADP-ribosyltransferase that targets elongation factor-2 (EF-2). EF-2 is an essential

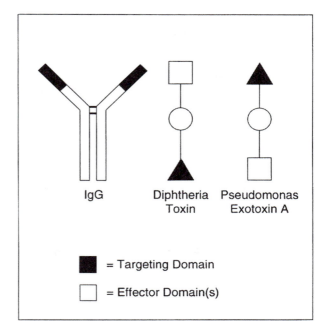

Figure 23-3. Targeting and effector domains of IgG and toxins.

element in the translational apparatus of the cell. Following ADP-ribosylation, EF-2 is inactivated and the intoxicated cell dies because it does not manufacture new cellular proteins. The extreme carboxy terminus of DT and the amino terminus of PEA function as receptor-binding elements and are responsible for the binding of the toxin to specific eukaryotic cell surface receptors (see Fig. 23-4). The third centrally located domain of both toxins serves as a translocating element and enables the intact toxin to traverse the target cell membrane, thereby permitting the toxin to enter the endosome and ensuring subsequent delivery of the toxophore to the cytosol (26–28).

IL-2 Fusion Toxins: DAB$_{486}$ IL-2 and DAB$_{398}$ IL-2

The genetic replacement of the receptor-binding domain of native DT or PEA with a cytokine (e.g., IL-2) or another growth factor has resulted in the development of a new class of biologic response modifiers—the fusion toxins (29–37).

IL-2 fusion toxins (DAB$_{486}$ IL-2 and DAB$_{398}$ IL-2), the first of this new class of targeted biologicals to be tested in the clinic, are specifically cytotoxic for IL-2R–expressing cells (31,32,34,35,37). The receptor binding domain of diphtheria toxin has been replaced by a specific targeting ligand, human interleukin-2 (see Fig. 23-4), creating a recombinant protein that kills activated IL-2R–expressing lymphocytes at 10^{-10} M to 10^{-11} M concentrations (31,32,34,35,37). DAB$_{486}$ IL-2 (67 kD) was the first fusion toxin to be evaluated clinically; DAB$_{398}$ IL-29, which has a higher affinity for the IL-2R than DAB$_{398}$ IL-2, is approximately 10 times more potent than DAB$_{486}$ IL-2.

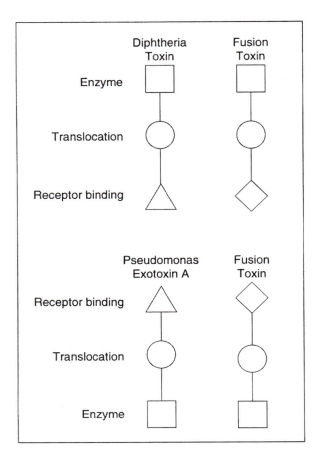

Figure 23-4. Structure-function relationships of native and fusion toxins.

Two of these fusion toxins, DAB_{486} IL-2 and DAB_{398} IL-2 (34,35), have been tested in several clinical circumstances.

IL-2 fusion toxins, once bound to the cell membrane IL-2 receptor, are rapidly internalized into an acidic endocytic vesicle. The toxic fragment then reaches the cell cytosol, initiating a cytotoxic event within 5 to 15 minutes. Protein synthesis is irreversibly inhibited as a result of ADP ribosylation of elongation factor-2, and cell death occurs over 36 to 72 hours (31,32,37).

This early clinical experience provides a basis for evaluation of DAB_{398} IL-2 in randomized, placebo-controlled clinical trials in patients with lymphoma (38) or psoriasis (39). DAB_{398} IL-2 produced five complete remissions (CRs) and eight partial responses (PRs) among 35 patients with cutaneous T-cell lymphoma, and one CR and two PRs were noted in 17 DAB_{398} IL-2 treated patients with non-Hodgkin's lymphoma. DAB_{398} IL-2 has been approved by the FDA for use in cutaneous T-cell lymphoma.

Summary

Recent clinical experience with modern anti-CD25 mAbs and IL-2 toxin fusion proteins has verified the utility of targeting the IL-2 receptor. As anticipated, highly selective and beneficial cell targeting of activated or malignant lymphoid cells is achieved.

References

1. Chatenoud L, Baudrihay MF, Chkoff N, et al. Restriction of the human *in vivo* immune response against the mouse monoclonal antibody OKT3. J Immunol 186;137(3):830–838.
2. Jaffers GJ, Fuller TC, Cosimi AB, et al. Monoclonal antibody therapy anti-idiotypic and non-anti-idiotypic antibodies to OKT3 arising despite intense immunosuppression. Transplantation 1986;41(5):572–578.
3. Thistlethwaite JR, Stuart JK, Mayes JT, et al. Monitoring and complications of monoclonal therapy: complications and monitoring of OKT3 therapy. Am J Kidney Dis 1988;11(2):112–119.
4. Morrison SL, Johnson MJ, Herzenberg LA, Oi VT. Chimeric human antibody molecules: mouse antigen-binding domains with human constant region domains. Proc Natl Acad Sci USA 1984;81:6851–6855.
5. Jones PT, Dear PH, Foote J, et al. Replacing the complementarity-determining regions in a human antibody with those from a mouse. Nature 1986;321(6069):522–525.
6. Smith KA. The two chain structure of high-affinity IL-2 receptors. Immunol Today 1987;8:11–13.
7. Cantrell PA, Smith KA. The interleukin-2 T-cell system: a new cell growth model. Science 1984;224:1312–1316.
8. Leonard WJ, Depper JM, Uchiyama T, et al. A mAb that appears to recognize the receptor for human T-cell growth factor; partial characterization of the receptor. Nature 1982;300:267–269.
9. Maddock EO, Maddock SW, Kelley VE, Strom TB. Rapid stereospecific stimulation of lymphocytic metabolism by interleukin-2. J Immunol 1985;135(6):4004–4008.
10. Tsudo M, Kozak RW, Goldman CK, Waldmann TA. Demonstration of a new peptide (non-Tac) that binds IL-2; a potential participant in a multichain IL-2 receptor complex. Proc Natl Acad Sci USA 1986;83(24):9694–9698.
11. Takeshita T, Asao H, Ohtani K, et al. Cloning of the gamma chain of the human IL-2 receptor. Science 1992;257:379–382.
12. Strom TB, Kelley VR, Murphy JR, et al. Interleukin-2 receptor-directed therapies: antibody- or cytokine-based targeting molecules. Annu Rev Med 1993;44:343–353.
13. Waldmann TA, O'Shea J. The use of antibodies against the IL-2 receptor in transplantation. Curr Opin Immunol 1998;10:507–512.
14. Kirkman RL, Shapiro ME, Carpenter CB, et al. Early experience with anti-Tac, an antihuman IL-2 receptor mAb. Transplantation 1989;21:1766–1768.
15. Soulillou JP, Peyronnet P, LeMauff B, et al. Prevention of rejection of kidney transplants by mAb directed against interleukin 2 (receptor). Lancet 1987;1:1339.

16. Soulillou JP, Cantarovich D, LeMauff B, et al. Randomized controlled trial of a monoclonal antibody against the interleukin-2 receptor (33B3.1) as compared with rabbit antithymocyte globulin for prophylaxis against rejection of renal allografts. N Engl J Med 1990;322:1175–1182.
17. Kirkman RL, Shapiro ME, Carpenter CB, et al. A randomized prospective trial of anti-tac monoclonal antibody in human renal transplantation. Transplantation 1991;51:107–113.
18. Van Gelder T, Zietse R, Mulder AH, et al. A variable blind study of uroclonal anti-interleukin-2 receptor antibody (BT563) administration to prevent acute rejection after kidney transplantation. Transplantation 1995;60:248–252.
19. Nashan B, Schlitt HJ, Schwinzer R, et al. Immunoprophylaxis with a monoclonal anti-IL-2 receptor antibody in liver transplant patients. Transplantation 1996;61:546–554.
20. Langren JM, Nussler NC, Neumann U, et al. A prospective randomized trial comparing interleukin-2 receptor antibody versus antithymocyte globulin as part of a quadruple immunosuppressive induction therapy following orthopic liver transplantation. Transplantation 1997;63:1772–1781.
21. Amlot PL, Rawslings E, Fernando ON, et al. Prolonged action of a chimeric interleukin-2 receptor [CD25] monoclonal antibody used in cadaveric renal transplantation. Transplantation 1995;60:748–756.
22. Queen C, Schneider WP, Selick HE, et al. A humanized antibody that binds to the interleukin 2-receptor. Proc Natl Acad Sci USA 1989;86:10029–10033.
23. Kahan BD, Rajagopalan PR, Hall M. Reduction of the occurrence of acute cellular rejection among renal allograft recipients treated with basiliximab, a chimeric anti-interleukin-2-receptor monoclonal antibody. United States Simulect Renal Study Group. Transplantation 1999 Jan 27;72(2):276–284.
24. Nashan B, Moore R, Amlot P, et al, for the CHIB 201 International Study Group. Randomised trial of basiliximab versus placebo for control of acute cellular rejection in renal allograft recipients. Lancet 1997;350:1193–1198.
25. Vincenti F, Kirkman R, Highe S, et al. Interleukin-2 receptor blockade with daclizumab to prevent acute rejection in renal transplantation. N Engl J Med 1998;338:161–165.
26. Choe S, Bennett MJ, Fugii G, et al. The crystal structure of diphtheria toxin. Nature 1992;357:216–222.
27. Pastan I, Willingham MC, FitzGerald DSP. Immunotoxins. Cell 1986;47:641–648.
28. Olsnes S, Sandrig K, Petersen OW, VanDeurs B. Immunotoxins—entry into cells and mechanisms of action. Immunol Today 1989;10:291–295.
29. Williams DP, Regier D, Akiyoshi D, et al. Design, synthesis and expression of a human interleukin-2 gene incorporating the codon usage bias found in highly expressed *Escherichia coli* genes. Nucleic Acids Res 1988;16:10453–10467.
30. Siegall CB, Chaudhary VK, Fitz-Gerald DJ, Pastan I. Cytotoxic activity of an interleukin-6 *Pesudomonas* exotoxin fusion protein on human myeloma cells. Proc Natl Acad Sci USA 1988;85:9738–9742.
31. Williams DP, Parker K, Bacha P, et al. Diphtheria toxin receptor binding domain substitution with interleukin-2: genetic construction and properties of a diphtheria toxin-related interleukin-2 fusion protein. Protein Eng 1987;1:493–498.
32. Williams DB, Snider CE, Strom TB, Murphy JR. Structure/function analysis of interleukin-2-toxin (DAB$_{486}$-IL-2). Fragment B sequences required for the delivery of fragment A to the cytosol of target cells. J Biol Chem 1990;265:1185–1189.
33. Lorberboum-Gaiski H, Fitz-Gerald D, Chaudhary V, et al. Cytotoxic activity of an interleukin-2 *Pseudomonas* exotoxin chimeric protein produced in *Escherichia coli*. Proc Natl Acad Sci USA 1988;85:1922–1926.
34. Murphy JR, Bishai W, Borowski A, et al. Genetic construction, expression, and melanoma-selective cytotoxicity of a diphtheria toxin-related alpha-melanocyte-stimulating hormone fusion protein. Proc Natl Acad Sci USA 1986;83:8258–8262.
35. Chaudhary VK, Fitz-Gerald DJ, Adhya S, Pastan I. Selective killing of HIV infected cells by recombinant human *CD4-Pseudomonas* exotoxin hybrid protein. Proc Natl Acad Sci USA 1987;84:4538–4542.
36. Chaudhary VK, Mizukami T, Fuerst TR, et al. Activity of a recombinant fusion protein between transforming growth factor type alpha and Pseudomonas toxin. Nature 1988;335:369–372.
37. Bacha P, Williams DP, Waters C, et al. Interleukin-2 receptor targeted cytotoxicity: interleukin-2 receptor mediated action of a diphtheria toxin-related interleukin-2 fusion protein. J Exp Med 1988;167(2):612–622.
38. LeMaistre CF, Saleh MN, Kuzel TM, et al. Phase I trial of a ligand fusion-protein (DAB$_{389}$IL-2) in lymphomas expressing the receptor for interleukin-2. Blood 1998;91:399–405.
39. Gottlieb SL, Gilicaudeau P, Johnson R, et al. The response of psoriasis to a lymphocyte selective toxin DAB389 IL-2 suggests a primary immune but not keratinocyte, pathogenic basis. Nat Med 1995;1(5):442–447.

Chapter 24

Monoclonal Antibodies to CD3

Lucienne Chatenoud

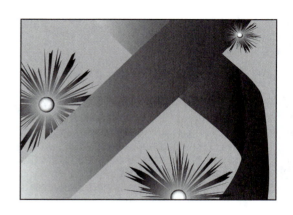

The first mouse hybridoma cell line producing a monoclonal antibody to human CD3 was reported by Kung et al in 1979 (1) and was named OKT3. Initial experiments disclosed that OKT3 defined a molecule expressed by all mature T cells and that it strongly inhibited in vitro proliferative responses in mixed lymphocyte cultures as well as the generation of alloreactive cytotoxic effectors. It was mostly on this basis that, since the early 1980s and long before both the molecular complexities and the key functional role of the CD3 molecule were discovered, OKT3 entered the clinical practice for the treatment and prevention of organ allograft rejection. From the first clinical trials, the strong immunosuppressive potency of OKT3 was evident, which explains the rapid expansion of its use and its availability on the market worldwide by 1984. Through the study of patients treated with OKT3, an enormous amount of knowledge was gained on the mode of action of murine anti–T-cell monoclonals and their side effects—knowledge that was invaluable for the design of more refined approaches.

Antibodies to human CD3 do not cross-react with lymphocytes from most commonly used nonhuman primates, such as rhesus or cynomolgus monkeys, although they may recognize chimpanzee cells. Fortunately, OKT3 was not the subject of conventional toxicologic studies, because the risk was high for this antibody to be excluded. In fact, it is quite evident that the main limitation to the use of CD3 antibodies in transplantation, as well as other clinical settings such as autoimmunity, has been the cytokine-mediated "flulike" syndrome, which we now know can be life threatening if high doses are used. This raises two major points. The first is an important word of caution about regulatory issues that, in the particular case of biologic agents, have to be considered with a sufficient degree of criticism to avoid stopping the development of potentially very useful drugs. The second point deals with the future of CD3 antibodies that, by definition, must be exclusively based on the use of humanized nonmitogenic antibodies. These new agents are well tolerated because they are relatively free of the deleterious cytokine-releasing capacity of conventional CD3 antibodies.

It is the aim of this brief review to present the data that have been collected so far on the use of CD3 antibodies and to discuss them in the context of the new clinically applicable therapeutic strategies to which they lead.

The CD3 Molecular Complex

The vast majority of T cells (90% to 95%) express specialized dimeric receptors, the T-cell receptor (TCR) α and β chains, that bind peptides presented in the context of major histocompatibility complex (MHC) molecules. The TCR α and β polypeptide chains include a constant portion and a variable portion; it is the variable portion that dictates antigen specificity. There is also another subset of T lymphocytes, less numerous, that express a distinct TCR heterodimer composed of the γ and δ chains. At variance with TCR $\alpha\beta$, TCR $\gamma\delta$ lymphocytes appear to recognize antigen directly without the requirement of MHC presentation.

The TCRs are expressed at the T-cell surface in association with a set of nonpolymorphic polypeptides constituting the CD3 molecular complex (Fig. 24-1). CD3 consists of five invariant membrane proteins designated γ, δ, ε, ζ, and η, which is a splicing variant of ζ (2). In some cases, the CD3 complex may also include the γ chain associated with FcεRI and FcγRIII (CD16). The γ, δ, and ε subunits are expressed as noncovalently linked γ–δ and γ–ε dimers; the ζ chain can disulfide bond to form homodimers $\zeta\zeta$ or heterodimers with either the η chain, especially in mouse T cells, or the γ chain associated with FcεRI and FcγRIII (CD16). Concerning the stoichiometry of the complex, current evidence favors the presence of at least two TCR heterodimers per CD3 cluster: $(\alpha\beta)_2 (\gamma\delta\varepsilon)_2 (\zeta\zeta)_4$ (3) (see Fig. 24-1).

CD3 plays a fundamental role in regulating the intracellular assembly and the expression of TCR at the T-cell surface and in transducing TCR $\alpha\beta$–mediated activation signals. In fact, the cytoplasmic domains of TCR $\alpha\beta$ are short (only five residues) and are unable to couple to the intracellular signal transducing machinery (3). The intracellular domains of CD3 polypeptides do not exhibit an intrinsic enzymatic activity but bear immunoreceptor tyrosine-based activation motifs (ITAMs) that once phosphorylated do interact with intracellular signaling proteins. One ITAM motif is present in the cytoplasmic portion of each of the

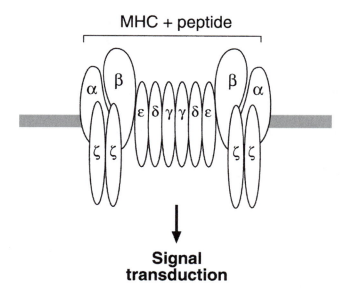

Figure 24-1. Schematic representation of the CD3/TCR molecular complex.

γ, δ, and ε chains of CD3; each ζ chain expresses three ITAM motifs.

Most of the CD3 antibodies that have been used in vitro for functional studies and in vivo, in both the experimental and clinical settings, are specific for the ε chain of the complex. This is particularly the case for OKT3, for the hamster monoclonal antibody 145 2C11 that is specific for murine CD3 and has been extensively used in mouse models (4), and also for the FN18 antibody that is specific for RhT3, the rhesus monkey CD3 molecule (5).

CD3 Antibodies in Clinical Transplantation

OKT3, a mouse IgG2a, was the first monoclonal antibody introduced into clinical practice in the early 1980s.

In the first pilot trial, which was conducted by the Cosimi group in Boston, OKT3 was administered to reverse ongoing early acute renal allograft rejection. Eight patients were enrolled who received escalating dosages of OKT3: 1–2 mg/day for 10 consecutive days in two cases, 3 mg/day for 14 days in two cases, and 4–5 mg/day for 14 to 20 days in four cases; the dosages of corticosteroids and azathioprine were reduced during OKT3 treatment (6,7). Reversal of rejection occurred within 2 to 4 days, and biopsy specimens showed that the dosage of 5 mg/day was needed to guarantee, in the majority of the patients, clearance of graft-infiltrating host leukocytes. Those patients who received the low OKT3 dosages were at higher risk of recurrent rejection. The dosage of 5 mg/day was then selected for all

subsequent trials, such as for the large, randomized, multicenter study conducted in 1984–1985, which involved a total of 123 patients and led to the licensing of OKT3 as a treatment for established rejection (8). OKT3 was also administered with great success to "rescue" patients from rejection episodes that were unresponsive to conventional high-dosage corticosteroids and polyclonal antilymphocyte globulins. Despite the fact that most of these studies were nonrandomized, some of them included very large numbers of patients and settled the validity of this clinical approach (9–11). Although the initial studies were conducted in renal transplantation, the use of OKT3 was rapidly applied with success in reversing rejection in liver and heart transplantation. In liver transplantation, OKT3 proved useful in rescuing steroid-resistant acute rejection episodes in 75% to 85% of cases in both adult and pediatric patients (12–14). This was also shown for heart transplants (15). The antibody has also been used as first-line treatment for acute rejection of liver transplants, but in this context some of the studies reported a higher incidence of early septic complications (74% versus 33%) (16).

In parallel to this use as a treatment for rejection, several centers included OKT3 in so-called prophylaxis or "induction" protocols with the aim of decreasing the incidence of acute rejection episodes and improving long-term allograft survival. The first prophylactic protocol was conducted in 1982 in our center by Kreis and coworkers (17–19). The particular design of this protocol, which for any ethical concern has to be considered in the context of the "immunosuppression" available in the early 1980s, was rich in very fundamental information. Six patients were enrolled, and they received OKT3 alone, at a dosage of 5 mg/day for 14 days, without any other treatment (17–19). For about 6 to 10 days, depending on the patient, effective circulating OKT3 levels were maintained and clinical signs of rejection were absent. Then, a massive anti-OKT3 humoral response developed that rapidly cleared the antibody and correlated with the onset of acute rejection, thus necessitating the institution of an alternative immunosuppression therapy (17–19). These results proved the very high immunosuppressive potency of OKT3, demonstrating that even alone this antibody could sustain the normal function of a mismatched human renal allograft. They also indicated that, despite this potent immunosuppression, a rapidly developing antiglobulin response totally precluded the use of OKT3 as the sole immunosuppressant.

Thus, in subsequent prophylactic protocols, OKT3 was administered for 10 to 14 consecutive days, starting on the day of transplantation, in association with corticosteroids and with azathioprine and cyclosporin, which were mostly applied by the end of OKT3 therapy. Various controlled, single-center studies demonstrated the efficacy of OKT3 in this setting when compared with conventional chemical immunosuppressant therapy (20–22). Moreover, the use of OKT3 in the early post-transplant period was an interesting approach to avoiding the complications linked to cyclosporin nephrotoxicity. Among the few studies that compared the prophylactic efficacy of

OKT3 with that of polyclonal anti–T cell antibodies, the one that used Minnesota ALG is particularly interesting (20). The data showed equivalent effects of the two drugs in terms of incidence of acute rejections, long-term survival, and infectious complications.

Prophylactic protocols using OKT3 were also conducted in liver transplantation, and results showed a lower incidence of rejection, a delay in onset of first rejection, and a decreased incidence of steroid-resistant rejection (23–25). Induction therapy with OKT3 in cardiac transplantation also showed a reduction in the incidence of acute rejection, and some authors also reported on a long-term beneficial effect resulting from a reduction in graft atherosclerosis (26).

Despite these data, most centers did not adopt OKT3 as a routine prophylactic treatment in transplant recipients, essentially for two reasons. The first was the risk of sensitization that could preclude reuse of the antibody for treating steroid-resistant rejection (16,24,27). This was particularly important in the pediatric population, in which the frequency of the OKT3-specific antiglobulin response was significantly higher than in adults (28). The second obstacle was the occurrence of the "flulike" syndrome that, in comparison with antithymocyte globulin (ATG) or conventional triple therapy with cyclosporin, could complicate the early management of the patients (25,29–31). In the particular case of heart transplant recipients, the syndrome could also generate serious hemodynamic complications. An additional problem was the risk of overimmunosuppression, which was particularly relevant in cardiac allograft recipients because OKT3 was applied mostly as part of a quadruple therapy (OKT3, high-dose cyclosporin, corticosteroids, and azathioprine), resulting in a very "heavy" regimen. This was, unfortunately, supported by the data from Swinnen et al, which showed an incidence of 11.4% (9/79) of virally induced B-cell lymphomas in OKT3-treated heart transplant recipients (32). Malignancies developed preferentially in the subgroup of patients who received a cumulative dose of OKT3 higher than 75 mg (i.e., a treatment longer than the usually recommended 14-day period, or more than one antibody course) or in those who were also treated with ATG in their post-transplant course. In clear contrast, between 1985 and 1991, the internal registry of the pharmaceutical company producing OKT3 (Johnson & Johnson) scored an incidence of 0.48% (192/40,000) of lymphomas. These figures were totally in keeping with our single-center experience in that same period of time—0.36% (1/274) (H. Kreis, personal communication). As a whole, these data support the notion that the frequency of malignancies in general, and of B-cell lymphomas in particular, tightly correlates with the potency of the overall immunosuppressive regimen administered rather than with the use of a particular immunosuppressive drug. Concerning OKT3, there has been no firm evidence that, using an adequate adaptation of the doses, there was an increased risk of lymphoma relative to that observed in patients receiving conventional antilymphocyte polyclonal antisera (25).

In Vivo Antigenic Modulation of the CD3/TCR: One Major Mode of Action of CD3 Antibodies

Most of the initial observations on the biologic effects elicited by the in vivo administration of CD3 antibodies were made on OKT3-treated patients and subsequently fully confirmed using equivalent antibodies in mice, rats, and monkeys.

After the first OKT3 injection, all T cells disappear from the peripheral blood within 30 to 60 minutes (18,19). This extremely rapid effect, seen only in the peripheral blood is attributable mostly to 1) the cytokine release, linked to the first antibody administration, that increases the adhesiveness of the activated vascular endothelium, which favors cell marginalization, and 2) cell trapping by the reticuloendothelial system (opsonization). Results obtained with mice receiving comparable doses of a CD3 antibody such as 145 2C11 confirmed that in the spleen and lymph nodes only 30% to 40% of CD3$^+$ cells were eliminated (33). At variance with what was initially expected, the in vivo monoclonal antibody–mediated cell destruction not only relies on the functional capacity of the constant Fc anti-body portion [i.e, complement-mediated depletion; antibody-dependent cell-mediated cytotoxicity (ADCC)] but also largely depends on the antibody fine specificity and on the density and distribution of the target cell antigen (34). Concerning CD3 antibodies, redirected T-cell lysis on bridging cytotoxic T cells to the target (35) and the induction of apoptosis are among the mechanisms potentially involved in antibody-mediated depletion. Apoptosis mediated through CD3/TCR signaling was initially demonstrated in immature thymocytes, but accumulating evidence indicates that it can also be triggered in activated mature peripheral T cells (36–38).

CD3$^+$ lymphocytes that are not depleted undergo antigenic modulation that is the reversible disappearance of a given cell receptor on binding to a specific ligand that promotes microaggregation of the complex, capping, and subsequent internalization or shedding (18,39). By the second to the fifth day of treatment, small but significant numbers of antigenically modulated T cells are present in lymphoid organs and in the circulation. They express the particular phenotype CD3-TCR-CD4$^+$ or CD3-TCR-CD8$^+$ (18,19,39). This phenomenon may be reversible within a few (8 to 12) hours if the antibody is cleared from the environment as may occur in vitro, if modulated cells are incubated in the absence of OKT3, or in vivo at cessation of treatment. CD3 antibody–modulated cells are fully unresponsive to antigen-specific or mitogen stimulation (18). This correlates with the profound in vivo immunosuppression exhibited even in patients treated with OKT3 alone in whom no allograft rejection was observed while T cells in the circulation did not express CD3 (6,17,25). Thus, the detection of CD3$^-$/TCR$^-$ cells in the circulation was an excellent parameter by which to monitor the effectiveness of OKT3 treatment. In patients receiving OKT3 for the treatment of a rejection episode, antigenic modulation also affected the cells infiltrating the rejecting allograft (40). CD3-mediated antigenic modulation does not occur in the absence of an efficient cross-linking of the receptor. Thus, monovalent CD3 antibodies did not promote antigenic modulation but improved the depletion of CD3$^+$ lymphocytes (41).

It is important to stress that neither the partial depletion nor the antigenic modulation accounts per se for the immunosuppressive effect of CD3 antibodies. In fact, antibodies to TCR such as BMA 031, which also modulate CD3/TCR, express, at least in the clinical setting, only a quite modest immunosuppressive capacity (42).

The Humoral Immune Response to Murine CD3 Antibodies

The occurrence of an antiglobulin response to the xenogeneic protein has been one of the major drawbacks in early trials using OKT3. Interestingly enough, most of the conclusions reached through the study of the antiglobulin response to OKT3 were fully applicable to most cell-binding antibodies that have been used not only in humans but also in the various experimental models.

We have already mentioned that when the antibody was administered alone, within 5 to 7 days, very high titers of anti-OKT3 IgM and IgG antibodies appeared (19). Immumochemical analysis of whole and chromatography-purified sera from OKT3-immunized patients suggested the exclusive presence of two components in the response—namely, an anti-isotypic component and an anti-idiotypic component (19). Anti-isotypic antibodies reacted with all mouse IgG2 immunoglobulins (OKT3 is a mouse IgG2a) irrespective of their fine specificity. Anti-idiotypic antibodies are specific for determinants located within the hypervariable regions and involved in the interaction with the antigen. Anti-idiotypic antibodies constitute the neutralizing component of the response because they compete with OKT3 for binding to the target antigen. From the clinical point of view, the abrogation of the therapeutic efficacy linked to anti-idiotypic antibodies has been the main deleterious consequence of the antiglobulin response (19,25). Anti-isotypic antibodies appear to be essentially non-neutralizing and to reinforce the modulating capacity of OKT3 (43).

One interesting practical consequence of the specificity restriction of the response is that hosts immunized to a given monoclonal antibody are still responsive to a second monoclonal expressing the same specificity but a different idiotype or an antibody of different specificity (i.e., distinct idiotypes). This was the case for recipients of renal allografts who mounted antiglobulin responses to a murine CD25 antibody they received for prophylaxis and were still fully responsive to OKT3 administered to treat ongoing acute rejection. Similarly, monkeys immunized to a murine CD4 antibody were successfully retreated with other murine CD4s expressing distinct idiotypes (44).

Studies performed on immunized patients and monkey sera using affinity purified anti-idiotypic antibodies showed that the response is oligoclonal (45). It thus appears that the neutralizing potential of the humoral response to monoclonal antibodies is more dependent on its specificity than on the overall amount of antibodies produced, because only a few specific clones are recruited. This may explain that, at variance to polyclonal antisera, sensitization to monoclonal antibodies never led to clinically overt immune complex disease (serum sickness), the amount of immune complexes formed probably being insufficient to allow sustained tissue deposition. The antiglobulin response may also include IgE antibodies associated with the potential risk of anaphylaxis, but in practice this has appeared to be an extremely rare observation (46).

Before the advent of humanized antibodies, one practical means of decreasing the sensitizing potential of murine monoclonals was their association with conventional immunosuppressants. In the case of OKT3, adding corticosteroids and azathioprine at adequate doses decreased the frequency of sensitization from 90–95% to 40–60%. Addition of cyclosporine further reduced it to 15–25%, and in most cases antibodies did not affect efficacy because they appeared only at the end of OKT3 treatment (47).

Monocyte Dependence of the Mitogenicity of CD3 Antibodies

CD3 antibodies are endowed with a potent mitogenic activity that drives T-cell proliferation and cytokine production (25,30,31). In vivo, this mitogenic activity translates, within the very first hours following the first CD3 antibody administration, into a massive though transient systemic release of several cytokines, including TNF, IFN-γ, IL-2, IL-3, IL-6, IL-10, and GM-CSF (25,31,48–52) as well as IL-4 (52,53). A transient expression of activation markers such as the α chain of the IL-2 receptor (CD25) and CD44 has also been observed at the T-cell surface. The cytokine release is responsible for one major side effect linked to administration of CD3 antibodies—the acute "flulike" syndrome (25,30,31). The main symptoms are high fever, chills, and headache, together with repeated episodes of vomiting and diarrhea; patients become prostrated through massive fluid and electrolyte loss. A low proportion of patients develop more severe and potentially life-threatening conditions, such as severe respiratory distress (related to pulmonary edema in patients with significant fluid overload), neurotoxicity, and hypotension. Like the cytokine release, this syndrome is self-limited; it resolves by the second to the third day of treatment.

The mitogenic capacity of CD3 antibodies is monocyte dependent and tightly correlated with the capacity of the Fc antibody portion to interact with Fc receptors on monocytes/macrophages that facilitates cross-linking. Thus, in vitro, CD3 F(ab′)2 fragments, which lack the Fc portion, are not mitogenic and the proliferative response varies according to the variable affinity of the murine isotype for human monocyte Fc receptors (IgG2a >> IgG1 >> IgG2b >> IgA) (54,55). This fully correlates with the pattern observed in vivo: murine CD3 antibodies of the IgA isotype did not promote massive cytokine release and were perfectly well tolerated (56); an identical pattern was observed using CD3 F(ab)′2 fragments in mice (55,57,58). These observations led to the design of humanized CD3 antibodies engineered to prevent them from binding to Fc receptors, thus eliminating their mitogenic potential (59,60). Importantly, both the experimental and clinical data confirmed that nonmitogenic CD3 antibodies fully retain their therapeutic activity (55,56,58,61–64).

Aside from the antibody Fc portion, the fine specificity, in terms of the epitope recognized within the CD3/TCR complex, also influences the mitogenic potential. This is well illustrated by the case of the human TCR antibody BMA 031 (mouse IgG2a). In vitro, BMA 031 is less mitogenic than OKT3, and in vivo it is very well tolerated. Like OKT3, BMA 031 induces TNF release, but no other cytokines are detected (65). These data also indirectly suggest that TNF alone is insufficient to produce the clinical syndrome and that synergy between cytokines is required.

In clinical practice, a single injection of high-dose corticosteroids, administered at least 1 hour prior to the first OKT3 injection, has been an effective means of significantly decreasing both the amount of cytokines released and the severity of the syndrome (30). Another approach that almost totally abolished the reaction in both mice and human patients was the pretreatment with monoclonal antibodies to TNF (66,67).

Of course, the availability of humanized engineered nonmitogenic CD3 antibodies represents by far a much more radical and sophisticated approach to circumventing this major side effect.

Humanized Nonmitogenic CD3 Antibodies

To reduce as much as possible the amount of xenogeneic sequences expressed, humanized chimeric or complementarity determining region (CDR)–grafted monoclonal antibodies were produced (68,69). Chimeric antibodies composed of the intact variable regions (Fab) from the parental rodent antibody coupled with a human immunoglobulin constant portion were initially produced by chemical procedures and subsequently by molecular engineering (69). Recombinant CDR-grafted antibodies express the parental hypervariable regions, which carry the antigen specificity, within human heavy and light chain immunoglobulin frameworks (68). In the case of both the chimeric and CDR-grafted antibodies, one may select for the desired human Fc fragment that will impact on the final antibody effector capacities [complement fixation, opsonization, and antibody-dependent cell-mediated cytotoxicity (ADCC)] and, as previously discussed, the mitogenic capacity.

There is now compelling evidence that the sensitization rate is very significantly decreased through the use of these humanized antibodies (70–73).

The risk of a deleterious anti-idiotypic response still occurring with these humanized antibodies is a valid concern. In fact, the clinical data available so far show that chimeric and reshaped humanized antibodies are immunogenic in some patients, especially those presenting with autoimmune diseases in whom the monoclonal is administered alone (in the absence of other immunosuppressants), and after more than 2 to 3 repeated antibody courses (71,74). At variance, several centers have now reported on the use of humanized monoclonal antibodies in clinical transplantation, where single antibody courses are given in association with other immunosuppressants, in the absence of sensitization (70,72,73).

Concerning CD3 antibodies, and as we have already discussed, the humanization offers the additional advantage of deriving nonmitogenic antibodies.

At present, two humanized nonmitogenic CD3 antibodies have been reported and are under study in pilot clinical trials.

One such antibody has been characterized by the group of H. Waldmann and is derived from the rat YTH 12.5 (59,75). YTH 12.5 was humanized, and a set of CD3 monoclonal antibodies with different H chain constant regions was derived from humanized IgG1 YTH 12.5. Among these was an antibody expressing a γ1 constant region that lacked the CH2 domain glycosylation site. Previous studies had shown that aglycosylated antibodies are unable to bind to Fc receptors or activate complement. A series of preclinical studies was performed on the aglycosylated human IgG1 YTH 12.5. The results (59) showed that:

1. Aglycosyl IgG1 YTH 12.5 failed to induce T-cell proliferation in the presence of human serum.
2. The ability of aglycosyl IgG1 YTH 12.5 to direct T cells to kill cells bearing human Fc receptors, in the absence of human serum, was reduced by a factor of 10 compared with the original human IgG1 antibody.
3. Aglycosyl IgG1 YTH 12.5 suppressed proliferation in a mixed lymphocyte reaction.

In addition, using transgenic mice that express the human CD3-ε chain, it was shown that the aglycosyl IgG1 YTH 12.5 antibody did not induce a significant TNF release, which was at variance with the original IgG1 CD3 antibody (59).

The second nonmitogenic humanized CD3 antibody was produced by the group of J. Bluestone and was derived from OKT3. This humanized γOKT3-5 antibody has been mutated in the Fc region and expresses a 100-fold decrease in its affinity for human Fc receptors as compared with the parental mono-clonal. The γOKT3-5 antibody is not mitogenic in vitro, and it did not show a significant in vivo cytokine-releasing capacity in an experimental model in which severe combined immunodeficient mice (hu-SPL-SCID mice) were inoculated with human splenocytes from cadaveric organ donors (60).

Importantly, similar prolongation of human allograft survival was achieved with both these anti-CD3 mAbs, indicating that they retained significant immunosuppressive properties in vivo.

Beyond Immunosuppression: CD3 Antibodies as Tolerance-Promoting Tools

The experimental and clinical experience in using polyclonal and some monoclonal anti–T-cell antibodies predominantly in transplantation, but also in autoimmunity, has clearly demonstrated their capacity to promote an acquired and durable state of antigen-specific unresponsiveness—namely, immune tolerance (57,76–85). For quite a long time the idea prevailed that only a few antibody specificities were able to afford robust tolerance, and in particular great attention was devoted to CD4 antibodies.

There is now compelling experimental evidence that antibodies to CD3 can also promote long-term specific unresponsiveness to both alloantigens and autoantigens. In the rat, a CD3 antibody induces permanent engraftment of histoincompatible vascularized heart grafts and permanent tolerance as assessed through the survival of donor skin grafts while third-party grafts are normally rejected (86).

This strategy was recently extended to nonhuman primates. A CD3 immunotoxin has been administered to rhesus monkeys associated with either donor bone marrow cells or 15-deoxyspergualin that induced long-term survival of completely mismatched renal allografts (87,88). The same authors implanted three monkeys presenting with spontaneous insulin-dependent diabetes with xenogeneic pancreatic islets under the cover of two injections of CD3 immunotoxin (on day 0 at 2 hours before transplantation and on day +1) supplemented with cyclosporine and steroids administered on days 0 through 4. No additional immunosuppression was given thereafter. All three islet recipients have remained euglycemic at 410, 255, and 100 days of follow-up despite recovery of peripheral T cells to normal levels (89).

Data from our laboratory have also shown the tolerogenic capacity of CD3 antibodies in an autoimmune experimental model—the nonobese diabetic (NOD) mouse. NOD mice develop a spontaneous form of autoimmune insulin-dependent diabetes mellitus that closely resembles the human disease (90,91). Autoreactive T lymphocytes play a major pathogenic role. Both CD4$^+$ T cells, which essentially belong to the IFN-γ–producing Th1 subset, and CD8$^+$ T cells have been implicated in the pathogenesis of the disease (92–97). Diabetogenic T cells, which transfer acute diabetes into immunoincompetent syngeneic recipients, are present in high frequency in the spleens of diabetic NOD mice (92,98). In parallel to these effector cells, there is substantial evidence showing the presence, especially in young prediabetic NOD mice, of a subset of T lymphocytes mediating "active tolerance"—namely, exerting an active control or a down-regulatory effect on diabetogenic lymphocytes or their precursors. Thus, cotransfer experiments have shown that CD4$^+$ T

splenocytes from prediabetic animals fully prevent the transfer of disease by diabetogenic cells (99,100).

A low-dose CD3 treatment applied in overtly diabetic NOD mice induced permanent remission by restoring self-tolerance (57,58). Thus, in mice presenting with full-blown diabetes (i.e., presence of glycosuria and glycemia of 4 g/L or more), a 5-consecutive-day treatment with low doses (5 to 20 μg) of the hamster anti-CD3 monoclonal antibody 145 2C11 induced, in 60% to 80% of mice, complete remission of disease—namely, a return to permanent normoglycemia in the absence of exogenous insulin supply (57,58). In order to ensure the metabolic reconstitution, the treatment had to be started while a significant β-cell mass was still present—that is, within 7 days of the detection of the first signs of overt diabetes. The remission was durable; mice were monitored for up to 8 months following treatment. Importantly, the effect was not related to generalized long-standing immunosuppression, because, at 8 to 10 weeks post anti-CD3 antibody treatment, the mice rejected histoincompatible skin grafts normally. Moreover, these animals, unlike control untreated overtly diabetic NOD females, did not destroy syngeneic islet grafts, thus showing that the anti-CD3 antibody–triggered unresponsiveness was specific for β-cell–associated antigens (57). Among the non–mutually exclusive immune mechanisms that may account for the remission of diabetes induced by anti-CD3 antibody treatment are the physical removal of at least part of the β-cell–specific autoreactive lymphocytes and/or their functional inhibition through a direct effect of the antibody to promote anergy, cytokine-mediated immune deviation of islet reactive cells, or induction of still ill-defined down-regulatory pathways that control the pathogenic potential of diabetogenic lymphocytes (91,99–101). In fact, at present our data argue against a massive deletion of autoreactive cells in protected animals while favoring the presence of immunoregulatory or dominant tolerance immune mechanisms that closely resemble those described in 6-to-8-week-old prediabetic NOD mice (57,58,91,99–102).

Just as do prediabetic NOD mice, anti-CD3–protected mice (20 to 40 weeks of age) present with an insulitis including CD3$^+$αβ$^+$CD4$^+$ and CD8$^+$ cells that remains confined to the periphery of the islets—that is, peripheral insulitis (57,58)—in great distinction to what is observed in untreated age-matched NOD mice that regularly exhibit an invasive/destructive type of insulitis. Moreover, cotransfer experiments could show the presence, in the spleens of protected mice, of CD3$^+$CD62L$^+$ cells that very effectively inhibit the transfer of diabetes by diabetogenic T lymphocytes.

Nonmitogenic F(ab')2 fragments of 145 2C11 were as effective as the whole mitogenic antibody in promoting permanent remission of overt diabetes (58). These results suggest that already available nonmitogenic engineered antibodies to human CD3 (59,103) could represent invaluable therapeutic tools for treating patients presenting with recent onset diabetes. They also present the prospect of using this same therapeutic strategy in other T-cell–dependent autoimmune diseases.

Conclusions

The advent of CD3 monoclonal antibodies almost 20 years ago was a major breakthrough in the field of immunosuppression that allowed the selective targeting of a T-cell surface receptor playing a major functional role. Both the clinical and experimental data accumulated have indicated that CD3 antibodies are probably among the more potent immunosuppressive agents presently available. Moreover, and perhaps more importantly, the recent evidence showing that a short-term course with CD3 antibodies may promote a durable and antigen-specific unresponsiveness opens the way to clinically applicable strategies in both transplantation and autoimmunity. This should be achievable in a not too distant future owing to the availability of humanized nonmitogenic CD3 antibodies that are totally devoid of the well-known toxicity displayed by the original murine CD3 antibodies (104,105).

References

1. Kung P, Goldstein G, Reinherz EL, Schlossman SF. Monoclonal antibodies defining distinctive human T cell surface antigens. Science 1979;206:347–349.
2. Clevers H, Alarcon B, Wileman T, Terhorst C. The T cell receptor/CD3 complex: a dynamic protein ensemble. Annu Rev Immunol 1988;6:629–662.
3. Davis MM, Chien YH. T cell antigen receptors. In: Paul WE, ed. Fundamental immunology. New York: Raven, 1999:341–366.
4. Leo O, Foo M, Sachs DH, et al. Identification of a monoclonal antibody specific for a murine T3 polypeptide. Proc Natl Acad Sci USA 1987;84:1374–1378.
5. Nooij FJ, Jonker M, Balner H. Differentiation antigens on rhesus monkey lymphocytes. II. Characterization of RhT3, a CD3-like antigen on T cells. Eur J Immunol 1986;16:981–984.
6. Cosimi AB, Colvin RB, Burton RC, et al. Use of monoclonal antibodies to T-cell subsets for immunologic monitoring and treatment in recipients of renal allografts. N Engl J Med 1981;305:308–314.
7. Cosimi AB, Burton RC, Colvin RB, et al. Treatment of acute renal allograft rejection with OKT3 monoclonal antibody. Transplantation 1981;32:535–539.
8. Ortho Multicenter Transplant Study Group. A randomized clinical trial of OKT3 monoclonal antibody for acute rejection of cadaveric renal transplants. N Engl J Med 1985;313:337–342.
9. Goldstein G. Overview of the development of Orthoclone OKT3: monoclonal antibody for therapeutic use in transplantation. Transplant Proc 1987;19:1–6.
10. Hricik DE, Zarconi J, Schulak JA. Influence of low-dose cyclosporine on the outcome of treatment with OKT3 for acute renal allograft rejection. Transplantation 1989;47:272–277.
11. Normal DJ, Barry JM, Bennett WM, et al. The use of OKT3 in cadaveric renal transplantation for rejection that is unresponsive to conventional anti-rejection therapy. Am J Kidney Dis 1988;11:90–93.
12. Colonna Jo II, Goldstein LI, Brems JJ, et al. A prospective study on the use of monoclonal anti-T3-cell antibody (OKT3) to treat steroid-resistant liver transplant rejection. Arch Surg 1987;122:1120–1123.
13. Woodle ES, Thistlethwaite JR Jr, Emond JC, et al. OKT3 therapy for hepatic allograft rejection. Differential response in adults and children. Transplantation 1991;51:1207–1212.
14. Goldstein G, Kremer AB, Barnes L, Hirsch RL. OKT3 monoclonal antibody reversal of renal and hepatic rejection in pediatric patients. J Pediatr 1987;111:1046–1050.
15. Gilbert EM, Dewitt CW, Eiswirth CC, et al. Treatment of refractory cardiac allograft rejection with OKT3 monoclonal antibody. Am J Med 1987;82:202–206.
16. Farges O, Samuel D, Bismuth H. Orthoclone OKT3 in liver transplantation. Transplant Sci 1992;2:16–21.
17. Vigeral P, Chkoff N, Chatenoud L, et al. Prophylactic use of OKT3 monoclonal antibody in cadaver kidney recipients. Utilization of OKT3 as the sole immunosuppressive agent. Transplantation 1986;41:730–733.
18. Chatenoud L, Baudrihaye MF, Kreis H, et al. Human in vivo antigenic modulation induced by the anti-T cell OKT3 monoclonal antibody. Eur J Immunol 1982;12:979–982.
19. Chatenoud L, Baudrihaye MF, Chkoff N, et al. Restriction of the human in vivo immune response against the mouse monoclonal antibody OKT3. J Immunol 1986;137:830–838.
20. Frey DJ, Matas AJ, Gillingham KJ, et al. Sequential therapy—a prospective randomized trial of MALG versus OKT3 for prophylactic immunosuppression in cadaver renal allograft recipients. Transplantation 1992;54:50–56.
21. Debure A, Chkoff N, Chatenoud L, et al. One-month prophylactic use of OKT3 in cadaver kidney transplant recipients. Transplantation 1988;45:546–553.
22. Abramowicz D, Goldman M, de Pauw L, et al. The long-term effects of prophylactic OKT3 monoclonal antibody in cadaver kidney transplantation—a single-center, prospective, randomized study. Transplantation 1992;54:433–437.
23. Farges O, Ericzon BG, Bresson-Hadni S, et al. A randomized trial of OKT3-based versus cyclosporine-based immunoprophylaxis after liver transplantation. Long-term results of a European and Australian multicenter study. Transplantation 1994;58:891–898.
24. Millis JM, McDiarmid SV, Hiatt JR, et al. Randomized prospective trial of OKT3 for early prophylaxis of rejection after liver transplantation. Transplantation 1989;47:82–88.
25. Eason JD, Cosimi AB. Biologic immunosuppressive agents. In: Ginns LC, Cosimi AB, Morris PJ, eds. Transplantation. Malden, MA: Blackwell Science, 1999:196–224.
26. Robbins RC, Oyer PE, Stinson EB, Starnes VA. The use of monoclonal antibodies after heart transplantation. Transplant Sci 1992;2:22–27.
27. Ericzon BG, Salmela K, Barkholt L, Hockerstedt K. OKT3 prophylaxis in liver transplantation: the Scandinavian experience. Transplant Proc 1990;22:223–224.
28. Niaudet P, Jean G, Broyer M, Chatenoud L. Anti-OKT3 response following prophylactic treatment in paediatric kidney transplant recipients. Pediatr Nephrol 1993;7:263–267.
29. Cosimi AB. Clinical development of Orthoclone OKT3. Transplant Proc 1987;19:7–16.
30. Chatenoud L, Legendre C, Ferran C, et al. Corticosteroid inhibition of the OKT3-induced cytokine-related syndrome—dosage and kinetics prerequisites. Transplantation 1991;51:334–338.

31. Abramowicz D, Schandene L, Goldman M, et al. Release of tumor necrosis factor, interleukin-2, and gamma-interferon in serum after injection of OKT3 monoclonal antibody in kidney transplant recipients. Transplantation 1989;47:606–608.

32. Swinnen LJ, Costanzo-Nordin MR, Fisher SG, et al. Increased incidence of lymphoproliferative disorder after immunosuppression with the monoclonal antibody OKT3 in cardiac-transplant recipients. N Engl J Med 1990; 323:1723–1728.

33. Hirsch R, Eckhaus M, Auchincloss H Jr, et al. Effects of in vivo administration of anti-T3 monoclonal antibody on T cell function in mice. I. Immunosuppression of transplantation responses. J Immunol 1988;140:3766–3772.

34. Isaacs JD, Clark MR, Greenwood J, Waldmann H. Therapy with monoclonal antibodies. An in vivo model for the assessment of therapeutic potential. J Immunol 1992;148:3062–3071.

35. Wong JT, Colvin RB. Selective reduction and proliferation of the CD4+ and CD8+ T cell subsets with bispecific monoclonal antibodies: evidence for inter-T cell-mediated cytolysis. Clin Immunol Immunopathol 1991;58:236–250.

36. Smith CA, Williams GT, Kingston R, et al. Antibodies to Cd3/T-cell receptor complex induce death by apoptosis in immature T cells in thymic cultures. Nature 1989;337: 181–184.

37. Wesselborg S, Janssen O, Kabelitz D. Induction of activation-driven death (apoptosis) in activated but not resting peripheral blood T cells. J Immunol 1993;150:4338–4345.

38. Choy EH, Adjaye, J Forrest L, et al. Chimaeric anti-CD4 monoclonal antibody cross-linked by monocyte Fc gamma receptor mediates apoptosis of human CD4 lymphocytes. Eur J Immunol 1993;23:2676–2681.

39. Chatenoud L, Bach JF. Antigenic modulation: a major mechanism of antibody action. Immunol Today 1984;5:20–25.

40. Caillat-Zucman S, Blumenfeld N, Legendre C, et al. The OKT3 immunosuppressive effect. In situ antigenic modulation of human graft-infiltrating T cells. Transplantation 1990; 49:156–160.

41. Routledge EG, Lloyd I, Gorman SD, et al. A humanized monovalent CD3 antibody which can activate homologous complement. Eur J Immunol 1991;21:2717–2725.

42. Smely S, Weschka M, Hillebrand G, et al. Prophylactic use of the new monoclonal antibody BMA 031 in clinical kidney transplantation. Transplant Proc 1990;22:1785–1786.

43. Baudrihaye MF, Chatenoud L, Kreis H, et al. Unusually restricted anti-isotype human immune response to KOT3 monoclonal antibody Eur J Immunol 1984;14:686–691.

44. Jonker M, Den Brok JH. Idiotype switching of CD4-specific monoclonal antibodies can prolong the therapeutic effectiveness in spite of host anti-mouse IgG antibodies. Eur J Immunol 1987;17:1547–1553.

45. Chatenoud L, Jonker M, Villemain F, et al. The human immune response to the OKT3 monoclonal antibody is oligoclonal. Science 1986;232:1406–1408.

46. Abramowicz D, Crusiaux A, Goldman M. Anaphylactic shock after retreatment with OKT3 monoclonal antibody. N Engl J Med 1992;327:736.

47. Hricik DE, Mayes JT, Schulak JA. Inhibition of anti-OKT3

48. Hirsch R, Gress RE, Pluznik DH, et al. Effects of in vivo administration of anti-CD3 monoclonal antibody on T cell function in mice. II. In vivo activation of T cells. J Immunol 1989;142:737–743.

49. Ferran C, Sheehan K, Dy M, et al. Cytokine-related syndrome following injection of anti-CD3 monoclonal antibody: further evidence for transient in vivo T cell activation. Eur J Immunol 1990;20:509–515.

50. Alegre M, Vandenabeele P, Flamand V, et al. Hypothermia and hypoglycemia induced by anti-CD3 monoclonal antibody in mice: role of tumor necrosis factor. Eur J Immunol 1990;20:707–710.

51. Durez P, Abramowicz D, Gerard C, et al. In vivo induction of interleukin 10 by anti-CD3 monoclonal antibody or bacterial lipopolysaccharide: differential modulation by cyclosporin A. J Exp Med 1993;177:551–555.

52. Yoshimoto T, Paul WE. CD4pos, NK1.1pos T cells promptly produce interleukin 4 in response to in vivo challenge with anti-CD3. J Exp Med 1994;179:1285–1295.

53. Flamand V, Abramowicz D, Goldman M, et al. Anti-CD3 antibodies induce T cells from unprimed animals to secrete IL-4 both in vitro and in vivo. J Immunol 1990;144:2875–2882.

54. Van Lier RA, Boot JH, de Groot ER, Aarden LA. Induction of T cell proliferation with anti-CD3 switch-variant monoclonal antibodies: effects of heavy chain isotype in monocyte-dependent systems. Eur J Immunol 1987;17: 1599–1604.

55. Hirsch R, Bluestone JA, de Nenno L, Gress RE. Anti-CD3 F(ab')2 fragments are immunosuppressive in vivo without evoking either the strong humoral response or morbidity associated with whole mAb. Transplantation 1990;49:1117–1123.

56. Parlevliet KJ, Ten Berge IJ, Young SL, et al. In vivo effects of IgA and IgG2a anti-CD3 isotype switch variants. J Clin Invest 1994;93:2519–2525.

57. Chatenoud L, Thervet E, Primo J, Bach JF. Anti-CD3 antibody induces long-term remission of overt autoimmunity in nonobese diabetic mice. Proc Natl Acad Sci USA 1994; 91:123–127.

58. Chatenoud L, Primo J, Bach JF. CD3 antibody-induced dominant self tolerance in overtly diabetic NOD mice. J Immunol 1997;158:2947–2954.

59. Bolt S, Routledge E, Lloyd I, et al. The generation of a humanized, nonmitogenic CD3 monoclonal antibody which retains in vitro immunosuppressive properties. Eur J Immunol 1993;23:403–411.

60. Alegre ML, Peterson LJ, Xu D, et al. A non-activating "humanized" anti-CD3 monoclonal antibody retains immunosuppressive properties in vivo. Transplantation 1994;57:1537–1543.

61. Hirsch R, Archibald J, Gress RE. Differential T cell hyporesponsiveness induced by in vivo administration of intact or F(ab')2 fragments of anti-CD3 monoclonal antibody. F(ab')2 fragments induce a selective T helper dysfunction. J Immunol 1991;147:2088–2093.

62. Hughes C, Wolos JA, Giannini EH, Hirsch R. Induction of T helper cell hyporesponsiveness in an experimental model

antibody generation by cyclosporine—results of a prospective randomized trial. Transplantation 1990;50:237–240.

of autoimmunity by using nonmitogenic anti-CD3 monoclonal antibody. J Immunol 1994;153:3319–3325.

63. Herold KC, Bluestone JA, Montag AG, et al. Prevention of autoimmune diabetes with nonactivating anti-CD3 monoclonal antibody. Diabetes 1992;41:385–391.

64. Johnson BD, McCabe C, Hanke CA, Truitt RL. Use of anti-CD3 epsilon F(ab')2 fragments in vivo to modulate graft-versus-host disease without loss of graft-versus-leukemia reactivity after MHC-matched bone marrow transplantation. J Immunol 1995;154:5542–5554.

65. Chatenoud L, Legendre C, Kurrle R, et al. Absence of clinical symptoms following the first injection of anti-T cell receptor monoclonal antibody (BMA 031) despite isolated TNF release. Transplantation 1993;55:443–445.

66. Ferran C, Dy M, Sheehan K, et al. Cascade modulation by anti-tumor necrosis factor monoclonal antibody of interferon-gamma, interleukin 3 and interleukin 6 release after triggering of the CD3/T cell receptor activation pathway. Eur J Immunol 1991;21:2349–2353.

67. Charpentier B, Hiesse C, Lantz O, et al. Evidence that anti-human tumor necrosis factor monoclonal antibody prevents OKT3-induced acute syndrome. Transplantation 1992;54:997–1002.

68. Riechmann L, Clark M, Waldmann H, Winter G. Reshaping human antibodies for therapy. Nature 1988;332:323–327.

69. Morrison SL, Johnson MJ, Herzenberg LA, Oi VT. Chimeric human antibody molecules: mouse antigen-binding domains with human constant region domains. Proc Natl Acad Sci USA 1984;81:6851–6855.

70. Lazarovits AI, Rochon J, Banks L, et al. Human mouse chimeric CD7 monoclonal antibody (SDZCHH380) for the prophylaxis of kidney transplant rejection. J Immunol 1993;150:5163–5174.

71. Elliott MJ, Maini RN, Feldmann M, et al. Repeated therapy with monoclonal antibody to tumour necrosis factor alpha (cA2) in patients with rheumatoid arthritis. Lancet 1994;344:1125–1127.

72. Vincenti F, Kirkman R, Light S, et al. Interleukin-2-receptor blockade with daclizumab to prevent acute rejection in renal transplantation. Daclizumab Triple Therapy Study Group [see comments]. N Engl J Med 1998;338:161–165.

73. Nashan B, Moore R, Amlot P, et al. Randomised trial of basiliximab versus placebo for control of acute cellular rejection in renal allograft recipients. CHIB 201 International Study Group [published erratum appears in Lancet 1997 Nov 15;350(9089):1484]. Lancet 1997;350:1193–1198.

74. Isaacs JD, Watts RA, Hazleman BL, et al. Humanised monoclonal antibody therapy for rheumatoid arthritis. Lancet 1992;340:748–752.

75. Routledge EG, Falconer ME, Pope H, et al. The effect of aglycosylation on the immunogenicity of a humanized therapeutic CD3 monoclonal antibody. Transplantation 1995;60:847–853.

76. Benjamin RJ, Waldmann H. Induction of tolerance by monoclonal antibody therapy. Nature 1986;320:449–451.

77. Gutstein NL, Seaman WE, Scott JH, Wofsy D. Induction of immune tolerance by administration of monoclonal antibody to L3T4. J Immunol 1986;137:1127–1132.

78. Cobbold SP, Qin S, Leong LY, et al. Reprogramming the immune system for peripheral tolerance with CD4 and CD8 monoclonal antibodies. Immunol Rev 1992;129:165–201.

79. Qin S, Cobbold SP, Pope H, et al. "Infectious" transplantation tolerance. Science 1993;259:974–977.

80. Isobe M, Yagita H, Okumura K, Ihara A. Specific acceptance of cardiac allograft after treatment with antibodies to ICAM-1 and LFA-1. Science 1992;255:1125–1127.

81. Lin H, Bolling SF, Linsley PS, et al. Long-term acceptance of major histocompatibility complex mismatched cardiac allografts induced by CTLA4Ig plus donor-specific transfusion. J Exp Med 1993;178:1801–1806.

82. Pearson TC, Madsen JC, Larsen CP, et al. Induction of transplantation tolerance in adults using donor antigen and anti-CD4 monoclonal antibody. Transplantation 1992;54:475–483.

83. Wofsy D, Seaman WE. Reversal of advanced murine lupus in NZB/NZW F1 mice by treatment with monoclonal antibody to L3T4. J Immunol 1987;138:3247–3253.

84. Wood KJ. Transplantation tolerance with monoclonal antibodies. Semin Immunol 1990;2:389–399.

85. Shizuru JA, Taylor-Edwards C, Banks BA, et al. Immunotherapy of the nonobese diabetic mouse: treatment with an antibody to T-helper lymphocytes. Science 1988;240:659–662.

86. Nicolls MR, Aversa GG, Pearce NW, et al. Induction of long-term specific tolerance to allografts in rats by therapy with an anti-CD3-like monoclonal antibody. Transplantation 1993;55:459–468.

87. Thomas JM, Neville DM, Contreras JL, et al. Preclinical studies of allograft tolerance in rhesus monkeys: a novel anti-CD3-immunotoxin given peritransplant with donor bone marrow induces operational tolerance to kidney allografts. Transplantation 1997;64:124–135.

88. Hamawy MM, Knechtle SJ. Strategies for tolerance induction in nonhuman primates. [Review] [26 refs.] Curr Opin Immunol 1998;10:513–517.

89. Thomas FT, Ricordi C, Contreras JL, et al. Reversal of naturally occurring diabetes in primates by unmodified islet xenografts without chronic immunosuppression. Transplantation 1999;67:846–854.

90. Castano L, Eisenbarth GS. Type-I diabetes: a chronic autoimmune disease of human, mouse, and rat. Annu Rev Immunol 1990;8:647–679.

91. Bach JF. Insulin-dependent diabetes mellitus as an autoimmune disease. Endocrine Rev 1994;15:516–542.

92. Bendelac A, Carnaud C, Boitard C, Bach JF. Syngeneic transfer of autoimmune diabetes from diabetic NOD mice to healthy neonates. Requirement for both L3T4+ and Lyt-2+ T cells. J Exp Med 1987;166:823–832.

93. Miller BJ, Appel MC, O'Neil JJ, Wicker LS. Both the Lyt-2+ and L3T4+ T cell subsets are required for the transfer of diabetes in nonobese diabetic mice. J Immunol 1988;140:52–58.

94. Yagi H, Matsumoto M, Kunimoto K, et al. Analysis of the roles of CD4+ and CD8+ T cells in autoimmune diabetes of NOD mice using transfer to NOD athymic nude mice. Eur J Immunol 1992;22:2387–2393.

95. Haskins K, Portas M, Bergman B, et al. Pancreatic islet-specific T-cell clones from nonobese diabetic mice. Proc Natl Acad Sci USA 1989;86:8000–8004.

96. Katz JD, Benoist C, Mathis D. T helper cell subsets in insulin-dependent diabetes. Science 1995;268:1185–1188.

97. Healey D, Ozegbe P, Arden S, et al. In vivo activity and in vitro specificity of CD4+ Th1 and Th2 cells derived from the

spleens of diabetic NOD mice. J Clin Invest 1995;95:2979–2985.

98. Wicker LS, Miller BJ, Mullen Y. Transfer of autoimmune diabetes mellitus with splenocytes from nonobese diabetic (NOD) mice. Diabetes 1986;35:855–860.

99. Boitard C, Yasunami R, Dardenne M, Bach JF. T cell-mediated inhibition of the transfer of autoimmune diabetes in NOD mice. J Exp Med 1989;169:1669–1680.

100. Hutchings PR, Cooke A. The transfer of autoimmune diabetes in NOD mice can be inhibited or accelerated by distinct cell populations present in normal splenocytes taken from young males. J Autoimmun 1990;3:175–185.

101. Delovitch TL, Singh B. The nonobese diabetic mouse as a model of autoimmune diabetes: immune dysregulation gets the NOD. Immunity 1997;7:727–738.

102. Yasunami R, Debray-Sachs M, Bach JF. Ontogeny of regulatory and effector T-cells in autoimmune NOD mice. In: Shafrir E, ed. Frontiers in diabetes research. Lessons from animal diabetes III. London: Smith-Gordon, 1990:88–93.

103. Alegre ML, Collins AM, Pulito VL, et al. Effect of a single amino acid mutation on the activating and immunosuppressive properties of a "humanized" OKT3 monoclonal antibody. J Immunol 1992;148:3461–3468.

104. Friend PJ, Hale G, Chatenoud L, et al. Phase I study of an engineered aglycosylated humanized CD3 antibody in renal transplant rejection. Transplantation 1999;68:1632–1637.

105. Woodle ES, Xu D, Zivin RA, et al. Phase I trial of a humanized, Fc receptor nonbinding OKT3 antibody, huOKT3 gamma 1 (Ala-Ala) in the treatment of acute renal allograft rejection. Transplantation 1999;68:608–616.

Chapter 25

Anti-IgE: Immunotherapy for Allergic Diseases

Donald MacGlashan, Jr.

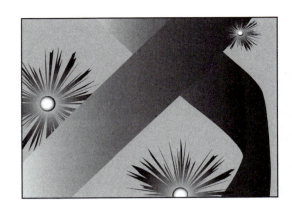

Once IgE was recognized in the 1960s to be a central and causative element in atopy, it has been a goal to develop the means to down-regulate its expression. Achieving this goal has required new information from many facets of immunobiology, and various approaches now exist that capitalize on the new understanding of the origins of the immune response that leads to generation of IgE. Current therapeutic approaches reach as far back into the process as modifying the "Th2ness" of the overall immune response (e.g., DNA vaccines [1]). However, an appealing general approach is based on the straightforward understanding that a large component of atopy results from the binding of IgE to its high-affinity receptor (FcεRI). There are a variety of ways to interfere with this interaction. For example, simple non-peptide organics or peptide antagonists that mimic IgE itself would compete for the high-affinity receptor binding site. This approach or its inverse, receptor mimetics that bind to IgE, are still in development and should be greatly aided by the recent publication of the x-ray crystallographic structure of the high-affinity receptor alpha subunit (2).

An alternative approach was considered decades ago—to use anti-IgE antibodies to clear IgE from the serum. However, it was immediately recognized that polyclonal antibodies not only would bind to IgE circulating in the serum but would attach to IgE bound to its high-affinity receptor on mast cells and basophils. Such binding would initiate mediator release from these cells, causing a severe anaphylactic reaction in the patient. After the development of techniques to generate monoclonal antibodies and the means to convert mouse antibodies into their human equivalents by "splicing" in the binding site amino acids (complementarity-determining regions) from the mouse monoclonal to an engineered human IgG, it became feasible to conceive of anti-IgE antibody as a therapeutic approach. The concept was to develop a monoclonal antibody that bound to the portion of IgE that is hidden in the receptor when IgE is bound to FcεRIα (3–6). With these constraints, the anti-IgE antibody could be safely administered to patients—it would bind only to free IgE antibody and thereby prevent its binding to any cells possessing FcεRI (and, as it turns out, also prevent binding to FcεRII). The characteristics of this kind of antibody are described in Figure 25-1. In the late 1980s and early 1990s, several antibodies were developed with these characteristics, and two of them, CGP51901 from Tanox/Novartis and E25 from Genentech, Inc., reached the level of clinical testing. Through a cooperative agreement between the two companies, E25 has progressed into phase III clinical trials.

There are valuable lessons to be learned from studies with these two antibodies in patients. If properly administered, these antibodies may provide the needed proof-of-concept for all approaches that seek to down-regulate the expression of IgE as a means to eliminate the atopic condition. However, even before the recent clinical testing of these antibodies, some biologic aspects raised concerns about the potential efficacy of such an approach. This chapter presents a review of recent clinical experience with anti-IgE antibodies, as well as the various biologic and immunologic constraints that may dictate how these new therapeutics should be managed.

Characteristics of the Problem

IgE binds to FcεRI with an extremely high affinity (7). Any agent that interferes with this association must also bind with a reasonably high affinity to IgE or else become impractical to use solely because the concentrations required would be prohibitive. Sufficient understanding exists about the sensitivity of human basophils and mast cells to make a prediction regarding the characteristics required of such agents. The goal is to reduce the effective, free-circulating IgE concentration sufficiently to suppress the mast cell or basophil response when these cells are challenged with antigens to which the individual is sensitive. The starting point for a prediction is the knowledge that most human basophils and mast cells require, on average, only 2000 to 3000 molecules of antigen-specific IgE on the surface of the cell to initiate an antigen-driven response that is half of the cell's maximal response (8,9). From physiologic studies, it is estimated that maximal smooth-muscle contraction in the human airway may result from the secretion by tissue mast cells of only 2% to 5% of the maximum possible amount of either histamine or sulfidopeptide leukotrienes. Therefore, secretion must be suppressed to 5% or less of the amount that the cell is capable of secreting. Because it is not known whether the level of release observed in tissue baths results from strong release in restricted locations of the tissue or weak release from all the cells of the tissue, the precise relationship between secretion and physiologic response is not yet fully defined. From the known physiologic data and the data regarding cellular sensitivity, one can estimate that fewer than 500 molecules of antigen-specific IgE must reside on the basophil or mast cell.

A typical circulating basophil in an atopic individual has approximately 250,000 FcεRI receptors on its plasma membrane

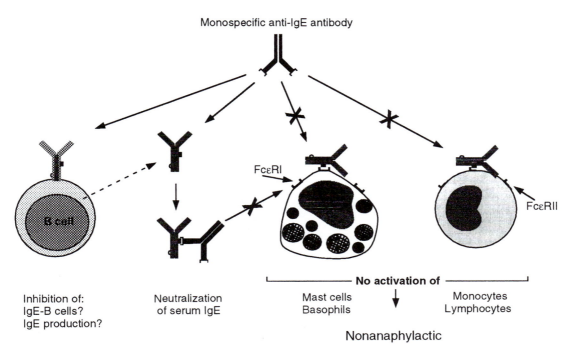

Figure 25-1. Characteristics of current, humanized, monoclonal anti-IgE antibodies.

surface. A typical serum IgE concentration might be 500ng/mL (225IU). The relationship between the occupancy of these receptors with IgE and the concentration of IgE follows a classic, ligand-binding curve whose midpoint is a function of the affinity of IgE for the receptor. Because the affinity of IgE is very high, this midpoint occurs well below the typical circulating IgE concentration in an atopic individual. The precise midpoint is not known because estimates of the affinity in the older literature may be artifactually low. Even with estimates of the affinity from the literature, the midpoint resides between 10 and 30ng/mL. Inasmuch as this represents the point of 50% occupancy, IgE concentrations need to be reduced 2000 to 10,000-fold (for typical aeroallergens, 10% of the circulating IgE may be specific for the antigens involved in the specific immune response). Such a reduction in IgE is a demanding requirement, and, based on the known affinities of the developed anti-IgE monoclonal antibodies, it would not be practically achievable.

A critical element not considered in the analysis above is the feedback loop between circulating IgE and the expression of FcεRI on basophils and mast cells (and possibly other cells that are now known to express this receptor). Studies by Malveaux and Lichtenstein in 1978 (10) demonstrated the log-linear relationship between serum IgE concentration and the density of FcεRI on peripheral blood basophils. Twenty years later, this relationship is understood to result from the ability of IgE to up-regulate the expression of FcεRI with its presence and to down-regulate the expression of FcεRI with its absence (7,11–15). The mechanism underlying this regulation is not yet known, although current evidence supports a view that IgE stabilizes the presence

of FcεRI on the plasma membrane of a cell that is a constitutively synthesizing receptor. An understanding of this mechanism may be highly relevant to the development of new therapeutics, including the use of anti-IgE antibody. However, the existence of this feedback loop changes the prediction noted in Figure 25-2. Now, as the IgE concentration drops, so does the cell-surface expression of FcεRI. These two events changing in concert allow a decrease of free-circulating IgE by about 100-fold to achieve a marked suppression of mediator release from basophils and mast cells. One of the clinical trials of E25 allowed this prediction to be verified experimentally. These same considerations have important implications for the implementation of these therapies.

Safety Considerations Related to the Biology of IgE

For any therapeutic approach that seeks to decrease free IgE levels in serum and tissue, concerns are raised that relate to the speculated protective effects of IgE. It has long been hypothesized that IgE provides protection in parasitic infections because serum IgE levels are markedly elevated in patients with these diseases. Depending on the model under study, in vitro or animal studies support or refute a role for IgE in parasite rejection, and correlative and epidemiologic studies in humans present a similarly confusing picture (16–18). However, parasite-specific IgE often accounts for only a small fraction of the total IgE, thus leading to the alternative hypothesis that the large rise in IgE is

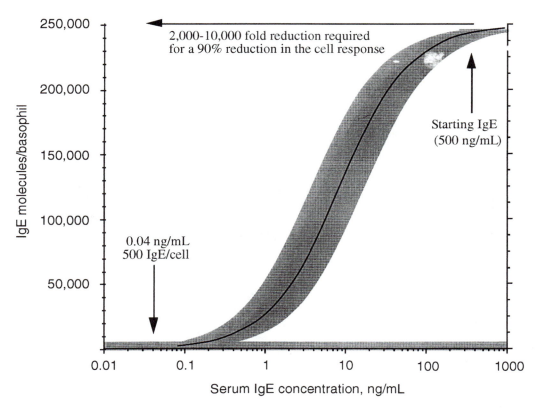

Figure 25-2. Titration of IgE binding to basophil or mast cell FcεRI. The simple ligand binding curve shown is representative of the situation for an atopic patient in the absence of any IgE-mediated regulation of the expression of FcεRI. Based on evidence for the sensitivity of human basophils to stimulation through FcεRI, cell-surface densities must be within the horizontal gray region shown along the x-axis. The gray region surrounding the ligand binding curve represents the ambiguity in the published observations about the affinity of IgE for FcεRI. As noted in the text, the nature of this curve is altered when feedback between serum IgE and cell-surface expression of FcεRI is included in the calculations.

indirectly driven by the parasite, so that the antiparasitic functions of IgE are effectively diluted as the ratio of specific to nonspecific IgE falls. Whatever the basis of the association, studies of a mouse model of *Shistosoma mansoni* infections demonstrated that the reduction of IgE to nondetectable levels (with a polyclonal antimouse IgE) resulted in *decreased* worm burden and egg production in the infected animals (19). It is not clear how to reconcile these results with the finding in IgE knockout mice that the absence of IgE leads to increased worm burdens (20). The precise role of IgE in human parasitic diseases will be understood only through long-term monitoring of patients who receive IgE-reducing therapy.

For nearly 25 years, IgE has been considered to have a protective role in the development of respiratory tract infections (21), but there is no evidence to support such a view. In an anecdotal report, Levy et al described a healthy individual with an isolated deficiency of IgE who had no other immunoglobulin abnormalities (22) and no identified increase in the incidence of infections. In the clinical trials of anti-IgE antibody thus far reported, there has been no observed incidence of increased infections.

Pharmacologic/Immunologic Properties of Anti-IgE Antibody

The two humanized antibodies that have been used in clinical trials were engineered to minimize the presence of immunogenic mouse sequences. E25 was engineered to exclude the complement binding site; CGP 51901 contains such a site, but has not been observed to activate complement. In early studies, the antibodies were administered by intravenous injection; subcutaneous injection was shown to be equally effective and has been used in recent phase III trials. Once injected, the antibodies form immune complexes with circulating IgE that appear to be limited in size (23,24). Depending on the relative concentrations of the two components, immune complexes range from cyclic trimers to hexamers of IgE and anti-IgE. Probably as a result of their small size, these complexes do not associate with cells expressing Fcγ receptors and therefore do not interact significantly with the reticuloendothelial system. The complexes and/or anti-IgE antibody remain associated with the blood compartment with no preferential association with tissues, including kidney (for a study period of 1 to 96 hours in cynomolgus monkeys) (23–25) and are eliminated primarily through urinary excretion.

Clinical Trials

Several clinical trials have been conducted in which the efficacy of anti-IgE antibodies to treat either allergic rhinitis or atopic asthma was studied, and the results have been published. In these trials, the doses of anti-IgE antibody were calculated on the basis of body weight alone, which has implications for the expected outcome. These trials assessed the relationship between the dose of anti-IgE antibody and the reduction in IgE and also demonstrated the dose relationship to the various clinical and laboratory indices examined.

A parallel group, randomized, placebo-controlled study of mild atopic patients with asthma was performed by Boulet et al (26). These patients were receiving only β2 agonists on an as-needed basis. Six doses of anti-IgE antibody (rhuMAb-E25) were administered intravenously, 2 weeks apart, with an initial dose of 2 mg/kg and subsequent doses of 1 mg/kg. Serum IgE levels in the actively treated group were reduced to approximately 10% of their starting levels (and those of the placebo group). Two clinical end points were examined: 1) allergen bronchial challenge four times before treatment, two times during treatment, and two times after treatment; and 2) methacholine bronchoprovocation challenge before, during, and after treatment. Skin testing to the relevant allergens was also performed. The results of these studies are summarized in Figure 25-3. Most notable was that by

day 27 of treatment, there was a reduction in the airway responsiveness to allergen challenge, measured as an increase in concentration of allergen, approximately 4-fold, required to induce a change in PC_{15}. This change persisted throughout treatment. Modest but statistically significant changes in the methacholine reactivity were reported. There were no changes in skin test reactivity to the relevant allergens.

In a similar randomized, placebo-controlled study performed by Fahy et al (27), patients with mild asthma received weekly intravenous doses of E25, 0.5 mg/kg, for 9 weeks. Pretrial serum IgE levels were $\leq$500 IU/mL (1100 ng/mL). Airway responsiveness was assessed by bronchial allergen challenge and methacholine reactivity (the effect of prior allergen on methacholine reactivity was also assessed by methacholine bronchoprovocation 24 hours after allergen challenge). Pulmonary function was assessed both early and late by following indices for 7 hours. Skin tests, sputum induction, and serum IgE levels were monitored. Free serum IgE levels were undetectable by the end of the study in six of the nine patients who received E25. Typically, IgE assays are sensitive to less than 0.25 ng/mL of IgE, but in early studies of E25, the assessment of free IgE was restricted to levels above 25 ng/mL of IgE. More recently, for example, in the phase I trial discussed below, minimum detectable levels were 3 to 5 ng/mL.

The salient features of the results are summarized in Figure 25-4. Treatment with E25 (bottom panel) caused significant reductions in both components of the airway response despite the fact that higher doses of allergen were required to elicit the 20% reduction observed in the treated individuals. Furthermore, methacholine reactivity did not increase after allergen challenge

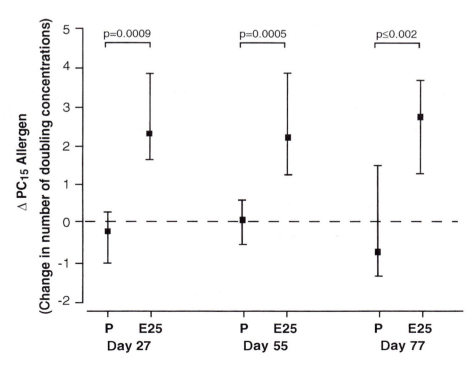

Figure 25-3. Effect of anti-IgE antibody (rhuMAb-E25) on acute airway responsiveness to allergen challenge. rhuMAb-E25 reduced acute airway responsiveness to allergen challenge by approximately two doubling doses in patients with asthma. The effects were similar for the 27th, 55th, and 77th days of treatment. The ordinate shows the change in allergen-induced PC_{15} from the pretreatment measurement in terms of the amount of allergen required to elicit the same PC_{15} response (i.e., a positive change means more allergen is required to elicit a change in lung function of 15%). Data shown are the median and the 25th to 75th quartiles, P, placebo; E25, rhuMAb-E25 anti-IgE treated. (Reprinted with permission from Boulet L, Chapman K, Cote J, et al. Inhibitory effects of an anti-IgE antibody E25 on allergen-induced early asthmatic responses. Am J Respir Crit Care Med 1997;155:1835–1840. Official journal of the American Thoracic Society. © American Lung Association.)

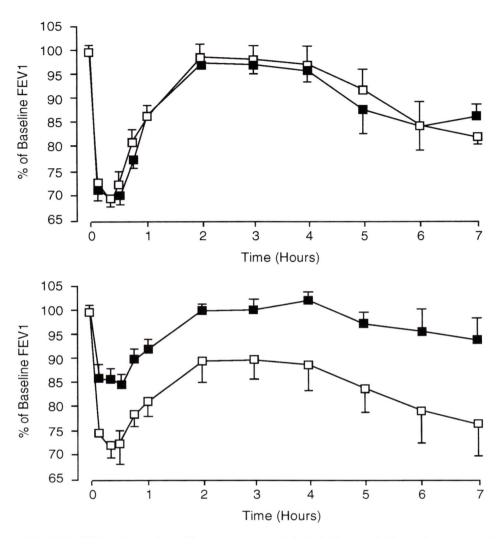

Figure 25-4. Effect of rhuMAb-E25 on the early and late responses to inhaled allergen challenge in patients with asthma. The pulmonary function parameter, FEV_1, as a percent of the baseline FEV_1 before challenge, is shown on the ordinate. Results (mean ± SD) are shown for nine patients treated with placebo (*top panel*) and nine patients treated with E25 (*bottom panel*) before (□) and after (■) the respective treatments. (Reprinted with permission from Fahy J, Fleming H, Wong H, et al. The effect of an anti-IgE monoclonal antibody on the early- and late-phase responses to allergen inhalation in asthmatic subjects. Am J Respir Crit Care Med 1997;155:1828–1834. Official Journal of the American Thoracic Society. © American Lung Association.)

of patients who had received E25. Although there was a trend toward a reduction in the number of eosinophils in sputum, it was not statistically significant. There were no changes in skin test reactivity.

There is one published report of an early trial of E25 in patients with seasonal allergic rhinitis (28). As with the studies discussed above, E25 was administered on the basis of body weight, and a population of 240 individuals was divided into four groups in a placebo-controlled, randomized, parallel group design. Each of the groups received treatments beginning 1 month before the ragweed season and every 2 weeks thereafter

for a total of eight treatments. Dosing included placebo, subcutaneous antibody at 0.15 mg/kg, the same dose intravenously, and a higher dose of 0.5 mg/kg intravenously. Free circulating IgE levels were suppressed not more than 60% in patients receiving the lower doses, and averaged only 70% in patients receiving the higher dose; in only a few patients was free circulating IgE undetectable, that is, ≤24 ng/mL. Although there were no statistically significant effects on symptoms of allergic rhinitis, the study did provide some insights into dosing regimens. This study suggested that subcutaneous and intravenous administrations should be equivalent in efficacy. In addition, it was possible to tease out of the data indications for a changed approach to dosing to account for the amount of circulating IgE before treatment. Thus, a phase I safety assessment of high doses of E25 given for a 1-year period was initiated in which various in vitro parameters of the atopic status of the patients were assessed.

Immunologic Effects of in vivo Treatment

The open-label, phase I safety trial of rhuMAb-E25, which lasted for nearly 1 year in 47 individuals with perennial allergic rhinitis and positive skin-prick tests to dust mites, used dosing that took into account the baseline serum IgE levels. The subjects were divided according to the baseline IgE level: high (251 to 550 IU/mL) and low (85 to 250 IU/mL). The dose of E25 was either 0.15 mg/kg/IU/mL or 0.03 mg/kg/IU/mL given intravenously.

In addition to a variety of safety outcomes, free and total IgE levels were monitored and skin test titrations were made before treatment and after 182 days. Some subjects were also examined by nasal provocation. For 15 patients, an extensive evaluation of several characteristics of peripheral blood basophils was made before treatment, 90 days into treatment, at the point just before the end of treatment, and at the end of a monitoring period that extended up to 1 year after treatment (12,29). The last assessment was made either when free serum IgE levels rose above 50% of the pretreatment levels or at 1 year, whichever occurred first.

For the basophil parameters, the response of the cells to stimulation with goat polyclonal anti-IgE antibody, *Dermatophagoides farinae* (DF) antigen, or the bacterial peptide, f-Met-Leu-Phe (FMLP), was examined. FMLP was used as an internal control because this stimulus activates basophils through a mechanism not dependent on FcεRI. In addition, the cell-surface density of FcεRI, both occupied and unoccupied, was examined by two techniques, so-called acetate stripping (where IgE is stripped from washed, enriched basophils of known number and measured by radioimmunoadsorbant test to calculate absolute cell-surface IgE density) or by flow cytometry (which gives a relative assessment of cell-surface IgE densities with a sensitivity that is somewhat poorer than the acetate strip method when the basophil purity is low). This study was included because earlier studies of basophil function suggested that changes in the expression of FcεRI would mirror the changes in free serum IgE. Furthermore, the relationship between changes in surface FcεRI/IgE and the response to antigenic challenge could be evaluated in the context of what was happening in vivo. Because the phase I trial included no placebo controls, two untreated mild atopic donors were followed during the same time frame. Although this number of controls was small, previous experience with examining basophil parameters longitudinally suggested that no gross changes in receptor expression would occur and that changes in histamine secretion would vary only modestly.

For the entire group, free-circulating IgE levels dropped approximately 100-fold within 24 hours of the first dose of E25

and remained at this low level throughout the first 180 days of treatment (Fig. 25-5). For three individuals, the kinetics of FcεRI expression on basophils was monitored every day for the first week of treatment and was found to decrease with an initial half-life of approximately 3 days. Within 5 weeks of treatment, the expression of FcεRI on the basophils of approximately 75% of subjects had decreased to below detection by flow cytometry. By 10 weeks, FcεRI expression on the basophils of all but one subject was undetectable by flow cytometry. With the acetate stripping method a 12-week time-point measurement showed that the average cell-surface expression of FcεRI had decreased from a pretreatment level of 220,000 per cell to 8000 per cell. The decrease in cell-surface IgE was greater, from a similar starting point of approximately 220,000 to less than 2200 (most often below the detection of this assay). This difference between FcεRI and IgE results from the fact that not only had the expression of FcεRI decreased, but the equilibrium at this concentration of free IgE ($\approx$5 ng/mL) meant that less than 25% of the available receptors were occupied. At the half-year point, the dosing of the E25 was changed so that 3- to 20-fold less E25 was administered every 2 weeks. Therefore, at the time for the measurements of FcεRI expression and basophil function (at the E25 termination point or about 1 year after the start of treatment) the subjects had experienced a modest rise in circulating free IgE concentration. Along with this increase in free IgE, the expression of FcεRI rose from the mean of 8000 per basophil at 12 weeks to 35,000 at 52 weeks. After E25 treatment ended, free IgE levels and the expression of FcεRI on basophils rose somewhat linearly with a doubling every 3 weeks. The final termination date for the study, which depended on reaching 50% of pretreatment levels of free IgE, occurred for most subjects within 6 months; a few were terminated because they had arrived at the 1-year mark without reaching 50% of pretreatment IgE levels. At the end of the study, however, the expression of basophil FcεRI was within statistical equivalence of pretreatment levels for all subjects (Fig. 25-6).

At 12 weeks, the median response of the subjects' basophils to stimulation with DF antigen was 10% of the pretreatment response. The response to stimulation with polyclonal anti-IgE antibody (which should cross-link/aggregate all available cell surface IgE) was decreased to 50% of pretreatment levels. With IgE densities hovering just below 1500 per basophil, the antigen-specific IgE density was probably well below 300 molecules per basophil. In contrast, 1500 molecules of IgE per basophil, stimulated with anti-IgE antibody, would be approximately the EC50 for secretion. The response to FMLP did not change over the course of the study, nor did the responses or FcεRI expression levels of the two nontreated subjects included in the study. These results were notable for supporting earlier estimates of the relationship between cell-surface expression of FcεRI (and therefore IgE) and the functional responses of the cell.

The telling observation in these studies is summarized in Figure 25-6. During the period between 90 and 360 days (probably because of the shift in dosing beginning at 180 days), both free-circulating IgE and FcεRI expression increased modestly. In contrast, the functional response of the cells became nearly the

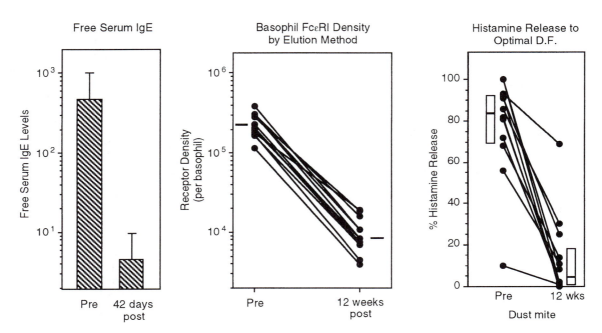

Figure 25-5. Changes in two characteristics of peripheral blood basophils from subjects treated with rhuMAb-E25. Left panel: Mean free serum IgE concentrations before and after treatment with E25. Levels of serum IgE were similar for days 1 through 180 (not shown). Middle panel: Change (pretreatment levels vs. levels at approximately 12 weeks of treatment) in cell-surface expression of FcεRI for a subset of 15 individuals. The horizontal bars represent the medians. Right panel: Change in histamine release (measured by in vitro challenge of enriched basophils with a predetermined optimal concentration of DF antigen) for the same individuals. Boxes indicate the medians and 25th to 75th quartiles.

same as that before treatment. The viewpoint of our group is expressed in panel C of Figure 25-6. When free IgE was suppressed approximately 100-fold, receptor expression was decreased on average 26-fold and cell-surface IgE fell below the EC50 for secretion. However, as evidenced by the results for anti-IgE antibody, the functional response hovered around the EC50 point. One would have predicted that from this starting point small rises in FcεRI/IgE would have a dramatic effect on secretion, and the results suggest that they did. By the end of the study (nearly 1 year after the last dose of E25 for some subjects), both anti-IgE and DF antigen–driven secretion had returned to pretreatment levels.

As an uncontrolled study, there were only anecdotal reports of the clinical effects of the treatment (which were often quite dramatic). However, skin tests demonstrated a marked suppression of mast cell secretion (30). On average the titration of antigen required for wheal and flare indicated a need for 32-fold more antigen. Such a result might lead to a confusion about antigen dosing in vitro versus in vivo. However, in vitro both experimental and theoretical studies demonstrate that the concentration of antigen that is optimal for secretion is not a function of cell-surface IgE density. Therefore, apparent suppression of the secretory response in vitro cannot be overcome by using more antigen if the concentration is already at the predetermined optimum (an increase in antigen concentration simply moves into the supraoptimal region of its biphasic dose response curve). In

the skin, the concentration of antigen used could very well be suboptimal for many cells. Furthermore, additional antigen may simply recruit a larger region of mast cells, giving the appearance of overcoming some suppression.

A potentially relevant correlation could be derived from this study. In Figure 25-7, the ratio of DF antigen–specific to total IgE is plotted against the ratio of histamine release induced by DF antigen for the 12-week treatment response/pretreatment response. Although the number of data points is small for a correlation of this kind, the trend indicates that if the starting DF antigen–specific to total IgE ratio is too high, suppression of the functional response is minimal. This result would be expected if treatment were sufficient only to suppress IgE levels to the point that basophil (or mast cell) secretion hovered at its threshold. Then, the ratio of antigen-specific IgE to total IgE influences the success of the treatment because at high ratios the fraction of cell surface IgE more closely approximates the total, which we know from the above study, provides a reasonable response. If suppression of free-circulating IgE were more complete, then the specific-to-total ratio would not be contributory because cells would not possess enough IgE (total or specific) to mount a secretory response. Consequently, these results suggest a somewhat paradoxical prediction that those patients with multiple antigen sensitivities might respond better to this therapy than those with single specificities (where the specific-to-total ratio may be high). Clearly, a central issue is that free-circulating IgE be suppressed

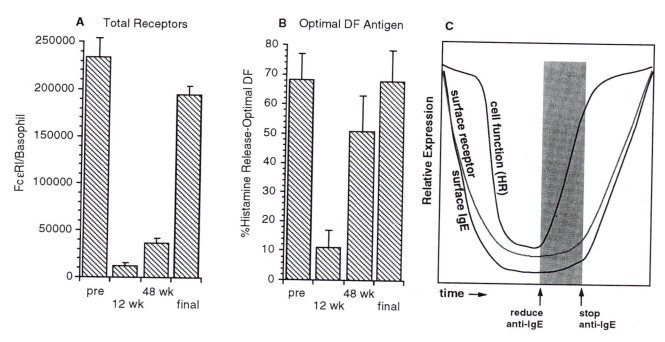

Figure 25-6. Synopsis of the changes in expression of FcεRI and the in vitro function of peripheral blood basophils from a sub-population of 15 patients in the year-long phase I trial of rhuMAb-E25. Panel A: Levels of FcεRI expression before treatment, 12 weeks into treatment, 48 weeks into treatment (just before cessation of treatment), and 4 to 12 months after treatment was stopped (final). Panel B: In vitro histamine release response for the same four periods of measurement. Panel C: General characteristics of the changes expected by the author to represent what is happening during treatment. The x-axis is not strictly linear in time. The gray region represents the time during which the amount of E25 administered was decreased 3- to 20-fold, leading to a small increase in free serum IgE, a small increase in the expression of basophil FcεRI, and therefore an increase in cell surface IgE. Consequently, the function of the cell changes more dramatically.

to levels below 5 to 10 ng/mL. If a patient begins with 100 ng/mL of IgE, of which 50% is specific for some one antigen, E25 given at doses used for more typically atopic individuals would still work, despite the high specific-to-total ratio, because the starting IgE level is low. Conversely, even a very low specific-to-total ratio may not allow a standard dosing of E25 to work if IgE levels begin above 10,000 ng/mL. For a typical atopic patient with IgE levels in the 500 to 1000 ng/mL range, the kinds of dosing schedules being suggested should have some effect, although success may be influenced by some of the less well studied aspects of basophil/mast cell secretion biology or modulation. For example, the basophils of one patient may require only 300 molecules of cell-surface IgE to mount a normal response, while those of another may require 30,000 (9).

Safety Considerations for Anti-IgE Antibody

A major concern for anti-IgE antibody therapy is the potential for inducing anaphylactic reactions. In the clinical trials of both CGP51901 and E25, the most common side effect has been the development of a small number of urticarial reactions, all of which occurred with the initial administration and were easily managed with appropriate intervention. For example, in the phase I toxicology trial discussed above, four of 47 patients reported such reactions. These patients proved negative to skin testing with E25 and were given an additional dose of intravenous E25. One patient experienced a reaction and withdrew from the study. Similar reactions are recognized with other initial infusions of monoclonal antibodies, and no evidence of mast cell/basophil mediator release or complement activation was found during the E25 or CGP51901 reactions. If the dose of antibody is high, spreading the initial infusion out over several days reduces the incidence of urticaria. The overall rate of urticarial reactions for E25 antibody is now reported to be approximately 2%.

With long-term administration of humanized antibodies comes concern that there will eventually be an immune response to the humanized antibody. Thus far, rhumAb-25 has not induced a detectable antibody response in humans. As noted above, the E25 antibody has been engineered to eliminate the complement binding site, and there has been no incidence or evidence of complement activation. There has also been no evidence of immune complex–mediated tissue damage (e.g., nephrotoxicity), and in

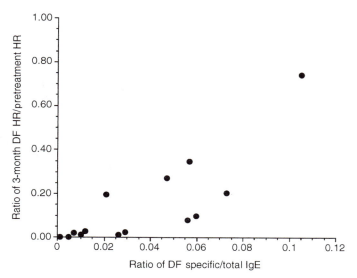

Figure 25-7. Relationship between the pretreatment DF (antigen–specific) to total IgE ratio and the subsequent reduction in the histamine release (HR) response of basophils on in vitro challenge. The ordinate is expressed as the ratio of posttreatment (12-week measurement) histamine release to pretreatment histamine release in response to an optimal concentration of DF antigen. The data show the correlation between the two parameters (i.e., the higher the ratio of antigen-specific IgE to total IgE, the smaller the reduction in in vitro histamine release). Note that DF antigen–specific IgE was measured with a standardized assay that has not been calibrated against the total IgE assay. Therefore, the ratios are useful in a relative sense only.

the long-term phase I study there was no evidence of increased sinopulmonary or other infections.

Summary

Recent clinical trials have demonstrated the potential for therapy designed to suppress circulating IgE levels. Proof-of-concept is now established for this approach. The ultimate success for diseases that have a clear dependence on IgE rests on a variety of practical issues. For diseases where the IgE component is probably not absolute (e.g., asthma), success is not yet fully demonstrated. As experience is gained about dosing and objective in vitro/in vivo measures of IgE-mediated function are carefully analyzed, it may be possible to make informed conclusions regarding the role of IgE in particular diseases. The relationship between IgE and the expression of FcεRI, which may extend to other cells that express this receptor, is probably a key piece of the biology that determines whether therapy that suppresses IgE is to be useful. Although the mechanism of stabilization of FcεRI expression by IgE is not currently known, such knowledge may be useful in designing therapies that cooperate with IgE suppression to suppress the functional responses of cells. Finally,

under the current schemes for dosing with anti-IgE antibodies, close attention should be paid to starting IgE levels and the ratio of specific-to-total IgE to develop a better sense of the kinds of patients that might benefit from this particular therapy.

Acknowledgments
With respect to the many in vitro studies that came from this division, I must acknowledge the contributions of Drs. Sarbjit Saini, Bruce Bochner, Alkis Togias, Robert Hamilton and Lawrence Lichtenstein at the JHU-Asthma and Allergy Center and Drs. Daniel Adelman and Paula Jardieu at Genentech, Inc.

References
1. Roman M, Spiegelberg HL, Broide D, Raz E. Gene immunization for allergic disorders. Springer Semin Immunopathol 1997;19:223–232.
2. Garman SC, Kinet JP, Jardetzky TS. Crystal structure of the human high-affinity IgE receptor. Cell 1998;95:951–961.
3. Chang TW, Davis FM, Sun N-C, et al. Monoclonal antibodies specific for human IgE-producing B cells: a potential therapeutic for IgE-mediated allergic diseases. Biotechnology 1990;8:122–126.
4. Jardieu P. Anti-IgE therapy. Curr Opin Immunol 1995; 7:779–782.
5. Saban R, Haak-Frendscho M, Zine M, et al. Human anti-IgE monoclonal antibody blocks passive sensitization of human and rhesus monkey bladder. J Urol 1997;157:689–693.
6. Presta LG, Lahr SJ, Shields RL, et al. Humanization of an antibody directed against IgE. J Immunol 1993;151:2623–2632.
7. MacGlashan DW Jr, White-Mckenzie J, Chichester K, et al. In vitro regulation of FceRIα expression on human basophils by IgE antibody. Blood 1998;91:1633–1643.
8. MacGlashan DW Jr, Peters SP, Warner J, Lichtenstein LM. Characteristics of human basophil sulfidopeptide leukotriene release: releasability defined as the ability of the basophil to respond to dimeric cross-links. J Immunol 1986;136:2231–2239.
9. MacGlashan DW Jr. Releasability of human basophils: cellular sensitivity and maximal histamine release are independent variables. J Allergy Clin Immunol 1993;91:605–615.
10. Malveaux EJ, Conroy MC, Adkinson NFJ, Lichtenstein LM. IgE receptors on human basophils. Relationship to serum IgE concentration. J Clin Invest 1978;62:176–181.
11. Hsu C, MacGlashan DW Jr. IgE Antibody up-regulates high affinity IgE binding on murine bone marrow derived mast cells. Immunol Lett 1996;52:129–134.
12. MacGlashan DW Jr, Bochner BS, Adelman DC, et al. Downregulation of FcεRI expression on human basophils during in vivo treatment of atopic patients with anti-IgE antibody. J Immunol 1997;158:1438–1445.
13. Yamaguchi M, Lantz CS, Oettgen HC, et al. IgE enhances mouse mast cell FcεRI expression in vitro and in vivo: evidence for a novel amplification mechanism in IgE-dependent reactions. J Exp Med 1997;185:663–672.
14. Lantz CS, Yamaguchi M, Oettgen HC, et al. IgE regulates mouse basophil FcεRI expression in vivo. J Immunol 1997;158:2517–2521.

15. Shaikh N, Rivera J, Hewlett BR, et al. Mast cell Fc epsilonRI expression in the rat intestinal mucosa and tongue is enhanced during *Nippostrongylus brasiliensis* infection and can be up-regulated by in vivo administration of IgE. J Immunol 1997;158:3805–3812.
16. Akue JP, Hommel M, Devaney E. High levels of parasite-specific IgG1 correlate with the amicrofilaremic state in *Loa loa* infection. J Infect Dis 1997;175:158–163.
17. Ogilvie BM, Parrott DM. The immunological consequences of nematode infection. Ciba Found Symp 1977;46:183–201.
18. Butterworth AE. Immunological aspects of human schistosomiasis. Br Med Bull 1998;54:357–368.
19. Amiri P, Haak-Frendscho M, Robbins K, et al. Antiimmunoglobulin E treatment decreases worm burden and egg production in *Schistosoma mansoni*-infected normal and interferon gamma knockout mice. J Exp Med 1994;180:43–51.
20. King CL, Xianli J, Malhotra I, et al. Mice with a targeted deletion of the IgE gene have increased worm burdens and reduced granulomatous inflammation following primary infection with *Schistosoma mansoni*. J Immunol 1997;158:294–300.
21. Cain WA, Amman AJ, Hong R, et al. IgE deficiency associated with chronic sinopulmonary infection. J Clin Invest 1969;48:12a–13a.
22. Levy D, Chen J. Healthy IgE-deficient person. N Engl J Med 1970;283:541–542.
23. Fox JA, Hotaling TE, Struble C, et al. Tissue distribution and complex formation with IgE of an anti-IgE antibody after intravenous administration in cynomolgus monkeys. J Pharmacol Exp Ther 1996;279:1000–1008.
24. Liu J, Lester P, Builder S, Shire SJ. Characterization of complex formation by humanized anti-IgE monoclonal antibody and monoclonal human IgE. Biochemistry 1995;34:10474–10482.
25. Racine-Poon A, Botta L, Chang TW, et al. Efficacy, pharmacodynamics, and pharmacokinetics of CGP 51901, an anti-immunoglobulin E chimeric monoclonal antibody, in patients with seasonal allergic rhinitis. Clin Pharmacol Ther 1997;62:675–690.
26. Boulet L, Chapman K, Cote J, et al. Inhibitory effects of an anti-IgE antibody E25 on allergen-induced early asthmatic responses. Am J Respir Crit Care Med 1997;155:1835–1840.
27. Fahy J, Fleming H, Wong H, et al. The effect of an anti-IgE monoclonal antibody on the early- and late-phase responses to allergen inhalation in asthmatic subjects. Am J Respir Crit Care Med 1997;155:1828–1834.
28. Casale T, Bernstein I, Busse W, et al. Use of an anti-IgE humanized monoclonal antibody in ragweed-induced allergic rhinitis. J Allergy Clin Immunol 1997;100:110–121.
29. Saini SS, MacGlashan DW Jr, Sterbinsky SA, et al. Down-regulation of human basophil IgE and FceRIa surface densities and mediator release by anti-IgE infusions is reversible in vitro and in vivo. J Immunol 1999;162:5623–5630.
30. Togias A, Corren J, Shapiro G, et al. Anti-IgE treatment reduces skin test (ST) reactivity. J Allergy Clin Immunol 1998;101:S171.

Chapter 26

Specific and Nonspecific Immunotherapy for Asthma and Allergic Diseases

M. Larché

A. B. Kay

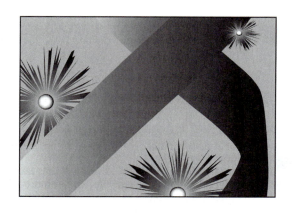

The increase in our understanding of the cellular and molecular mechanisms in allergic diseases has resulted in both a reappraisal of the mode of action of traditional treatment and the opportunity to develop novel strategies. In this chapter we discuss various allergen-specific and nonspecific approaches for down-regulating the allergic response on the basis of recently acquired knowledge. Traditional specific allergen injection immunotherapy (SIT) has been used for almost 90 years. Evidence suggests that this form of treatment may have several effects on the immune system, including modification of T-cell function. Several novel immunotherapeutic strategies have been proposed, or are being evaluated, which are based on the Th2 hypothesis of allergy. Thus, as explained in the relevant section, SIT may produce "immune deviation" from a Th2 to a Th1 phenotype, induction of tolerance, anergy or hyporesponsiveness, and/or the production of cells with active suppressor function. There is considerable current interest in the induction of hyporesponsiveness by allergen-specific peptides, as well as methods of redirection to a Th1 response by the combination of allergen with Th1-inducing cytokines, or the use of altered peptide ligands. Another new approach is the incorporation of allergen peptides into appropriate adjuvants, or the concept of plasmid (allergen epitope) gene therapy. Nonspecific Th2-based immunotherapeutic approaches may include the targeting of Th2 transcription factors such as STAT6 or the neutralization of IL-4 and IL-5 by soluble receptors, humanized antibody, or mutant proteins. Similarly, IgE may be targeted by humanized nonanaphylactic antibody.

Other potential nonspecific therapies include the use of potent and safe immunosuppressant drugs, anti–T-cell antibodies, and methods of inhibiting cell adhesion molecules. Finally, because the eosinophil is believed to be a major effector cell in allergic tissue injury, some antieosinophil strategies are also discussed.

We believe that consideration of the mode of action of successful SIT is both a useful and a logical starting point for a discussion of immunotherapy in general. This traditional form of treatment for allergic disease needs to be safer and more effective. Current attempts to achieve this goal range from approaches that are at present only concepts or ideas to those that have been validated by animal experiments or have "proof of principle" in humans. Only time will tell what will eventually become established in the treatment of allergic disease.

Specific Immunotherapy

Allergen Injection Immunotherapy

The practice of administering gradually increasing quantities of an allergen extract to an allergic individual to ameliorate symptoms associated with subsequent exposure to causative allergen arose before World War I, when Noon and Freeman at St. Mary's Hospital, London, introduced desensitizing vaccines to treat summer hayfever (1,2). This procedure, referred to variously as allergen injection immunotherapy, specific immunotherapy (SIT), hyposensitization, or desensitization, has been used worldwide to treat allergic diseases caused by inhalant allergens and Hymenoptera venoms. It is generally considered to be efficacious in venom hypersensitivity, seasonal or perennial allergic rhinitis, and, probably, mild allergic asthma. In seasonal allergic rhinitis, and to a lesser extent perennial rhinitis, SIT is extremely effective and long lasting, especially when treatment is maintained for several years (3). The role of allergen immunotherapy in the treatment of allergic disease, together with guidelines for its use were recently summarized in a WHO Position Paper (4).

In the United Kingdom specific allergen injection immunotherapy is given on a routine basis only to patients with seasonal allergic rhinitis caused by grass pollen (hayfever) who have failed to respond adequately to antiallergic drugs and to patients with anaphylaxis resulting from wasp or bee venom hypersensitivity. Only high-quality, standardized allergen extracts licensed under the provision of the UK Medicines Act and associated European Directives are recommended (5). All allergen extracts (for skin testing, as well as immunotherapy) are biologically standardized, and changes from the products of one company to those of another during the course of treatment should be avoided.

Mechanisms and Mode of Action of Immunotherapy

The immunologic changes after immunotherapy that lead to clinical improvement may not necessarily be the same in insect venom–induced anaphylaxis and in allergic rhinitis/asthma associated with inhalant allergens. Both are associated with inappropriate expression of type 2 cytokines and increases in specific IgE.

Here they are considered together in terms of possible mechanisms involved.

Antibody Response. The concept of SIT-induced IgG that prevents access of specific allergen to mast cell- or basophil-bound IgE is termed the "blocking antibody theory" and has been popular for many years. More recent data suggest that the binding of allergen by IgG is unlikely to be the main mechanism of protection in specific immunotherapy (6). Although serum IgE concentrations are elevated initially during conventional immunotherapy and gradually decrease to normal over a period of months, target organ sensitivity may decrease in the face of these elevations in serum IgE. In contrast, there are marked increases in IgG1 and IgG4 antibodies specific for the allergen used for immunotherapy. Thus, although serum levels of both isotypes increase during the early phase of treatment, the ratio of specific IgE to IgG4 decreases by 10- to 100-fold (7). In bee-venom hypersensitivity interleukin (IL)-10 is a potent suppressor of both total and phospholipase A (PLA)–specific IgE and simultaneously increases IgG4 formation (8). Increases in serum, allergen-specific IgG concentrations after immunotherapy may be related to increases in IL-10 and IL-12, both of which are increased after SIT. IL-12, however, induces a Th1-type cytokine response and favors IgG4 synthesis of allergen-specific T-cell clones (9,10). IgG may down-regulate the allergic response by competition with IgE for allergen binding (classical blocking antibody theory), prevention of aggregation of FcεRI-bound IgE through steric hindrance, or interference with antigen trapping and focusing by IgE bound to antigen-presenting cells (6).

Mediators, Inflammatory Cells, and the Late-Phase Allergic Reaction. Immunotherapy is associated with decreases in inflammatory mediators after SIT. For example, the antigen-induced increases in the concentrations of histamine, TAME-esterase, and prostaglandin D_2 in nasal lavage fluid are significantly lowered by immunotherapy (11).

The late-phase allergic reaction (LPR) in the skin, the nose, and the lung is an established model of IgE-dependent inflammation. Successful immunotherapy characteristically inhibits, often dramatically, the LPR, and this event in turn is associated with decreases in the numbers of mast cells, basophils, and eosinophils in blood and target organs (12–14). Neutrophil numbers are not decreased. IL-10 may play a critical role in decreasing mast-cell numbers and reactivity, as well as down-regulating eosinophil function through a variety of mechanisms, which include increased apoptosis, reduction of priming, or inhibition of the production of activating agents such as tumor necrosis factor-alpha (TNF-α), granulocyte macrophage colony–stimulating factor (GM-CSF), and IL-6 (8,15). IL-10 inhibits GM-CSF production and CD40 expression by activated eosinophils (16).

T Lymphocytes. Although IL-4 (and probably IL-13) is required for isotype switch to Cε and Cγ4, at later stages antigen-specific IgE antibody production by memory B cells depends on

IL-4 and IL-13. This production is suppressed by interferon-γ (IFN-γ) and IL-10, whereas specific IgG4 synthesis requires IFN-γ and is enhanced by IL-10 (Fig. 26-1). In in vitro experiments, immunotherapy inhibited the proliferation of peripheral blood T cells and their production of IL-4 and IFN-γ; the addition of IL-2 or IL-15 to cultures restored cell proliferation and IFN-γ production but not IL-4 production (17).

Current views suggest that immunotherapy is associated with profound modulation of T-cell function, with immune deviation from a Th2 to Th1 phenotype, anergy, or both. There is some evidence, mostly from experimental animals, that CD8+ T cells with suppressor activity may also be induced by SIT (18). SIT results in a decrease in antigen-induced recruitment to tissues of CD4+ T cells and eosinophils, with concomitant increases in cells expressing HLA-DR and CD25 (13). This situation may be the result of augmentation of HLA-DR and CD25 by IFN-γ derived from Th1 cells. Thus, immunotherapy is associated with a decrease in the recruitment of CD4 cells, possible enhancement of CD8+ cell function, down-regulation of IL-4 and IL-5, and increases in IL-10 and IL-12.

Interleukin-10 has been studied mainly in bee-venom SIT with the major allergen PLA (8). IL-10 levels increased fairly rapidly for 7 days after SIT and plateaued at 4 weeks. IL-10 was increased not only in T cells but also in monocytes and B cells. Naturally anergized beekeepers have increased numbers of IL-10–producing, activated T cells and monocytes. IL-10 inhibits the proliferation and cytokine responses of both Th1 and Th2 cells and also blocks costimulatory pathways in T cells. In vitro IL-10 induces a long-term, antigen-specific anergic state in human CD4+ T cells and can give rise to a regulatory IL-10–producing population termed Tr1 cells (19).

Allergen immunotherapy may initially establish a state of specific hyporesponsiveness of peripheral T cells, as shown by a decreased proliferative response and T-cell cytokine release together with simultaneous increases in IL-10 production (see Fig. 26-1). The autocrine elaboration of IL-10 by T cells maintains the hyporesponsive state. These events suppress specific IgE and enhance IgG4 production and in turn down-regulate activation, priming, and survival of effector inflammatory cells. When anergic cells enter the tissue, they either adopt the Th1 phenotype under the influence of IL-2 and IL-15, producing IgG4 as in successful immunotherapy, or are reactivated by IL-4 to produce Th2 cells, which in turn initiate IgE synthesis (unsuccessful SIT) (15).

Other factors that appear critical in the development of T-cell anergy/tolerance include the concentration of allergen in the establishment of MHC class II/peptide/TCR complexes (20). Thus, increasing antigen concentrations favor a Th1 phenotype, whereas IL-4 is decreased at high antigen doses. This finding indicates that Th1/Th2 cell do not represent stable phenotypes, but can be modulated by the dose of antigen. Therefore, in specific immunotherapy the concentration of antigen may be critical in determining IgE or IgG formation, which results in either hypersensitivity or immunity.

The induction of hyporesponsiveness in Th2 cells by IL-10 is believed to be an active process; although these cells do not have

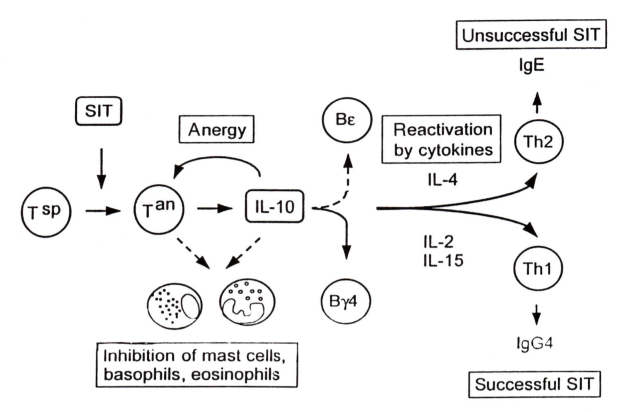

Figure 26-1. Immunologic mechanisms of specific immunotherapy (SIT). Continuous treatment with high doses of allergen establishes a state of allergen-specific anergy in peripheral T cells (T^{an}), which is characterized by suppressed proliferative and cytokine responses, together with an increase in IL-10 production. IL-10 suppresses specific T cells (T^{sp}) in an autocrine fashion. It also suppresses IgE production and enhances IgG4 production. Subsequent activation, priming, and survival of allergic inflammatory effector cells are down-regulated. The anergic T cell can be reactivated by cytokines from the tissue microenvironment. In successful SIT, anergic T cells recover under the influence of microenvironmental IL-2 and/or IL-15 to produce Th0/Th1 cytokines. In an atopic individual, IL-4 may reconstitute a Th2 cytokine pattern and reactivate an allergic response. (Figure courtesy of Dr. K. Blaser, SIAF, Davos, Switzerland.)

increased tyrosine phosphorylation of p56^{lck} and ZAP-70 kinases when stimulated with anti-CD3, they do have increased levels of basal tyrosine kinase, cytokine production, and CD25 up-regulation (21,22).

It has been proposed that SIT, as with other forms of immune modulation, also involves immunologic tricks in which nonresponsiveness induced to one epitope of a molecule confers "tolerance" either to the whole molecule (linked suppression) or adjacent molecules (bystander tolerance), or is passed to the next generation of regulatory T cells (infectious tolerance) (23).

Allergoids

The concept of reducing the allergenicity of allergen preparations has been expounded for decades (24). Modification of antibody-binding epitopes on the outer surface of allergens has most frequently been achieved with formaldehyde, which modifies lysine residues and results in the cross-linking of amino acid side chains,

destroying three-dimensional epitopes in the process. Because the treatment does not effect cleavage of the protein, linear T-cell epitopes are thought to be maintained. Extensive clinical evaluation has been carried out with a variety of allergoid preparations, including ragweed (25,26), grass pollen (27–31), parietaria (32), and mite allergens (33,34); ragweed was evaluated with an allergoid preparation prepared by modification with pyridine. Routes of administration and treatment regimens have varied in line with unmodified allergen immunotherapy and have included RUSH protocols (27–30) and sublingual/oral administration (34).

Naturally Occurring Allergen Isoforms

Whole allergen immunotherapy is occasionally associated with general (sometimes fatal) anaphylaxis induced by the triggering of mast cells through IgE-independent mechanisms. Studies on allergens derived from plants and trees have identified naturally occurring isoforms of allergens that have a reduced capacity to bind IgE (35). The relative lack of interaction with IgE is caused by amino acid substitutions or deletions within the IgE-binding site or at sites that induce conformational changes in the molecule, thus preventing IgE binding. These observations have led to suggestions that immunotherapy performed with hypoallergenic isoforms might allow the use of higher doses, thereby providing a more effective method of modulating the T-cell response to allergens. From studies investigating immunoreactivity to isoforms of common allergens (36,37) contained within immunotherapy extracts, it has become clear that some individuals develop isoform-specific IgE during the course of whole allergen–extract immunotherapy. The consequences of such antiisoform IgE induction during therapy are not yet understood.

Recombinant Allergens

At present, the diagnosis of immediate hypersensitivity is still made with whole-allergen extracts known to contain large numbers of contaminating proteins and multiple allergens. Because of the difficulty of standardizing such "crude" extracts for content of individual allergens, concern has been expressed about the sensitivity and accuracy of current skin-testing methods. The use of recombinant, purified allergens has been proposed to circumvent this problem since recombinant technology allows expression and purification of a large number of major allergens and allows batch variation to be excluded. Recent studies have described the use of recombinant proteins for the diagnosis of immediate hypersensitivity by skin-prick testing.

The introduction of recombinant DNA technology has enabled investigators to clone, sequence, and express allergen proteins in the laboratory. Detailed analysis of IgE-binding epitopes has resulted in mapping of IgE-binding sites for a number of the major allergens. More recently, these findings, together with earlier observations concerning the relative lack of immunogenicity associated with some allergen isoforms, have been exploited by the use of in vitro mutagenesis to create allergen proteins in which single amino acids have been modified, or deletions introduced, to produce molecules with dramatically reduced IgE-binding capacity (38).

The major peanut allergen Ara h 2 has been recently modified by single alanine substitutions in four of its ten linear IgE-binding epitopes (39). Sixteen subjects were skin tested with the modified recombinant protein. Twelve individuals demonstrated dramatically reduced skin-test reactivity, three showed no change in IgE reactivity, and one had increased reactivity. Allergens from mites have also become the target of strategies to reduce IgE binding. Smith and Chapman (40) produced engineered isoforms of the major, house-dust-mite allergen Der p 2 and demonstrated reduced IgE-binding activity. A subtly different approach to amino acid substitutions in allergen sequences has recently been reported by Takai et al (41), who substituted cysteine residues involved in the three disulfide bonds in the mite allergen Der f 2. While all substitutions reduced IgE binding from patient sera, those involving the C8/C119 disulfide bond proved to be particularly suitable targets, with substitutions of serine at C8 and/or

C119 dramatically reducing skin-test reactivity while T-cell reactivity was retained in vitro.

Recombinant variants of the grass allergen Phl p 5b have recently been generated and their IgE-binding characteristics investigated (42). In addition to point mutations in the allergen molecule, deletions of part or parts of the allergen molecule were used to generate point and deletion mutants. IgE reactivity was reduced in certain deletion mutants but, in contrast to data obtained with the tree-pollen allergens described earlier, point mutations were relatively ineffective at reducing IgE binding, as assessed with biochemical techniques. In common with other allergen-engineering approaches, no single mutant molecule was found to be completely devoid of IgE-binding activity, indicating a more complex scenario than originally had been anticipated. Clearly, for recombinant allergens to be effective and safe clinically, skin-prick tests or other IgE-binding measurements need to be made in individual patients before use in immunotherapy.

In addition to point mutations and deletions of regions of the allergen molecule, some groups have developed recombinant allergens with short sequences from the allergen rearranged to produce a molecule (43) that has little or no IgE-binding activity but retains the T-cell epitopes believed necessary for the success of immunotherapy. More recently, Vrtala et al (44) have generated two recombinant polypeptides from Bet v 1a that effectively divide the molecule in two. The two polypeptides lack natural Bet v 1 conformational determinants and fail to bind IgE.

Together, these approaches toward allergen engineering offer the prospect of purified, standardized allergen reagents for the diagnosis and therapy of allergic diseases. However, as more data become available, problems may be encountered with this approach because of the large numbers of isoforms that occur naturally, particularly for plant and tree allergens. A successful approach to unequivocal diagnosis of IgE-mediated hypersensitivity with these reagents must take this factor into account and ensure that a sufficiently large panel of isoforms is used.

T-Cell Epitope Vaccines

Strategies to target allergen-specific T lymphocytes in the relative absence of interaction with IgE have included the development of chemically modified allergens, the selection of allergen isoforms with reduced IgE-binding capacity, the engineering of recombinant allergens to reduce IgE binding, and the production of large polypeptide fragments of allergens that demonstrate reduced three-dimensional conformation. An alternative approach is that of peptide-based immunotherapy, which has pioneered in animal model systems and has recently been evaluated for human immunotherapy. Dominant T-cell epitopes have been identified in both murine and human systems. Peptides based on these epitopes have been shown to prevent the induction of disease and to modulate ongoing disease in murine models of diseases after subcutaneous, intranasal, and intravenous administration. Peptide-induced tolerance has been demonstrated in models of experimental autoimmune encephalomyelitis (EAE) (45,46), collagen-induced arthritis (47,48), and diabetes (49), and more recently, in models of allergic disease. Briner et al sensitized mice to the cat allergen Fel d 1 and subsequently demonstrated the ability of allergen-derived peptides to inhibit T-cell cytokine and antibody production (50). Hoyne et al (51) demonstrated the ability of peptides from the house-dust-mite allergen Der p 2 to down-regulate T-cell and antibody responses to challenge with intact protein and also to prevent sensitization by prior administration (51).

Concerns have been raised about the relevance of studies performed in inbred animal strains, where peptide epitopes and their restriction elements are well defined. The polymorphism displayed by both the human major histocompatibility complex (MHC) and many allergen genes has given rise to the view that peptide immunotherapy for allergic diseases in humans is impractical because the large number of potential epitope-MHC combinations involved in disease pathogenesis cannot possibly be accommodated. The problem of polymorphism is particularly pertinent to the allergic diseases because, unlike many autoimmune diseases, there are few, strong, human leukocyte antigen (HLA) disease associations. The same is not true of diseases such as multiple sclerosis (MS), where clear associations between HLA haplotype and disease are seen. The identification of immunodominant T-cell peptide epitopes restricted by HLA-DR2 has led to a peptide from myelin basic protein (MBP) being administered to patients with MS in phase I clinical trials (52,53). Despite these reservations in allergic diseases, peptide-based immunotherapy has recently been evaluated in individuals with allergic disease induced by either cat or ragweed allergens. Two relatively large peptides from the major cat allergen Fel d 1 were evaluated by Norman et al (54). After four injections of peptide in three dose groups, clinical efficacy was observed only at the highest dose of peptide ($4 \times 750\,\mu g$). A relatively modest improvement in mainly subjective symptom scores resulted in cat and ragweed vaccines being withdrawn from clinical trials.

More recently, three T-cell peptide epitopes have been identified in the bee venom phospholipase A_2 (PLA2) molecule and have been used to desensitize five allergic individuals (55). The peptides were well tolerated; despite the different MHC backgrounds of the subjects. T-cell responses to all three peptides occurred. Thus, the use of peptide immunotherapy in an outbred population such as humans may not present as much of a problem as has been envisaged in the past.

Broad patterns of peptide reactivity have also been reported by Haselden et al (56), who investigated responses to three peptides derived from the cat allergen Fel d 1. In this study, peptides were administered intradermally to cat-allergic individuals with asthma. Isolated, late, asthmatic reactions were induced in a proportion of the individuals. Each of the three peptides was capable of inducing peripheral-blood, mononuclear-cell proliferation in some of the subjects. The ability to induce isolated, late, asthmatic reactions did not correlate with peptide-induced proliferative responses, because the latter may be dose-dependent and the dose administered in the study was the lowest dose demonstrated to induce a late asthmatic reaction. T-cell responses to two of the three peptides were MHC-restricted, and those individuals experiencing a late asthmatic reaction expressed HLA-DR molecules associated with peptide restriction. The authors reported promis-

cuous binding of peptides to more than one DR microvariant and, in the case of one peptide, to more than one DR specificity. The ability of certain peptide epitopes to bind to many HLA molecules has become increasingly well documented and has led to the designation of HLA supertypes to which certain peptide sequences bind promiscuously (57). Thus, peptides designed on the basis of MHC class II restriction have potential for greater efficacy on a population basis.

DNA Vaccines

In contrast to strategies that employ whole proteins or peptides to modify the immune response to allergens, recent interest has focused on direct immunization with DNA encoding allergen proteins. A number of variations of the theme of DNA vaccination have been investigated. Unmethylated CpG motifs (ACGT) have been used to induce Th1 immune responses either alone or in combination with allergen proteins. Additionally, plasmid vectors encoding whole-protein allergen genes have been injected directly into animals either before or after allergen challenge (58).

Palindromic nucleotide sequences containing the motif ACGT are found in microbial DNA. They have been shown to induce the production of interferons in human peripheral blood mononuclear cells (59), to activate B cells (60), and to stimulate the production of Th1-enhancing cytokines such as IL-12, IFNγ, and TNF-α in mice (61,62).

Oligonucleotides containing CpG motifs have been evaluated in murine models of asthma. The inhibition of IL-5 resulted in failure to release eosinophils from the bone marrow and was characterized by an inhibition of airways eosinophilia accompanied by modulation of airways inflammation and hyperresponsiveness (63,64).

Nearly a decade ago, transfer and expression of genes directly into murine muscle cells in vivo opened the possibility that immunization with "naked" plasmid DNA could be an effective method for inducing protective immunity to a multitude of exogenous pathogen-derived proteins (65). After a single administration, injected plasmid DNA and expressed product have been demonstrated for periods as long as 19 months (66). Direct comparison of murine immune responses to whole-protein immunization or administration of plasmid DNA encoding the same proteins (β-galactosidase and influenza nucleoprotein) demonstrated that, while immunization with whole protein in either saline or with alum adjuvant induced IL-4 and IL-5 in the relative absence of IFNγ, plasmid vaccination induced strong IFNγ responses in the absence of Th2-type cytokines (67). Mice were sensitized with recombinant Der p 5 after immunization with plasmid DNA encoding the allergen under the control of a CMV promoter (or empty-vector control). Allergen-specific IgE levels were 90% lower in mice immunized with the Der p 5 construct. In addition, Der p 5–specific CD8 T cells produced high levels of IFNγ and could adoptively transfer suppression of IgE responses (68).

In a rat model of asthma, immunization with plasmid constructs encoding a house-dust-mite allergen prevented IgE

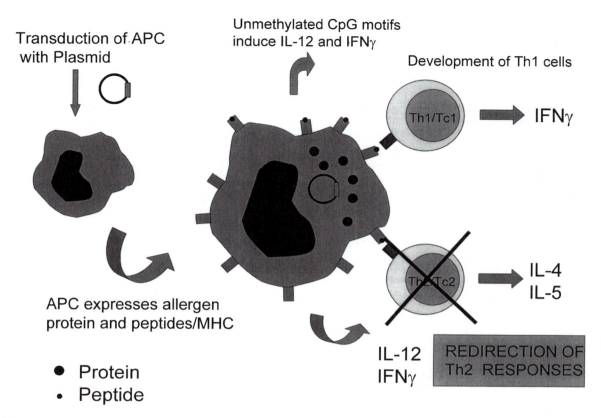

Figure 26-2. Mechanisms of immune deviation by plasmid DNA vaccination. After intradermal or subcutaneous administration of plasmid DNA containing unmethylated CpG motifs (immunostimulatory sequences) and encoding an antigen or antigen peptide (or in certain cases, cytokine), antigen presenting cells (APC) are transduced. APC become activated and produce IL-12, IL-18, IFNα, and IFNγ in response to immunostimulatory sequences. Proteins (peptides or cytokines) encoded by the plasmid insert are transcribed and translated. Peptide fragments bind to MHC molecules and are presented to specific T cells at the APC surface. Cytokines induced by immunostimulatory sequences encourage Th1/Tc1 development and antagonize Th2/Tc2 development and effector function.

synthesis, histamine release in the lung, and airways hyperresponsiveness induced by allergen challenge (69).

In addition to immunization with plasmid vectors encoding allergen proteins, mucosal Th2-type immune responses have also been inhibited after cytokine gene transfer. Li et al (70) expressed IFNγ in the airway epithelium of mice after gene transfer and observed inhibition of both allergen- and T-cell–induced airways eosinophilia.

To induce allergen gene expression in the intestinal epithelium, mice were immunized orally with DNA nanoparticles generated by complexing plasmid vector containing the gene encoding the major peanut allergen Ara h 2 with the polysaccharide chitosan. Mice receiving DNA nanoparticles exhibited secretory IgA and serum IgG2a production in contrast to mice receiving uncomplexed plasmid vector or no immunization. Furthermore, mice displayed a reduction in allergen-induced anaphylaxis concomitant with reduced levels of IgE (71).

Thus, strategies to abrogate Th2-type cytokine production by immunization with DNA motifs or plasmids encoding allergen

and cytokine genes hold promise for the therapy of allergic disease, including asthma (Fig. 26-2). However, most data collected in this area to date have come from murine models of disease. A cautionary note has recently been sounded by Li et al (72), who demonstrate distinct, strain-dependent antibody isotype responses to plasmid-encoded Ara h 2. The authors highlight the importance of selecting appropriate animal strains for investigation of DNA vaccines ultimately intended for human use.

Viruslike Particles (VLPs)

In a comparative study of delivery systems for the induction of cytotoxic T-cell responses to a single T-cell epitope, Allsopp et al (73) found that a single inoculation of mice with a yeast-derived Ty viruslike particle (VLP) resulted in consistently strong lytic responses. Other studies have confirmed the ability of VLPs expressing engineered fusion proteins to generate strong Th1-type T-cell responses to antigen (74,75). Recently, Harris et al (76) expressed the Der p 1 peptide 111–139 in a Ty VLP and used the construct to prime mice. The sequence 111–139 contains both a CD8 and a CD4 epitope in the context of H-2[b]. In the absence of adjuvant, they observed the induction of strong Tc1-type CD8 responses characterized by high levels of IFNγ and low levels of IL-5 and IL-6. However, in the presence of alum adjuvant, CD4 responses predominated and were of the Th1 phenotype. These results support the notion that the route of administration of antigen is critically important in determining the Th1 or Th2 outcome of antigen responses. These results also suggest that VLPs may have potential for modulating Th2 responses in allergic individuals. Ty-VLPs have been administered to healthy human volunteers with no detectable adverse reactions (77,78).

Nonspecific Immunotherapy

Immunosuppression in Chronic Asthma

Acute asthma results from the immediate release of bronchoconstrictor mediators such as histamine and leukotrienes by mast cells through the interaction of IgE and antigen and results in rapid airways obstruction. Chronic asthma is characterized by an inflammatory cellular infiltrate and, in particular, increased numbers of airway eosinophils and activated T lymphocytes (79). There is increasing evidence that the asthma process is "driven" and maintained by the persistence of a subset of chronically activated T-memory cells sensitized against allergenic, occupational, or viral antigens, which "home" to the lung after antigen exposure or viral infection. In general, allergens induce a CD4 T helper (Th)–cell response, whereas viruses recognize CD8+ cytotoxic (Tc) cells. In the asthmatic airways there are CD4+ cells, and to a lesser degree CD8+ cells, with a type-2 cytokine phenotype (i.e., Th-2 and Tc-2 types). These cells produce IL-5, IL-3, and GM-CSF, which recruit, mobilize, and activate eosinophils for subsequent mucosal damage; they also produce IL-4, an essential cofactor for local or generalized IgE production. This production leads to epithelial shedding, mucus hypersecretion, and bronchial muscle contraction. Thus, although the eosinophil may damage the mucosal surfaces in asthma, its function appears to be under T-cell control. Support for this hypothesis includes the following points:

1. The identification of activated T cells and their products in biopsies from the major variants of the disease (atopic, nonatopic, and occupational asthma)
2. The colocalization of mRNA for type-2 cytokines to CD4+ and CD8+ cells in atopic and nonatopic asthma
3. The presence of activated cytokine-producing T cells in corticosteroid-resistant asthma
4. The association of disease severity with type-2 cytokines, especially IL-5
5. The capacity of T-cell peptide epitopes to induce IgE-dependent, MHC class II–restricted, late asthmatic reactions (Fig. 26-3) (56)

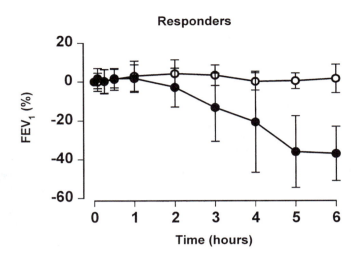

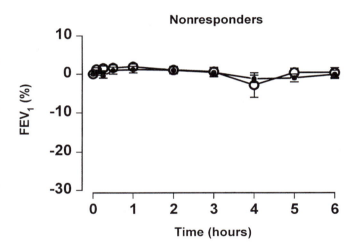

Figure 26-3. Induction of isolated, late asthmatic reactions by intradermal injection of peptides derived from Fel d 1. The mean percent changes in FEV_1 after the intradermal administration of Fel d 1 chain 1 peptides (FC1P; closed circles) and during a control day (open circles) of nine responders (*top*) and thirty-one nonresponders (*bottom*). Area-under-the-curve analysis to compare the percentage change in FEV_1 on control days and FC1P days in the 9 responders was statistically significant at $P = .0004$. Error bars denote standard error from the mean (SEM).

A schematic representation of the proposed inflammatory cells and cytokine network involved in acute and chronic asthma is shown in Figure 26-4.

In addition to a wide variety of effects on proinflammatory cells, corticosteroids significantly inhibit T-lymphocyte activation and proliferation. The use of inhaled corticosteroids is now established in international and national guidelines for asthma management and has significantly reduced the number of patients who require long-term, oral corticosteroids. However, a small

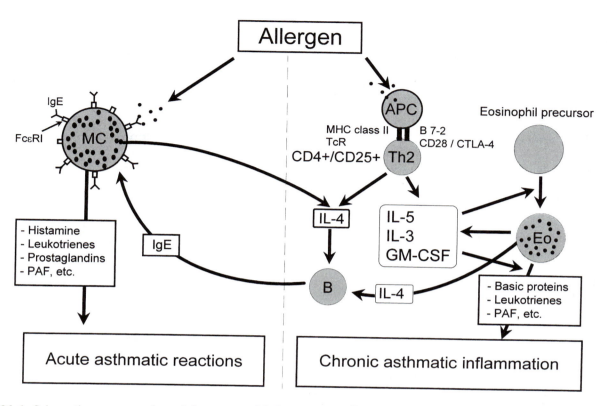

Figure 26-4. Schematic representation of the proposed inflammatory cell and cytokine network involved in acute and chronic asthma. MC, mast cell; Eo, eosinophil.

proportion of the asthmatic population still requires such treatment ("steroid-dependent" asthmatics). Many such patients suffer from the side effects of the corticosteroids (such as diabetes, hypertension, and osteoporosis) and also from poorly controlled disease. High-dose inhaled corticosteroid treatment may cause nonpulmonary side-effects because of systemic absorption. There are also patients who have corticosteroid-resistant asthma and who may therefore require alternative anti-inflammatory treatment. Given these reasons and the accumulating evidence for an inflammatory basis to the pathogenesis of chronic asthma, considerable interest has been evoked in immunosuppressive or immunomodulatory strategies that enable both the reduction or elimination of oral corticosteroids and improved asthma control. In particular, inhibitors and/or antagonists directed against more precise, T-cell–associated molecular targets hold promise for the future treatment of chronic asthma.

After the demonstration that a number of low-dose cytotoxic agents are of benefit in inflammatory diseases requiring oral corticosteroids such as rheumatoid arthritis, the usefulness of these agents was studied in the treatment of asthma. In general, the results of these studies were disappointing. In retrospect, it is likely that there were insufficient numbers of patients and that treatment was given over too short a period. Interest in this topic was revived after Mullarkey et al (80) demonstrated that

methotrexate is an effective corticosteroid-sparing agent in asthma. The best-studied agents to date are methotrexate (80,81), gold (82–84), and cyclosporin A (85,86). All of the immunosuppressants that have been investigated for the treatment of asthma have potentially serious side effects. No controlled study has proceeded for more than 1 year, so it is difficult to judge whether the reduction in the oral corticosteroid dose outweighs the deleterious effect of the immunosuppressant agent. Furthermore, no study has yet compared the relative effects of different corticosteroid-sparing agents. At present these drugs should be used either in clinical trials or on an individual-patient basis, with the clinician attempting to weigh the relative benefits and risks of treatment. They should be used only after other avenues of treatment, particularly with high-dose, inhaled corticosteroids, have proved inadequate and after full discussion of the advantages and disadvantages with the patient.

Cyclosporin A

Cyclosporin A (CsA) is a lipophilic, cyclic undecapeptide derived from the fungus *Tolypocladium inflatum Gams*. CsA (complexed to its immunophilin, cyclophilin) inhibits calcineurin phosphatase activity, which in turn is required for translocation of the cytoplasmic component of the nuclear factor of activated T cells (NF-AT) to the nucleus. It arrests T-lymphocyte division in the G0 or early G1 phase of the cell cycle and inhibits cell activation by decreasing interleukin-2 (IL-2) and IL-2 receptor expression (87). CsA has an established role in the treatment of organ transplant rejection; low-dose CsA is used extensively to treat autoimmune diseases and inflammatory conditions in which activated T lymphocytes appear to be involved, particularly psoriasis, atopic dermatitis, Crohn's disease, and rheumatoid arthritis. CsA suppresses IL-5 and GM-CSF mRNA transcription and translation by CD4+ T lymphocytes in individuals with asthma (88,89). Although the predominant effect of CsA is on the T lymphocyte, it also affects the rapid release of preformed and de novo synthesized mediators from human mast cells in vitro and basophils ex vivo. In addition, it affects the production of cytokines by eosinophils, mast cells, and monocytes and also affects antigen-presenting cell function.

Three controlled clinical trials of CsA in severe asthma have been reported. In a placebo-controlled crossover study of oral corticosteroid-dependent patients with asthma, Alexander et al (85) found a 12% improvement in the morning peak expiratory flow rate and an 18% improvement in the forced expiratory volume in 1 second (FEV_1) in patients receiving 5 mg/kg/day of CsA over those receiving placebo. In patients treated with CsA there was also a decrease in the number of exacerbations of asthma requiring an increase in the dose of oral corticosteroids. The same group (86) demonstrated in a follow-up, parallel group design study of 39 subjects that the same dose of CsA allowed a significant decrease in the required oral corticosteroid dose over the course of 36 weeks (median reduction of 62%) with an increase in lung function and a trend toward fewer disease exacerbations. During the wash-out period corticosteroid requirements returned to baseline values. Nizankowska et al (90) have shown a smaller decrease in the oral corticosteroid requirement in patients treated with CsA over the trial period in a parallel group design study. Although the final corticosteroid dose reduction in patients receiving CsA compared with those receiving placebo was not significantly different, these investigators did demonstrate a significant reduction in night-time symptoms and inhaled β-agonist use in the CsA-treated individuals. In a small open study of corticosteroid-dependent patients with asthma, Fukuda et al (91) demonstrated a decrease in bronchial hyper-responsiveness and T-cell activation markers after CsA therapy and therefore provided further evidence to implicate the mode of action of CsA in patients with severe asthma as being primarily on the T lymphocyte. More recently, a double-blind, placebo-controlled study by Sihra et al (92) in an allergen challenge model in patients with mild asthma demonstrated a 50% reduction in the late asthmatic reaction by pretreatment with two doses of CsA with no effect on the early-phase response. This finding likely reflects the predominant effect of CsA on the T lymphocyte rather than on mast-cell degranulation.

Side effects in the studies in asthma were those predictable for CsA with an increase in diastolic blood pressure and decrease in renal function. Other side effects include hepatic dysfunction, hypertrichosis, tremor, gingival hyperplasia, and paraesthesia. De novo malignancies secondary to CsA and the occurrence of lymphoproliferative disorders are rare in low-dose CsA treatment.

Inhalation of drugs in asthma improves the therapeutic index by allowing the drug to act locally in the lung without systemic toxicity. In the short term, inhaled CsA is tolerated and effective in lung allograft recipients (93), and therefore the administration of CsA by inhalation may be of use in asthma.

Other Potential Novel Immunosuppressants

New immunosuppressive agents continue to be assessed, particularly in the field of transplantation medicine, with a view to achieving more effective immunosuppression with fewer toxic effects. Some of these novel compounds may also serve as effective corticosteroid-sparing agents in severe asthma.

FK506 (tacrolimus), a macrolide produced from *Streptomyces tsukubaensis*, is already being used in transplantation medicine and has a mode of action similar to that of CsA by binding to the immunophilin FKBP, thereby blocking cytokine gene transcription (94). In lung transplantation, FK506 may be more effective than CsA in reducing persistent rejection (94). It inhibits the transcription of IL-2, IL-3, IL-4, IL-5, GM-CSF, IFN-γ, and TNF-α from both mononuclear cells and mast cells and can inhibit IgE-dependent histamine release from basophils and mast cells. Therefore, FK506 has a role in the treatment of asthma.

Rapamycin, another macrolide derived from *Streptomyces hygroscopius*, inhibits signal transduction mediated by IL-2 and other cytokines and targets cells only late in the G1 phase of cell cycle (95). Therefore, it inhibits cells that are already activated and is likely to have a more rapid immunomodulatory effect. Rapamycin inhibits immunoglobulin synthesis. Because of its binding to FKBP, it also offers the possibility of synergism with CsA. There is also in vitro evidence that rapamycin inhibits IL-5–induced eosinophil survival and degranulation (96).

Similarly, leflunomide (97), through its metabolite A77 1726, functions as a protein tyrosine kinase inhibitor and inhibits T- and B-cell responses to IL-2. Because of the resulting inhibition of T- and B-cell proliferation, immunoglobulin production, and smooth muscle proliferation, leflunomide is a potentially useful agent in the treatment of asthma and has already been studied in animal models of allergic disease with promising results (98). Although stimulation of the T cell through the CD28 pathway is insensitive to the effects of CsA and FK506, rapamycin and leflunomide are capable of blocking this pathway.

Mycophenolate mofetil limits de novo purine synthesis through inhibition of inosine monophosphate dehydrogenase and therefore selectively inhibits proliferation of activated T and B lymphocytes. It appears to be effective in preventing acute rejection in transplants in combination with CsA and has a relatively good toxicity profile (99). Brequinar sodium also inhibits de novo pyrimidine synthesis. Deoxyspergualin, a semisynthetic polyamine appears to have effects on the differentiation and proliferation of T lymphocytes, but also inhibits antigen-presenting cells and B cells.

The sites of action in the cell cycle of these various agents are summarized in Figure 26-5.

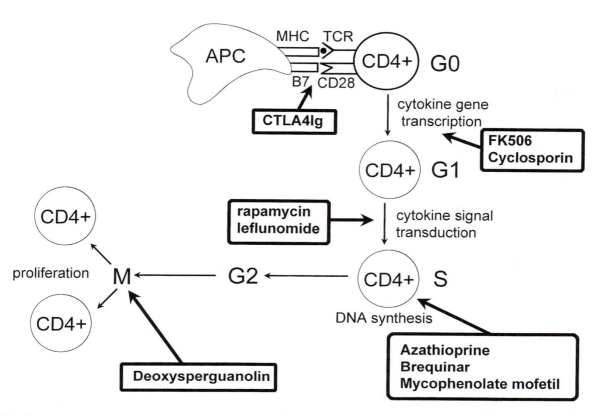

Figure 26-5. Schematic representation of the sites of action of various immunosuppressive agents. CTLA, cytolytic T lymphocyte-associated antigen.

Anti-CD4 Monoclonal Antibody Therapy

Anti-CD4 monoclonal antibody (mAb) therapy has been used in other diseases associated with activated T lymphocytes such as organ transplantation rejection, rheumatoid arthritis, nephritis, systemic lupus erythematosus, psoriasis, inflammatory bowel disease, and Wegener's granulomatosis. The effects of a single intravenous infusion of Keliximab (IDEC CE9.1), a chimeric (PRIMATIZED®) anti-CD4 mAb, was recently evaluated in patients with severe corticosteroid-dependent asthma (100). In a small, randomized, placebo-controlled, double-blind, dose-ranging study, patients receiving 3.0 mg/kg had a significant increase from baseline values in the morning and evening peak expiratory flow rate from day 1 to day 14 (Fig. 26-6). These patients also showed a trend toward an improvement in symptom scores. Significant transient reductions in CD4 counts occurred in all three active dosing cohorts (0.5, 1.5, and 3.0 mg/kg), but the highest dosing cohort appeared to have a longer period of decrease in CD4 counts. In this study a single infusion was used, and it may be that repeated doses may have a more prolonged beneficial effect. There were no serious adverse effects related to treatment.

Previous studies of anti-CD4 mAb in rheumatoid arthritis, even with prolonged depletion of CD4+ lymphocytes and in com-bination with other immunosuppressant therapy, have not demonstrated any significant increase in the risk of opportunistic infections or neoplasms. However, the use of these agents in the treatment of asthma should still be regarded as experimental and will require further large trials to substantiate whether anti-CD4 therapy may be a safe and effective adjunctive treatment for severe asthma.

Inhibitors of Costimulatory Molecules

Ligation of the T-cell receptor (TcR) of naive T cells in the absence of costimulation leads to abortive activation and, subsequently, anergy or cell death. A number of molecules have costimulatory capabilities in T-cell activation, including IL-1, LFA-1, CD40 ligand, and, most commonly, CD28 (Fig. 26-7). Allergen-specific T-cell responses, including those of airway T cells with memory phenotype, depend on costimulation through the CD28/CD86 pathway (101,102). In murine models of allergic disease, CD80 (103) and CD86 (104) have been shown to be required for the induction of pulmonary eosinophilia and altered airway responsiveness, respectively. In a study evaluating the effects of administration of monoclonal blocking antibodies to either CD80 or CD86, Keane-Myers et al (105) demonstrated that anti-CD86 antibodies could abolish allergen-induced

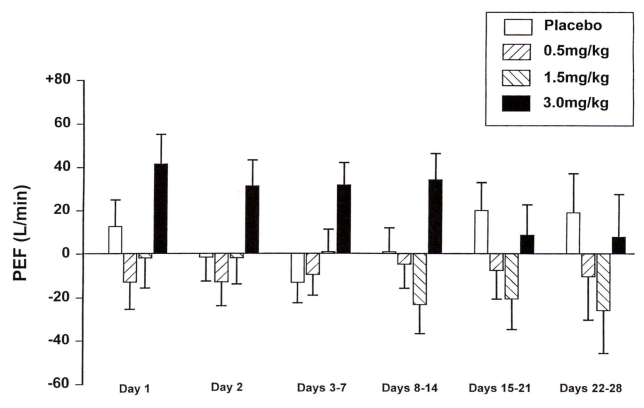

Figure 26-6. Changes from baseline value in morning peak expiratory flow rate (PEF) in chronic, severe, corticosteroid-dependent patients with asthma after infusion with an anti-CD4 mAb Keliximab. Error bars denote SEM. The area-under-the-curve change from baseline for days 1 to 14 in the patients receiving 3.0 mg/kg was significantly different from that of those receiving placebo ($P = .0174$).

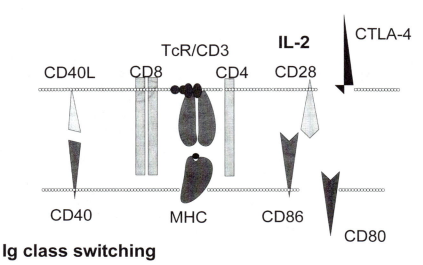

Figure 26-7. Schematic representation of costimulatory molecules involved in T-cell activation. CD28 is expressed constitutively on T cells and initially interacts with CD86, which is constitutively expressed on APC. The expression of CTLA-4 on T cells and CD80 on APC increases after cellular activation. Costimulation through CD28 is important in regulation of the synthesis of IL-2 and other cytokines. Expression of CD40L is up-regulated on T cells after activation. Ligation of CD40 and CD40L provides essential costimulatory signals for Ig isotype switching in B cells.

airways hyperresponsiveness, pulmonary eosinophilia, and elevations in serum IgG1 and IgE in ovalbumin-sensitized mice. In contrast, antibodies to CD80 had no effect on antibody levels or airway hyperresponsiveness, but did significantly diminish airway eosinophilia after allergen challenge (105). Taken together, these and other studies implicate both CD80 and CD86 in the induction and maintenance of allergic diseases.

CTLA4, a molecule closely related to CD28 in terms of gene sequence and genomic organization, acts as an additional ligand for both CD80 and CD86. Although some controversy remains about the function of CTLA4 in T-cell activation, the current consensus opinion is that, whereas CD28 acts to amplify the T-cell response, ligation of CTLA4 has the opposite effect. The observed dependence of T-cell activation on CD80 and CD86 has led a number of groups to develop strategies to block costimulation with the use of mAbs or genetically engineered proteins such as the soluble CTLA4-Ig molecule (see Fig. 26-5).

The use of CTLA4-Ig to block T-cell responses in a number of models of murine asthma has resulted in a general ability to block both airway hyperresponsiveness and pulmonary eosinophilia, together with system-dependent down-regulation of IgE and cellular infiltration into the lung after allergen challenge (106–108).

Recently, a number of groups have studied the requirement for blockade of another costimulatory pathway, the CD40/CD40L axis. Murine models of transplantation (109–112), autoimmunity (113), and immune responses to adenoviral vectors administered to the airways (114) have revealed that optimal responses to antigen at least partially depend on costimulation through CD40L.

In addition to the CD28 and CD40L pathways, the interaction of LFA-1 with its ligands ICAM-1 and 2 regulates the production of Th2 cytokines. However, in contrast to the down-regulatory effects of antibodies or soluble ligands to CD80, CD86, and CD40, the blockade of LFA-1 signaling during T-cell activation was shown to result in a 100 to 1000-fold increase in the production of Th2 cytokines (115). Using a small-molecule inhibitor of VLA-4–mediated fibronectin binding, Abraham et al showed a decrease in the early antigen-induced bronchial response of 40% in sheep sensitized to Ascaris. More strikingly, the late-phase bronchial response in this model was reduced by 88% (116). These findings raise the possibility that combined intervention in both the CD28 and CD40L costimulatory pathways, the active induction of LFA-1 signaling, or the blockade of VLA-4 may provide a useful therapeutic approach to allergic disease. However, as with all nonspecific forms of therapy, the generalized immunosuppressive effects of such approaches may preclude their use in humans.

Anti-IgE

Since the discovery of IgE in the late 1960s, various strategies have been considered that would enable selective inhibition of IgE antibody function or formation (see chapter by D. MacGlashan). The concept of an inhibitor of IgE that blocks binding to high-affinity IgE receptors but lacks the ability to trigger degranulation of IgE synthesized cells has been realized by the generation of nonanaphylactogenic anti-IgE antibodies (117). These antibodies have no effect on IgM or IgG production; inhibit IgE production by B cells; neutralize IgE in blood; and do not activate mast cells, basophils, or monocytes (i.e., they are nonanaphylactic). A humanized anti-IgE (rhuMAB-E25) was well tolerated in phase I studies and was shown to reduce symptoms of allergic rhinitis and to inhibit the early- and late-phase asthmatic reaction (118). MAB-E25 was recently shown to improve lung function, and to reduce both symptoms and corticosteroid usage in chronic asthma (119). Thus, although this approach clearly represents a potentially important advance, it is unclear whether anti-IgE will become established in the treatment of a relatively mild disease such as allergic conjunctivorhinitis because of issues of cost and the uncertainty of the effects of long-term depletion of IgE.

Cytokines and Their Inhibitors

Interleukin-1

The biologic activities of IL-1 are complex. IL-1α and β and their precursor forms are involved in multiple aspects of inflammation and host defense (120). Within this family of gene products there is also a naturally occurring receptor antagonist, IL-1ra, as well as related receptor proteins that have differential signaling functions and activities. IL-1 enhances basophil histamine release and is up-regulated during late-phase allergic reactions in the skin and nose. IL-1 receptor antagonists have been shown to reduce airway hyperresponsiveness in experimental animals (121). However, clinical studies of recombinant human IL-1ra in the treatment of asthma have been disappointing.

Interferon-γ

Interferon-γ down-regulates IgE production and inhibits the Th2 phenotype. The administration of interferon-γ to patients with asthma by nebulization was not effective, although it is uncertain whether high enough concentrations were obtained locally in the airways (122).

Interleukin-10

As discussed above under allergen-specific immunotherapy, IL-10 has a wide range of effects on allergic inflammation, which include inhibition of IgE production, mediator release from mast cells, eosinophil development, cytokine production, and IL-5 production by Th2 cells. For these reasons IL-10 might have potential in the treatment of allergy and asthma. However, the administration of IL-10 to humans was associated with "flulike symptoms," which may restrict its development (16). Although IL-10 has potential applications in inflammatory bowel disease and graft-versus-host disease, its usefulness in allergic inflammation is uncertain.

Interleukin-12

IL-12 promotes the development of naive T cells into Th1 effector cells, and in experimental animals it inhibits allergic inflammation and allergen sensitization (123). Its effect is through the release of endogenous interferon-γ. The ability of IL-12 to down-regulate Th2 responses and enhance Th1 responses may have important therapeutic implications. Recombinant human IL-12 has been administered to humans, but there are no current data about its usefulness in the treatment of allergic disease. Theoretically, early treatment with IL-12, possibly in combination with allergen, may favor a balance toward Th1 cells and away from Th2.

Interleukin-4

Interleukin-4 is essential for the development and maintenance of allergic diseases through its promotion of the Th2 response and the production of IgE (124). The production of IgE is clearly central to the development of atopic diseases. IL-4 is expressed by T cells, mast cells, basophils, and eosinophils. IL-4 exerts pleitropic effects, acting on T cells, B cells, macrophages, and endothelial cells. Thus, IL-4 directs the development of the Th2 phenotype, leading to the production of IL-4, IL-5, and IL-13. IL-4 has a number of effects on B cells, including production of IgE and IgG4, up-regulation of CD23, MHC class II, IL-4R, CD40, and IL-2Rβ.

Macrophages also respond to IL-4 by increasing CD23 and enhanced antigen presentation. IL-4 also increases the expression of VCAM-1 on endothelial cells, thereby promoting preferential adhesion of eosinophils and basophils.

The IL-4 receptor (IL-4R) consists of a functional alpha (α) chain and a common cytokine gamma (γ) chain. Theoretically, IL-4Rα can be targeted by soluble IL-4Rα (125), IL-4 mutant proteins, IL-4δ2 (an alternative splice mRNA of hIL-4 in which exon 2 of the hIL-4 gene is omitted (126), anti–IL-4Rα antibody (127), and ligand toxin (e.g., an IL-4/diptheria toxin fusion protein) (128). Soluble recombinant IL-4 receptor was shown to improve moderate atopic asthma in a placebo-controlled trial (129). Several antagonistic mutant proteins of IL-4 have also been developed (130,131). For example, site-directed mutagenesis has revealed two sites important for receptor interaction on IL-4. Site 1 mediates binding to the IL-4Rα subunit, whereas site 2 is involved in signal transduction through the receptor complex. Specific site-2 mutants have been shown to bind to the receptor with high affinity, but have little or no agonist activity (130). They are therefore potentially effective inhibitors of IL-4 action. One such IL-4 mutant protein has a tyrosine residue at position 124 placed by aspartic acid (IL-4, Y124D) (131).

The IL-4 receptor is widely expressed on many cell types, including T cells, B cells, mast cells, endothelial cells, and macrophages. The IL-4R uses multiple intracellular domains for binding of Janus family kinases (JAK) and for binding and activation of insulin receptor substrates-1 and -2 (IRS-1, IRS-2) and signal transducer and activator of transcription (STAT)-6 proteins through tyrosine phosphorylation (124). In fact, many biologic activities result from the activation of JAK-1, JAK-3, and STAT-6 (132). Members of the suppressor of cytokine signaling (SOCS) family of protein can inhibit JAK-STAT signaling. For example, SOCS-1 potently inhibits the activation of JAK-1 kinase and STAT-6 in response to IL-4 (133). Another transcription

factor involved in IL-4 signaling is c-maf, which may also be an attractive molecular therapeutic target (134).

Several animal studies indicate that an anti–IL-4 or soluble IL-4R may have efficacy in allergic diseases (135). Results vary according to protocols, but in mice CD4+ T cells were able to mediate the pathogenic changes that occur in human asthma through IL-4–dependent mechanisms independently of IL-5, IgE, or both (136). An anti–IL-4 was shown to inhibit a local Th2 response in the development of eosinophilic infiltration in the lung. However, it was suggested that sequential involvement of IL-4 and IL-5, with IL-4 committing naive T cells to the Th2 phenotype, may be involved; on activation by aerosol provocation these cells secrete IL-5, resulting in eosinophilic inflammation (137).

Anti–IL-5

Eosinophil leukocytes are generally considered to be major proinflammatory cells in causing tissue damage in atopic allergic diseases, including asthma, as well as having a role in adaptive immunity to infection with helminthic parasites. A key molecule that controls eosinophil formation, function, and fate is IL-5. IL-5 specifically promotes terminal differentiation of eosinophil precursors, releases mature (and possibly immature) eosinophils from bone marrow, primes and activates the tissue eosinophil for effector functions, and delays programmed cell death (apoptosis), thereby enhancing tissue survival. Some of these properties are also shared with the related cytokines, IL-3 and GM-CSF.

The importance of IL-5 and IL-5Rα in asthma was emphasized by the demonstration of elevated mRNA in bronchoalveolar lavage fluid and bronchial biopsies and the correlation with clinical features, including lung function and the degree of airway hyperresponsiveness (138–141). Furthermore, there was up-regulation of IL-5 after allergen-provoked asthma (142) and down-regulation after successful treatment with corticosteroids (143). IL-5 mRNA colocalized mainly to CD4+ cells in bronchial biopsies from patients with both atopic and nonatopic asthma at baseline, although other cell types such as CD8+ cells, mast cells, and eosinophils were also mRNA+ to a lesser degree (144). In nonhuman primates an anti–IL-5 almost completely abrogated eosinophilia and airway hyperresponsiveness in an Ascaris model of asthma (145). CD34+/IL-5Rα+ cells (putative eosinophil precursors) have also been observed in bronchial biopsies from patients with asthma, and their numbers correlated with the degree of airflow obstruction (140).

Whereas IL-5 is mainly involved in eosinophil maturation, the critical molecules for selective eosinophil migration into the sites of allergic tissue reactions are believed to be the CC chemokines, particularly eotaxin. In experimental animals IL-5 and eotaxin appear to act synergistically at the bone marrow and tissue levels to produce a pronounced blood and tissue eosinophilia (146,147).

To demonstrate that a bioactive mediator is of importance in a disease such as asthma, it is necessary to fulfill certain criteria. First, as described above, the level of the agent must be elevated in the disease, and the concentrations should correlate with the disease activity. Second, the agent should also produce characteristic features of the disease when administered to susceptible individuals. This criterion has been partially demonstrated by Shi et al (148), who observed that inhalation of IL-5 by humans with asthma was accompanied by increases in eosinophils in sputum and enhanced airway hyperresponsiveness. Third, it is essential to show that the disease is attenuated or ameliorated by a specific antagonist (e.g., anti–IL-5). SB240563 is a high-affinity, humanized mAb (IgG1) that has recently been shown to be well tolerated and to reduce the numbers of eosinophils in blood and allergen-induced sputum in patients with mild asthma. Recent preliminary studies in mild asthma have shown that SB240563 abolished blood eosinophils and reduced sputum eosinophils but, surprisingly, had no apparent effect on the late asthmatic reaction or airway hyperresponsiveness (149). Long-term studies, in which total inhibition of tissue eosinophilia is achieved, will be required to establish conclusively the role of eosinophils and IL-5 in chronic atopic allergic disease and asthma.

BCG and Other Forms of Stimulating Th1 Patterns of Immunity

The explanation for the increasing prevalence of atopic disease in developed countries in recent decades has remained enigmatic. Among the many potential contributing factors is the relative reduction of childhood exposure to infectious diseases after the introduction of antibiotics and widespread vaccination program (150). Epidemiologic studies have suggested that an inverse correlation exists between the numbers of older siblings and the incidence of allergic rhinitis, implying that the increased number of childhood infections contracted from siblings may protect against the development of atopic responses (151).

Shaheen et al (152) studied the incidence of atopy in a West African community in relation to previous active measles infection. They found that active infection, when compared with immunization, protected against the development of atopy as assessed by positive skin-prick test to house dust mite. Shirakawa et al (153) have described an inverse relationship between tuberculin responses and atopy in Japanese children. However, a similar study in Swedish school children failed to establish a protective link with BCG vaccination in children with atopic heredity (154).

The effect of mycobacterial vaccination on the development of atopic responses has been evaluated in animal models. Prior immunization of BALB/c mice with BCG resulted in increased IFN-γ responses and reduced proliferative responses to ovalbumin. Albumin-specific IgG1 and IgE were reduced, while IgG2a levels increased. Furthermore, BCG immunization prevented bronchial hyperresponsiveness and reduced levels of IL-4 and IL-5 in bronchial lavage fluid (155). A similar study with heat-killed *Mycobacterium vaccae* showed similar but less impressive results (156). Hetzel et al (157) have expressed peptides from Der p 1 in the superoxide dismutase gene of both *Mycobacterium bovis* and *Mycobacterium vaccae* and demonstrated peptide-specific IFN-γ responses in mice (157). Phase II clinical trials of a heat-killed preparation of *Mycobacterium vaccae* are currently under way in atopic individuals.

Anti–Adhesion Molecules

Cell adhesion molecules include those of the immunoglobulin superfamily, that is, ICAM-1, ICAM-2, and ICAM-3, as well as leukocyte integrins, which are homodimers consisting of alpha and beta subunits. A mAb to ICAM-1 prevented eosinophil infiltration and airway responsiveness after allergen exposure in sensitized primates (158). Thus ICAM-1 blockers may have therapeutic potential in asthma. Antibodies against the β1-integrin $\alpha_4\beta_1$ (very late antigen [VLA-4]) may be more selective since VLA-4 is expressed on eosinophils but not neutrophils. An anti–VLA-4 (HP1/2) inhibited eosinophil infiltration in the skin and in allergic sheep and guinea pigs after exposure to allergen (159,160). Several small nonpeptide VLA-4 inhibitors are also under development.

Eosinophil Inhibitors

In addition to anti–IL-5 and anti–VLA-4 antibodies, another possible mechanism of eosinophil inhibition includes blockage of the eotaxin receptor CCR3 (161,162). Eosinophil migration appears to depend largely on the elaboration of CC chemokines, particularly eotaxin, eotaxin-2, MCP-3, MCP-4, and RANTES, all of which engage CCR3 and are believed to be critical for eosinophil migration from the vasculature to the tissues. Thus, blockade of CCR3 would seem a logical antiasthma approach. A further strategy for decreasing eosinophil-mediated tissue injury is to accelerate apoptosis or, conversely, to prevent the action of eosinophil survival factors such as IL-5, IL-3, and GM-CSF.

Glucocorticosteroids increase eosinophil apoptosis by unknown mechanisms. Local anesthetics (e.g., lidocaine) also have similar effects (163). Nitric oxide donors increase eosinophil survival, suggesting that nitric oxide synthase inhibitors might also decrease eosinophil survival (164).

Conclusions

Immunologically specific and nonspecific approaches to the treatment of asthma and allergic diseases are discussed. The expectation is reasonable that, in the foreseeable future, safe and effective strategies will be available for inducing some form of allergen-specific, T-cell hyporesponsiveness or tolerance. Particularly promising approaches include the use of allergen isoforms, recombinant allergens, MHC class II–based T-cell epitope vaccines, and DNA vaccines. In situations where the role of allergens is uncertain such as chronic asthma, or where several allergens are operative, more global nonspecific approaches are required. Many novel approaches such as nonanaphylactogenic anti-IgE, novel immunosuppressant drugs, anti–cytokine antibodies, and anti–adhesion molecules hold promise for future therapy. Validated new and effective immunologically based treatments for asthma and allergy are a realistic hope within the next decade.

References

1. Noon L. Prophylactic inoculation against hay fever. Lancet 1911;1:1572.
2. Freeman J. Vaccination against hay fever: report of results during the first three years. Lancet 1914;1:1178.
3. Durham SR, Walker SM, Varga EM, et al. Long-term clinical efficacy of grass-pollen immunotherapy. N Engl J Med 1999;341:468–475.
4. Allergen Immunotherapy: Therapeutic vaccines for allergic diseases. WHO Position Paper. Allergy 1998;54(suppl 53):1–42.
5. Position Paper on Allergen Immunotherapy. Report of a BSACI Working Party. Clin Exp Allergy 1993;23(suppl 3):1–44.
6. Durham SR, Till SJ. Immunologic changes associated with allergen immunotherapy. J Allergy Clin Immunol 1998;102:157–164.
7. Akdis CA, Blesken T, Akdis M, et al. Induction and differential regulation of bee venom phospholipase A_2-specific human IgE and IgG4 antibodies in vitro requires allergen-specific and nonspecific activation of T and B cells. J Allergy Clin Immunol 1997;99:345–353.
8. Akdis CA, Blesken T, Akdis M, et al. Role of interleukin 10 in specific immunotherapy. J Clin Invest 1998;102:98–106.
9. Manetti R, Parronchi P, Giudizi MG, et al. Natural killer cell stimulatory factor (interleukin 12 (IL-12)) induces T helper type 1 (Th1)-specific immune responses and inhibits the development of IL-4-producing Th cells. J Exp Med 1993;177:1199–1204.
10. Yamashita N, Takeno M, Kaneko S, et al. Therapeutic effects of preferential induction of mite-specific T helper 0 clones. Clin Exp Immunol 1997;109:332–341.
11. Creticos PS, Adkinson NF Jr, Kagey Sobotka A, et al. Nasal challenge with ragweed pollen in hay fever patients. Effect of immunotherapy. J Clin Invest 1985;76:2247–2253.
12. Nish WA, Charlesworth EN, Davis TL, et al. The effect of immunotherapy on the cutaneous late phase response to antigen. J Allergy Clin Immunol 1994;93:484–493.
13. Varney VA, Hamid QA, Gaga M, et al. Influence of grass pollen immunotherapy on cellular infiltration and cytokine mRNA expression during allergen-induced late-phase cutaneous responses. J Clin Invest 1993;92:644–651.
14. Furin MJ, Norman PS, Creticos PS, et al. Immunotherapy decreases antigen-induced eosinophil cell migration into the nasal cavity. J Allergy Clin Immunol 1991;88:27–32.
15. Akdis CA, Blaser K. IL-10-induced anergy in peripheral T cell and reactivation by microenvironmental cytokines: two key steps in specific immunotherapy. FASEB J 1999;13:603–609.
16. Borish L. IL-10: evolving concepts. J Allergy Clin Immunol 1998;101:293–297.
17. Akdis CA, Akdis M, Blesken T, et al. Epitope-specific T cell tolerance to phospholipase A_2 in bee venom immunotherapy and recovery by IL-2 and IL-15 in vitro. J Clin Invest 1996;98:1676–1683.
18. Renz H, Lack G, Saloga J, et al. Inhibition of IgE production and normalization of airways responsiveness by sensitized CD8 T cells in a mouse model of allergen-induced sensitization. J Immunol 1994;152:351–360.
19. Groux H, O'Garra A, Bigler M, et al. A CD4+ T-cell subset inhibits antigen-specific T-cell responses and prevents colitis. Nature 1997;389:737–742.
20. Blaser K, Carballido JM, Faith A, et al. Determinants and mechanisms of human immune responses to bee venom phospholipase A_2. Int Arch Allergy Immunol 1998;117:1–10.
21. Faith A, Akdis CA, Akdis M, et al. Defective TCR stimulation in anergized type 2 T helper cells correlates with abrogated $p56^{lck}$ and ZAP-70 tyrosine kinase activities. J Immunol 1997;159:53–60.
22. Faith A, Akdis CA, Akdis M, et al. An altered peptide ligand specifically inhibits Th2 cytokine synthesis by abrogating TCR signaling. J Immunol 1999;162:1836–1842.
23. Larché M. Allergen isoforms for immunotherapy: diversity, degeneracy and promiscuity. Clin Exp Allergy 1999;29:1588–1590.
24. Marsh DG, Lichtenstein LM, Campbell DH. Studies on "allergoids" prepared from naturally occurring allergens. I. Assay of allergenicity and antigenicity of formalinized rye group component. Immunology 1970;18:705–722.
25. Norman PS, Lichtenstein LM, Marsh DG. Studies on allergoids from naturally occurring allergens. IV. Efficacy and safety of long-term allergoid treatment of ragweed hay fever. J Allergy Clin Immunol 1981;68:460–470.
26. Norman PS, Lichtenstein LM, Kagey-Sobotka A, Marsh DG. Controlled evaluation of allergoid in the immunotherapy of ragweed hay fever. J Allergy Clin Immunol 1982;70:248–260.
27. Bousquet J, Hejjaoui A, Skassa-Brociek W, et al. Double-blind, placebo-controlled immunotherapy with mixed grass-pollen allergoids. I. Rush immunotherapy with allergoids and standardized orchard grass-pollen extract. J Allergy Clin Immunol 1987;80:591–598.
28. Bousquet J, Maasch H, Martinot B, et al. Double-blind, placebo-controlled immunotherapy with mixed grass-pollen allergoids. II. Comparison between parameters assessing the efficacy of immunotherapy. J Allergy Clin Immunol 1988;82:439–446.
29. Bousquet J, Maasch HJ, Hejjaoui A, et al. Double-blind, placebo-controlled immunotherapy with mixed grass-pollen allergoids. III. Efficacy and safety of unfractionated and high-molecular-weight preparations in rhinoconjunctivitis and asthma. J Allergy Clin Immunol 1989;84:546–556.
30. Bousquet J, Hejjaoui A, Soussana M, Michel FB. Double-blind, placebo-controlled immunotherapy with mixed grass-pollen allergoids. IV. Comparison of the safety and efficacy of two dosages of a high-molecular-weight allergoid. J Allergy Clin Immunol 1990;85:490–497.
31. Pastorello EA, Pravettoni V, Incorvaia C, et al. Clinical and immunological effects of immunotherapy with alum-absorbed grass allergoid in grass-pollen-induced hay fever. Allergy 1992;47:281–290.
32. Tari MG, Mancino M, Ghezzi E, et al. Immunotherapy with an alum-adsorbed Parietaria-pollen allergoid: a 2-year, double-blind, placebo-controlled study. Allergy 1997;52:65–74.
33. Pecoud A, Nicod L, Badan M, et al. Effects of one-year hyposensitization in allergic rhinitis. Comparison of two house dust mite extracts. Allergy 1990;45:386–392.
34. Passalacqua G, Albano M, Fregonese L, et al. Randomised controlled trial of local allergoid immunotherapy on

allergic inflammation in mite-induced rhinoconjunctivitis. Lancet 1998;351:629–632.

35. Ferreira F, Hirtenlehner K, Jilek A, et al. Dissection of immunoglobulin E and T lymphocyte reactivity of isoforms of the major birch pollen allergen Bet v 1: potential use of hypoallergenic isoforms for immunotherapy. J Exp Med 1996;183:599–609.

36. Breiteneder H, Ferreira F, Hoffmann-Sommergruber K, et al. Four recombinant isoforms of Cor a I, the major allergen of hazel pollen, show different IgE-binding properties. Eur J Biochem 1993;212:355–362.

37. Schenk S, Hoffmann-Sommergruber K, Breiteneder H, et al. Four recombinant isoforms of Cor a 1, the major allergen of hazel pollen, show different reactivities with allergen-specific T-lymphocyte clones. Eur J Biochem 1994;224:717–722.

38. Ferreira F, Ebner C, Kramer B, et al. Modulation of IgE reactivity of allergens by site-directed mutagenesis: potential use of hypoallergenic variants for immunotherapy. FASEB J 1998;2:231–242.

39. Stanley JS, King N, Burks AW, et al. Identification and mutational analysis of the immunodominant IgE binding epitopes of the major peanut allergen Ara h 2. Arch Biochem Biophys 1997;342:244–253.

40. Smith AM, Chapman MD. Reduction in IgE binding to allergen variants generated by site-directed mutagenesis: contribution of disulfide bonds to the antigenic structure of the major house dust mite allergen Der p 2. Mol Immunol 1996;33:399–405.

41. Takai T, Yokota T, Yasue M, et al. Engineering of the major house dust mite allergen Der f 2 for allergen-specific immunotherapy. Nat Biotechnol 1997;15:754–758.

42. Schramm G, Kahlert H, Suck R, et al. "Allergen engineering": variants of the timothy grass pollen allergen Phl p 5b with reduced IgE-binding capacity but conserved T cell reactivity. Immunol 1999;162:2406–2414.

43. Rogers BL, Bond JF, Craig SJ, et al. Potential therapeutic recombinant proteins comprised of peptides containing recombined T cell epitopes. Mol Immunol 1994;31:955–966.

44. Vrtala S, Hirtenlehner K, Vangelista L, et al. Conversion of the major birch pollen allergen, Bet v 1, into two nonanaphylactic T cell epitope-containing fragments: candidates for a novel form of specific immunotherapy. J Clin Invest 1997;99:1673–1681.

45. Clayton JP, Gammon GM, Ando DG, et al. Peptide-specific prevention of experimental allergic encephalomyelitis. J Exp Med 1989;169:1681–1691.

46. Gaur A, Wiers B, Liu A, et al. Amelioration of experimental autoimmune encephalomyelitis by myelin basic protein synthetic peptide-induced anergy. Science 1992;258:1491–1494.

47. Ku G, Kronenberg M, Peacock DJ, et al. Prevention of experimental autoimmune arthritis with a peptide fragment of type II collagen. Eur J Immunol 1993;23:591–599.

48. Staines NA, Harper N, Ward FJ, et al. Mucosal tolerance and suppression of collagen-induced arthritis (CIA) induced by nasal inhalation of synthetic peptide 184–198 of bovine type II collagen (CII) expressing a dominant T cell epitope. Clin Exp Immunol 1996;103:368–375.

49. Vaysburd M, Lock C, McDevitt H. Prevention of insulin-dependent diabetes mellitus in non-obese diabetic mice by immunogenic but not tolerated peptides. J Exp Med 1995;182:897–902.

50. Briner TJ, Kuo MC, Keating KM, et al. Peripheral T-cell tolerance induced in naive and primed mice by subcutaneous injection of peptides from the major cat allergen Fel d I. Proc Natl Acad Sci USA 1993;90:7608–7612.

51. Hoyne GF, O'Hehir RE, Wraith DC, et al. Inhibition of T cell and antibody responses to house dust mite allergen by inhalation of the dominant T cell epitope in naive and sensitized mice. J Exp Med 1993;178:1783–1788.

52. Karin N, Binah O, Grabie N, et al. Short peptide-based tolerogens without self-antigenic or pathogenic activity reverse autoimmune disease. J Immunol 1998;160:5188–5194.

53. Warren KG, Catz I, Wucherpfennig KW. Tolerance induction to myelin basic protein by intravenous synthetic peptides containing epitope P85 VVHFFKNIVTP96 in chronic progressive multiple sclerosis. J Neurol Sci 1997;152:31–38.

54. Norman PS, Ohman JL Jr, Long AA, et al. Treatment of cat allergy with T-cell reactive peptides. Am J Respir Crit Care Med 1996;154:1623–1628.

55. Muller U, Akdis CA, Fricker M, et al. Successful immunotherapy with T-cell epitope peptides of bee venom phospholipase A2 induces specific T-cell anergy in patients allergic to bee venom. J Allergy Clin Immunol 1998;101:747–754.

56. Haselden BM, Kay AB, Larché M. IgE-independent MHC-restricted T cell peptide epitope-induced late asthmatic reactions. J Exp Med 1999;189:1885–1894.

57. Southwood S, Sidney J, Kondo A, et al. Several common HLA-DR types share largely overlapping peptide binding repertoires. J Immunol 1998;160:3363–3373.

58. Tighe H, Corr M, Roman M, Raz E. Gene vaccination: plasmid DNA is more than just a blueprint. Immunol Today 1998;19:89–97.

59. Yamamoto T, Yamamoto S, Katakota T, et al. Synthetic oligonucleotides with certain palindromic sequences stimulate interferon production of human peripheral blood lymphocytes in vitro. Jpn J Cancer Res 1994;85:775–779.

60. Krieg AM, Yi AK, Matson S, et al. CpG motifs in bacterial DNA trigger direct B cell activation. Nature 1995;374:546–549.

61. Halpern MD, Kurlander RJ, Pisetsky DS. Bacterial DNA induces murine interferon-gamma production by stimulation of interleukin-12 and tumor necrosis factor-alpha. Cell Immunol 1996;167:72–78.

62. Klinsman DM, Yi AK, Beaucage SL, et al. CpG motifs present in bacterial DNA rapidly induce lymphocytes to secrete interleukin 6, interleukin 12 and interferon-γ. Proc Natl Acad Sci USA 1996;93:2879–2883.

63. Kline JN, Waldschmidt TJ, Businga TR, et al. Modulation of airway inflammation by CpG oligodeoxynucleotides in a murine model of asthma. J Immunol 1998;160:2555–2559.

64. Broide D, Schwarze J, Tighe H, et al. Immunostimulatory DNA sequences inhibit IL-5, eosinophilic inflammation and airway hyperresponsiveness in mice. J Immunol 1998;161:7054–7062.

65. Wolff JA, Malone RW, Williams P, et al. Direct gene transfer into mouse muscle in vivo. Science 1990;247:1465–1468.

66. Wolff JA, Ludtke JJ, Acsadi G, et al. Long term persistance of plasmid DNA and foreign gene expression in mouse muscle. Hum Mol Genet 1992;1:363–369.

67. Raz E, Tighe H, Sato Y, et al. Preferential induction of a Th1 immune response and inhibition of specific IgE antibody formation by plasmid DNA immunization. Proc Natl Acad Sci USA 1996;93:5141–5145.

68. Hsu CH, Chua KY, Tao MH, et al. Inhibition of specific IgE response in vivo by allergen-gene transfer. Int Immunol 1996;8:1405–1411.

69. Hsu CH, Chua KY, Tao MH, et al. Immunoprophylaxis of allergen-induced immunoglobulin E synthesis and airway hyperresponsiveness in vivo by genetic immunization. Nat Med 1996;2:540–544.

70. Li XM, Chopra RK, Chou TY, et al. Mucosal IFN-gamma gene transfer inhibits pulmonary allergic responses in mice. J Immunol 1996;157:3216–3219.

71. Roy K, Mao HQ, Huang SK, Leong KW. Oral gene delivery with chitosan-DNA nanoparticles generates immunologic protection in a murine model of peanut allergy. Nat Med 1999;5:387–391.

72. Li X, Huang CK, Schofield BH, et al. Strain-dependent induction of allergic sensitization caused by peanut allergen DNA immunization in mice. J Immunol 1999;162:3045–3052.

73. Allsopp CE, Plebanski M, Gilbert S, et al. Comparison of numerous delivery systems for the induction of cytotoxic T lymphocytes by immunization. Eur J Immunol 1996; 26:1951–1959.

74. Lo-Man R, Rueda P, Sedlik C, et al. A recombinant virus-like particle system derived from parvovirus as an efficient antigen carrier to elicit a polarized Th1 immune response without adjuvant. Eur J Immunol 1998;28:1401–1407.

75. Plebanski M, Gilbert SC, Schneider J, et al. Protection from Plasmodium berghei infection by priming and boosting T cells to a single class I-restricted epitope with recombinant carriers suitable for human use. Eur J Immunol 1998;28: 4345–4355.

76. Harris SJ, Roth JF, Savage N, et al. Prediction of murine MHC class I epitopes in a major house dust mite allergen and induction of T1-type CD8+ T cell responses. Int Immunol 1997;9:273–280.

77. Martin SJ, Vyakarnam A, Cheingsong-Popov R, et al. Immunization of human HIV-seronegative volunteers with recombinant p17/p24:Ty virus-like particles elicits HIV-1 p24-specific cellular and humoral immune responses. AIDS 1993;7:1315–1323.

78. Weber J, Cheinsong-Popov R, Callow D, et al. Immunogenicity of the yeast recombinant p17/p24:Ty virus-like particles (p24-VLP) in healthy volunteers. Vaccine 1995;13: 831–834.

79. Kay AB, Frew AJ, Corrigan CJ, Robinson DS. The T cell hypothesis of chronic asthma. In: Kay AB, ed. Allergy and allergic diseases. Vol. 2. Oxford: Blackwell Science, 1997:1379–1394.

80. Mullarkey MF, Blumenstein BA, Andrade WP, et al. Methotrexate in the treatment of corticosteroid-dependent asthma. A double-blind crossover study. N Engl J Med 1988;318:603–607.

81. Shiner RJ, Nunn AJ, Chung KF, Geddes DM. Randomised, double-blind, placebo-controlled trial of methotrexate in steroid-dependent asthma. Lancet 1990;336:137–140.

82. Bernstein IL, Bernstein DI, Dubb JW, et al. A placebo-controlled multicenter study of auranofin in the treatment of patients with corticosteroid-dependent asthma. Auranofin Multicenter Drug Trial. J Allergy Clin Immunol 1996;98:317–324.

83. Muranaka M, Miyamoto T, Shida T, et al. Gold salt in the treatment of bronchial asthma—a double-blind study. Ann Allergy 1978;40:132–137.

84. Nierop G, Gijzel WP, Bel EH, et al. Auranofin in the treatment of steroid dependent asthma: a double blind study. Thorax 1992;47:349–354.

85. Alexander AG, Barnes NC, Kay AB. Trial of cyclosporin in corticosteroid-dependent chronic severe asthma. Lancet 1992;339:324–328.

86. Lock SH, Kay AB, Barnes NC. Double-blind, placebo-controlled study of cyclosporin A as a corticosteroid-sparing agent in corticosteroid-dependent asthma. Am J Respir Crit Care Med 1996;153:509–514.

87. Kahan BD. Cyclosporine. N Engl J Med 1989;321:1725–1738.

88. Mori A, Suko M, Nishizaki Y, et al. IL-5 production by CD4+ T cells of asthmatic patients is suppressed by glucocorticoids and the immunosuppressants FK506 and cyclosporin A. Int Immunol 1995;7:449–457.

89. Sano T, Nakamura Y, Matsunaga Y, et al. FK506 and cyclosporin A inhibit granulocyte/macrophage colony-stimulating factor production by mononuclear cells in asthma. Eur Respir J 1995;8:1473–1478.

90. Nizankowska E, Soja J, Pinis G, et al. Treatment of steroid-dependent bronchial asthma with cyclosporin. Eur Respir J 1995;8:1091–1099.

91. Fukuda T, Asakawa J, Motojima S, Makino S. Cyclosporine A reduces T lymphocyte activity and improves airway hyperresponsiveness in corticosteroid-dependent chronic severe asthma. Ann Alllergy Asthma Immunol 1995;75:65–72.

92. Sihra BS, Kon OM, Durham SR, et al. Effect of cyclosporin A on the allergen-induced late asthmatic reaction. Thorax 1997;52:447–452.

93. O'Riordan TG, Iacono A, Keenan RJ, et al. Delivery and distribution of aerosolized cyclosporine in lung allograft recipients. Am J Respir Crit Care Med 1995;151:516–521.

94. Schreiber SL, Crabtree GR. The mechanism of action of cyclosporin A and FK506. Immunol Today 1992;13:136–142.

95. Bonham CA, Thomson AW. Immunosuppressants (drugs and monoclonal antibodies). In: Kay AB, ed. Allergy and allergic diseases. Oxford: Blackwell Science, 1997:642–666.

96. Meng Q, Ying S, Corrigan CJ, et al. Effects of rapamycin, cyclosporin A, and dexamethasone on interleukin 5-induced eosinophil degranulation and prolonged survival. Allergy 1997;52:1095–1101.

97. Fox RI. Mechanism of action of leflunomide in rheumatoid arthritis. J Rheumatol Suppl 1998;53:20–26.

98. Eber E, Uhlig T, McMenamin C, Sly PD. Leflunomide, a novel immunomodulating agent, prevents the development of allergic sensitization in an animal model of allergic asthma. Clin Exp Allergy 1998;28:376–384.

99. Sollinger HW. Update on preclinical and clinical experience with mycophenolate mofetil. Transplant Proc 1996;28(6 suppl 1):24–29.

100. Kon OM, Sihra BS, Compton CH, et al. Randomised, dose-ranging, placebo-controlled study of chimeric antibody to

CD4 (keliximab) in chronic severe asthma. Lancet 1998;352: 1109–1113.

101. Van Neerven RJ, Van de Pol MM, Van der Zee JS, et al. Requirement of CD28–CD86 costimulation for allergen-specific T cell proliferation and cytokine expression. Clin Exp Allergy 1998;28:808–816.

102. Larché M, Till SJ, Haselden B-M, et al. Co-stimulation through CD86 is involved in airway presenting cell and T cell responses to allergen in atopic asthmatics. J Immunol 1998;161:6375–6382.

103. Harris N, Peach R, Naemura J, et al. CD80 costimulation is essential for the induction of airway eosinophilia. J Exp Med 1997;185:177–182.

104. Tsuyuki S, Tsuyuki J, Einsle K, et al. Costimulation through B7-2 (CD86) is required for the induction of a lung mucosal T helper cell 2 (TH2) immune response and altered airway responsiveness. J Exp Med 1997;185:1671–1679.

105. Keane-Myers AM, Gause WC, Finkelman FD, et al. Development of murine allergic asthma is dependent upon B7-2 costimulation. J Immunol 1998;160:1036–1043.

106. Krinzman SJ, De Sanctis GT, Cernadas M, et al. Inhibition of T cell costimulation abrogates airway hyperresponsiveness in a murine model. J Clin Invest 1996;98:2693–2699.

107. Keane-Myers A, Gause WC, Linsley PS, et al. B7-CD28/CTLA-4 costimulatory pathways are required for the development of T helper cell 2-mediated allergic airway responses to inhaled antigens. J Immunol 1997;158:2042–2049.

108. Van Oosterhout AJ, Hofstra CL, Shields R, et al. Murine CTLA4-IgG treatment inhibits airway eosinophilia and hyperresponsiveness and attenuates IgE upregulation in a murine model of allergic asthma. Am J Respir Cell Mol Biol 1997;17:386–392.

109. Kirk AD, Harlan DM, Armstrong NN, et al. CTLA4-Ig and anti-CD40 ligand prevent renal allograft rejection in primates. Proc Natl Acad Sci USA 1997;94:8789–8794.

110. Konieczny BT, Dai Z, Elwood ET, et al. IFN-gamma is critical for long-term allograft survival induced by blocking the CD28 and CD40 ligand T cell costimulation pathways. J Immunol 1998;160:2059–2064.

111. Li Y, Zheng XX, Li XC, et al. Combined costimulation blockade plus rapamycin but not cyclosporine produces permanent engraftment. Transplantation 1998;66:1387–1388.

112. Stuber E, von Freier A, Folsch UR. The effect of anti-gp39 treatment on the intestinal manifestations of acute murine graft-versus-host disease. Clin Immunol 1999;90:334–339.

113. Daikh DI, Finck BK, Linsley PS, et al. Long-term inhibition of murine lupus by brief simultaneous blockade of the B7/CD28 and CD40/gp39 costimulation pathways. J Immunol 1997;159:3104–3108.

114. Scaria A, St George JA, Gregory RJ, et al. Antibody to CD40 ligand inhibits both humoral and cellular immune responses to adenoviral vectors and facilitates repeated administration to mouse airway. Gene Ther 1997;4:611–617.

115. Salomon B, Bluestone JA. LFA-1 interaction with ICAM-1 and ICAM-2 regulates Th2 cytokine production. J Immunol 1998;161:5138–5142.

116. Abraham WM, Ahmed A, Sielczak MW, et al. Blockade of late-phase airway responses and airway hyperresponsiveness in allergic sheep with a small-molecule peptide inhibitor of VLA-4. Am J Respir Crit Care Med 1997;156: 696–703.

117. Heusser C, Jardieu P. Therapeutic potential of anti-IgE antibodies. Curr Opin Immunol 1997;9:805–814.

118. Demoly P, Bousquet J. Anti-IgE therapy for asthma. Am J Respir Crit Care Med 1997;155:1825–1827.

119. Milgrom H, Fick RB, Su JQ, et al. Treatment of allergic asthma with monoclonal anti-IgE antibody. N Engl J Med 1999;341:1966–1973.

120. Rosenwasser LJ. Biologic activities of IL-1 and its role in human disease. J Allergy Clin Immunol 1998;102:344–350.

121. Selig W, Tocker J. Effect of interleukin-1 receptor antagonist on antigen-induced pulmonary responses in guinea pigs. Eur J Pharmacol 1992;213:331–336.

122. Boguniewicz M, Martin RJ, Gibson U, Celniker A. The effects of nebulized recombinant interferon-γ in asthmatic airways. J Allergy Clin Immunol 1995;95:133–135.

123. Gavett SH, O'Hearn DJ, Li X, et al. Interleukin 12 inhibits antigen-induced airway hyperresponsiveness, inflammation and Th2 cytokine expression in mice. J Exp Med 1995;182: 1527–1536.

124. Ryan JJ. Interleukin-4 and its receptor: essential mediators of the allergic response. J Allergy Clin Immunol 1997;99: 1–5.

125. Fanslow WC, Clifford K, Vandenbos T, et al. A soluble form of the interleukin 4 receptor in biological fluids. Cytokine 1990;2:398–401.

126. Sorg RV, Enczmann J, Sorg UR, et al. Identification of an alternatively spliced transcript of human interleukin-4 lacking the sequence encoded by exon 2. Exp Hematol 1993;21:560–563.

127. Gavett SH, O'Hearn DJ, Karp CL, et al. Interleukin-4 receptor blockade prevents airway responses induced by antigen challenge in mice. Am J Physiol 1997;272:L253–L261.

128. Kreitman RJ, Puri RK, Pastan I. Increased antitumor activity of a circularly permuted interleukin-4 toxin in mice with interleukin 4 receptor-bearing human carcinoma. Cancer Res 1995;55:3357–3363.

129. Borish L, Nelson HS, Lanz MJ, et al. Interleukin-4 receptor in moderate atopic asthma. A phase I/II randomized, placebo-controlled trial. Am J Respir Crit Care Med 1999;160:1816–1823.

130. Duschl A, Muller T, Sebald W. Antagonistic mutant proteins of interleukin-4. Behring Inst Mitt 1995;96:87–94.

131. De Vries JE, Yssel H. Modulation of the human IgE response. Eur Respir J Suppl 1996;22:58s–62s.

132. Hou J, Schindler U, Henzel WJ, et al. An interleukin-4–induced transcription factor IL-4 stat. Science 1994;265: 1701–1706.

133. Losman JA, Chen XP, Hilton D, et al. SOCS-1 is a potent inhibitor of IL-4 signal transduction. J Immunol 1999;162: 3770–3774.

134. Ho IC, Hodge MR, Rooney JW, Glimcher LH. The proto-oncogene c-maf is responsible for tissue-specific expression of interleukin-4. Cell 1996;85:973–983.

135. Renz H, Bradley K, Enssle K, et al. Prevention of the development of immediate hypersensitivity and airway hyperresponsiveness following in vivo treatment with soluble IL-4 receptor. Int Arch Allergy Immunol 1996;109:167–176.

136. Corry DB, Gruenig G, Hadeiba H, et al. Requirements for allergen-induced airway hyperreactivity in T and B cell-deficient mice. Mol Med 1998;4:344–355.

137. Coyle AJ, Le Gros G, Bertrand C, et al. Interleukin-4 is

required for the induction of lung Th2 mucosal immunity. Am J Respir Cell Mol Biol 1995;13:54–59.

138. Foster PS, Hogan SP, Ramsay AJ, et al. Interleukin 5 deficiency abolishes eosinophilia, airways hyperreactivity, and lung damage in a mouse asthma model. J Exp Med 1996;183:195–201.

139. Sehmi R, Wood LJ, Watson R, et al. Allergen-induced increases in IL-5Rα subunit expression on bone-marrow derived CD34+ cells from asthmatic subjects. J Clin Invest 1997;100:2466–2475.

140. Robinson DS, Damia R, Zeibecoglou K, et al. CD34+/IL-5Rα mRNA+ cells in the bronchial mucosa in asthma: potential airway eosinophil progenitors. Am J Respir Cell Mol Biol 1999;20:9–13.

141. Sehmi R, Wardlaw AJ, Cromwell O, et al. Interleukin-5 (IL-5) selectively enhances the chemotactic response of eosinophils obtained from normal but not eosinophilic subjects. Blood 1992;79:2952–2959.

142. Bentley AM, Meng Q, Robinson DS, et al. Increases in activated T lymphocytes, eosinophils and cytokine messenger RNA for IL-5 and GM-CSF in bronchial biopsies after allergen inhalation challenge in atopic asthmatics. Am J Respir Cell Mol Biol 1993;8:35–42.

143. Bentley AM, Hamid Q, Robinson DS, et al. Prednisolone treatment in asthma: reduction in the numbers of eosinophils, T cells, tryptase-only positive mast cells (MC$_T$) and modulation of interleukin-4, interleukin-5 and interferon-gamma cytokine gene expression within the bronchial mucosa. Am J Respir Crit Care Med 1996;153:551–556.

144. Ying S, Humbert M, Barkans J, et al. Expression of IL-4 and IL-5 mRNA and protein product by CD4+ and CD8+ T cells, eosinophils and mast cells in bronchial biopsies obtained from atopic and non-atopic (intrinsic) asthmatics. J Immunol 1997;158:3539–3544.

145. Mauser PJ, Pitman AM, Fernandez X, et al. Effects of an antibody to interleukin-5 in a monkey model of asthma. Am J Respir Crit Care Med 1995;152:467–472.

146. Mould AW, Matthaei KI, Young IG, Foster PS. Relationship between interleukin-5 and eotaxin in regulating blood and tissue eosinophilia in mice. J Clin Invest 1997;99:1064–1071.

147. Collins PD, Marleau S, Griffiths JD, et al. Cooperation between interleukin-5 and the chemokine Eotaxin to induce eosinophil eosinophil accumulation *in vivo*. J Exp Med 1995;182:1169–1174.

148. Shi HZ, Xiao CQ, Zhong D, et al. Effect of inhaled interleukin-5 on airway hyperreactivity and eosinophilia in asthmatics. Am J Respir Crit Care Med 1998;157:204–209.

149. Leckie MJ, ten Brinke A, Lordan J, et al. SB 240563, a humanised anti-IL-5 monoclonal antibody: initial single dose safety and activity in patients with asthma. Am J Respir Crit Care Med 1999;159:A624.

150. Rook GA, Stanford JL. Give us this day our daily germs. Immunol Today 1998;19:113–116.

151. Strachan DP. Hay fever, hygiene and household size. BMJ 1989;229:1259–1260.

152. Shaheen SO, Aaby P, Hall AJ, et al. Measles and atopy in Guinea-Bissau. Lancet 1996;347:1792–1796.

153. Shirakawa T, Enomoto T, Shimazu S, Hopkin JM. The inverse association between tuberculin responses and atopic disorder. Science 1997;275:77–79.

154. Alm JS, Lilja G, Pershagen G, Scheynius A. Early BCG vaccination and development of atopy. Lancet 1997;350:400–403.

155. Herz U, Gerhold K, Gruber C, et al. BCG infection suppresses allergic sensitization and development of increased airway reactivity in an animal model. J Allergy Clin Immunol 1998;102:867–874.

156. Wang C-C, Rook GAW. Inhibition of an established allergic response to ovalbumin in BALB/c mice by killed *Mycobacterium vaccae*. Immunology 1998;93:307–313.

157. Hetzel C, Janssen R, Ely SJ, et al. An epitope delivery system for use with recombinant mycobacteria. Infect Immun 1998;66:3643–3648.

158. Wegner CD, Gundel R, Reilly P, et al. Intracellular adhesion molecule-1 (ICAM-1) in the pathogenesis of asthma. Science 1990;247:456–459.

159. Abraham WM, Sielczak MW, Ahmed A, et al. Alpha 4-integrin mediate antigen-induced late bronchial responses and prolonged airway hyperresponsiveness in sheep. J Clin Invest 1994;93:776–787.

160. Pretolani M, Ruffie C, Lapa ER, et al. Antibody to very late activation antigen 4 prevents antigen-induced bronchial hyperreactivity and cellular infiltration in the guinea pig airways. J Exp Med 1994;180:795–805.

161. Kitaura M, Nakajima T, Imai T, et al. Molecular cloning of human eotaxin, an eosinophil-selective CC chemokine, and identification of a specific eosinophil eotaxin receptor, CC chemokine receptor 3. J Biol Chem 1996;271:7725–7730.

162. Daugherty BL, Siciliano SJ, De Martino JA, et al. Cloning, expression, and characterisation of the human eosinophil eotaxin receptor. J Exp Med 1996;183:2349–2354.

163. Ohnishi T, Kita H, Mayeno AN, et al. Lidocaine in bronchoalveolar lavage fluid (BALF) is an inhibitor of eosinophil-active cytokines. Clin Exp Immunol 1996;104:325–331.

164. Beauvais F, Michel L, Dubertret L. The nitric oxide donors, azide and hydroxylamine, inhibit the programmed cell death of cytokine-deprived eosinophils. FEBS Lett 1995;361:229–232.

Chapter 27

Treatment of Allergy to Insect Stings

Martin D. Valentine

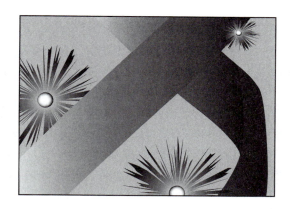

Historic Perspective

Approximately fifty individuals die each year in the United States from anaphylaxis caused by allergy to the venom of stinging insects (order Hymenoptera). In the larger number who experience such reactions and survive, prevention of future reactions is a physician's principal concern. Although counseling about the avoidance of stings is the cornerstone of prevention, it is not always sufficient to prevent potentially fatal stings. In the first quarter of the 20th century, Braun (1) used a regimen of immunization with an extract prepared from the "posterior 1/8 inch of the insect" to treat a woman allergic to honeybee stings. Later, Benson and Semenov (2) thought they had found an "intrinsic bee protein" throughout the entire bodies of the insects and reasoned that an extract of the entire creature could successfully protect patients from sting reactions if used as a vaccine. This work led to the practice of immunization of sting-allergic patients with an extract of "mixed stinging insects" prepared from a filtrate of crushed, whole insect bodies. Although the crudity of this procedure seems analogous to treating diabetic patients with crushed whole pig in the hope that porcine insulin would survive the process and persist in quantity sufficient to lower a patient's blood sugar, most allergists were content to use this crude preparation of whole insect bodies to immunize sting-sensitive patients. They chose to ignore the logic of Dr. Mary Loveless (3), who advocated the use of unadulterated venom, either collected and administered from a syringe or from naturally delivered stings.

Venom collection from honeybees was facilitated by the development in 1964 of an electric stimulation technique (4). With this method, large quantities of honeybee venom could be collected without harm to the bees, who reflexively expelled droplets of venom onto an electrically charged collecting plate. Honeybee venom contains an alarm pheromone that leads other honeybees to deposit their venom at a single, focused site, further facilitating venom collection. The dried venom droplets were eventually gleaned from the collecting plate. For a number of reasons, this technique has resisted successful adaptation to the collection of other Hymenopteran venoms. The latter has remained almost a "cottage" industry: venom sac dissectors are supplied with nests collected from the wild, which are frozen and then thawed for the extraction of venom from the venom sacs of individual insect bodies. A separation process that allowed centrifugal extraction of venom of high purity from vespid venom sacs with a β-alanine buffer was perfected by Simon and Benton

in 1969 (5). Using venoms collected by these methods, scientists in the laboratory of Lichtenstein found that if peripheral blood basophils from venom-allergic patients were exposed to nontoxic concentrations of venoms, they would release histamine in a dose-dependent fashion (6). The importance of this observation was the recognition that "high" concentrations of venom cause nonspecific, toxic histamine release from all mast cells and basophils, but lower concentrations elicit histamine release only from the cells of sensitized individuals. It was then shown that this reaction depends on the presence and participation of venom-specific IgE antibodies. Other, clinical observations have been made regarding toxic, rather than immunologic, effects in humans (7).

Schwartz had noted the ambiguity of test results when he used the irritating extracts made from whole insect bodies (whole body extract, WBE) (8). Venoms were shown to initiate allergen-specific histamine release from basophils in vitro, and testing in vivo soon followed. The safety and efficacy of skin-testing with dilute venom solutions in human volunteers was shown by Lichtenstein's group (9,10) and others. In addition to the failure of WBE extracts in diagnosis, "treatment failures"—that is, failure of WBE immunotherapy to prevent major or even fatal sting reactions—were reported (11,12). The need for a radical reassessment of WBE treatment efficacy was brought to light in the first contemporary report of venom treatment of a sting-sensitive person. Treatment with WBE extract of a child was a failure, as it had been for his deceased sister before him (13). After 3 months of honeybee venom immunotherapy, the immunized child developed a titer of venom-specific blocking antibody comparable to that of his bee-venom immune father (a frequently-stung, professional beekeeper). An in-hospital challenge sting was then administered to the child, resulting in a few shed tears but no allergic reaction. This was the first instance in which the development of "blocking" IgG antibodies was correlated with the development of immunity to a sting. The criterion for the quantity of "blocking" antibody that was expected to be protective was empirically derived from the values found in patients who were immunized with venoms and then successfully stung (without systemic reaction), and this quantity amounted to a doubling of the individual's baseline blocking antibody (14). Later, the functional assay for the measurement of blocking antibody was replaced by an immunoassay for venom-specific IgG (15–18). In 1978 the results of a placebo-controlled trial of venom immunotherapy were published; the study showed that venom immunotherapy was 97% effective in reducing the risk of future sting reactions and that WBE therapy was no more effective than placebo (19). In 1979 venoms were licensed for commercial use.

More recent research has focused on the criteria for the selection of patients for venom immunotherapy (VIT), on tests for determining the efficacy of VIT, and on determining when VIT may be discontinued. As is discussed below, the means by which immunotherapy protects patients from sting reactions is unclear and is a subject of great interest.

Immunotherapy with specific venom(s) reduces the risk and severity of future reactions to insect stings in patients who have previously experienced systemic allergic reactions to stings from the same species of insect (19,20). Insect venoms that have been evaluated include those from honeybee, yellow jacket, white-faced hornet (black hornet), yellow hornet, and Polistes paper wasps (21). Sensitivity to stings from the imported fire ant (genus Solenopsis) has been successfully treated with extracts prepared from whole ant bodies, presumably because the ratio of relevant venom protein to irrelevant body protein in these extracts is relatively large (22,23). In all of the Hymenoptera, only females can sting. The males are relegated to more mundane tasks, with the name "drone" being applied to male honeybees.

Pathophysiology

The insects most frequently responsible for allergic reactions in humans are yellow jackets, honeybees, wasps, hornets, and ants. An abbreviated classification of the taxonomic relationship of the insects of most importance in venom allergy is shown in Figure 27-1. The relationships in this figure are reflected by immuno-chemical relationships of the constituents of the venoms of these insects, which are discussed below.

Hymenoptera venoms contain a number of biologically interesting constituents. Honeybee venom contains proteins (that are functionally phospholipase A_2, hyaluronidase, and acid phosphatase), and polypeptides called mellitin (which has detergent-like activity), apamin (a neurotoxin), and mast cell-degranulating peptide. Vespids have proteins that are similar in enzyme function but are immunochemically distinct. They include a phospholipase A_1, hyaluronidase, acid phosphatase, and a material called antigen 5, which is neurotoxic for some invertebrate marine animals. Vespids also have a kinin in their venoms. Although honeybees originated in Europe and have both phospholipase and hyaluronidase activities in their venom, the proteins bearing the same enzymatic functions in vespid venoms are immunochemically different. This may be an example of convergent evolution, since these functional activities represent proteins with little structural homology (for example, between honeybee hyaluronidase and yellow jacket hyaluronidase). It was found in antibody-inhibition studies on sera from mice immunized with purified venom allergens that extensive cross-reactivity exists between white-faced hornet, yellow hornet, and yellow jacket for hyaluronidase and antigen 5, but not phospholipase (24–27). Thus, although a degree of cross-sensitization to hyaluronidase and antigen 5 is observed between the vespids, and to a lesser extent with Polistes wasp (between wasp, yellow hornet, and white-faced hornet for hyaluronidase and between wasp and yellow jacket for antigen 5), there is limited cross-reactivity between honeybee, vespid, and fire ant venoms (28).

The dried weight of the venom deposited by a honeybee that has been induced to "sting" a plastic film is approximately 50 µg, which includes all nonvolatile solids (29). A single sting from one of the Vespoidea delivers an estimated 10 to 100 µg of protein. The protein content of venoms is probably overstated because

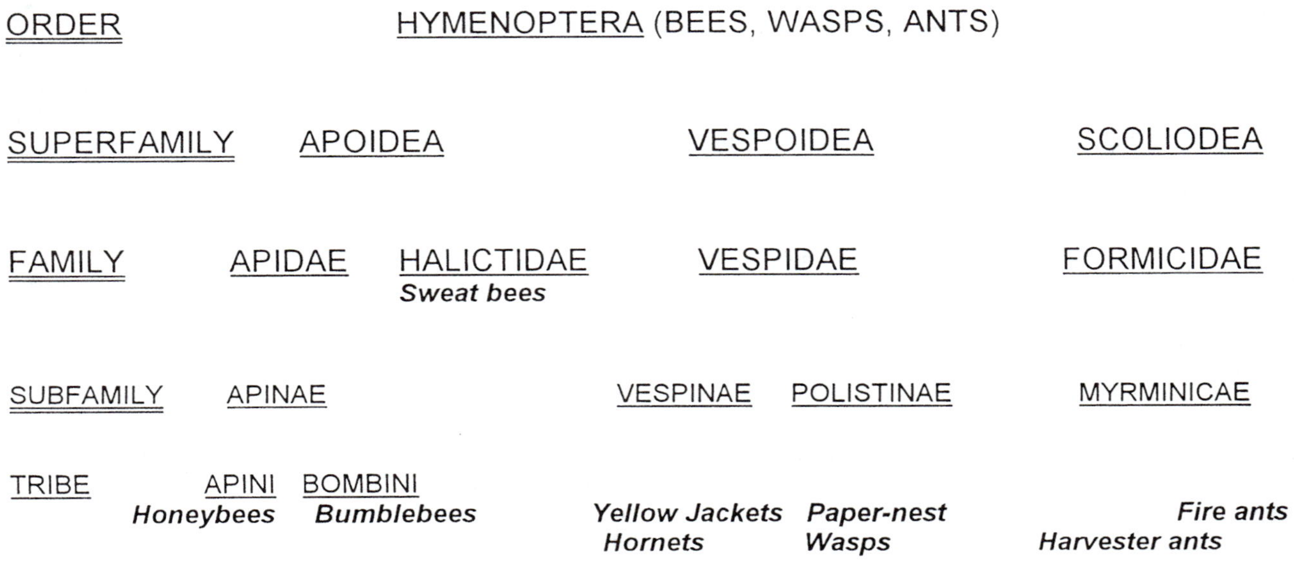

ORDER	HYMENOPTERA (BEES, WASPS, ANTS)			
SUPERFAMILY	APOIDEA		VESPOIDEA	SCOLIODEA
FAMILY	APIDAE	HALICTIDAE *Sweat bees*	VESPIDAE	FORMICIDAE
SUBFAMILY	APINAE		VESPINAE POLISTINAE	MYRMINICAE
TRIBE	APINI *Honeybees*	BOMBINI *Bumblebees*	*Yellow Jackets Paper-nest Hornets Wasps*	*Fire ants Harvester ants*

Figure 27-1. Abridged classification of stinging insects.

the micro-Kjeldahl assay used to estimate protein in such materials does not discriminate between proteins and small polypeptides; the sum of individually assayed proteins such as hyaluronidase and phospholipase falls short of the overall "protein" found by the micro-Kjeldahl estimate. Thus, the individual, larger protein allergens in a vial of commercially prepared "venom" may represent as little as 10% of the stated content on the vial label (King TP, personal communication).

The barbs along the shaft of the honeybee stinger cause it to remain embedded in the flesh of the sting recipient. As it flies away, the honeybee that has stung kills itself through evisceration. The eviscerated bee's venom sac, still attached to the stinger in the victim's skin, contracts spasmodically. Contrary to common "wisdom," there is no evidence that the "contractions" are anything other than agonal, nonfunctional twitches of the already empty venom sac. Leaving the stinger behind at the sting site is called *autotomy* (30). This process distinguishes the honeybee from the other stinging Hymenoptera, whose stingers are rarely left at the sting site, and which therefore can sting repeatedly. Other interspecies differences are seen not only in behavior but also in the chemical constituents of the venoms.

Spectrum of Reactions

Normal
A sting from one of the Hymenoptera usually results in local redness, swelling, pruritus, and/or pain, all of which are transient and are caused by proinflammatory chemicals or substances in the venoms. This reaction begins seconds to minutes after the sting and fades within a few hours. It is distinguished from the IgE antibody–mediated, large, local reaction, which begins hours after a sting and peaks 12 to 48 hours later.

Systemic Allergic Reactions
Systemic allergic reactions come in many shapes and sizes. Those that occur within seconds or minutes after allergen exposure are regarded as one or another variety of anaphylaxis, even though the clinical manifestations may be mild and non–life-threatening; one such reaction consists solely of generalized urticaria. An unwarranted forecast often made by emergency physicians or other health care providers when evaluating a sting victim is that the severity of ensuing reactions will inevitably be worse than prior reactions. Thus, the patient who appears in an emergency room covered with hives is usually told, "your next reaction may be your last." This assumption is contrary to observations made during both in-hospital sting-challenges and natural, "field" stings. Only between 25% and 60% of patients with histories of prior systemic sting reactions will react again on deliberate sting challenge (19,31). When an unimmunized patient experiences a reaction from a subsequent sting, it is most likely to be similar qualitatively and in severity to previous reactions. Only a small number of sting reactions are fatal. Rarely, in a patient without an immediate reaction, a significant systemic allergic reaction may be seen hours after a sting. No certain explanation has been found for this event.

Systemic allergic reactions may have cutaneous, vascular, or respiratory components. Generalized urticaria, angioedema, or flushing, usually with pruritus, are varieties of cutaneous sting reactions. The pattern of eruption and pruritus may conform to the pattern of increased skin mast-cell distribution at skin folds (wrists, elbows, axillae, neck, knees, and the inguinal area). The most common vascular reaction to stings appears as hypotension, usually with tachycardia. Although this reaction may be difficult to distinguish from a "vasovagal" reaction, the latter is usually accompanied by bradycardia. Rarely, hypertension may occur, presumably because of the release of endogenous sympathomimetic amines (32). Dyspnea and wheezing may result from bronchospasm; inspiratory stridor may signal laryngeal edema.

Urticaria, fever, proteinuria, lymphadenopathy, and arthropathy have been described as occurring as a result of a sting, usually after an acute systemic reaction. This reaction has been termed "serum sickness" despite the imperfect analogy with "classic" serum sickness. Although one might be concerned that serum sickness will recur when venom immunotherapy is initiated in such patients (to prevent anaphylaxis), it has not been reported. However, a boy treated with WBE experienced fever, arthralgia, malaise, and lymphadenopathy after each injection (33); these symptoms did not occur when he was later immunized with venom.

Various atypical reactions after insect stings include nausea, vomiting, diarrhea, myasthenia gravis, and peripheral neuropathies (34,35). The mechanism of these reactions is unclear; when considering whether to employ immunotherapy in patients who have experienced these reactions, one must always consider the possibility of immunotherapy causing harm rather than benefit.

Large Local Reactions
Delayed cutaneous reactions, areas of erythema and firm induration contiguous with the site of a sting, generally peaking 48 to 72 hours after a sting, are termed "large local reactions." Although at one time they were considered examples of Arthus reactions in which the participation of IgG antibodies and complement caused a local inflammatory response, they are now considered to be IgE-mediated, late-phase reactions (36). As such, the inflammatory tissue component is responsive to the administration of corticosteroids, whereas purely immediate reactions are considered to be unaffected by corticosteroids. Approximately 10% of patients with this type of reaction history will have a systemic allergic reaction with a future sting. Most physicians do not use immunotherapy unless such a patient has also experienced a systemic reaction. However, it is appropriate to equip such patients with emergency, epinephrine, self-treatment kits to use if a systemic reaction should occur. Some have suggested that paramedical personnel and even camp counselors, lifeguards, and others who work in areas where the risk of stings is high, be equipped with epinephrine kits and instructed in their appropriate use if they observe an unexpected anaphylactic reaction (37).

Epidemiology

There are no data regarding the number of people who have been stung in the past, the number of those who are stung in any given season, or what proportion of those who are stung experience any reaction out of the ordinary. Attempts to derive such data from population samples were undertaken in Rhode Island, where allergists examined the frequency of Hymenoptera sensitivity in populations of college students and in their office practices (38,39), as well as in a summer Boy Scout encampment (40). The Boy Scout figures probably should be regarded as *incidence*, since allergists looked at how many youngsters reacted in a given period. The answers to these questions have been pursued worldwide (41–43). Settipane (44) found a proportion of about 0.4%, which is much smaller than the percentage arrived at by Golden et al (45,46) in the evaluation of a random sample of a population of workers at a factory in a Baltimore suburb. Nearly 5% of the latter had a history of more than a "normal" reaction to a sting. Moreover, there was skin-test and/or RAST-test evidence of the presence of venom-specific IgE antibodies in nearly 25% of these workers, even in those without a history of unusual sting reactions.

Mortality from Sting Reactions

Stinging insect allergy is a worldwide problem. In the United States, about 50 deaths each year are attributed to insect sting reactions (47). Additional deaths have been reported abroad (48,49). About 20 sting-induced deaths occur annually in Europe and a smaller number in Asia. In all countries, an unknown number of additional deaths may be incorrectly attributed to an acute cardiovascular or central nervous system event. In a survey of postmortem sera from individuals dying from no known cause, a significant number had clinically relevant levels of IgE antibodies to one or more Hymenoptera (50,51).

More men than women die from insect sting reactions. The risk of death increases with age. Despite the observation that the typical individual who experiences a systemic reaction is a male child, most systemic reactions in childhood consist predominantly of urticaria, and only one or two children experience fatal reactions each year. In 50% of those who die from sting reactions, there may be no prior history of difficulty with insect stings.

Insect Morphology and Behavior

Honeybees are small, fuzzy-appearing insects with alternating tan and dark-brown stripes. To the person just stung or the casual observer, they may seem to be indistinguishable from the yellow-and black-striped yellow jackets or some striped wasps. They are often seen gathering nectar from attractive flowers, while the hairs on their back legs accumulate pollen grains. Although there are pollen allergens in honey, there are none in venom; nor are there any venom allergens in honey. Although honeybees may become aggressive or excessively defensive in very wet or very dry weather, they are relatively noncombative while they are grazing for nectar and generally sting only when caught underfoot.

Until recently, all of the honeybees in the United States were of European descent (imported deliberately by colonists from Europe). Africanized honeybees (so-called "killer" bees) are the result of escaped offspring from interbreeding between established colonies of European honeybees and African honeybees brought to Brazil to improve honey production. The "killer" bees do not have unusual venom potency, but do have a tendency to attack "en masse" (52,53). They have steadily advanced northward and in 1994 reached the middle of Texas. In 1999 a colony was identified in Florida. Bumblebees are large, slow-moving, noisy bees with hairy bodies of alternating yellow and black stripes. They are nonaggressive and account for only a small fraction of stings, but they have been reported to cause problems in certain occupations (54). "Sweat bees" belong to another family (Halictidae), but also are said to be capable of causing anaphylaxis with stings (55).

Ground-nesting yellow jackets are identified by alternating yellow and black body stripes. Although they too appreciate a sip of nectar, they are omnivorous scavengers. They are often seen darting around picnic tables and garbage cans. Some regard the yellow hornets as aerial-nesting yellow jackets, Their globular nests may be found hanging from low tree branches or in shrubs. The back (white- or bald-faced) hornets are found in similar locations. Usually, a single entrance to the football-sized nest can be seen in a dependent location. The nest is constructed of a paper-like material made from wood masticated by the insects; the color of the paper reflects the color of the wooden source, but all are shades of grey. The yellow jacket nest is typically subterranean, sometimes beginning as an enlargement of an old mouse or other animal burrow. Although not visible until unearthed, the yellow jacket nest is also made of paper manufactured by the insects. Rows of cells, where eggs are laid and develop into pupae, are neatly arranged in layers in a roughly spherical form. This nest is similar ot the hornet nest, with the exception that the hornet nests have an extra paper sheath around the entire structure. The locations of the nests pose particular problems to lawn cutters, landscapers, and tree and bush trimmers who may unwittingly encounter a nest and be subjected to dozens of stings. The nests of the narrow-waisted paper wasps (*Polistinae*) are built in the eaves of buildings, under air conditioners, in outdoor light sockets, or in mail boxes; they have a characteristic appearance in which the hexagonal cells, where eggs are laid, hatched, and pupated, are not enclosed in a paper envelope.

The imported fire ants appear to have been inadvertently launched from a visiting freighter at the port of Mobile, Alabama, earlier this century. They have gradually extended their distribution in the Gulf Coast states and continue to enlarge their territory (56). Although they cannot tolerate cold temperatures, they have been found attempting to tunnel north under the warm pavement of interstate highways. They build 2- to 3-foot-high mounds containing thousands of ants, which are very aggressive (22). When they sting, they seize the skin of their victim with their jaws and pivot about, inflicting a circle of stings with their abdominal stinger. The pain of their sting probably results from the piperidine alkaloid content of their venom, which is also said to cause the characteristic rosette of sterile pustules at sting sites 1 to 2 days after the sting (23). Fire ants present a special hazard to children who may fall on a mound and receive dozens or even hundreds of stings. Their venoms also contain traces of the immunogenic proteins found in vespid venoms and thus are also responsible for allergic reactions to the venom proteins. Atypical (neurologic) sequelae to stings have also been reported (57).

Tests for Insect-Specific or Venom-Specific IgE Antibodies

"Anaphylaxis" is a term generically applicable to a spectrum of systemic allergic reactions ranging from mild, cutaneous reactions such as urticaria to potentially fatal bronchospasm, obstructive edema of the upper airway, and hypotension refractory to treatment with simple measures. Schwartz et al (58) have found significant levels of mast cell tryptase in serum after anaphylaxis. Blood eosinophilia may also be present, and urinary metabolites of histamine may be increased (59). Blood histamine has been elevated in patients with hypotensive sting reactions (60).

Skin Tests

Cautious titration of skin reactivity to a panel of venoms usually helps to narrow the field of suspects (9). Although an epicutaneous test (prick/puncture) is usually recommended before intradermal tests are performed, most allergists have never seen a positive epicutaneous test with venom, possibly because most individuals would react on prick-puncture only to a concentration of venom of 1000 μg/mL or greater. Commercially prepared venoms can successfully be reconstituted only to about 200 μg/mL.

In practice, intracutaneous skin tests are begun with a concentration in the range of 0.001 to 0.1 μg/mL, the weaker concentrations being preferable for those whose reactions have been fairly recent and/or extremely severe. Approximately 0.02 mL (enough to raise a tiny bleb) is placed very superficially on the flexor aspect of the forearm, with positive and negative controls on the same arm. If the lower concentrations cause no reaction, 10-fold increases in concentration, up to a maximum of 1.0 μg/mL, are tested. Although the argument has been made that the 1.0 μg/mL concentration is too strong for highly specific results (61) (i.e., positive tests that are correlated with the severity of a patient's reaction), the 0.1 μg/mL concentration is not sufficiently sensitive to detect more than 80% of patients with prior systemic reactions (9). Some have pushed the maximum skin-test concentration of venom to 3.0 μg/mL, but even at this concentration not enough antigen is introduced in the skin-testing procedure to result in an increase in serum or cell-bound IgE venom antibodies.

There is some question about choosing a suitable time for skin testing (62). The theory has been advanced that a systemic allergic reaction may result in a temporary refractory state, such that tests performed soon after a reaction may be falsely negative. This refractory state is believed to resemble the condition of a patient after a successful, rapid desensitization procedure (such as might be done with penicillin in a penicillin-allergic patient). In the case of rapid desensitization, the patient is considered to become "desensitized" (or refractory to allergen challenge) by one or more of several mechanisms: 1) Saturation of all cell-bound antigen-specific IgE antibodies with antigen tightly bound from the prior reaction; 2) depletion of intracellular mediators during the preceding reaction, so that the quantities of mediators that remain are not sufficient to support a clinically apparent reaction; or 3) down-regulation of the signal transduction mechanisms, resulting in failure of the mediator secretory process. It is thought that one or more of these conditions may exist in the patient who has recently experienced a systemic allergic reaction.

As noted above, the venoms of different members of the vespid superfamily contain structurally homologous proteins that have extensive immunologic cross-reactivity. Whether crossed sensitization can result in clinically relevant cross-reactivity has not been established. Patients whose sting reactions were caused by yellow jackets may exhibit positive skin tests when tested with other vespid venoms, presumably because of the homology of the authentic with the cross-reacting antigens. Whether this degree of cross-reactivity is sufficient to result in clinically relevant cross-reactivity to accidental stings is not really known. What is known is that patients who have positive skin tests to yellow jacket and to Polistes and whose Polistes RAST test is inhibited by the addition of yellow jacket venom fail to react to a Polistes challenge after immunization solely with yellow jacket venom (63) (see below).

RAST Testing

The RAST (radioallergosorbent) test is a legitimate serologic test that may be applied to venom allergy if appropriate reagents, duplicates, and controls are used. Hamilton and Adkinson have developed a variant of this test, which provides the clinician with information that is not only qualitative, but quantitative and reproducible (17).

The technique of RAST inhibition, in which authentic antigen (e.g., yellow jacket venom) is allowed to react with the patient's antibody-containing serum before addition of the possibly cross-reacting venom (e.g., Polistes wasp), enables the practitioner to eliminate one or more venoms from a patient's immunotherapy prescription (63). In the example given, Polistes antigen would be prevented from binding to the patient's serum because of prior binding of yellow jacket antigens to the antibodies in the test mixture. In other words, if the binding of patient serum to the Polistes venom–labeled substrate in the performance of the Polistes RAST could be reduced by 90% or more through the addition of yellow jacket venom, this result could be interpreted to mean that the vast majority of the binding of Polistes antigen to patient serum was the result of cross-reactivity.

A small number of patients with negative venom skin tests but positive histories for insect sting reactions have been reported to have subsequently reacted to accidental stings (64). It is not known whether those particular patients would have had positive RAST tests at the time of their negative skin tests. In other reports, up to 10% of history-positive, skin-test–negative patients had positive RAST tests or venom-induced basophil histamine release in vitro. In general, venom-induced basophil histamine release correlates well with skin testing (6).

Acute Treatment of Sting Reactions

The expected minor local swelling and pruritus can be treated with ice and antihistamines. If present, the imbedded stinger should be flicked off with a scraping motion. Some authorities feel that one should not grasp the fleshy venom sac to extract the stinger since more venom might then be injected through the stinger. However, Schumacher et al (65) showed that essentially the entire honeybee venom load is injected in less than 20 seconds.

If a generalized reaction occurs, epinephrine is the keystone of management. Epinephrine halts the further release of mediators and reverses many of the effects of released mediators. Other measures commonly used in the treatment of anaphylaxis include oxygen, inhaled sympathomimetics, intravenous fluids, pressor agents, and antiarrhythmic agents.

Most systemic allergic reactions are reversed promptly after the administration of a single, subcutaneously injected dose of epinephrine. The adult dose is 0.3 mg (0.3 mL of a 1:1000 dilution). Although a larger dose may be required if the patient is taking a β-receptor–blocking agent, it is usually better to repeat the 0.3 mg dose in 10 to 15 minutes if the first dose does not appear effective or if there is no effect on the pulse rate. Larger initial doses usually add nothing except unpleasant side effects, which may lead a patient to claim that he or she is "allergic" to epinephrine. Epinephrine, even administered intravenously in a 1:10,000 concentration, may be ineffective in profound anaphylactic shock, unless the functional hypovolemia of this state is corrected with intravenous fluid (60) (oxygenation in the presence of laryngeal edema is maintained by intubation). Some authorities have suggested that "military" antishock trousers, which help to reverse peripheral blood pooling, may be useful if epinephrine is ineffective (66). The pediatric dose of epinephrine is 0.01 mg/kg body weight, up to a maximum of 0.3 mg. Over-the-counter epinephrine inhalers are sold for self-treatment of self-diagnosed asthma. Although inhaled epinephrine may reach the systemic circulation, it is doubtful whether the 0.1-mg (per puff) inhaled dose, or two or three puffs, would be sufficient to reverse the signs of systemic anaphylaxis. Glucagon administration, which stimulates secretion of endogenous catecholamines, has been suggested for use in patients with pharmacologic blockade of their β-receptors and for any patient unresponsive to subcutaneous epinephrine (67,68).

In older adults, who may have significant, sometimes undiagnosed, cardiovascular disease, the potential risk of adverse cardiovascular side effects from epinephrine must be weighed against the consequences of inadequately treated anaphylaxis. It is inadvisable to improvise an emergency kit from a disposable, plastic syringe with a premeasured dose of epinephrine, as the epinephrine in such extemporaneously prepared "kits" will likely oxidize within minutes or hours; the epinephrine in the commercial kits is packed under nitrogen to prevent premature spoilage. Pharmacologic β-receptor blockade presents a problem: very often the patient who needs a beta-blocker also needs immunotherapy with the possibility that epinephrine might be required in the event of a reaction to therapy (69).

Meridian Laboratories distributes the Epi-Pen (0.3 mg epinephrine) and Epi-Pen Jr (0.15 mg epinephrine); these are spring-actuated auto-injectors originally manufactured by Survival Technology, a firm experienced in the manufacture of lidocaine and atropine auto-injectors. A new variation is the EpiEZPen, said to be preferred by some because of ease of use. The Ana-Kit and Ana-Guard (Hollister-Stier) provide a syringe loaded with two doses of 0.3 mg of epinephrine; although these kits require self-injection, they also permit the administration of second and fractional doses. The physician who prescribes a self-injectable epinephrine kit should ensure that the individual understands the indications for and technique of its use.

Prevention of Future Sting Reactions

Sensitized individuals must be advised to take positive steps to avoid stings. Such measures include avoidance of areas where insect nests are known to exist, use of fragrance-free cosmetics and toiletries, and avoidance of uniformly dark clothing or clothing with floral prints. Patients should avoid eating outdoors and being near garbage-disposal areas. Hands, feet, and other body parts should not be placed where the eyes have not first looked for insects or insect nests. Closed shoes are preferred to bare feet, open-toed shoes, or sandals. Known nests near a patient's residence should be removed or exterminated professionally.

Venom Immunotherapy (VIT)

Selection of Patients

Positive Tests for Venom-Specific IgE Antibodies
Evidence for the presence of IgE antibody against one or more insect venoms, either in vivo by skin tests or in vitro by RAST testing, is a prerequisite for recommending VIT. Although a sting-induced, large, local reaction involves the participation of IgE antibodies, and thus has an allergic mechanism (85% have a positive venom skin test), VIT is rarely recommended for patients with large local reactions because the risk of a subsequent systemic reaction is low (2% to 10%), and the morbidity of large local reactions is usually not severe enough to warrant the atten-

dant risks of VIT (but see above regarding risk factors). A positive venom skin test or RAST without a history of a sting-induced generalized allergic reaction is not an indication for VIT. Golden has found that as many as one-fourth of the population may have evidence of IgE antibodies to venom. This condition is probably transient, but the appropriate prospective studies that would predict risk have not been done.

History of a Systemic Reaction to a Sting

Patients selected for prophylactic VIT should have had at least one prior systemic reaction to a sting. In a controlled trial (19), 60% of patients who had reacted previously and who did not receive VIT reacted systemically to laboratory stings. Because not all previously reacting patients react when stung again, some (31) have advocated including a positive reaction to a challenge sting in the list of prerequisites for venom immunotherapy.

Age

Valentine et al demonstrated that children who have mild systemic reactions, that is, cutaneous reactions such as itching, hives, or angioedema, have only a 5% to 10% risk of any reaction to a future sting and thus do not require VIT (70). However, most physicians feel that if a child's prior reaction had been vascular or respiratory, immunotherapy should be recommended. Some practitioners have applied the pediatric experience to young adults with insect allergy and recommend withholding VIT from young, otherwise healthy adults whose systemic reactions to stings have been limited to the skin. This practice is not based on controlled observation; studies have been carried out in children but not in young adults.

Multiple Stings

Individuals reacting systemically only after multiple stings may do so because of the large allergen burden received and might not react to the amount of venom in a single sting. Although there are no hard data on this point, patients have been observed for whom this conclusion seems to hold true, and who have done well without the intervention of immunotherapy.

Challenge Stings

In a study carried out in the Netherlands (31), 25% of skin-test positive, unimmunized vespid-sensitive patients reacted to deliberate challenge stings in a protected environment. Because of this finding, the authors suggested that only patients reacting systemically to challenge stings be treated with VIT. A recent exchange of letters in the pages of the Journal of Allergy and Clinical Immunology underscored the sharp differences of opinion that still exist on this topic, primarily because of the concern on the one hand that some patients might be needlessly treated, and on the other, that a challenge sting in an unimmunized patient might have dire consequences (71–74). Other Dutch investigators, employing a similar protocol, found that a significant proportion of patients who tolerated a first challenge sting without a systemic reaction, did react to a second challenge (75). Despite

these differences, the consensus now favors selecting patients for treatment without performing a challenge sting.

Selection of Venoms

Because the immune response to insect stings is relatively specific for the venom proteins of particular species of Hymenoptera, it is appropriate medically and financially to narrow the choice of venoms as much as possible. It may be difficult for a patient to identify which type of insect has just stung him; nonetheless, the details of the history of the patient's sting may help incriminate a specific species. The geographic locale of the sting, as well as the appearance and location of the insect nest, may be useful in classifying the type of insect responsible for a sting reaction. For example, honeybees are common causes of stings among agricultural workers and in commercial or amateur gardens; house painters and air-conditioner service people often disturb nests of Polistes wasps; yellow-jacket nests are usually found buried in soil, compost, or mulch or in niches in masonry walls; hornet nests are found in shrubs or suspended from the lower branches of trees. Polistes wasp stings are more common in the deep South, as are fire ant stings. Other stinging insects are found in more exotic locations, for example, *Polistes metricus* on Kwajalein Island in the Pacific and in southern Asia (Miles Guralnick [Vespa Laboratories], personal communication). Positive identification by an entomologist is most helpful whenever possible.

The exception to the statement made earlier in this chapter about the usefulness of venom therapy versus treatment with WBE is that extracts of imported fire-ant bodies are effective in treating individuals with anaphylactic sensitivity to stings from these aggressive insects.

Regimens of Immunotherapy

Although the venom package insert suggests a series of 15 weekly injections commencing at a dose of 0.05μg and progressing gradually to the usual maintenance dose of 100μg of each venom prescribed, in practice several different regimens are employed. All venoms are administered separately except for mixed vespid venom, which is a combination of equal amounts of yellow jacket, yellow hornet, and white-faced hornet venoms; the usual maintenance dose for the mixture of three vespid venoms is 300μg. Hunt et al (19) devised a "modified rush" protocol in which several doses were given at each of the first two visits. The purpose was to achieve a therapeutic venom dose while sufficient insects were still available, before a frost, for challenge stings. This protocol was well tolerated and served to shorten the build-up phase; the maintenance dose was achieved in 6 weeks. Since that report, modifications of this regimen have proven practical for most patients. With the level of venom-specific serum IgG as a guide, the interval between maintenance injections is increased by 1-week increments to 4 weeks. If IgG levels are maintained, booster injections are given every 4 weeks for the first 6 to 12 months. Using the same criterion, the interval between venom injections is lengthened to 6 or 8 weeks in the second year. If the

IgG level drops below 3.5 μg/mL, the interval between venom doses is reduced.

In Israel, Goldberg and colleagues studied 28 children and adults in whom the VIT injection interval was increased to 3 months after they had received monthly injections for a mean duration of 17 months (76). Nineteen honeybee-allergic individuals tolerated a challenge sting after 6 to 38 months (mean = 18 months) of 3-month injection intervals. Although Yunginger et al (77) reported unsatisfactory results with a rush immunotherapy protocol in which 11 of 20 patients required treatment with epinephrine for injection-induced reactions (77), variations on this theme have been popular in Europe, particularly when a patient presents for evaluation shortly before the next stinging season (78). Some protocols have combined the administration of venom-antibody–rich sera with rush VIT (79–82). Recently, Bernstein et al extended their observations on rush VIT (83). Seventy-seven patients received a cumulative dose of 58.55 μg of venom on treatment day 1, followed by doses of 70, 80, 90, and 100 μg on treatment days 3, 7, 14, and 21, respectively. Only four patients had reactions on day 1; all were mild.

The maintenance dose of venom has been the subject of debate. The origin of the notion that 100 μg of venom is an appropriate "maintenance" or target immunotherapy dose was based on observations made in preparation for immunization of the child described by Lichtenstein et al (13). When dried "stings" from honeybees were collected after bees were individually induced to deposit their venom on plastic wrap, the dried droplets had a mean weight of 50 μg (29). It was reasoned that if an immunized patient could tolerate twice the venom in a single sting, then that patient could be considered relatively immune. Whereas Reisman and Livingston felt that "satisfactory" results are obtained with a 50-μg maximum dose (84,85), Golden et al (86) found that only 79% of individuals who were brought to a 50-μg target dose were protected from challenge-sting–induced systemic reactions.

Antigen (venom)-specific IgG, "blocking" antibodies appear in the serum of most venom-immunized patients. The binding of venom antigens to IgG antibodies in the circulation, and thus de facto inactivation of venom proteins as circulating antigens, remains the most likely mechanism by which VIT leads to lessening of a patient's susceptibility to a reaction to a sting, at least early in the course of treatment (86). Other theories have been advanced, dealing with the possibility that the development of autoantibodies (87) or anti-idiotypic antibodies (88) during the course of VIT might be beneficial. Studies of passive immunotherapy support the IgG hypothesis: Lessof et al (81) identified five honeybee-allergic individuals who suffered systemic reactions ranging from angioedema to respiratory distress when subjected to subcutaneous injections of honeybee venom in doses of 10 to 100 μg. Soon after the intramuscular or intravenous administration of the gamma globulin fraction of pooled beekeepers' serum containing a high, anti-honeybee-venom–blocking antibody titer, the same individuals tolerated one and a half to five times the previous symptom-eliciting venom dose without reactions.

Efficacy of Treatment

Ninety-seven percent of patients treated with venoms are protected from significant systemic allergic reactions as judged by their response to a challenge sting. However, a placebo-controlled trial of VIT found that more than half of previously reacting patients fail to react to challenge stings without benefit of immunotherapy. Among immunized patients, those who continue to react to stings generally have smaller increases in their venom-specific IgG antibodies (89). Early detection of such a paucity of IgG antibodies can usually be remedied by an increase in venom dosage (1.5 to 2 times the usual dose) or frequency of administration. Since there are so few treatment failures with VIT, it has been argued that it is not cost-effective to perform venom IgG antibody assays on all immunized patients (90). However, most patients prefer to know whether they are among those patients who are at greater risk of reactions to stings despite VIT. Patients occasionally wish to have a challenge sting in the clinic setting to demonstrate immunity. If undertaken, this procedure should be done with all the precautions taken as if it were assumed the challenge would result in a life-threatening reaction. Several investigators have observed that neither skin-test reactivity to venom nor serum IgE or IgG antivenom antibodies bear any relation to immunity to stings in patients who have undergone prolonged (>4 years) VIT (91) (see below). In immunized patients, there is a gradual shift toward the selective production of IgG₄ antibodies (92).

Duration of Therapy

The optimal duration of venom treatment for prophylaxis of recurrent, sting-induced, systemic reactions has not been determined. When VIT was first introduced and found to be extremely effective, it was assumed that it would be administered indefinitely. However, it was eventually observed that there might be a relatively favorable outcome of stings in individuals who had stopped VIT for reasons of cost or inconvenience. Those reports suggest an intermediate risk of sting-induced systemic reactions of about 25% in patients who prematurely discontinue VIT. This risk contrasts with the 1% to 3% risk in patients treated for 4 or more years and the 40% to 60% risk in patients never treated.

Various indications for stopping VIT have been considered. Loss of allergic sensitization determined either by venom skin test or measurement of venom-specific IgE levels occurs in some patients. Over time, the venom skin test may become negative in 5% to 29% of patients. When VIT was discontinued in patients whose venom-specific IgE levels had fallen to insignificant levels, the patients experienced a 5% reaction rate per sting (93). Most authorities consider the ablation of allergic sensitization to be the most obvious indication for stopping VIT. However, as noted, not all patients develop a negative venom skin test or unmeasurable levels of venom-specific IgE. Therefore, many researchers have selected a specific duration for treatment. Golden and colleagues at Johns Hopkins prospectively studied 30 patients who agreed to stop VIT after 5 or more years of injections. Sting challenges performed after 12 months without VIT resulted in no systemic reactions to 29 yellow jacket and three honeybee stings (94). A follow-up report of 74 patients who had been treated with venom injections for 5 to 8 years and then repeatedly subjected to challenge stings every 1 to 2 years noted sting reactions in seven (10%) of the patients (95–97). Of 74 patients who were stung after stopping VIT of 5 or more years' duration, systemic symptoms occurred in eight of 270 stings (3% of stings) and seven of 74 patients (9% of patients). All of the eight systemic reactions included pruritus and erythema; one patient had urticaria and angioedema, one had scattered urticaria, and two had solitary urticarial lesions. Seven patients had subjective symptoms only. Schuberth et al reported similar results in children (98). Researchers at the Mayo Clinic studied 51 patients age 9 to 67 years who stopped VIT after 2 to 10 years (mean 5 years) of treatment (99). All patients had tolerated a challenge sting(s) at the conclusion of therapy. One year later, challenge stings caused systemic reactions in two of the 51 patients. One patient had only itching of the face and neck, but the other suffered hypotension and difficulty breathing. VIT was resumed in both. Both patients who reacted had had the most severe grade of reaction before VIT and received VIT for shorter than average lengths of time (2 and 4 years). Subsequently, 16, 11, 2, and 2 patients underwent sting challenges 2, 3, 4, and 5 years, respectively, after VIT was discontinued. No further reactions occurred.

European researchers have also investigated the outcome of deliberately discontinuing VIT (100). Haugaard et al (101) studied 25 primarily yellow-jacket-sensitive adults treated with VIT for 36 to 83 months (mean = 43 months). No systemic reactions resulted from 21 yellow jacket and seven honeybee challenge stings administered 12 to 36 months (mean = 25 months) after the conclusion of VIT. Müller et al reported on 86 honeybee-sensitive children and adults with severe reactions before VIT who received VIT for 3 to 10 years (102). A challenge sting 10 to 24 months (mean = 13 months) later resulted in only normal local reactions in 71 patients (83%).

Currently, there are no accepted guidelines for practicing allergists concerning the discontinuation of VIT. In several groups of venom-immunized patients, Golden found that among those who stopped treatment after several years, 90% had persistent immunity regardless of their IgG antibody levels (103). A report from a multi-specialty group practice setting suggests that VIT should be continued indefinitely in only a small minority of patients (104). Of 204 patients in whom VIT was initiated between 1978 and 1986, only 12 (6%) were still receiving venom injections in 1992 when the population was surveyed. Approximately equal proportions of patients off VIT had discontinued treatment because of patient preference or physician recommendation. Several researchers have found that patients with severe reactions before VIT are more likely to react to stings after VIT has been discontinued. It has been suggested that VIT should be continued indefinitely, especially for a patient with a history of a more severe reaction. If venom maintenance injections can be spaced 2 to 3 months apart, the associated inconvenience would be greatly diminished. When VIT is stopped after 5 or more years, the risk of a sting reaction increases from the range of 1% to 3% to about 5% to 10%. Whether that degree of an increased reaction rate warrants further administration of VIT is a decision best made jointly by the patient and physician after a consideration of the severity of the reaction before VIT, age, occupation, and other factors.

Reactions to Venom Immunotherapy

Many expect a substance called "venom" to result in more frequent or more severe reactions when used in immunotherapy. However, the range of reactions is no different with VIT than with immunotherapy with other allergens, nor are reactions more frequent (105,106). Venom immunotherapy during pregnancy was found by Schwartz et al (107) to compromise neither the mother nor the fetus. However, although it seems safe and probably even desirable for the pregnant woman to maintain her venom immunity by continuing an established regimen of venom injections, it may be prudent to avoid initiating any type of immunotherapy during a known pregnancy, thereby avoiding the occasional, systemic, allergic reactions that may occur with any immunotherapy regimen.

Occasionally, a patient will react adversely to nearly every attempt at VIT. If any immunotherapy reaction is potentially life-threatening, very careful consideration must be given to discontinuing therapy and placing reliance instead on sting avoidance and prompt use of an emergency kit if an accidental sting occurs. Before therapy is stopped, the treatment regimen may be modified to provide smaller increases in venom dosage than in the usual regimen. Although there is no ultimate advantage to any particular regimen, there are fewer total reactions to therapy if the faster regimen is used. An intermediate position is to attempt to block the symptoms of a reaction by pretreatment of the patient with mediator antagonists and steroids, as is recommended in anticipation of a reaction to the intravenous administration of iodinated, radiographic contrast materials. H_1 and H_2 histamine receptor blockers, with or without prednisone, are given 13 hours before treatment, 60 minutes before treatment, and 11 hours after treatment, if needed (108,109). Another tactic employed in special circumstances in honeybee-sensitive patients was suggested by the studies of combined active and passive immunotherapy, with IgG antibodies from beekeepers' serum (see above). When such measures fail to prevent reactions, the benefit of VIT must be weighed against the risk of morbidity.

References
1. Braun LIB. Notes on desensitization of a patient hypersensitive to bee stings. S Afr Med Rec 1925;23:408.
2. Benson RL, Semenov H. Allergy in its relation to the bee sting. J Allergy 1930;1:105.
3. Loveless MH. Immunization in wasp-sting allergy through venom repositories and periodic insect stings. J Immunol 1962;89:204.
4. Benton AW, Morse RA, Stewart JD. Venom collection from honeybees. Science 1963;142:228.

5. Simon RP, Benton A. A method for mass collection of wasp venoms. Ann Entomol Soc Am 1969;62:277–278.

6. Sobotka AK, Valentine MD, Benton AW, Lichtenstein LM. Allergy to insect stings. I. Diagnosis of IgE-mediated hymenoptera sensitivity by venom-induced histamine release. J Allergy Clin Immunol 1974;53:170–184.

7. Bousquet J, Huchard G, Michel FB. Toxic reactions induced by hymenoptera venom. Ann Allergy 1984;52:371–374.

8. Schwartz HJ. Skin sensitivity in insect allergy. JAMA 1965; 194:113.

9. Hunt KJ, Valentine MD, Sobotka AK, Lichtenstein LM. Diagnosis of allergy to stinging insects by skin testing with Hymenoptera venoms. Ann Intern Med 1976;85:56–59.

10. Zeleznick LD, Hunt KJ, Sobotka AK, et al. Diagnosis of Hymenoptera hypersensitivity by skin testing with Hymenoptera venoms. J Allergy Clin Immunol 1997;59:2–9.

11. Torsney PJ. Treatment failures: insect desensitization. J Allergy Clin Immunol 1973;52:303–306.

12. Reisman RE. Stinging insect allergy—treatment failures. J Allergy Clin Immunol 1973;52:257–258.

13. Lichtenstein LM, Valentine MD, Sobotka AK. A case for venom treatment in anaphylactic sensitivity to Hymenoptera sting. N Engl J Med 1974;290:1223–1227.

14. Golden DB, Meyers DA, Kagey-Sobotka A, et al. Clinical relevance of the venom-specific immunoglobulin G antibody level during immunotherapy. J Allergy Clin Immunol 1982;69:489–493.

15. Golden DBK, Valentine MD. Allergen-specific IgG antibody measurements in the management of immediate hypersensitivity to Hymenoptera venoms. J Clin Immunoassay 1983;6:172–176.

16. Golden DBK, Valentine MD. Allergen-specific IgG antibody measurements in the management of immediate hypersensitivity to Hymenoptera venoms. J Clin Immunoassay 1983;6:172–176.

17. Hamilton RG, Adkinson NF Jr. Clinical laboratory methods for the assessment and management of human allergic diseases. Clin Lab Med 1986;6:117–138.

18. Sobotka AK, Valentine MD, Ishizaka K, Lichtenstein LM. Measurement of IgG blocking antibodies: development and application of a radioimmunoassay. J Immunol 1976;117:84–90.

19. Hunt KJ, Valentine MD, Sobotka AK, et al. A controlled trial of immunotherapy in insect hypersensitivity. N Engl J Med 1978;299:157–161.

20. Valentine MD. Allergy to stinging insects. Ann Allergy 1993;70:427–432.

21. Thueson DO, Rahr R, Findlay SR, et al. Diagnosis of Polistes sensitivity. J Allergy Clin Immunol 1979;63:136.

22. deShazo RD, Butcher BT, Banks WA. Reactions to the stings of the imported fire ant. N Engl J Med 1990;323:462–466.

23. deShazo RD, Griffing C, Kwan TH, et al. Dermal hypersensitivity reactions to imported fire ants. J Allergy Clin Immunol 1984;74:841–847.

24. King TP. Insect venom allergens. Monogr Allergy 1990;28:84–100.

25. King TP, Valentine MD. Allergens of hymenopteran venoms. Clin Rev Allergy 1987;5:137–148.

26. Lu G, Kochoumian L, King TP. Sequence identity and antigenic cross-reactivity of white face hornet venom allergen, also a hyaluronidase, with other proteins. J Biol Chem 1995;270:4457–4465.

27. Lu G, Villalba M, Coscia MR, et al. Sequence analysis and antigenic cross-reactivity of a venom allergen, antigen 5, from hornets, wasps, and yellow jackets. J Immunol 1993;150:2823–2830.

28. Hoffman DR, Dove DE, Moffitt JE, Stafford CT. Allergens in Hymenoptera venom. XXI. Cross-reactivity and multiple reactivity between fire ant venom and bee and wasp venoms. J Allergy Clin Immunol 1988;82:828–834.

29. Sobotka AK. Diagnosis of insect hypersensitivity. J Allergy Clin Immunol 1977;60:213–214.

30. Mulfinger L, Yunginger J, Styer W, et al. Sting morphology and frequency of sting autotomy among medically important vespids (Hymenoptera: Vespidae) and the honey bee (Hymenoptera: Apidae). J Med Entomol 1992;29:325–328.

31. van der Linden PW, Hack CE, Struyvenberg A, van der Zwan JK. Insect-sting challenge in 324 subjects with a previous anaphylactic reaction: current criteria for insect-venom hypersensitivity do not predict the occurrence and the severity of anaphylaxis. J Allergy Clin Immunol 1994; 94:151–159.

32. van der Linden PWG, Struyvenberg A, Kraaijenhagen RJ, et al. Anaphylactic shock after insect-sting challenge in 138 persons with a previous insect-sting reaction. Ann Intern Med 1993;11:161–168.

33. Hunt KJ, Sobotka AK, Valentine MD, et al. Sensitization following Hymenoptera whole body extract therapy. J Allergy Clin Immunol 1978;61:48–53.

34. Light WC, Reisman RE, Shimizu M, Arbesman CE. Unusual reactions following insect stings. Clinical features and immunologic analysis. J Allergy Clin Immunol 1977;59:391–397.

35. Mazza JA, Moote DW, Gamble JB, Young GB. Memory loss and pneumonitis after anaphylaxis due to an insect sting. Can Med Assoc J 1991;144:175–176.

36. Graft DF, Schuberth KC, Kagey-Sobotka A, et al. A prospective study of the natural history of large local reactions after Hymenoptera stings in children. J Pediatr 1984;104:664–668.

37. Fortenberry JE, Laine J, Shalit M. Use of epinephrine for anaphylaxis by emergency medical technicians in a wilderness setting. Ann Emerg Med 1995;25:785–787.

38. Chafee FH. The prevalence of bee sting allergy in an allergic population. Acta Allergol (Copenh) 1970;25:292.

39. Settipane GA, Newstead GJ, Boyd GK. Frequency of Hymenoptera allergy in an atopic and normal population. J Allergy Clin Immunol 1972;50:146.

40. Settipane GA, Boyd GK. Prevalence of bee sting allergy in 4992 Boy Scouts. Acta Allergol (Copenh) 1970;25:286.

41. Birnbaum J, Vervloet D, Charpin D. Atopy and systemic reactions to Hymenoptera stings. Allergy Proc 1994;15:49–52.

42. Charpin D, Birnbaum J, Lanteaume A, Vervloet D. Prevalence of allergy to Hymenoptera stings in different samples of the general population. J Allergy Clin Immunol 1992; 90:331–334.

43. Shimizu T, Hori T. Evaluation of venom specific IgE and total serum IgE among forest administration workers. Arerugi 1990;39:654–661.

44. Settipane GA, Chafee FH. Natural history of allergy to Hymenoptera. Clin Allergy 1979;9:385–390.

45. Golden DB. Epidemiology of allergy to insect venoms and stings. Allergy Proc 1989;10:103–107.

46. Golden DB, Marsh DG, Kagey-Sobotka A, et al. Epidemiology of insect venom sensitivity. JAMA 1989;262:240–244.

47. Barnard JH. Studies of 400 Hymenoptera sting deaths in the United States. J Allergy Clin Immunol 1973;52:259.

48. Fernandez J, Rodes F, Marti J, Blanca M. Wasp sting anaphylaxis as a cause of death: a case report. Allergol Immunopathol (Madrid) 1992;20:40–41.

49. Sasvary T, Muller U. Fatalities from insect stings in Switzerland 1978 to 1987. Schweiz Med Wochenschr 1994;124:1887–1894.

50. Schwartz HJ, Squillace DL, Sher TH, et al. Studies in stinging insect hypersensitivity: postmortem demonstration of antivenom IgE antibody in possible sting-related sudden death. Am J Clin Pathol 1986;85:607–610.

51. Yunginger JW, Nelson DR, Squillace DL, et al. Laboratory investigation of deaths due to anaphylaxis. J Forensic Sci 1991;36:857–863.

52. Franca FO, Benvenuti LA, Fan HW, et al. Severe and fatal mass attacks by "killer" bees (Africanized honey bees—*Apis mellifera scutellata*) in Brazil: clinicopathological studies with measurement of serum venom concentrations. Q J Med 1994;87:269–282.

53. Schumacher MJ, Schmidt JO, Egen NB, Lowry JE. Quantity, analysis, and lethality of European and Africanized honey bee venoms. Am J Trop Med Hyg 1990;43:79–86.

54. Kochuyt AM, Van Hoeyveld E, Stevens EA. Occupational allergy to bumble bee venom. Department of Internal Medicine, University Hospital of Leuven, Belgium. Clin Exp Allergy 1993;23:190–195.

55. Pence HL, White AF, Cost K, et al. Evaluation of severe reactions to sweat bee stings. Ann Allergy 1991;66:399–404.

56. Freeman TM. Imported fire ants: the ants from hell! Allergy Proc 1994;15:11–15.

57. Candiotti KA, Lamas AM. Adverse neurologic reactions to the sting of the imported fire ant. Int Arch Allergy Immunol 1993;102:417–420.

58. Schwartz LB, Yunginger JW, Miller J, et al. Time course of appearance and disappearance of human mast cell tryptase in the circulation after anaphylaxis. J Clin Invest 1989;83:1551–1555.

59. Stephan V, Zimmermann A, Kuhr J, Urbanek R. Determination of N-methylhistamine in urine as an indicator of histamine release in immediate allergic reactions. J Allergy Clin Immunol 1990;86:862–868.

60. Smith PL, Kagey-Sobotka A, Bleecker ER, et al. Physiologic manifestations of human anaphylaxis. J Clin Invest 1980;66:1072.

61. Georgitis JW, Reisman RE. Venom skin tests in insect-allergic and insect-nonallergic populations. J Allergy Clin Immunol 1985;76:803–807.

62. Golden DB. Guidelines for venom immunotherapy. Ann Allergy 1988;61:159–161.

63. Hamilton RG, Wisenauer JA, Golden DB, et al. Selection of Hymenoptera venoms for immunotherapy on the basis of patient's IgE antibody cross-reactivity. J Allergy Clin Immunol 1993;92:651–659.

64. Selcow JE, Mendelson LM, Rosen JP. Anaphylactic reactions in skin test–negative patients. J Allergy Clin Immunol 1980;65:400. Letter.

65. Schumacher MJ, Tveten MS, Egen NB. Rate and quantity of delivery of venom from honeybee stings. J Allergy Clin Immunol 1994;93:831–835.

66. Granata AV, Halickman JF, Borak J. Utility of military antishock trousers (MAST) in anaphylactic shock—a case report. J Emerg Med 1985;2:349–351.

67. Perkin RM, Anas NG. Mechanisms and management of anaphylactic shock not responding to traditional therapy. Ann Allergy 1985;54:202–208.

68. Pollack CV Jr. Utility of glucagon in the emergency department. J Emerg Med 1993;11:195–205.

69. Kivity S, Yarchovsky J. Relapsing anaphylaxis to bee sting in a patient treated with beta-blocker and Ca blocker. J Allergy Clin Immunol 1990;85:669–670. Letter.

70. Valentine MD, Schuberth KC, Kagey-Sobotka A, et al. The value of immunotherapy with venom in children with allergy to insect stings. N Engl J Med 1990;323:1601–1603.

71. van der Linden PWG, Hack CE, Struyvenberg A, van der Zwan JC. (Comment on Novey H. J Allergy Clin Immunol 1995;96:703.). J Allergy Clin Immunol 1995;96:703–704.

72. Novey H. Sting challenges as criteria for venom immunotherapy. J Allergy Clin Immunol 1995;96:703. Letter.

73. Reisman RE. Insect sting challenges: do no harm. J Allergy Clin Immunol 1995;96:702. Letter.

74. Lichtenstein LM. (Comment on Reisman RE. J Allergy Clin Immunol 1995;96:702). J Allergy Clin Immunol 1995;96:702–703.

75. Franken HH, Dubois AEJ, Minkena ITJ, et al. Lack of reproducibility of a single negative sting challenge response in the assessment of anaphylactic risk in patients with suspected yellow jacket sensitivity. J Allergy Clin Immunol 1994;93:431–436.

76. Goldberg A, Confino-Cohen R, Mekori YA. Deliberate bee sting challenge of patients receiving maintenance venom immunotherapy at 3-month intervals. J Allergy Clin Immunol 1954;93:997–1001.

77. Yunginger JW, Paull BR, Jones RT, Santrach PJ. Rush venom immunotherapy program for honeybee venom sensitivity. J Allergy Clin Immunol 1979;63:340–347.

78. Berchtold E, Maibach R, Müller U. Reduction of side effects with rush-immunotherapy with honeybee venom by pretreatment with terfenadine. Clin Exp Allergy 1992;22:59–65.

79. Bousquet J, Fontez A, Aznar R, et al. Combination of passive and active immunization in honeybee venom immunotherapy. J Allergy Clin Immunol 1987;79:947–954.

80. Lessof MH, Sobotka AK, Lichtenstein LM. Effects of passive antibody in bee venom anaphylaxis. Johns Hopkins Med J 1978;142:1–7.

81. Lessof MH, Sobotka AK, Lichtenstein LM. Protection against anaphylaxis in Hymenoptera-sensitive patients by passive immunization. J Allergy Clin Immunol 1976;57:246.

82. Müller U, Morris T, Bischof M, et al. Combined active and passive immunotherapy in honeybee-sting allergy. J Allergy Clin Immunol 1986;78:115–122.

83. Bernstein DI, Mittman RJ, Kagen SL, et al. Clinical and immunologic studies of rapid venom immunotherapy in

Hymenoptera-sensitive patients. J Allergy Clin Immunol 1989;84:951–959.

84. Reisman RE, Livingston A. Venom immunotherapy: 10 years of experience with administration of single venoms and 50 micrograms maintenance doses. J Allergy Clin Immunol 1992;89:1189–1195.

85. Reisman RE. Venom hypersensitivity. J Allergy Clin Immunol 1994;94:651–658.

86. Golden DB, Kagey-Sobotka A, Valentine MD, Lichtenstein LM. Dose dependence of Hymenoptera venom immunotherapy. J Allergy Clin Immunol 1981;67:370–374.

87. Kemeny DM, Tomioka H, Tsutsumi A, et al. The relationship between anti-IgE auto-antibodies and the IgE response to wasp venom during immunotherapy. Clin Exp Allergy 1990;20:67–69.

88. Khan RH, Szewczuk MR, Day JH. Bee venom anti-idiotypic antibody is associated with protection in beekeepers and bee sting-sensitive patients receiving immunotherapy against allergic reactions. J Allergy Clin Immunol 1991;88:199–208.

89. Golden DB, Lawrence ID, Hamilton RG, et al. Clinical correlation of the venom-specific IgG antibody level during maintenance venom. J Allergy Clin Immunol 1992;90:386–393.

90. Reisman RE. Should routine measurements of serum venom-specific IgG be a standard of practice in patients receiving venom immunotherapy? (Comment on: J Allergy Clin Immunol 1992;90:386–393.) J Allergy Clin Immunol 1992;90:282–284.

91. Kemeny DM, Lessof MH, Patel S, et al. IgG and IgE antibodies after immunotherapy with bee and wasp venom. Int Arch Allergy Appl Immunol 1989;88:247–249.

92. Urbanek R, Kemeny DM, Richards D. Sub-class of IgG anti-bee venom antibody produced during bee venom immunotherapy and its relationship to long-term protection from bee stings and following termination of venom immunotherapy. Clin Allergy 1986;16:317–322.

93. Randolph CC, Reisman RE. Evaluation of decline in serum venom-specific IgE as a criterion for stopping venom immunotherapy. J Allergy Clin Immunol 1986;77:823–827.

94. Golden DBK, Kwiterovich KA, Kagey-Sobotka A, et al. Discontinuing venom immunotherapy (VIT): determinants of clinical reactivity. J Allergy Clin Immunol 1989;83:273. Abstract.

95. Golden DBK, Kwiterovich KA, Kagey-Sobotka A, et al.

96. Golden DBK, Kwiterovich KA, Valentine MD, et al. Risk and benefit of discontinuing venom immunotherapy (VIT) after 5 years. J Allergy Clin Immunol 1991;87:237. Abstract.

97. Golden DBK, Johnson K, Addison BI, et al. Clinical and immunologic observations in patients who stop venom immunotherapy. J Allergy Clin Immunol 1986;77:435–442.

98. Schuberth KC, Kwiterovich KA, Kagey-Sobotka A, et al. Starting and stopping venom immunotherapy (VIT) in children with insect allergy. J Allergy Clin Immunol 1988;81:200. Abstract.

99. Keating MU, Kagey-Sobotka A, Hamilton RG, Yunginger JW. Clinical and immunologic follow-up of patients who stop venom immunotherapy. J Allergy Clin Immunol 1991;88:339–348.

100. Oei HD, Stroes ES, Beukema WP, van der Zwan JC. [When can desensitization with bee and wasp venom be stopped?] Ned Tijdschr Geneeskd 1991;135:719–720.

101. Haugaard L, Norregard OFH, Dahl R. In-hospital sting challenge in insect venom-allergic patients after stopping venom immunotherapy. J Allergy Clin Immunol 1991;87:699.

102. Müller U, Berchtold E, Helbling A. Honeybee venom allergy: results of a sting challenge 1 year after stopping successful venom immunotherapy in 86 patients. J Allergy Clin Immunol 1991;87:702–709.

103. Golden DB. Discontinuation of venom immunotherapy. J Allergy Clin Immunol 1998;102:703–704.

104. Graft DF, Schoenwetter WF. Insect sting allergy: analysis of a cohort of patients who initiated venom immunotherapy from 1978 to 1986. Ann Allergy 1994;73:481–485.

105. Levine MI. Systemic reactions to immunotherapy. J Allergy Clin Immunol 1979;63:209.

106. Lockey RF, Benedict LM, Turbeltaub PC, Bubantz SC. Fatalities from immunotherapy and skin testing. J Allergy Clin Immunol 1987;79:660.

107. Schwartz HJ, Golden DB, Lockey RF. Venom immunotherapy in the Hymenoptera-allergic pregnant patient. J Allergy Clin Immunol 1990;85:709–712.

108. Greenberger PA. Contrast media reactions. J Allergy Clin Immunol 1984;74:600–605.

109. Greenberger PA, Halwig JM, Patterson R, Wallemark CB. Emergency administration of radiocontrast media in high-risk patients. J Allergy Clin Immunol 1986;77:630–634.

Chapter 28

The CD28 T-Cell Costimulatory Pathway: Pharmacologic Inhibition and Augmentation

Carl H. June
Jeffrey A. Ledbetter

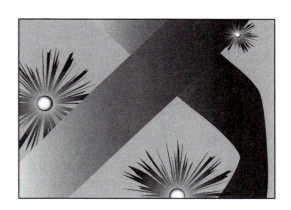

Unlike B-cell immunoglobulin receptors that can bind native antigens directly, T-cell receptors (TCRs) bind both antigen fragments and major histocompatibility complex (MHC) molecules. In addition, antigen recognition by the TCR requires accessory molecules, either CD4 or CD8, to enhance the avidity of the TCR for the antigen/MHC complex and the non-covalently associated CD3 chains to transduce the antigen-specific signal. Thus, the "signal 1" delivered to the T cell via the TCR is actually dependent on a multicomponent receptor complex involving the TCR binding to Ag/MHC but also CD4 (or CD8) binding directly to nonpolymorphic parts of either class II or class I MHC molecules. In addition to this antigen-specific recognition, antigen nonspecific or costimulatory ("signal 2") interactions between the T cell and the antigen-presenting cells (APCs) are required for optimal immune responses to T-cell–dependent antigens (1). The best characterized costimulatory molecules on APCs are the structurally related glycoproteins CD80 (B7-1) and CD86 (B7-2). The receptors for B7 molecules on the T cell are CD28 and CD152 (CTLA-4), which are structurally related members of the immunoglobulin superfamily. Because of their importance for immune responses, these pairs of receptors and counter-receptors, and the signaling pathways they trigger, offer new targets for development of therapeutic immune regulators. Blocking of the CD28/B7 pathway could result in immunosuppression, with implications for the treatment of autoimmune diseases, organ transplantation, and graft-versus-host disease (GVHD). Activation of the CD28/B7 pathway could be useful for inducing the immune system to recognize and eliminate tumors and viruses that evade the immune system. Finally, the CD28/B7 pathway could be involved in maintaining immune tolerance, because recent studies suggest that the preferential binding of the B7-CTLA-4 pathway results in the down-regulation of the responding T cells. Thus, development of pharmacologic agonists and antagonists of the B7/CD28/CTLA-4 pathway has the potential for inducing tolerance and for both positively and negatively regulating immune responses.

CD28 and B7 Receptor Family

The CD28 receptor was discovered with a monoclonal antibody (mAb) called 9.3 produced at the Fred Hutchinson Cancer Research Center in 1980 (2). The 9.3 mAb remained unique for several years, and the antigen recognized by 9.3 was not clustered until the Third International Leukocyte Workshop (3), where it was designated CD28. Studies published prior to 1987 called the antigen 9.3 or Tp44, referring to the structure of the antigen as a 44-kD homodimer expressed by T cells (Fig. 28-1).

The early reports focused on functional and phenotypic experiments using the 9.3 mAb. The first study of 9.3 function reported that the mAb blocked the autologous and allogeneic mixed lymphocyte reaction (MLR) (4), and yet this activity was not well recognized or understood until much later. The ability of 9.3 to stimulate, rather than inhibit, T-cell proliferation responses when added with phorbol ester (PMA) or anti-CD3 was reported later, and captured more attention from T-cell biologists (5–7). CD28 cross-linking was later found to be a key factor in signal transduction, and 9.3 was shown to either stimulate or inhibit CD28 signals depending on the degree of receptor cross-linking (8,9). Bivalent F(ab')$_2$ fragments of 9.3 could stimulate partial CD28 signals, whereas monovalent Fab fragments of 9.3 did not stimulate CD28 signals but retained inhibitory activity. Optimal stimulation of CD28 with 9.3 is now generally done with highly multivalent cross-linking using mAb immobilized on plastic or beads, or is expressed on the cell surfaces after gene transduction of cDNA encoding the 9.3 single chain Fv (scFv) (see below). When T cells were activated with anti-CD3, the costimulatory signal through the CD28 receptor was shown to increase production of IL-2 (10), and coordinately to increase the production of several other cytokines, including IFN-γ, GM-CSF, and TNF-α (11).

Early studies with human peripheral blood T cells showed that expression of CD28 defines functional T-cell subpopulations within both the CD4$^+$ and CD8$^+$ compartments. The CD8$^+$CD28$^-$ T cells contained suppressors of alloantigen-specific T-cell responses and B-cell immunoglobulin synthesis, whereas the CD8$^+$CD28$^+$ T cells contained precursors of alloantigen-specific cytotoxic lymphocytes (12–14). CD4$^+$CD28$^-$ T cells also have been detected and found to respond poorly to alloantigen and to express a restricted repertoire as assessed by TCR β chain expression (15). CD28 and CD11b are expressed on reciprocal, nonoverlapping subsets of T cells, and the CD28-negative T cells are CD11b$^+$, a marker shared with monocytes, NK cells,

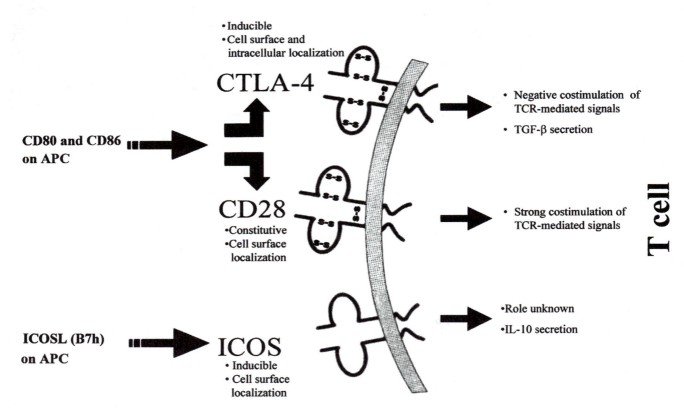

Figure 28-1. Summary of structure and properties of the CD28 family of T cell receptors. CD28, CTLA-4, and ICOS are shown as homodimeric molecules comprising a single immunoglobulin superfamily variable-like domain in their extracellular regions. Approximate locations of inter- and intrachain disulfide bonds are depicted (178;179). (APC = antigen-presenting cell; TCR = T-cell receptor).

and granulocytes (16). The mechanism of alloantigen-specific suppression by the CD8+CD28− T-cell population may be related to their inability to express CD154, the ligand for CD40, resulting in a failure to generate the CD40 signal during contact with APC (17).

The frequency of CD4+CD28− T cells increases with aging, and activation of this population is associated with high levels of production of IL-2 and IFN-γ, but a lack of expression of CD154 (18). The CD4+CD28− cells are reactive to autoantigens in vitro and may be involved in the skewing toward autoreactive responses and away from responses against exogenous antigens that occurs with aging. Increased proportions of CD28− T cells occur in situations of chronic immune stimulation, and as T cells reach proliferative senescence in culture after multiple rounds of cell division (19,20). Stimulation of CD28 results in transient down-regulation of CD28 expression and prolonged unresponsiveness to CD28 signals (21). In elderly patients, studies of nuclear extracts from their CD28-deficient T cells show the loss of two noncompeting binding activities within a 67-bp segment of the minimal promoter (22). Together, these facts suggest that

prolonged stimulation of the CD28 receptor may lead to loss of CD28 expression and alterations in T-cell activation conditions and function.

The importance of the CD28 receptor in T-cell biology was widely recognized following the discovery of a natural ligand, first termed B7/BB1, that is expressed as a cell surface glycoprotein on activated B cells (23). Thus, it became clear that natural activation of CD28 during an antigen-specific immune response occurs by the binding of T cells to antigen-presenting cells (APCs) (24). B7/BB1, later named CD80, is a member of the butyrophilin family of receptors and is expressed by B cells and APCs after activation (25,26). Several signals stimulate expression of CD80, including cross-linking of MHC class II and CD40 (27–29). A third member of the B7 family termed B7h has recently been identified (30). It is likely that this receptor is a ligand for ICOS, and the function of this putative receptor pair remains unknown.

CD28 is expressed on plasma cells from myeloma patients but not on normal plasma cells (31,32). The CD28 receptor family has limited expression on nonlymphoid cells. Hypereosinophilic

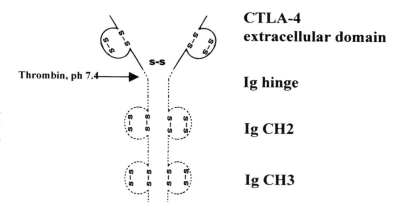

Figure 28-2. Structure of CTLA4Ig. A schematic representation of human CTLA4Ig depicting its domain structure is shown. The CTLA-4 portion of the molecule is shown in solid lines and the Fc portion in broken lines. Intrachain disulfide bonds are indicated, as is the interchain disulfide bond from CTLA-4. Also indicated is a thrombin cleavage site in the Fc hinge region used to produce the soluble CTLA-4 dimer, CTLA-4T.

patients express membrane CD28 and CD86 but not CD80 on the eosinophil surface. CD28 ligation but not CD86 ligation on the eosinophil results in IL-2 and IFN-γ secretion (33). Recent studies indicate that CD80 is also expressed in mouse embryonic stem (ES) cells, and this suggests that the early embryonic environment may utilize cellular signaling systems analogous to those seen in the immune system (34).

CTLA-4, also termed CD152, is a receptor expressed by T cells after activation that is structurally related to CD28 and is encoded by a closely linked gene (35,36). CTLA-4 is expressed as a soluble molecule with a human IgG Fc tail (hinge, CH2, and CH3 domains) and, like CD28, has been found to bind CD80 (Fig. 28-2). However, CTLA4Ig binds with higher affinity to CD80 than does CD28-Ig, and soluble CTLA4Ig inhibits T-cell responses that are dependent on signals from CD28 (37). A second ligand for CD28 and CTLA-4 was discovered by expression cloning with CTLA4Ig. This molecule, termed B7-2 or CD86, is structurally related to CD80 and is another member of the butyrophilin family (38,39). Like CD80, CD86 is expressed by activated APCs, but is induced sooner after activation. The binding affinities of CD80 and CD86 to CTLA-4 and CD28 are similar, and they differ in their binding kinetics. CD86 exhibits a higher on rate and a higher off rate binding to CTLA-4 than CD80 (40). Although the significance of the distinct binding kinetics of CD80 and CD86 to CD28 and CTLA-4 is not fully understood, it is possible that this property controls the rate or degree of receptor cross-linking and thus the balance of signals between CD28 and CTLA-4. This could account for the differences between CD80 and CD86 that have been found in their ability to generate costimulatory signals in some assays. It has been proposed that B7 genes and the MHC class I and class II genes were once linked and that B7-1 and B7-2 or their ancestral genes were translocated away from the MHC locus during evolution (26).

CTLA-4 knockout mice exhibit a severe T-cell lymphoproliferative disease that is lethal by about 8 to 12 weeks of age (41,42). The T-cell proliferation results in the predominant accumulation of CD4⁺ T cells (43). T-cell proliferation in these mice is dependent on CD28 signals, because mice that also contain a defective CD28 gene do not exhibit the lymphoproliferative disorder. In addition, treatment with CTLA4Ig prevents lymphoproliferation in the CTLA-4 knockout mice. Similarly, CTLA-4 knockout mice that also have defective CD80 and CD86 genes do not suffer from T-cell lymphoproliferation (44). Thus, CTLA-4 is essential for inhibition of T-cell responses to CD28 stimulation. Although CTLA-4 seems to inhibit CD28 activation when these two receptors are coexpressed, one recent report showed that transfer of normal syngeneic T cells into CTLA-4 knockout mice prevented lethal T-cell lymphoproliferation (45). Thus, the expression of CTLA-4 on a few T cells prevented the uncontrolled proliferation of large numbers of CTLA-4 negative T cells. Stimulation of CTLA-4 on CD4⁺ T cells can induce the production of TGF-β (46), and it was proposed that TGF-β production by T cells after CTLA-4 stimulation is essential for controlling proliferation of CTLA-4 negative T cells. This hypothesis is supported by the phenotype of TGF-β knockout mice, because these mice also suffer early lethality as a result of a multifocal inflammatory disease (47,48).

Stimulation of CD28 in vivo by injection of anti-CD28 mAb does not result in T-cell proliferation in normal mice. However, the same treatment of mice lacking functional expression of CD80 and CD86 results in T-cell lymphoproliferation (44). Therefore, the negative signal from CD80 and CD86 binding to CTLA-4 prevents the T-cell response to CD28 activation, even when the CD28 signal is given with an mAb specific for CD28, rather than from the natural ligand CD80 or CD86.

A third member of the CD28 family of receptors was recently discovered (49). This molecule, termed ICOS, for inducible costimulator, is expressed by activated but not resting T cells. Structural homology among CD28, CD152, and ICOS is significant, and yet ICOS differs from CD28 and CD152 in the MYPPPY homology domain involved in binding to CD80 and CD86. ICOS is functionally active, because binding of an mAb to ICOS costimulates T-cell proliferation as potently as binding to

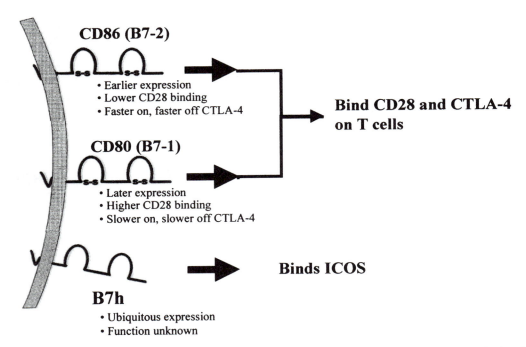

Figure 28-3. Summary of the structure and properties of the B7 family of molecules. These receptors are depicted as single-chain molecules, comprising (N-terminal) immunoglobulin superfamily variable-like and constant-like domains. Predicted intrachain disulfide bonds are indicated. B7h is a ligand for ICOS. See text for details.

CD28, without the accompanying increase in production of IL2. Instead, anti-ICOS induces production of large amounts of IL-10. Expression of ICOS is high on T cells from tonsillar germinal centers, suggesting that ICOS may have a specialized function in regulating B-cell differentiation (49). ICOS-Ig, a soluble molecule composed of the ICOS extracellular domain fused with human IgG1 hinge, CH2, and CH3 domains, has been created and expressed (submitted for publication). This molecule binds with high affinity to activated dendritic cells, B-cell lymphoblastoid cell lines, and activated monocytes, but does not bind to CD80 or CD86 expressed on CHO cells. The ligand for ICOS has not yet been reported, but based on homology with CD28 and CTLA-4, the ligand is speculated to be another member of the butyrophilin family. T-cell proliferative responses to alloantigen are inhibited by ICOS-Ig by up to 50%, confirming that ICOS is functionally active in T cell/APC interactions. Based on these data, we propose a model in which T cells express ICOS after activation to promote signals that are not inhibited by CTLA-4 (Figs. 28-1 and 28-3).

CD28 and CTLA-4 Signal Transduction

The functional importance of the CD28 receptor was recognized from studies with anti-CD28 mAb before the discovery of the natural ligands for CD28 (5,7,10,50–52). The early studies showed that CD28 cross-linking was important for these functional effects. Fab fragments of anti-CD28 mAb 9.3 were unable to cooperate with anti-CD3 mAb-generated signals to drive T-cell proliferation (6). Soluble bivalent mAb 9.3 enhanced IL-2 secretion by mitogen-stimulated T cells by prolonging IL-2 mRNA half-life (11). The CD28 response was distinct from stimulation through the TCR because it was resistant to inhibition by the immunosuppressive drug cyclosporine (53). Because cyclosporine inhibits a calcium-dependent phosphatase (54), CD28 therefore signals, at least in part, through a calcium-independent pathway. In agreement with this, bivalent mAb 9.3 triggering does not increase cytoplasmic calcium concentration (55). The functional synergy between CD28 receptor activation and the CD2 (56,57) or CD3-TCR pathways supports the idea that the CD28 signaling pathway is distinct, as does the observation that CD28 up-regulates responses from pharmacologic stimulation with calcium ionophore plus phorbol ester (58). The potential importance of calcium-independent signaling via CD28 has been reviewed (59).

The idea that CD28 provides a positive signal during T-cell activation was challenged when it was found that soluble 9.3 did not up-regulate responses of T cells stimulated by APCs but instead blocked these responses unless CD28 was further cross-linked using a second-step antiglobulin (8). Under these conditions of multivalent cross-linking, CD28 activated tyrosine

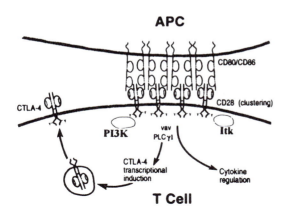

Figure 28-4. CD28 signal transduction requires clustering. CD80 or CD86 binds with a 2:1 stoichiometry to homodimeric CD28. CD28 signal transduction leads to cytokine and other gene expression, and also to induction of CTLA-4 expression. Oligomerization of CD80/CD86 is required for high-avidity CTLA-4 binding. CTLA-4 binds with low avidity to monomeric CD86 (63).

phosphorylation (60) and increased cytoplasmic calcium concentration through tyrosine kinase-dependent activation of phospholipase Cγl (PLC-γ) (61). We now understand that activation of CD28 by engagement with a natural ligand (B7-1 or B7-2) during contact with APC is more similar to activation by cross-linked mAb 9.3 and that the effects of soluble mAb 9.3 reflect partial CD28 activation. The 2:1 stoichiometry of B7-1 binding to CTLA-4 or CD28 homodimers (62,63) favors multivalent cross-linking during cell-cell interaction (Fig. 28-4). Soluble CD28 mAb 9.3 can thus be thought of as both a partial agonist and a partial antagonist because it blocks the binding of natural ligand while triggering a subset of CD28-linked signals.

The biochemical basis of the CD28 signaling pathways remains poorly understood. Many of the events that occur after CD28 signaling also occur after TCR triggering. The activation of tyrosine phosphorylation (60) and the src-family kinase p56^{lck} by CD28 cross-linking (64) suggests that these tyrosine kinases are involved in the CD28 response and that some of the enzymes activated in the cytoplasm are a subset of those that mediate the response from TCR triggering, including PLC-γl and vav (65). The more recent description of direct tyrosine phosphorylation of CD28 with CD28 triggering and the association of PI-3K with CD28 by an SH2-dependent interaction (66,67) have further argued for CD28 signals that overlap with TCR signals. The role of PI-3K in CD28 signal transduction is controversial (68). Another common element in CD28 signaling is the induction of NFκ-B-like transcriptional response elements (69–71) and the Iκ-B kinases (72).

The structural elements of CD28 that mediate signal transduction are still being defined. The highly conserved cytosolic domain of CD28 is required for costimulatory signal transduction. The cytoplasmic domain of CD28 contains four tyrosine

residues, and a single residue appears necessary for stimulation in Jurkat T cells (73). Both vav and a 62-kD phosphoprotein are tyrosine phosphorylated after CD28 stimulation, and recent studies indicate that distinct domains with the CD28 cytoplasmic tail are responsible for these activities (65).

One of the most specific biochemical changes described following CD28 ligation is stabilization of a variety of mRNAs, including cytokines (11) and several glycoproteins such as CTLA-4 and CD40L (74,75). The mechanism reported for this effect may involve the c-Jun NH-terminal kinase (JNK) pathway (76,77). Early studies showed that CD28 stimulation was associated with a decrease in the ratio of cAMP to cGMP cytosolic concentrations (55), and recent studies indicate that another downstream kinase in the CD3 and CD28 pathway is the cAMP-specific phosphodiesterase-7 (PDE7) (78). Because expression of the PDE7 protein is T cell specific, this may represent a good target for development of selective inhibitors of T-cell activation.

How then does the CD28 receptor provide functional responses that synergize with TCR activation and up-regulate expression of multiple cytokines? Most likely, the CD28 receptor contributes to TCR-linked signals by prolonging the kinetics of tyrosine kinase activation, but it may also recruit distinct cytoplasmic response elements. The Tec protein-tyrosine kinase family includes Btk, Itk/Tsk/Emt, Tec, Rlk/Txk, and Bmx, which are involved in signals mediated by various cytokines or antigen receptors. Inducible T-cell kinase (Itk) is relatively specific in T-cell expression, is tightly bound to CD28 before ligation of the receptor, and is activated by binding of soluble mAb 9.3 (79). The role of Itk in calcium-independent signaling requires further elucidation, because more recent studies from Itk-deficient mice found that whereas the CD3-mediated proliferative response was severely compromised in the absence of Itk, the calcineurin-independent CD28-mediated response was significantly elevated when compared with cells from control animals (80). Overexpression of Tec but not Itk can enhance IL-2 promoter activity mediated by CD28 stimulation (81). The present results suggest that Tec and/or Itk have distinct roles in the CD3 versus the CD28 signaling pathways.

A principal controversy in the nature of costimulatory signal transduction concerns the general mechanisms involved. One argument is that CD28 operates signal transduction that is biochemically distinct from that initiated by the TCR/CD3 complex (82,83). Another argument is that costimulation is merely a quantitative phenomenon and that CD28 lowers the threshold of TCR-CD3 signals required for activation (84). The fact that CD28 cytosolic domain does not encode any of the signaling motifs found in the TCR/CD3 complex is one line of evidence used to support the first argument. Evidence in support of the latter hypothesis is the demonstration that costimulation triggers the accumulation of signaling molecules at the interface of the T cell and APC into lipid raft microdomains (85,86). Thus, CD28 may exert its costimulatory action by facilitating the assembly of an effective scaffold of signaling elements within the TCR complex. It is likely that both arguments are correct in that costimulation through CD28 leads to the assembly of a signaling scaffold that generates signals that are temporally and biochemically distinct from those generated by the TCR alone. Furthermore, Berridge has proposed a signal transduction model to account for self-tolerance in which absence of costimulation through CD28 would result in the assembly of a defective scaffold that would reverse slowly and thus might induce a state of unresponsiveness responsible for peripheral T-cell tolerance (87).

The expression of CD28 and its coupling to the T-cell signal transduction machinery are regulated during T-cell activation. CD28 signals are potent when they are received simultaneously with or after TCR triggering, but CD28 signals received by resting T cells without TCR signals can inhibit subsequent responses from TCR activation (21). This process of CD28 desensitization is reflected in the regulation of CD28 expression, because TCR triggering up-regulates CD28 expression whereas CD28 triggering down-regulates CD28 expression (21). These observations further emphasize the importance of the regulation of B7 expression during activation of APC.

While CD28 transmits costimulatory signals that enhance T-cell activation, CTLA-4 transmits inhibitory signals that are essential for turning off T-cell proliferation (88). The mechanisms of CTLA-4 signal transduction are also controversial and complex. Unlike CD28, CTLA-4 has highly regulated intracellular trafficking and cell surface expression that is necessary for its function, and this occurs by a post-translational mechanism that is based on a tyrosine-based motif. Current evidence indicates that CTLA-4 mediates its inhibitory functions by means of two distinct mechanisms. First, CTLA-4 acts as a decoy for B7, and by virtue of its higher affinity for B7 than that of CD28, CTLA-4 can divert signaling from CD28 by receptor competition. Therefore, some functions of CTLA-4 appear not to require the cytosolic tail (89). Second, CTLA-4 appears to mediate direct signal transduction because ligation of CTLA-4 can induce TGF-β (46). The cytoplasmic tail of CTLA-4 associates with a protein tyrosine phosphatase, SHP-2, that dephosphorylates the CD3 chains associated with the T-cell receptor (90,91). CTLA-4 cross-linking induces an association with SHP-2 but not with PI3-K, in contrast to CD28 activation, which results in the recruitment of PI3-K but not SHP-2 (92).

CD28 Pathway Inhibition

The biologic and specific control of the rejection process has been the central goal of immunologists for decades, and this search has been termed the Holy Grail of Immunology. It is possible that new immunomodulatory agents that block costimulatory pathways will permit the development of immunologic tolerance. Since the development of the first reagents to block CD28 costimulation in 1992, many studies have bolstered the hope for the potentially broad therapeutic utility of this approach (Table 28-1).

It is likely that soluble agents that block CD28:B7 interactions, as well as intracellular small molecule compounds, will eventually be developed for CD28 pathway inhibition. Currently,

Table 28-1. Potential Uses of Costimulatory Blockade

Application	Reference(s)
Immunosuppression or tolerance induction for organ allografts and xenografts	(100)
Treatment/prevention of GVHD	(104,136)
Therapy of autoimmune disorders	(106)
Therapy of allergic disorders	(137,138)
Use for gene therapy: induction of tolerance to vector product	(139)

most experience is with CTLA4Ig, the first agent to provide potent inhibition of CD28 signal transduction. Antibodies that bind B7 with higher affinity than does CTLA4Ig are also under current development, but the preclinical studies of these reagents are not yet as extensive as of CTLA4Ig.

CTLA4Ig is a potent inhibitor of CD28:CTLA-4–B7 interactions (see Fig. 28-2). It has a novel mechanism of action and also has several attractive features for an immunosuppressive drug, including low toxicity, long serum half-life, and in some cases the ability to induce long-lasting antigen-specific immune suppression (tolerance) after therapy. CTLA4Ig thus represents a prototype of a new class of immunosuppressive drugs that function by blocking T-cell costimulation through the CD28 receptor. Results from numerous animal studies demonstrate that CTLA4Ig has efficacy in animal models of transplantation, autoimmune disease, and gene therapy (Table 28-2). Many of these studies used human CTLA4Ig (human CTLA-4–human Ig). This molecule has impaired Fc effector functions, partly as a result of mutation of the disulfide bonds in the hinge region. Although this molecule has shown efficacy in rodent models, it is not optimal for use because it elicits a delayed but vigorous murine anti-CTLA4Ig antibody response (93). Murine CTLA4Ig is less immunogenic (94) and is more effective in rodent studies than human CTLA4Ig (95). Thus, the studies presented in Table 28-2 using human CTLA4Ig probably underestimated its true potency as an immunosuppressive agent.

CTLA4Ig and anti-B7 antibodies have been tested in several transplantation models. CTLA4Ig delayed rejection of rat cardiac allografts but did not induce transplantation tolerance in most treated animals (96). Refinements in the dosing schedule using this model showed that the best results were obtained when recipient rats were pretreated with donor spleen cells [donor-specific transfusion (DST)] plus CTLA4Ig (97). When DST was administered at the time of transplantation followed by a single dose of CTLA4Ig 2 days later, all animals had long-term graft survival. Responses to donor, but not third-party, skin grafts were also delayed in these animals, and donor-matched second cardiac allografts were also tolerated. Thus, combinations of DST and CTLA4Ig induced prolonged, often indefinite, cardiac allograft acceptance in rodents. Human CTLA4Ig treatment alone induced classic transplantation tolerance in a murine cardiac

Table 28-2. Use of CD28 Pathway Inhibitors in Animal Models

Model	Reagent	Species	Results	Reference(s)
Organ transplantation	CTLA4Ig	Mouse, rat	Prolonged graft survival of islet, cardiac, renal, hepatic, lung, and skin allografts and induction of tolerance in some cases. CTLA4Ig alone fails to reverse acute rejection.	(96–99,140)
Organ transplantation	Anti-B7 antibodies	Mouse	Prolongation of cardiac and islet allografts. Combination treatment with anti-CD80 plus CD86 is more effective than either agent alone.	(102,103,141)
Graft-versus-host disease	CTLA4Ig, anti-CTLA-4 antibody	Mouse	In vivo treatment of the host with CTLA4Ig solely during the initial period of donor alloactivation can completely abort the subsequent development of GVH reaction. CTLA-4 antibody injection exacerbates GVHD.	(136,142,143)
Graft-versus-host disease	Anti-B7 antibodies	Mouse	Abort or ameliorate acute GVHD. Combination treatment with anti-CD80 plus CD86 is more effective than either agent alone.	(144,145)
Autoimmune disease	CTLA4Ig, anti-B7 antibodies	Mouse, rat	Prevent or treat a variety of acute induced and spontaneous autoimmune diseases. Depending on time of treatment, EAE can be exacerbated by CTLA4Ig.	(93,94,146–151)
Antibody responses to T-cell-dependent antigens	CTLA4Ig, anti-B7 antibodies	Mouse, monkey	Blocked responses; antigen-specific unresponsiveness induced; germinal center formation prevented.	(152–154)
Gene therapy: organ transplantation, autoimmune disease	Adenoviral CTLA4Ig	Mouse, rat	Adenovirus-mediated expression of CTLA-4 prevents allograft rejection or ameliorates EAE and diabetes.	(155–157)
Gene therapy: prevention of vector-specific immunity	CTLA4Ig	Mouse	CTLA4Ig prolonged expression of adenovirus and adeno-associated vectors. Combination therapy with cyclosporine or anti-CD40L is more effective.	(139,158–162)
Kidney allograft	hCTLA4Ig, anti-hB7	Monkey	CTLA4Ig monotherapy prolongs rejection. Anti-B7 antibodies delay or prevent rejection.	(111,163); Kirk et al, unpublished
Islet cell allograft	hCTLA4Ig	Monkey	CTLA4Ig monotherapy delays islet cell allograft rejection.	(101)
Delayed type hypersensitivity	CD28 phosphorothioate oligonucleotides	Mouse	Oligonucleotide-mediated inhibition of CD28 function in vitro and in vivo.	(164,165)
Mixed lymphocyte reaction	NP1835-2	Human T cells	NP1835-2, isolated from a microbial extract, inhibits T-cell activation. Together at suboptimal concentrations, NP1835-2 and cyclosporine were able to impair T-cell activation in an additive fashion.	(166)

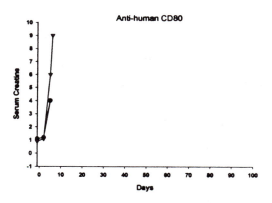

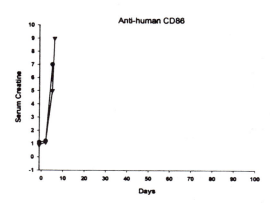

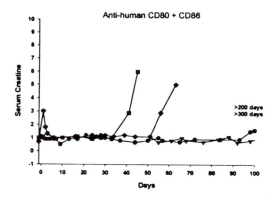

Figure 28-5. Combination anti-B7 antibody therapy delays or prevents mismatched primate renal allograft rejection. Rhesus renal allografts were performed as previously reported (111). Allograft survival as measured by serum creatinine is shown following mismatched allogeneic renal transplantation following therapy with humanized anti-CD80 (B71) alone, humanized anti-CD86 alone, or following therapy with humanized anti-human CD80 plus CD86 antibodies (4 animals each). The graft survival of unmodified rejection is shown for 5 animals. Animals were loaded with 20 mg/kg of the antibodies and then treated with 5 mg/kg weekly doses for 8 weeks. (Unpublished data courtesy of AD Kirk and GG Gray.)

transplantation model (98) and in pancreatic islet cell xenografts (99). In primates, CTLA4Ig prolongs the survival but does not prevent rejection of renal and pancreatic islet allografts (100,101). However, human CTLA4Ig given as monotherapy is not sufficient to induce tolerance to allografts in primates. It is possible that primate CTLA4Ig might be more effective in rhesus allograft models. CTLA4Ig has not yet been tested for efficacy in human organ allotransplantation.

Anti-B7 antibodies also prolong the survival of cardiac and islet cell allografts in rodents (102,103). Combination therapy with both anti-CD80 plus anti-CD86 blockade appears necessary, because the blockade of either CD80 or CD86 alone is generally not sufficient to prevent rejection. Recent data (A. D. Kirk, G. Gray, et al, unpublished data) indicate that humanized anti-B7 antibodies, when given in combination to provide simultaneous blockade of CD80 and CD86, are able to provide prolonged acceptance of renal allografts in a primate model (Fig. 28-5). To date, there are no published results comparing the efficacy of CTLA4Ig to B7 blockade with anti-B7 antibodies. These preliminary results with organ allografts in nonhuman primates achieved with blockade of B7 alone are very encouraging, and are superior to those observed with the highest tolerated doses of conventional immunosuppressants such as cyclosporine and tacrolimus. Previously it was not possible for any single agent to prevent rejection in a rigorous transplant model in primates unless combination immunosuppressive therapy was administered.

Beneficial effects of CD28 blockade were also obtained in studies of the effects of CTLA4Ig and anti-B7 antibodies on lethal graft-versus-host disease (GVHD) induced by allogeneic bone marrow transplantation in mice (see Table 28-2). Recent clinical studies indicate that ex vivo incubation of human donor and lethally irradiated recipient marrow in the presence of CTLA4Ig, followed by infusion of the marrow mixture, may be a promising approach for bone marrow or stem cell transplantation (104). The initial results from this novel approach indicate that ex vivo CTLA4Ig treatment permits the engraftment of histoincompatible marrow and that this therapy may ameliorate the severity of the expected GVHD.

Ectopic or aberrant expression of B7 can lead to loss of self-tolerance and to autoimmune disorders in mice (105). The ability of CTLA4Ig and anti-B7 antibodies to inhibit T-cell–dependent antibody responses suggested that these reagents might be an effective treatment for autoimmune diseases in which pathogenic effects are at least partly due to T-cell–dependent antibodies. This has been borne out by initial studies on the use of CD28 blockade for autoimmune disease in a variety of rodent models (see Table 28-2). In humans, the potential role of CTLA4Ig in psoriasis was recently reported (106). Forty-three patients were treated in a 26-week, phase I, open-label dose-escalation study. Forty-six percent of all study patients achieved 50% or greater sustained improvements in clinical disease activity, with progressively greater effects observed in the highest-dosing cohorts. Striking improvements in cutaneous lesions were observed in some patients (Fig. 28-6). Improvement in these patients was associated with quantitative reduction in epidermal hyperplasia, which correlated with quantitative reduction in skin-infiltrating T

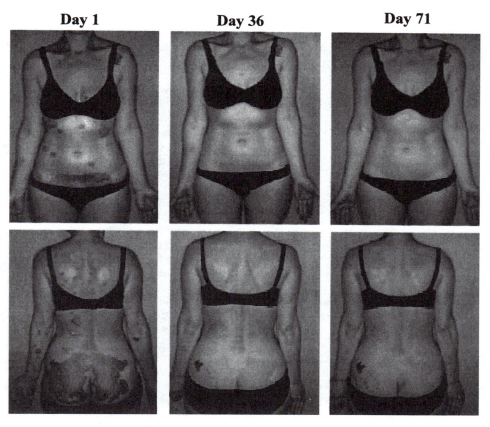

Figure 28-6. Effect of CTLA4Ig therapy on psoriasis. Serial photographs of a patient obtained at baseline, day 36, and day 71. CTLA4Ig was administered as a 1-hour intravenous infusion starting on day 1, and repeated on days 3, 16, and 19 at 50mg/kg as previously described (106). (Photographs courtesy of Susan Kelley, M.D., Bristol-Myers Squibb and Sewon Kang, M.D., University of Michigan.)

cells. CTLA4Ig therapy diminished the antibody responses to T-cell–dependent neoantigens in this study, but immunologic tolerance to these antigens was not demonstrated. Bristol-Myers Squibb is continuing to test CTLA4Ig for autoimmune disorders, and currently has an ongoing trial in patients with rheumatoid arthritis (M. Stewart and J. C. Becker, Bristol-Myers Squibb, personal communication).

The results from many studies that are now available indicate that blocking of B7:CD28-dependent T-cell costimulation leads to substantial prolongation of transplant survival, and that in many instances donor-specific tolerance is achieved. There are several areas that future research will likely address. First, the optimal schedule of administration of costimulation blockade needs to be further resolved. In many studies, CTLA4Ig is most effective if its administration is delayed until after transplantation (107). This may reflect the fact that cycling T cells are more susceptible to the absence of costimulatory signals than resting T cells. Second, the effectiveness of CTLA4Ig is limited by its relatively rapid off-rate from B7. It is likely that second-generation compounds or monoclonal antibodies can

be engineered that will have longer dwell times. Third, the most effective reagent will be one that selectively binds to CD28 and prevents CD28 signal transduction, because CTLA4Ig or anti-B7 reagents prevent the delivery of both CD28 and CTLA-4 signals. Recent studies indicate that CTLA-4 function may be required for the induction of tolerance (108). Fourth, it is likely that combination therapies that block alternative costimulatory pathways will be most effective (109). Recently, the CD40:CD40 ligand pathway, initially described as having a role in B-cell activation, has been recognized as a key pathway for T-cell activation as well. Prolonged mismatched renal allograft acceptance in primates is possible with anti-CD40L and CTLA4Ig therapy (110,111).

CD28 Pathway Augmentation

It is likely that some pathogens have evolved strategies to escape or delay immune elimination by decreasing costimulation. Simi-

Table 28-3. Reagents in Development for Augmentation of CD28 Costimulation

Reagent	Reference(s)
Anti-CD28 antibodies	(112,114)
Anti-CTLA-4 monoclonal antibodies	(131)
Bispecific anti-CD28 antibody conjugates	(115,116)
Anti-CD28 single chain Fv (scFv) antibodies	(118,122,167)
B7-modified tumor cells	(124)
B7Ig fusion protein	(134,135)
DNA vaccines using B7 cDNA	(168,169)
Recombinant viruses expressing B7	(127)

larly, many tumors are poorly immunogenic because they do not express B7 molecules. Tumors that lack costimulatory ligands may be ignored by the immune system or may be poor stimulators of immune effector cells. Therefore, the immunogenicity of pathogens and tumors could be increased by augmentation of costimulatory signals. Three general approaches are being used to increase costimulation: 1) systemic administration of reagents that activate CD28 or limit CTLA-4 signaling, 2) genetic modification of tumor cells and pathogens to express B7, and 3) vaccination with cDNA or recombinant viruses that express B7 (Fig. 28-7). Therefore, a variety of reagents are being developed for therapeutic augmentation of CD28 costimulation (Table 28-3).

The most direct method of enhancing costimulation would be to coinject antigen:MHC complexes with a CD28 ligand or with a small-molecule compound that activates CD28 signal transduction. Another technically less demanding approach has been to inject CD28 antibodies alone. Some CD28 antibodies stimulate T-cell proliferation directly, without a requirement for a TCR signal (112–114). The reason why only a subset of antibodies are directly mitogenic has not yet been fully explained and does not appear to be attributable simply to binding site differences, because some CD28 antibodies that cross-block each other

display direct activating properties while others exhibit the more typical costimulatory functional activity. As shown in Table 28-4, a variety of functional effects have been reported in rodents following injection of CD28 antibodies. The mechanisms behind these effects probably are complex and relate in part to distinct functional effects of the antibodies. In some systems, the effects of intact and fab fragments of CD28 antibodies are similar, implying that both forms of antibody interfere with the delivery of B7:CD28 signals. It is also likely that, depending on the experimental model, some antibodies are agonistic in vivo and others are inhibitory or have partial agonist properties. This would be expected from the observations that CD28 signaling functions optimally when coligated with the TCR; thus, CD28 antibody in the absence of antigen stimulation may have antagonistic effects. In triple knockout mice that lack B7-1, B7-2, and CTLA-4, injection of anti-CD28 causes marked T-cell proliferation, but wild type mice are unaffected by the same treatment (44). This suggests in some cases that the inhibitory effects of CTLA-4 are preventing the agonistic effects of anti-CD28.

Another approach currently being tested for cancer immunotherapy is to target CD28 ligands to tumor cells with bispecific anti-CD28 antitumor mAb conjugates (115,116). These experiments showed that T-cell cytotoxic activity is enhanced by ligation of CD28, in agreement with results following B7-1 transfection into a cytotoxic T-cell tumor target (117). More recently, the approach has been refined with the construction of bispecific single chain Fv (scFv) molecules specific for the CD28 receptor and a tumor antigen that are capable of binding and generating costimulatory signals to activate T cells (118,119). ScFv molecules represent the smallest functional fragments of an Ab that maintain the complete specificity of the entire Ab. They are heterodimers composed of V_H and V_L domains bound together and stabilized by a flexible peptide linker. These constructs have been used to express a CD28-specific scFv in tumor cells with a transmembrane domain and cytoplasmic tail from CD80. In a related approach, minigenes were created that encode a scFv specific for a tumor antigen fused to CD80 or CD86 ligands to deliver CD80 or CD86 to the tumor cell. The recombinant mol-

Table 28-4. Summary of Results in Rodents Following In Vivo Injection of CD28 Antibodies

Effect Following Anti-CD28 Injection	Reference
Increased the number of single positive T cells in the thymus and led to enlargement of peripheral lymphoid organs with expansion of B cells in mice.	(170)
Prevented superantigen-mediated septic shock in mice.	(171)
Induced proliferation of most CD4 T cells and, indirectly, of B cells in rats.	(114)
Prolonged cardiac allograft survival in rats.	(172)
CD28 antibody fab fragments prevented experimental autoimmune encephalomyelitis in mice.	(173)
Prevented insulitis and protected onset of diabetes in NOD female mice.	(174)
Intact and fab fragments of anti-CD28 antibody blocked bacterial superantigen-induced proliferation of T cells in mice.	(175)
Induced T-cell proliferation in vivo in mice lacking CTLA-4, B7-1, and B7-2, but not in wild type mice.	(44)

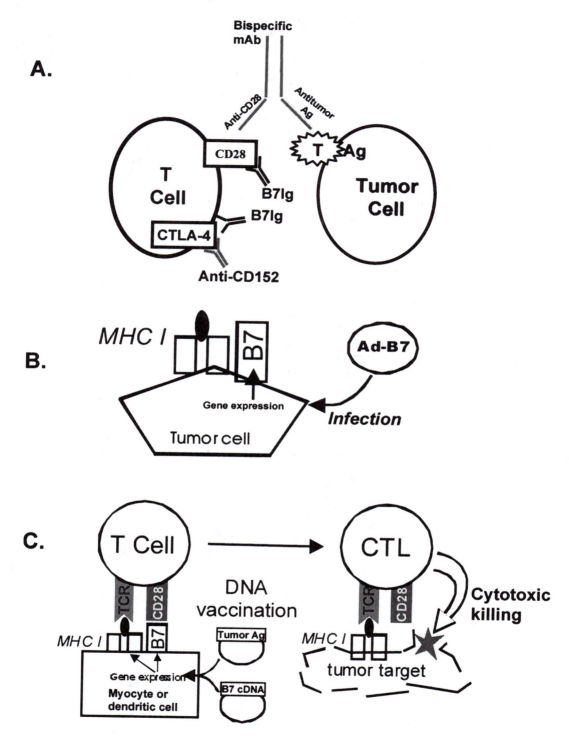

Figure 28-7. Three general in vivo approaches to augmentation costimulation. (*A*) Systemic administration of reagents that promote CD28 signaling or limit CTLA-4 signaling. (*B*) Genetic modification of tumor cells to express B7 with recombinant adenovirus. (*C*) Vaccination with cDNA to express B7 and tumor antigens. (B7Ig = B7-IgG fusion protein; Ad-B7 = adenovirus B7).

ecules have been tested as soluble bispecific constructs or transduced into tumors as approaches to generating costimulatory effects resulting in T-cell activation (118,120,121). ScFv chimeric receptors, or T-bodies, have also been introduced into T cells with intracellular sequences comprising the cytosolic domain of CD28 (122). In some models, antitumor effects may be improved by engineering the cytosolic domain to encode intracellular sequences for CD28 in tandem with the zeta chain from the TCR complex (123). To date, there is limited clinical experience with these engineered costimulatory antibody reagents. In settings in which multiple administration will be required, the antibodies will require humanization in order to limit neutralizing antibody responses. Even then, it is possible that anti-idiotype responses will still limit the eventual utility of this approach.

Tumors engineered to express B7 are being studied as potential vaccines by several groups (124–127). Ectopic B7-1 expression on murine tumors induced recognition and rejection by host T cells. Even tumors at remote sites that do not express CD80 or CD86 can be destroyed, demonstrating that initiation of the immune response may be dependent on CD28 activation, whereas the effector phase is not. Tumor destruction initiated by immunization with CD80- or CD86-positive tumor cells is dependent on CD8$^+$ CTL activation, although CD4 helper T cells can also play a role in some tumor models. In one study, expression of an antigen on the tumor cells that T cells were capable of recognizing was required for tumor rejection (128), so that forms of gene therapy using B7-modified tumor may be effective for only the subset of human tumors that are antigenic.

CTLA-4 blockade enhances T-cell responses in vivo. One strategy for improving tumor gene therapy with CD80 or CD86 is to inject anti-CTLA-4 mAb to block the CTLA-4 receptor and thus shift the balance toward the CD28 activation. In mice, injection of anti-CTLA-4 antibody increases T-cell proliferation and cytokine release that is provoked by staphylococcal enterotoxin B (129). Autoreactivity is also enhanced because a nonlethal and spontaneously resolving form of experimental allergic encephalomyelitis can be converted to a lethal illness by the administration of a single injection of anti-CTLA-4 antibody (130). Allison and colleagues have demonstrated that prophylactic and therapeutic antitumor immunotherapy is possible in several types of rodent tumors that previously were refractory to other forms of immunotherapy (131,132). CTLA-4 antibody therapy appears to enhance anti-tumor immunity by an effect distinct from preventing the induction of tolerance to tumor antigens (133).

O'Toole and coworkers have tested B7Ig, a fusion protein comprised of the extracellular domains of B7-1 or B7-2 fused with immunoglobulin (Ig) Fc domains (134,135). Similar antitumor effects were observed following the injection of either B7-1Ig or B7-2Ig, and the therapeutic effects were equivalent to those reported with anti-CTLA-4 antibodies. It is surprising that B7Ig appears to have adjuvant efficacy similar to that of anti-CTLA-4 antibody. This is a paradox, because B7Ig should transmit both positive and negative signals through CD28 and CTLA-4, while anti-CTLA-4 administration presumably acts by preventing the generation of inhibitory signals through B7:CTLA-4. The latter notion is supported by the fact that both intact and fab fragments of anti-CTLA-4 have similar in vivo activity in most models. Human testing of these new forms of tumor immunotherapy using anti-CTLA-4 or B7Ig is imminent.

Summary

The results from many animal models demonstrate a variety of promising therapeutic applications of costimulation blockade or augmentation. Several approaches have already reached the clinic (Table 28-5). Results from early clinical trials already show that CTLA4Ig blockade has little apparent toxicity and may exhibit substantial clinical activity in transplantation and autoimmune diseases. Upcoming clinical trials are awaited to determine the potential clinical utility of costimulation for augmentation of tumor immunotherapy.

Modulation of the immune response by regulation of costimulation promises to increase the specificity of therapy for autoimmune disease, transplantation, and cancer, resulting in lower toxicity and increased effectiveness. It is likely that second

Table 28-5. Examples of Ongoing or Completed Clinical Trials of CD28 Pathway Reagents

Disease	Status	Approach	Location (Reference)
Hematologica malignancy	Phase I	Ex vivo use of CTLA4Ig for prevention of graft-versus-host disease.	Boston, MA (104)
Psoriasis, rheumatoid arthritis	Phase I/II	Systemic CTLA4Ig (BMS-188667).	Bristol-Myers Squibb (106)
Metastatic colon cancer	Phase I	ALVAC CEA-B7 Canarypox virus vaccine	Bronx, NY; Philadelphia, Bethesda (176)
Metastatic ovarian carcinoma	Phase I	Adoptive autologous immunotherapy with bispecific anti-CD3/28-coated T cells.	Milan (177)
Glioblastoma	Phase I	Gene therapy with adenovirus–mediated B7 infection of tumor cells.	Philadelphia (Eck et al, unpublished)

generation costimulation reagents will be developed that display increased potency. Determination of the ultimate clinical utility of these reagents will require further research and development. Concerns about cost of therapy should eventually be overcome as costimulation therapy achieves long-lasting effects such as transplantation tolerance or tumor immunity.

References

1. Bretscher P, Cohn M. A theory of self-nonself discrimination. Science 1970;169(950):1042–1049.
2. Hansen JA, Martin PJ, Nowinski RC. Monoclonal antibodies identifying a novel T-cell antigen and Ia antigens of human lymphocytes. Immunogenetics 1980;10:247–260.
3. McMichael AJ, Gotch F. T-cell antigens: new and previously defined clusters. In: McMichael AJ, ed. Leukocyte Typing III. London: Oxford University Press, 1987:33–62.
4. Damle NK, Hansen JA, Good RA, Gupta S. Monoclonal antibody analysis of human T lymphocyte subpopulations exhibiting autologous mixed lymphocyte reaction. Proc Natl Acad Sci USA 1981;78:5096–5098.
5. Hara T, Fu SM, Hansen JA. Human T cell activation. II. A new activation pathway used by a major T cell population via a disulfide-bonded dimer of a 44 kilodalton polypeptide (9.3 antigen). J Exp Med 1985;161:1513–1524.
6. Ledbetter JA, Martin PJ, Spooner CE, et al. Antibodies to Tp67 and Tp44 augment and sustain proliferative responses of activated T cells. J Immunol 1985;135:2331–2336.
7. Weiss A, Manger B, Imboden J. Synergy between the T3/antigen receptor complex and Tp44 in the activation of human T cells. J Immunol 1986;137:819–825.
8. Damle NK, Doyle LV, Grosmaire LS, Ledbetter JA. Differential regulatory signals delivered by antibody binding to the CD28 (Tp44) molecule during the activation of human T lymphocytes. J Immunol 1988;40:1753–1761.
9. Ledbetter JA, Imboden JB, Schieven GL, et al. CD28 ligation in T-cell activation: evidence for two signal transduction pathways. Blood 1990;75:1531–1539.
10. Martin PJ, Ledbetter JA, Morishita Y, et al. A 44 kilodalton cell surface homodimer regulates interleukin 2 production by activated human T lymphocytes. J Immunol 1986;136:3282–3287.
11. Lindsten T, June CH, Ledbetter JA, et al. Regulation of lymphokine messenger RNA stability by a surface-mediated T cell activation pathway. Science 1989;244:9333–9343.
12. Damle NK, Mohagheghpour N, Hansen JA, Engleman EG. Alloantigen-specific cytotoxic and suppressor T lymphocytes are derived from phenotypically distinct precursors. J Immunol 1983;131:2296–2300.
13. Lum LG, Orcutt-Thordarson N, Seigneuret MC, Hansen JA. In vitro regulation of immunoglobulin synthesis by T-cell subpopulations defined by a new human T-cell antigen (9.3). Cell Immunol 1982;72:122–129.
14. Liu Z, Tugulea S, Cortesini R, Suciu-Foca N. Specific suppression of T helper alloreactivity by allo-MHC class I-restricted CD8+CD28– T Cells. Int Immunol 1998;10(6):775–783.
15. Morishita Y, Sao H, Hansen JA, Martin PJ. A distinct subset of human CD4+ cells with a limited alloreactive T cell receptor repertoire. J Immunol 1989;143:2783–2789.
16. Yamada H, Martin PJ, Bean MA, et al. Monoclonal antibody 9.3 and anti-CD11 antibodies define reciprocal subsets of lymphocytes. Eur J Immunol 1985;15:164–168.
17. Liu Z, Tugulea S, Cortesini R, et al. Inhibition of CD40 signaling pathway in antigen presenting cells by T suppressor cells. Hum Immunol 1999;60(7):568–574.
18. Weyand CM, Brandes JC, Schmidt D, et al. Functional properties of CD4+ CD28– T cells in the aging immune system. Mech Ageing Dev 1998;102(2–3):131–147.
19. Effros RB. Loss of CD28 expression on T lymphocytes: a marker of replicative senescence. Dev Comp Immunol 1997;21(6):471–478.
20. Vallejo AN, Brandes JC, Weyand CM, Goronzy JJ. Modulation of CD28 expression: distinct regulatory pathways during activation and replicative senescence. J Immunol 1999;162(11):6572–6579.
21. Linsley PS, Bradshaw J, Urnes M, et al. CD28 engagement by B7/BB-1 induces transient down-regulation of CD28 synthesis and prolonged unresponsiveness to CD28 signaling. J Immunol 1993;150:3161–3169.
22. Vallejo AN, Nestel AR, Schirmer M, et al. Aging-related deficiency of CD28 expression in CD4+ T cells is associated with the loss of gene-specific nuclear factor binding activity. J Biol Chem 1998;273(14):8119–8129.
23. Linsley PS, Clark EA, Ledbetter JA. T-cell antigen CD28 mediates adhesion with B cells by interacting with activation antigen B7/BB-1. Proc Natl Acad Sci USA 1990;87:5031–5035.
24. Linsley PS, Brady W, Grosmaire L, et al. Binding of the B cell activation antigen B7 to CD28 costimulates T cell proliferation and interleukin 2 mRNA accumulation. J Exp Med 1991;173:7217–7230.
25. Freeman GJ, Freedman AS, Segil JM, et al. B7, a new member of the Ig superfamily with unique expression on activated and neoplastic B cells. J Immunol 1989;143:2714–2722.
26. Henry J, Miller MM, Pontarotti P. Structure and evolution of the extended B7 family. Immunol Today 1999;20(6):2852–2888.
27. Nabavi N, Freeman GJ, Gault A, et al. Signaling through the MHC class II cytoplasmic domain is required for antigen presentation and induces B7 expression. Nature 1992;360:266–268.
28. Ranheim EA, Kipps TJ. Activated T cells induce expression of B7/BB1 on normal or leukemic B cells through a CD40-dependent signal. J Exp Med 1993;177(4):925–935.
29. Watts TH, Alaverdi N, Wade WF, Linsley PS. Induction of costimulatory molecule B7 in M12 B lymphomas by cAMP or MHC-restricted T cell interaction. J Immunol 1993;150(6):2192–2202.
30. Swallow MM, Wallin JJ, Sha WC. B7h, a novel costimulatory homolog of B7.1 and B7.2, is induced by TNFα Immunity 1999;11:423–432.
31. Kozbor D, Moretta A, Messner HA, et al. Tp44 molecules involved in antigen-independent T cell activation are expressed on human plasma cells. J Immunol 1987;138:4128–4132.
32. Pellat Deceunynck C, Bataille R, Robillard N, et al. Expression of CD28 and CD40 in human myeloma cells: A comparative study with normal plasma cells. Blood 1994;84:2597–2603.

33. Woerly G, Roger N, Loiseau S, et al. Expression of CD28 and CD86 by human eosinophils and role in the secretion of type 1 cytokines (interleukin 2 and interferon gamma): inhibition by immunoglobulin A complexes. J Exp Med 1999;190(4):487–495.

34. Ling V, Munroe RC, Murphy EA, Gray GS. Embryonic stem cells and embryoid bodies express lymphocyte costimulatory molecules. Exp Cell Res 1998;241(1):55–65.

35. Harper K, Balzano C, Rouvier E, et al. CTLA-4 and CD28 activated lymphocyte molecules are closely related in both mouse and human as to sequence, message expression, gene structure, and chromosomal location. J Immunol 1991; 147:1037–1044.

36. Buonavista N, Balzano C, Pontarotti P, et al. Molecular linkage of the human CTLA-4 and CD28 Ig-superfamily genes in yeast artificial chromosomes. Genomics 1992; 13:856–861.

37. Linsley PS, Brady W, Urnes M, et al. CTLA-4 is a second receptor for the B cell activation antigen B7. J Exp Med 1991;174:561–569.

38. Freeman GJ, Borriello F, Hodes RJ, et al. Uncovering of functional alternative CTLA-4 counter-receptor in B7-deficient mice. Science 1993;262:907–909.

39. Freeman GJ, Borriello F, Hodes RJ, et al. Murine B7-2, an alternative CTLA-4 counter-receptor that costimulates T cell proliferation and interleukin-2 production. J Exp Med 1993;178:2185–2192.

40. Linsley PS, Greene JL, Brady W, et al. Human B7-1 (CD80) and B7-2 (CD86) bind with similar avidities but distinct kinetics to CD28 and CTLA-4 receptors. Immunity 1994;1:793–801.

41. Waterhouse P, Penninger JM, Timms E, et al. CTLA-4 deficiency causes lymphoproliferative disorder with early lethality. Science 1995;270:985–988.

42. Tivol EA, Borriello F, Schweitzer AN, et al. Loss of CTLA-4 leads to massive lymphoproliferation and fatal multiorgan tissue destruction, revealing a critical negative regulatory role of CTLA-4. Immunity 1995;3(5):541–547.

43. Chambers CA, Sullivan TJ, Allison JP. Lymphoproliferation in CTLA-4-deficient mice is mediated by costimulation-dependent activation of CD4+ T cells. Immunity 1997;7(6):885–895.

44. Mandelbrot DA, McAdam AJ, Sharpe AH. B7-1 or B7-2 is required to produce the lymphoproliferative phenotype in mice lacking cytotoxic T lymphocyte-associated antigen 4 (CTLA-4). J Exp Med 1999;189(2):435–440.

45. Bachmann MF, Kohler G, Ecabert B, et al. Cutting edge: lymphoproliferative disease in the absence of CTLA-4 is not T cell autonomous. J Immunol 1999;163(3):1128–1131.

46. Chen W, Jin W, Wahl SM. Engagement of cytotoxic T lymphocyte-associated antigen 4 (CTLA-4) induces transforming growth factor beta (TGF-beta) production by murine CD4(+) T cells. J Exp Med 1998;188(10):1849–1857.

47. Shull MM, Ormsby I, Kier AB, et al. Targeted disruption of the mouse transforming growth factor-beta 1 gene results in multifocal inflammatory disease. Nature 1992;359(6397):693–699.

48. Kulkarni AB, Huh CG, Becker D, et al. Transforming growth factor beta 1 null mutation in mice causes excessive inflammatory response and early death. Proc Natl Acad Sci USA 1993;90(2):770–774.

49. Hutloff A, Dittrich AM, Beier KC, et al. ICOS is an inducible T-cell co-stimulator structurally and functionally related to CD28. Nature 1999;397(6716);263–266.

50. Thompson CB, Lindsten T, Ledbetter JA, et al. CD28 activation pathway regulates the production of multiple T-cell-derived lymphokines/cytokines. Proc Natl Acad Sci USA 1989;86:1333–1337.

51. Moretta A, Pantaleo G, Lopez-Botet M, Moretta L. Involvement of T44 molecules in an antigen-independent pathway of T cell activation. Analysis of the correlations to the T cell antigen-receptor complex. J Exp Med 1985;162:823–838.

52. Gmünder H, Lesslauer W. A 45-kDa human T-cell membrane glycoprotein functions in the regulation of cell proliferative responses. Eur J Biochem 1984;142:153–160.

53. June CH, Ledbetter JA, Gillespie MM, et al. T-cell proliferation involving the CD28 pathway is associated with cyclosporine-resistant interleukin 2 gene expression. Mol Cell Biol 1987;7:4472–4481.

54. Bierer BE, Hollander G, Fruman D, Burakoff SJ. Cyclosporin A and FK506: molecular mechanisms of immunosuppression and probes for transplantation biology. Curr Opin Immunol 1993;5:763–773.

55. Ledbetter JA, Parsons M, Martin PJ, et al. Antibody binding to CD5 (Tp67) and Tp44 T cell surface molecules: effects on cyclic nucleotides, cytoplasmic free calcium, and cAMP-mediated suppression. J Immunol 1986;137:3299–3305.

56. Cerdan C, Razanajaona D, Martin Y, et al. Contributions of the CD2 and CD28 T lymphocyte activation pathways to the regulation of the expression of the colony-stimulating factor (CSF-1) gene. J Immunol 1992;149:373–379.

57. van Lier RA, Brouwer M, Aarden LA. Signals involved in T cell activation. T cell proliferation induced through the synergistic action of anti-CD28 and anti-CD2 monoclonal antibodies. Eur J Immunol 1988;18:167–172.

58. June CH, Ledbetter JA, Lindsten T, Thompson CB. Evidence for the involvement of three distinct signals in the induction of IL-2 gene expression in human T lymphocytes. J Immunol 1989;143:153–161.

59. June CH, Ledbetter JA, Linsley PS, Thompson CB. Role of the CD28 receptor in T-cell activation. Immunol Today 1990;11:211–216.

60. Vandenberghe P, Freeman GJ, Nadler LM, et al. Antibody and B7/BB1-mediated ligation of the CD28 receptor induces tyrosine phosphorylation in human T cells. J Exp Med 1992;175:951–960.

61. Ledbetter JA, Linsley PS. CD28 receptor crosslinking induces tyrosine phosphorylation of PLCgamma$_1$. Adv Exp Med Biol 1992;323:23–27.

62. Linsley PS, Nadler SG, Bajorath J, et al. Binding stoichiometry of the cytotoxic T lymphocyte-associated molecule-4 (CTLA-4). A disulfide-linked homodimer binds two CD86 molecules. J Biol Chem 1995;270(25):15417–15424.

63. Greene JL, Leytze GM, Emswiler J, et al. Covalent dimerization of CD28/CTLA-4 and oligomerization of CD80/CD86 regulate T cell costimulatory interactions. J Biol Chem 1996;271(43):26762–26771.

64. August A, Dupont B. Activation of src family kinase lck following CD28 crosslinking in the Jurkat leukemic cell line. Biochem Biophys Res Commun 1994;199:1466–1473.

65. Klasen S, Pages F, Peyron JF, et al. Two distinct regions of the CD28 intracytoplasmic domain are involved in the tyro-

sine phosphorylation of Vav and GTPase activating protein-associated p62 protein. Int Immunol 1998;10(4):481–489.

66. Pages F, Ragueneau M, Rottapel R, et al. Binding of phosphatidylinositol-3-OH kinase to CD28 is required for T-cell signaling. Nature 1994;369:327–329.

67. Prasad KV, Cai YC, Raab M, et al. T-cell antigen CD28 interacts with the lipid kinase phosphatidylinositol 3-kinase by a cytoplasmic Tyr(P)-Met-Xaa-Met motif. Proc Natl Acad Sci USA 1994;91(7):2834–2838.

68. Hutchcroft JE, Bierer BE. Signaling through CD28/CTLA-4 family receptors: puzzling participation of phosphatidyl-inositol-3 kinase. J Immunol 1996;156(11):4071–4074.

69. Verweij CL, Geerts M, Aarden LA. Activation of inter-leukin-2 gene transcription via the T-cell surface molecule CD28 is mediated through an NF-kB-like response element. J Biol Chem 1991;266:14179–14182.

70. Ghosh P, Tan TH, Rice NR, et al. The interleukin 2 CD28-responsive complex contains at least three members of the NF kappa B family: c-Rel, p50, and p65. Proc Natl Acad Sci USA 1993;90:1696–1700.

71. Fraser JD, Irving BA, Crabtree GR, Weiss A. Regulation of interleukin-2 gene enhancer activity by the T cell accessory molecule CD28. Science 1991;251:313–316.

72. Harhaj EW, Sun SC. IkappaB kinases serve as a target of CD28 signaling. J Biol Chem 1998;273(39):25185–25190.

73. Sadra A, Cinek T, Arellano JL, et al. Identification of tyro-sine phosphorylation sites in the CD28 cytoplasmic domain and their role in the costimulation of Jurkat T cells. J Immunol 1999;162(4):1966–1973.

74. Finn PW, He H, Wang Y, et al. Synergistic induction of CTLA-4 expression by costimulation with TCR plus CD28 signals mediated by increased transcription and mes-senger ribonucleic acid stability. J Immunol 1997;158(9):4074–4081.

75. Johnson-Leger C, Christensen J, Klaus GG. CD28 co-stim-ulation stabilizes the expression of the CD40 ligand on T cells. Int Immunol 1998;10(8):1083–1091

76. Su B, Jacinto E, Hibi M, et al. JNK is involved in signal inte-gration during costimulation of T lymphocytes. Cell 1994;77:727–736.

77. Chen CY, Gatto-Konczak F, Wu Z, Karin M. Stabilization of interleukin-2 mRNA by the c-Jun NH2-terminal kinase pathway. Science 1998;280(5371):1945–1949.

78. Li L, Yee C, Beavo JA. CD3- and CD28-dependent induc-tion of PDE7 required for T cell activation. Science 1999;283(5403):848–851.

79. August A, Gibson S, Kawakami Y, et al. CD28 is associated with and induces the immediate tyrosine phosphorylation and activation of the Tec family kinase ITK/EMT in the human Jurkat leukemic T-cell line. Proc Natl Acad Sci USA 1994;91:9347–9351.

80. Liao XC, Fournier S, Killeen N, et al. Itk negatively regulates induction of T cell proliferation by CD28 costimulation. J Exp Med 1997;186(2):221–228.

81. Yang WC, Ghiotto M, Barbarat B, Olive D. The role of Tec protein-tyrosine kinase in T cell signaling. J Biol Chem 1999;274(2):607–617.

82. June CH, Bluestone JA, Nadler LM, Thompson CB. The B7 and CD28 receptor families. Immunol Today 1994;15:321–331.

83. Rudd CE. Upstream-downstream: CD28 cosignaling pathways and T cell function. Immunity 1996;4(6):527–534.

84. Viola A, Lanzavecchia A. T cell activation determined by T cell receptor number and tunable thresholds. Science 1996;273(5271):104–106.

85. Wulfing C, Davis MM. A receptor/cytoskeletal movement triggered by costimulation during T cell activation. Science 1998;282(5397):2266–2269.

86. Viola A, Schroeder S, Sakakibara Y, Lanzavecchia A. T lymphocyte costimulation mediated by reorganization of membrane microdomains. Science 1999;283(5402):680–682.

87. Berridge MJ. Lymphocyte activation in health and disease. Crit Rev Immunol 1997;17(2):155–178.

88. Walunas TL, Lenschow DJ, Bakker CY, et al. CTLA-4 can function as a negative regulator of T cell activation. Immunity 1994;1(5):405–413.

89. Nakaseko C, Miyatake S, Iida T, et al. Cytotoxic T lympho-cyte antigen 4 (CTLA-4) engagement delivers an inhibitory signal through the membrane-proximal region in the absence of the tyrosine motif in the cytoplasmic tail. J Exp Med 1999;190:765–774.

90. Lee KM, Chuang E, Griffin M, et al. Molecular basis of T cell inactivation by CTLA-4. Science 1998;282(5397):2263–2266.

91 Marengere LE, Waterhouse P, Duncan GS, et al. Regulation of T cell receptor signaling by tyrosine phosphatase SYP association with CTLA-4. Science 1996;272(5265):1170–1173.

92. Chuang E, Lee KM, Robbins MD, et al. Regulation of cyto-toxic T lymphocyte-associated molecule-4 by Src kinases. J Immunol 1999;162(3):1270–1277.

93. Nishikawa K, Linsley PS, Collins AB, et al. Effect of CTLA-4 chimeric protein on rat autoimmune anti-glomerular basement membrane glomerulonephritis. Eur J Immunol 1994;24:1249–1254.

94. Finck BK, Linsley PS, Wofsy D. Treatment of murine lupus with CTLA4Ig. Science 1994;265:1225–1227.

95. Wallace PM, Johnson JS, MacMaster JF, et al. CTLA4Ig treatment ameliorates the lethality of murine graft-versus-host disease across major histocompatibility complex barriers. Transplantation 1994;58:602–610.

96. Turka LA, Linsley PS, Lin H, et al. T-cell activation by the CD28 ligand B7 is required for cardiac allograft rejection in vivo. Proc Natl Acad Sci USA 1992;89:11102–11105.

97. Lin H, Bolling SF, Linsley PS, et al. Long-term acceptance of major histocompatibility complex mismatched cardiac allografts induced by CTLA4Ig plus donor-specific transfu-sion. J Exp Med 1993;178:1801–1806.

98. Pearson TC, Alexander DZ, Winn KJ, et al. Transplantation tolerance induced by CTLA4Ig. Transplantation 1994;57:1701–1706.

99. Lenschow DJ, Zeng Y, Thistlethwaite JR, et al. Long-term survival of xenogeneic pancreatic islet grafts induced by CTLA4Ig. Science 1992;257:789–792.

100. Kirk AD, Harlan DM, Armstrong NN, et al. CTLA4Ig and anti-CD40 ligand prevent renal allograft rejection in primates. Proc Natl Acad Sci USA 1997;94(16):8789–8794.

101. Levisetti MG, Padrid PA, Szot GL, et al. Immunosuppres-sive effects of human CTLA4Ig in a non-human primate model of allogeneic pancreatic islet transplantation. J Immunol 1997;159(11):5187–5191.

102. Woodward JE, Bayer AL, Chavin KD, et al. T-cell alter-ations in cardiac allograft recipients after B7 (CD80 and CD86) blockade. Transplantation 1998;66(1):14–20.

103. Lenschow DJ, Zeng Y, Hathcock KS, et al. Inhibition of transplant rejection following treatment with anti-B7-2 and anti-B7-1 antibodies. Transplantation 1995;60(10): 1171–1178.

104. Guinan EC, Boussiotis VA, Neuberg D, et al. Transplantation of anergic histoincompatible bone marrow allografts. N Engl J Med 1999;340(22):1704–1714.

105. Harlan DM, Hengartner H, Huang ML, et al. Mice expressing both B7-1 and viral glycoprotein on pancreatic beta cells along with glycoprotein-specfic transgenic T cells develop diabetes due to a breakdown of T-lymphocyte unresponsiveness. Proc Natl Acad Sci USA 1994;91:3137–3141.

106. Abrams JR, Lebwohl MG, Guzzo CA, et al. CTLA4Ig-mediated blockade of T-cell costimulation in patients with psoriasis vulgaris. J Clin Invest 1999;103(9):1243–1252.

107. Sayegh MH, Akalin E, Hancock WW, et al. CD28-B7 blockade after alloantigenic challenge in vivo inhibits Th1 cytokines but spares Th2. J Exp Med 1995;181:1869–1874.

108. Perez VL, Van Parijs L, Biuckians A, et al. Induction of peripheral T cell tolerance in vivo requires CTLA-4 engagement. Immunity 1997;6(4):411–417.

109. Watts TH, DeBenedette MA, T cell co-stimulatory molecules other than CD28. Curr Opin Immunol 1999; 11(3):286–293.

110. Kirk AD, Burkly LC, Batty DS, et al. Treatment with humanized monoclonal antibody against CD154 prevents acute renal allograft rejection in nonhuman primates. Nat Med 1999;5(6):686–693.

111. Kirk AD, Harlan DM, Armstrong NN, et al. CTLA4Ig and anti-CD40 ligand prevent renal allograft rejection in primates. Proc Natl Acad Sci USA 1997;94(16): 8789–8794.

112. Nunes J, Klasen S, Franco MD, et al. Signaling through CD28 T-cell activation pathway involves an inositol phospholipid-specific phospholipase C activity. Biochem J 1993;293:835–842.

113. Siefken R, Kurrle R, Schwinzer R. CD28-mediated activation of resting human T cells without costimulation of the CD3/TCR complex. Cell Immunol 1997;176(1):59–65.

114. Tacke M, Hanke G, Hanke T, Hunig T. CD28-mediated induction of proliferation in resting T cells in vitro and in vivo without engagement of the T cell receptor: evidence for functionally distinct forms of CD28. Eur J Immunol 1997;27(1):239–247.

115. Jung G, Ledbetter JA, Muller-Eberhard HJ. Induction of cytotoxicity in resting human T lymphocytes bound to tumor cells by antibody heteroconjugates. Proc Natl Acad Sci USA 1987;84:4611–4615.

116. Renner C, Jung W, Sahin U, et al. Cure of xenografted human tumors by bispecific monoclonal antibodies and human T cells. Science 1994;264:833–835.

117. Azuma M, Cayabyab M, Phillips JH, Lanier LL. Requirements for CD28-dependent T cell-mediated cytotoxicity. J Immunol 1993;150:2091–2101.

118. Hayden MS, Grosmaire LS, Norris NA, et al. Costimulation by CD28 sFv expressed on the tumor cell surface or as a soluble bispecific molecule targeted to the L6 carcinoma antigen. Tissue Antigens 1996;48(4 Pt 1):242–254.

119. Gerstmayer B, Altenschmidt U, Hoffmann M, Wels W. Costimulation of T cell proliferation by a chimeric B7-2 antibody fusion protein specifically targeted to cells expressing the erbB2 proto-oncogene. J Immunol 1997; 158(10):4584–4590.

120. Guo YJ, Che XY, Shen F, et al. Effective tumor vaccines generated by in vitro modification of tumor cells with cytokines and bispecific monoclonal antibodies. Nat Med 1997;3(4):451–455.

121. Holliger P, Manzke O, Span M, et al. Carcinoembryonic antigen (CEA)-specific T-cell activation in colon carcinoma induced by anti-CD3 x anti-CEA bispecific diabodies and B7 x anti-CEA bispecific fusion proteins. Cancer Res 1999;59(12):2909–2916.

122. Krause A, Guo HF, Latouche JB, et al. Antigen-dependent CD28 signaling selectively enhances survival and proliferation in genetically modified activated human primary T lymphocytes. J Exp Med 1998;188(4):619–626.

123. Finney H, Lawson A, Bebbington C, Weir A. Chimeric receptors providing both primary and costimulatory signaling in T cells from a single gene product. Personal communication, 1998.

124. Chen L, Ashe S, Brady WA, Hellstrom I, et al. Costimulation of antitumor immunity by the B7 counterreceptor for the T lymphocyte molecules CD28 and CTLA-4. Cell 1992;71:1093–1102.

125. Baskar S, Nabavi N, Glimcher LH, Ostrand-Rosenberg S. Tumor cells expressing major histocompatibility complex class II and B7 activation molecules stimulate potent tumor-specific immunity. J Immunother 1993;14:209–215.

126. Brunschwig EB, Levine E, Trefzer U, Tykocinski ML. Glycosylphosphatidylinositol-modified murine B7-1 and B7-2 retain costimulator function. J Immunol 1995;155(12): 5498–5505.

127. Hodge JW, Abrams S, Schlom J, Kantor JA. Induction of antitumor immunity by recombinant vaccinia viruses expressing B7-1 or B7-2 costimulatory molecules. Cancer Res 1994;54(21):5552–5555.

128. Chen L, McGowan P, Ashe S, et al. Tumor immunogenicity determines the effect of B7 costimulation on T cell-mediated tumor immunity. J Exp Med 1994;179:523–532.

129. Krummel MF, Sullivan TJ, Allison JP. Superantigen responses and co-stimulation: CD28 and CTLA-4 have opposing effects on T cell expansion in vitro and in vivo. Int Immunol 1996;8(4):519–523.

130. Perrin PJ, Maldonado JH, Davis TA, et al. CTLA-4 blockade enhances clinical disease and cytokine production during experimental allergic encephalomyelitis. J Immunol 1996;157(4):1333–1336.

131. Leach DR, Krummel MF, Allison JP. Enhancement of antitumor immunity by CTLA-4 blockade. Science 1996;271(5256):1734–1736.

132. Hurwitz AA, Yu TF, Leach DR, Allison JP. CTLA-4 blockade synergizes with tumor-derived granulocyte-macrophage colony-stimulating factor for treatment of an experimental mammary carcinoma. Proc Natl Acad Sci USA 1998; 95(17):10067–10071.

133. Sotomayor EM, Borrello I, Tubb E, et al. In vivo blockade of CTLA-4 enhances the priming of responsive T cells but fails to prevent the induction of tumor antigen-specific tolerance. Proc Natl Acad Sci USA 1999;96(20): 11476–11481.

134. Fields PE, Finch RJ, Gray GS, et al. B7.1 is a quantitatively stronger costimulus than B7.2 in the activation of naive

CD8+ TCR-transgenic T cells. J Immunol 1998;161(10): 5268–5275.

135. Swiniarski H, Sturmhoefel K, Lee K, et al. Immune response enhancement by in vivo administration of B7.2Ig, a soluble costimulatory protein. Clin Immunol 1999;92(3):235–245.

136. Blazar BR, Taylor PA, Linsley PS, Vallera DA. In vivo blockade of CD28/CTLA-4: B7/BB1 interaction with CTLA4Ig reduces lethal murine graft-versus-host disease across the major histocompatibility complex barrier in mice. Blood 1994;83:3815–3825.

137. Tang A, Judge TA, Nickoloff BJ, Turka LA. Suppression of murine allergic contact dermatitis by CTLA4Ig. Tolerance induction of Th2 responses requires additional blockade of CD40-ligand. J Immunol 1996;157(1):117–125.

138. Krinzman SJ, De Sanctis GT, Cernadas M, et al. Inhibition of T cell costimulation abrogates airway hyperresponsiveness in a murine model. J Clin Invest 1996;98(12): 2693–2699.

139. Wilson CB, Embree LJ, Schowalter D, et al. Transient inhibition of CD28 and CD40 ligand interactions prolongs adenovirus-mediated transgene expression in the lung and facilitates expression after secondary vector administration. J Virol 1998;72(9):7542–7550.

140. Sayegh HM, Turka LA. The role of T-cell costimulatory activation pathways in transplant rejection. N Engl J Med 1998;338(25):1813–1821.

141. Lin H, Rathmell JC, Gray GS, et al. Cytotoxic T lymphocyte antigen 4 (CTLA-4) blockade accelerates the acute rejection of cardiac allografts in CD28-deficient mice: CTLA-4 can function independently of CD28. J Exp Med 1998;188(1):199–204.

142. Hakim FT, Cepeda R, Gray GS, et al. Acute graft-versus-host reaction can be aborted by blockade of costimulatory molecules. J Immunol 1995;155:1757–1766.

143. Blazar BR, Taylor PA, Panoskaltsis-Mortari A, et al. Opposing roles of CD28:B7 and CTLA-4:B7 pathways in regulating in vivo alloresponses in murine recipients of MHC disparate T cells. J Immunol 1999;162(11): 6368–6377.

144. Blazar BR, Sharpe AH, Taylor PA, et al. Infusion of ant-B7.1 (CD80) and anti-B7.2 (CD86) monoclonal antibodies inhibits murine graft-versus-host disease lethality in part via direct effects on CD4+ and CD8+ T cells. J Immunol 1996;157(8):3250–3259.

145. Saito K, Sakurai J, Ohata J, et al. Involvement of CD40 ligand-CD40 and CTLA-4-B7 pathways in murine acute graft-versus-host disease induced by allogeneic T cells lacking CD28. J Immunol 1998;160(9):4225–4231.

146. Milich DR, Linsley PS, Hughes JL, Jones JE. Soluble CTLA-4 can suppress autoantibody production and elicit long term unresponsiveness in a novel transgenic model. J Immunol 1994;153:429–435.

147. Perrin PJ, Scott D, Quigley L, et al. Role of B7:CD28/CTLA-4 in the induction of chronic relapsing experimental allergic encephalomyelitis. J Immunol 1995;154:1481–1490.

148. Daikh D, Wofsy D, Imboden JB. The CD28-B7 costimulatory pathway and its role in autoimmue disease. J Leukoc Biol 1997;62(2):156–162.

149. Hurwitz AA, Sullivan TJ, Krummel MF, et al. Specific blockade of CTLA-4/B7 interactions results in exacerbated clinical and histologic disease in an actively-induced model of experimental allergic encephalomyelitis. J Neuroimmunol 1997;73(1–2):57–62.

150. Knoerzer DB, Karr RW, Schwartz BD, Mengle-Gaw LJ. Collagen-induced arthritis in the BB rat. Prevention of disease by treatment with CTLA4Ig. J Clin Invest 1995; 96(2):987–993.

151. Nakajima A, Azuma M, Kodera S, et al. Preferential dependence of autoantibody production in murine lupus on CD86 costimulatory molecule. Eur J Immunol 1995; 25(11):3060–3069.

152. Linsley PS, Wallace PM, Johnson J, et al. Immunosuppression in vivo by a soluble form of the CTLA-4 T cell activation molecule. Science 1992;257:792–795.

153. Daikh DI, Wofsy D. Effects of anti-B7 monoclonal antibodies on humoral immune responses. J Autoimmun 1999;12(2):101–108.

154. Ronchese F, Hausmann B, Hubele S, Lane P. Mice transgenic for a soluble form of murine CTLA-4 show enhanced expansion of antigen-specific CD4+ T cells and defective antibody production in vivo. J Exp Med 1994;179:809–817.

155. Wood KJ. Gene therapy and allotransplantation. Curr Opin Immunol 1997;9(5):662–668.

156. Croxford JL, O'Neill JK, Ali RR, et al. Local gene therapy with CTLA-4 immunoglobulin fusion protein in experimental allergic encephalomyelitis. Eur J Immunol 1998;28(12):3904–3916.

157. Uchikoshi F, Yang ZD, Rostami S, et al. Prevention of autoimmune recurrence and rejection by adenovirus-mediated CTLA4Ig gene transfer to the pancreatic graft in BB rat. Diabetes 1999;48(3):652–657.

158. Halbert CL, Standaert TA, Wilson CB, Miller AD. Successful readministration of adeno-associated virus vectors to the mouse lung requires transient immunosuppression during the initial exposure. J Virol 1998;72(12):9795–9805.

159. Guibinga GH, Lochmuller H, Massie B, et al. Combinatorial blockade of calcineurin and CD28 signaling facilitates primary and secondary therapeutic gene transfer by adenovirus vectors in dystrophic (mdx) mouse muscles. J Virol 1998;72(6):4601–4609.

160. Jooss K, Turka LA, Wilson JM. Blunting of immune responses to adenoviral vectors in mouse liver and lung with CTLA4Ig. Gene Ther 1998;5(3):309–319.

161. Olthoff KM, Judge TA, Gelman AE, et al. Adenovirus-mediated gene transfer into cold-preserved liver allografts: survival pattern and unresponsiveness following transduction with CTLA4Ig. Nat Med 1998;4(2):194–200.

162. Schowalter DB, Meuse L, Wilson CB, et al. Constitutive expression of murine CTLA4Ig from a recombinant adenovirus vector results in prolonged transgene expression. Gene Ther 1997;4(8):853–860.

163. Ossevoort MA, Ringers J, Boon L, et al. Blocking of costimulation prevents kidney graft rejection in rhesus monkeys. Transplant Proc 1998;30(5):2165–2166.

164. Tam RC, Wu-Pong S, Pai B, et al. Increased potency of an aptameric G-rich oligonucleotide is associated with novel functional properties of phosphorothioate linkages [In Process Citation]. Antisense Nucleic Acid Drug Dev 1999;9(3):289–300.

165. Tam RC, Phan UT, Milovanovic T, et al. Oligonucleotide-mediated inhibition of CD28 expression induces human T cell hyporesponsiveness and manifests impaired

contact hypersensitivity in mice. J Immunol 1997;158(1): 200–208.

166. Fine JS, Macosko HD, Justice L, et al. An inhibitor of CD28-CD80 interactions impairs CD28-mediated costimulation of human CD4 T cells. Cell Immunol 1999;191(1):49–59.

167. de Ines C, Cochlovius B, Schmidt S, et al. Apoptosis of a human melanoma cell line specifically induced by membrane-bound single-chain antibodies. J Immunol 1999; 163(7):3948–3956.

168. Horspool JH, Perrin PJ, Woodcock JB, et al. Nucleic acid vaccine-induced immune responses require CD28 costimulation and are regulated by CTLA-4. J Immunol 1998;160(6):2706–2714.

169. Kim JJ, Bagarazzi ML, Trivedi N, et al. Engineering of in vivo immune responses to DNA immunization via codelivery of costimulatory molecule genes. Nat Biotechnol 1997;15(7):641–646.

170. Shi Y. Radvanyi LG, Sharma A, et al. CD28-mediated signaling in vivo prevents activation-induced apoptosis in the thymus and alters peripheral lymphocyte homeostasis. J Immunol 1995;155(4):1829–1837.

171. Wang R, Fang Q, Zhang L, Radvany L, et al. CD28 ligation prevents bacterial toxin-induced septic shock in mice by inducing IL-10 expression. J Immunol 1997;158(6):2856–2861.

172. Dengler TJ, Szabo G, Sido B, et al. Prolonged allograft survival but no tolerance induction by modulating CD28 antibody JJ319 after high-responder rat heart transplantation. Transplantation 1999;67(3):392–398.

173. Perrin PJ, June CH, Maldonado JH, et al. Blockade of CD28 during in vitro activation of encephalitogenic T cells or after disease onset ameliorates experimental autoimmune encephalomyelitis. J Immunol 1999;163:1704–1710.

174. Arreaza GA, Cameron MJ, Jaramillo A, et al. Neonatal activation of CD28 signaling overcomes T cell anergy and prevents autoimmune diabetes by an IL-4-dependent mechanism. J Clin Invest 1997;100(9):2243–2253.

175. Krummel MF, Sullivan TJ, Allison JP. Superantigen responses and co-stimulation: CD28 and CTLA-4 have opposing effects on T cell expansion in vitro and in vivo. Int Immunol 1996;8(4):519–523.

176. Zhu MZ, Marshall J, Cole D, et al. Specific cytolytic T-cell responses to human CEA from patients immunized with recombinant avipox-CEA vaccine. Clin Cancer Res 2000;6(1):24–33.

177. Canevari S, Mezzanzanica D, Mazzoni A, et al. Approaches to implement bispecific antibody treatment of ovarian carcinoma. Cancer Immunol Immunother 1997;45(3–4): 187–189.

178. Metzler WJ, Bajorath J, Fenderson W, et al. Solution structure of human CTLA-4 and delineation of a CD80/CD86 binding site conserved in CD28. Nat Struct Biol 1997;4(7):527–531.

179. Peach RJ, Bajorath J, Brady W, et al. Complementarity determining region 1 (CDR1)-and CDR3-analogous regions in CTLA-4 and CD28 determine the binding to B7-1. J Exp Med 1994;180(6):2049–2058.

Chapter 29

Bacterial Vaccines

Hilde-Kari Guttormsen
Dennis L. Kasper

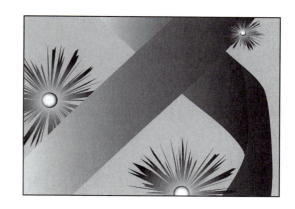

The function of bacterial vaccines is to induce a protective immune response (humoral and/or cellular) either systemically or at the mucosal effector sites. A protective response neutralizes exotoxins or prevents colonization and/or invasive disease. While pure polysaccharide vaccines do not induce immunologic memory, protein vaccines induce B- and T-cell memory, which results in an anamnestic immune response including a brisk and greatly enhanced immune response on future encounters with the organism or recall vaccination. For some vaccines, the induced protective responses might not be of the same levels as those induced during natural infection (1).

Circulating antibodies as well as antibodies in the tissue and at mucosal sites are of great importance in preventing or attenuating disease caused by extracellular pathogens, including toxin-producing organisms (2). In contrast, even though antibodies might be important in preventing the initial attachment and invasion by intracellular bacteria, cell-mediated immunity is the major protective immune response against infection with intracellular pathogens (2).

Many bacterial vaccines used for routine immunizations (mainly inactivated whole-cell vaccines or detoxified exotoxins) have been developed empirically (3). Recent advances in microbial genetics and immunology have greatly enhanced our understanding of microbial pathogenesis and of host defense mechanisms. Defining the molecular basis of bacterial virulence and identifying antigens essential for the induction of protective host defense mechanisms are necessary for construction of successful vaccines. New vaccine strategies based on knowledge of protective immune responses have resulted in highly effective typhoid, acellular pertussis, and polysaccharide-conjugate vaccines (Table 29-1).

Immunologic adjuvants are substances that enhance the immune response to an antigen. In addition, adjuvants can direct the immune response to enhanced systemic or mucosal humoral immunity and/or cell-mediated immunity (5).

Experimental DNA-mediated vaccines in which a gene for a putative protective antigen is inserted into a bacterial expression plasmid or another delivery vector (6–9) elicit antibodies and CD4+ T-cell responses in animals as well as antigen-specific cytotoxic T lymphocytes (10). DNA vaccines are therefore potentially useful against both extracellular and intracellular bacteria and are discussed in Chapter 31 (11).

This chapter focuses on bacterial vaccine development in relation to the relevant protective immune effector mechanisms(s). Parenteral vaccines against extracellular bacteria, including exotoxin-producing bacteria and intracellular bacteria, are discussed separately. The recently licensed mucosal vaccines are also discussed.

Immunity to Extracellular Bacteria

Extracellular bacteria, which replicate outside host cells, normally gain entry into the human host by attaching to and colonizing mucosal membranes of the nasopharynx (*Haemophilus influenzae, Streptococcus pneumoniae, Neisseria meningitidis, Corynebacterium diphtheriae, Bordetella pertussis*) or of the gastrointestinal or urogenital tract [*Vibrio cholerae, Streptococcus agalactiae* or group B streptococci (GBS), *Escherichia coli, Neisseria gonorrhoeae*] or through breaching of the skin (group A streptococci, *Clostridium tetani*).

Extracellular bacteria produce several virulence factors that allow them to attach to human cells, invade, and cause tissue damage (see Fig. 29-1). Adhesins mediate attachment of bacteria to eukaryotic cells and are categorized as fimbrial (pili and fimbriae) and afimbrial. Extracellular bacteria may produce exotoxins (*C. diphtheriae* and *C. tetani*) or endotoxins or LPSs (lipopolysaccharides, which are a major constituent of the outer membranes of gram-negative bacteria). LPS, peptidoglycan (a major constituent of the outer membrane of gram-positive bacteria), and other glycosyl-based microbial polymers activate monocytes and macrophages through interaction with circulating LPS-binding protein, CD14, and toll-like receptors 2 and 4 (cell surface coreceptors for CD14) (12–15), leading to the production of endogenous inflammatory mediators such as tumor necrosis factor alpha (TNF-α), interleukin 1 (IL-1), and IL-6—substances ultimately responsible for the phlogistic responses to these organisms (16).

Immune responses to extracellular bacteria are aimed at neutralizing the effects of their toxins and/or eliminating the bacteria. Clearance of the bacteria can be achieved through inhibition of adherence to mucosal surfaces by antibodies directed to the structures mediating attachment to eukaryotic cells or by opsonophagocytic or bactericidal antibodies that promote killing

Table 29-1. Licensed Bacterial Vaccines (in the United States)

Vaccine	Year	Type of Immunizing Agent	Protective Mechanism	Route of Administration	Indications	Efficacy	Adverse Events
Anthrax	1970	Inactivated avirulent bacteria	Not known	SQ	For high risk of exposure	nd	No serious adverse effects known
BCG	1950	Living bacteria (attenuated *Mycobacterium bovis*)	Not known	ID	PPD-negative; exposed to active TB patient	>80% against miliary and meningitic TB; 0–80% against pulmonary TB	Regional adenitis, disseminated BCG infections, osteitis
Cholera	1914	Inactivated bacteria	Antibodies to polysaccharide O-antigens	SQ or IM	Not recommended for public health use	50% (short-lived)	Frequent fever, local pain, swelling
DT Td	1949 1955	Toxoid	Diphtheria- and tetanus-neutralizing antitoxins, ≥0.1 IU/mL each	IM	Routine Routine >7 years old	D: 95% T: 95%	Local reactions, hypersensitivity to tetanus toxoid
Hib	1987	Bacterial polysaccharide protein conjugate	Antibody to capsular polysaccharide, 0.15 μg/mL	IM	Routine	90%	Few local, no serious reactions
Lyme	1998	Lipidated recombinant OspA	Antibodies to OspA	IM	At risk for exposure to infected vector ticks; 15–70 years old	50% (2 doses), 78% (3 doses); duration unknown	Transient arthralgia and myalgia
Meningococcus A, C, Y, W135	1981	Bacterial polysaccharide of 4 serogroups	Antibody to capsular polysaccharide	SQ	Military personnel; travelers to epidemic areas	90% for 2–3 years	Rare
Pertussis	1949	Killed whole-cell vaccine	Not known	IM	Routine	35–80%, short-lived	Local reactions (75%); mild systemic reactions (30%); severe, irreversible reactions (rare)
Acellular pertussis	1993 1996	Inactivated bacterial antigen Acellular (DTaP)	Not known	IM	Routine, recommended	80%	Reduced local reactions compared with whole-cell vaccines; no serious reactions reported
Plague	1911	Inactivated bacteria	Not known	IM	Laboratory workers	nd	10% local reactions; rare sterile abscesses and hypersensitivity
Pneumococcus	1983	Bacterial polysaccharide of 23 types	Antibody to capsular polysaccharide	IM or SQ	Chronic disease; >65 years old	60–80%	Local reactions; rare anaphylaxis
Typhoid: Killed	1952	Killed whole bacteria	Not known	IM	Travelers and contacts of carriers	50–70%, short-lived	Frequent fever, local swelling, pain
Ty21a	1992	Live mutant bacteria	Not known	Oral	Travelers and contacts of carriers	50–70%	None
Vi	1995	Vi capsular polysaccharide	Antibody to capsular polysaccharide	IM	Travelers	70–75%	Local reactions

BCG, bacille Calmette-Guérin; DT, diphtheria and tetanus toxoids, adsorbed; Td, tetanus and diphtheria toxoids, adsorbed, for adult use; aP, acellular pertussis; Hib, *Haemophilus influenzae* type b; SQ, subcutaneous; ID, intradermal; IM, intramuscular; nd, not determined; PPD, purified protein derivative used in intradermal test for tuberculosis; TB, tuberculosis; OspA, outer-surface protein A.
Adapted from Tables 122–4 and 122–5 in (4).

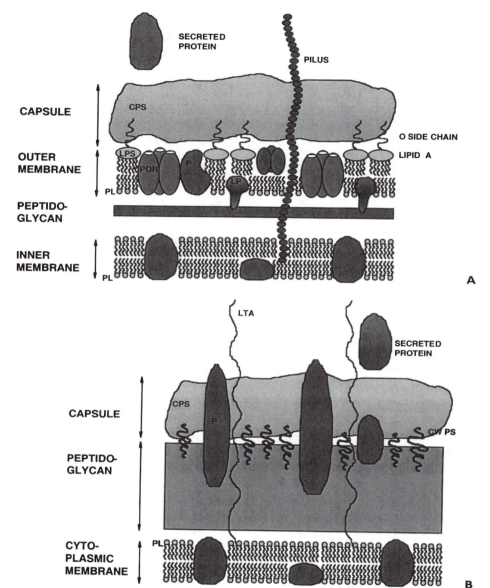

Figure 29-1. (A) Major structures of the gram-negative cell wall, including extracellular capsular polysaccharide (CPS); inner and outer membranes with their phospholipid (PL) bilayers and associated proteins; periplasm containing peptidoglycan; and outer membrane containing outer-membrane proteins (P), including trimeric porin molecules (POR), phospholipids, lipoproteins (LP), and lipid A and O side chain components of lipopolysaccharide (LPS). One pilus anchored in the inner membrane extends through the capsule layer and into the extracellular space, where secreted proteins can also be found. (B) Major structures of the gram-positive cell wall, including extracellular capsular polysaccharide (CPS); cytoplasmic membrane with its PL bilayer and associated proteins; a substantial peptidoglycan layer; and the polysaccharide capsule layer with associated proteins (P). The cell wall polysaccharide (CW PS) is associated with and may bridge the peptidoglycan and the capsular polysaccharide. Lipoteichoic acid (LTA) extends from the inner membrane into the extracellular space, where secreted proteins can also be found.

of the invading pathogen (17). Bactericidal antibodies and complement components deposited on the bacteria promote direct bacteriolysis of some gram-negative organisms (18). Opsonophagocytic antibodies and specific complement component fragments (opsonins) coat gram-positive and serum-resistant gram-negative organisms. Polymorphonuclear and mononuclear phagocytic cells recognize and bind to opsonized bacteria to cause phagocytosis and killing of the pathogens (17).

Protection Mediated by Antitoxin-Neutralizing Antibodies

Diphtheria

Diphtheria is a noninvasive infection of the nasopharyngeal tissues caused by toxigenic strains. The diphtheria toxin (DT) is the major virulence factor and the major protective antigen. DT causes local necrotic lesions and local inflammation as well as systemic effects resulting from its inhibition of protein synthesis.

Proteolytic cleavage of DT results in an amino-terminal A fragment and a carboxy-terminal B fragment linked through a disulfide bond (19). The toxin consists of three functional domains (20), with the catalytic domain (C domain) located in the A fragment, the translocation domain (T domain) in the N-terminal part of the B fragment, and the receptor-binding domain (R domain) in the carboxy-terminal part of the B fragment. DT binds to receptors of susceptible eukaryotic cells through its R domain and is internalized by receptor-mediated endocytosis, with subsequent translocation of the A fragment into the cytosol, where it blocks protein synthesis and thereby causes cell death. The majority of the neutralizing antibodies bind to the R domain (19).

Detoxified DT vaccine has been used for mass immunization since the 1920s, when safe detoxification methods using formaldehyde were developed. Before the introduction of mass vaccination, 75% of the population was immune to diphtheria without having had clinical disease (21). Antibodies to DT protect against disease, and a booster dose of the toxoid is needed every 10 years to maintain protective levels of these antibodies (diphtheria-neutralizing antibodies $\geq 0.1 \, IU/mL$). Adults frequently have adverse reactions to toxoid vaccines (diphtheria-tetanus) owing to high levels of preexisting antibodies, and a reduced dose is recommended for booster vaccination after the age of 7 (21). It is generally believed that antibodies to DT can neutralize only toxin that has not bound to the tissue. Equine diphtheria antitoxin is available for treating infected nonimmune individuals or for preventing disease in exposed susceptible individuals (22).

Diphtheria is still endemic in a few densely populated countries. Of additional concern is the high number of adults in industrialized countries who do not have protective levels of antibodies to DT (22–24), possibly because of a lack of "natural boosting of immunity" as a result of the disappearance of the disease and of the carriage of toxigenic strains among healthy individuals. The risk of diphtheria outbreaks is increasing, and several outbreaks have occurred in Europe following importation of toxigenic strains (23,24).

Tetanus

Spores of *C. tetani* are ubiquitous in the environment and can be introduced into humans through breaches of the skin or through the umbilici of newborn infants. The spores germinate in an anaerobic environment and produce the heterodimeric tetanus toxin (TT), which is responsible for the disease. The heavy chain of the toxin mediates binding to nerve-cell receptors and entry into the cells, and the light chain blocks neurotransmitter release, resulting in increased muscle tone and spasms. Symptoms can occur locally at the site of infection or can be more generalized (25), as classically described for "lockjaw." TT is the major virulence factor of this organism and a protective antigen. Like DT, TT consists of catalytic (C), translocation (T), and receptor-binding (R) domains. Antibodies that neutralize the effects of the toxin are mainly directed toward its R domain (26).

Detoxified TT vaccines induce protective immunity, and a boost every 10 years is recommended to ensure protective

antibody levels (tetanus-neutralizing antibodies $\geq 0.1 \, IU/mL$). Patients recovering from infection with *C. tetani* do not develop protective levels of antibodies because immunity is not induced by the small amounts of toxin that produce the disease (25). Neonatal tetanus is usually attributable to poor hygienic conditions during delivery. This devastating illness can be prevented by immunizing all previously unimmunized women of childbearing age, including pregnant women. Maternal antibodies to TT are transferred across the placenta to protect the infant. Human and equine tetanus-specific immunoglobulins are available for treating infected nonimmune individuals or preventing disease in exposed susceptible individuals.

Protection Mediated by Antiattachment, Opsonizing, and/or Bactericidal Antibodies: Pertussis

Pertussis, or whooping cough, is a highly contagious respiratory disease caused by *B. pertussis*. Before mass vaccination with heat-killed whole-cell vaccines, 60% of children had clinical disease before school age (27). The bacteria attach to and colonize the upper respiratory tract and cause both local and systemic disease (28). Natural infection is thought to induce lifelong immunity, but the protective immune response and protective antigens are not well defined (27).

Inactivated whole-cell pertussis vaccines have been given as part of childhood vaccination programs and have greatly reduced disease rates (27,29,30). Even though the vaccine-induced protection is not lifelong (27), the licensed whole-cell vaccines cannot be used to boost the immune response beyond 7 years of age because of increased reactogenicity (28). Public fear about adverse effects of pertussis immunization (rare side effects such as seizures and hypotonic hyporesponsive episodes) has lessened the use of this vaccine. As a result, the number of susceptible individuals and the incidence of pertussis have been rising steadily in recent years (27,31). In order to decrease the rate of reactions, vaccines based on purified *B. pertussis* antigens have been developed (27).

Many pertussis antigens, such as filamentous hemagglutinin (FHA), pertactin, pertussis toxin (PT), and fimbriae 2 and 3, are protective in an animal respiratory infection model (27). In addition to the obligatory role for pertussis-specific B cells and their products, interferon-gamma (IFN-γ) is important for preventing atypical disseminated disease in mice (32,33). In fact, adoptive transfer of IFN-γ-producing CD4 $T_H 1$ cells alone confers protective immunity against pertussis in an animal model of pertussis infection (33).

In humans, there is a direct correlation between the levels of antibodies to pertactin, fimbriae 2 and 3, and PT at exposure and protection against clinical disease (34). A protective, inactivated, whole-cell vaccine induced substantial levels of antibodies to defined bacterial structures such as FHA, pertactin, and fimbriae 2 and 3 but not to PT in infants (30). A new generation of acellular pertussis vaccines containing only purified *B. pertussis* antigens has been proven safe, immunogenic, and efficacious (29,30,

35). Several recent clinical trials in Europe have suggested that protection, especially against mild disease, increases with the number of vaccine components (29,30,35).

A recent report from the Netherlands suggests that long-term vaccination (40 years or more) with a whole-cell pertussis vaccine can select for clinical pertussis strains that contain polymorphism (differences in the amino acid sequence) in virulence factors and immunogens such as pertactin and PT (36). At the introduction of the whole-cell vaccine in 1949, pertactin and PT isolated from the disease-causing strains were 100% identical at the amino acid level to those of the vaccine strain and the recently used acellular pertussis vaccines, while now the percentage of clinical isolates with identical amino acid structures varies. For example, in the Netherlands only 10% of case strains are identical at the amino acid level to those included in the whole-cell vaccine and in the acellular pertussis vaccine (36). This finding may have substantial implications for the long-term efficacy of both whole-cell and acellular pertussis vaccines.

Capsular Polysaccharide–Based Vaccines

Despite the availability of effective antibiotics, infections with many encapsulated bacteria (e.g., *N. meningitidis*, *Salmonella typhi*, *S. pneumoniae*, and GBS) remain major health problems throughout the world. The capsular polysaccharide renders such bacteria resistant to ingestion and killing by phagocytes (17). The increasing threat of antibiotic resistance among some of these species has accelerated the pace of research into new vaccines to prevent infections.

Purified polysaccharides from these organisms are T-cell–independent antigens that bind to polysaccharide-specific (PS-specific) B cells and stimulate production of PS-specific antibodies without recruitment of T-cell help or induction of immunologic memory to the polysaccharide (2,37). Such antibodies can prevent attachment of encapsulated bacteria (Vi polysaccharide of *S. typhi*; see Immunity Induced at Mucosal Sites) or can promote bactericidal killing (in some gram-negative bacteria) and/or opsonophagocytic killing (in both gram-positive and gram-negative bacteria) of encapsulated bacteria, thereby protecting against disease. Antibodies directed to the capsule are specific for the polysaccharide type; depending on the number of disease-causing serotypes existing for each bacterial species, a protective polysaccharide-based vaccine may consist of one serotype, as in the *H. influenzae* type b (Hib) vaccine, or a mixture of many serotypes, as in the licensed pneumococcal vaccine.

Covalent coupling of a polysaccharide to an immunogenic protein carrier results in an enhanced immune response with 1) high levels of PS-specific antibodies, 2) rapid kinetics, 3) induction of immunologic memory, and 4) isotype switching of the PS-specific antibodies (IgM to IgG) on booster vaccination or subsequent encounter with the polysaccharide as presented on the bacteria (37,38). The enhanced immune response to a polysaccharide conjugated to a protein in comparison with the polysaccharide alone indicates a shift from a thymus-independent to a thymus-dependent response (37–39). Studies of mice deficient in molecules critical for stimulatory, cognate B-/T-cell interactions and normal mice treated with pathway antagonists have demonstrated that several stimulatory molecules are critical for recruitment of T-cell help by the glycoconjugate vaccines to the PS-specific B cells (40). As for classic T-cell–dependent protein antigens (41,42), the activation of T-helper cells is dependent on two signals: signal 1, conferring carrier specificity [i.e., presentation of the T-cell epitopes from the processed carrier molecule in the context of class II major histocompatibility complex (MHC) molecules on the B cell to the T-cell receptor (TCR) on the T-helper cell]; and signal 2, providing optimal T-cell activation through increased and sustained TCR-induced phosphorylation (interaction of the costimulatory molecules B7-1 and/or B7-2 on B cells with CD28 on the T-helper cell) (40,43). In addition, B-cell stimulation through interaction of CD40 on B cells with CD40L on activated T-helper cells is critical for the immune responses to glycoconjugate vaccines in vivo (40). T cells activated by a glycoconjugate vaccine also play a pivotal role in determining the magnitude of the IgM response to the polysaccharide (40).

The licensed pneumococcal vaccine will be described as the prototype of polysaccharide vaccines and Hib conjugated to a carrier protein as the prototype for a glycoconjugate vaccine.

Purified Pneumococcal Polysaccharide Vaccines

Streptococcus pneumoniae is a major cause of bacterial pneumonia and a significant cause of bacterial meningitis. Older people (70 years or older) and children under 2 years of age, in addition to patients with severe chronic debilitating diseases or cerebrospinal fluid leakage, are at high risk of serious pneumococcal infections (44,45). Ninety serotypes exist, each containing a unique polysaccharide capsule that renders the bacteria resistant to ingestion and killing by phagocytes. *S. pneumoniae* colonizes the nasopharynx after initial attachment via bacterial adhesins to epithelial cell receptors containing the disaccharide GlcNAcβ1-4Gal and is part of the normal flora (45). Pneumococci can be isolated from 5% to 10% of healthy adults and from 20% to 40% of healthy children (44). Inhalation or aspiration of the organisms to the lungs results in activation of complement, cytokine production, and invasion of polymorphonuclear leukocytes. A large bacterial load, concurrent viral infection, lack of type-specific protective opsonophagocytic antibodies, and/or compromised phagocyte function can result in invasive disease. Individuals with asplenia (anatomic or functional) cannot clear the organisms efficiently and risk developing overwhelming fatal pneumococcal bacteremia (45). Type-specific antibodies to pneumococcal capsular polysaccharide appear naturally after colonization and disease (44).

The licensed vaccine against pneumococcal disease consists of a mixture of purified capsular polysaccharides of various pneumococcal serotypes. A 14-valent vaccine consisting of purified polysaccharides of the most prevalent disease-causing serotypes was licensed in 1977; its efficacy was 67% in a case-control study in high-risk patients (46). The 14-valent vaccine was replaced in 1983 by a 23-valent vaccine in which several serotypes were added on the basis of the epidemiology of the disease. Pneumococcal polysaccharide vaccine is recommended for healthy persons over 65 years of age and for adults with chronic diseases associated with increased frequency or severity of pneumococcal disease (45). Vaccination stimulates a greater than twofold increase in antibodies to most serotypes in most recipients over 2 years of age (44). However, the immune response varies with serotype and the underlying disease (45). The protection rate for the 23-valent vaccine is 85% in persons under 55 years old, and the protection lasts for at least 5 years. However, with increasing age the protection rate and duration decrease significantly. In those at highest risk for disease (i.e., immunocompromised persons or those with severe chronic disease), the effect of the vaccine is questionable (44). Protection induced by unconjugated polysaccharides used as vaccines depends on the level of type-specific antibodies at the mucosal surface or in the circulation at the time of infection, because no anamnestic or memory response will be induced by the capsular polysaccharide as presented on an invading organism. The concentration of vaccine-induced antibodies decreases over time, and the antibodies are relatively short lived (44,45).

Polysaccharide-Protein Conjugate Vaccines

Haemophilus influenzae type b (Hib) is an encapsulated bacterium that causes both local and serious systemic disease in infants and young children. Of the known serotypes (based on their capsular polysaccharide), only type b is virulent and causes systemic disease. Type-specific bactericidal and opsonophagocytic antibodies are protective against disease (47). However, neither systemic disease nor immunization with pure type b capsular polysaccharide (a T-cell–independent type 2 antigen) induces protective antibodies in susceptible infants and young children (48,49). Therefore, the capsular polysaccharide (polyribosyl-ribitol phosphate, or PRP) has been conjugated to various carrier proteins (*N. meningitidis* outer-membrane protein, or OMP; CRM_{197}, a diphtheria toxin derivative; tetanus toxoid, or TT) in an effort to enhance the immune response to the polysaccharide (50,51). These glycoconjugate vaccines induce higher levels of PS-specific IgG antibodies in infants and adults than purified polysaccharides, and, in contrast to the response to unconjugated polysaccharide, the conjugates elicit booster responses in infants (52). The three Hib conjugate vaccines that are licensed for use in infants less than 15 months old in the United States differ in their immunokinetic profiles. PRP-OMP, which induces protective antibodies after one injection, does not reach as high a peak concentration after a full course as does either PRP-CRM_{197} or PRP-TT. These latter vaccines induce a more gradual acquisition of antibody that reaches protective levels after two or three doses (53). All licensed Hib glycoconjugate vaccines have been proven to be efficacious in preventing invasive disease (49,54), are now used routinely for childhood immunization in industrialized countries, and have nearly eliminated invasive Hib disease in children less than 5 years old (55–57).

An additional feature of the Hib glycoconjugate vaccines is their effect on Hib colonization in the immunized population (49,58). A marked decrease in oropharyngeal carriage of Hib in vaccinated children reduces transmission to unvaccinated children (herd immunity), thereby lowering the incidence of invasive disease in both vaccinated and unvaccinated children (59). However, the licensed Hib glycoconjugate vaccines differ in their effects on oropharyngeal carriage in unique populations (59). Immunization of Navajo children and Alaska natives, who are at high risk for invasive Hib disease (60), with PRP-OMP virtually eliminated invasive disease but did not eliminate carriage of Hib (59). In contrast, widespread vaccination with a PRP-DT vaccine in Finland and with PRP-TT in Atlanta has nearly eliminated Hib carriage (61) as well as invasive disease. The mechanism (or mechanisms) responsible for the effect of glycoconjugate vaccines on acquisition of oropharyngeal colonization with Hib is not known.

In contrast to Hib disease, in which invasive disease is caused by one serotype, invasive group B streptococcal, pneumococcal, and meningococcal diseases are caused by organisms of different serotypes (GBS, pneumococcus) or serogroups (meningococcus). To protect against disease caused by these encapsulated organisms, the candidate conjugate vaccines must contain a mixture of the capsular polysaccharides from the serotypes that most frequently cause invasive disease. Several pneumococcal and meningococcal candidate vaccines have been developed in which purified polysaccharides from several serotypes/serogroups are conjugated individually to carrier proteins and given as a multivalent vaccine (62–69). Most of these glycoconjugate vaccine candidates have used routine childhood vaccine antigens such as diphtheria or tetanus toxoids as carrier proteins. Multivalent glycoconjugate pneumococcal and meningococcal vaccines have been shown to be immunogenic in infants and children under 2 years of age (70–74), but the efficacies against invasive pneumococcal and meningococcal diseases are not known.

Immunity to Intracellular Bacteria

Several types of bacteria are able to survive and replicate within host cells. An important mechanism for survival of intracellular bacteria is their ability to resist elimination by phagocytes. Natural immunity can therefore be quite ineffective in controlling infection by and spread of these organisms. Chronic and latent infections occur frequently (2,75). Some intracellular bacteria escape to the cytosol by lysing of the phagosomal membrane by bacterial encoded proteins (i.e., *Listeria monocytogenes*), while others inhibit phagolysosomal fusion (i.e., *Mycobacterium tuberculosis* and *Legionella pneumophila*) (2).

Intracellular bacteria that reside in lysosomal compartments primarily stimulate CD4 T-helper cells through antigen presentation in the context of MHC class II molecules. Those residing in the cytoplasm are primarily recognized by CD8 T cells through MHC class I antigen presentation. Some bacterial pathogens such as *M. tuberculosis* stimulate both CD4 and CD8 T cells (76).

Intracellular bacteria also activate natural killer (NK) cells directly or through IL-12 secreted by activated macrophages. IFN-γ secreted by NK cells in turn activates macrophages and promotes killing of phagocytosed bacteria. Adoptive cell transfer studies have demonstrated that the major form of protective immunity against intracellular bacteria is cell mediated (77).

Individuals deficient in cell-mediated immunity are extremely susceptible to infections with intracellular bacteria (78). The major effector mechanisms against intracellular organisms are killing by macrophages activated by cytokines (IFN-γ) secreted by activated antigen-specific CD4 T_H1 cells and by NK cells (79) and lysis of infected cells by cytolytic CD8 T cells (2). Indeed, immunity to tuberculosis can be compromised by excessive release of inflammatory cytokines or T_H2 activity (80). In an animal model of tuberculosis, a T_H2 cytokine pattern is found during latent disease, with a shift to a T_H1 cytokine pattern during reactivation of tuberculosis (81). The macrophage activation in response to the infections can cause tissue damage, and persistent antigens can result in chronic stimulation of T cells and macrophages, causing granuloma formation (82).

BCG Vaccine Against Mycobacterium Tuberculosis

Although the bacille Calmette-Guérin (BCG) vaccine for controlling tuberculosis is the most widely used vaccine in the world, the protective antigens are not known. A recent meta-analysis of BCG vaccine trials and case-control studies demonstrated that the protective efficacy of BCG vaccination against serious forms (meningitis or disseminated) of tuberculosis in children is greater than 80% (83). However, the estimates of efficacy against pulmonary tuberculosis in adolescents and adults, which is the most prevalent form of the disease, vary from no protection to 85% (83). The various live BCG vaccines that exist throughout the world, which are all derived from the original attenuated *Mycobacterium bovis* strain, vary in efficacy, presumably owing to genetic differences in the vaccine, the host population, or the infecting *M. tuberculosis* strains (80).

The lymphoproliferative responses of BCG-vaccinated individuals are more efficient on stimulation with live than with inactivated vaccine (84). Secreted, extracellular proteins of *M. tuberculosis* are therefore considered candidate components of subunit vaccines against tuberculosis. Purified extracellular proteins alone or in combinations induced strong cell-mediated immune responses and substantial protective immunity in an animal model of pulmonary tuberculosis (85). Immunization of mice with plasmid DNA constructs encoding a secreted protein of *M. tuberculosis* induced substantial humoral and cell-mediated immune responses and conferred significant protection against challenge with live *M. tuberculosis* (86). This approach is now used in an effort to define the protective antigens of *M. tuberculosis* and may lead to the development of a second generation of more effective vaccines against tuberculosis.

Immunity Induced at Mucosal Sites

Secretory IgA (sIgA) antibodies are pivotal for protective mucosal immunity against pathogenic bacteria (87). The mucosa-associated lymphoid tissue (MALT) consists of specialized epithelial M (membrane) cells with underlying pockets filled with antigen-presenting cells and T cells localized over organized lymphoid follicles (87). Several bacterial pathogens have a predilection for M cells (88), which sample live and dead luminal particles nonspecifically or by receptor-mediated uptake (89). The foreign materials are actively transported through the M cells and delivered to the underlying M-cell pocket, where presumably the initial B- and T-cell stimulation takes place (89). Primed antigen-specific B cells at the mucosal inductive sites in the gut epithelium home via the lymph or peripheral blood to mucosal effector sites, where they proliferate and undergo terminal differentiation into plasma cells in the mucosal lamina propria. This process results in secretion of sIgA and sIgM and passive diffusion of IgG into the lumen (89).

Studies of protective mucosal immune mechanisms have emphasized the importance of sIgA antibodies for protection against noninvasive, enterotoxigenic infections such as cholera and enterotoxigenic *E. coli* (ETEC) diarrhea (90–92). For invasive dysenteric and enteric-fever infections caused by such organisms as *Shigella* and *Salmonella*, optimal protection may depend on a combination of mucosal and systemic immunity (93,94). On the basis of this knowledge, several new vaccines have been developed and proven to be efficacious in large field trials.

Vaccines Against Noninvasive, Enterotoxigenic Infections: Cholera

Ideally, a cholera vaccine should be safe and should induce long-term immunity against both overt disease and asymptomatic intestinal carriage of *Vibrio cholerae* (the latter being responsible for the majority of infections in endemic areas) (90). Mucosal immunity (sIgA) appears to be a critical feature of natural protective immunity from cholera (90). The toxin-coregulated pilus (TCP) is a critical colonization factor (95,96), and the serogroup- and serotype-specific lipopolysaccharide O antigens are primary targets of protective immunity to cholera (90). There are 140 recognized serogroups based on the carbohydrate determinants of their O antigens, of which only two have been identified in disease isolates (O1 and O139) (97). Once bound, the bacterium excretes a potent enterotoxin, the cholera toxin. The B subunit of the toxin binds to the GM_1 ganglioside receptor on the enterocyte, and the enzymatically active A subunit (ADP-ribosylating activity) causes the voluminous diarrhea characteristic of the disease.

Parenterally administered cholera vaccines (killed whole-cell, lipopolysaccharide, and toxoid) have been largely abandoned because these vaccines induce only weak and short-lived immunity (90) with no local mucosal immune response in immunologically naive individuals (98).

The intestinal immune system is thought to be better stimulated with oral administration of antigens, which primes for immunologic memory; repeated oral administration boosts sIgA (98). Hence, the vaccine candidates currently being developed and evaluated are designed for oral administration. Several vaccine formulations are being tried, such as killed whole-cell toxoid vaccine; a bacterial fraction (subunit) vaccine; a killed, highly piliated whole-cell vaccine (WC); live attenuated *V. cholerae* strains; and *S. typhi* strains carrying *V. cholerae* antigens.

Three doses of a combination vaccine consisting of a whole-cell component containing four killed serogroup O1 strains of different biotypes (classic and El Tor) and serotypes and the purified B subunit of the cholera toxin (BS-WC) evoke antibacterial as well as antitoxic intestinal immunity (99,100). This monovalent vaccine was safe but protected against cholera for only 3 years in a 5-year follow-up study (101,102). The efficacy was lower against El Tor strains, and the vaccine did not block intestinal carriage of these strains (90). Field trials are ongoing in Peru to test whether booster doses of the vaccine can extend the duration of protection against El Tor strains (102). The monovalent vaccine also confers substantial, although shorter-lasting, immunity to diarrhea caused by ETEC, presumably because of the shared epitopes of the B subunits of cholera toxin and the heat-labile enterotoxin of ETEC. Epidemiologic and laboratory studies suggest that natural immunity to *V. cholerae* O1 is not protective against *V. cholerae* O139 (103), a new serogroup that appeared in Asia in 1992 (104); therefore, a bivalent BS-WC cholera vaccine is now being developed.

Live attenuated *V. cholerae* vaccines may offer some advantages over inactivated vaccines (105,106) because they are likely to induce immune responses that best mimic natural convalescence from cholera (90). Until the advent of recombinant DNA technology, attenuated live oral cholera vaccines consisting of naturally occurring environmental or chemically mutagenized strains were tested and shown to stimulate anticolonizing and antitoxic immunity to cholera (98). However, because of relatively high reactogenicity (mild diarrhea in almost 25% of volunteers) and the possibility of reversion to toxigenicity, these vaccine constructs have been supplanted by genetically attenuated vaccine strains. A live attenuated vaccine containing the genetically manipulated *V. cholerae* O1 strain CVD 103-HgR protected adult volunteers against challenge with *V. cholerae* (107). However, results of a large-scale field trial carried out in Indonesia for 4 years have shown surprisingly low protection (108).

Presently, new vaccine strains are being constructed by mutagenesis of motility and chemotaxis genes in order to reduce reactogenicity of the vaccines (90). Another safety concern associated with live cholera vaccine is a possible horizontal gene transfer and recombination event that causes reversion to virulence. Therefore, potential vaccine strains have been generated in which the CTX genetic element (a site-specific transposon containing all cholera toxin genes), its chromosomal target site for insertion, and the recombinase A gene have been removed, thereby inactivating both site-specific and homologous recombination in the vaccine strain. Such constructs offer an extremely high level of safety in terms of recombinational reversion (90).

Vaccines Against Invasive Dysenteric and Enteric-Fever Infections: Salmonella

Typhoid fever, an acute infection of the reticuloendothelial system, the lymphoid tissue of the intestine, and the gall bladder, is caused by the encapsulated *S. typhi*. Two to five percent of patients become chronic gall bladder carriers. Fimbriae mediate the initial adherence of typhoid bacilli to enterocytes or to M cells in the small intestine. The attachment activates a bacterially encoded type III protein secretion system that delivers several bacterial proteins into the host cytosol, thereby causing membrane ruffling through actin cytoskeleton rearrangement and bacterial internalization by micropinocytosis. Inside the epithelial cell, *Salmonella* removes its vacuole from the normal endocytic route, produces proteins that neutralize lysosomal killing mechanisms, and transverses the intestinal membrane to enter macrophages in the lamina propria. *Salmonella* resides in intracytoplasmic vacuoles, where it replicates, induces apoptosis, and escapes to invade other macrophages and the bloodstream.

Two new vaccines against *Salmonella* infections have now been developed and licensed—a live attenuated whole-cell vaccine and a polysaccharide-based vaccine. Newer typhoid vaccines undergoing clinical testing include recombinant attenuated *S. typhi* strains and Vi polysaccharide/carrier-protein conjugate vaccines.

Salmonella typhi Ty21a is a Vi polysaccharide– and Gal E–deficient mutant that is derived by chemical mutagenesis. O antigen (polysaccharide chain of the LPS)–specific antibody-secreting cells (ASCs) in the peripheral blood have been used as a reflection of the mucosal immune response to Ty21a vaccine (109). Specific ASCs appear temporarily in human blood as a response to both oral and parenteral vaccination (110). O antigen–specific ASCs (IgA dominating) are found in humans vaccinated with live oral or killed oral *S. typhi* Ty21a vaccine; however, the response to the live vaccine is significantly stronger and lasts longer (110). The route of administration influences the antigenic specificity of the vaccine response; the response after oral vaccination is almost exclusively directed to the surface O antigen, whereas after parenteral vaccination an equally strong response is directed to the O antigen, to the lipopolysaccharide core, and to flagella (110). The gut-induced Ty21a-specific ASCs home to the gut (i.e., their final effector site), while the parenterally induced ASCs home mostly to the systemic compartment, although some express mucosal homing receptors (111). In a 7-year follow-up study of the live attenuated Ty21a vaccine in Chile (a three-dose regimen, with doses given 2 days apart), 67% of school-age children were protected against bacteriologically confirmed typhoid fever (112).

An alternative parenteral vaccine is based on purified polysaccharide (Vi) from *S. typhi* (113,114). Even though the great majority of patients recovering from typhoid fever do not develop high titers of Vi-specific antibodies (115), a single dose of Vi polysaccharide provided up to 72% protection after 2 years and up to 55% protection after 5 years (116,117). The polysaccharide vaccine induced a significant increase in Vi-specific serum antibodies that lasted for at least 12 months (116). The serologic correlate of protection (antibodies to Vi) was estimated to be 1 μg/mL in an endemic area (118).

Several experimental vaccines, such as single-dose oral vaccines produced by genetic engineering and Vi polysaccharide conjugate vaccines, are under development.

References

1. Abrutyn E. Tetanus. In: Fauci AS, Braunwald E, Isselbacher KJ, eds. Harrison's principles of internal medicine. 14th ed. New York: McGraw-Hill, 1998:901–904.
2. Janeway CAJ, Travers P. Immunobiology: the immune system in health and disease. 3rd ed. New York: Current Biology/Garland, 1997.
3. Lambert PH, Siegrist CA. Science, medicine, and the future. Vaccines and vaccination. BMJ 1997;315(7122):1595–1598.
4. Keusch GT, Bart KJ. Immunization principles and vaccine use. In: Fauci AS, Braunwald E, Isselbacher KJ, eds. Harrison's principles of internal medicine. 14th ed. New York: McGraw-Hill, 1998:758–771.
5. Furlong ST, David JR. Adjuvants. In: Austen KF, Burakoff SJ, Rosen FS, Strom TB, eds. Therapeutic immunology. Cambridge: Blackwell Science, 1996:605–614.
6. Wolff JA, Malone RW, Williams P, et al. Direct gene transfer into mouse muscle in vivo. Science 1990;247(4949 Pt 1):1465–1468.
7. Tang DC, DeVit M, Johnston SA. Genetic immunization is a simple method for eliciting an immune response. Nature 1992;356(6365):152–154.
8. Ulmer JB, Donnelly JJ, Parker SE, et al. Heterologous protection against influenza by injection of DNA encoding a viral protein [see comments]. Science 1993;259(5102):1745–1749.
9. Wang R, Doolan DL, Le TP, et al. Induction of antigen-specific cytotoxic T lymphocytes in humans by a malaria DNA vaccine. Science 1998;282(5388):476–480.
10. Donnelly JJ, Ulmer JB, Shiver JW, Liu MA. DNA vaccines. Annu Rev Immunol 1997;15:617–648.
11. Robinson H. DNA vaccines. In: Austen KF, Burakoff SJ, Rosen FS, Strom TB, eds. Therapeutic immunology. 2nd ed. Cambridge: Blackwell Science, 2000:430–440.
12. Chow JC, Young DW, Golenbock DT, et al. Toll-like receptor-4 mediates lipopolysaccharide-induced signal transduction. J Biol Chem 1999;274(16):10689–10692.
13. Kirschning CJ, Wesche H, Merrill Ayres T, Rothe M. Human toll-like receptor 2 confers responsiveness to bacterial lipopolysaccharide. J Exp Med 1998;188(11):2091–2097.
14. Rietschel ET, Schletter J, Weidemann B, et al. Lipopolysaccharide and peptidoglycan: CD14-dependent bacterial inducers of inflammation. Microb Drug Resist 1998;4(1):37–44.
15. Yoshimura A, Lien E, Ingalls RR, et al. Cutting edge: recognition of gram-positive bacterial cell wall components by the innate immune system occurs via toll-like receptor 2. J Immunol 1999;163:1–5.
16. Ulevitch RJ, Tobias PS. Receptor-dependent mechanisms of cell stimulation by bacterial endotoxin. Annu Rev Immunol 1995;13:437–457.
17. Pier GB, Kasper DL. Bacteria. In: Frank MM, Austen KF, Claman HN, Unanue ER, eds. Samter's immunologic diseases. 5th ed. Boston: Little, Brown and Company, 1995:1393–1412.
18. Goldschneider I, Gotschlich EC, Artenstein MS. Human immunity to the meningococcus. I. The role of humoral antibodies. J Exp Med 1969;129(6):1307–1326.
19. Lobeck K, Drevet P, Leonetti M, et al. Towards a recombinant vaccine against diphtheria toxin. Infect Immun 1998;66(2):418–423.
20. Bennett MJ, Eisenberg D. Refined structure of monomeric diphtheria toxin at 2.3 Å resolution. Protein Sci 1994;3(9):1464–1475.
21. Gross R, Rappuoli R. Diphtheria. In: Cryz SJ Jr, ed. Vaccines and immunotherapy. New York: Pergamon, 1991:1–12.
22. Holmes RK. Diphtheria, other corynebacterial infections, and anthrax. In: Fauci AS, Braunwald E, Isselbacher KJ, eds. Harrison's principles of internal medicine. 14th ed. New York: McGraw-Hill, 1998:892–899.
23. Galazka AM, Robertson SE, Oblapenko GP: Resurgence of diphtheria. Eur J Epidemiol 1995;11(1):95–105.
24. Galazka AM, Robertson SE. Diphtheria: changing patterns in the developing world and the industrialized world. Eur J Epidemiol 1995;11(1):107–117.
25. Habig WH, Tankersley DL. Tetanus. In: Cryz SJ Jr, ed. Vaccines and immunotherapy. New York: Pergamon, 1991:13–19.
26. Umland TC, Wingert LM, Swaminathan S, et al. Structure of the receptor binding fragment HC of tetanus neurotoxin [letter]. Nat Struct Biol 1997;4(10):788–792.
27. Granstrom M, Blennow M, Winberry L. Pertussis vaccine. In: Cryz SJ Jr, ed. Vaccines and immunotherapy. New York: Pergamon, 1991:20–35.
28. Siber GR, Samore MH. Pertussis. In: Fauci AS, Braunwald E, Isselbacher KJ, eds. Harrison's principles of internal medicine. 14th ed. New York: McGraw-Hill, 1998:933–936.
29. Greco D, Salmaso S, Mastrantonio P, et al. A controlled trial of two acellular vaccines and one whole-cell vaccine against pertussis. Progetto Pertosse Working Group [see comments]. N Engl J Med 1996;334(6):341–348.
30. Olin P, Rasmussen F, Gustafsson L, et al. Randomised controlled trial of two-component, three-component, and five-component acellular pertussis vaccines compared with whole-cell pertussis vaccine. Ad Hoc Group for the Study of Pertussis Vaccines [see comments] [published erratum appears in Lancet 1998 Feb 7;351(9100):454]. Lancet 1997;350(9091):1569–1577.
31. Scott PT, Clark JB, Miser WF. Pertussis: an update on primary prevention and outbreak control. Am Fam Physician 1997;56:1121–1128.
32. Mahon BP, Sheahan BJ, Griffin F, et al. Atypical disease after *Bordetella pertussis* respiratory infection of mice with targeted disruptions of interferon-gamma receptor or immunoglobulin mu chain genes. J Exp Med 1997;186(11):1843–1851.
33. Mills KH, Barnard A, Watkins J, Redhead K. Cell-mediated immunity to *Bordetella pertussis*: role of Th1 cells in bacterial clearance in a murine respiratory infection model. Infect Immun 1993;61(2):399–410.
34. Storsaeter J, Hallander HO, Gustafsson L, Olin P. Levels of anti-pertussis antibodies related to protection after household exposure to *Bordetella pertussis* [see comments]. Vaccine 1998;16(20):1907–1916.
35. Gustafsson L, Hallander HO, Olin P, et al. A controlled trial of a two-component acellular, a five-component acellular, and a whole-cell pertussis vaccine [see comments] [pub-

lished erratum appears in N Engl J Med 1996 May 2;334(18):1207]. N Engl J Med 1996;334(6):349–355.

36. Mooi FR, van Oirschot H, Heuvelman K, et al. Polymorphism in the *Bordetella pertussis* virulence factors P.69/pertactin and pertussis toxin in the Netherlands: temporal trends and evidence for vaccine-driven evolution. Infect Immun 1998;66(2):670–675.

37. Guttormsen H-K, Wetzler LM, Finberg RW, Kasper DL. Immunologic memory induced by a glycoconjugate vaccine in a murine adoptive lymphocyte transfer model. Infect Immun 1998;66:2026–2032.

38. Garner CV, Pier GB. Immunologic considerations for the development of conjugate vaccines. In: Cruse JM, Lewis REJ, eds. Conjugate vaccines. Vol. 10. Basel: Karger, 1989:11–17.

39. Stein KE. Glycoconjugate vaccines. What next? Int J Technol Assess Health Care 1994;10:167–176.

40. Guttormsen H-K, Sharpe AH, Chandraker AK, et al. Cognate stimulatory B-/T-cell interactions are critical for T-cell help recruited by glycoconjugate vaccines. Infect Immun 1999 (in press).

41. Schweitzer AN, Sharpe AH. The complexity of the B7-CD28/CTLA-4 costimulatory pathway. Agents Actions Suppl 1998;49:33–43.

42. Sharpe AH. Analysis of lymphocyte costimulation in vivo using transgenic and "knockout" mice. Curr Opin Immunol 1995;7(3):389–395.

43. Viola A, Schroeder S, Sakakibara Y, Lanzavecchia A. T lymphocyte costimulation mediated by reorganization of membrane microdomains [see comments]. Science 1999;283(5402):680–682.

44. Musher DM. Pneumococcal infections. In: Fauci AS, Braunwald E, Isselbacher KJ, eds. Harrison's principles of internal medicine. 14th ed. New York: McGraw-Hill, 1998:869–875.

45. Shapiro ED. Pneumococcal vaccine. In: Cryz SJ Jr, ed. Vaccines and immunotherapy. New York: Pergamon, 1991:127–139.

46. Shapiro ED, Clemens JD. A controlled evaluation of the protective efficacy of pneumococcal vaccine for patients at high risk of serious pneumococcal infections. Ann Intern Med 1984;101(3):325–330.

47. Santosham M, Reid R, Ambrosino DM, et al. Prevention of *Haemophilus influenzae* type b infections in high-risk infants treated with bacterial polysaccharide immune globulin. N Engl J Med 1987;317(15):923–929.

48. Smith DH, Peter G, Ingram DL, et al. Responses of children immunized with the capsular polysaccharide of *Hemophilus influenzae*, type b. Pediatrics 1973;52(5):637–644.

49. Robbins JB, Schneerson R, Anderson P, Smith DH. The 1996 Albert Lasker Medical Research Awards. Prevention of systemic infections, especially meningitis, caused by *Haemophilus influenzae* type b. Impact on public health and implications for other polysaccharide-based vaccines. JAMA 1996;276(14):1181–1185.

50. Schneerson R, Barrera O, Sutton A, Robbins JB. Preparation, characterization, and immunogenicity of *Haemophilus influenzae* type b polysaccharide-protein conjugates. J Exp Med 1980;152(2):361–376.

51. Anderson P. Antibody responses to *Haemophilus influenzae* type b and diphtheria toxin induced by conjugates of oligosaccharides of the type b capsule with the nontoxic protein CRM197. Infect Immun 1983;39(1):233–238.

52. Anderson P, Pichichero ME, Insel RA. Immunization of 2-month-old infants with protein-coupled oligosaccharides derived from the capsule of *Haemophilus influenzae* type b. J Pediatr 1985;107(3):346–351.

53. Granoff DM, Anderson EL, Osterholm MT, et al. Differences in the immunogenicity of three *Haemophilus influenzae* type b conjugate vaccines in infants. J Pediatr 1992;121(2):187–194.

54. Eskola J, Peltola H, Takala AK, et al. Efficacy of *Haemophilus influenzae* type b polysaccharide-diphtheria toxoid conjugate vaccine in infancy. N Engl J Med 1987;317(12):717–722.

55. Adams WG, Deaver KA, Cochi SL, et al. Decline of childhood *Haemophilus influenzae* type b (Hib) disease in the Hib vaccine era [see comments]. JAMA 1993;269(2):221–226.

56. Peltola H, Kilpi T, Anttila M. Rapid disappearance of *Haemophilus influenzae* type b meningitis after routine childhood immunisation with conjugate vaccines. Lancet 1992;340(8819):592–594.

57. Booy R, Heath PT, Slack MP, et al. Vaccine failures after primary immunisation with *Haemophilus influenzae* type-b conjugate vaccine without booster [see comments] [published erratum appears in Lancet 1997 May 31;349(9065):1630]. Lancet 1997;349(9060):1197–1202.

58. Barbour ML, Mayon-White RT, Coles C, et al. The impact of conjugate vaccine on carriage of *Haemophilus influenzae* type b. J Infect Dis 1995;171(1):93–98.

59. Galil K, Singleton R, Levine OS, et al. Reemergence of invasive *Haemophilus influenzae* type b disease in a well-vaccinated population in remote Alaska. J Infect Dis 1999;179(1):101–106.

60. Ward JI, Margolis HS, Lum MK, et al. *Haemophilus influenzae* disease in Alaskan Eskimos: characteristics of a population with an unusual incidence of invasive disease. Lancet 1981;1(8233):1281–1285.

61. Barbour ML. Conjugate vaccines and the carriage of *Haemophilus influenzae* type b. Emerg Infect Dis 1996;2(3):176–182.

62. Vella PP, Marburg S, Staub JM, et al. Immunogenicity of conjugate vaccines consisting of pneumococcal capsular polysaccharide types 6B, 14, 19F, and 23F and a meningococcal outer membrane protein complex. Infect Immun 1992;60(12):4977–4983.

63. Steinhoff MC, Edwards K, Keyserling H, et al. A randomized comparison of three bivalent *Streptococcus pneumoniae* glycoprotein conjugate vaccines in young children: effect of polysaccharide size and linkage characteristics. Pediatr Infect Dis J 1994;13(5):368–372.

64. Kayhty H, Ahman H, Ronnberg PR, et al. Pneumococcal polysaccharide-meningococcal outer membrane protein complex conjugate vaccine is immunogenic in infants and children. J Infect Dis 1995;172(5):1273–1278.

65. Kayhty H, Eskola J. New vaccines for the prevention of pneumococcal infections. Emerg Infect Dis 1996;2(4):289–298.

66. Peltola H. Meningococcal vaccines. Current status and future possibilities. Drugs 1998;55(3):347–366.

67. Al'Aldeen AA, Cartwright KA. *Neisseria meningitidis*: vaccines and vaccine candidates. J Infect 1996;33(3):153–157.

68. Anderson EL, Bowers T, Mink CM, et al. Safety and immunogenicity of meningococcal A and C polysaccharide

conjugate vaccine in adults. Infect Immun 1994;62(8): 3391–3395.

69. Lieberman JM, Chiu SS, Wong VK, et al. Safety and immunogenicity of a serogroups A/C *Neisseria meningitidis* oligosaccharide-protein conjugate vaccine in young children. A randomized controlled trial. JAMA 1996;275(19): 1499–1503.

70. Anderson EL, Kennedy DJ, Geldmacher KM, et al. Immunogenicity of heptavalent pneumococcal conjugate vaccine in infants. J Pediatr 1996;128(5 Pt 1):649–653.

71. Dagan R, Melamed R, Zamir O, Leroy O. Safety and immunogenicity of tetravalent pneumococcal vaccines containing 6B, 14, 19F and 23F polysaccharides conjugated to either tetanus toxoid or diphtheria toxoid in young infants and their boosterability by native polysaccharide antigens. Pediatr Infect Dis J 1997;16(11):1053–1059.

72. Rennels MB, Edwards KM, Keyserling HL, et al. Safety and immunogenicity of heptavalent pneumococcal vaccine conjugated to CRM197 in United States infants. Pediatrics 1998;101(4 Pt 1):604–611.

73. Ahman H, Kayhty H, Lehtonen H, et al. *Streptococcus pneumoniae* capsular polysaccharide-diphtheria toxoid conjugate vaccine is immunogenic in early infancy and able to induce immunologic memory. Pediatr Infect Dis J 1998; 17(3):211–216.

74. Richmond P, Borrow R, Miller E, et al. Meningococcal serogroup C conjugate vaccine is immunogenic in infancy and primes for memory. J Infect Dis 1999;179(6):1569–1572.

75. Madoff LC, Kasper DL. Introduction to infectious diseases: host-parasite interaction. In: Fauci AS, Braunwald E, Isselbacher KJ, eds. Harrison's principles of internal medicine. 14th ed. New York: McGraw-Hill, 1998:749–754.

76. Kaufmann SH, Hess J. Impact of intracellular location of and antigen display by intracellular bacteria: implications for vaccine development. Immunol Lett 1999;65(1–2):81–84.

77. Bhardwaj V, Kanagawa O, Swanson PE, Unanue ER. Chronic *Listeria* infection in SCID mice: requirements for the carrier state and the dual role of T cells in transferring protection or suppression. J Immunol 1998;160(1):376–384.

78. Hopewell PC. Impact of human immunodeficiency virus infection on the epidemiology, clinical features, management, and control of tuberculosis. Clin Infect Dis 1992; 15(3):540–547.

79. Flynn JL, Chan J, Triebold KJ, et al. An essential role for interferon gamma in resistance to *Mycobacterium tuberculosis* infection. J Exp Med 1993;178(6):2249–2254.

80. Anonymous. Proceedings of a symposium on genetics and tuberculosis. Cape Town, South Africa, 18–20 November 1997. Novartis Foundation Symposium 1998;217:1–269.

81. Howard AD, Zwilling BS. Reactivation of tuberculosis is associated with a shift from type 1 to type 2 cytokines. Clin Exp Immunol 1999;115(3):428–434.

82. Raviglione MC, O'Brien RJ. Tuberculosis. In: Fauci AS, Braunwald E, Isselbacher KJ, eds. Harrison's principles of internal medicine. 14th ed. New York: McGraw-Hill, 1998;1004–1014.

83. Colditz GA, Brewer TF, Berkey CS, et al. Efficacy of BCG vaccine in the prevention of tuberculosis. Meta-analysis of the published literature [see comments]. JAMA 1994;271 (9):698–702.

84. Esin S, Batoni G, Kallenius G, et al. Proliferation of distinct human T cell subsets in response to live, killed or soluble extracts of *Mycobacterium tuberculosis* and *Myco. avium*. Clin Exp Immunol 1996;104(3):419–425.

85. Horwitz MA, Lee BW, Dillon BJ, Harth G. Protective immunity against tuberculosis induced by vaccination with major extracellular proteins of *Mycobacterium tuberculosis*. Proc Natl Acad Sci USA 1995;92(5):1530–1534.

86. Huygen K, Content J, Denis O, et al. Immunogenicity and protective efficacy of a tuberculosis DNA vaccine [see comments]. Nat Med 1996;2(8):893–898.

87. Mayer L. Current concepts in mucosal immunity. I. Antigen presentation in the intestine: new rules and regulations. Am J Physiol 1998;274(1 Pt 1):G7–G9.

88. Neutra MR. Current concepts in mucosal immunity. V. Role of M cells in transepithelial transport of antigens and pathogens to the mucosal immune system. Am J Physiol 1998;274(5 Pt 1):G785–G791.

89. Brandtzaeg P, Baekkevold ES, Farstad IN, et al. Regional specialization in the mucosal immune system: what happens in the microcompartments? Immunol Today 1999;20(3): 141–151.

90. Mekalanos JJ, Sadoff JC. Cholera vaccines: fighting an ancient scourge. Science 1994;265(5177):1387–1389.

91. Jertborn M, Ahren C, Holmgren J, Svennerholm AM. Safety and immunogenicity of an oral inactivated enterotoxigenic *Escherichia coli* vaccine. Vaccine 1998;16(2–3):255–260.

92. Ahren C, Wenneras C, Holmgren J, Svennerholm AM. Intestinal antibody response after oral immunization with a prototype cholera B subunit-colonization factor antigen enterotoxigenic *Escherichia coli* vaccine. Vaccine 1993;11 (9):929–934.

93. Bloom PD, Boedeker EC. Mucosal immune responses to intestinal bacterial pathogens. Semin Gastrointest Dis 1996;7(3):151–166.

94. Holmgren J, Svennerholm AM. Bacterial enteric infections and vaccine development. Gastroenterol Clin North Am 1992;21(2):283–302.

95. Parsot C, Taxman E, Mekalanos JJ. ToxR regulates the production of lipoproteins and the expression of serum resistance in *Vibrio cholerae*. Proc Natl Acad Sci USA 1991;88(5):1641–1645.

96. DiRita VJ, Parsot C, Jander G, Mekalanos JJ. Regulatory cascade controls virulence in *Vibrio cholerae*. Proc Natl Acad Sci USA 1991;88(12):5403–5407.

97. Keusch GT, Deresiewicz RL. Cholera and other vibrioses. In: Fauci AS, Braunwald E, Isselbacher KJ, eds. Harrison's principles of internal medicine. 14th ed. New York: McGraw-Hill, 1998;962–968.

98. Kaper JB, Levine MM. Cholera. In: Cryz SJ Jr, ed. Vaccines and immunotherapy. New York: Pergamon, 1991:73–85.

99. Black RE, Levine MM, Clements ML, et al. Protective efficacy in humans of killed whole-vibrio oral cholera vaccine with and without the B subunit of cholera toxin. Infect Immun 1987;55(5):1116–1120.

100. Holmgren J, Clemens J, Sack DA, Svennerholm AM. New cholera vaccines. Vaccine 1989;7(2):94–96.

101. Clemens JD, Sack DA, Harris JR, et al. Field trial of oral cholera vaccines in Bangladesh: results from three-year follow-up [see comments]. Lancet 1990;335(8684): 270–273.

102. van Loon FP, Clemens JD, Chakraborty J, et al. Field trial of inactivated oral cholera vaccines in Bangladesh: results from 5 years of follow-up. Vaccine 1996;14(2):162–166.

103. Clemens J, Sack D, Rao M, et al. The design and analysis of cholera vaccine trials: recent lessons from Bangladesh. Int J Epidemiol 1993;22(4):724–730.

104. Large epidemic of cholera-like disease in Bangladesh caused by *Vibrio cholerae* O139 synonym Bengal. Cholera Working Group, International Centre for Diarrhoeal Diseases Research, Bangladesh [see comments]. Lancet 1993; 342(8868):387–390.

105. Levine MM, Noriega F. A review of the current status of enteric vaccines. PNG Med J 1995;38(4):325–331.

106. Levine MM. Oral vaccines against cholera: lessons from Vietnam and elsewhere [comment] [see comments]. Lancet 1997;349(9047):220–221.

107. Levine MM, Kaper JB, Herrington D, et al. Safety, immunogenicity, and efficacy of recombinant live oral cholera vaccines, CVD 103 and CVD 103-HgR. Lancet 1988;2 (8609):467–470.

108. Fournier JM, Villeneuve S. [Cholera update and vaccination problems]. Med Trop (Mars) 1998;58(2):32–35.

109. Kantele A, Arvilommi H, Jokinen I. Specific immunoglobulin-secreting human blood cells after peroral vaccination against *Salmonella typhi*. J Infect Dis 1986;153 (6):1126–1131.

110. Kantele A, Arvilommi H, Kantele JM, et al. Comparison of the human immune response to live oral, killed oral or killed parenteral *Salmonella typhi* TY21A vaccines. Microb Pathog 1991;10(2):117–126.

111. Kantele A, Kantele JM, Savilahti E, et al. Homing potentials of circulating lymphocytes in humans depend on the site of activation: oral, but not parenteral, typhoid vaccination induces circulating antibody-secreting cells that all bear homing receptors directing them to the gut. J Immunol 1997;158(2):574–579.

112. Levine MM, Ferreccio C, Black RE, Germanier R. Large-scale field trial of Ty21a live oral typhoid vaccine in enteric-coated capsule formulation. Lancet 1987;1(8541):1049–1052.

113. Levin DM, Wong KH, Reynolds HY, et al. Vi antigen from *Salmonella typhosa* and immunity against typhoid fever. 11. Safety and antigenicity in humans. Infect Immun 1975;12(6): 1290–1294.

114. Robbins JD, Robbins JB. Reexamination of the protective role of the capsular polysaccharide (Vi antigen) of *Salmonella typhi*. J Infect Dis 1984;150(3):436–449.

115. Levine MM, Hone DM. Typhoid fever. In: Cryz SJ Jr, ed. Vaccines and immunotherapy. New York: Pergamon, 1991:59–72.

116. Klugman KP, Gilbertson IT, Koornhof HJ, et al. Protective activity of Vi capsular polysaccharide vaccine against typhoid fever. Lancet 1987;2(8569):1165–1169.

117. Acharya IL, Lowe CU, Thapa R, et al. Prevention of typhoid fever in Nepal with the Vi capsular polysaccharide of *Salmonella typhi*. A preliminary report. N Engl J Med 1987;317 (18):1101–1104.

118. Klugman KP, Koornhof HJ, Robbins JB, Le Cam NN. Immunogenicity, efficacy and serological correlate of protection of *Salmonella typhi* Vi capsular polysaccharide vaccine three years after immunization. Vaccine 1996;14(5): 435–438.

Chapter 30

Viral Vaccines

Ronald W. Ellis

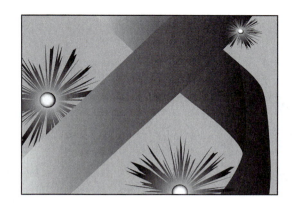

Immunization has had a tremendous impact on public health over the last century. With the possible exception of clean water, immunization has had more impact on reducing mortality and enabling population growth than any other health measure. Moreover, immunization against smallpox virus resulted in the eradication of a human disease, the first disease ever eliminated from our planet. Poliovirus vaccine is so effective in immunization programs that polio may become the second human disease to be eradicated. Several other viral vaccines are contributing significantly to the worldwide control of disease. This chapter begins with a presentation of the major technologies used for currently licensed and key experimental viral vaccines and then reviews key aspects of the design of each major viral vaccine, immunogenicity and efficacy, prospects for improvement or further development, and (for licensed vaccines) current recommendations for use.

All licensed viral vaccines are prophylactic (i.e., preventive). In the cases of hepatitis B virus (HBV), human immunodeficiency virus type 1 (HIV-1), human papilloma virus (HPV), and herpes simplex virus (HSV), there are therapeutic vaccines under development for the treatment of chronically infected individuals. However, until the first therapeutic viral vaccine is licensed, such vaccines will remain significant challenges for development.

The focus in this chapter will be on *active* vaccines, which are defined as vaccines that stimulate an immune response. There also are *passive* vaccines, which are preparations of antibodies that can be used for the short-term prevention of infection in at-risk individuals. Passive vaccines generally are used in cases where there is acute exposure to a virus, such that antibodies provide an immediate immunologic benefit more rapidly than an active vaccine could elicit an immune response. Alternatively, a passive vaccine may be used for prophylaxis in at-risk individuals when an active vaccine is not available, as in the case of the recently licensed monoclonal antibody preparation for immunoprophylaxis of infections by respiratory syncytial virus (RSV) in premature infants (1).

There may be an immune response to a particular vaccine that correlates with its protective efficacy. Ideally, such an immune response is quantitatively or qualitatively absent or low in individuals who are susceptible to disease or infection and is present or at higher levels through naturally acquired immunity or in those who are protected following prior immunization. The laboratory parameter that is used to measure such an immune response associated with protection is called an *immunologic correlate of efficacy* (2). The best correlate of efficacy is one for which there is a clearly identified assay, known as a *surrogate assay*. A defined level of antibodies (or measurement of another type of immune response) associated with protection is known as the *seroprotective level* of antibodies, although it should be noted that a seroprotective level generally is relative, not absolute. For some infectious diseases, especially those with relatively long incubation periods, induction of seroconversion by vaccines is paralleled by the induction of immunologic memory, the latter providing a mechanism for long-term protection even if antibody titers wane or disappear.

Technologies for Making Viral Vaccines

There are three general types of active vaccines. *Live* vaccines are able to replicate in host cells. Such vaccines are developed from viruses isolated in vivo. *Subunit* (including *inactivated*) vaccines consist of protein components and are unable to replicate in host cells. *Nucleic acid* vaccines are nucleic acids that stimulate the synthesis of the viral vaccine antigen only on entry into host cells. In addition, there are numerous enabling technologies that complement these three types of vaccines.

Live Vaccines

Live viral vaccines are able to infect the host and induce an immune response that is often as broad as that induced by the wild-type virus. Live viruses isolated from humans are pathogenic. Therefore, such viruses must be attenuated (i.e., weakened in their infectivity) in order to develop live vaccines. Historically, this has been done by passaging the viruses in cell culture. Since most viruses lack suitable animal models for evaluating infectivity and pathogenicity, attenuation can be proven definitively only in humans. Other live vaccines are derived from related animal viruses. Although such viruses are naturally attenuated for humans, further passage in cell culture may be required for full attenuation. Another type of live viral vaccine, especially developed for influenza and RSV vaccines, is cold-adapted (*ca*) by passage in culture at reduced temperature. A further mechanism of attenuation is to use recombinant DNA (rDNA) techniques to eliminate particular viral genes required for infectivity or pathogenicity. A virus attenuated by any of the above means may be used as a live vector for the expression of a foreign antigen derived from another virus. For this purpose, the gene encoding the foreign antigen is integrated at a nonessential point in the viral genome under the control of a viral promoter, such that the foreign antigen is expressed in the course of viral infection. Viral vectors may be DNA or RNA viruses. Following infection, viral vectors may replicate productively in the host or may induce an abortive infection in a single round without yielding progeny virus. In either case, the foreign antigen may trigger an antibody- and/or cell-based immune response.

Subunit and Inactivated Vaccines

Subunit and inactivated vaccines are unable to replicate in the host. They act as immunogens that induce immune responses (generally antibody-based responses) against their respective pathogens. Subunit viral vaccines consist of purified viral proteins, almost always recombinant-derived. The commonly used recombinant host cells include bacteria cells (*Escherichia coli*), yeast cells (*Saccharomyces cerevisiae, Pichia pastoris*), insect cells (infected by recombinant baculovirus), and mammalian cells [Chinese hamster ovary (CHO) cells]. More recently, plants, such as tomatoes, tobacco, and potatoes, have been used as recombinant host systems (3). Vaccine antigens may be purified from such plants, or the entire plant or its parts can be fed per se. Other nonreplicating vaccines are inactivated whole viruses or their parts (split vaccine). Inactivated whole viral vaccines may be especially potent immunologically by virtue of their presenting highly antigenic conformational epitopes. The expression in eukaryotic cells of the genes encoding certain viral structural proteins may result in the formation of virus-like particles (VLPs). This was shown first for HBV, and then subsequently of HPV, rotavirus, and parvovirus, as discussed below. Recombinant VLPs, like inactivated whole viruses, have been shown to be highly immunogenic. In some cases, VLPs have been used to display immunogenic epitopes from surface proteins of other viruses, with the goal of eliciting a protective immune response against the second virus as well. Peptides constituting B- and/or T-cell epitopes from protein antigens also have been used as candidate vaccines, although such vaccines generally require modifications or adjuvantation in order to enhance their immunogenicity.

Nucleic Acid Vaccines

Such vaccines are based on nucleic acids that are taken up by cells, in which they direct the synthesis of vaccine antigens that are directed to the surface of the cell; the antigen then stimulates antibody- and/or cell-based immune responses (4). Such vaccines are usually DNA molecules that are constructed as plasmids containing a eukaryotic transcriptional promoter, the gene encoding the vaccine antigen of interest, and a transcriptional terminator. The prototype genetic vaccine consists of purified plasmid DNA molecules. Attention is now focused on ways in which to facilitate the uptake of DNA by cells and thereby increase the level of vaccine antigen. There are chemical formulations in which the

DNA is mixed with and/or bound by other molecules. Another approach, which is a hybrid between a nucleic acid vaccine and a live vaccine, is based on a DNA plasmid being delivered by a nonreplicating virus or bacteria. Alternatively, RNA encoding a vaccine antigen can be delivered by an RNA virus. Such vaccines have been evaluated in early clinical trials and represent a very promising new approach to developing new vaccines.

Enabling Technologies

Many subunit vaccine antigens are not sufficiently immunogenic to be used by themselves as vaccines. Therefore, these antigens are formulated with other components—namely, adjuvants and/or delivery systems—in order to increase immunogenicity or to enable them to be presented through routes of administration other than injection. The one group of vaccine adjuvants that are broadly licensed, and used in most subunit/inactivated vaccines, are aluminum salts (hydroxide/phosphate/hydroxyphosphate) and calcium phosphate. The only other licensed vaccine adjuvant is MF59, an oil-in-water emulsion (5), which is licensed in Europe in an influenza vaccine. There are approximately 25 other adjuvants that have been evaluated in clinical studies (not yet licensed), including plant-derived saponins, inactivated toxins, emulsions, cytokines, and other immunomodulators (6). Several delivery systems have been designed to present antigens to certain dendritic or Langerhans' cells in order to increase immunogenicity (7). Other systems, including microparticles, may be used for intranasal (IN) or oral administration of vaccines and enable the antigen to be presented more efficiently to the mucosal immune system.

Adjuvants and delivery systems also have been used with live vaccines and genetic vaccines (4). Cytokines and immunomodulators have been used to influence the intensity and balance of immune response between antibody-mediated and cell-mediated and are included in formulations according to what is needed for the particular immunologic application. Purified DNA has been formulated with cationic lipids and other binding complexes to facilitate uptake by cells and nuclei, thereby increasing levels of gene expression and, by extension, the degree of immunogenicity.

Combination Vaccines

Given the increasing number of vaccines indicated for administration at the same time (e.g., at 2, 4, and 6 months in infants), the successful development and commercialization of combination vaccines is very beneficial for ensuring improved compliance with immunization programs. A combination vaccine is defined as a mixture of individual vaccines blended before administration in vivo so that multiple vaccines are combined in an individual injection (or by another route of administration) (8). There are two types of combination vaccines. Some are mixtures of vaccines already licensed for different diseases (e.g., measles-mumps-rubella and hepatitis A–hepatitis B). Such *multidisease combinations* are preferentially mixed at the time of manufacturing and filling into a single vial or syringe; alternatively, mixing can be

Table 30-1. Licensed Viral Vaccines

Vaccine[a]	Type[b]	Indication	Licensed[c]
Adenovirus	Live (bivalent)	Military	1980
Hepatitis A	Inactivated whole	Traveler or endemic	1995
Hepatitis A–hepatitis B	Inactivated whole + VLP[d] (mixed)	Diverse	1997
Hepatitis B	VLP[d]	Infant, child, adult	1987
Influenza	Inactivated whole or split (trivalent)	All, especially elderly	1945
Japanese encephalitis	Inactivated whole	Traveler or endemic	1992
Measles	Live	Universal toddler	1963
Measles-mumps-rubella	Live	Universal toddler	1971
Mumps	Live	Universal toddler	1967
Polio	Inactivated whole or live (trivalent)	Universal infant	1956, 1963
Rabies	Inactivated whole	Postexposure, high-risk	1980
Rotavirus	Live reassortant (quadrivalent)	Infant	1998[e]
Rubella	Live	Universal toddler	1969
Varicella	Live	Toddler	1995
Yellow fever	Live	Traveler or endemic	1953

[a] Arranged alphabetically.
[b] As described under Technologies for Making Viral Vaccines.
[c] In the United States, except for Hepatitis A–Hepatitis B in EU.
[d] Recombinant virus-like particle.
[e] Withdrawn from distribution in 1999.

performed at the time of injection. Some vaccines for a particular disease are multivalent in that the pathogen has multiple serotypes (e.g., polio, influenza, and rotavirus). Such *multivalent combinations* are mixed at the time of manufacturing into single vaccines. Formulating all such combination vaccines presents numerous challenges in terms of the technology for developing stable formulations, in addition to analytical, clinical, regulatory, and manufacturing challenges (9).

Key Viral Vaccines

Most viral vaccines that have been licensed and used worldwide, in both developed and developing countries, are live vaccines. These vaccines have had generally excellent profiles of safety and efficacy. However, most viruses for which vaccines are in preclinical or clinical phases are not amenable to a live vaccine strategy. Furthermore, issues concerning potential vaccine liabilities have discouraged many companies from developing new live attenuated vaccines except for selected applications. Therefore, most newer vaccines in development are subunit/inactivated or nucleic acid in nature. Except when stated otherwise, all the following vaccines are administered by injection, either intramuscularly (IM) or subcutaneously (SC).

Currently Licensed Vaccines

Several of the vaccines discussed below—especially the first seven—have been in widespread use for decades and have made substantial contributions to human health worldwide through the reduction of widespread morbidity and mortality. Two of these

vaccines—hepatitis A and rotavirus—were introduced for the first time in any country only in the 1990s. These vaccines are discussed in the approximate order of their licensure and availability in the United States. Salient features of the licensed vaccines are summarized in Table 30-1.

Influenza

These enveloped viruses, with segmented RNA genomes, can cause a severe respiratory disease that is highly contagious. The commonly used influenza vaccines are inactivated vaccines, which are indicated for annual immunization of older individuals. These vaccines, which have been available in the United States since 1945, are prepared following the growth of influenza virus in chicken eggs, collection of fluids, inactivation with formalin, and dilution. The vaccine is trivalent and may be either a whole-virus or (following incubation with a detergent such as deoxycholate) a split-virus vaccine. The composition of the vaccine is selected each year to contain three influenza virus serotypes (two type A and one type B) based on prevalent serotypes of the virion surface glycoprotein hemagglutinin (HA) in sentinel areas worldwide (10). The potency of the vaccine is quantified on the basis of the amount of each of the three viral HA proteins (10). Because these vaccines do not elicit group-common immunity and because serotypes can vary each year, annual single-dose immunization is indicated. However, the rate of vaccine efficacy has not been consistently higher than 70% to 80%, as has been the case for most viral vaccines. Antibodies to HA are quantified by the hemagglutination inhibition (HI) assay using red blood cells and the same antigens as those in the vaccine being evaluated (11). The titer is defined as the final serum dilution inhibiting a given number of HA units of virus. Serologic analyses also have employed a virus neutralization (Nt) assay (12). The HI and Nt assays have been used as surrogate assays for measuring anti-HA or antivirion antibodies as correlates of efficacy. The protective level of HI antibodies has been estimated at 1:32 on a calibrated scale in some studies (13,14), Each HA serotype strain protects against the homologous serotype only.

Three areas in which the inactivated vaccine can be improved are the method of cell culture production, increased immune responses to provide for higher rates of clinical efficacy, and route of administration. Growth of the virus in eggs entails logistic difficulties, lack of complete assuredness of yearly supply, and the ability of the viral HA sequence to mutate. Therefore, groups have turned to developing cell culture systems—e.g., a dog cell line (MDCK)—for growing influenza virus in bioreactors (15).

Influenza vaccines have been the objects of the largest number of vaccine studies with novel adjuvants and delivery systems, owing to the need to provide for higher rates of efficacy as wells as the widespread supply of vaccine antigens from many different manufacturers. Oil-in-water emulsions such as MF59 (5), as well as ISCOMs (Immune Stimulating COMplexes), a delivery system containing saponins as adjuvants, have been shown to increase immune responses in clinical (5) and preclinical (16) studies. Other approaches have been taken to the development of IN formulations, including the use of microparticles (17), with the goal of avoiding the use of needlesticks.

A second type of influenza vaccine, live attenuated *ca* vaccine, has been developed as an IN vaccine, with the immunologic objective that replication in the nasal cavity will mimic natural virus infection and induce significant nasal (mucosal) immune responses (18). The original virus strain was attenuated by passage in chick kidney cells at progressively lower temperatures down to 25°C (19). The potency of the virus is quantified on the basis of egg infectious doses. The resultant *ca* donor virus, adapted to efficient growth in vitro, and new virus strains selected annually are used to coinfect cells for creating *ca* reassortants that are plaque-purified for virus production in eggs. The trivalent live attenuated *ca* vaccine induces mucosal IgA, consistent with its mucosal replication. This vaccine has been shown to be efficacious in phase 3 trials (20), although a serologic correlate of protection is not yet apparent.

Nucleic acid immunization has been investigated, with the goal of eliciting a group-common immune response. It was demonstrated that immunization of mice with DNA-encoding nucleoprotein, an internal viral protein, was able to protect mice against challenge with a heterologous (with respect to HA) strain of virus (21).

Yellow Fever

Yellow fever virus (YFV) is an enveloped arbovirus with a genomic RNA encoding a single polyprotein gene product. Mosquitoes are the known vectors for virus transmission, which can result in hepatic and renal injury as well as hemorrhage and a high rate of lethality. The 17D strain, having been recommended by the World Health Organization (WHO) as the source strain for all vaccine strains (22), is the source of most commonly used vaccines. This strain was isolated from a disease case, then passaged serially in rhesus monkeys, *Aedes aegypti* mosquitoes, whole mouse embryonic tissue culture, and minced chick embryos (23). Increased passage was shown to result in a lower level of neurotropism for monkeys and mice (24). Rigorous safety testing was shown to be required, given the variation in neurovirulence observed among different substrains of 17D, including plaque variants observed on passage in Vero cells (25). The live attenuated vaccine, which was licensed in the United States in 1953, is grown for production in fertilized hens' eggs derived from a pathogen-free flock. A minimum human immunizing dose has been defined, above which there are satisfactory seroconversion rates. Because the 17D strain had been isolated and developed into a vaccine in the 1920s, double-blind, placebo-controlled efficacy studies were not run to establish a rate of efficacy. However, experience from the immunization of more than 600,000 individuals in Colombia showed more than 95% effectiveness in preventing yellow fever (26). Long-term persistence of immunity appears to be excellent (27). The vaccine is recommended as a single SC dose for travelers to or residents in endemic areas, which are mostly in tropical areas of South America and Africa.

Polio

Infection with poliovirus, a picornavirus, can result in paralytic disease. There are two types of polio vaccines that have been in widespread use for universal immunization, beginning in infants. One type, oral polio vaccine (OPV), is a trivalent mixture of live attenuated viruses grown in culture (28) and has been used in the United States since 1963. The strategy behind the use of a live vaccine was to mimic the immunobiology of natural infection and thereby stimulate longer-lasting protection against reinfection, because the natural infection confers lifelong immunity. Attenuation was made possible by the passage of polioviruses in tissues other than those from the nervous system. This resulted in a loss of the capability to replicate in the nervous system, thereby losing virulence (29). Potency of each component of the vaccine is quantified by infectious units in cell culture (30). These viruses interfere with one another in vivo, hence the full regimen of three doses is required for full immunization. Having been used worldwide for decades, OPV is on its way to potentially eradicating polio worldwide by the middle of the next decade. Immunization at 2, 4, and 6 months of age with OPV elicits serum-neutralizing antibodies in nearly 100% of infants and children following three doses (31). Immunization also elicits immunity in the gut, based on secretory IgA, which may exist even when levels of serum antibody are low (32). Given the relative ease of measuring serum antibodies as opposed to antibodies in gut secretions, the presence of detectable serum-neutralizing antibodies is accepted as the serologic correlate of protection, as commonly measured by a micro-Nt assay (33).

The second type of vaccine, inactivated polio vaccine (IPV), is made by growing and collecting poliovirus, which then is purified and inactivated with formalin (34). Like OPV, this vaccine is trivalent. Changes in the original production process (used since 1956) resulted in an enhanced IPV (eIPV), which became available in 1987 (35). Potency of IPV is quantified in vitro in terms of D-antigen units and also can be tested in animals relative to an international vaccine reference (35). One advantage of the use of IPV in developed countries is that its use does not result in vaccine-associated polio paralysis, which is a rare complication associated with the use of initial doses of OPV. The recent recommendation for polio vaccination in the United States is the use of IPV at 2 and 4 months and OPV at 6 and 15 months of age (36). Immunization at 2, 4, and 6 months of age with IPV elicits neutralizing antibodies after the first dose in nearly 100% of infants and children and secretory IgA following the second and third doses (37). There also is long-term persistence of neutralizing antibodies and priming for long-term memory (38). As with OPV, the micro-Nt assay is used as a surrogate assay for the detection of serum-neutralization antibodies, the correlate of efficacy (29). IPV has been combined with diphtheria-tetanus-pertussis (DTP) with or without hepatitis B (HB) and *Haemophilus influenzae* type *b* (Hib) vaccines into a pediatric multidisease combination vaccine.

Measles

Measles virus, a paramyxovirus (RNA genome), causes a severe skin rash that can have serious dermatologic and neurologic sequelae. The vaccine consists of live attenuated measles virus grown in cells in culture, usually chicken embryo fibroblasts (39,40). The virus is collected in culture medium and diluted in stabilizer to its final use level, then lyophilized. The potency of the vaccine is quantified on the basis of in vitro infectivity in appropriate indicator cells, in assays that measure plaque-forming units (pfu) or tissue-culture-infectious doses ($TCID_{50}$). The vaccine, first available in the United States in 1963, is indicated for immunization at 12 to 18 months of age. Some countries with a high incidence of disease in early childhood immunize children as early as 9 months of age, with some experimental vaccines having been tested as early as 6 months of age (41). The accepted immunologic correlate of efficacy is the titer of antivirion antibodies, with neutralizing antibodies being most directly related to clinical protection (42). Surrogate assays either are Nt assays or are based on the detection of such antibodies and comparison with neutralizing antibody titrations (40) utilizing a range of serologic techniques including HI, complement fixation (CF), and enzyme-linked immunosorbent assay (ELISA), with seroprotective levels defined according to the particular assay (42). There have been many measles strains evaluated clinically and used throughout the world. The vaccine has an excellent track record of safety and efficacy, as a result of which there has been very little exploration of alternative vaccine approaches.

Mumps

Mumps virus, a paramyxovirus, causes swelling of the parotid glands. The vaccine, licensed in the United States in 1967, consists of live attenuated mumps virus grown in cells in culture, usually chicken embryo fibroblasts (43). The virus is produced and its potency quantified as for measles vaccine. Primary immunization is indicated at 12 to 18 months of life. As with measles vaccine,

the immunologic correlate of efficacy against mumps has been accepted to be antibodies directed against the virion, especially virus-neutralizing antibodies. Surrogate assays either are Nt assays or are based on the detection of such antibodies and demonstration of correlation with neutralizing antibody titrations (44), utilizing serologic techniques including HI and ELISA with seroprotective levels defined accordingly. There have been only a few mumps strains developed into vaccines. Because of its excellent safety and efficacy record, there have been practically no attempts to make mumps vaccines through means other than live attenuated.

Rubella

Rubella virus, a togavirus (RNA genome), is the cause of German measles, a skin rash. The virus is highly teratogenic and has been responsible for serious birth defects in infants infected in utero. The vaccine consists of live attenuated rubella virus grown in cells in culture, usually human diploid fibroblasts (45). The virus is produced and its potency quantified as for measles vaccine. The vaccine, licensed in the United States in 1969, is indicated for immunization at 12 to 18 months of life. Some countries have focused their immunization practice on teenage girls, with the goal of establishing a high level of rubella-specific antibodies during the child-bearing period [which can be transmitted transplacentally to the fetus in order to minimize the likelihood of in utero infection with rubella virus and its teratogenic consequences (46)]. However, this strategy has proven suboptimal for control. As with measles and mumps vaccines, the immunologic correlate of efficacy has been accepted to be antibodies directed against the virion, especially virus-neutralizing antibodies. Surrogate assays either are Nt assays or are based on the detection of such antibodies (47) utilizing serologic techniques including HI, CF, and ELISA with seroprotective levels defined according to each assay. As has been documented for measles and mumps vaccines, the excellent safety and efficacy record of rubella vaccine has effectively precluded investigation of alternative vaccine approaches.

Measles-Mumps-Rubella

The three live virus vaccines have been developed as a multidisease combination vaccine (MMR), first available in the United States in 1971. The three bulk viruses in their harvested growth media are mixed to their appropriate use levels in stabilizer, then lyophilized. This vaccine is given in developed countries as a two-dose series, with primary immunization at 12 to 18 months of age and the booster dose on entry to primary or secondary school (36,48). This vaccine has been responsible for a reduction of more than 99% in the incidence of the three diseases and is very highly cost-effective. Use of the MMR vaccine may be able to eradicate the three diseases in areas where there is an intensive immunization program, such as Finland (49).

Rabies

Rabies virus, an enveloped rhabdovirus (bullet-shaped), contains a single nonsegmented RNA genome. The virus is transmitted to humans following a bite from a rabies-infected animal. Following an incubation period of 10 to 60 days, infection develops in the central nervous system and is almost uniformly 100% fatal. The modern history of this vaccine began with the classical story of Louis Pasteur's vaccine and its first field test on a boy who had been bitten by a rabid dog. The original crude vaccination method, while successful, was used only during the first half of the twentieth century. Vaccines used worldwide, based on inactivated rabies virus propagated in the brains of animals, induced significant adverse reactions owing to their crude nature and residual nervous system components. Nevertheless, such vaccines have continued to be used in developing countries because of their very low cost. Propagation of rabies virus in cell culture, followed by inactivation of culture supernatants with β-propiolactone (50), has resulted in the development of safer vaccines. The vaccine currently used in most developed countries (available in the United States since 1980) is propagated in human diploid cells. Vaccinated individuals efficiently develop virus-neutralizing antibodies, and those vaccinated subsequent to animal bites are protected from disease and death (51). For preexposure prophylaxis, the vaccine is recommended as a three-dose regimen (weeks 0, 1, and 4) administered IM. For postexposure prophylaxis, rabies immune globulin is given on day 0 and the vaccine on days 0, 3, 7, 14, and 28.

The high cost of the human diploid cell vaccine had led to the use of continuous cell lines or primary cell substrates for propagating rabies virus, followed by inactivation with β-propiolactone (52,53). Newer vaccines have been based on expression of the viral G glycoprotein in viral vectors. One such vector, recombinant poxvirus expressing G glycoprotein, has been licensed as an oral "bait" vaccine for prevention of rabies in animals (54). More recently, G glycoprotein has been expressed in a recombinant plant virus on infection of tobacco plants (55). A vaccine based on a homogenate of infected tobacco leaves (or other plant species) could be given orally and, if effective, could be a very low-cost and safe vaccine for developing countries.

Adenovirus

The adenoviruses are nonenveloped DNA viruses with an icosahedral structure. There are 47 serotypes of adenovirus, of which 14 have been associated most commonly with disease. Infection can result in pathology of the respiratory, ocular, and gastrointestinal systems. Noteworthy among associated diseases are acute respiratory disease (ARD), pneumonia, pharyngitis, and tonsillitis. Such infections are most serious in infants, children, military recruits, and immunocompromised individuals. Inactivated vaccines developed in the 1950s showed a very highly variable rate of protective efficacy (56). Because adenovirus can proliferate in the gut and induce protective antibodies, subsequent attention has focused on the development of oral live attenuated vaccines. The wild-type viruses were attenuated by passage in human cells. Although adenovirus types 4 and 7 (Ad4 and Ad7) cultivated in human embryonic kidney cells were oncogenic in hamsters, strains cultivated in WI-38 human diploid fibroblasts were not (57); therefore, available vaccine strains have been grown in WI-38 cells. Initial live vaccines were formulated in liquid or

encapsulated form. Subsequently, a tablet was developed in order to optimize virus stability in storage and during passage through gastric juice. The innermost core of the tablet contains the lyophilized vaccine strains at more than 10^5 TCID$_{50}$, which is the quantitative parameter for potency. The next layer consists of starch and binders for protection. The outermost level is an enteric coating that releases the virus only in the intestines, in which the virus stimulates a mucosal immune response. The bivalent Ad4-Ad7 vaccine shows no interference between serotypes following immunization, based on immunogenicity data. Following extensive studies in military recruits, immunization with adenovirus resulted in a 95% reduction in the incidence of ARD (58). The currently licensed vaccine, available since 1980, is bivalent and is used only in military personnel.

Adenoviruses have been developed into live vaccine vectors for expressing antigens of other viruses. A live vector expressing HBsAg from HBV (59) has been tested clinically, and a live vector expressing the core protein region of HIV-1 has been evaluated preclinically (60).

Hepatitis B

The HB virus (HBV), a hepadnavirus, can cause acute infection of the liver, which resolves in the majority of adults but in only a minority of children and infants. Unresolved infections become chronic, leading to reverse transcription and integration of HBV genomic DNA. Up to 25% of chronic infections can develop further into cirrhosis or hepatocellular carcinoma. HBV is the most common cause of infectious hepatitis that is spread perinatally, sexually, or by blood. The major envelope protein is the surface (S) protein or antigen. During HBV infection, excess S protein is secreted from infected cells as 20-nm noninfectious particles known as HB surface antigen (HBsAg) particles. These HBsAg particles were the basis for the first-generation plasma-derived HB vaccine (licensed in 1981 but no longer available commercially in the United States), which still is produced and distributed in some areas of the world, especially Asia. The S gene subsequently was expressed as recombinant proteins in the form of 20-nm particles in eukaryotic cells, particularly bakers' yeast (*Saccharomyces cerevisiae*). These particles are the basis for the second-generation recombinant-derived HB vaccine available in the United States since 1987 (61). Although smaller than HBV virions, these 20-nm particles are VLPs in that they display the major antigenic determinants of the virion. The HBsAg vaccine antigen is quantified for potency on the basis of its protein content, with dosage levels in the range of 5 to 20 μg. The vaccines are typically given to all age groups in most countries in a three-dose regimen at a schedule such as 0, 1, and 6 months, where the third dose serves to establish long-term immunologic memory following the two priming doses. The HB vaccine has been combined with Hib and with DTP + IPV + Hib into pediatric combination vaccines. The use of HB vaccine in Taiwan has resulted in a decrease in the incidence of hepatocellular carcinoma (62). This is the first example of a vaccine that can prevent the development of a type of cancer by preventing an infection.

Both types of HBsAg particles display a major conformational epitope (*a* epitope) that elicits anti-HBsAg antibodies that do not recognize individual S polypeptides. Anti-HBsAg antibodies (anti-HBs) were shown to be associated with protection against HBV infection, and efficacy studies with the plasma-derived HB vaccine demonstrated that following immunization the presence of at least 10 mIU anti-HBs/mL of serum [quantified by radioimmunoassay (RIA) and subsequently by ELISA as surrogate assays, relative to an international reference standard] confers protection against clinical infection (63). Subsequent studies demonstrated that immunization with recombinant-derived HB vaccine elicits a similar level of protective immunity as does the plasma-derived vaccine (64), as well as biologically equivalent antibodies (65). Thus, the induction of 10 mIU anti-HBs/mL or more has become accepted as the correlate of efficacy for HB. Despite waning levels of anti-HBs (<10 mIU/mL down even to undetectable levels) at 5 to 12 years after immunization, there have been very few reports of clinical HB disease among vaccinees who achieved the seroprotective level of 10 mIU anti-HBs/mL or more after primary immunization (66).

The extents of morbidity and mortality associated with chronic hepatitis B have spawned significant interest in developing a therapeutic vaccine whose goal is to clear the virus infection, as detected by the seroconversion from positivity for HBsAg to positivity for anti-HBs. Conventional HB vaccines, which are effective at eliciting anti-HBsAg antibodies, have not been shown to be effective in treating chronic HB. Some approaches have sought to induce a cytotoxic T cell (CTL) response. One of these approaches focuses on the use of peptides containing T-cell epitopes from the hepatitis B core antigen, which was shown capable of eliciting CTL responses in mice (67). Nucleic acid vaccines also are under investigation as both prophylactic and therapeutic HB vaccines.

Japanese Encephalitis

Japanese encephalitis virus (JEV), an enveloped flavivirus (RNA genome), is transmitted by mosquitoes. There are 50,000 infections per year, primarily in Asia, with a 25% rate of mortality and a high rate of neurologic sequelae. There is a single major serotype of JEV. The virus has an envelope glycoprotein (E) and membrane protein (M), both of which have been shown to elicit protective immune responses (68). Whereas recombinant vaccines based on these proteins have been evaluated recently as experimental vaccines, the licensed vaccines in widespread use are based on whole JEV, both inactivated and live attenuated. The JEV strains isolated from clinical disease cases were used to provide the prototype virus strains used for vaccine production. The most widely available vaccine is prepared by propagating the Nakayama virus strain in mouse brain, followed by enrichment, inactivation with formalin, and final purification (69). Special attention is paid to controlling the residual level of myelin basic protein at less than 2 ng/mL, which is well below the level considered to be encephalitogenic in a guinea pig test system. Licensed in the United States in 1992, the vaccine is distributed either in liquid form or lyophilized, for reconstition with sterile water. A second inactivated vaccine is prepared following propagation of the P3 virus strain in primary hamster kidney (PHK) cells (70). A live attenuated vaccine consists of the SA-14-14-2

strain propagated in PHK cells (71). The latter two vaccines are produced and distributed only in China. For the assessment of immunogenicity, a neutralizing antibody titer greater than 1:10 is considered a marker of seroconversion and a correlate of efficacy. The inactivated mouse brain vaccine has shown an approximately 90% rate of efficacy (72). However, the persistence of immunity is limited, such that an initial booster is indicated 1 year after the two-dose priming period, with further boosters indicated at 3-year intervals. There are no established efficacy data on the inactivated PHK cell vaccine. The efficacy of the live attenuated vaccine has been generally greater than 90% (73). These vaccines are indicated for residents in endemic areas, especially young children in rural areas, and for travelers to such areas and to Asia in general.

Varicella

Varicella-zoster virus (VZV), an α-herpesvirus with a large DNA genome, is the causative agent of chickenpox. Following acute infection, VZV usually causes a latent infection of neuronal cells that can persist for a lifetime and become reactivated as zoster (shingles). Varicella (chickenpox) vaccine, licensed in the United States in 1995, consists of live attenuated VZV grown in human diploid fibroblasts (74). Very little infectious virus is secreted into culture medium. Thus, the infected cells are lysed in buffer and sonicated, diluted in stabilizer to the final use level, and lyophilized. The potency of the varicella vaccine (VV) is quantified by pfu following infection of human diploid fibroblasts in vitro. For combination with other live attenuated vaccines (measles, mumps, rubella) as an experimental vaccine, the VZV-infected cell lysate is diluted appropriately, mixed with diluted culture media containing the other viruses, and lyophilized. The VV is indicated as a single dose for routine administration in children over 15 months of age, although it would not be unexpected that the vaccine be indicated in the future for a second dose later in childhood at a time similar to that for MMR vaccine. The immune response to VV in most U.S. clinical trials has been measured by an ELISA using VZV-infected cell glycoproteins (gp) as solid-phase antigen. Because the neutralizing antibody response against VZV is directed at VZV envelope gp, serum titers measured by this *gpELISA* have shown good correlation with neutralizing antibody titers (75). For VV, 1% to 3% per year of immunized children develop a mild breakthrough infection, known as modified varicella-like syndrome (MVLS), following significant exposure to wild-type VZV (76). MVLS is characterized by a reduced number of lesions (usually less than 50) and little fever exceeding 38°C compared with hundreds of lesions and a high rate of fever following natural varicella. The initial anti-VZV IgG response following VV immunization shows a rough overall correlation with protection against infection during the next 2 years (77). There are general inverse relationships both between gpELISA titer and rate of breakthrough to the development of MVLS as well as between gpELISA titer and the median number of lesions in breakthrough cases. Thus, gpELISA or another assay qualified in a similar fashion would appear to be a useful general immunologic correlate of efficacy for VV. However, this is only a trend rather than a solid correlation as in the cases of other vaccines such as HB and some live virus vaccines.

Owing to the complexity of VZV immunity, subunit vaccine approaches have not yet advanced to the clinic. The VZV vaccine strain has been developed into a live vector for the expression of antigens of other viruses (78).

Hepatitis A

The HA virus (HAV) causes acute, but not chronic, hepatitis. HAV is a picornavirus that is spread enterically, sometimes in epidemics, especially through contaminated food and water. Like poliovirus, HAV has been developed as an inactivated whole-virus vaccine; alternative technical approaches have not been successful to date. HAV is not efficiently released by cells in culture and therefore is purified from infected mammalian cells grown in vitro. The virus is inactivated by treatment with a chemical such as formalin (79). The vaccine antigen is quantified for potency on the basis of protein content or units of reactivity in a specific ELISA. The vaccine, which has been available in the United States since 1995, is indicated for immunization of those living in or traveling to endemic areas. HA vaccine is administered as a two-dose series, where the first priming dose is followed 6 months later by a dose that should establish long-term immunologic memory. The major epitopes on HAV are conformational and are not present on the individual capsid polypeptides. Anti-HAV antibodies (anti-HA) specific to such epitopes have been quantified by RIA. It first was demonstrated that passive protection against HAV infection was conferred by immune globulin (IG), because minute levels of anti-HAV IG (levels below the limits of detectability of current assays) confer protection. There is only a partially quantified correlation with the presence of detectable anti-HA (80); however, any individual with a postvaccinal detectable titer (>10 mIU anti-HA/mL) is considered protected. Immunization with inactivated HA vaccine then was demonstrated to elicit protective efficacy against HAV disease, which also was shown to correlate with the appearance of RIA-detectable anti-HA (81) and parallel induction of immunologic memory (82). As has been shown for HB vaccine, despite waning levels of anti-HA postvaccination, immunologic memory can be documented by the rapid anti-HA response following booster vaccination (83). The extent to which long-term memory is established by primary immunization with HA vaccine will be established following long-term studies of vaccinees, given that HA vaccines have been available for only a few years. Thus, RIA for the detection of anti-HA is considered a surrogate assay for the correlate of efficacy. The HA vaccine may be the most potent immunogen among all vaccines tested to date. A single dose of 50 ng was able to seroconvert most adults and to be efficacious (81,83).

Hepatitis A–Hepatitis B

This vaccine, a combination of HA and HB vaccines, was licensed in the European Union (EU) in 1997 for both adults and children. Although the two vaccines are indicated for individuals of different epidemiologic groups, this combination vaccine can be used as a convenience in giving a second important vaccine to an individual who is being immunized primarily for either HA or HB. Both vaccines consist of aluminum-adsorbed vaccine antigens that proved to be compatible on mixing, such that developing the combination proved to be relatively straightforward. Immunization with the combination vaccine in a schedule of months 0, 1, and 6 elicits levels of anti-HA and anti-HB titers comparable to those elicited by the vaccines administered at different sites (84).

Rotavirus

Rotavirus, which was discovered only 25 years ago, is the primary cause of severe dehydrating diarrhea in children and is responsible for nearly 1 million deaths worldwide per year. The rotavirus genome consists of nine double-stranded RNA segments, each of which encodes a viral protein. The oral rotavirus vaccine consists of live attenuated rotavirus grown in subhuman primate cells in culture. The virus, which has a segmented genome, is collected from culture media, diluted in stabilizer, and lyophilized. The potency of the vaccine is quantified on the basis of infectious units of each virus type in a primate cell line such as Vero (85,86). Clinical trials typically have employed a schedule of three oral doses in the first year of life, all given at the same time as other childhood vaccines such as DTP, polio, and Hib conjugate vaccine. Early vaccines consisted of rhesus (85) or bovine (86) rotaviruses, which are naturally attenuated in their infectivity for humans. These vaccines showed highly variable levels of efficacy in clinical trials and were not developed further.

There are two types of live oral vaccines. Multivalent reassortant rotaviruses consist of rhesus or bovine rotaviruses that, through genetic reassortment following coinfection with human rotavirus, contain a human rotavirus segment encoding VP7 or VP4, the virion surface proteins. Given that there are four VP7 types and one VP4 type that cause more than 90% of infections in infants, such live vaccines are multivalent mixtures of four or five reassortant rotavirus types (87,88). The quadrivalent reassortant rhesus rotavirus vaccine, licensed in the United States in 1998, was indicated for routine immunization of infants at 2, 4, and 6 months of age. It has been shown to provide approximately 50% efficacy against all rotavirus disease, 80% efficacy against serious disease, and more than 90% efficacy against the most severe rotavirus disease (87,89). However, this vaccine was withdrawn from distribution in 1999 due to an increased rate of intussusception observed postvaccination. The second type of vaccine in development is a live attenuated human rotavirus (or mixture of human rotaviruses) grown in primate cells in culture (90). In the more than 10 years during which rotavirus clinical trials have been conducted, no clear correlate of efficacy has been found (89,91).

An alternative technical approach employs the recombinant expression of rotavirus VP2 + VP4 + VP6 + VP7 or VP2 + VP4 + VP6 in eukaryotic cells to achieve the formation of rotavirus VLPs, which could be developed as an inactivated injected vaccine (92). These VLPs are morphologically highly similar to native rotavirus virions and display the neutralization epitopes of VP4 and VP7.

Table 30-2. Viral Vaccines in Development

Vaccine[a]	Type[b]
Arenavirus	Live vector[c], subunit[d]
Cytomegalovirus	Subunit, live
Dengue	Subunit, live
Epstein-Barr virus	Subunit
Filovirus	Subunit
Hepatitis A	Inactivated virosome formulation[e]
Hepatitis B	Peptides, VLP[f], VLP carrier[g], nucleic acid, therapeutic
Hepatitis C	Subunit, nucleic acid
Hepatitis E	Subunit
Herpes simplex virus	Subunit, live, nucleic acid, therapeutic
Human immunodeficiency virus type 1	Subunit, inactivated, live vector, peptide, nucleic acid, therapeutic
Human immunodeficiency virus type 2	Inactivated, subunit, nucleic acid
Human papilloma virus	VLP, live vector, therapeutic
Human T-cell leukemia virus type 1	Subunit
Influenza	Live cold-adapted, inactivated intranasal, new cell substrate, subunit, nucleic acid
Parainfluenza	Live cold-adapted, subunit, nucleic acid
Parvovirus	VLP, VLP carrier
Rabies	Live vector, plants as antigen source
Respiratory syncytial virus	Subunit, live cold-adapted, nucleic acid
Rotavirus	Live human virus, VLP
Varicella	Subunit, live vector

[a] Major vaccines in preclinical or clinical development, arranged alphabetically.
[b] As described under Technologies for Making Viral Vaccines; representative examples are not all-inclusive.
[c] Live recombinant virus expressing protein from virus of interest.
[d] Recombinant protein.
[e] Liposome-virus mixture.
[f] Recombinant virus-like particle.
[g] Expressing epitopes of another virus.

Experimental Vaccines

The vaccine candidates described in the following sections have been evaluated in advanced preclinical studies or in clinical trials, some of which have advanced to phase 3. Table 30-2 summarizes some of the significant approaches being taken to develop new vaccines or to develop alternative or improved versions of existing licensed vaccines.

Human Immunodeficiency Virus Type I

The research and development of HIV-1 vaccine arguably constitute the most challenging among all vaccines and may be considered the "Holy Grail of Vaccinology." The virus infects cells of the immune system and causes impairment of immune responses. Once infection occurs, the viral genomic RNA is reverse-transcribed and integrated, resulting in lifelong chronic infection. Furthermore, owing to an error-prone reverse transcriptase, the viral sequences mutate significantly in the course of infecting the host, resulting in an immunologic diversification that is a probable mechanism for immune evasion. There has been no clear consensus on whether inducing neutralizing antibodies or T-cell immunity (especially CTLs), or both, should be the immunobiologic objective for an HIV-1 vaccine. The major envelope glycoprotein gp120/160 has hypervariable domains that elicit neutralizing antibodies. Because an effective vaccine needs to elicit group-common immunity, combinations of gp120/160 antigens have been considered for subunit vaccines. Recombinant gp120 expressed in CHO cells is now in phase 3 clinical studies. However, some breakthrough HIV-1 infections have been observed in phase 1–2 studies, which has raised concern as to whether this subunit vaccine approach will be sufficient per se for an effective vaccine (93). Another approach that has received significant effort is the use of avipoxvirus as a vector for expressing HIV-1 genes, including envelope, core, protease, and polymerase. Avipoxvirus is the avian counterpart of human variola virus (smallpox); it is able to infect human cells but cannot produce infectious progeny. Thus, it may be useful for eliciting CTL responses to its vectored genes (i.e., HIV-1 genes) with minimal reactogenicity in humans. Several clinical trials also have examined priming with recombinant avipoxvirus vectors expressing gp120/160 followed by boosting with gp120/160 (94). This prime-boost approach appears to give better combined antibody and CTL responses than the use of either approach separately as well as long-term immunologic memory. Other approaches being used for HIV-1 vaccines include inactivated whole virus, live vectors, peptides, VLPs, and nucleic acid immunization. An effective HIV-1 vaccine may be recommended for use in individuals of all ages, especially at-risk adults.

Therapeutic immunization for HIV-1 remains especially challenging given the ability of HIV to integrate into the host genome and to initiate latent infection for essentially the lifetime of the infected individual. Progress on a therapeutic HIV-1 vaccine requires insights into the development of effective prophylactic HIV vaccines as well as useful correlates of immunity ascertained through preclinical models and long-term clinical observations.

Herpes Simplex Virus

There are two types of herpes simplex viruses—type 1 (HSV-1) and type 2 (HSV-2)—which, respectively, cause predominantly oral and genital herpes, starting in young adults. Following replication at mucosal surfaces, the virus can establish latent infection of dorsal root ganglia, which can persist for a lifetime. Once infection becomes latent, reactivation can occur at any time, resulting in local replication and evidence of vesicles or ulcers. Early investigations of live vaccines resulted in some suggestions of efficacy but also evidence of recurrent infection (95). Subsequent studies of inactivated viruses showed discrepant levels of efficacy and likewise were abandoned (96). Most recent studies have focused on subunit vaccines composed of recombinant viral glycoproteins. Among the 11 HSV glycoproteins, gB and gD have received the most attention because these glycoproteins efficiently elicit virus-neutralizing antibodies. These glycoproteins have been expressed in CHO cells in a form in which their hydrophobic anchor domain has been removed; the resultant protein is secreted by CHO cells into the growth media for ease of purification. Recombinant gB and gD have been evaluated separately and together in clinical trials, often formulated with novel adjuvants. There has been a report of protection against HSV disease as well as of the possible alleviation of the frequency of recurrent infection (97). Phase 3 trials have been undertaken to establish the efficacy profile of these subunit vaccines, although negative results have been reported following the conclusion of one of these trials (98). An effective vaccine may be useful for the immunization of young adults.

There also have been attempts to develop live genetically attenuated HSV vaccines. One such vaccine, created by deleting loci responsible for neurovirulence and recombining HSV-1 and -2 sequences, was shown to be attenuated but only weakly immunogenic in humans (99). Another live vaccine was developed by deleting the gene for gH. The resultant virus is grown in a recombinant cell that expresses the gH gene in trans, resulting in the production of a gH⁻ virus that carries gH on its surface. This DISC (disabled inactivated single cycle) virus can infect cells by virtue of its surface gH but cannot spread without genetically encoded gH (100), thus apparently combining the advantage of live infection for eliciting a broad immune response with the attenuating phenotype of lack of spread in vivo.

The goal of therapeutic HSV immunization is to prevent recurrent infections and associated symptoms. Feasibility has been demonstrated in animal models, although further progress depends on successes in the development of effective prophylactic HSV vaccines.

Respiratory Syncytial Virus

A member of the paramyxovirus family, RSV is a major cause of viral respiratory tract disease that can result in hospitalization and death in young children and infants, with disease incidence peaking at 2 months of age. Thus, universal immunization of infants has been perceived as desirable. There are two major virus serogroups, A and B, based on the antigenic divergence of the G glycoprotein. Because infection leads to disease in infants as young as 2 months of age, immunization should be initiated before that age in order to optimize the rate of disease prevention. Many infants at that age have maternal anti-RSV antibody, which can blunt the immunogenicity of certain vaccines. Because natural infection induces only incomplete protection against reinfection in infants, it seems likely that multiple doses of vaccine will be required for optimal protection. The results of a clinical trial run during the 1960s retarded progress in the field of vaccine development for decades. It was observed that immunization with a formalin-inactivated RSV vaccine resulted in the paradoxical enhancement of disease in vaccinated children. There has been considerable investigation of this phenomenon, with the explanation that enhanced disease may have been a pulmonary delayed-type hypersensitivity reaction mediated by CD4⁺ T cells (101). Nevertheless, as a consequence of this early clinical study, there has been much caution in vaccine development, especially with respect to clinical studies in seronegative infants.

Most attention in RSV vaccine development has been directed toward live attenuated vaccines, which would be expected to elicit an immune response resembling that of wild-type virus and to be effective in the presence of maternal antibodies in young infants while avoiding the issue of enhanced disease observed with inactivated vaccines. As for influenza virus, *ca* live attenuated RSV vaccines have been investigated extensively in animal models as well as in some clinical studies (102). Such viruses have been created through low-temperature in vitro passage in cell culture as well as following chemical mutagenesis. Two surface glycoproteins of RSV, F (fusion) and G (attachment), have been shown to elicit neutralizing antibodies that are protective in animal challenge models (103). Recombinant F and G glycoproteins as well as an FG chimeric fusion protein were expressed in mammalian cells or baculovirus-infected insect cells; these proteins are generally weakly immunogenic (104,105). Because multiple doses or immunization with adjuvants or delivery systems may be required for successful immunization, such preparations might not be useful for seronegative infants. Furthermore, there needs to be a very high level of assurance that the use of such vaccines would not entail the risk of enhanced disease. However, the ability of a single dose of purified F glycoprotein vaccine to stimulate serum neutralizing in seropositive subjects suggests that this vaccine may be useful as a boost to those previously infected with RSV and at risk for reinfection (106).

Parainfluenza

Parainfluenza virus type 3 (PIV3), like RSV, is a paramyxovirus that causes respiratory tract disease. The peak incidence of disease is somewhat later than that caused by RSV, and immunization should be initiated by 6 months of age. Because PIV3 is a member of the same virus family as RSV and measles virus, the observation of enhanced disease following immunization with inactivated RSV or measles vaccine also has slowed down the field of PIV3 vaccine development. The two main approaches taken have been live attenuated and recombinant subunit vaccines. Bovine PIV3 virus (BPIV3), which is serologically cross-reactive with PIV3, has been used as a naturally attenuated vaccine strain by virtue of its animal origin. BIPV3 vaccine was shown to be well tolerated in children and able to elicit HI antibodies in seronegative children (107). A PIV3 virus strain was attenuated and cold-adapted by passage in primary monkey kidney cells. This live attenuated *ca* vaccine was well tolerated and seroconverted approximately 80% of seronegative children (108). As has been done for RSV F and G glycoproteins, recombinant F and HN surface glycoproteins have been shown to be immunogenic and protective in animal models. Interestingly, the FHN fusion protein was shown to have greater efficacy than F and HN used separately (109).

Cytomegalovirus

Cytomegalovirus (CMV), a β-herpesvirus, is widely detected in humans. Infections usually are benign. However, in utero infection of fetuses can result in lasting neurologic sequelae. Also, allograft recipients are at risk for a range of diseases. Therefore, vaccination would be desirable to prevent infections in utero and in seronegative transplantees. A live attenuated vaccine (Towne strain) was developed following propagation in human embryo fibroblasts (110). A double-blind, placebo-controlled efficacy study in seronegative renal transplant recipients showed that the vaccine induced partial protection against CMV infection (111). Because the major use of a CMV vaccine would be to prevent congenital CMV infectious, approaches other than live attenuated virus have been considered. The major CMV viral glycoprotein gB has been expressed in different vector systems as an approach to a recombinant viral subunit vaccine (112).

Hepatitis C

HAV and HBV were identified in the middle of the twentieth century as the major causes of enteric and blood-borne infectious hepatitides, respectively. Following the discovery of HAV and HBV, there remained a large number of cases of infectious hepatitis, both enteric and blood-borne, for which no etiologic agent could be identified. Such putative viruses were referred to collectively as non-A, non-B (NANB) hepatitis viruses. This remained the case until the late 1980s, when recombinant DNA (rDNA) technology was applied to the identification of new viral agents. This led to the identification of hepatitis C virus (HCV) as the major cause of blood-borne NANB hepatitis (113). HCV is a flavivirus, although it is not serologically cross-reactive with JEV or dengue virus. The E1 and E2 surface glycoproteins have been investigated as vaccine candidates. Immunization of chimpanzees with an oligomer of recombinant E1/E2 was shown to confer protection against HCV challenge (114). As for HIV, the hypervariability of glycoprotein epitopes is a significant hurdle to vaccine development. Immunization of young children in endemic areas, sexually active young adults, and those exposed to blood would be desirable.

Hepatitis E

In parallel with the discovery of HCV, rDNA technology was applied to enterically transmitted hepatitis. This resulted in the identification of hepatitis E virus (HEV) as the major cause of enteric infectious NANB and the cloning and sequencing of its full genome (115). A subunit vaccine consisting of the major viral capsid protein (ORF2) was shown to elicit protective immunity in rhesus monkeys following challenge with HEV (116). A vaccine composed of ORF2 is in the early stages of clinical development. Immunization of residents of and travelers to endemic areas would be desirable.

Dengue

Dengue virus is a mosquito-borne flavivirus that causes millions of infections worldwide per year, especially in tropical areas. Associated sequelae that occur in a minority of cases include severe headache and fever, hemorrhage, and shock. There are four serotypes of dengue virus, denoted as types 1 to 4. Infection with one virus serotype results in strong homotypic protection but not heterotypic protection. Most vaccine development has been concentrated on live attenuated vaccines. Clinical isolates have been cultured in primary dog kidney cells for various numbers of passages in order to achieve attenuation. Some attenuated strains then are cultured in fetal rhesus kidney cells for vaccine production. Individual serotype vaccines have been evaluated in initial clinical studies, with the strategy being to combine the optimal monovalent strains into a quadrivalent vaccine. Achieving the proper level of attenuation has been an empirical exercise in that there is no animal model for attenuation. Thus, only studies in small groups of volunteers can establish whether a strain is appropriately attenuated. Some candidate vaccines have been shown to be underattenuated, such that immunized volunteers have experienced dengue-like illnesses (117). Other strains have shown a better balance between immunogenicity and safety (118). Immunization of travelers to and residents of endemic areas would be desirable.

Human Papilloma Virus

The human papilloma viruses (HPVs) are a genomically diverse group of viruses that cause a range of epithelial cell infections and diseases. These viruses have been classified on the basis of DNA sequence homologies into approximately 60 consecutively numbered genotypes. Some types cause skin and plantar warts, another group causes premalignant lesions in epidermodysplasia verruciformis, and yet another group infects laryngopharyngeal epithelial and mucosal surfaces. However, the most significant infections in terms of morbidity and mortality are those of genital mucosal epithelial cells. Immunization of young adults, particularly women, is perceived as highly desirable for preventing this sexually transmitted disease. Following acute infection, the viral genomic DNA can integrate, resulting in chronic infection with the risk of neoplastic progression. Infections with HPV-16, -18,

-31, and -45 are associated with the development of high-grade precancerous disease and invasive squamous cell (cervical) carcinoma. Infections with HPV-6 and -11 predispose to low-grade dysplasia and genital warts, which usually regress without becoming invasive. The virion is a capsid composed of proteins L1 and L2. The L1 proteins show significant antigenic diversity, which appears generally to cotrack with virus genotype. The recombinant expression of L1 or L1 + L2 in eukaryotic cells results in the expression of VLPs that morphologically are highly similar to HPV virions (119). Multivalent recombinant VLPs are in early clinical studies as candidate prophylactic vaccines. Chronic HPV infections, especially those predisposing to cervical carcinoma, may be ameliorated through therapeutic vaccination. The E6 and E7 proteins are logical therapeutic targets (120), because 80% to 90% of cervical cancers express these proteins from HPV-16, -18, -33, or -45 (121). Different strategies have been investigated for the proper immunologic presentation of E6 and E7.

Epstein-Barr Virus

Epstein-Barr virus (EBV), a γ-herpesvirus, causes infectious mononucleosis. As a sequel of latent infection, EBV also is the etiologic agent of Burkitt's lymphoma and nasopharyngeal carcinoma, although it is believed that there are cofactors that contribute to the development of these cancers. It was observed that the major viral envelope glycoprotein, gp350, elicited the production of virus neutralizing antibodies. This glycoprotein is one of the most heavily glycosylated proteins characterized; its molecular mass is more than 50% glycan by weight. The gene for gp350 was identified, cloned, and expressed. Immunization with recombinant gp350 has been shown to elicit protective immunity in preclinical simian models of EBV infection (122). A recombinant gp350 vaccine is in the early stages of clinical development and may be useful for immunization of populations in areas where they are at risk for the development of these cancers.

Parvovirus

B19 parvovirus causes the common childhood rash known as fifth disease. The virus infects cells of the erythroid lineage, which can result in anemia. The icosahedral virion has a capsid shell composed of 60 copies of the major capsid protein VP2 with a single-stranded DNA genome. The recombinant gene for VP2 can be expressed in eukaryotic cells, in which the recombinant VP2 proteins assemble into VLPs that are immunologically and morphologically similar to natural virions (123). The ability of such VLPs to elicit the formation of virus-neutralizing antibodies makes these recombinant particles a vaccine candidate. In addition, it has been shown that a gene encoding a foreign antigen can be spliced into a truncated VP1 gene, such that expression of the resultant VP2-VP1-chimeric gene in baculovirus-infected insect cells elicits the production of VLPs with the foreign antigen on the surface (124). This chimeric antigen could be a useful antigen-presentation vehicle.

Human Immunodeficiency Virus Type 2

The close relative of HIV-1, HIV-2 has been shown to cause AIDS in humans, although at a lower rate of prevalence. Because HIV-2 and its close relatives are endogenous to several species, of monkeys, there have been many preclinical studies of candidate HIV-2 vaccines. These approaches have included live attenuated vaccines that would be very difficult from a safety perspective to consider for evaluation in humans. As a prototype vaccine that is amenable to development for humans, an inactivated whole-virus HIV-2 vaccine was coupled to ISCOMs. Cynomolgus monkeys that had been immunized with this vaccine were shown to be protected against HIV-2 followed by rechallenge 12 to 18 months later (125). An HIV-2 vaccine might be used for the same target groups as those for an HIV-1 vaccine.

Human T-Cell Leukemia Virus Type I

The lymphotropic human T-cell leukemia virus type 1 (HTLV-1) is a retrovirus that has been shown to be associated with the development of T-cell lymphoma and uveitis in certain populations, especially in Japan. A range of approaches to the development of an HTLV-1 vaccine have been taken. Pig-tailed macaques immunized with an HTLV-1 subunit vaccine were protected against challenge with simian T-cell lymphotropic virus type 1 (126), a close relative of HTLV-1. Achieving such heterologous protection augurs well for the development of an effective HTLV-1 vaccine, which could be used in geographic areas where individuals are at risk of lymphoma and uveitis.

Hemorrhagic Disease Viruses: Arenaviruses and Filoviruses

The arenaviruses and filoviruses are distinct classes of RNA viruses that can cause fatal hemorrhagic disease. Vaccines against such viruses would be useful for residents of and travelers to endemic areas, although the highly sporadic nature of the appearance of these rare viruses might complicate the strategy for effective vaccination in the field.

Although immunization with inactivated vaccines for Lassa fever virus (LFV), a pathogenic arenavirus, have not been shown to be protective in animal models, immunization with a recombinant vaccinia virus expressing LFV glycoproteins protected rhesus monkeys challenged with LFV (127). For Marburg virus (MBGV), a filovirus, immunization with either inactivated adjuvanted whole virus or recombinant MBGV glycoprotein was shown to protect guinea pigs against MBGV challenge (128).

Other Vaccines

Human herpesvirus 6 (HHV-6) has been implicated as the causative agent for exanthema subitum (129). This lymphotropic γ-herpesvirus, which can infect many of the same cell types as HIV-1, also has been associated with acute lymphocytic leukemia and infectious mononucleosis. An envelope glycoprotein of HHV-6, by analogy to other human herpesviruses (HSV, CMV, EBC, VZV), may be useful as an HHV-6 vaccine candidate.

HHV-8 may be the etiologic agent of Kaposi's sarcoma (KS), because HHV-8 DNA and antibodies are detected at about the time of clinical development of KS (130). An envelope glycoprotein-based vaccine may be a useful vaccine candidate. An effective vaccine may be useful in HIV-1–infected subjects for the prevention of KS.

Hepatitis G virus (HGV) was discovered in 1995 using rDNA technology (131). This flavivirus has not been clearly associated with liver pathology to date. Therefore, there has not yet been much interest in developing an HGV vaccine.

HTLV-2 is a retrovirus related to HTLV-1 and has been shown to exist in at least two major subtypes (132). However, because infection with HTLV-2 is not clearly identified with any recognized disease etiology, there has been relatively little interest to date in developing an HTLV-2 vaccine.

Future Developments

A wide range of technologies continue to be applied to development of new vaccines, especially for viral infections for which no vaccines are currently licensed. For live vaccines, making precise genetic attenuations based on identifying viral genes involved in pathogenesis should continue to be an active area. Such attenuated viruses also will continue to be developed as viral vectors. Although most activities to date in the live vector field have involved DNA viruses owing to their larger genomes, increased attention is being placed on RNA virus vectors and approaches such as alphavirus replicons (133), which are hybrids between live viruses and nucleic acid vaccines. For subunit and inactivated vaccines, much work continues in the development of novel adjuvants and delivery systems that are both safe and effective in eliciting improved immune responses. Modulating immune responses to different immunologic compartments is also important, as in the case of stimulating mucosal immune responses to viruses that infect mucosal tissues (e.g., nasal). For nucleic acid vaccines, new formulations are being developed that would increase uptake of DNA by cells and/or nuclei in order to increase the amount of viral antigen synthesized by the transfected cells. Finally, as more viral vaccines are licensed for use in the same age groups (e.g., pediatric), developing new multidisease combination vaccines will continue to be important for improving compliance with immunization policies and ensuring the highest level of use of new vaccines.

References

1. The IMpact-RSV Study Group. Palivizumab, a humanized respiratory syncytial virus monoclonal antibody, reduces hospitalization from respiratory syncytial virus infection in high-risk infants. Pediatrics 1998;102:531–537.
2. Ellis RW. Immunological correlates of efficacy. In: Ellis RW, ed. Combination vaccines. Totawa, NJ: Humana, 1999: 107–153.
3. Thanavala Y, Young Y-F, Lyons P, et al. Immunogenicity of transgenic plant-derived hepatitis B surface antigen. Proc Natl Acad Sci USA 1994;92:3358–3361.
4. Donnelly JJ, Ulmer JB, Shiver JW, Liu MA. DNA vaccines. Ann Rev Immunol 1997;15:617–648.
5. Higgins DA, Carlson JR, van Nest G. MF59 adjuvant enhances the immunogenicity of influenza vaccine in both young and old mice. Vaccine 1996;14:478–484.
6. Cox JC, Coulter AR. Adjuvants—a classification and review of their modes of action. Vaccine 1997;15:248–256.
7. Mestecky J, Moldoveanu Z, Michalek SM, et al. Current options for vaccine delivery systems by mucosal routes. J Controlled Release 1997;48:243–257.
8. Goldenthal KL, Burns DL, McVittie LD, et al. Overview—combination vaccines and simultaneous administration. Past, present and future. In: Williams JC, Goldenthal KL, Burns DL, Lewis BP, eds. Combined vaccines and simultaneous administration: current issues and perspectives. Ann NY Acad Sci 1995;754:xi–xv.
9. Ellis RW, Brown KR. Combination vaccines. In: August JT, Anders MW, Murad F, Coyle JT, eds. Advances in pharmacology. San Diego: Academic, 1997:393–423.
10. Kilbourne ED. Inactivated influenza vaccines. In: Plotkin SA, Mortimer EA, eds. Vaccines. 2nd ed. Philadelphia: WB Saunders, 1994:565–581.
11. Dowdle WN, Kendall AP, Nable GR. Influenza viruses. In: Lennart EH, Schmidt NJ, eds. Diagnostic procedures for viral, rickettsial and chlamydial infections. 5th ed. Washington: American Public Health Association, 1979:603–605.
12. Frank AL, Puck J, Hughes BJ, Cate TR. Microneutralization test for influenza A and B and parainfluenza 1 and 2 viruses that uses continuous cell lines and fresh serum enhancement. J Clin Microbiol 1980;12:426–432.
13. Quinnan GV, Schooley R, Doli R, et al. Serologic responses and systemic reactions in adults after vaccination with monovalent A/USSR/77 and trivalent A/USSR/77, A/Texas/77 and B/HongKong/72 influenza vaccines. Rev Infect Dis 1983;5:748–757.
14. Belshe RB, van Voris LP, Bartram J, Crookshank FK. Live attenuated influenza A virus vaccines in children: results of a field trial. J Infect Dis 1984;150:834–840.
15. Halperin SA, Nestruck AC, Eastwood BJ. Safety and immunogenicity of a new influenza vaccine grown in mammalian cell culture. Vaccine 1998;16:1331–1335.
16. Deliyannis G, Jackson DC, Dyer W, et al. Immunopotentiation of humoral and cellular responses to inactivated influenza vaccines by two different adjuvants with potential for human use. Vaccine 1998;16:2058–2068.
17. Higaki M, Takase T, Igarashi R, et al. Enhancement of immune response to intranasal influenza HA vaccine by microparticle resin. Vaccine 1998;16:741–745.
18. Wright PF, Johnson PR, Karzon DT. Clinical experience with live, attenuated vaccines in children. In Kendal AP, Patriarca PA, eds. Options for the control of influenza: proceedings of a Viratek-UCLA symposium. New York: Alan R. Liss, 1986.
19. Maassab HF, DeBorde DC. Development and characterization of cold-adapted viruses for use as live virus vaccines. Vaccine 1985;3:355–369.
20. Belshe RB, Mendelman PM, Treanor J, et al. The efficacy of live attenuated, cold-adapted, trivalent, intranasal influenza virus vaccine in children. New Eng J Med 1998;888:1405–1412.
21. Donnelly JJ, Friedman A, Martinez D, et al. Preclinical efficacy of a prototype DNA vaccine: enhanced protection against antigenic drift in influenza virus. Nat Med 1995;1:583–587.
22. World Health Organization. Expert Committee on Biological Standardization. World Health Org Tech Rep 1976;594.
23. Lloyd W, Theiler M, Ricci NI. Modification of the virulence of yellow fever virus by cultivation in tissues in vitro. Trans R Soc Trop Med Hyg 1936;29:481–529.

24. Theiler M, Smith HH. The effect of prolonged cultivation in vitro upon the pathogenicity of yellow fever virus. J Exp Med 1937;65:767–786.

25. Liprandi F. Isolation of plaque variants differing in virulence from the 17D strain of yellow fever virus. J Gen Virol 1981;56:363–370.

26. Bugher JC, Gast-Galvis A. The efficacy of vaccination in the prevention of yellow fever in Colombia. Am J Hyg 1944;39:58–66.

27. Rosenzweig EC, Babione RW, Wisseman CL. Immunological studies with group B arboviruses. IV. Persistence of yellow fever antibodies following vaccination with 17D strain yellow fever vaccine. Am J Trop Med Hyg 1963;12:230–235.

28. Sabin AB. Properties and behavior of orally administered attenuated poliovirus vaccine. J Am Med Assoc 1957;164:1216–1223.

29. Enders JF, Robbins FC, Weller TH. The cultivation of the poliomyelitis viruses in tissue culture. Les Prix Nobel 1954, Stockholm, Sweden.

30. Melnick JL, Benyesh-Melnick M, Brennan JC. Studies on live poliovirus vaccine. Its neurotropic activity in monkeys and its increased neurovirulence after multiplication in vaccinated children. J Am Med Assoc 1959;171:1165–1172.

31. World Health Organization Consultative Group. Evidence on the safety and efficacy of live poliovirus vaccines currently in use, with special reference to type 3 poliovirus. Bull WHO 1969;40:925–945.

32. Sabin AB, Michaels RH, Ziring P, et al. Effect of oral poliovirus vaccine in newborn children. II. Intestinal resistance and antibody response at 6 months in children fed type 1 vaccine at birth. Pediatrics 1963;31:641–650.

33. Grenier B, Hamza B, Biron G, et al. Seroimmunity following vaccination in infants by an inactivated poliovirus preparation on Vero cells. Rev Infect Dis 1984;6:545–547.

34. Salk J, Gori GB. A review of theoretical, experimental, and practical considerations in the use of formaldehyde for the inactivation of poliovirus. Ann NY Acad Sci 1960;83:609–637.

35. Montagnon B, Fanget B, Vincent-Falquet JC. Industrial-scale production of inactivated poliovirus vaccine prepared by culture of Vero cells and microcarrier. Rev Infect Dis 1984;6:S341–S344.

36. Centers for Disease Control. Recommended childhood immunization schedule—United States, 1998. MMWR 1998;47:8–12.

37. Carlsson B, Zaman S, Mellander L, et al. Secretory and serum immunoglobulin class-specific antibodies to poliovirus after immunization. J Infect Dis 1985;152:1238–1244.

38. Salk J. Persistence of immunity after administration of formalin-treated poliovirus vaccine. Lancet 1960;2:715–723.

39. Schwartz AJF, Anderson JT. Immunization with a further attenuated live measles vaccine. Arch Virusforsch 1965;16:273–278.

40. Hilleman MR, Buynak EB, Weibel RE, et al. Development and evaluation of the Moraten measles virus vaccine. JAMA 1968;206:587–590.

41. Expanded Programme on Immunization. Safety of high-titre measles vaccines. Wkly Epidemiol Rec 1991;67:357–361.

42. Black FL. Measles. In: Evans AS, ed. Viral infections of humans, epidemiology and control. 3rd ed. New York: Plenum, 1989:451–465.

43. Buynak EB, Hilleman MR. Live attenuated mumps virus vaccine. 1. Vaccine development. Proc Soc Exp Biol Med 1966;123:768–775.

44. Shehab ZM, Brunell PA, Cobb E. Epidemiological standardization of a test for the susceptibility to mumps. J Infect Dis 1984;149:810–812.

45. Plotkin SA, Buser F. History of RA27/3 rubella vaccine. Rev Infect Dis 1985;7:77–78.

46. Dudgeon JA. Selective immunization: protection of the individual. Rev Infect Dis 1980;7:S185–S190.

47. Weibel RE, Villarejos VM, Klein EB, et al. Clinical and laboratory studies of live attenuated RA27/3 and HPV-77DE rubella virus vaccines. Proc Soc Exp Biol Med 1980;165:44–49.

48. Paunio M, Virtanen M, Peltola H, et al. Increase of vaccination coverage by mass media and individual approach: intensified measles, mumps and rubella prevention program in Finland. Am J Epidemiol 1991;133:1152–1160.

49. Davidkin I, Valle M. Vaccine-induced measles virus antibodies after two doses of combined measles, mumps and rubella vaccine: a 12-year follow-up in two cohorts. Vaccine 1998;16:2052–2057.

50. Plotkin SA. Rabies vaccine prepared in human cell cultures: progress and perspectives. Rev Infect Dis 1980;2:433–447.

51. Bahmanyar M, Fayaz A, Nour-Salehi S, et al. Successful protection of humans exposed to rabies infection. Postexposure treatment with the new human diploid cell rabies vaccine and antirabies serum. JAMA 1976;236:2751–2754.

52. Montagnon BJ. Polio and rabies vaccines produced in continuous cell lines: a reality for Vero cell line. Dev Biol Stand 1989;70:27–47.

53. Bijok U, Vodopija I, Smerdel S, et al. Purified chick embryo cell (PCEC) rabies vaccine for human use: clinical trials. Behring Inst Mitt 1984;76:155–164.

54. Brochier B, Kieny MP, Costy F, et al. Large-scale eradication of rabies using recombinant vaccinia-rabies vaccine. Nature 1991;354:520–522.

55. Modelska A, Dietzschold B, Sleysh N, et al. Immunization against rabies with plant-derived antigen. Proc Natl Acad Sci USA 1998;95:2481–2485.

56. Buescher EL. Respiratory diseases and the adenoviruses. Med Clin North Am 1967;51:769–779.

57. Rubin BA, Minecci LC, Tint H. Karyologic characteristics of the WI-38 diploid cell system—general comments. Nat Cancer Inst Monograph 1968;29:97–104.

58. Top FH, Dudding BA, Russell PK, Buescher EL. Control of respiratory disease in recruits with types 4 and 7 adenovirus vaccines. Am J Epidemiol 1971;94:141–146.

59. Morin JE, Lubeck MD, Barton JE, et al. Recombinant adenovirus induces antibody response to hepatitis B virus surface antigen in hamsters. Proc Natl Acad Sci USA 1987;84:4626–4630.

60. Prevec L, Christie BC, Laurie KE, et al. Immune response to HIV-1 gag antigens induced by recombinant adenovirus vectors in mice and rhesus macaque monkeys. J Acquir Immune Defic Syndr 1991;4:568–576.

61. Krugman S, Stevens CE. Hepatitis B vaccine. In: Plotkin SA, Mortimer EA, eds. Vaccines. 2nd ed. Philadelphia: WB Saunders, 1992;419–438.

62. Chang MH, Chen CJ, Lai MS, et al. Universal hepatitis B vaccination in Taiwan and the incidence of hepatocellular carcinoma in children. Taiwan Childhood Hepatoma Study Group. N Engl J Med 1997;336:1855–1859.

63. Szmuness W, Steven CE, Zang EA, et al. A controlled clinical trial of the efficacy of the hepatitis B vaccine (Heptavax B): a final report. Hepatology 1981;1:377–385.

64. West DJ. Clinical experience with hepatitis B vaccines. Am J Infect Control 1989;17:172–180.

65. Emini EA, Ellis RW, Miller WJ, et al. Production and immunological analysis of recombinant hepatitis B vaccine. J Infect 1986;13A:3–9.

66. West DA, Calandra GB. Vaccine-induced immunologic memory for hepatitis B surface antigen: implications for policy on booster vaccination. Vaccine 1996;14:1019–1027.

67. Livingston BD, Crimi C, Grey H, et al. The hepatitis B virus-specific CTL responses induced in humans by lipopeptide vaccination are comparable to those elicited by acute viral infection. J Immunol 1997;159:1383–1392.

68. Yasuda A, Kimura-Kuroda J, Ogimoto M, et al. Induction of protective immunity in animals vaccinated with recombinant vaccinia viruses that express preM and E glycoproteins of Japanese encephalitis virus. J Virol 1990;64:2788–2795.

69. Oya J. Japanese encephalitis vaccine. Acta Ped Jpn 1988;30:175–184.

70. Gu PW, Ding ZF. Japanese encephalitis vaccine made in hamster cell culture (a review). JE and HPRS Bull 1987;2:1–26.

71. Yu YX, Wu PF, Ao J, et al. Selection of a better immunogenic and highly attenuated live vaccine virus strain of JE. Some biological characteristics of SA-14-14-2 mutant. Chin J Microbiol Immunol 1981;1:77–84.

72. Hoke CH, Nisalak A, Sangawhipa N, et al. Protection against Japanese encephalitis by inactivated vaccines. N Engl J Med 1988;319:608–614.

73. Regional Antiepidemic Station, Hueyang G. Preliminary observation on epidemiological effectiveness of JE live vaccine. Bull Biol Prod 1978;7:111–114.

74. Takahashi M. Vaccine development. In: Ellis RW, White CJ, eds. Varicella vaccine. Philadelphia: WB Saunders, 1996: 469–488.

75. Provost PJ, Krah DL, Kuter BJ, et al. Antibody assays suitable for assessing responses to live varicella vaccine. Vaccine 1991;9:111–116.

76. Bernstein HH, Rothstein EP, Watson BM, et al. Clinical survey of natural varicella compared with breakthrough varicella after immunization with live attenuated Oka/Merck varicella vaccine. Pediatrics 1993;92:833–837.

77. White CJ, Kuter BJ, Ngai A, et al. Modified cases of chickenpox after varicella vaccination: correlation of protection with antibody response. Pediatr Infect Dis J 1992;11:19–23.

78. Lowe RS, Keller PM, Keech BJ, et al. Varicella-zoster virus as a live vector for the expression of foreign genes. Proc Natl Acad Sci USA 1987;84:3896–3900.

79. Provost PJ, Hughes JV, Miller WJ, et al. An inactivated hepatitis A vaccine of cell culture origin. J Med Virol 1986;19:23–31.

80. Conrad ME, Lemon SM. Prevention of icteric viral hepatitis by administration of immune serum gamma globulin. J Infect Dis 1987;156:56–63.

81. Werzberger A, Mensch B, Kuter B, et al. A controlled trial of a formalin-inactivated hepatitis A vaccine in healthy children. New Engl J Med 1992;327:453–457.

82. Werzberger A, Kuter B, Nalin D. Six years follow-up after hepatitis A vaccination. New Engl J Med 1998;338:1160.

83. Nalin DR. Hepatitis A vaccine, purified inactivated. Drugs of the Future 1995;20:24–29.

84. Reutter J, Bart PA, Francioli P, et al. Production of antibody to hepatitis A virus and hepatitis B surface antigen measured after combined hepatitis A/hepatitis B vaccination in 242 adult volunteers. J Viral Hepat 1998;5:205–211.

85. Gothefors L, Wadell G, Juto P, et al. Prolonged efficacy of rhesus rotavirus vaccine in Swedish children. J Infect Dis 1989;159:753–757.

86. Clark HF, Borian FE, Bell LM, et al. Protective effect of WC3 vaccine against rotavirus diarrhea in infants during a predominantly serotype 1 rotavirus season. J Infect Dis 1988;158:570–587.

87. Bernstein DI, Glass RI, Rodgers G, et al, US Rotavirus Vaccine Efficacy Group. Evaluation of rhesus rotavirus monovalent and tetravalent reassortant vaccines in US children. JAMA 1995;273:1191–1196.

88. Clark HF, Offit PA, Ellis RW, et al. WC3 reassortant vaccines in children. Brief review. Arch Virol 1996;12:187–198.

89. Ward RL, Knowlton DR, Zito ET, et al, US Rotavirus Vaccine Efficacy Group. Serological correlates of immunity in a tetravalent reassortant rotavirus vaccine trial. J Infect Dis 1997;176:570–577.

90. Bernstein DI, Smith VE, Sherwood JR, et al. Safety and immunogenicity of live, attenuated human rotavirus vaccine 89-12. Vaccine 1998;16:381–387.

91. Ward RL, Bernstein DI, US Rotavirus Efficacy Group. Lack of correlation between serum rotavirus antibody titers and protection following vaccination with reassortant RRV vaccines. Vaccine 1995;13:1226–1232.

92. Crawford SE, Labbe M, Cohen J, et al. Characterization of virus-like particles produced by the expression of rotavirus capsid proteins in insect cells. J Virol 1994;68:5945–5952.

93. Connor RI, Korber BT, Graham BS, et al. Immunological and virological analyses of persons infected by human immunodeficiency virus type 1 while participating in trials of recombinant gp120 vaccines. J Virol 1998;72:1552–1576.

94. Fleury B, Janvier G, Pialoux G, et al. Memory cytotoxic T lymphocyte responses in human immunodeficiency virus type 1 (HIV-1)-negative volunteers immunized with a recombinant canarypox expressing gp160 of HIV-1 and boosted with a recombinant gp160. J Infect Dis 1996; 174:734–738.

95. Blank H, Haines HG. Experimental human reinfection with herpes simplex virus. J Invest Dermatol 1973;61:223–225.

96. Kern AB, Schiff BL. Vaccine therapy in recurrent herpes simplex. Arch Dermatol 1964;89:844–845.

97. Straus SE, Corey L, Burke RL, et al. Placebo-controlled trial of vaccination with recombinant glycoprotein D of herpes simplex virus type 2 for immunotherapy of genital herpes. Lancet 1994;343:1460–1463.

98. Corey L, Langenberg AGM, Ashley R, et al. Recombinant glycoprotein vaccine for the prevention of genital HSV-2 infection: two randomized controlled trials. JAMA 1999;282: 331–340.

99. Cadoz M, Micoud M, Seignerurin JM, et al. Phase I trial of R7020: a live attenuated recombinant herpes simplex (HSV) candidate vaccine. Interscience Conference on Antimicrobial Agents and Chemotherapy, Anaheim, CA, October 11–14, 1992.

100. McLean CS, Ni Challanain D, Duncan I, et al. Induction of a protective immune response by mucosal vaccination with a DISC HSV-1 vaccine. Vaccine 1996;14:987–992.

101. Murphy BR, Hall SL, Kulkarni AB, et al. An update on approaches to the development of respiratory syncytial virus (RSV) and parainfluenza virus type 3 (PIV3) vaccines. Virus Res 1994;32:13–36.

102. Chanock RM, Murphy BR. Past efforts to develop safe and effective RSV vaccines. In: Meignier B, Murphy B, Ogra P, eds. Animal models of respiratory syncytial virus infections. Merieux Foundation, 1991:35–42.

103. Connors M, Collins PL, Firestone CY, Murphy BR. Respiratory syncytial virus (RSV) F, G, M2 (22K), and N proteins each induce resistance to RSV challenge, but resistance induced by M2 and N proteins is relatively short-lived. J Virol 1991;65:1634–1637.

104. Connors M, Collins PL, Firestone CY, et al. Cotton rats previously immunized with a chimeric RSV FG glycoprotein develop enhanced pulmonary pathology when infected with RSV, a phenomenon not encountered following immunization with vaccinia-RSV recombinants or RSV. Vaccine 1992;10:475–484.

105. Murphy BR, Sotnikov A, Paradiso PR, et al. Immunization of cotton rats with the fusion (F) and large (G) glycoproteins of respiratory syncytial virus (RSV) protects against RSV challenge without potentiating RSV disease. Vaccine 1989;7:533–540.

106. Paradiso PR, Hildreth SW, Hogerman DA, et al. Safety and immunogenicity of a subunit respiratory syncytial virus vaccine in children 24–48 months old. Pediatr Infect Dis J 1994;13:792–798.

107. Clements ML, Belshe RB, King J, et al. Evaluation of bovine, cold-adapted human, and wild-type human parainfluenza type 3 viruses in adult volunteers and in chimpanzees. J Clin Microbiol 1991;29:1175–1182.

108. Karron RA, Wright PF, Newman FK, et al. A live attenuated human parainfluenza type-3 vaccine is attenuated and immunogenic in healthy infants and children. J Infect Dis 1995;72:1445–1450.

109. Lehman DJ, Roof LL, Brideau RJ, et al. Comparison of soluble and secreted forms of human parainfluenza virus type 3 glycoproteins expressed from mammalian and insect cells as subunit vaccines. J Gen Virol 1993;74:459–469.

110. Yamane Y, Furukawa T, Plotkin SA. Supernatant virus release as a differentiating marker between low passage and vaccine strains of human cytomegalovirus. Vaccine 1983;1: 23–34.

111. Plotkin S, Starr S, Friedman H, et al. Effect of Towne live virus vaccine on cytomegalovirus disease after renal transplant. Ann Intern Med 1991;114:525–531.

112. Plotkin SA, Starr SE, Friedman HM, et al. Vaccines for the prevention of human cytomegalovirus infection. Rev Infect Dis 1990;12:827–838.

113. Choo Q-L, Kuo G, Weiner AJ, et al. Isolation of a cDNA clone derived from a blood-borne non-A, non-B viral hepatitis genome. Science 1989;244:359–362.

114. Choo Q-L, Kuo G, Ralston R, et al. Vaccination of chimpanzees against infection by the hepatitis C virus. Proc Natl Acad Sci USA 1994;91:1294–1298.

115. Tam AW, Smith MM, Guerra ME, et al. Hepatitis E virus (HEV): molecular cloning and sequencing of the full-length genome. Virology 1991;185:120–131.

116. Tsarev SA, Tsareva TS, Emerson SU, et al. Recombinant vaccine against hepatitis E: dose response and protection against heterologous challenge. Vaccine 1997;15:1834–1838.

117. McKee KT Jr, Bancroft WH, Eckels KH, et al. Lack of attenuation of a candidate dengue 1 vaccine (45AZ5) in human volunteers. Am J Trop Med Hyg 1987;36:435–442.

118. Khin MM, Jirakanjanakit N, Yoksan S, Bhamarapravati N. Infection, dissemination, transmission and biological attributes of dengue-2 PDK 53 candidate vaccine virus after oral infection in Aedes aegypti. Am J Trop Med Hyg 1994;51: 864–869.

119. Zhou J, Sun X-Y, Stenzel DJ, Fraser IH. Expression of vaccinia recombinant HPV-16 11 and 12 ORF proteins in epithelial cells is sufficient for assembly of HPV virion-like particles. Virology 1991;185:251–257.

120. Ji H, Chang EY, Lin KY, et al. Antigen-specific immunotherapy for murine lung metastatic tumors expressing human papillomavirus type 16 E7 oncoprotein. Int J Cancer 1998; 78:41–45.

121. Beaudenon S, Kremsdorf D, Croissant O, et al. A novel type of human papillomavirus associated with genital neoplasias. Nature 1986;321:246–249.

122. Finerty S, Tarlton J, Mackett M, et al. Protective immunization against Epstein-Barr virus-induced disease in cottontop tamarins using the virus envelope glycoprotein gp340 produced from a bovine papillomavirus expression vector. J Gen Virol 1992;73:449–453.

123. Kajigawa S, Fujii H, Field AM, et al. Self-assembled B19 parvovirus capsids, produced in a baculovirus system, are antigenically and immunogenically similar to native virions. Proc Natl Acad Sci USA 1991;88:4646–4650.

124. Miyamura K, Kajigaya S, Momoeda M, et al. Parvovirus particles as platforms for protein presentation. Proc Natl Acad Sci USA 1994;91:8507–8511.

125. Putkonen P, Bjorling E, Akerblom L, et al. Long-standing protection of macaques against cell-free HIV-2 with a HIV-2 ISCOM vaccine. J Acquir Immune Defic Syndr 1994;7: 551–559.

126. Dezzutti CS, Frazier DE, Olsen RG. Efficacy of an HTLV-1 subunit vaccine in prevention of a STLV-1 infection in pig-tailed macaques. Dev Biol Stand 1990;72:287–296.

127. Fisher-Hoch SP, McCormick JB, Auperin D, et al. Protection of rhesus monkeys from fatal Lassa fever by vaccination with recombinant vaccinia virus containing the Lassa virus glycoprotein gene. Proc Natl Acad Sci USA 1989;86:317–321.

128. Hevey M, Negley D, Geisbert J, et al. Antigenicity and vaccine potential of Marburg virus glycoprotein ex-

pressed by baculovirus recombinants. Virology 1997;239: 206–211.

129. Sumiyoshi Y, Akashi K, Kikuchi M. Detection of human herpes virus 6 (HHV-6) in the skin of a patient with primary HHV-6 infection and erythroderma. J Clin Pathol 1994;47: 762–763.

130. Moore PS, Kingsley LA, Holmberg SD, et al. Kaposi's sarcoma-associated herpesvirus infection prior to the onset of Kaposi's sarcoma. AIDS 1996;10:175–180.

131. Simons JN, Leary TP, Dawson GJ, et al. Isolation of novel virus-like sequences associated with human hepatitis. Nat Med 1995;1:564–569.

132. Eiraku N, Novoa P, da Costa Ferreira M, et al. Identification and characterization of a new and distinct molecular subtype of human T-cell lymphotropic virus type 2. J Virol 1996;70:1481–1492.

133. Peroulis I, Mills J, Meanger J. Respiratory syncytial virus G glycoprotein expressed using the Semliki Forest virus replicon is biologically active. Arch Virol 1999;144:107–116.

Chapter 31

DNA Vaccines

Harriet L. Robinson

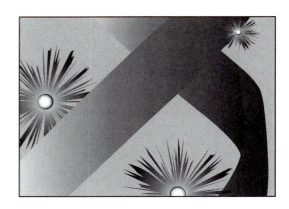

DNA-based vaccines use bacterial plasmids to express protein immunogens in vaccinated hosts (Fig. 31-1). Recombinant DNA technology is used to clone cDNAs encoding immunogens of interest into eukaryotic expression plasmids. Vaccine plasmids are then amplified in bacteria, purified, and directly inoculated into the hosts being vaccinated. DNA can be inoculated by a saline-needle injection or by a gene gun device, which delivers DNA-coated gold beads into skin. The plasmid DNA is taken up by host cells, the vaccine protein is expressed, processed, and presented in the context of self–major histocompatibility complex (MHC) class I and class II molecules, and an immune response against the DNA-encoded immunogen is generated.

History

The historical foundations of DNA vaccines emerged concurrently from studies on gene therapy and studies using retroviral vectors. Gene therapy studies on DNA delivery into muscle revealed that pure DNA was as effective as liposome-encapsulated DNA at mediating transfection of skeletal muscle cells (1). This unencapsulated DNA was termed "naked DNA," a fanciful term that has become popular for the description of the pure DNA used for nucleic acid vaccinations. Gene therapy studies also used gene guns, which had been developed to deliver DNA into plant cells, to deliver DNA into skin. In a series of experiments testing the ability of plasmid-expressed human growth hormone to alter the growth of mice, it was realized that the plasmid inoculations, which had failed to alter growth, had elicited antibody (2). This was the first demonstration of the raising of an immune response by an inoculated plasmid DNA. At the same time, in experiments using retroviral vectors, we realized that very few infected cells (on the order of 10^4 to 10^5) could raise protective immune responses. This led us to direct testing of the replication-defective proviral DNA that had been used to produce infectious forms of the immunizing retroviral vector for vaccination. These experiments in an influenza model in chickens resulted in the first demonstration of protective immunizations (3). Classic references for DNA vaccines include the first demonstration of the raising of an immune response (2); the first demon-

stration of cytotoxic T-cell (Tc)–mediated immunity (4); the first demonstration of the protective efficacy of intradermal (ID), intramuscular (IM), intravenous (IV), intranasal (IN), and gene gun immunizations (3,5); the first use of genetic adjuvants (6); the first use of library immunizations (7); the first demonstration of immunomodulatory unmethylated deoxycytosine deoxygunosine (CpG) motifs (8); and the first demonstration of the ability to modulate the T-helper type of immune response by the method of DNA delivery (9). A highly useful website for DNA vaccines can be found at http://www.genweb.com/Dnavax/dnavax.html.

Advantages and Disadvantages

DNA-based immunizations have several advantages, as well as disadvantages, in comparison with more classic methods of immunization (Table 31-1). The major immunologic advantage is the ability of the immunogen to be presented by both class I and class II MHC molecules. Endogenously synthesized proteins readily enter processing pathways for the loading of peptide epitopes onto MHC I as well as MHC II molecules. MHC I–presented epitopes raise cytotoxic T (Tc) cells whereas MHC II–presented epitopes raise helper T (Th) cells. By contrast, immunogens that are not synthesized in cells are largely restricted to the loading of MHC II epitopes and the raising of Th but not Tc cells. When compared with live attenuated vaccines or recombinant viral vectors that produce immunogens in cells and raise both Th and Tc cells, DNA vaccines have the advantages of not being infectious and of focusing the immune response on only those antigens desired for immunization. DNA vaccines also have the advantage that they can be manipulated relatively easily to raise type 1 or type 2 T-cell help. This allows a vaccine to be tailored for the type of immune response that will be mobilized to combat an infection or disease (see below). DNA vaccines also have the advantage that they are cost effective. This cost effectiveness results from the ease with which plasmids can be constructed using recombinant DNA technology, the ability to use a generic method for vaccine production (growth and purification of plasmid DNA), and the stability of DNA over a wide range of temperatures. Disadvantages of DNA vaccines include

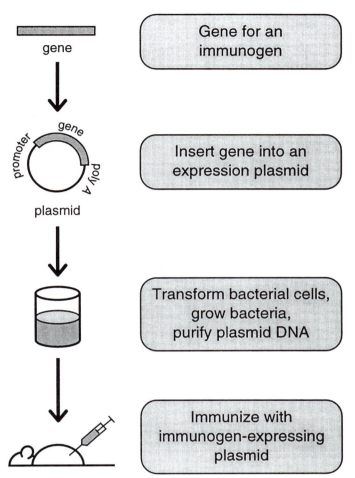

gene

promoter gene poly A

plasmid

Gene for an immunogen

Insert gene into an expression plasmid

Transform bacterial cells, grow bacteria, purify plasmid DNA

Immunize with immunogen-expressing plasmid

Figure 31-1. Schematic of the construction, production, and inoculation of a DNA vaccine. Adapted with permission from Robinson HL, Ginsberg HS, Davis HL, et al. The scientific future of DNA for immunization. Washington: American Academy of Microbiology, 1997.

the limitation of immunizations to protein immunogens and the potential for atypical processing of bacterial and parasitic proteins by eukaryotic cells.

Plasmid Vectors and Delivery

The best immune responses are achieved using highly active expression vectors modeled on those developed for the production of recombinant proteins (10). The most frequently used transcriptional control elements include a strong promoter, such as the cytomegalovirus immediate early promoter, and a strong polyadenylation signal, such as the bovine growth hormone or rabbit β globin signals (11–15). The cytomegalovirus immediate early promoter can be used with or without intron A (11). The

Table 31-1. Advantages and Disadvantages of DNA Vaccines Compared with Classic Immunization Methods

Advantages of DNA Vaccines

Subunit immunization with no risk for infection
Antigen presentation by both class I and class II MHC molecules
Ability to raise type 1 or type 2 T-cell help
Focused immune response
Ease of development and production
Stability of vaccine

Disadvantages of DNA Vaccines

Limited to protein immunogens
Potential for atypical processing of bacterial and parasitic proteins

presence of intron A increases the expression of many antigens from RNA viruses, bacteria, and parasites, presumably by providing the expressed RNA with sequences that support processing and function as a eukaryotic mRNA. Expression also can be enhanced by optimizing the codon usage of prokaryotic mRNAs for eukaryotic cells (16,17). Multicistronic vectors can be used to express more than one immunogen or an immunogen and an immunostimulatory protein (18,19). Plasmids expressing up to 4000 member DNA libraries have been successfully used to raise protective immunity (7). The potential for library immunizations is a tribute to the power of the immune system to recognize and respond to very few antigen-expressing cells.

The two most broadly used approaches to DNA delivery are injection of DNA in saline using a hypodermic needle and gene gun delivery of DNA-coated gold beads (Fig. 31-2). Saline injections deliver DNA into extracellular spaces, whereas gene gun deliveries bombard DNA directly into cells. The saline injections require much larger amounts of DNA (100 to 1000 times more) than the gene gun (5). These two types of delivery also differ in that saline injections bias responses toward type 1 T-cell help whereas gene gun deliveries bias responses toward type 2 T-cell help (9). The most frequent routes of vaccination by saline injection are IM and ID. Gene gun deliveries target the epidermal layer of the skin. Immunization by mucosal delivery of DNA has been less uniformly successful than immunizations using parenteral routes of inoculation. However, some success has been achieved using liposomes (20), microspheres (21,22), and recombinant shigella vectors (23,24). Methods and routes of DNA delivery that are effective at raising immune responses in mice have been effective in other species.

Immunostimulatory CpG Sequences

At least part of the efficacy of DNA-based immunizations has been attributed to the ability of plasmid DNA to serve as an adjuvant as well as the source of the encoded immunogen (8). This adjuvant activity appears to be a general property of unmethylated CpG motifs in bacterial-derived DNA [for reviews, see (25,26)]. CpG motifs in bacterial DNA distinguish themselves

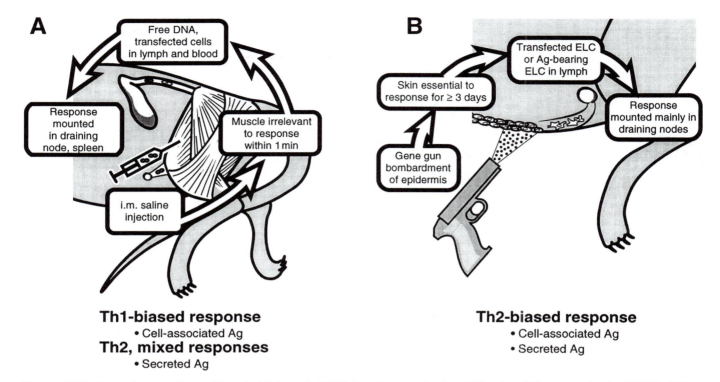

Figure 31-2. Role of target site and lymphoid tissue in DNA-based immunizations following different methods of DNA delivery. *A*, Saline injection of DNA. *B*, Gene gun delivery of DNA. The predominant Th types of responses raised by different methods of DNA delivery and different forms of DNA-expressed antigen are summarized below the schematics. (Adapted with permission from Robinson HL, Pertmer TM. DNA vaccines for viral infections: basic studies and applications. Virus Res 2000 (in press).

from those in eukaryotic DNAs by being both unmethylated and more frequent. In certain nucleotide sequence contexts, termed CpG-stimulatory (CpG-S), CpG sequences trigger innate immune defenses, the production of Th1 cytokines, and the activation of dendritic cells (25,27,28). These innate responses synergize with acquired immune responses against the DNA-expressed protein. In other base contexts, termed CpG-neutralizing (CpG-N), CpG sequences inhibit activation of innate immune responses, potentially providing a mechanism for a microbe to evade host immune defenses. CpG-N sequences are over-represented in the human genome, where CpG-N motifs are two to five times more frequent than CpG-S motifs (27). The manipulation of CpG-S and CpG-N sequences in vaccine vectors can improve the efficiency of immunization (27). Complicating the issues of CpG motifs are apparent differences in the sequence motifs that are immunostimulatory for rodents and primates.

Mechanistic Basis for DNA-Raised Immune Responses

DNA vaccines generate immune responses with nanogram levels of expressed protein. Initial skepticism about DNA vaccines was rooted in the belief that such low levels of expressed protein—about 1000 times lower than those in killed whole-virus or protein vaccines—could not possibly raise immune responses. So why do DNA vaccines work? The answer is likely to lie in the high efficiencies of antigen presentation that are achieved by the direct transfection of professional antigen-presenting cells (APCs) (29–32). The adjuvant activity of unmethylated CpG sequences in plasmid DNA also may contribute to the efficiency of DNA vaccines (33) (see above).

The firmest knowledge of how DNA vaccines work comes from studies in chimeric mice. These studies demonstrate that antigen presentation is by bone marrow–derived cells. Bone marrow–derived cells include the dendritic cells, macrophages, and B cells that are specialized for antigen presentation and termed professional APCs. For studies on antigen presentation, F1 mice were bred and their bone marrow destroyed by irradiation. The irradiated mice were reconstituted with the marrow of one parent. The reconstituted mice were then immunized and tested for the MHC restriction of the raised Tc response. Following both gene gun and IM immunizations, the haplotype specificity of the Tc response was restricted to that of the reconstituting marrow (34–36). This restriction held in the presence of cotransfected DNAs expressing the B7.2 costimulatory molecule or granulocyte-macrophage colony-stimulating factor (GM-CSF) plus interleukin-12 (IL-12) (35). Thus, the addition of molecules associated with antigen presentation to keratinocytes or muscle cells was not sufficient to support antigen presentation.

The site of antigen presentation and the nature of the APC have been tracked further using reporter plasmids and sorted cells (see Fig. 31-2). Following gene gun immunizations, reporter-plasmid-bearing epidermal Langerhans' cells migrate to the draining lymph node (29,31), where they present antigen (31). Approximately 60 directly transfected epidermal Langerhans-derived dendritic cells were observed in the draining node following the delivery of four gene gun shots to the abdominal skin (31). Following IM and ID saline injections of DNA, dendritic cells in the draining lymph node also have been found to carry vaccine DNA and to present antigen (30). Approximately 0.4% of the dendritic cells in the draining node were estimated to be presenting vaccine antigen following IM DNA immunizations (30). Given that the number of dendritic cells in a lymph node ranges from 15,000 to 40,000, this would suggest that between 60 and 160 directly transfected APCs are present in the draining nodes of IM-inoculated mice.

Cross-priming of dendritic cells or macrophages could also account for antigen presentation. Cross-priming occurs when a bone marrow–derived cell (such as a dendritic cell) presents peptides derived from proteins synthesized in another cell (37). Cross-priming has been demonstrated to prime CD8+ Tc responses following injection of transfected myoblasts (38). Cross-priming also has been demonstrated following IM immunization of SCID mice followed by infusion of a competent bone marrow (39). Following gene gun immunizations, the temporal dependence of Tc responses on the skin target site suggests that cross-priming is important for the realization of a full primary response (40).

Role of Antigen Expression at the Target Site

The skin and muscle targets for DNA delivery play different roles in the initiation of DNA-raised immune responses (see Fig. 31-2). The highest densities of transfected cells are found at the sites of DNA delivery, with the most frequent expressing cells being keratinocytes in skin (41–43) and striated muscle cells in muscle (1,44). Temporal ablation studies of gene gun–bombarded skin have revealed that the skin plays an essential role in the mounting of both antibody and Tc responses (40,45). By contrast, ablation of the muscle target revealed that both antibody and Tc responses were independent of the injected muscle within minutes of DNA delivery (40). These two different patterns of target site dependence held for DNAs that expressed plasma membrane, secreted, or intracellular antigens (40). These results suggest that following gene gun inoculations, both directly transfected epidermal Langerhans' cells and antigen expression by keratinocytes contribute to primary antibody responses. They also suggest that following intramuscular immunizations, the immunologically important transfection events occur at distal sites or in trafficking lymphoid cells.

DNA-Raised Memory

A characteristic of DNA-raised immune responses is the generation of effective memory. Normal mechanisms for the development of immunologic memory as well as unique aspects of DNA-based immunization are likely to contribute to this phenomenon. An immunologic mechanism for sustaining the viability and differentiation of activated B cells is the display of antigen-antibody complexes by follicular dendritic cells (FDCs). FDCs are non–bone marrow–derived cells that reside in the germinal centers of lymph nodes and display both Fc and complement receptors (32,46). These cells are potent stimulators of B-cells. A second type of immune-complex-bearing germinal center dendritic cell can serve as a potent stimulator of T cells (47). This second type of germinal center dendritic cell may serve a function for the maintenance and differentiation of activated T cells similar to that served by FDCs for B cells. Following both gene gun and IM deliveries of DNA, DNA vaccines result in antigen presentation for several weeks (39,39a). This length of time for antigen presentation overlaps the appearance of generated antibody. Thus, there is the potential for the generation of FDC-displayed immune complexes between the newly appearing antibody and the still-expressed antigen. This phenomenon could account for the ability of single DNA immunizations to raise long-lasting memory responses.

Immune Responses Raised by DNA

T-Cell Help

One of the unique features of DNA vaccines is the relative ease with which immunizations can be manipulated to bias the type of raised T-cell help toward type 1 or type 2 (9). Both the method of DNA delivery and the expressed immunogen affect the predominant type of T-cell help that is raised by a DNA immunization (Table 31-2; see Fig. 31-2). In general, saline injections of DNA raise immune responses that are biased toward type 1 help, whereas gene gun deliveries of DNA raise immune responses that are biased toward type 2 help (9,48) (see Fig. 31-2). These patterns of raised help hold for intracellular and plasma membrane–bound forms of DNA-expressed antigens (see Fig. 31-2). However, for secreted antigens, both IM and gene gun inoculations tend to raise type 2 help (49–52) (see Fig. 31-2). The Th2-biased response observed for secreted antigens is the same type of response observed for inoculated proteins. Some exceptions to these generalizations have been reported. For example, Th1-biased responses are raised by a secreted form of the hepatitis C nucleocapsid protein (53). Also, certain MHC backgrounds affect the T-helper type of response for certain antigens (51). For most DNA-raised responses, the type of raised T-cell help is stable over time. Furthermore, the type of DNA-primed help is maintained in the face of challenge infections or subsequent immunizations that would raise the opposite type of help in a naive animal (9,48).

Table 31-2. Time Line for DNA Vaccines

1992	Demonstration of immunogenicity
1993	Early protective studies
1994	Naming of technology, WHO
1995	First phase 1 human trial
1996	FDA points to consider
1998	HIV-1, malaria, influenza, herpes, and hepatitis B in human trials

The mechanism by which DNA immunizations raise different types of T-cell help is not understood. A popular hypothesis as to why IM immunizations raise Th1-biased immune responses is that the large amounts of DNA used for these immunizations trigger type 1 help (see above). By using 100 to 1000 times more DNA for saline than for gene gun inoculations, one inoculates many more "immunostimulatory" CpG sequences during a saline injection than during a gene gun bombardment. Tests of this hypothesis for a membrane-associated antigen have revealed no difference in the types of responses raised by different doses of DNA (9). However, for a secreted antigen, larger doses of DNA can move a Th2-biased response toward a Th1-biased response (S. Johnston, personal communication). This is consistent with the Th1 adjuvant activity of CpG sequences for protein immunizations (54,55).

Cytotoxic T Cells

A forte of DNA vaccines is their inability to raise cytotoxic T cells. Attachment of ubiquitination signals to a DNA-expressed protein can increase Tc responses (56–58). Recombinant DNA molecules encoding a string of MHC epitopes from different pathogens can elicit Tc responses to a variety of pathogens (59). These strings of Tc epitopes are most effective if they also include a Th epitope (60,61). Most analyses for DNA-raised Tc have been done in bulk assays following in vivo or in vitro restimulation. However, more recently, limiting dilution analyses have been undertaken to define precursor frequencies more rigorously. These analyses reveal similar frequencies of Tc raised by IN immunizations with Sendai virus and gene gun DNA immunizations (62). Similar frequencies of Tc were also observed following IM immunization with a ubiquitinated minigene for lymphocytic choriomeningitis virus (LCMV) and intraperitoneal (IP) immunizations with the Armstrong strain of LCMV (56). In this latter instance, a sixfold lower frequency of Tc had been raised by the nonubiquitinated form of the minigene (56). In the Sendai model, similar frequencies of responses were mounted to dominant and subdominant epitopes by the DNA immunization and the natural infection (62). In the LCMV model, the T-cell receptors (TCRs) on the DNA-raised and infection-raised Tc had similar affinities as measured by the ability to lyse targets coated with 0.1 to 1000 nm peptide (56). Interestingly, TCRs raised by a herpesvirus minigene may have had lower affinities than those raised by natural infection (63). This was suggested by a good ability to lyse peptide-pulsed targets but a poor ability to lyse virus-infected targets (64,65). The high levels of expression of a minigene epitope may have resulted in lower-affinity receptors just as high levels of peptide during selection of T-cell lines selects for clones with low-affinity receptors (64).

Studies in the LCMV model have revealed DNA-raised Tc causing immunopathology as well as protection. In these studies, a suboptimal nucleoprotein-expressing DNA vaccine raised precursor frequencies of Tc to approximately 1 in 90,000. On challenge with the Armstrong strain of virus, some mice exhibited accelerated disease whereas others were protected. The Armstrong strain of LCMV does not kill infected cells. Thus, the enhancement of disease presumably reflected failure of Tc to control the LCMV infection sufficiently to prevent spread of virus and consequent Tc-mediated cell destruction.

Interferons

Cytotoxic as well as helper T cells also control viral infection by the suppressive activity of interferons for viral infections. For DNA vaccines, nondestructive IFN-γ–mediated control of an infection has been observed for hepatitis B virus (HBV). Immunization of transgenic mice that replicated the HBV genome and sustained the HBV life cycle with a DNA expressing the HBV surface antigen raised CD8+ cells that abolished HBV gene expression and viral replication while killing only a small fraction of the HBV-expressing hepatocytes (66). Studies of this phenomenon using transfer of HBV surface antigen–specific clones of Tc into the transgenic mice revealed that the antiviral effect was mediated by IFN-γ and TNF-α (67). Interestingly, researchers have not been able to replicate these cytokine-mediated effects in vitro, and in vivo experiments (68) have been required.

Antibody

DNA-raised antibody responses differ in several ways from those raised by protein inoculations or viral infections. These differences presumably reflect differences in the timing, longevity, and amounts of the immunizing antigen. DNA immunizations are accomplished with nanogram levels of protein expression whereas protein immunizations are accomplished with microgram levels of protein. Following protein immunizations, protein is available for only a short period. The initial protein immunization initiates a primary immune response characterized by the presence of IgM. A second protein immunization initiates the secondary response during which IgG is generated and the antibody undergoes affinity maturation. Following DNA immunizations or viral infections, active antigen presentation takes place for several weeks (see above). This prolonged presence of antigen serves to support both primary and secondary phases of antibody responses. Raised antibody undergoes avidity maturation (69), and antibody-secreting cells (ASCs) migrate to the bone marrow for long-term production of antibody (70,71). As do viral infections, DNA-raised antibody responses have plateau levels of expression. In murine models, these plateaus are frequently similar to the level of antibody raised by an infection (72–75).

DNA-raised antibody responses have proven to be a powerful approach not only for vaccination but also for the production of needed reagents. DNA immunizations have been used by several investigators to raise polyclonal (76,77) as well as monoclonal (78) antibodies. For the production of monoclonals, responses can be primed with DNA and then boosted with less pure antigen, such as an antigen-expressing cell line or a partially purified protein, to achieve large numbers of B cells to be used for fusions with myeloma cells.

Increasing the Efficiency of DNA-Based Immunizations

Adjuvants for DNA Vaccines

In addition to the CpG-S sequences in plasmids that act as endogenous adjuvants for DNA vaccines, both conventional and genetic adjuvants have been explored for their ability to increase, or change, the Th bias of DNA-raised immune responses. Conventional adjuvants have included gel-type adjuvants such as alum and calcium phosphate, bacterial adjuvants such as monophosphoryl lipid A (79,80) and cholera toxin (81,82), cationic (83,84) and mannan-coated (85,86) liposomes, emulsifier-based adjuvants such as QS-21 (87), and synthetic adjuvants such as carboxymethylcellulose and Ubenimex (88). All of these adjuvants have had some effect on immunization.

Studies on genetic adjuvants, or DNAs expressing an immunomodulatory molecule, have focused on the cotransfection of plasmids expressing lymphokines, chemokines, or costimulatory molecules [for a review, see (89)]. The vast majority of experiments have been conducted with the native forms of lymphokines or costimulatory molecules by codelivery of DNAs expressing the genetic adjuvant and the immunogen. In general the coinoculated genetic adjuvants have had the expected effects: signature lymphokines for Th1 differentiation have increased Tc responses and signature lymphokines for Th2 responses have increased antibody responses. In general, increases in the magnitudes of immune responses have been fairly minor, with most increases being only two- to threefold. One of the best of the increases (about eightfold) occurred in a study with cotransfected CD40 ligand (90).

Alternative Boosts

Both protein and recombinant viruses have been used to boost DNA-primed responses. Protein boosts have been used to increase neutralizing antibody responses to the HIV-1 Env (91,92). Recombinant pox virus boosts have proved to be a highly successful method of boosting DNA-primed CD8+ cell responses (93–97). Following the pox virus boost, antigen-specific CD8 cells have been increased by as much as 10-fold in DNA-primed mice or macaques. Studies testing the order of immunizations reveal that the DNA must be delivered first (94). This has been hypothesized to reflect the DNA priming focusing the immune response on the desired immunogens. The larger increases in specific CD8+ cell responses following pox virus compared with DNA boosts have been hypothesized to reflect the larger amount of antigen expressed by the pox virus vector, as well as pox virus–induced cytokines augmenting immune responses (94,96).

Enhanced Immunizations Using Alpha Virus Vectors

DNA forms of alpha virus–based vectors can increase the efficiency of DNA-based immunizations by 100- to 1000-fold (98,99). Alpha virus DNA vectors use an RNA polymerase II promoter to express a self-replicating alpha virus RNA. The RNA replicon comprises nonstructural replicase genes, the 5′ and 3′ ends required in cis for replication, and the vaccine insert that has been substituted for structural genes. Expression of the vaccine insert is achieved by linking it to the alpha virus subgenomic promoter. Both Sindbis virus (98) and Semliki Forest virus (99) have been used to build DNAs expressing alpha virus replicons. The alpha virus vectors are unlike conventional plasmid DNA immunizations in that they kill transfected cells and are only transiently expressed. They also are unlike conventional DNA vaccines in that they express foreign proteins (the alphavirus replicase genes) in addition to the vaccine insert.

The high ability of alpha virus replicons to raise immune responses was originally thought to reflect the high levels of protein expression by the self-replicating RNA vector (98). However, further studies with vectors that express lower levels of protein have revealed that the high ability to immunize is not attributable solely to high levels of protein expression. Rather, it may reflect additional factors such as replicon-induced cytokine responses, or possibly replicon-induced apoptosis [which facilitates antigen uptake by dendritic cells (100)]. Irrespective of how DNA-based alpha virus vectors elicit such high immune responses, this new approach to DNA immunization holds much promise for the future.

Designer Proteins

Another approach to increasing immune responses has been to fuse immunogens to immunotargeting molecules. To date, the most successful of these fusions have targeted secreted immunogens to APCs or lymph nodes (101). Fusion of a secreted form of human IgG with cytotoxic T lymphocyte antigen 4 (CTLA-4) elicited more than a 1000-fold increase in antibody responses to the IgG and changed the bias of the response from complement (C′)-dependent to C′-independent antibodies. This very effective fusion was hypothesized to increase the delivery of the immunogen to APC by the CTLA-4 fusion partner directing the protein to the B7.1 and B7.2 receptors of APC. Binding of the fusion protein also may have increased antibody responses by activating the costimulatory activity of B7.1 and B7.2. Fusions of human IgG with L-selectin also increased antibody responses, but did not change the C′ binding characteristics of the raised antibody (101). The immunogen fused with L-selectin was presumably delivered by the binding of L-selectin ligands to the high endothelial venules, which serve as portals for venous cells or molecules to lymph nodes. A lymphoma-specific single-chain immunoglobulin (sFv) has been fused to interferon-inducible protein 10 (IP-10) or monocyte chemotactic protein-3 (MCP-3) (102). These fusions increased antibody responses by about 100-fold and raised apparently cell-mediated protection against tumor challenges. The authors hypothesized that these effects were attributable to the proinflammatory chemokines targeting the sFv fusion to professional APCs.

Applications

To date, DNA vaccines have been tested for at least 40 different viral infections, nine different bacterial infections, and nine different parasitic infections and prions (103). Thirty-four of 40 viral models, eight of nine bacterial models, and four of nine parasitic models have reported protection. The vast majority of these studies have been done in mice. However, the vaccines have also been effective in nonhuman primates (97,104,105), cows (106,107), and trout (108).

The ability to polarize T-cell help by DNA-based immunizations has been applied to preclinical models for allergies and autoimmune diseases. In allergies, the goal has been to shift the allergic Th2 response (and the associated production of IgE) to nonallergic Th1 responses. In autoimmune diseases, the goal has been to shift the response from a self-destructive Th1 response to a nondestructive Th2 response. In both models, predisease priming of responses for the desired Th type has prevented or ameliorated the induction of disease (109,110). Shifting the pattern of T-cell help for established disease also has had some success (111). DNA vaccines are also achieving success in preclinical cancer models (112–115).

Safety Issues

Regulatory agencies considering the application of DNA vaccines for human and veterinary use have identified several areas of concern. These areas include chance integration of the vaccine plasmid causing a cancer-inducing mutation, the potential induction of immune tolerance to the vaccine antigen, the potential induction of autoimmunity, and the potential induction of antibodies to the vaccine DNA. To date, none of these concerns has been realized in preclinical or clinical trials (116,117).

Future Promise

With the explosion of interest in the use of DNA vaccines (see Table 31-2), what promise does this novel technology truly hold for the development of needed vaccines? Successful vaccinations in inbred populations of mice are not equivalent to successful vaccinations in real-world populations of humans and domestic animals. Indications that DNA vaccines will be successful in human populations come from a phase 1 trial in which IM inoculations of a DNA expressing a malaria circumsporozoite protein raised Tc responses higher than those typically observed in naturally infected humans or in humans exposed to irradiated circumsporozoites (the current best vaccine) (118). In this study, Tc responses were directed against all 10 peptides tested and were restricted by six human MHC I alleles. Responses included Tc cells that were restricted by more than one allele in one individual. These highly promising results suggest that protective Tc responses will be able to be raised by DNA immunizations in humans. Indications that protective antibody responses will also be able to be raised come from a phase 1 trial in which gene gun inoculations were used to deliver an HBV surface antigen–expressing DNA (see DNA Vaccine website: http://www.genweb.com/Dnavax/dnavax.html). All 11 of the inoculated individuals seroconverted to antibody levels that confer protection against HBV disease. Other promising, as well as less hopeful, results have been presented at meetings. Thus, there has been variability in the success of early human trials. However, some trials are working, a portent that DNA vaccines, with development, will provide needed human and animal vaccines.

DNA vaccines also hold promise in their empowerment of the ability of basic scientists to manipulate and study immune responses. Microbiologists for the first time are able to screen the protective effects of multiple genes or combinations of genes from microbes. For the first time, the relative efficacy of the protection provided by Th1 or Th2 responses can be readily approached. Immunologists are empowered by the ability to use the in vivo delivery of designer genes for the study of the molecular and cellular biology of immune responses. Much has been learned in the short but already productive life span of DNA vaccines, but much more needs to be accomplished using this novel approach to raising immune responses.

Acknowledgements

Portions of the text as well as Tables 31-1 and 31-2 were adapted with permission from Robinson and Pertmer (103). We would like to thank H. Drake-Perrow for invaluable administrative assistance. This work was supported in part by Public Health Service Grants R01 AI 34946, R01 AI 34241, R01 AI 35149, and P01 AI 43045.

References

1. Wolff JA, Malone RW, Williams P, et al. Direct gene transfer into mouse muscle in vivo. Science 1990;247(4949 Pt 1):1465–1468.
2. Tang DC, De Vit M, Johnston SA. Genetic immunization is a simple method for eliciting an immune response. Nature 1992;356(6365):152–154.
3. Robinson HL, Hunt LA, Webster RG. Protection against a lethal influenza virus challenge by immunization with a haemagglutinin-expressing plasmid DNA. Vaccine 1993; 11(9):957–960.
4. Ulmer JB, Donnelly JJ, Parker SE, et al. Heterologous protection against influenza by injection of DNA encoding a viral protein. Science 1993;259(5102):1745–1749.
5. Fynan EF, Webster RG, Fuller DH, et al. DNA vaccines: protective immunizations by parenteral, mucosal, and gene-gun inoculations. Proc Natl Acad Sci USA 1993;90(24):11478–11482.

6. Xiang Z, Ertl HC. Manipulation of the immune response to a plasmid-encoded viral antigen by coinoculation with plasmids expressing cytokines. Immunity 1995;2(2): 129–135.

7. Barry MA, Lai WC, Johnston SA. Protection against mycoplasma infection using expression-library immunization. Nature 1995;377(6550):632–635.

8. Sato Y, Roman M, Tighe H, et al. Immunostimulatory DNA sequences necessary for effective intradermal gene immunization. Science 1996;273(5273):352–354.

9. Feltquate DM, Heaney S, Webster RG, Robinson HL. Different T helper cell types and antibody isotypes generated by saline and gene gun DNA immunization. J Immunol 1997;158(5):2278–2284.

10. Robinson HL, Pertmer TM. Nucleic acid immunizations. In: Coico R, ed. Current protocols in immunology. New York: John Wiley & Sons, 1998:2.14.1–2.14.19.

11. Chapman BS, Thayer RM, Vincent KA, Haigwood NL. Effect of intron A from human cytomegalovirus (Towne) immediate-early gene on heterologous expression in mammalian cells. Nucleic Acids Res 1991;19(14):3979–3986.

12. Bohm W, Kuhrober A, Paier T, et al. DNA vector constructs that prime hepatitis B surface antigen-specific cytotoxic T lymphocyte and antibody responses in mice after intramuscular injection. J Immunol Meth 1996;193(1):29–40.

13. Montgomery DL, Shiver JW, Leander KR, et al. Heterologous and homologous protection against influenza A by DNA vaccination: optimization of DNA vectors. DNA Cell Biol 1993;12(9):777–783.

14. Hartikka J, Sawdey M, Cornefert-Jensen F, et al. An improved plasmid DNA expression vector for direct injection into skeletal muscle. Hum Gene Ther 1996; 7(10):1205–1217.

15. Manthorpe M, Cornefert-Jensen F, Hartikka J, et al. Gene therapy by intramuscular injection of plasmid DNA: studies on firefly luciferase gene expression in mice. Hum Gene Ther 1993;4(4):419–431.

16. Andre S, Seed B, Eberle J, et al. Increased immune response elicited by DNA vaccination with a synthetic gp120 sequence with optimized codon usage. J Virol 1998; 72(2):1497–1503.

17. Uchijima M, Yoshida A, Nagata T, Koide Y. Optimization of codon usage of plasmid DNA vaccine is required for the effective MHC class I-restricted T cell responses against an intracellular bacterium. J Immunol 1998;161(10):5594–5599.

18. Iwasaki A, Stiernholm BJ, Chan AK, et al. Enhanced CTL responses mediated by plasmid DNA immunogens encoding costimulatory molecules and cytokines. J Immunol 1997;158(10):4591–4601.

19. Wild J, Gruner B, Metzger K, et al. Polyvalent vaccination against hepatitis B surface and core antigen using a dicistronic expression plasmid. Vaccine 1998;16(4):353–360.

20. McCluskie MJ, Chu Y, Xia JL, et al. Direct gene transfer to the respiratory tract of mice with pure plasmid and lipid-formulated DNA [In Process Citation]. Antisense Nucleic Acid Drug Dev 1998;8(5):401–414.

21. Jones DH, Corris S, McDonald S, et al. Poly(DL-lactide-co-glycolide)-encapsulated plasmid DNA elicits systemic and mucosal antibody responses to encoded protein after oral administration. Vaccine 1997;15(8):814–817.

22. Chen SC, Jones DH, Fynan EF, et al. Protective immunity induced by oral immunization with a rotavirus DNA vaccine encapsulated in microparticles. J Virol 1998;72(7): 5757–5761.

23. Sizemore DR, Branstrom AA, Sadoff JC. Attenuated shigella as a DNA delivery vehicle for DNA-mediated immunization. Science 1995;270(5234):299–302.

24. Sizemore DR, Branstrom AA, Sadoff JC. Attenuated bacteria as a DNA delivery vehicle for DNA-mediated immunization. Vaccine 1997;15(8):804–807.

25. Krieg AM, Yi AK, Schorr J, Davis HL. The role of CpG dinucleotides in DNA vaccines. Trends Microbiol 1998; 6(1):23–27.

26. Pisetsky DS. Immune activation by bacterial DNA: a new genetic code. Immunity 1996;5(4):303–310.

27. Krieg AM, Wu T, Weeratna R, et al. Sequence motifs in adenoviral DNA block immune activation by stimulatory CpG motifs. Proc Natl Acad Sci USA 1998;95(21): 12631–12636.

28. Jakob T, Walker PS, Krieg AM, et al. Activation of cutaneous dendritic cells by CpG-containing oligodeoxynucleotides: a role for dendritic cells in the augmentation of Th1 responses by immunostimulatory DNA. J Immunol 1998;161(6): 3042–3049.

29. Condon C, Watkins SC, Celluzzi CM, et al. DNA-based immunization by in vivo transfection of dendritic cells. Nat Med 1996;2(10):1122–1128.

30. Casares S, Inaba K, Brumeanu TD, et al. Antigen presentation by dendritic cells after immunization with DNA encoding a major histocompatibility complex class II-restricted viral epitope. J Exp Med 1997;186(9):1481–1486.

31. Porgador A, Irvine KR, Iwasaki A, et al. Predominant role for directly transfected dendritic cells in antigen presentation to CD8+ T cells after gene gun immunization. J Exp Med 1998;188(6):1075–1082.

32. Banchereau J, Steinman RM. Dendritic cells and the control of immunity. Nature 1998;392(6673):245–252.

33. Klinman DM, Yi AK, Beaucage SL, et al. CpG motifs present in bacteria DNA rapidly induce lymphocytes to secrete interleukin 6, interleukin 12, and interferon gamma. Proc Natl Acad Sci USA 1996;93(7):2879–2883.

34. Corr M, Lee DJ, Carson DA, Tighe H. Gene vaccination with naked plasmid DNA: mechanism of CTL priming. J Exp Med 1996;184(4):1555–1560.

35. Iwasaki A, Torres CA, Ohashi PS, et al. The dominant role of bone marrow-derived cells in CTL induction following plasmid DNA immunization at different sites. J Immunol 1997;159(1):11–14.

36. Fu TM, Ulmer JB, Caulfield MJ, et al. Priming of cytotoxic T lymphocytes by DNA vaccines: requirement for professional antigen presenting cells and evidence for antigen transfer from myocytes. Mol Med 1997;3(6):362–371.

37. Carbone FR, Bevan MJ. Class I-restricted processing and presentation of exogenous cell-associated antigen in vivo. J Exp Med 1990;171(2):377–387.

38. Ulmer JB, Deck RR, De Witt CM, et al. Expression of a viral protein by muscle cells in vivo induces protective cell-mediated immunity. Vaccine 1997;15(8):839–841.

39. Doe B, Selby M, Barnett S, et al. Induction of cytotoxic T lymphocytes by intramuscular immunization with plasmid

DNA is facilitated by bone marrow-derived cells. Proc Natl Acad Sci USA 1996;93(16):8578–8583.

39a. Boyle CM, Robinson HL. Basic mechanisms of DNA-raised antibody responses to intramuscular and gene gun immunizations. DNA Cell Biol 2000;19(3):157–165.

40. Torres CA, Iwasaki A, Barber BH, Robinson HL. Differential dependence on target site tissue for gene gun and intramuscular DNA immunizations. J Immunol 1997; 158(10):4529–4532.

41. Eisenbraun MD, Fuller DH, Haynes JR. Examination of parameters affecting the elicitation of humoral immune responses by particle bombardment-mediated genetic immunization. DNA Cell Biol 1993;12(9):791–797.

42. Raz E, Carson DA, Parker SE, et al. Intradermal gene immunization: the possible role of DNA uptake in the induction of cellular immunity to viruses. Proc Natl Acad Sci USA 1994;91(20):9519–9523.

43. Hengge UR, Chan EF, Foster RA, et al. Cytokine gene expression in epidermis with biological effects following injection of naked DNA. Nat Genet 1995;10(2):161–166.

44. Davis HL, Whalen RG, Demeneix BA. Direct gene transfer into skeletal muscle in vivo: factors affecting efficiency of transfer and stability of expression. Hum Gene Ther 1993;4(2):151–159.

45. Klinman DM, Sechler JM, Conover J, et al. Contribution of cells at the site of DNA vaccination to the generation of antigen-specific immunity and memory. J Immunol 1998;160(5):2388–2392.

46. Liu YJ, Grouard G, de Bouteiller O, Banchereau J. Follicular dendritic cells and germinal centers. Intl Rev Cytology 1996;166:139–179.

47. Grouard G, Durand I, Filgueira L, et al. Dendritic cells capable of stimulating T cells in germinal centres. Nature 1996;384(6607):364–367.

48. Pertmer TM, Roberts TR, Haynes JR. Influenza virus nucleoprotein-specific immunoglobulin G subclass and cytokine responses elicited by DNA vaccination are dependent on the route of vector DNA delivery. J Virol 1996;70(9):6119–6125.

49. Boyle JS, Koniaras C, Lew AM. Influence of cellular location of expressed antigen on the efficacy of DNA vaccination: cytotoxic T lymphocyte and antibody responses are suboptimal when antigen is cytoplasmic after intramuscular DNA immunization. Int Immunol 1997;9(12):1897–1906.

50. Lewis PJ, Cox GJ, van Drunen Littel-van den Hurk S, Babiuk LA. Polynucleotide vaccines in animals: enhancing and modulating responses. Vaccine 1997;15(8):861–864.

51. Sallberg M, Townsend K, Chen M, et al. Characterization of humoral and CD4+ cellular responses after genetic immunization with retroviral vectors expressing different forms of the hepatitis B virus core and e antigens. J Virol 1997;71(7):5295–5303.

52. Haddad D, Liljeqvist S, Stahl S, et al. Comparative study of DNA-based immunization vectors: effect of secretion signals on the antibody responses in mice. FEMS Immunol Med Microbiol 1997;18(3):193–202.

53. Inchauspe G, Vitvitski L, Major ME, et al. Plasmid DNA expressing a secreted or a nonsecreted form of hepatitis C virus nucleocapsid: comparative studies of antibody and

T-helper responses following genetic immunization. DNA Cell Biol 1997;16(2):185–195.

54. Chu RS, Targoni OS, Krieg AM, et al. CpG oligodeoxynucleotides act as adjuvants that switch on T helper 1 (Th1) immunity. J Exp Med 1997;186(10):1623–1631.

55. Davis HL, Weeranta R, Waldschmidt TJ, et al. CpG DNA is a potent enhancer of specific immunity in mice immunized with recombinant hepatitis B surface antigen. J Immunol 1998;160(2):870–876.

56. Rodriguez F, Zhang J, Whitton JL. DNA immunization: ubiquitination of a viral protein enhances cytotoxic T-lymphocyte induction and antiviral protection but abrogates antibody induction. J Virol 1997;71(11):8497–8503.

57. Tobery TW, Siliciano RF. Targeting of HIV-1 antigens for rapid intracellular degradation enhances cytotoxic T lymphocyte (CTL) recognition and the induction of de novo CTL responses in vivo after immunization. J Exp Med 1997;185(5):909–920.

58. Wu Y, Kipps TJ. Deoxyribonucleic acid vaccines encoding antigens with rapid proteasome-dependent degradation are highly efficient inducers of cytolytic T lymphocytes. J Immunol 1997;159(12):6037–6043.

59. Hanke T, Schneider J, Gilbert SC, et al. DNA multi-CTL epitope vaccines for HIV and Plasmodium falciparum: immunogenicity in mice. Vaccine 1998;16(4):426–435.

60. Maecker HT, Umetsu DT, DeKruyff RH, Levy S. Cytotoxic T cell responses to DNA vaccination: dependence on antigen presentation via class II MHC [In Process Citation]. J Immunol 1998;161(12):6532–6536.

61. Thomson SA, Sherritt MA, Medveczky J, et al. Delivery of multiple CD8 cytotoxic T cell epitopes by DNA vaccination. J Immunol 1998;160(4):1717–1723.

62. Chen Y, Webster RG, Woodland DL. Induction of CD8+ T cell responses to dominant and subdominant epitopes and protective immunity to Sendai virus infection by DNA vaccination. J Immunol 1998;160(5):2425–2432.

63. Yu Z, Karem KL, Kanangat S, et al. Protection by mini-genes: a novel approach of DNA vaccines. Vaccine 1998;16(17):1660–1667.

64. Alexander-Miller MA, Leggatt GR, Berzofsky JA. Selective expansion of high- or low-avidity cytotoxic T lymphocytes and efficacy for adoptive immunotherapy. Proc Natl Acad Sci USA 1996;93(9):4102–4107.

65. Speiser DE, Kyburz D, Stubi U, et al. Discrepancy between in vitro measurable and in vivo virus neutralizing cytotoxic T cell reactivities. Low T cell receptor specificity and avidity sufficient for in vitro proliferation or cytotoxicity to peptide-coated target cells but not for in vivo protection. J Immunol 1992;149(3):972–980.

66. Mancini M, Hadchouel M, Davis HL, et al. DNA-mediated immunization in a transgenic mouse model of the hepatitis B surface antigen chronic carrier state. Proc Natl Acad Sci USA 1996;93(22):12496–12501.

67. Guidotti LG, Ishikawa T, Hobbs MV, et al. Intracellular inactivation of the hepatitis B virus by cytotoxic T lymphocytes. Immunity 1996;4(1):25–36.

68. Heise T, Guidotti LG, Cavanaugh VJ, Chisari FV. Hepatitis B virus RNA-binding proteins associated with cytokine-induced clearance of viral RNA from the liver of transgenic mice. J Virol 1999;73(1):474–481.

69. Boyle JS, Silva A, Brady JL, Lew AM. DNA immunization: induction of higher avidity antibody and effect of route on T cell cytotoxicity. Proc Natl Acad Sci USA 1997;94 (26):14626–14631.

70. Boyle CM, Morin M, Webster RG, Robinson HL. Role of different lymphoid tissues in the initiation and maintenance of DNA-raised antibody responses to the influenza virus H1 glycoprotein. J Virol 1996;70(12):9074–9078.

71. Slifka MK, Antia R, Whitmire JK, Ahmed R. Humoral immunity due to long-lived plasma cells. Immunity 1998;8(3):363–372.

72. Robinson HL, Boyle CA, Feltquate DM, et al. DNA immunization for influenza virus: studies using hemagglutinin- and nucleoprotein-expressing DNAs. J Infect Dis 1997; 176(suppl 1):S50–S55.

73. Xiang J, Koropatnick J, Qi Y, et al. Production of a bifunctional hybrid molecule B72.3/metallothionein-1 by protein engineering. Immunology 1993;78(4):574–581.

74. Michel ML, Davis HL, Schleef M, et al. DNA-mediated immunization to the hepatitis B surface antigen in mice: aspects of the humoral response mimic hepatitis B viral infection in humans. Proc Natl Acad Sci USA 1995; 92(12):5307–5311.

75. Deck RR, De Witt CM, Donnelly JJ, et al. Characterization of humoral immune responses induced by an influenza hemagglutinin DNA vaccine. Vaccine 1997;15(1): 71–78.

76. Sundaram P, Xiao W, Brandsma JL. Particle-mediated delivery of recombinant expression vectors to rabbit skin induces high-titered polyclonal antisera (and circumvents purification of a protein immunogen). Nucleic Acids Res 1996;24(7):1375–1377.

77. Robinson WH, Prohaska SS, Santoro JC, et al. Identification of a mouse protein homologous to the human CD6 T cell surface protein and sequence of the corresponding cDNA. J Immunol 1995;155(10):4739–4748.

78. Barry MA, Barry ME, Johnston SA. Production of monoclonal antibodies by genetic immunization. Biotechniques 1994;16(4):616–618, 620.

79. Sasaki S, Tsuji T, Hamajima K, et al. Monophosphoryl lipid A enhances both humoral and cell-mediated immune responses to DNA vaccination against human immunodeficiency virus type 1. Infect Immun 1997;65(9):3520–3528.

80. Sasaki S, Hamajima K, Fukushima J, et al. Comparison of intranasal and intramuscular immunization against human immunodeficiency virus type 1 with a DNA-monophosphoryl lipid A adjuvant vaccine. Infect Immun 1998;66(2):823–826.

81. Kuklin N, Daheshia M, Karem K, et al. Induction of mucosal immunity against herpes simplex virus by plasmid DNA immunization. J Virol 1997;71(4):3138–3145.

82. Ban EM, van Ginkel FW, Simecka JW, et al. Mucosal immunization with DNA encoding influenza hemagglutinin. Vaccine 1997;15(8):811–813.

83. Gregoriadis G, Saffie R, de Souza JB. Liposome-mediated DNA vaccination. FEBS Lett 1997;402(2–3):107–110.

84. Ishii N, Fukushima J, Kaneko T, et al. Cationic liposomes are a strong adjuvant for a DNA vaccine of human immunodeficiency virus type 1. AIDS Res Hum Retroviruses 1997;13(16):1421–1428.

85. Sasaki S, Fukushima J, Arai H, et al. Human immunodeficiency virus type-1-specific immune responses induced by DNA vaccination are greatly enhanced by mannan-coated diC14-amidine. Eur J Immunol 1997;27(12): 3121–3129.

86. Toda S, Ishii N, Okada E, et al. HIV-1-specific cell-mediated immune responses induced by DNA vaccination were enhanced by mannan-coated liposomes and inhibited by anti-interferon-gamma antibody. Immunology 1997;92(1): 111–117.

87. Sasaki S, Sumino K, Hamajima K, et al. Induction of systemic and mucosal immune responses to human immunodeficiency virus type 1 by a DNA vaccine formulated with QS-21 saponin adjuvant via intramuscular and intranasal routes. J Virol 1998;72(6):4931–4939.

88. Sasaki S, Fukushima J, Hamajima K, et al. Adjuvant effect of Ubenimex on a DNA vaccine for HIV-1. Clin Exp Immunol 1998;111(1):30–35.

89. Cohen AD, Boyer JD, Weiner DB. Modulating the immune response to genetic immunization [In Process Citation]. Faseb J 1998;12(15):1611–1626.

90. Mendoza RB, Cantwell MJ, Kipps TJ. Immunostimulatory effects of a plasmid expressing CD40 ligand (CD154) on gene immunization. J Immunol 1997;159(12):5777–5781.

91. Letvin NL, Montefiori DC, Yasutomi Y, et al. Potent, protective anti-HIV immune responses generated by bimodal HIV envelope DNA plus protein vaccination. Proc Natl Acad Sci USA 1997;94(17):9378–9383.

92. Richmond JF, Lu S, Santoro JC, et al. Studies of the neutralizing activity and avidity of anti-human immunodeficiency virus type 1 Env antibody elicited by DNA priming and protein boosting. J Virol 1998;72(11):9092–9100.

93. Hanke T, Blanchard TJ, Schneider J, et al. Enhancement of MHC class I-restricted peptide-specific T cell induction by a DNA prime/MVA boost vaccination regime. Vaccine 1998;16(5):439–445.

94. Schneider J, Gilbert SC, Blanchard TJ, et al. Enhanced immunogenicity for CD8+ T cell induction and complete protective efficacy of malaria DNA vaccination by boosting with modified vaccinia virus Ankara. Nat Med 1998;4 (4):397–402.

95. Irvine KR, Chamberlain RS, Shulman EP, et al. Enhancing efficacy of recombinant anticancer vaccines with prime/boost regimens that use two different vectors. J Natl Cancer Inst 1997;5:89.

96. Kent SJ, Zhao A, Best SJ, et al. Enhanced T-cell immunogenicity and protective efficacy of a human immunodeficiency virus type 1 vaccine regimen consisting of consecutive priming with DNA and boosting with recombinant fowlpox virus. J Virol 1998;72(12):10180–10188.

97. Robinson HL, Montefiori DC, Johnson RP, et al. Neutralizing antibody-independent containment of immunodeficiency virus challenges by DNA priming and recombinant pox virus booster immunization. Nat Med 1999;5:526–534.

98. Hariharan MJ, Driver DA, Townsend K, et al. DNA immunization against herpes simplex virus: enhanced efficacy using a Sindbis virus-based vector. J Virol 1998;72 (2):950–958.

99. Berglund P, Smerdou C, Fleeton MN, et al. Enhancing immune responses using suicidal DNA vaccines [see comments]. Nat Biotechnol 1998;16(6):562–565.

100. Albert ML, Sauter B, Bhardwaj N. Dendritic cells acquire antigen from apoptotic cells and induce class I-restricted CTLs. Nature 1998;392(6671):86–89.

101. Boyle JS, Brady JL, Lew AM. Enhanced responses to a DNA vaccine encoding a fusion antigen that is directed to sites of immune induction. Nature 1998;392(6674):408–411.

102. Biragyn A, Tani K, Grimm MC, et al. Genetic fusion of chemokines to a self tumor antigen induces protective, T-cell dependent antitumor immunity [In Process Citation]. Nat Biotechnol 1999;17(3):253–258.

103. Robinson HL, Pertmer TM. DNA vaccines for viral infections: basic studies and applications. Adv Virus Res 2000 (in press).

104. Donnelly JJ, Friedman A, Martinez D, et al. Preclinical efficacy of a prototype DNA vaccine: enhanced protection against antigenic drift in influenza virus. Nat Med 1995;1(6):583–587.

105. Prince AM, Whalen R, Brotman B. Successful nucleic acid based immunization of newborn chimpanzees against hepatitis B virus. Vaccine 1997;15(8):916–919.

106. Cox GJ, Zamb TJ, Babiuk LA. Bovine herpesvirus 1: immune responses in mice and cattle injected with plasmid DNA. J Virol 1993;67(9):5664–5667.

107. Schrijver RS, Langedijk JP, Keil GM, et al. Immunization of cattle with a BHV1 vector vaccine or a DNA vaccine both coding for the G protein of BRSV. Vaccine 1997;15(17–18):1908–1916.

108. Anderson ED, Mourich DV, Fahrenkrug SC, et al. Genetic immunization of rainbow trout (Oncorhynchus mykiss) against infectious hematopoietic necrosis virus. Mol Mar Biol Biotechnol 1996;5(2):114–122.

109. Waisman A, Ruiz PJ, Hirschberg DL, et al. Suppressive vaccination with DNA encoding a variable region gene of the T-cell receptor prevents autoimmune encephalomyelitis and activates Th2 immunity. Nat Med 1996;2(8):899–905.

110. Hsu CH, Chua KY, Tao MH, et al. Immunoprophylaxis of allergen-induced immunoglobulin E synthesis and airway hyperresponsiveness in vivo by genetic immunization. Nat Med 1996;2(5):540–544.

111. Raz E, Tighe H, Sato Y, et al. Preferential induction of a Th1 immune response and inhibition of specific IgE antibody formation by plasmid DNA immunization. Proc Natl Acad Sci USA 1996;93(10):5141–5145.

112. Syrengelas AD, Chen TT, Levy R. DNA immunization induces protective immunity against B-cell lymphoma. Nat Med 1996;2(9):1038–1041.

113. Chen Y, Hu D, Eling DJ, et al. DNA vaccines encoding full-length or truncated Neu induce protective immunity against Neu-expressing mammary tumors. Cancer Res 1998;58(9):1965–1971.

114. King CA, Spellerberg MB, Zhu D, et al. DNA vaccines with single-chain Fv fused to fragment C of tetanus toxin induce protective immunity against lymphoma and myeloma [see comments]. Nat Med 1998;4(11):1281–1286.

115. Conry RM, White SA, Fultz PN, et al. Polynucleotide immunization of nonhuman primates against carcinoembryonic antigen. Clin Cancer Res 1998;4(11):2903–2912.

116. Nichols WW, Ledwith BJ, Manam SV, Troilo PJ. Potential DNA vaccine integration into host cell genome. Ann NY Acad Sci 1995;772:30–39.

117. Mor G, Singla M, Steinberg AD, et al. Do DNA vaccines induce autoimmune disease? Hum Gene Ther 1997;8(3):293–300.

118. Wang R, Doolan DL, Le TP, et al. Induction of antigenspecific cytotoxic T lymphocytes in humans by a malaria DNA vaccine. Science 1998;282(5388):476–480.

119. Robinson HL, Ginsberg HS, Davis HL, et al. The scientific future of DNA for immunization. Washington: American Academy of Microbiology, 1997.

Chapter 32

Blockade of the CD40L/CD40 Pathway

Leonard Chess

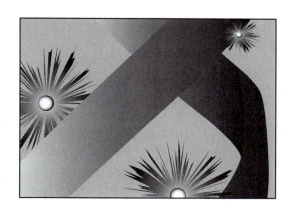

Immune responses are initiated when resting precursor CD4+ T cells are triggered by MHC/peptide complexes in concert with costimulatory molecules on the surface of antigen-presenting cells (APCs) (1–3). As a consequence of this triggering, the CD4+ T cells proliferate, begin to secrete cytokines (IL-2, IFN-γ, IL-4, etc.), and express important cell-surface molecules, including the IL-2 receptor (CD25), CTLA-4, and CD40 ligand. In addition, CD4+ T cells interact with a variety of cells to further induce immune and inflammatory responses. For example, CD4+ T cells interact with B lymphocytes and play pivotal roles in "helping" B cells to differentiate into antibody-secreting cells (4–7). Moreover, CD4+ T cells interact with antigen-presenting cells (APCs), including macrophages and dendritic cells to induce the expression of cell-surface costimulatory molecules important in T-cell activation, as well as to induce the secretion of cytokines and chemokines, which effect inflammation and immune responses (3,8–10). Further, CD4+ T cells also interact with mesenchymal elements, including fibroblasts and endothelial cells. The CD4+ T-cell–fibroblast interaction induces fibroblast activation, proliferation, and the release of cytokines important in fibrosis, whereas the interaction with endothelial cells governs in part the expression of cell-surface molecules involved in hemostasis, as well as the migration of immune cells to the sites of inflammation. A key molecule involved in all of these inducer functions has been found to be a 30 Kd protein, termed CD40 ligand (CD40L or CD154), that is expressed transiently following T-cell receptor (TCR) activation on the surface of CD4+ T cells. CD40L interacts with CD40 expressed on B cells, macrophages, dendritic cells, fibroblasts, and endothelial cells to induce and effect immune responses.

The important biologic role of the CD40L/CD40 pathway has been firmly established because, in vivo, deletion or mutations of the CD40L molecule lead to severe immunodeficiency in both man and mouse characterized by hypogammaglobulinemia, as well as T-cell defects in cell-mediated immunity. Moreover, blockade of the CD40L/CD40 pathway by antibodies to CD40L has been used in experimental animals to effectively prevent and treat a variety of autoimmune diseases as well as allograft rejection without inducing generalized immune suppression. As a consequence of these preclinical animal studies, antibodies to CD40L are currently in clinical trials to treat immunologically induced disease in man. In this chapter we will first briefly review the immunobiology of the CD40L/CD40 pathway that directly bears

on therapeutic strategies and then review the preclinical experimental evidence that strongly suggests that blockade of the CD40L/CD40 pathway may provide a novel form of therapy for immune-mediated disease. Finally, we will discuss the current projections for clinical use and potential complications of antibodies to CD40L in the treatment of human immune disease.

The Discovery of the CD40L/CD40 Pathway

It was discovered in the late 1960s and early 1970s that interactions between thymus-derived T cells (termed helper T cells) and B cells were required to generate effective antibody responses (11–13). By the early 1980s evidence emerged that specialized subsets of T cells distinguished by the CD4 cell-surface molecule carried out this T-cell helper function (14–16). Although the precise molecular mechanisms involved in T-B interaction were unknown, it was thought that the process by which T cells help B cells to differentiate could be divided into two distinct phases: the inductive or cognitive phase and the effector phase. In the inductive phase, antigen-specific CD4+ T cells contact antigen-primed B cells, and this association allows clonotypic T-cell receptors (TCR) to interact with class II MHC/peptide antigen complexes expressed on the surface of B cells. The affinity of this interaction is enhanced by CD4 coreceptor molecules, which bind to MHC class II and permit the formation of stable T-B cognate pairs and bidirectional T- and B-cell activation (17,18). In the effector phase, clear evidence emerged that the set of effector molecules released by the CD4+ T cells that mediate B-cell help were lymphokines (including IL-4, IL-5, and IL-6). Moreover, several lines of evidence suggested that non–antigen-specific T-cell surface molecules become expressed on activated CD4+ T cells and that these surface molecules in concert with lymphokines were required for full B-cell activation and differentiation (17,18). In addition, an important finding by Banchereau et al was that a key B-cell surface molecule involved in B-cell activation was a molecule designated as CD40 (19,20). Triggering of CD40 on the surface of B cells by antibodies induced B-cell proliferation and activation. Furthermore, ligation of CD40 in the presence of IL-4 induced Ig class switching and Ig synthesis in vitro, suggesting a role of CD40 in the normal physiology of B-cell activation. The cDNA encoding CD40 was isolated and found to be a member of the TNF receptor family of molecules (21). These genetic studies suggested that the natural ligand for CD40 would probably be a key effector molecule of T-B interaction, and the search for the CD40L began.

Two distinct lines of experimental studies led to the identification of the CD40 ligand (CD40L) as a key molecule mediating the contact-dependent effector phase of T-B collaboration and help. In the first line of studies, a mutant of the functionally competent Jurkat T-cell line, termed D1.1, was isolated that constitutively activated human B cells to secrete immunoglobulin in conventional in vitro assays of T-cell help (22). This helper function depended on cell-cell contact. Moreover, a monoclonal antibody, termed 5c8, was raised to D1.1 and specifically reacted with the immunizing D1.1 cell line but not with the parental Jurkat T-cell line. The 5c8 antibody immunoprecipitates a 30 Kd surface protein that was shown to be expressed on activated, normal, human CD4+ T cells, but was not detectable on a variety of other lymphocyte populations and was not expressed on resting CD4+ T-cells (23). Also, the 5c8 antibody specifically inhibited helper function of CD4+ T cells, including the capacity to induce B cells to secrete IgG, IgA, and IgE in vitro. The 30 Kd surface protein detected by 5c8 was initially termed T-B-cell activating molecule or T-BAM and was later found to identify the CD40L structure (23–26). In a second line of studies, investigators employed molecular cloning strategies to isolate the cDNA's encoding proteins that bind CD40 (27–29). Structurally, the CD40L cDNA sequence was homologous to the TNF family of genes that now includes TNF, lymphotoxin (LT)-α, LT-β, Fas ligand, CD27L, CD30L, OX40L, TRANCE, and TNF-related apoptosis-inducing ligand (TRAIL) (30,31). Functionally, recombinant CD40L together with IL-4 was shown to drive normal B cells to proliferate, class switch, and secrete IgG, IgA, and IgE antibodies. Moreover, a cDNA clone isolated from D1.1 was identical to CD40L by sequence and drives the expression of a 5c8 reactive protein on transfected cells, formally demonstrating that the antigen recognized by the 5c8 antibody is CD40L (26).

The definitive evidence that the CD40L molecule is essential for human T-helper function and for Ig class switching in vivo was provided by the finding that mutant CD40L genes encode dysfunctional proteins in patients with the X-linked hyper-IgM syndrome (HIMS) (29,32–34). HIMS is a serious, congenital, immunodeficiency disorder characterized by the inability of patients to mount an appropriate antibody response and the absence of germinal centers. Patients have elevated serum IgM levels but low or absent serum IgG, IgA, and IgE and, if untreated with pooled human Ig, succumb from pyogenic infections. In addition, these patients are susceptible to opportunistic infections, including *Pneumocystis carinii* pneumonia. Although patients show abnormal antibody responses, their B cells in vitro are capable of producing normal antibodies when cocultured with normal T-helper (Th) cells, indicating that the defect lies in the inability of T cells to activate B cells (35). Indeed, activated CD4+ T cells from HIM patients are not reactive with 5c8 or other anti-CD40L antibodies, and the Ig secreting defect in HIM is overcome in vitro by recombinant soluble CD40L (29,33,34).

These data demonstrate that defects in CD40L account for the HIM syndrome and unequivocally demonstrate the critical and nonredundant role of the CD40L/CD40 pathway in normal antibody responses in humans. Moreover, about this time a crystal structure of a soluble extracellular fragment of human CD40L was determined (36). Although the molecule was observed to form a trimer, similar to that found for other members of the TNF family such as TNF-α and lymphotoxin-α, and to exhibit a similar overall fold, there were considerable differences in several loops, including those predicted to be involved in CD40 binding. Interestingly, analysis of the structure with respect to the mutations found in the HIM syndrome suggested that most of the hyper-IgM syndrome mutations affect the folding and stability of the molecule rather than the CD40-binding site directly. Moreover, despite the fact that the hyper-IgM syndrome mutations are dispersed in the primary sequence, a large fraction of them are clustered in space in the vicinity of a surface loop, close to the predicted CD40-binding site (36).

These in vivo data in humans were confirmed in murine studies with the isolation of cDNAs encoding murine CD40L, the creation of knockout mice with a CD40L–/– genotype, and the preparation of an antibody (termed MR1) that recognizes murine CD40L (8,37,38). The MR1 antibody given in vivo to normal mice inhibits primary and secondary antibody responses and inhibits Ig isotype switching and germinal-center formation. Moreover, CD40L–/– gene knockout mice, similar to HIM patients, lack CD40 ligand (expressed on activated T cells), do not generate germinal centers, and are unable to make IgG, IgA, or IgE antibody responses (37). It has been assumed that the clinical phenotype in the HIM syndrome and in the CD40–/– mice is the result of an absence of signals to B cells through CD40. However, there is evidence that, in addition, signaling to T cells through CD40 ligand may contribute to some of the functional abnormalities. Thus, the administration of soluble CD40 in vivo to CD40 knockout mice initiates germinal-center formation, presumably by restoring the missing signal through CD40 ligand (39). Furthermore, T cells primed in the absence of CD40 (in CD40–/– mice) are unable to help normal B cells to class switch or to form germinal centers. These results are consistent with the idea that costimulation of T cells through CD40 ligand may play a role in their differentiation into cells that help B cells to make mature antibody responses.

Biologic Properties of CD40L Molecule Relevant to Therapeutic Strategies

The Tissue Distribution and Cell-Surface Expression of CD40L

As described above, CD40L was originally identified on antigen-activated CD4+ T cells. Later CD40L was found to be expressed on stimulated mast cells, basophils, and platelets (40,41). However, significant levels of CD40L are not usually expressed on other lymphoid tissues, including activated CD8+ T cells or B cells, and

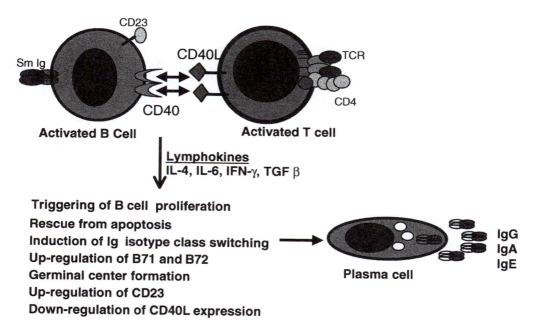

Figure 32-1. Final phases of B-cell differentiation are mediated by contact-depend CD40L signals and lymphokines.

CD40L is not expressed on macrophages or dendritic cells. Moreover, CD40L is not detected in normal, nonlymphoid tissues or mesenchymal structures (24), and although there have been reports of surface expression of CD40L on endothelial cells in vitro, the significance of these findings is not clear (42,43). In fact, even in lymphoid organs the percentage of CD40L-expressing cells is small and limited to activated CD4+ T cells parked in regions associated with germinal centers (44,45). In addition to the limited tissue distribution of CD40L, it is of interest that CD40L is not expressed on resting CD4+ T cells and that the molecule is only transiently expressed following T-cell activation by MHC/peptide complexes (23). For example, following T-cell-receptor triggering of CD4+ T cells in vitro, CD40L surface expression is maximal from 6 to 8 hours following activation. Subsequently, the surface expression of CD40L is rapidly down-regulated and is absent by 24 hours following stimulation (46). This transient expression of CD40L may provide a molecular solution to limiting nonspecific B-cell activation. Thus, the transient expression of CD40L in the localized milieu of antigen-specific cognate T-B pairs may channel the antigen/MHC-unrestricted activating function of CD40L only to appropriate B-cell clones in germinal centers. The tissue and functional specificity of CD40L, together with the transient nature of its expression coincident with antigen triggering, offers the real possibility that blocking CD40L action would predominately target CD4+ T cells being activated at the time of blockade. This might provide preferential blocking of T cells being constitutively activated in vivo by either autoantigens or alloantigens. This type of specificity is not possible with therapeutic strategies directed at more ubiquitously expressed molecules or molecules whose expression is independent of antigen triggering.

The Consequences of CD40L Signaling of B Cells

The interaction of CD40L expressed on activated helper CD4+ T cells gives the essential effector signal to CD40 expressed on the surface of naïve B cells, which promotes B-cell growth, survival, Ig isotype switching, and differentiation to plasma cells (Fig. 32-1). The precise functional consequences of CD40L/CD40 interactions to B cells include 1) the rescue of B cells from apoptosis induced by Fas (CD95) or by surface immunoglobulin M (IgM) cross-linking by antigen (44,47–50); 2) the up-regulation of the key costimulator molecules B7-1 (CD80) and B7-2 (CD86) (51–54), which interact with CD28 and CD152 (CTLA-4) on the surface of activated T cells; 3) the increased expression of other cell-surface activation molecules CD23, CD54, and CD95 (55–57) and lymphotoxin-α (LT-α) (58); and 4) the induction of immunoglobulin isotype class switching (25,59,60). When considering this key role of the CD40L/CD40 pathway in antibody formation, it suggests that blockade of this pathway may provide a novel means of inhibiting pathogenic autoantibodies or unwanted antibodies that may arise during the exogenous administration of foreign antigens.

The signal transduction pathways triggered by ligation of CD40 have been extensively studied. As noted above, CD40 is a member of the TNF receptor (TNFR) family of molecules, and it is of interest that a number of intracellular proteins that belong to the family of TNFR-associated cytoplasmic factors (TRAFs), have been found to associate with the cytoplasmic domain of CD40 (61–65). Thus, CD40 ligation activates NFκB/Rel family members by inducing the recruitment of TRAFs to the CD40 cytoplasmic domain (66,67). The activation and nuclear trans-location of different NF-B/Rel family members regulate the CD40-dependent, germ-line transcription of CH genes by binding critical DNA elements located within the corresponding upstream promoter (68). Moreover, CD40 engagement contributes to this preferential isotype production by activating NF-kappaB/Rel to induce germ-line γ1 transcripts, which are essential for class IgG switch recombination. In addition, CD40 ligand induces production of endogenous TGF-β and IL-10, expression of germ-line Iα1-Cα1 and Iα2-Cα2 transcripts, mature VHDJH-Cα1 and VHDJH-Cα2 transcripts, and IgA secretion. In concert with IL-4, CD40L induces ε transcription and switching to IgE. In summary, the key role of CD40, the triggering of NFκB/Rel proteins, is intimately involved in activating the transcriptional machinery for class switching to IgG, IgA, and IgE (20,25,69).

With respect to the further regulation of Ig class switching, it is of interest that CD30 signaling interferes with the CD40-mediated, NF-κB–dependent transcriptional activation of down-stream C(H) genes. In addition, CD40L signals to CD40 induce CD30 expression on B cells, suggesting a potential homeostatic loop for the control of isotype switching. Furthermore, although CD30 triggering interferes with those CD40-mediated signaling pathways that are related to Ig class switching, it does not interfere with other CD40-mediated, B-cell responses, including proliferation; enhancement of IgM secretion; or CD23, CD54, CD80, CD86, and CD95 up-regulation (55–57). In addition to activation of NFκB, engagement of CD40 activates protein tyrosine kinases (PTKs) and serine/threonine kinases (70–72) that are important in CD40-mediated, B-cell activation. It was shown that CD40 ligation on the surface of B lymphocytes leads to the tyrosine phosphorylation and activation of the PTK Jak3 and of STAT3 (57). Importantly, Jak3 was constitutively associated with CD40, and functional studies strongly suggest that Jak3 is involved in CD40 induction of expression of CD23, ICAM-1, and lymphotoxin β genes in B cells. Earlier studies showed that TRAF3 was also involved in CD23 expression and Ig class switching. Taken together, the emerging evidence suggests that the Jak3-STAT3 signaling pathway and the TRAF signaling pathways, which include TRAF2-mediated activation of NF-B and TRAF3, may synergize to activate switch recombination (57).

The Consequences of CD40L Signaling of APCs Other Than B Cells

Although the primary in vivo function of CD40 ligand (CD40L) was initially believed to be in the regulation of T-B interactions and the T-cell induction of humoral immunity, it is now appreciated that CD40L-induced triggering of CD40 at the surface of other antigen-presenting cells, including dendritic cells and macrophages, may ultimately control both the afferent phases of immune recognition by T cells, as well as important effector mechanisms of cell-mediated immunity (8,73,74) (Fig. 32-2). For example, CD40 triggering augments the antigen-presenting functions of dendritic cells by inducing maintenance of high levels of MHC class II antigens and marked up-regulation of accessory molecules, including CD58 (LFA-3). In addition, CD40L triggering induces up-regulation of the key costimulatory molecules

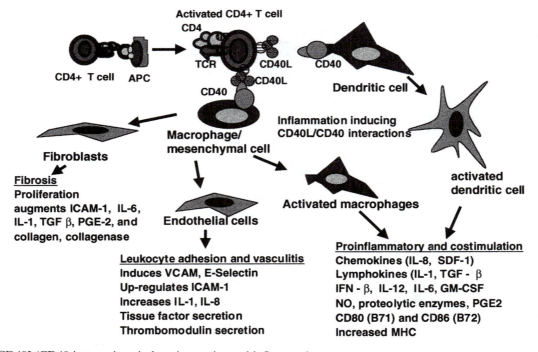

Figure 32-2. CD40L/CD40 interactions induce immunity and inflammation.

CD80 (B7-1) and CD86 (B7-2), which interact with CD28 to provide the essential second signal to T cells that, in concert with triggering of the T-cell receptor, is required for full T-cell activation. Thus, in the absence of B7-1 and B7-2 triggering of CD28, anergy or tolerance rather than T-cell activation ensues as a consequence of antigen triggering (3,75–77). These data suggest that the CD40L/CD40 pathway may ultimately influence whether the consequence of TCR triggering by MHC/peptide complexes will be immunity or tolerance. In this regard, recent in vivo studies in mice have strongly suggested that blockade of CD40L-CD40 interactions by antibody is tolerogenic. For example, the anti-CD40L mAb (MR1) alone has allowed indefinite islet allograft survival in recipient mice and significantly inhibits heart, skin, and kidney allograft rejection (see below) (78–81). Moreover, CD40L blockade induces tolerance in murine models of contact sensitivity (82), and the induction of tolerance may play a role in the potent effects of CD40L blockade in EAE, collagen-induced arthritis, and SLE murine models (see below).

In addition to the role of CD40L/CD40 signals to antigen-presenting cells in controlling the afferent phases of T-cell activation, these signals also control other aspects of immune and inflammatory reactions. For example, CD40L-CD40 interactions induce dendritic cells to secrete an important set of cytokines and chemokines, including IL-12, TNF-α, IL-8, and macrophage inflammatory protein 1 alpha (MIP-1α) (83). The effect of CD40 ligation on IL-12 secretion is of interest because IL-12 itself up-regulates CD40L expression on T cells and synergizes with IL-2, as well as with other costimulatory interactions, including B7-1 and B7-2, to maximize CD40L expression (84). In addition, IL-12 functions as a major cytokine governing the differentiation of CD4+ T-cell subsets by promoting the differentiation of the Th1 subsets, and it has been shown that CD40L-CD40 interactions are crucial for the IL-12–dependent priming of Th1 T cells in vivo (85). Interestingly, blockade of the CD40L/CD40 pathway prevents a variety of immune disorders in mice mediated by Th1 CD4+ T cells, including type I collagen-induced arthritis, experimental autoimmune encephalitis, and the NOD model of diabetes mellitus (see below).

In addition to the effects on dendritic cells, CD40L-CD40 interactions also induce macrophages to produce an array of cytokines and chemokines, including IL-1, IL-6, IL-8, IL-10, IL-12, TNF-α, and MIP-α, that are important in effecting and controlling inflammatory responses. Moreover, CD40L-CD40 interactions also induce macrophages to produce other proinflammatory molecules, including nitric oxide (NO) and prostaglandins (see Fig. 32-2). For example, T cells derived from CD40L–/– "knockout" mice are fourfold less effective than CD40L+/+ wild-type T cells in activating the nitric oxide response in allogeneic macrophages. Moreover, CD40L signals also control the expression of chemokine receptors, which govern the chemotactic functions of chemokines and thus control the migration of inflammatory cells to the site of inflammation. For example, CD40L induces down-regulation of the two main chemokine receptors expressed by these macrophages, CCR1 and CCR5, and abrogates chemotaxis to their ligands. Concomitantly, the expression of CCR7 and the migration to its ligand MIP-3b, a chemokine expressed in lymphoid organs, are strongly up-regulated. Rapid inhibition of responsiveness to chemoattractants present at sites of inflammation and immune reaction may be permissive for leaving peripheral tissues. Conversely, the slower acquisition of responsiveness to MIP-3b may guide subsequent localization of dendritic cells in lymphoid organs (86).

The Role of the CD40L/CD40 Pathway in the Induction of CD8+ Cytotoxic T-Lymphocyte (CTL) Responses: a Consequence of Dendritic-Cell Activation

The in vivo priming of CD8+ cytotoxic T lymphocytes (CTLs) responding to virally infected cells, as well as allogeneic or tumor cells, generally requires the participation of CD4+ T-helper lymphocytes. During the last several years, the nature of this help has been further defined and shown to involve CD40L signals. For example, as noted above, following MHC/peptide triggering of the TCR expressed on CD4+ T cells, the T cells begin to express CD40L. This CD40L interacts with CD40 expressed on DCs, which induces the DCs to express more MHC, as well as the essential costimulatory molecules CD80 and CD86 (87). This sequence of events "licenses" the DCs to activate CD8+ precursors (88). How CDs present protein antigen endogenously expressed inside other cells (like viral antigens, tumor associated antigens or cellular autoantigens) was not clear until recent studies by Albert et al (89,90). In these studies, it was shown that DCs specifically recognize and engulf whole apoptotic cells. The DCs that have been licensed by CD40L signals then efficiently cross-present MHC/peptide complexes that trigger CD8+ T-cell precursors. Thus, it is envisioned that following antigen activation, CD4+ T-cell clones provide CD40L signals to DCs that not only augment antigen processing and presentation to T cells but also may enable the capacity of DCs to engulf apoptotic cells. In fact, it was shown that signaling through CD40 can replace CD4+ T-helper cells in priming of helper-dependent CD8+ CTL responses. Moreover, blockade of CD40L inhibits CTL priming, and this inhibition is overcome by signaling through CD40. Taken together, these results support the view that CD40-CD40L interactions are vital in the delivery of T-cell help for CTL priming (88,91,92).

The Biologic Consequences of CD40L Signaling of CD40 on the Surface of Fibroblasts, Endothelial Cells, and Platelets

Another important aspect of the biology of CD40L-CD40 interactions in the control of immunity and inflammation is the mounting data that CD40L can mediate functional interactions of CD4+ T cells with other cells that express CD40, including fibroblasts, synovial cells, and endothelial cells (93,94) (see Fig. 32-2). Thus, CD40L-CD40 interactions induce fibroblast CD54 (intercellular adhesion molecule-1 [ICAM-1]) and CD106 (vascular cell adhesion molecule-1 [VCAM-1]) up-regulation. Moreover, ligation of fibroblast CD40 augments IL-6 production, triggers collagenase and collagen production, and induces fibroblasts to proliferate. Together, these functional effects suggest that CD40L signals may be involved in the induction of fibrosis associated with immune responses and autoimmunity.

In addition, similar to TNF-α and interleukin-1 (IL-1), CD40L-CD40 interactions induce endothelial cells to express CD62E (E-selectin), CD106, and CD54. These adhesion molecules are thought to be involved in the binding of inflammatory cells to endothelium and the subsequent migration of cells to sites of inflammation. Further, functional studies have provided further evidence that CD40L blockade will retard migration of leukocytes through endothelial-cell barriers. In this regard, it is of interest that, in vivo, antibodies to CD40L block the appearance of inflammatory cells at the site of inflammation in a variety of animal models of autoimmunity. Moreover, CD40L-CD40 interactions on the endothelial-cell surfaces induce secretion of tissue factor and expression of thrombomodulin (95). These procoagulant effects are of interest because clotting is often an important by-product of the vasculitis associated with delayed-type hypersensitivity responses in general and autoimmune-induced vasculitis in particular. Interestingly, in addition to expressing CD40, as noted above, endothelial cells also have been reported to express CD40L. Although the precise biologic function of CD40L expression on endothelial cells is not known, it is of major interest that blockade of the CD40L/CD40 pathway can inhibit animal models of atherosclerosis (see below). Also, it has recently been reported that platelets express CD40L within seconds of thrombin activation in vitro and in the process of thrombus formation in vivo. CD40L on platelets induces endothelial cells to secrete chemokines and to express adhesion molecules, thereby generating signals for the recruitment and extravasation of leukocytes at the site of injury. These results indicate that platelets are not only involved in hemostasis but that they also may directly initiate an inflammatory response of the vessel wall that may be susceptible to blockade of the CD40L/CD40 pathway.

Blockade of the CD40L/CD40 Pathway in Animal Models of Disease

The biologic effects of in vivo administered antibodies to CD40L in normal mice are summarized in Table 32-1. In addition to abrogating antigen-induced germinal-center formation and isotype class switching to IgG, IgA, and IgE, antibody blockade of CD40L-CD40 interactions also significantly abrogates cell-mediated immune responses and inflammatory responses. These effects will be illuminated below where we will discuss the effects of anti-CD40L therapy on immune-mediated disease in animal models. In principle, the effects of anti-CD40L therapy in immune disease could affect distinct cellular events and pathways during the development of immune injury. For example, one could envision that anti-CD40L might ameliorate immune disease by the following means:

1. Inhibiting the activation of autoreactive or alloreactive CD4+ T cells
2. Skewing the differentiation of pathogenic CD4+ TH cells from TH1 to TH2 cells
3. Altering the T-cell receptor (TCR) repertoire of antigen-specific CD4+ T cells
4. Inducing tolerance to autoantigens or alloantigens
5. Preventing the migration of pathogenic CD4+ T cells into the CNS
6. Facilitating the cellular events in the induction or effector phases of CD4+ or CD8+ regulatory T cells that specifically down-regulate CD4+ TH1 pathogenic clones

Below we will discuss these mechanisms with reference to treatment of specific syndromes (Table 32-2).

SLE-like Syndromes

A common feature of SLE in both mice and humans is the unusual propensity to produce immunoglobulin G (IgG) autoantibodies with specificities directed to a variety of nuclear antigens, including certain protein–nucleic-acid complexes, notably chromatin, the U1 and Sm small nuclear ribonucleoprotein (snRNP) particles, and the Ro/SSA and La/SSB RNP complexes (96–98). A separate group of autoantibodies in SLE are directed to phospholipids (complexed to β2 glycoprotein 1) and/or cell-surface molecules (99). The phospholipid antibodies are associated with clotting phenomenon in SLE, and the cell-surface antibodies are thought to account for the hemolytic anemia, thrombocytopenia, and leukopenia associated with SLE. However, the IgG autoantibodies to dsDNA play the prominent role in the immune complex of glomerulonephritis and vasculitis of SLE (99–101). In addition, immune complex formation induced by IgG autoantibodies is thought to play a major role in the arthritis, serositis, and vasculitis associated with SLE. In this regard, the key role of the CD40L/CD40 pathway in antibody formation suggests that

Table 32-1. Biologic Effects of Antibodies to CD40L In Vivo

- Markedly reduced IgG, IgA, and IgE synthesis to recently administered antigens
- Absence of newly formed germinal centers
- Impaired macrophage activation and function
- Impaired T-cell priming and reduced IFN-γ– and IL-12–driven Th1 responses and skewing of responses toward Th2
- Reduced follicular dendritic-cell network and function
- Impaired expression of costimulatory molecules and induction of tolerance to select antigens, including alloantigens

Table 32-2. Anti-CD40L Therapy in Animal Models of Immunologic Disease

SLE models

- Anti-CD40 ligand antibody treatment prevents the development of lupus-like nephritis in NZB/NZW and SNF1 SLE mice (104).
- Treatment of SNF1 mice with anti-CD40 ligand antibody reverses established nephritis and preserves kidney function (102,103).

Multiple sclerosis models (EAE in rodents)

- Specific blockade of CD40L at the time of immunization markedly suppresses the incidence, mortality, day of onset, and clinical scores of EAE in B10P1L and (PLJ × SJL) F1 mice induced by either MBP or PLP myelin antigens (119,144,145).

RA models (collagen-induced arthritis)

- Anti-CD40L blocks the development of joint inflammation, serum antibody titers to collagen, the infiltration of inflammatory cells into the subsynovial tissue, and the erosion of cartilage and bone in collagen-induced arthritis (110).

Insulin-dependent type I diabetes models

- The nonobese diabetic (NOD) mouse spontaneously develops T-cell–dependent autoimmune diabetes. Anti-CD40L mAb treatment of 3- to 4-week-old NOD females (the age at which insulitis typically begins) completely prevented the insulitis and diabetes. Cytokine analysis revealed a dramatic decrease in IFN-γ and IL-2 release without a concomitant increase in IL-4 production by T cells from anti-CD40L–treated mice (144).

Inhibition of allograft and xenograft transplant rejection

- Anti-CD40L prevents the development *renal rejection* of fully allogeneic grafts in mice (79).
- Moreover, the survival of renal allografts transplanted into nephrectomized rhesus monkeys is markedly prolonged by anti-CD40L therapy alone (80).
- Similarly, anti-CD40L therapy has prevented graft rejection of *skin, islet cells, and cardiac transplants*, as well as GVH disease in rodents (131).

blockade of this pathway may provide an effective means of inhibiting the production of pathogenic autoantibodies. This is especially the case in SLE where the pathogenic antibodies are usually IgG and thus require class switching, known to depend on CD40L signals. Therefore, it is not surprising that in murine models of SLE, anti-CD40L monoclonal antibodies have been shown to effectively prevent and treat disease.

For example, initial studies of the role of CD40L-CD40 interactions in the development of glomerulonephritis in lupus mice demonstrated that lupus mice had much higher percentages of CD40L+ T cells in their spleens even at the preautoimmune age of 1 month and that the pathogenic, autoantibody-inducing ability of Th clones and splenic Th cells from lupus mice could be blocked in vitro by the hamster antimurine CD40L Ab, MR1 (102). Acceleration of lupus nephritis by the transfer of pathogenic, autoantibody-inducing Th clones in vivo could also be completely blocked by anti-CD40L Ab. Importantly, treatment of lupus mice with the MR1 Ab had a sustained beneficial effect on their spontaneous disease long after the Ab had been cleared from their systems. Only three injections of MR1 given to prenephritic lupus mice at 3 months of age markedly delayed and reduced the incidence of lupus nephritis up to 12 months of age, by which time almost all the control mice had developed severe glomerulonephritis. Moreover, pathogenic Th cells were left intact in these MR1-treated mice, but their B cells could not produce pathogenic autoantibodies even 9 months after cessation of therapy (102). It was subsequently shown that anti-CD40L

treatment of mice with established lupus nephritis prolonged survival and decreased the incidence of severe nephritis. In the anti-CD40L treated mice, but not in controls, there was a decline in proteinuria, and histologic examination of kidneys revealed dramatically diminished inflammation, sclerosis/fibrosis, and vasculitis. Spleens from anti-CD40L–treated mice also exhibited markedly reduced inflammation and fibrosis compared with controls. Together, these results show that treatment of nephritic mice with long-term, anti-CD40L immunotherapy significantly prolongs survival; reduces the severity of nephritis; and diminishes associated inflammation, vasculitis, and fibrosis (103).

In other studies, anti-CD40L Ab treatment of lupus-prone mice reduced anti-DNA autoantibody production and renal disease, and pathologic examination verified the absence of significant renal damage or immune complex deposition in responding mice. In addition, long-term survivors mounted a substantial Ab response to keyhole limpet hemocyanin after completion of anti-CD40L Ab treatment, suggesting that some of the immunosuppressive effects of the anti-CD40L may be reversible (104). Interestingly, it was shown that MR1 treatment significantly augmented the survival of lupus-prone mice treated with blockade of the B7/CTLA-4 pathway and that brief simultaneous blockade of the B7/CD28 and CD40L/CD40 costimulation pathways produces benefit that lasts long after treatment has been discontinued (105). Important clinical observations during these murine studies were that, although the anti-CD40L therapy was effective in preventing and treating SLE prone mice, there was no evidence of generalized immunosuppression or evidence of increased incidence of infections.

With respect to the role of the CD40L/CD40 pathway in SLE, it is important to note that interruption of the CD40 ligand–dependent pathway by antibody blockade could downmodulate SLE activity by acting at the distal level of the cognitive T-B interaction involved in IgG autoantibody production or at the induction and regulation of autoreactive T-cell clones. Moreover, these effects of antibody blockade could result from interference with T-cell interaction with B cells or with dendritic cells and macrophages. In addition, there is evidence that ligation of CD40L by CD40 (during the interaction of T cells with antigen-presenting cells) may deliver signals to CD4+ T cells and induce functional changes. These more proximal mechanisms for anti-CD40L treatment could diminish the number of autoreactive cells in the T-cell repertoire.

Murine Models of Collagen-Induced Arthritis

Injecting genetically susceptible strains of mice with cartilage constituents such as collagen type II in complete Freund's adjuvant induces an arthritis with synovitis and erosions histologically resembling rheumatoid arthritis (RA) (106,107). Moreover, similar to human RA, susceptibility to collagen-induced arthritis is MHC class II–restricted, and the disease process is induced by CD4+ cells. However, both T-cell and B-cell activation are important in collagen-induced arthritis. Cytokines of both Th1 (IFN-γ–secreting) and Th2 (IL-4–secreting) cells are produced, and at disease onset a Th1 profile predominates. In fact, adoptive transfer of Th1 collagen reactive Vβ8.2+ CD4+ T cells can induce disease. Moreover, transgenic animals expressing the Vβ8.2 collagen–reactive T-cell receptor develop arthritis when given collagen II (108,109). Antibodies against lymphocyte surface markers such as CD4, CD40L, and MHC class II have been shown to suppress disease progression. The role of CD40L-CD40 interactions in collagen-induced arthritis was investigated in vivo with the use of the MR1 anti-CD40L antibody. Arthritis induced in mice by immunization with type II collagen was dramatically inhibited by MR1. The MR1 antibody not only blocked the antibody response to collagen but also markedly reduced the development of joint inflammation. Thus, there was almost complete reduction in the infiltration of inflammatory cells into the subsynovial tissue (110). Moreover, the subsequent erosion of cartilage and bone was abrogated. These studies strongly suggest that blockade of CD40L-CD40 interactions may have therapeutic potential in the treatment of inflammatory arthritis, including rheumatoid arthritis (110).

Murine Models of Multiple Sclerosis: Experimental Autoimmune Encephalomyelitis (EAE)

Mice immunized with myelin basic protein (MBP) peptides generate encephalitogenic MBP–reactive CD4+ T-cell clones that migrate to the central nervous system (CNS) and induce an autoimmune neurologic disease in mice, termed experimental autoimmune encephalomyelitis (EAE), that is highly analogous to multiple sclerosis (MS) in humans (111–113). The CNS histopathology in EAE, similar to MS, is characterized by an inflammatory infiltrate that surrounds venules and extends into the myelin sheath and CNS parenchyma, which is comprised of CD4+, CD8+, and γ,δ T cells, as well as activated macrophages. During the evolution of EAE there is an initial expansion of disease, inducing Th1 CD4+ T cells (secreting IFN-γ) with a subsequent shift of the Th phenotype of MBP-reactive CD4+ T-cell clones from Th1 to Th2 (secreting IL-4 and IL-5) (114, 115).

The effector mechanisms by which Th1 CD4+ myelin–reactive T cells induce tissue injury in the CNS is thought to involve many of the general mechanisms operative in delayed-type hypersensitivity (DTH) reactions. Thus, myelin-reactive T cells express CD40L and other activation molecules and release IL-2 and IFN-γ. IL-2 induces and triggers the clonal outgrowth of the myelin-reactive T cells, and the IFN-γ activates macrophages, which subsequently release TNF-α and IL-1, as well as other proinflammatory cytokines and chemokines (116). The activated T cells also express CD40L, which further induces macrophages and dendritic cells to release proinflammatory cytokines, as well as NO (117,118). In addition, CD40L also induces endothelial cells to express CD62E, CD106, and CD54 molecules thought to be involved in the migration of cells to the site of inflammation (94). The obligate role of CD40L in EAE pathogenesis was determined in studies of CD40L-deficient mice that carried a transgenic T-cell receptor specific for myelin basic protein (119). These mice failed to develop EAE after priming with antigen, and CD4+ T cells remained quiescent and produced no IFN-γ.

Because of the developing evidence that the CD40L/CD40 pathway was involved in T-cell–dendritic-cell interactions and in the differentiation of Th1 cells, the potential role of the pathway in EAE was directly studied. First, the CNS of EAE animals, but not normal mice, contained CD40L-expressing CD4+ T cells, and the expression of CD40L in the CNS was increased during clinical attacks. Moreover, treatment with anti-CD40L monoclonal antibody (MR1) completely prevented the development of disease. Furthermore, the administration of anti-CD40L monoclonal antibody, even after disease onset, shortly before maximum disability score was reached, led to dramatic disease reduction. Importantly, the disease suppression was not associated with generalized immunosuppression or deletion of autoreactive T cells, but was accompanied by a drastic alteration of their cytokine profiles. The production of IFN-γ was markedly suppressed, while that of IL-4 enhanced. These results suggest that CD40-CD40L interactions play important roles in the differentiation of autoreactive Th1 versus Th2 cells in vivo and that CD40L blockade is effective in preventing autoimmune encephalomyelitis. Thus, anti-CD40L therapy in this animal model indicates that blockade of CD40-CD40L–mediated cellular interactions may be a method for interference in active human MS.

Murine Experimental Autoimmune Thyroiditis (EAT)

Murine experimental autoimmune thyroiditis (EAT) is a T-cell–mediated disease induced in SJL mice with repeated administration of thyroglobulin (Tg) and adjuvant. Recently, the role of CD40L in the induction of EAT was studied in vivo. Mice received Tg and adjuvant induction in the presence of either the anti-CD40L antibody MR1 or control hamster Ig. Control mice developed severe thyroiditis with diffuse cellular infiltration of the thyroid, whereas the MR1-treated mice exhibited very low levels of focal cellular infiltration (120). On restimulation with Tg in vitro, lymph node cells from Tg-primed, MR1-treated mice proliferated less strongly and secreted significantly lower amounts of IL-2 and IFN-γ than T cells from untreated or control mice. These results suggest that in vivo blockade of CD40L suppresses EAT by inhibiting the priming of inflammatory, Tg-specific Th1 CD4+ T cells.

Hapten-Induced Colitis in Mice

The rectal application of low doses of the hapten, trinitrobenzene sulfonic acid (TNBS), in BALB/c and SJL/J mice results in a chronic transmural colitis with severe diarrhea, weight loss, and rectal prolapse, an illness that mimics some characteristics of Crohn's disease in humans. The colon of TNBS-treated mice on day 7 was marked by infiltration of CD4+ Th1 cells expressing high levels of IFN-γ. The administration of monoclonal anti–IL-12 antibodies to the TNBS-treated mice, both early (at 5 days) and late (at 20 days) after induction of colitis, led to a striking improvement in both the clinical and histopathologic aspects of the disease and frequently abrogated the established colitis completely, suggesting a pivotal role of IL-12 and IFN-γ in this murine model of chronic intestinal inflammation (121). The potential role the CD40L/CD40 pathway in the hapten-induced colitis was also investigated (122). The administration of the anti-CD40L antibody, MR1, during the induction phase of the Th1 response prevented IFN-γ production by lamina propria CD4+ T cells and also prevented clinical and histologic evidence of disease. In contrast, the secretion of IL-4, a Th2-type cytokine, was increased after anti-CD40L treatment with MR1. In further studies, when MR1 was given after the disease was established, no effect on the disease activity was observed. These studies imply that CD40L-CD40 interaction is crucial for the in vivo priming of Th1 T cells through the stimulation of IL-12 secretion by antigen-presenting cells (APC) and thus suggest a potential role for CD40L blockade in preventing relapses of Crohn's disease in humans.

Atherosclerosis and Coronary Artery Disease

Considerable evidence supports the involvement of inflammation and immunity in atherogenesis, and atherosclerosis can be characterized in part as a chronic, inflammatory, fibroproliferative disease of the vessel wall. The attachment of monocytes and T lymphocytes to the injured endothelium, followed by their migration into the intima, is one of the first and most crucial steps in lesion development (123). The colocalization of CD4+ T cells and macrophages in the lesion, the abundant expression of HLA class II molecules, and the costimulatory molecule CD40 and its ligand (CD40L) indicate a contribution of cell-mediated immunity to atherogenesis (123,124). As noted above, ligation of CD40 on endothelial cells and other atheroma-associated cells in vitro activates functions related to atherogenesis, including induction of proinflammatory cytokines, matrix metalloproteinases, adhesion molecules, and tissue factor (94,95,125,126). Recently, it has been shown that interruption of CD40 signaling influences atherogenesis in vivo in hyperlipidemic mice (124). Treatment with the MR1 limited atherosclerosis in mice that lacked the receptor for low-density lipoprotein (LDL) and that had been fed a high-cholesterol diet for 12 weeks. MR1 treatment reduces the size of aortic atherosclerotic lesions, as well as the lipid content. Furthermore, atheroma of mice treated with anti-CD40L antibody contained significantly fewer macrophages and T lymphocytes, and these mice exhibited decreased expression of vascular-cell adhesion molecule-1. These data support the involvement of inflammatory pathways in atherosclerosis and indicate a role for CD40 signaling during atherogenesis in hyperlipidemic mice. Moreover, support for this idea has emerged from studies showing that enhanced levels of soluble and membrane-bound CD40 ligand are found in patients with unstable angina. These data could reflect the role of T lymphocyte and/or platelet involvement in the pathogenesis of acute coronary syndromes (127,128).

Transplantation-Induced Allograft Rejection

A number of studies have shown that the CD40L/CD40 pathway plays an important role in allograft rejection, and anti-CD40L therapy has been shown to markedly prolong survival of allografts. For example, it was initially shown that anti-CD40L by itself allowed indefinite islet allograft survival in 40% of recipient mice (79). Moreover, addition of small lymphocytes expressing donor antigens to the anti-CD40L treatment regimen increased islet survival to greater than 90%. Subsequently, it has been shown that anti-CD40L therapy can prolong allograft survival of renal (80,129), cardiac (78,130–132), skin (78,133), and bone marrow transplants (134–136). In addition, anti-CD40L therapy prevents neonatal induction of transplantation tolerance (137).

The ability of CD40L signals to induce CD80 (B7-1) and CD86 (B7-2) expression on antigen-presenting cells (APCs) has led to the hypothesis that the role of CD40-CD40L interactions in transplant rejection might be indirect, that is, to promote the costimulatory capacity of APCs (79,130,135). Thus, the role of CD40L in the up-regulation of CD80 (B71) and CD86 (B72) molecules suggests that CD40L-CD40 interactions may ultimately control the initial afferent phases of immune recognition by T cells and the ultimate decision of whether activation or tolerance ensues. B7 triggering of CD28 and/or CTLA-4 is known to regulate T-cell activation or anergy induction, and blockade of

B7/CD28 interactions promotes T-cell tolerance. Moreover, in vivo studies in mice have strongly suggested that blockade of CD40L-CD40 interactions is also tolerogenic (82,136–138). For example, in a murine, vascularized, cardiac allograft model, treatment of the recipients with donor splenocytes and a single dose of anti-CD40L mAb induces long-term graft survival (>100 days). This is associated with marked inhibition of intragraft Th1 cytokine (IFN-γ) and IL-12 expression with reciprocal up-regulation of Th2 cytokines (IL-4 and IL-10). In untreated allograft recipients, CD86 is strongly expressed on endothelial cells and infiltrating mononuclear cells of the graft within 24 hours. In contrast, CD80 expression is not seen until 72 hours after engraftment. However, animals treated with anti-CD80 mAb or with a mutated form of CTLA4Ig (which does not bind to CD86) rejected their cardiac allografts, indicating that blockade of CD80 alone does not mediate the graft-prolonging effects of anti-CD40L mAb. These data support the idea that the role of CD40/CD40L in transplant rejection is not solely to promote CD80 or CD86 expression, but rather that this pathway can directly and independently costimulate T cells. These data also suggest that long-term graft survival can be achieved without blockade of either T-cell-receptor–mediated signals or CD28-CD86 engagement (130). However, blockade of both the CD40L/CD40 pathway and CD28-CD86 engagement appears more effective than blockade of either pathway alone.

The synergism observed in simultaneous blockade of these pathways for effective inhibition of alloimmunity indicates that, although they are interrelated, the CD28 and CD40 pathways are critical, independent regulators of allograft responses (78,139). Finally, in terms of the mechanisms that ultimately account for the dramatic effects of CD40L blockade in preventing allograft rejection, it is possible that interference with the generation of alloreactive CTL may play a role. Thus, as reviewed above, the in vivo priming of CD8+ cytotoxic T lymphocytes (CTLs) that respond to allogenic cells generally requires the participation of CD4+ T-helper lymphocytes. During the last several years, the nature of this help has been further defined and shown to involve CD40L interaction with CD40 expressed on DCs, which induces the DCs to express more MHC, as well as the essential costimulatory molecules CD80 and CD86 (87). As discussed above, this sequence of events could "license" the DCs to activate CD8+ precursor alloreactive CTL (88).

In recent studies the dramatic effects of CD40L blockade have been extended to determine whether CD40L blockade would induce long-term acceptance of allografted tissues in primates (80,129,132,140,141). For example, in one study the combined effects of CTLA4-Ig and the CD40L-specific monoclonal antibody 5C8 were tested in rhesus monkeys. Renal allografts were transplanted into nephrectomized rhesus monkeys disparate at major histocompatibility complex class I and class II loci. Control animals rejected their allografts in 5 to 8 days. Brief induction treatment with CTLA4-Ig or 5C8 alone significantly prolonged rejection-free survival (20 to 98 days). Two of four animals treated with both agents experienced extended (>150 days) rejection-free allograft survival. Two animals treated with 5C8 alone and one animal treated with both 5C8 and CTLA4-Ig experienced late, biopsy-proven rejection, but a repeat course of their induction regimen successfully restored normal graft function. Neither drug affected peripheral T-cell or B-cell counts, and there were no clinically evident side effects or rejections during treatment. Recently, these studies have been extended to show that administration of the CD40L-specific monoclonal antibody (hu5C8) alone permits renal allotransplantation in outbred, MHC-mismatched rhesus monkeys without acute rejection. The effect persisted for more than 10 months after therapy termination, and no additional drug was required to achieve extended graft survival. Monkeys treated with antibody against CD40L remained healthy during and after therapy, and the mechanism of action does not involve global depletion of T or B cells (141).

Blockade of the CD40L/CD40 Pathway in Human Immune Disease

The basic studies reviewed above, as well as the preclinical evaluation of anti-CD40L blockade in a variety of autoimmune diseases in addition to the setting of allorejection, strongly suggest that this form of therapy may of value in the treatment of human immune disease. The major potential targets for anti-CD40L therapy are indicated in Table 32-3. For example, the key and nonredundant role of the CD40L/CD40 pathway in Ig class switching and in the normal production of IgG, IgA, or IgE antibodies suggests that anti-CD40L antibodies may be of value in human diseases mediated, at least in part, by antibodies of these Ig isotypes, including SLE, idiopathic thrombocytopenic purpura, drug-induced autoimmunity, and allergic phenomenon. In addition, the prominent role of CD40L signals in the induction and activation of dendritic-cell and macrophage function leading to the clonal outgrowth of Th1 cells suggests that blockade of CD40L may prevent Th1 differentiation and skew Th differentiation toward Th2. This could be of clinical value in diseases medi-

Table 32-3. Potential Targets for Anti-CD40L Antibody Therapy

- Autoimmune diseases (including SLE, ITP, multiple sclerosis, rheumatoid arthritis, type 1 diabetes, scleroderma, thyroiditis)
- Treatment and prevention of organ and bone marrow transplant rejection
- Inhibition of immune responses to exogenous foreign antigens (factor 8 therapy in hemophilia, gene therapy, foreign monoclonal antibodies, drug-induced autoimmunity, allergic phenomenon)
- Complications of vascular disease associated with atherosclerosis
- Tumor cells expressing CD40L

ated by predominately by Th1 cells, including rheumatoid arthritis, multiple sclerosis, thyroiditis, and type 1 diabetes mellitus. The role of CD40L signals in the activation of fibroblasts (including synovial cells) suggests a potential role of anti-CD40L therapy in the treatment of systemic sclerosis (scleroderma), as well as in the therapy of chronic synovitis associated with rheumatoid arthritis, Lyme disease, or with the spondyloarthropathies. In addition, the role of CD40L signals in the activation of endothelial cells suggests that anti-CD40L therapy may have a role in many vasculitic disorders, including SLE, polyarteritis nodosa, and Wegeners granulomatosis. In addition, the intriguing results in animal models of atherosclerosis suggest a potential role of CD40L blockade in the inhibition of atheroma formation. Finally, the important role of the CD40L pathway in the induction of co-stimulatory molecules (CD80 and CD86) suggested that the CD40L blockade could be used to induce tolerance and could be particularly effective in prevention of allograft responses. As reviewed above, this has been borne out in animal studies of allograft rejection.

On the basis of the preclinical trials that demonstrate that antibodies to CD40L can be used to safely treat immune disease in animals models, including nonhuman primates, clinical trials were initiated within the last 2 years. For example, a trial was initiated by Biogen that focused on idiopathic thrombocytopenic purpura (ITP), an autoimmune disease characterized by the presence of IgG antiplatelet antibodies, marked thrombocytopenia, and a severe bleeding diathesis. Because the CD40L/CD40 pathway is central to the production of IgG antibodies, it was hypothesized that the humanized monoclonal antibody to the CD40 ligand (Hu5c8) may block antiplatelet antibody productions and may be therapeutically useful in patients with chronic ITP. A phase I, multi-center, randomized, single-dose, double-blind, controlled, dose-escalation study to evaluate the safety of and the effect on platelet count of Hu5c8 was initiated in patients with chronic refractory ITP. The study, which was recently reported at the American Society of Hematology meetings, evaluated four doses of Hu5c8, given as intravenous infusions of 0.3, 1, 3, or 10mg/kg (142). Eighteen patients with refractory ITP entered the study with platelet counts less than 30,000. All patients were followed for 115 days after entry; none were lost to follow-up. None of the patients died or developed severe infection, and the drug was well tolerated. Three patients given Hu5c8 had mild to moderate upper respiratory infection (none were considered likely or definitely related to study drug). There were no significant trends observed on counts of lymphocytes or lymphocyte subsets. One patient developed major bleeding from a ruptured ovarian cyst at 12 weeks during follow-up. However, two of six patients given Hu5c8 at 10mg/kg had increased platelet counts from less than 30,000 to 100,000 or more 6 weeks following treatment. It was concluded from this encouraging preliminary study that further studies of the safety and effectiveness of repeated doses of 10mg/kg of Hu5c8 were warranted (142).

In addition, within the last year two trials of anti-CD40L therapy were initiated to evaluate the safety and efficacy of treating patients with SLE. For example, in one phase I trial Biogen initiated a randomized, double-blind, controlled, multiple-dose,

dose-escalation study to evaluate the efficacy and safety of the humanized 5c8 anti-CD40L antibody in 25 subjects with SLE with proliferative glomerulonephritis who had failed conventional therapy. The majority of patients were receiving high-dose steroids. There were no serious infections, and the antibody was generally well tolerated. However, three patients developed thromboembolic signs and symptoms, and the study was halted to further evaluate the significance of this complication. Because thromboembolic complications are part of the natural history of SLE, the precise interpretation of this data is not clear. In a second trial the IDEC corporation initiated a single-center, single-dose, dose-escalating, phase I trial to investigate the safety, tolerability, and pharmacology of IDEC-131, a humanized, anti-CD40L, monoclonal antibody in 23 patients with symptomatic SLE. The results of this trial were reported at the American College of Rheumatology meetings in November 1999 (143). The majority of patients were also receiving concomitant therapy for SLE, including NSAIDs, hydroxychloroquine, and/or corticosteroids. An overall favorable safety profile was observed, and no thromboembolic phenomenon were reported. Most adverse events were mild or moderate in severity and included events such as asthenia, dizziness, nausea, and headache. No serious adverse events were reported. All reported infections (predominantly URI) were mild to moderate in severity and were considered unrelated to treatment. Flow cytometric analysis revealed that there was no evidence of treatment-related T-cell depletion. There were no clinical features indicative of a cytokine-mediated infusion syndrome, nor was an anti-IDEC-131 antibody response detected. Because the anti-CD40L antibody was well tolerated in this single-dose study, a multiple-dose phase II study in SLE patients is currently under way (143). We are obviously only at the earliest stages of investigations to determine whether anti-CD40L therapy will be safe and/or useful for the treatment of human autoimmune disorders.

Summary

A decade ago, several lines of evidence suggested that T-cell surface molecules become expressed on antigen-activated CD4+ T cells in vitro, and that these surface molecules in concert with lymphokines were required for full B-cell activation and differentiation (17,18). However, these molecules were not identified, and there was no evidence that these contact-dependent CD4+ surface molecules were critical for antibody formation in vivo. In the early 1990s the key molecule that becomes expressed on activated CD4+ T cells and that induces B-cell differentiation was identified to be a novel member of the TNF family of molecules, termed CD40 ligand (CD40L). It has been quite gratifying to witness the rapid evolution of our knowledge of the CD40L molecule and CD40L/CD40 pathway since that time. For example, the monoclonal antibodies to CD40L, as well as the delineation of cDNA sequence, permitted analysis of patients with the hyper-IgM syndrome (HIMS) and the finding that mutant CD40L genes encode dysfunctional proteins in patients with the X-linked

HIMS (29,32–34). These studies provided definitive evidence that the CD40L molecule is essential for human T-helper function and Ig class switching in vivo. Subsequently, studies in both mice and humans showed that, by virtue of the interaction of CD40L with CD40 expressed on dendritic cells, macrophages, endothelial cells, and fibroblasts, the CD40L/CD40 pathway was also critical to a variety of cell-mediated immune responses and in the induction of inflammation. Moreover, studies of a variety of murine and nonhuman primate models of immune-mediated disease provided direct evidence that blockade of the CD40L/CD40 pathway using monoclonal antibodies to CD40L may be useful in the prevention or treatment of a wide variety of immune diseases, including autoimmune syndromes and allograft rejection. On the basis of these studies, clinical trials in humans of the safety and effectiveness of anti-CD40L therapy were recently initiated. Thus, within a decade studies of the CD40L/CD40 pathway have proceeded from concept to bench to bedside. It is hoped that, as the basic and clinical studies evolve, further useful approaches to the blockade of the CD40L/CD40 pathway will emerge and lead to the safe and effective treatment of immunologically induced disease in humans.

References

1. Mueller DL, Jenkins MK, Schwartz RH. Clonal expansion versus functional clonal inactivation: a costimulatory signalling pathway determines the outcome of T cell antigen receptor occupancy. [Review] [140 refs]. Annu Rev Immunol 1989;7:445–480.
2. Janeway C Jr, Bottomly K. Signals and signs for lymphocyte responses. [Review]. Cell 1994;76:275–285.
3. Lenschow DJ, Walunas TL, Bluestone JA. CD28/B7 system of T cell costimulation. Annu Rev Immunol 1996;14:233–258.
4. Claman HN, Chaperon EA, Triplett RF. Thymus-marrow cell combinations-synergism in antibody formation. Proc Soc Exp Biol Med 1966;122:1167–1171.
5. Miller JF, Mitchell GF. Cell to cell interaction in the immune response. I. Hemolysin-forming cells in neonatally thymectomized mice reconstituted with thymus or thoracic duct lymphocytes. J Exp Med 1968;128:801–820.
6. Mitchell GF, Miller JF. Cell to cell interaction in the immune response. II. The source of hemolysin-forming cells in irradiated mice given bone marrow and thymus or thoracic duct lymphocytes. J Exp Med 1968;128:821–837.
7. Nossal GJ, Cunningham A, Mitchell GF, Miller JF. Cell to cell interaction in the immune response. III. Chromosomal marker analysis of single antibody-forming cells in reconstituted, irradiated, or thymectomized mice. J Exp Med 1968;128:839–853.
8. Durie FH, Foy TM, Masters SR, et al. The role of CD40 in the regulation of humoral and cell-mediated immunity. [Review]. Immunol Today 1994;15:406–411.
9. Klaus SJ, Pinchuk LM, Ochs HD, et al. Costimulation through CD28 enhances T cell-dependent B cell activation via CD40-CD40L interaction. J Immunol 1994;152:5643–5652.
10. Koulova L, Clark EA, Shu G, Dupont B. The CD28 ligand B7/BB1 provides costimulatory signal for alloactivation of CD4+ T cells. J Exp Med 1991;173:759–762.
11. Cooper MD, Raymond DA, Peterson RD, et al. The functions of the thymus system and the bursa system in the chicken. J Exp Med 1966;123:75–102.
12. Dent PB, Good RA. Absence of antibody production in the bursa of Fabricius. Nature 1965;207:491–493.
13. Miller JF, Mitchell GF. The thymus and the precursors of antigen reactive cells. Nature 1967;216:659–663.
14. Kung P, Goldstein G, Reinherz EL, Schlossman SF. Monoclonal antibodies defining distinctive human T cell surface antigens. Science 1979;206:347–349.
15. Thomas Y, Sosman J, Irigoyen O, et al. Functional analysis of human T cell subsets defined by monoclonal antibodies. I. Collaborative T-T interactions in the immunoregulation of B cell differentiation. J Immunol 1980;125:2402–2408.
16. Dialynas DP, Quan ZS, Wall KA, et al. Characterization of murine T cell surface molecule, designated L3T4, identified by monoclonal antibody GK1.5: similarity of L3T4 to the human Leu-3/T4 molecule. J Immunol 1983;131:2445–2451.
17. Parker DC. T cell-dependent B cell activation. [Review] [159 refs]. Annu Rev Immunol 1993;11:331–360.
18. Parker DC. T cell-dependent B cell activation. Annu Rev Immunol 1993;11:331–360.
19. Banchereau J, de Paoli P, Valle A, et al. Long-term human B cell lines dependent on interleukin-4 and antibody to CD40. Science 1991;251:70–72.
20. Banchereau J, Bazan F, Blanchard D, et al. The CD40 antigen and its ligand. [Review] [233 refs]. Annu Rev Immunol 1994;12:881–922.
21. Banchereau J, Bazan F, Blanchard D, et al. The CD40 antigen and its ligand. Annu Rev Immunol 1994;12:881–922.
22. Yellin MJ, Lee JJ, Chess L, Lederman S. A human CD4– T cell leukemia subclone with contact-dependent helper function. J Immunol 1991;147:3389–3395.
23. Lederman S, Yellin MJ, Krichevsky A, et al. Identification of a novel surface protein on activated CD4+ T cells that induces contact-dependent B cell differentiation (help). J Exp Med 1992;175:1091–1101.
24. Lederman S, Yellin MJ, Inghirami G, et al. Molecular interactions mediating T-B lymphocyte collaboration in human lymphoid follicles. Roles of T cell-B-cell-activating molecule (5c8 antigen) and CD40 in contact-dependent help. J Immunol 1992;149:3817–3826.
25. Lederman S, Yellin MJ, Covey LR, et al. Non-antigen signals for B-cell growth and differentiation to antibody secretion. Curr Opin Immunol 1993;5:439–444.
26. Covey LR, Cleary AM, Yellin MJ, et al. Isolation of cDNAs encoding T-BAM, a surface glycoprotein on CD4+ T cells mediating contact-dependent helper function for B cells: identity with the CD40-ligand. Mol Immunol 1994;31:471–484.
27. Graf D, Korthauer U, Mages HW, et al. Cloning of TRAP, a ligand for CD40 on human T cells. Eur J Immunol 1992;22:3191–3194.
28. Armitage RJ, Fanslow WC, Strockbine L, et al. Molecular and biological characterization of a murine ligand for CD40. Nature 1992;357:80–82.
29. Aruffo A, Farrington M, Hollenbaugh D, et al. The CD40 ligand, gp39, is defective in activated T cells from patients with X-linked hyper-IgM syndrome. Cell 1993;72:291–300.

30. Gruss HJ. Molecular, structural, and biological characteristics of the tumor necrosis factor ligand superfamily. [Review] [238 refs]. Int J Clin Lab Res 1996;26:143–159.

31. Josien R, Wong BR, Li HL, et al. TRANCE, a TNF family member, is differentially expressed on T cell subsets and induces cytokine production in dendritic cells. J Immunol 1999;162:2562–2568.

32. Callard RE, Smith SH, Herbert J, et al. CD40 ligand (CD40L) expression and B cell function in agammaglobulinemia with normal or elevated levels of IgM (HIM). Comparison of X-linked, autosomal recessive, and non-X-linked forms of the disease, and obligate carriers. J Immunol 1994;153:3295–3306.

33. Puck JM. Molecular and genetic basis of X-linked immunodeficiency disorders. [Review] [51 refs]. J Clin Immunol 1994;14:81–89.

34. Aruffo A, Hollenbaugh D, Wu LH, Ochs HD. The molecular basis of X-linked agammaglobulinemia, hyper-IgM syndrome, and severe combined immunodeficiency in humans. Curr Opin Hematol 1994;1:12–18.

35. Mayer L, Kwan SP, Thompson C, et al. Evidence for a defect in "switch" T cells in patients with immunodeficiency and hyperimmunoglobulinemia M. N Engl J Med 1986;314:409–413.

36. Karpusas M, Hsu YM, Wang JH, et al. A crystal structure of an extracellular fragment of human CD40 ligand. Structure 1995;3:1031–1039.

37. Grewal IS, Xu J, Flavell RA. Impairment of antigen-specific T-cell priming in mice lacking CD40 ligand. Nature 1995;378:617–620.

38. Noelle RJ, Roy M, Shepherd DM, et al. A 39-kDa protein on activated helper T cells binds CD40 and transduces the signal for cognate activation of B cells. Proc Natl Acad Sci USA 1992;89:6550–6554.

39. van Essen D, Kikutani H, Gray D. CD40 ligand-transduced co-stimulation of T cells in the development of helper function. Nature 1995;378:620–623.

40. Gauchat JF, Henchoz S, Mazzei G, et al. Induction of human IgE synthesis in B cells by mast cells and basophils. Nature 1993;365:340–343.

41. Henn V, Slupsky JR, Grafe M, et al. CD40 ligand on activated platelets triggers an inflammatory reaction of endothelial cells. Nature 1998;391:591–594.

42. Mach F, Schonbeck U, Sukhova GK, et al. Functional CD40 ligand is expressed on human vascular endothelial cells, smooth muscle cells, and macrophages: implications for CD40-CD40 ligand signaling in atherosclerosis. Proc Natl Acad Sci USA 1997;94:1931–1936.

43. Reul RM, Fang JC, Denton MD, et al. CD40 and CD40 ligand (CD154) are coexpressed on microvessels in vivo in human cardiac allograft rejection. Transplantation 1997;64:1765–1774.

44. Lederman S, Yellin MJ, Cleary AM, et al. T-BAM/CD40-L on helper T lymphocytes augments lymphokine-induced B cell Ig isotype switch recombination and rescues B cells from programmed cell death. J Immunol 1994;152:2163–2171.

45. MacLennan IC. Germinal centers. [Review] [139 refs]. Annu Rev Immunol 1994;12:117–139.

46. Yellin MJ, Sippel K, Inghirami G, et al. CD40 molecules induce down-modulation and endocytosis of T cell surface T cell-B cell activating molecule/CD40-L. Potential role in regulating helper effector function. J Immunol 1994;152:598–608.

47. Garrone P, Neidhardt EM, Garcia E, et al. Fas ligation induces apoptosis of CD40-activated human B lymphocytes. J Exp Med 1995;182:1265–1273.

48. Cleary AM, Fortune SM, Yellin MJ, et al. Opposing roles of CD95 (Fas/APO-1) and CD40 in the death and rescue of human low density tonsillar B cells. J Immunol 1995;155:3329–3337.

49. Tsubata T, Wu J, Honjo T. B-cell apoptosis induced by antigen receptor crosslinking is blocked by a T-cell signal through CD40. Nature 1993;364:645–648.

50. Valentine MA, Licciardi KA. Rescue from anti-IgM-induced programmed cell death by the B cell surface proteins CD20 and CD40. Eur J Immunol 1992;22:3141–3148.

51. Ranheim EA, Kipps TJ. Elevated expression of CD80 (B7/BB1) and other accessory molecules on synovial fluid mononuclear cell subsets in rheumatoid arthritis [see comments]. Arthritis Rheum 1994;37:1637–1646.

52. Yellin MJ, Sinning J, Covey LR, et al. T lymphocyte T cell-B cell-activating molecule/CD40-L molecules induce normal B cells or chronic lymphocytic leukemia B cells to express CD80 (B7/BB-1) and enhance their costimulatory activity. J Immunol 1994;153:666–674.

53. Goldstein MD, Debenedette MA, Hollenbaugh D, Watts TH. Induction of costimulatory molecules B7-1 and B7-2 in murine B cells. The CBA/N mouse reveals a role for Bruton's tyrosine kinase in CD40-mediated B7 induction. Mol Immunol 1996;33:541–552.

54. Kaneko Y, Hirose S, Abe M, et al. CD40-mediated stimulation of B1 and B2 cells: implication in autoantibody production in murine lupus. Eur J Immunol 1996;26:3061–3065.

55. Ranheim EA, Kipps TJ. Activated T cells induce expression of B7/BB1 on normal or leukemic B cells through a CD40-dependent signal. J Exp Med 1993;177:925–935.

56. Schattner EJ, Elkon KB, Yoo DH, et al. CD40 ligation induces Apo-1/Fas expression on human B lymphocytes and facilitates apoptosis through the Apo-1/Fas pathway. J Exp Med 1995;182:1557–1565.

57. Hanissian SH, Geha RS. Jak3 is associated with CD40 and is critical for CD40 induction of gene expression in B cells. Immunity 1997;6:379–387.

58. Worm M, Geha RS. CD40 ligation induces lymphotoxin alpha gene expression in human B cells. Int Immunol 1994;6:1883–1890.

59. Clark EA, Ledbetter JA. How B and T cells talk to each other. Nature 1994;367:425–428.

60. Noelle RJ, Ledbetter JA, Aruffo A. CD40 and its ligand, an essential ligand-receptor pair for thymus-dependent B-cell activation. [Review] [27 refs]. Immunol Today 1992;13:431–433.

61. Cheng G, Cleary AM, Ye ZS, et al. Involvement of CRAF1, a relative of TRAF, in CD40 signaling. Science 1995;267:1494–1498.

62. Ishida TK, Tojo T, Aoki T, et al. TRAF5, a novel tumor necrosis factor receptor-associated factor family protein, mediates CD40 signaling. Proc Natl Acad Sci USA 1996;93:9437–9442.

63. Ishida T, Mizushima S, Azuma S, et al. Identification of TRAF6, a novel tumor necrosis factor receptor-associated factor protein that mediates signaling from an amino-

terminal domain of the CD40 cytoplasmic region. J Biol Chem 1996;271:28745–28748.

64. Mosialos G, Birkenbach M, Yalamanchili R, et al. The Epstein-Barr virus transforming protein LMP1 engages signaling proteins for the tumor necrosis factor receptor family. Cell 1995;80:389–399.

65. Nakano H, Oshima H, Chung W, et al. TRAF5, an activator of NF-kappaB and putative signal transducer for the lymphotoxin-beta receptor. J Biol Chem 1996;271:14661–14664.

66. Rothe M, Sarma V, Dixit VM, Goeddel DV. TRAF2-mediated activation of NF-kappa B by TNF receptor 2 and CD40. Science 1995;269:1424–1427.

67. Kehry MR. CD40-mediated signaling in B cells. Balancing cell survival, growth, and death. [Review] [77 refs]. J Immunol 1996;156:2345–2348.

68. Lin SC, Stavnezer J. Activation of NF-kappaB/Rel by CD40 engagement induces the mouse germ line immunoglobulin Cgammal promoter. Mol Cell Biol 1996;16:4591–4603.

69. Gray D, Siepmann K, Wohlleben G. CD40 ligation in B cell activation, isotype switching and memory development. [Review] [44 refs]. Semin Immunol 1994;6:303–310.

70. Faris M, Gaskin F, Parsons JT, Fu SM. CD40 signaling pathway: anti-CD40 monoclonal antibody induces rapid dephosphorylation and phosphorylation of tyrosine-phosphorylated proteins including protein tyrosine kinase Lyn, Fyn, and Syk and the appearance of a 28-kD tyrosine phosphorylated protein. J Exp Med 1994;179:1923–1931.

71. Ren CL, Morio T, Fu SM, Geha RS. Signal transduction via CD40 involves activation of lyn kinase and phosphatidylinositol-3-kinase, and phosphorylation of phospholipase C gamma 2. J Exp Med 1994;179:673–680.

72. Uckun FM, Gajl-Peczalska K, Myers DE, et al. Temporal association of CD40 antigen expression with discrete stages of human B-cell ontogeny and the efficacy of anti-CD40 immunotoxins against clonogenic B-lineage acute lymphoblastic leukemia as well as B-lineage non-Hodgkin's lymphoma cells. Blood 1990;76:2449–2456.

73. Noelle RJ. The role of gp39 (CD40L) in immunity. [Review]. Clin Immunol Immunopathol 1995;76:S203–S207.

74. Noelle RJ, Mackey M, Foy T, et al. CD40 and its ligand in autoimmunity. [Review] [32 refs]. Ann N Y Acad Sci 1997;815:384–391.

75. Linsley PS, Ledbetter JA. The role of the CD28 receptor during T cell responses to antigen. Annu Rev Immunol 1993;11:191–212.

76. Jenkins MK, Johnson JG. Molecules involved in T-cell co-stimulation. Curr Opin Immunol 1993;5:361–367.

77. Boussiotis VA, Freeman GJ, Gribben JG, Nadler LM. The role of B7-1/B7-2:CD28/CLTA-4 pathways in the prevention of anergy, induction of productive immunity and down-regulation of the immune response. Immunol Rev 1996;153:5–26.

78. Larsen CP, Elwood ET, Alexander DZ, et al. Long-term acceptance of skin and cardiac allografts after blocking CD40 and CD28 pathways. Nature 1996;381:434–438.

79. Parker DC, Greiner DL, Phillips NE, et al. Survival of mouse pancreatic islet allografts in recipients treated with allogeneic small lymphocytes and antibody to CD40 ligand. Proc Natl Acad Sci USA 1995;92:9560–9564.

80. Kirk AD, Harlan DM, Armstrong NN, et al. CTLA4-Ig and anti-CD40 ligand prevent renal allograft rejection in primates. Proc Natl Acad Sci USA 1997;94:8789–8794.

81. Larsen CP, Pearson TC. The CD40 pathway in allograft rejection, acceptance, and tolerance. Curr Opin Immunol 1997;9:641–647.

82. Tang A, Judge TA, Turka LA. Blockade of CD40-CD40 ligand pathway induces tolerance in murine contact hypersensitivity. Eur J Immunol 1997;27:3143–3150.

83. Dubois B, Massacrier C, Vanbervliet B, et al. Critical role of IL-12 in dendritic cell-induced differentiation of naive B lymphocytes. J Immunol 1998;161:2223–2231.

84. Peng X, Remacle JE, Kasran A, et al. IL-12 up-regulates CD40 ligand (CD154) expression on human T cells. J Immunol 1998;160:1166–1172.

85. Kelsall BL, Stuber E, Neurath M, Strober W. Interleukin-12 production by dendritic cells. The role of CD40-CD40L interactions in Th1 T-cell responses. Ann N Y Acad Sci 1996;795:116–126.

86. Sozzani S, Allavena P, D'Amico G, et al. Differential regulation of chemokine receptors during dendritic cell maturation: a model for their trafficking properties. J Immunol 1998;161:1083–1086.

87. Caux C, Massacrier C, Vanbervliet B, et al. Activation of human dendritic cells through CD40 cross-linking. J Exp Med 1994;180:1263–1272.

88. Ridge JP, Di Rosa F, Matzinger P. A conditioned dendritic cell can be a temporal bridge between a CD4+ T-helper and a T-killer cell [see comments]. Nature 1998;393:474–478.

89. Albert ML, Sauter B, Bhardwaj N. Dendritic cells acquire antigen from apoptotic cells and induce class I-restricted CTLs. Nature 1998;392:86–89.

90. Albert ML, Pearce SF, Francisco LM, et al. Immature dendritic cells phagocytose apoptotic cells via alphavbeta5 and CD36, and cross-present antigens to cytotoxic T lymphocytes. J Exp Med 1998;188:1359–1368.

91. Schoenberger SP, Toes RE, van der Voort EI, et al. T-cell help for cytotoxic T lymphocytes is mediated by CD40-CD40L interactions [see comments]. Nature 1998;393:480–483.

92. Bennett SR, Carbone FR, Karamalis F, et al. Help for cytotoxic-T-cell responses is mediated by CD40 signalling [see comments]. Nature 1998;393:478–480.

93. Yellin MJ, Winikoff S, Fortune SM, et al. Ligation of CD40 on fibroblasts induces CD54 (ICAM-1) and CD106 (VCAM-1) up-regulation and IL-6 production and proliferation. J Leukoc Biol 1995;58:209–216.

94. Yellin MJ, Brett J, Baum D, et al. Functional interactions of T cells with endothelial cells: the role of CD40L-CD40-mediated signals. J Exp Med 1995;182:1857–1864.

95. Miller DL, Yaron R, Yellin MJ. CD40L-CD40 interactions regulate endothelial cell surface tissue factor and thrombomodulin expression. J Leukoc Biol 1998;63:373–379.

96. Hoffman RW, Takeda Y, Sharp GC, et al. Human T cell clones reactive against U-small nuclear ribonucleoprotein autoantigens from connective tissue disease patients and healthy individuals. J Immunol 1993;151:6460–6469.

97. Bockenstedt LK, Gee RJ, Mamula MJ. Self-peptides in the initiation of lupus autoimmunity. J Immunol 1995;154:3516–3524.

98. Okubo M, Kokubun M, Nishimaki T, et al. T cell epitope mapping of U1-A RNP. Arthritis Rheum 1995;38:1170–1172.

99. Cabral AR, Alarcon-Segovia D. Autoantibodies in systemic lupus erythematosus [in process citation]. Curr Opin Rheumatol 1998;10:409–416.

100. Spronk PE, Horst G, Van Der Gun BT, et al. Anti-dsDNA production coincides with concurrent B and T cell activation during development of active disease in systemic lupus erythematosus (SLE). Clin Exp Immunol 1996;104:446–453.

101. Datta SK, Patel H, Berry D. Induction of a cationic shift in IgG anti-DNA autoantibodies. Role of T helper cells with classical and novel phenotypes in three murine models of lupus nephritis. J Exp Med 1987;165:1252–1268.

102. Mohan C, Shi Y, Laman JD, Datta SK. Interaction between CD40 and its ligand gp39 in the development of murine lupus nephritis. J Immunol 1995;154:1470–1480.

103. Kalled SL, Cutler AH, Datta SK, Thomas DW. Anti-CD40 ligand antibody treatment of SNF1 mice with established nephritis: preservation of kidney function. J Immunol 1998;160:2158–2165.

104. Early GS, Zhao W, Burns CM. Anti-CD40 ligand antibody treatment prevents the development of lupus-like nephritis in a subset of New Zealand black x New Zealand white mice. Response correlates with the absence of an anti-antibody response. J Immunol 1996;157:3159–3164.

105. Daikh DI, Finck BK, Linsley PS, et al. Long-term inhibition of murine lupus by brief simultaneous blockade of the B7/CD28 and CD40/gp39 costimulation pathways. J Immunol 1997;159:3104–3108.

106. Courtenay JS, Dallman MJ, Dayan AD, et al. Immunisation against heterologous type II collagen induces arthritis in mice. Nature 1980;283:666–668.

107. Staines NA, Wooley PH. Collagen arthritis—what can it teach us? [Review] [106 refs]. Br J Rheumatol 1994;33:798–807.

108. Osman GE, Toda M, Kanagawa O, Hood LE. Characterization of the T cell receptor repertoire causing collagen arthritis in mice. J Exp Med 1993;177:387–395.

109. Osman GE, Cheunsuk S, Allen SE, et al. Expression of a type II collagen-specific TCR transgene accelerates the onset of arthritis in mice. Int Immunol 1998;10:1613–1622.

110. Durie FH, Fava RA, Foy TM, et al. Prevention of collagen-induced arthritis with an antibody to gp39, the ligand for CD40. Science 1993;261:1328–1330.

111. Martin R, McFarland HF, McFarlin DE. Immunological aspects of demyelinating diseases. Annu Rev Immunol 1992;10:153–187.

112. Stinissen P, Medaer R, Raus J. Myelin reactive T cells in the autoimmune pathogenesis of multiple sclerosis. Mult Scler 1998;4:203–211.

113. Lehmann PV, Forsthuber T, Miller A, Sercarz EE. Spreading of T-cell autoimmunity to cryptic determinants of an autoantigen. Nature 1992;358:155–157.

114. Jensen MA, Arnason BG, Toscas A, Noronha A. Global inhibition of IL-2 and IFN-gamma secreting T cells precedes recovery from acute monophasic experimental autoimmune encephalomyelitis. J Autoimmun 1996;9:587–597.

115. Howard LM, Miga AJ, Vanderlugt CL, et al. Mechanisms of immunotherapeutic intervention by anti-CD40L (CD154) antibody in an animal model of multiple sclerosis. J Clin Invest 1999;103:281–290.

116. Steinman L. Multiple sclerosis: a coordinated immunological attack against myelin in the central nervous system. Cell 1996;85:299–302.

117. Stout RD, Suttles J, Xu J, et al. Impaired T cell-mediated macrophage activation in CD40 ligand-deficient mice. J Immunol 1996;156:8–11.

118. Zhou P, Seder RA. CD40 ligand is not essential for induction of type 1 cytokine responses or protective immunity after primary or secondary infection with histoplasma capsulatum. J Exp Med 1998;187:1315–1324.

119. Grewall IS, Foellmer HG, Grewall KD, et al. Requirement for CD40 ligand in costimulation induction, T cell activation, and experimental allergic encephalomyelitis. Science 1996;273:1864–1867.

120. Carayanniotis G, Masters SR, Noelle RJ. Suppression of murine thyroiditis via blockade of the CD40-CD40L interaction. Immunology 1997;90:421–426.

121. Neurath MF, Fuss I, Kelsall BL, et al. Antibodies to interleukin 12 abrogate established experimental colitis in mice. J Exp Med 1995;182:1281–1290.

122. Stuber E, Strober W, Neurath M. Blocking the CD40L-CD40 interaction in vivo specifically prevents the priming of T helper 1 cells through the inhibition of interleukin 12 secretion. J Exp Med 1996;183:693–698.

123. Schmitz G, Herr AS, Rothe G. T-lymphocytes and monocytes in atherogenesis. Herz 1998;23:168–177.

124. Mach F, Schonbeck U, Sukhova GK, et al. Reduction of atherosclerosis in mice by inhibition of CD40 signalling. Nature 1998;394:200–203.

125. Laman JD, de Smet BJ, Schoneveld A, van Meurs M. CD40-CD40L interactions in atherosclerosis. [Review] [31 refs]. Immunol Today 1997;18:272–277.

126. Schonbeck U, Mach F, Sukhova GK, et al. Expression of stromelysin-3 in atherosclerotic lesions: regulation via CD40-CD40 ligand signaling in vitro and in vivo [in process citation]. J Exp Med 1999;189:843–853.

127. Lee Y, Lee W, Lee S, et al. CD40 activation in circulating platelets in patients with acute coronary syndrome. Cardiology 2000;92:11–16.

128. Aukrust P, Muller F, Ueland T, et al. Enhanced levels of soluble and membrane-bound CD40 ligand in patients with unstable angina. Possible reflection of T lymphocyte and platelet involvement in the pathogenesis of acute coronary syndromes. Circulation 1999;100:614–620.

129. Ossevoort MA, Ringers J, Boon L, et al. Blocking of costimulation prevents kidney graft rejection in rhesus monkeys. Transplant Proc 1998;30:2165–2166.

130. Hancock WW, Sayegh MH, Zheng XG, et al. Costimulatory function and expression of CD40 ligand, CD80, and CD86 in vascularized murine cardiac allograft rejection. Proc Natl Acad Sci USA 1996;93:13967–13972.

131. Larsen CP, Alexander DZ, Hollenbaugh D, et al. CD40-gp39 interactions play a critical role during allograft rejection. Suppression of allograft rejection by blockade of the CD40-gp39 pathway. Transplantation 1996;61:4–9.

132. Chang AC, Blum MG, Blair KS, et al. Prolonged anti-CD40 ligand therapy improves primate cardiac allograft survival. Transplant Proc 1999;31:95.

133. Markees TG, Phillips NE, Noelle RJ, et al. Prolonged survival of mouse skin allografts in recipients treated with donor splenocytes and antibody to CD40 ligand. Transplantation 1997;64:329–335.

134. Blazar BR, Taylor PA, Panoskaltsis-Mortari A, et al. Blockade of CD40 ligand-CD40 interaction impairs CD4+ T cell-mediated alloreactivity by inhibiting mature donor T cell expansion and function after bone marrow transplantation. J Immunol 1997;158:29–39.

135. Lu L, Li W, Fu F, et al. Blockade of the CD40-CD40 ligand pathway potentiates the capacity of donor-derived dendritic cell progenitors to induce long-term cardiac allograft survival. Transplantation 1997;64:1808–1815.

136. Saito K, Sakurai J, Ohata J, et al. Involvement of CD40 ligand-CD40 and CTLA4-B7 pathways in murine acute graft-versus-host disease induced by allogeneic T cells lacking CD28. J Immunol 1998;160:4225–4231.

137. Flamand V, Donckier V, Demoor FX, et al. CD40 ligation prevents neonatal induction of transplantation tolerance. J Immunol 1998;160:4666–4669.

138. Tang A, Judge TA, Nickoloff BJ, Turka LA. Suppression of murine allergic contact dermatitis by CTLA4Ig. Tolerance induction of Th2 responses requires additional blockade of CD40-ligand. J Immunol 1996;157:117–125.

139. Elwood ET, Larsen CP, Cho HR, et al. Prolonged acceptance of concordant and discordant xenografts with combined CD40 and CD28 pathway blockade. Transplantation 1998;65:1422–1428.

140. Pierson RN 3rd, Chang AC, Blum MG, et al. Prolongation of primate cardiac allograft survival by treatment with ANTI-CD40 ligand (CD154) antibody. Transplantation 1999;68:1800–1805.

141. Kirk AD, Burkly LC, Batty DS, et al. Treatment with humanized monoclonal antibody against CD154 prevents acute renal allograft rejection in nonhuman primates [see comments]. Nat Med 1999;5:686–693.

142. George J, Raskob G, Lichtin A, et al. Safety and effect on platelet count of single-dose monoclonal antibody to CD40 ligand in patients with chronic ITP. Blood 1998;92(suppl 1):707A.

143. Davis J, Totoritis MC, Sklenar TA, et al. Results of a phase I, single-dose, dose-escalating trial of a humanized anti-CD40L monoclonal antibody (IDEC-131) in patients with systemic lupus erythematosus (SLE). Arthritis Rheum 1999;42(suppl):S281.

144. Balasa B, Krahl T, Patstone G, et al. CD40 ligand-CD40 interactions are necessary for the initiation of insulitis and diabetes in nonobese diabetic mice. J Immunol 1997;159: 4620.

145. Gerritse K, Laman JD, Noelle RJ, et al. CD40-CD40 ligand interactions in experimental allergic encephalomyelitis and multiple sclerosis. Proc Natl Acad Sci USA 1996;93: 2499.

146. Laman JD, Maassen CB, Schellekens MM, et al. Therapy with antibodies against CD40L (CD154) and CD44-variant isoforms reduces experimental autoimmune encephalomyelitis induced by a proteolipid protein peptide [In Process Citation]. Mult Scler 1998;4:147.

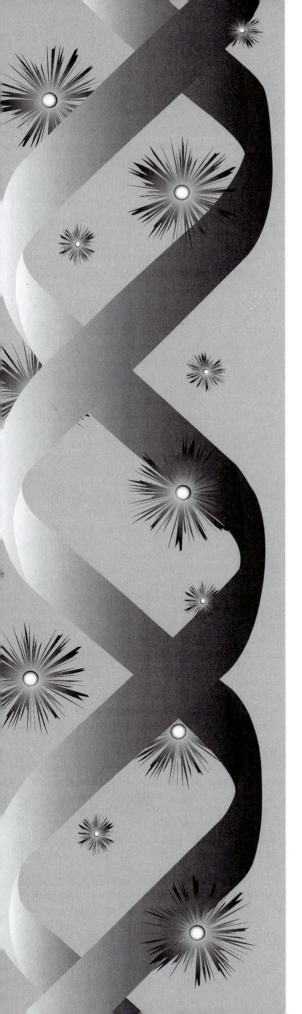

IV

Maneuvers

Transplantation

Cellular Therapy

Gene Therapy

Additional Interventions

Drug Therapy for HIV Infection

Chapter 33

Renal Transplantation

Manikkam Suthanthiran
Terry B. Strom

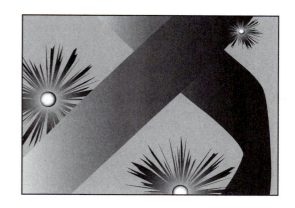

Renal transplantation is the treatment of choice for patients with end-stage renal disease (ESRD). A better comprehension of the antiallograft response, improved preservation of organs, judicious use of immunosuppressive drugs, application of antilymphocyte agents for the treatment of rejection, and adaptation of infection prophylaxis protocols have all contributed to the recent short-term, as well as long-term, improvements in the outcome following renal transplantation.

Current Status

Transplantation results in better long-term survival and fuller rehabilitation compared with dialytic therapy. Given the limited supply of organs, transplantation, however, should be reserved for patients likely to obtain meaningful rehabilitation with engraftment. Other individuals with ESRD not considered for transplantation are the elderly (>75 years), those with a recent history of malignancy (less than 2 years), those with active glomerulonephritis, HIV infection, or active sepsis, and those in whom chronic infection might be reactivated by immunosuppressive treatment.

Excellent patient and graft outcomes following renal transplantation have been accomplished (Table 33-1). Repeat transplants have also benefited with recent advances in transplant patient management (1). The 1-year graft survival rate of transplants performed during 1995 to 1996 was 87.3% for primary transplants (n = 12,494), and 83.2% for repeat transplants (n = 2013) (see Table 33-1). The excellent results, the shortage of organs, and the lack of adverse medical consequences following renal donation have all led to the broadening of the "rules" regarding organ donors. Since there are no significant differences in outcomes of living-donor transplants using unrelated and partially HLA-mismatched donors, many transplant teams now consider not only genetically related individuals as living donors but also emotionally related (e.g., spouse) as suitable living donors (see Table 33-1).

Organ Shortage

The waiting list for renal transplantation in the United States has grown from 13,943 patients in 1988 to 38,270 patients in 1997 (see Table 33-1) (2). The median waiting time has also increased from 400 days in 1988 to 962 days by 1995. In 1997, 2009 deaths occurred while awaiting transplantation. The shortage of organs for transplantation will not be resolved without new initiatives.

Characteristics of the Kidney Donors and Recipients

Because of the shortage in organs for transplantation, the proportion of cadaver kidneys from donors in the United States over age 45 rose from 24% in 1991 to 33% in 1997 (1). The age of the recipient has also increased over the last 7 years from 42.4 years to 46.1 years for recipients of cadaver-donor kidneys and from 33.7 years to 39.6 years for recipients of living-donor grafts. About 15% of the transplants are repeat transplants. Organs from HIV- or HBV-seropositive individuals are not used. In some centers HCV carriers are utilized as organ donors, especially for HCV-positive recipients.

Surgical Procedure and Complications

In adults, the graft is placed extraperitoneally in the iliac fossa through an oblique lower abdominal incision and, in children, retroperitoneally through a midline abdominal incision (3). The renal artery is usually anastomosed end-to-end to the recipient's hypogastric artery. The renal vein is anastomosed to the iliac vein (adults) or to the inferior vena cava (children). Renal artery or renal vein thrombosis is a rare complication (3,4). The donor ureter is inserted by creating a submucosal tunnel into the recipient's bladder. Urinary leak occurs in 2% of recipients and is usually the result of technical problems (3,4).

Lymphocele (2% to 5% incidence) is caused by leakage of lymph from the recipient's lymphatics. Symptomatic lymphoceles (obstruction of the ureter or the venous drainage) are relieved by percutaneous aspiration and/or by drainage into the peritoneal cavity (3,4).

Costs

An ESRD patient with a functioning graft at 3 years posttransplantation represents a net financial saving to the Medicare program (5).

Table 33-1. Current Status of Renal Transplantation in the United States

Survival Rates	5-Year Survival Rate (%) and Half-life ($T^1/_2$ Yrs)			
	Patient	$T^1/_2$	Graft	$T^1/_2$
Type and number of transplants[a]				
Living donor (n = 20,258)	90	>30	77	15.3
Cadaver donor (n = 50,291)	82	21.2	63	9.4

	Graft Survival Rate (%)	
	1 year	5 years
Previous transplants (cadaver)[b]		
No (primary, n = 12,494)	87.3	61.0
Yes (repeat, n = 2103)	83.2	55.7
Previous transplants (living donor)[b]		
No (primary, n = 5911)	93.5	76.6
Yes (repeat, n = 551)	91.1	72.5
Relation of living donor to recipient[b]		
Parent (n = 1337)	93.8	73.7
Offspring (n = 905)	92.0	71.8
Sibling (n = 2572)	94.6	79.9
Other relative (n = 303)	92.4	74.9
Spouse (n = 506)	91.8	75.6
Other unrelated (n = 274)	94.8	71.3

	$T^1/_2$ (Years)	
Additional Factors[b]	Living	Cadaver
Race		
White	17.0	11.1
Black	8.7	6.2
Asian	15.3	16.7
Previous transplant		
None	15.5	9.5
One	13.1	9.3
More than one	14.0	7.0
Presensitization		
0–10%	15.5	9.7
11–50%	15.2	8.7
>50%	12.7	8.8

Waiting List[c]	No.
Number of patients awaiting transplantation	38,270
Median waiting time (days)	962
Number of deaths while awaiting transplantation	2009

[a] Five-year survival rates and half-lives derived by analyses of kidney transplants reported to the UNOS Scientific Transplant Registry during 1991–1997 (1).
[b] Transplants reported to the UNOS Scientific Registry during 1995–1996 (2).
[c] UNOS OPTN waiting list on the last day of 1997 (2).

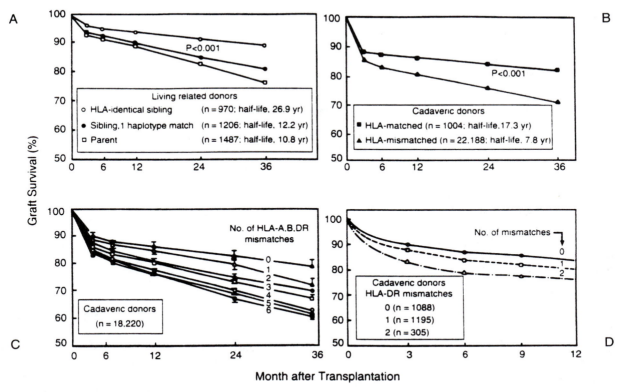

Figure 33-1. Effect of HLA matching on renal allograft survival rates. Panel A shows the effect of haplotype matching in renal transplantation from living related donors. (Graft-survival data are from Cecka and Terasaki [8].) Panel B shows the superior results obtained with HLA-matched (for A, B, and DR antigens), cadaveric renal grafts as compared with mismatched grafts. (Data are from Takemoto et al [9].) Panel C shows the effect of different degrees of HLA-A, B, and DR mismatching on the survival of cadaveric grafts. (Data are from Terasaki et al [10].) Panel D shows the stepwise improvement in the survival of cadaveric grafts after matching for the HLA-DR antigens identified by DNA typing. (Data are from Opelz et al [11].) (From Suthanthiran M, Strom TB. Renal transplantation. N Engl J Med 1994;331:365–376. Copyright © 1994 Massachusetts Medical Society. All rights reserved.)

Factors Affecting Transplant Outcome

A number of factors influence renal transplantation outcome. The adverse factors include early graft dysfunction, repeat transplantation, age less than 15 years or greater than 50 years, and presence of anti-HLA antibodies in the serum of the prospective recipient, prolonged ex vivo preservation time, rejection episodes, and race (1). Black recipients have a reduced rate of engraftment using either cadaver or living kidney donors (1,6). The discontinuation of cyclosporine, because of financial reasons, contributes to graft loss in blacks (7).

The clinical benefits of HLA-matching are illustrated in Figure 33-1 (8–11). The effect of matching for HLA in cadaveric graft recipients has been examined in a prospective study (9) in which kidneys were shared nationally on the basis of matching for HLA-A, B, and DR antigens. All transplantation centers in the United States participated in this study. The 1-year graft survival rate was 88% for HLA-matched kidneys and 79% for mismatched kidneys, and the estimated half-life of the HLA-matched graft was 17.3 years and that of mismatched allografts,

7.8 years. Current registry data continue to show a strong benefit for receiving a well-matched cadaver donor kidney, as well as improved half-life allograft survival times in all typing categories.

A potential problem of national sharing—prolongation of cold ischemia time resulting from the time required for the transportation of the grafts—was also examined in this study (9). The cold ischemia time was prolonged by 4 hours by sharing; more importantly, graft survival rate was higher for HLA-matched kidneys for each of the cold ischemia periods examined. These data confirm and extend collaborative transplant study data, which show that graft survival rates of zero-antigen–mismatched kidneys with cold ischemia times that are up to 48 hours are superior to those of four-antigen–mismatched grafts with cold ischemia times that are less than 24 hours (12). However, an increase in cold ischemia times is detrimental to the outcome of cadaver donor transplants that are HLA mismatched (13).

DNA-based molecular techniques are being explored for the finer resolution of the HLA system. Existing molecular methodologies have already helped to resolve the discrepancies associated with the often-faulty serologic identification of HLA-DR

Table 33-2. Mechanism of Action of Immunosuppressive Drugs

Agent	Mode of Action
Cyclosporine—FK-506	Blocks Ca^{++}-dependent T-cell activation pathway by binding to calcineurin
Corticosteroids	Blocks NFκB-dependent immune gene expression
Azathioprine	Inhibits purine synthesis
Mycophenolate mofetil	Inhibits a lymphocyte-selective guanosine synthesis pathway
Rapamycin	Inhibits the mTOR-dependent response to antigen-activated lymphocytes to growth factors

antigens. Molecular typing has also permitted appreciation of a stepwise increase in the survival of cadaveric transplants matched for 0, 1, or 2 HLA-DR antigens (11).

Currently, there is no dispute in the transplantation community regarding the preference of a two-haplotype–matched over a one-haplotype– or zero-haplotype–matched, living, related renal graft. With respect to cadaver source renal grafts, a national policy of mandatory sharing for six-antigen–matched or phenotypically identical (zero mismatch for HLA) kidneys currently exists, and the excellent results found justify its continuation.

Cross-Match

Cross-match testing is performed routinely prior to renal transplantation. The test consists of incubating the recipient's serum with the donor's lymphocytes in the presence of rabbit serum as the source of complement. The presence of donor-specific, class I HLA antibodies (positive T-cell cross-match) in the recipient's serum is an absolute contraindication since 80% to 90% of transplants performed in the presence of a positive test are rapidly and irreversibly rejected (14).

Immunosuppressive Regimens

Immunologic considerations, including antirejection therapy, are organized around a few general principles. The first consideration is careful patient preparation and selection of the best available ABO-compatible, human leukocyte antigen (HLA) match in the event that several potential living donors are available for organ donation. The second is a multitiered approach to immunosuppressive therapy similar in principle to that used in chemotherapy; several agents are used simultaneously, each of which is directed at a different molecular target within the allograft response (Table 33-2). Additive-synergistic effects are achieved through application of each agent at a relatively low dose, thereby limiting the toxicity of each individual agent while increasing the total immunosuppressive effect. The third principle is that higher immunosuppressive drug doses or more individual immunosuppressive drugs are required to gain early engraftment and to treat established rejection than are needed to maintain immunosuppression in the long term. Hence, intensive induction and lower-dose maintenance drug protocols are used. The fourth principle involves careful investigation of each episode of post-transplantation graft dysfunction, with the realization that most

of the common causes of graft dysfunction, including rejection-drug toxicity and infections, can (and frequently do) coexist. Successful therapy, therefore, involves several simultaneous therapeutic maneuvers. The fifth principle involves the appropriate reduction or withdrawal of an immunosuppressive drug when that drug's toxicity exceeds its therapeutic benefit.

Therapy Designed to Prevent Rejection

All posttransplantation immunosuppressive protocols use at least two agents, each directed at a discrete site in the T-cell activation cascade (see Table 33-2). In the United States three drug protocols are in routine use. In patients at high risk to suffer immunologic graft failure a course of treatment with a polyclonal or monoclonal anti–T-cell antibody is often used as an adjunct in the immediate posttransplant period.

Immunopharmacology of Allograft Rejection

Cyclosporine and Tacrolimus (FK506)

Cyclosporine, a small, neutral, hydrophobic, cyclic peptide of fungal origin, and tacrolimus (FK506), a water-soluble, macrolide lactone produced by *Streptomyces tsukubaenis*, block the Ca^{2+}–dependent T-cell activation pathway (15–18). The immunosuppressive effects of cyclosporine and FK506 depend on the formation of heterodimeric complexes that consist of the drug (cyclosporine or FK506) and its respective cytoplasmic "immunophilin" receptor protein, cyclophilin (19) or FK-binding protein (FKBP) (20,21). Both cyclosporine-cyclophilin and FK506-FKBP complexes bind calcineurin, a calcium-sensitive and calmodulin-sensitive phosphatase, and inhibit its enzymatic activity (see Table 33-2) (22,23). Cyclosporine-FK506–mediated inhibition of calcineurin's phosphatase activity prevents the dephosphorylation of cytoplasmic NF-AT and thereby impedes subsequent import of this deoxyribonucleic acid (DNA)–binding protein into the nucleus (24,25). Calcineurin inhibitors block the expression of not only NF-AT but also the activities of other DNA-binding proteins such as NF-κB and activated protein-1

(AP-1) factors (26–28). The phosphorylation status of transcription factors affects not only their nuclear import but also their DNA-binding ability and interaction with the cellular transcriptional machinery (e.g., *c-jun*) (29). As a consequence, treatment with calcineurin inhibitors dampens the expression of numerous T-cell–activation genes.

It is also significant that cyclosporine, in striking contrast to its inhibitory activity on the induced expression of IL-2, enhances the expression of transforming growth factor-β_1 (TGF-β_1) (30). This effect is operative in human subjects treated with cyclosporine (31). Because TGF-β_1 is a potent inhibitor of IL-2–stimulated T-cell proliferation and generation of antigen-specific cytotoxic T lymphocytes, enhanced expression of TGF-β_1 is likely to contribute to the immunosuppressive activity of cyclosporine. This novel effect of cyclosporine suggests also a mechanism for some of the complications (e.g., renal fibrosis, malignancy) of cyclosporine therapy since TGF-β_1 is a fibroblast growth factor (32,33) and can promote tumor growth (34).

Corticosteroids

Corticosteroids were first used in clinical transplantation to reverse acute rejection reactions in patients treated with maintenance doses of azathioprine. It is now customary to use modest doses of a corticosteroid in maintenance drug protocols. A short course of corticosteroids in increased doses is often used to treat acute rejection episodes. Corticosteroids inhibit T-cell proliferation, macrophage activation, T-cell–dependent immunity, and cytokine gene transcription (including IL-1, IL-2, IL-6, IFN-α, and tumor necrosis factor genes) (see Table 33-2) (35–37). Although no individual cytokine can totally reverse the inhibitory effects of corticosteroids on mitogen-stimulated T-cell proliferation, a combination of cytokines is effective (38). The effects of corticosteroids on gene activation events are complex and include interference with the activities of DNA-binding proteins (39–41).

Inhibitors of Purine Metabolism: Azathioprine and Mycophenolate Mofetil

Azathioprine is the 1-methyl-4-nitro-5-imidazolyl derivative of 6-mercaptopurine (42,43). This purine analog functions as a purine antagonist and inhibits cellular proliferation (see Table 33-2). Allopurinol blocks the catabolism of azathioprine, causing a dramatic increase in bone marrow suppression. Azathioprine has been used in conjunction with cyclosporine or tacrolimus and corticosteroids in maintenance protocols. Although application of azathioprine diminishes the incidence and intensity of rejection episodes, it is not valuable in the therapy of ongoing rejection.

Mycophenolate mofetil (MMF) blocks purine metabolism through its inhibitory effect on inosine monophosphate dehydrogenase, an enzyme in the de novo purine biosynthetic pathway (44) (see Table 33-2). MMF has replaced azathioprine in most centers since it is superior to azathioprine in reducing the incidence of early, acute, rejection episodes. Long-term engraftment, however, has not dramatically improved with MMF use (45,46).

Rapamycin

The efficacy of rapamycin, an agent that inhibits the proliferative signal imparted by T-cell growth factors IL-2, IL-4, IL-7, or IL-15 to antigen-activated T cells, as well as a variety of other tissue-specific growth factors, has been evaluated in triple-therapy regimens as a substitute for azathioprine or mycophenolate mofetil or in combination with corticosteroids as a replacement for cyclosporine (47,48). The drug has proved effective in preventing acute rejection episodes and was approved for use by the FDA in September 1999.

Alternative Approaches

Sequential Immunotherapy

Following the lead of Soulillou et al (49), many centers have adopted an alternative approach to antirejection prophylaxis. OKT3, anti-CD25 mAb, or polyclonal antilymphocyte antibodies are used in many transplant centers as induction therapy in the immediate posttransplantation period. These protocols establish an immunosuppressive umbrella that enables initial engraftment without immediate use of high-dose nephrotoxic calcineurin period. The incidence of early rejection episodes is reduced by the prophylactic usage of these antilymphocyte antibodies (49–53). This protocol is particularly beneficial long term for patients at high risk for immunologic graft failure (e.g., broadly presensitized or retransplant patients, pediatric recipients, or African-Americans) (50).

OKT3 mAb

The multimeric CD3 complex proteins are noncovalently associated to the alpha and beta chains of the T-cell receptor (TCR) for antigen. This complex is expressed on the surface of all functionally competent T lymphocytes. OKT3 mAb binds to the epsilon-chain of the CD3 complex; OKT3 binding to T cells leads to modulation of all components of the TCR-CD3 complex from the T-cell surface, either by shedding or internalization. Moreover, T cells virtually disappear from the peripheral blood after the administration of OKT3 mAb. In a randomized clinical trial, OKT3 mAb was found to be superior to corticosteroids in reversing acute rejection of renal allografts (51).

Anti-CD25 mAb

While OKT3 interacts with all T cells, antibodies directed against the CD25 proteins, the alpha chain of the trimolecular, high-affinity IL-2–receptor complex, are far more selective. CD25 is expressed on recently activated T cells and other activated mononuclear leukocytes, but CD25 is not expressed on resting or memory T cells. Thus, anti-CD25 mAb is specific for the small population of activated T cells engaged in the allograft response. Both the chimeric mouse human [Simulect] and hyperchimeric humanized [Zenapax] anti-CD25 mAbs are available for use (52,53). Administration of these antibodies reduces the incidence and severity of early allograft rejection episodes. Treatment with either has proven rather safe. These antibodies do not cause the troublesome symptoms frequently associated with the first several doses of OKT3.

Maintenance Immunosuppressive Regimens

The basic immunosuppressive protocol used in most transplant centers involves the use of multiple drugs; for example, a calcineurin inhibitor plus corticosteroids with or without mycophenolate mofetil or rapamycin, each directed at a discrete site in the T-cell activation cascade (see Table 33-2) and each with distinct side effects. Cyclosporine, FK506, azathioprine, corticosteroids, mycophenolate mofetil, and rapamycin are approved by the Food and Drug Administration.

Therapy Designed to Treat Established Rejection

Low-dose prednisone, a calcineurin inhibitor, and a purine blocker or rapamycin maintenance drug therapy are effective in the prevention of acute cellular rejection; each drug blocks a different facet of T-cell activation. Their proximal sites of activity, however, render these regimens ineffective in blocking the activity of already activated T cells or late-acting elements of the allograft response that no longer require helper T-cell input. Thus, these agents do not readily abrogate an established acute rejection episode or totally prevent chronic rejection. Treatment of established rejection requires the use of agents that act against already fully activated T cells. Thus, high-dose corticosteroids, polyclonal antilymphocyte antibodies, or OKT3 are often used for the treatment of acute cellular rejection.

Approximately, two-thirds of acute cellular rejections will respond to high-dose corticosteroid boluses. Steroid-sensitive rejection episodes are typically characterized by a dense infiltration of T cells in the medullary regions of the graft. We often treat the first kidney allograft rejection episode with a bolus of intravenous methylprednisolone (500 mg to 1000 mg) daily for 3 consecutive days. Most centers use antilymphocytic antibodies (e.g., ATG, OKT3) for the treatment of steroid-refractory rejection or an extremely aggressive first rejection episode. In patients treated with cyclosporine, a switch from cyclosporine to FK506 is often undertaken. While the calcineurin inhibitors share a similar mode of drug action, they differ greatly in their composition and pattern of distribution.

Polyclonal antilymphocyte antibody preparations are derived from animals immunized with human lymphocytes. The antibodies are directed against both lymphocyte-specific antigens and more broadly expressed antigens. More than 80% of steroid-resistant, first rejection episodes will respond to these polyclonal antibodies. Patients are pretreated before each dose with diphenhydramine and steroids. Antilymphocyte antibodies are administered daily by slow intravenous infusion for approximately 10 days. Adverse reactions include anaphylaxis; hemolysis; thrombocytopenia; neutropenia; dyspnea; chills; fever; hypotension; chemical phlebitis; pruritus; serum sickness; and chest, flank, and back pain. Unlike the complications noted with the first dose of OKT3, the severity of anaphylactoid side effects to these polyclonal antilymphocyte preparations can increase with subsequent doses. Frank anaphylaxis can occur anytime during treatment. The use of polyclonal antilymphocyte antibodies has increased in the United States because an effective preparation, long used in Europe, has become available and is very effective in reversing or preventing rejection.

We rarely treat a kidney transplant recipient for more than three rejection episodes in the early posttransplantation period because third and fourth rejections tend to be vasculitic forms that are therapeutically resistant, and the risks to the patient from overzealous immunosuppression are unacceptably high by that point.

Although current drug protocols are far superior to those used a decade ago, the situation is far from ideal. Most allografts eventually succumb to chronic rejection. Long-term immunosuppressive therapy is mandatory.

Adjunctive Vasodilation Therapy

Acute cyclosporine/FK506 nephrotoxicity is caused at least in part by intense intrarenal vasospasm. Moreover, renal allografts are subject to calcium-dependent ischemic and reperfusion injury. These considerations have fostered trials of adjunctive vasodilating agents such as calcium antagonists or fish oil during the early posttransplantation period. Supplementation of a standard drug protocol with nifedipine, diltiazem, or verapamil has reduced the rate of early graft dysfunction and enhanced graft survival rate (54,55).

Preclinical trials of fish oil have demonstrated immunosuppressive effects—effects that synergize with cyclosporine (56)—and an ability to mitigate cyclosporine-mediated nephrotoxicity (57). A reduction in the incidence of rejection, improved renal blood flow and function, and lower arterial pressure in recipients of renal allografts have been reported with fish oil supplementation of a cyclosporine and prednisolone regimen (58).

Infection Prophylaxis

Perioperative antimicrobial therapy with a broad-spectrum antibiotic has diminished infection in the immediate postoperative period and has contributed to the decline in the morbidity and mortality following renal transplantation (59). Prophylactic trimethoprim-sulfamethoxazole, introduced to prevent urinary tract infection, also reduces the incidence of *Pneumocystis carinii* pulmonary infection (60). Routine antiviral (61,62) and antifungal prophylaxis is currently prescribed during the early posttransplantation period when the dosage of immunosuppressants is high. Cytomegalovirus (CMV)–negative recipients of kidneys from CMV-positive donors are particularly susceptible to life-threatening sequelae of primary CMV infection. Although acyclovir is not effective for treating active CMV disease, prophylactic treatment with acyclovir or ganciclovir to recipients harboring latent virus or non–CMV-immune recipients receiving a graft from a CMV-positive donor reduces the rate of active disease posttransplantation (62). Symptomatic CMV disease is also frequent and virulent in CMV-positive recipients treated with antilymphocyte antibodies, and preemptive ganciclovir therapy is beneficial in this population at high risk for CMV disease (62).

Hyperacute Rejection

If a transplant recipient bears circulating antibodies against donor class I HLA determinants HLA-A or HLA-B prior to transplantation, hyperacute rejection often occurs promptly following kidney transplantation. These anti–class I HLA antibodies result from sensitization by previous blood transfusions, multiple pregnancies, or a previously rejected graft. Hyperacute rejection is an untreatable, catastrophic type of vasculitis and often requires emergency transplant nephrectomy. Fortunately, the routine application of careful pretransplant cross-matching usually identifies presensitized patients, and the incidence of hyperacute rejection is now extremely low.

Acute Rejection: Cellular and Humoral

The incidence of acute rejection is greatest in the first 3 months, less in the next 6, and relatively uncommon 1 year following transplantation in drug-compliant patients. Acute rejection is characterized by a decrease in renal function and blood flow. Clinically, the most common signs are fever, graft enlargement, and tenderness, but acute rejection is often a subtle, clinical process identified only by the biochemical indices of decreased glomerular filtration.

Acute cellular rejection is characterized by a dense, interstitial, graft infiltrate consisting of a lymphocyte-rich population of mononuclear leukocytes. Cellular rejection is usually graded using pathologic criteria based on the extent and cytodestructive sequelae.

The infiltrate consists predominantly of T cells (80% to 90%); the majority of tubular-interstitial, infiltrating T cells are $CD8^+$ (cellular rejection). A low or inverted CD4/CD8 ratio among the perivascular infiltrate was a correlate of poor prognosis in a study of 20 allograft biopsies (63). Recent analyses of intragraft gene-expression events demonstrate that numerous T-cell–activation genes are expressed during acute rejection. Particularly common is the expression of granzyme B, perforin, fas ligand, IL-10, and IL-15 (64,65).

During advanced humoral rejection, the vascular endothelium of the graft is the target of antibody-mediated immune attack. Severe vascular rejection is noted in recipients who elaborate antibodies posttransplantation against donor class I MHC antigens (66–68). Thrombosis of renal arterioles, which causes progressive renal ischemia and leukocytic infiltration of the perivascular tissues, probably results from complement-related chemotactic factors. Endothelial-cell swelling is followed by endothelial-cell proliferation and, finally, fibrosis. The sequelae of this process such as mesangial-cell proliferation, increased mesangial matrix, glomerular capillary collapse or thrombosis, interstitial fibrosis, and tubular atrophy are often evident.

Early vascular rejection, manifested by perivascular infiltrates, endothelial-cell swelling, and modest proliferation, can often be successfully treated. In patients with donor-specific antibody, plasma exchange may be useful (69). In contrast, late humoral rejection (thrombosis and fibrosis) and hyperacute rejection are refractory to therapy.

Chronic Rejection

Chronic rejection is caused by inflammatory vascular injury to the graft. Current immunologic strategies have little impact on retarding the progression of chronic rejection, the most common cause of failure of long-term allografts. Antigen-specific cellular and humoral immunity and additional cellular elements, including macrophages and platelets (and their secretory products, eicosanoids and growth factors), hypertension, reduced renal mass, and dyslipidemia have been hypothesized as pathogenetic factors (70,71). TGF-β_1, a profibrotic cytokine, is hyperexpressed in human renal allografts displaying histologic features of chronic rejection (72). Recently, a link between heretofore undiscovered subclinical episodes of acute rejection and the development of chronic rejection has been discovered (73). Vascular smooth-muscle-cell proliferation, increased extracellular matrix, interstitial fibrosis, and glomerular sclerosis are all characteristics of this process and are of prognostic value (74).

Recurrence

Original disease recurs in 10% to 20% of grafts (75). Graft loss as a result of recurrence, however, is rare (<2%). Most causes of renal failure are not contraindications to renal transplantation, nor do they require special considerations. However, combined liver and renal transplantation might be more appropriate in type I hyperoxaluria; cadaveric rather than live-donor grafts are more appropriate in focal segmental glomerulosclerosis and hemolytic uraemic syndrome; and a 1- to 2-year waiting period is recommended in the case of rapidly progressive renal failure. Patients whose original disease is focal glomerulosclerosis are at the greatest risk of all kidney transplant recipients to suffer rapid and serious recurrent kidney disease. Through early detection and early treatment with plasmapheresis (76) or extracorporeal plasma protein absorption (77), the incidence and severity of nephrotic range proteinuria and azotemia can be reduced.

Malignancy

Basal cell carcinoma, Kaposi's sarcoma, carcinoma of the vulva and perineum, non-Hodgkin's lymphoma, squamous cell carcinoma, hepatobiliary carcinoma, and in-situ carcinoma of the uterine cervix are all more frequent in graft recipients compared with the general population (78,79). High-dose immunosuppression, especially multiple courses of treatment with antilymphocyte antibodies, is a risk factor. Interestingly, the common types of cancers—carcinoma of the breast, lung, prostate, and colon—are not increased in the transplant population. Patients successfully treated for cancer can be transplanted after a 2-year waiting period (79).

Rehabilitation

Measurable improvements in the quality of life following renal transplantation have been observed consistently in cross-sectional and longitudinal studies. A 20% increase in full-time work status has also been reported. A survey of 226 recipients of primary cadaveric renal grafts has revealed the following: 1) whereas 46% of the patients stayed indoors 1 year prior to transplantation because of poor health, only 13.5% of recipients with functioning grafts experienced such physical limitation; 2) 66.6% of the nondiabetics and 49% of the diabetics with functioning grafts perceived their health to be excellent or good; and 3) 74% of the nondiabetics and 34.7% of the diabetics were able to work full- or part-time following transplantation (80).

Conclusion

Renal transplantation, the forerunner of other life-saving organ replacement therapies, represents the fruition of the dedicated efforts of basic scientists, clinicians, and allied personnel. An excellent paradigm for the effective application of knowledge gained by basic research to the alleviation of life-threatening illness, renal transplantation also affords unparalleled opportunities for the investigation of the systemic basis for renal disease independent of organ-specific mechanisms. We anticipate clinical application in the near future of more refined immunosuppressive regimens and synergistic therapeutic protocols that target discrete steps in antigen recognition, signal transduction, and effector immunity. We are optimistic regarding the inducibility of antigen-specific tolerance in the clinical setting. Finally, the ultimate prize of transplantation would be that the basic principles learned would facilitate the prevention of the disease that necessitated transplantation in the first place.

Acknowledgement
The authors are grateful to Ms. Frances C. Pechenick and Ms. Linda Stackhouse for their meticulous help in the preparation of this chapter.

References

1. Cecka JM. The UNOS Scientific Renal Transplant Registry. In: Cecka JM, Terasaki PI, eds. Clinical transplants 1998. Los Angeles: UCLA Tissue Typing Laboratory, 1999:1–16.
2. 1998 Annual Report of the U.S. Scientific Registry for Transplant Recipients and the Organ Procurement and Transplantation Network: Transplant Data: 1988–1997. U.S. Department of Health and Human Services, Health Resources and Services Administration, Office of Special Programs, Division of Transplantation, Rockville, MD; UNOS, Richmond, VA.
3. Belzer FO, Salvatierra O. Renal transplantation, organ procurement, preservation and surgical management. In: Brenner BM, Rector FC, eds. The kidney. Vol 2. Philadelphia: WB Saunders, 1976:1796–1818.
4. Sagalowsky AI, Dawidson I. Surgical complications of renal transplantation. In: Jacobson HR, Striker GE, Klahr S, eds. The principles and practice of nephrology. Philadelphia: BC Decker, 1991:846–848.
5. Eggers PW. Effect of transplantation on the Medicare end-stage renal disease program. N Engl J Med 1988;318:223–229.
6. Opelz G, Wujclak T, Mytilineos J, et al. The Collaborative Transplant Study. Collaborative transplant study analysis of graft survival in blacks. Transplant Proc 1993;5:2443–2445.
7. Sanders CE, Curtis JJ, Julian BA, et al. Tapering or discontinuing cyclosporine for financial reasons—a single-center experience. Am J Kidney Dis 1993;21:9–15.
8. Cecka JM, Terasaki PI. The UNOS Scientific Renal Transplant Registry—1991. In: Terasaki PI, ed. Clinical transplants 1991. Los Angeles: UCLA Tissue Typing Laboratory, 1991:1–11.
9. Takemoto S, Terasaki PI, Cecka JM, et al. Survival of nationally shared, HLA-matched kidney transplants from cadaveric donors. N Engl J Med 1992;327:834–839.
10. Terasaki PI, Cecka JM, Lim E, et al. UCLA and UNOS registries: overview. In: Terasaki PI, ed. Clinical transplants 1991. Los Angeles: UCLA Tissue Typing Laboratory, 1991: 409–430.
11. Opelz G, Mytilineos J, Scherer S, et al. Survival of DNA HLA-DR typed and matched cadaver kidney transplants. Lancet 1991;338:461–463.
12. Opelz G. The Collaborative Transplant Study. The benefit of exchanging donor kidneys among transplant centers. N Engl J Med 1988;318:1289–2992.
13. Held PJ, Kahan BD, Hunsicker LG, et al. The impact of HLA mismatches on the survival of first cadaveric kidney transplants. N Engl J Med 1994;331:765–770.
14. Williams GM, Hume DM, Hudson RP, et al. "Hyperacute" renal homograft rejection in man. N Engl J Med 1968; 279:611.
15. Schreiber SL. Chemistry and biology of the immuniphilins and their immunosuppressive ligands. Science 1991;251: 283–287.
16. Schreiber SL. Immunophilin-sensitive protein phosphatase activation in cell signalling pathways. Cell 1992;70:365–368.
17. Schreiber SL, Crabtree GR. The mechanism of action of cyclosporin A and FK506. Immunol Today 1992;13:136–142.
18. Baumann G. Molecular mechanism of immunosuppressive agents. Transplant Proc 1992;24(suppl 2):4–7.
19. Handschumacher RE, Harding MW, Rice J, Drugge RJ. Cyclophilin: a specific cytosolic binding protein for cyclosporin A. Science 1984;226:544–547.
20. Harding MW, Galat A, Uchling DE, Schreiber SL. A receptor for the immunosuppressant FK506 is cis-transpeptidylprolyl isomerase. Nature 1989;342:758–760.
21. Siekierka JJ, Hung SHY, Poe M, et al. A cytosolic binding protein for the immunosuppressant FK506 has peptidylprolyl isomerase activity but is distinct from cyclophilin. Nature 1989;341:755–757.
22. Liu J, Farmer JD Jr, Lane WS, et al. Calcineurin is a common target of cyclophilin-cyclosporin A and FKBP-FK506 complexes. Cell 1991;66:807–815.
23. Fruman DA, Klee CB, Bierer BE, Burakoff SI. Calcineurin phosphatase activity in T lymphocytes is inhibited by FK506 and cyclosporin A. Proc Natl Acad Sci USA 1992;89: 3686–3690.
24. Emmel EA, Verweij CL, Durand DB, et al. Cyclosporin A specifically inhibits function of nuclear proteins involved in T cell activation. Science 1989;246:1617–1620.

25. Flanagan WM, Corthesy B, Brown RJ, Crabtree GR. Nuclear association of a T-cell transcription factor blocked by FK506 and cyclosporine. Nature 1991;352:802–807.
26. Granelli-Piperno A, Nolan P, Inaba K, Steinman RM. The effect of immunosuppressive agents on the induction of nuclear factors that bind to sites on the interleukin-2 promoter. J Exp Med 1990;172:1869–1872.
27. Kang S-M, Tran C-A, Grilli M, Lenardo MJ. NF-KB subunit regulation in non-transformed CD4+ T lymphocytes. Science 1992;256:1452–1456.
28. Sehajpal PK, Sharma VK, Inguili E, et al. Synergism between the CD3 antigen and CD2 antigen derived signals: exploration at the level of induction of DNA binding proteins and characterization of the inhibitory activity of cyclosporine. Transplantation 1993;55:1118–1124.
29. Hunter T, Karin M. The regulation of transcription by phosphorylation. Cell 1992;70:375–387.
30. Li B, Sehajpal PK, Khanna A, et al. Differential regulation of transforming growth factor β and interleukin-2 genes in human T cells: demonstration by usage of novel competitor DNA constructs in the quantitative polymerase chain reaction. J Exp Med 1991;174:1259–1262.
31. Shin GT, Khanna A, Ding R, et al. In vivo expression of transforming growth factor-beta1 in humans: stimulation by cyclosporine. Transplantation 1998;65:313–318.
32. Massague J. The transforming growth factor-β family. Annu Rev Cell Biol 1990;6:597–641.
33. Roberts AB, Sporn MB. Physiological actions and clinical applications of transforming growth factor-β (TGF-β). Growth Factors 1993;8:1–9.
34. Hojo M, Morimoto T, Maluccio M, et al. Cyclosporine induces cancer progression by a cell-autonomous mechanism. Nature 1999;397:530–554.
35. Arya SK, Wong-Staal F, Gallo RC. Dexamethasone mediated inhibition of T-cell growth factor and gamma interferon messenger RNA. J Immunol 1984;133:273–276.
36. Knudsen PJ, Dinaretio CA, Strom TB. Glucocorticoids inhibit transcription and post-transcriptional expression of interleukin-1. J Immunol 1987;139:4129–4134.
37. Zanker B, Walz G, Wieder KJ, Strom TB. Evidence that glucocorticosteroids block expression of the human IL-6 gene by accessory cell. Transplantation 1990;49:198–201.
38. Almawi WY, Hadro ET, Strom TB, et al. Abrogation of glucocorticosteroid-mediated inhibition of T cell proliferation by the synergistic action of IL-1, IL-6, and IFN. J Immunol 1991;146:3523–3527.
39. Vacca A, Felli MP, Farina AR, et al. Glucocorticoid receptor-mediated suppression of the interleukin-2 gene expression through impairment of the cooperativity between nuclear factor of activated T cells and AP-I enhancer elements. J Exp Med 1992;175:637–646.
40. Yang-Yen HF, Chambard JC, Sun YL, et al. Transcriptional interference between *c-jun* and the glucocorticoid receptor: mutual inhibition of DNA binding due to direct protein-protein interaction. Cell 1990;62:1205–1215.
41. Palvogianni F, Raptis A, Ahuja SS, et al. Negative transcriptional regulation of human interleukin-2 (IL-2) gene by glucocorticoids through interference with nuclear transcription factors AP-I and NF-AT. J Clin Invest 1993;91:1481–1487.
42. Elion GB. Biochemistry and pharmacology of purine analogues. Fed Proc 1967;26:898–904.
43. Bach J-F, Strom TB. The mode of action of immunosuppressive agents. In: Bach J-F, Strom TB, eds. Research monographs in immunology. Vol. 9. 2nd ed. Amsterdam: Elsevier, 1986:105–158.
44. Franklin TJ, Cook JM. The inhibition of nucleic acid synthesis by mycophenolic acid. Biochem J 1969;113:515.
45. European Mycophenolate Mofetil Cooperative Study Group. Mycophenolate mofetil in renal transplantation: 3-year results from the placebo-controlled trial. Transplantation 1999;68:391–396.
46. Mathew TH. The Tricontinental Mycophenolate Mofetil Renal Transplantation Study. A blinded, long-term, randomized multicenter study of mycophenolate mofetil in cadaveric renal transplantation: results at three years. Transplantation 1998;65:2450–2454.
47. Kahan BD, Podbielski J, Nappoli KL, et al. Immunosuppressive effects and safety of a sirolimus/cyclosporine combination regimen for renal transplantation. Transplantation 1998;66:1040–1046.
48. Groth CG, Backman L, Morales JM, et al. The Sirolimus European Renal Transplant Study Group. Sirolimus (rapamycin)-based therapy in human renal transplantation: similar efficacy and different toxicity compared with cyclosporine. Transplantation 1999;67:1036–1042.
49. Hourmant M, Soulillou JP, Remi JP, et al. Use of cyclosporin A after anti-lymphocyte serum in renal transplantation. Presse Med 1985;14:2093–2096.
50. Cecka JM, Cho YW, Terasaki PI. Analysis of the UNOS scientific renal transplant registry at three years—early events affecting transplant success. Transplantation 1992;53:59–64.
51. Ortho Multicenter Transplant Study Group. A randomized clinical trial of OKT3 monoclonal antibody for acute rejection of cadaveric renal transplants. N Engl J Med 1985;313:337–342.
52. Kahan BD, Rajagopalan PR, Hall M. The United States Simulect Renal Study Group. Reduction of the occurrence of acute cellular rejection among renal allograft recipients treated with basilisimab, a chimeric anti-interleukin-2–receptor monoclonal antibody. Transplantation 1999;67:276–284.
53. Vincenti F, Kirkman R, Light S, et al. The Daclizumab Triple Therapy Study Group. Interleukin-2 receptor blockade with daclizumab to prevent acute rejection in renal transplantation. N Engl J Med 1998;338:161–165.
54. Neumayer H-H, Kunzendorf U, Schreiber M. Protective effects of calcium antagonists in human renal transplantation. Kidney Int 1992;41:S87–S93.
55. Suthanthiran M, Haschemeyer RH, Riggio RR, et al. Excellent outcome with a calcium channel blocker supplemented immunosuppressive regimen in cadaveric renal transplantation: a potential strategy to avoid antibody induction protocols. Transplantation 1993;55:1008–1013.
56. Kelley VE, Kirkman RL, Bastos M, et al. Enhancement of immunosuppression by substitution of fish oil for olive oil as a vehicle for cyclosporine. Transplantation 1989;48:98–102.
57. Rogers TS, Elzinga L, Bennett WM, et al. Selective enhancement of thromboxane in macrophages and kidneys in cyclosporine-induced nephrotoxicity. Dietary protection by fish oil. Transplantation 1988;45:153–156.
58. Van Der Heide JJH, Bilo HJG, Donker JM, et al. Effect of dietary fish oil on renal function and rejection in cyclosporine-treated recipients of renal transplants. N Engl J Med 1993;329:769–773.

59. Tilney NL, Strom TB, Vineyard GC, et al. Factors contributing to the declining mortality rate in renal transplantation. N Engl J Med 1978;299:1321.

60. Fox BC, Sollinger HW, Belzer FO, et al. A prospective, randomized, double-blind study of trimethoprim-sulfamethoxazole for prophylaxis of infection in renal transplantation: clinical efficacy, absorption of trimethoprim-sulfamethoxazole, effects on the microflora, and the cost-benefit of prophylaxis. Am J Med 1990;89:255–274.

61. Balfour HH Jr, Bean B, Laskin OL, et al. Acyclovir halts progression of herpes zoster in immunocompromised patients. N Engl J Med 1983;308:1448–1453.

62. Turgeon N, Fishman JA, Basgoz N, et al. Effect of oral acyclovir or ganciclovir therapy after preemptive intravenous ganciclovir therapy to prevent cytomegalovirus disease in cytomegalovirus seropositive renal and liver transplant recipients receiving antilymphocyte antibody therapy. Transplantation 1998;66:1780–1786.

63. van Es A, Meyer CJ, Oljans PJ, et al. Mononuclear cells in renal allografts: correlation with peripheral blood T lymphocyte subpopulations and graft prognosis. Transplantation 1984;37:134–139.

64. Strehlau J, Pavlakis M, Lipman M, et al. Quantitative detection of immune activation transcripts as a diagnostic tool in kidney transplantation. Proc Natl Acad Sci USA 1997;94: 695–700.

65. Suthanthiran M. Molecular analyses of human renal allografts: differential intragraft gene expression during rejection. Kidney Int 1997;51(suppl 58):S15–S21.

66. Suthanthiran M, Garavoy MR. Immunologic monitoring of the renal transplant recipient. Urol Clin North Am 1983;10:315–325.

67. Halloran PF, Schlaut J, Solez K, Srinivasa NS. The significance of the anti–class I response. II. Clinical and pathologic features of renal transplants with anti–class I-like antibody. Transplantation 1992;53:550–555.

68. Trpkov K, Campbell P, Pazderka F, et al. Pathologic features of acute renal allograft rejection associated with donor-specific antibody. Analysis using the Banff grading schema. Transplantation 1996;61:1586–1592.

69. Pascual M, Saidman S, Tolkoff-Rubin N, et al. Plasma exchange and tacrolimus-mycophenolate rescue for acute humoral rejection in kidney transplantation. Transplantation 1998;66:1460–1464.

70. Tilney NL, Whitley WD, Diamond JR, et al. Chronic rejection—an undefined conundrum. Transplantation 1991;52: 389–398.

71. Terasaki PI, Koyama H, Cecka JM, Gjertson DW. The hyperfiltration hypothesis in human renal transplantation. Transplantation 1994;57:1450–1454.

72. Sharma VK, Bologa RM, Xu G-P, et al. Intragraft TGF-β_1 mRNA: a correlate of interstitial fibrosis and chronic allograft nephropathy. Kidney Int 1996;49:1297–1393.

73. Nickerson P, Jeffery J, Gough J, et al. Effect of increasing baseline immunosuppression on the prevalence of clinical and subclinical rejection: a pilot study. J Am Soc Nephrol 1999;19:1801–1805.

74. Kasiske BL, Kalil RSN, Lee HS, et al. Histopathologic findings associated with a chronic, progressive decline in renal allograft function. Kidney Int 1991;40:514–524.

75. Mathew TH. Recurrence of disease following renal transplantation. Am J Kidney Dis 1988;12:85–96.

76. Artero M, Biava C, Amend W, et al. Recurrent focal glomerulosclerosis: natural history and response to therapy. Am J Med 1992;92:375–383.

77. Dantal J, Bigot E, Bogers W, et al. Effect of plasma protein adsorption on protein excretion in kidney-transplant recipients with recurrent nephrotic syndrome. N Engl J Med 1994;330:7–14.

78. Penn I. The effect of immunosuppression on pre-existing cancers. Transplantation 1993;55:742–747.

79. Penn I. Occurrence of cancers in immunosuppressed organ transplant recipients. In: Cecka JM, Terasaki PI, eds. Clinical transplants 1998. Los Angeles: UCLA Tissue Typing Laboratory, 1999:147–158.

80. Manninen DL, Evans RW, Dugan MK. Work disability, functional limitations, and the health status of kidney transplantation recipients post-transplant. In: Terasaki P, ed. Clinical transplants 1991. Los Angeles: UCLA Tissue Typing Laboratory, 1992:193–203.

Chapter 34

Pancreas Transplantation

Michael E. Shapiro

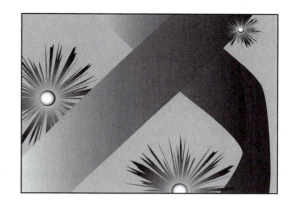

Rigorous control of hyperglycemia may mitigate the relentless progression of secondary complications in diabetes (1). Nonetheless, control of blood glucose by the exogenous administration of insulin has failed to achieve true normoglycemia despite intensive efforts by patients with type I diabetes mellitus and their caregivers. Even intensive insulin therapy by pump or multiple daily insulin injections fails to maintain normal levels of HbA1c (1,2). Thus, it is to provide for normal glucose homeostasis that pancreas transplantation has been developed as a therapy for type I diabetes.

The first pancreatic transplants for diabetes were performed at the University of Minnesota in 1966 (3). One of the first two patients rapidly became normoglycemic and remained so for months. Over the next 20 years, small numbers of pancreatic allografts were performed, mostly at Minnesota, with generally poor results. The 1-year graft survival for cadaveric pancreas transplants as recently as 1982 was below 20% (4). Since that time, because of changes in immunosuppressive protocols and operative techniques, major improvements in patient and graft outcomes have occurred, with results equal to that of kidney transplantation (5). For this reason, in many centers combined pancreas-renal transplantation is now considered the standard of care in appropriate patients with type I diabetes who require a kidney transplant (6).

Patient Selection

Pancreas transplants are currently indicated only for patients with type I diabetes mellitus. There has been recent debate concerning whether patients with type II diabetes would benefit from a pancreatic graft, as their underlying problem relates primarily to insulin resistance rather than pancreatic endocrine insufficiency. It has been suggested that the hyperinsulinemia following systemically drained pancreas transplantation might overcome this insulin resistance. In most instances, there is little question of the form of a patient's diabetes, based on age of onset and history of progression. In those cases where the etiology of a patient's diabetes is not clear, C-peptide levels should be determined to verify the absence of endogenous insulin production.

One major issue has been the appropriate timing of pancreatic transplantation in relation to the natural history of diabetes. Ideally, one would like to perform a pancreas transplant prior to the development of serious secondary diabetic complications. However, because current technology requires lifelong immunosuppression for allograft survival, early pancreatic transplantation trades the ravages of diabetes for those of prolonged immunosuppression. For that reason, the vast majority of pancreatic grafts have been performed simultaneously with a renal transplant (SPK) in patients with uremic diabetes. Increasingly, patients with diabetes who have preexisting renal transplants such as from living donors may subsequently receive a pancreas transplant at a later time (PAK). This is particularly useful at centers where the wait for cadaveric kidneys is particularly long. By performing a living-donor renal transplantation early, followed by a subsequent PAK, one avoids the excess mortality experienced by patients with diabetes who are on dialysis (7). Some centers have performed isolated pancreas transplantations in patients before the onset of frank uremia. The need for nephrotoxic calcineurin inhibitors (cyclosporine or tacrolimus) as part of the immunosuppressive regimen requires that these patients have excellent renal function.

The proper selection of patients who are likely to benefit from pancreas transplantation has resulted in major improvements in outcome. Series as recently as 10 years ago reported operative mortality as high as 10% following SPK; nearly all of these deaths were cardiovascular in nature (8). Thus, careful examination for evidence of coronary artery disease is crucial in the preoperative evaluation of patients with diabetes, whether for SPK or kidney transplant alone. The presence of autonomic neuropathy with the potential for silent myocardial ischemia makes the history notoriously unreliable in these patients (9). Patients able to exercise should be evaluated by exercise-thallium scintigraphy. Many uremic diabetics have little exercise tolerance, however, and these patients should, at a minimum, have either dipyridamole-thallium or dobutamine echo testing (9,10). Those patients with suggestions of ischemia on such testing or those with an inadequate stress-thallium scan should undergo coronary angiography prior to transplantation. It is still debated whether patients with correctable coronary lesions should be candidates for pancreas transplantation after revascularization.

Another area of concern in patients with long-standing diabetes is the effects of autonomic neuropathy on urinary bladder and gastrointestinal function. Many of these patients have poor sensation of bladder distension and poor bladder emptying as well. This is of particular concern if the pancreas is to be drained to the bladder. Urodynamic studies should be performed in all such pancreas recipients, and enteric drainage is preferred for those with inadequate urodynamic function. Patients with severe gastroparesis or diabetic enteropathy may have difficulty with absorption of immunosuppression and may also have more difficulty with enteric drainage of pancreatic secretions.

An overall assessment needs to be made of a patient's likelihood of benefit from an undertaking as daunting as combined pancreas-renal transplantation. Clearly, patients with far-advanced secondary complications are unlikely to note any improvement in quality of life from a pancreas transplant. Patients with severe nutritional deficiencies may have increased difficulty with wound healing and increased rates of postoperative complications. Those with severe coronary artery disease, even if surviving the perioperative period, may have a limited life expectancy and should not be considered for transplantation.

Technique

Transplantation of the pancreas (as opposed to isolated islets) requires a technique for management of the pancreatic exocrine secretions in addition to providing vascular connections for the islet tissue; there have been problems with exocrine drainage that have proved most vexing until recently. In the United States, most pancreatic allografts consist of the whole pancreas with an attached segment of duodenum containing the ampulla of Vater that is used for the exocrine-drainage anastomosis. Enteric drainage to the small intestine was initially used, but required entering the gastrointestinal tract at a time of maximal immunosuppression and therefore with the expected risk of infection. Bladder drainage of the duodenal segment was popularized by Sollinger (11) and Nghiem (12) in the mid-1980s and became the technique of choice for whole-organ transplants. In addition to allowing for a safe method of exocrine drainage, monitoring of exocrine secretion in the urine (urinary amylase) permits evaluation of pancreatic function.

Over the past few years, however, increasing problems with bladder drainage have been noted, including an increased rate of urinary tract infection, "reflux" pancreatitis, and bladder or urethral inflammation resulting from activated pancreatic enzymes. Additionally, the value of measuring urinary amylase as a marker for pancreatic rejection has been called into question because of its low sensitivity and specificity, particulary in the case of an SPK transplant where the kidney may serve as an early marker of allograft rejection. For those reasons, in many centers it has been found necessary to convert many bladder-drained pancreases to enteric drainage, and there they have returned to enteric drainage of the pancreas as an initial approach (13).

In Europe, many groups utilize segmental pancreatic grafts, which are either drained into the intestine (14) or duct-occluded with polymer (15). Early problems with graft thrombosis, which led to creative techniques such as creation of distal splenic arteriovenous fistulas, have lessened in the past few years, possibly because of better graft preservation and the use of anticoagulants.

Immunosuppression

Immunosuppressive approaches for organ allografts have been dealt with elswhere in detail (Chapter 32) and will be discussed only briefly. Maintenance immunosuppression for most SPK or PAK allografts consists of combination therapy, usually cyclosporine or tacrolimus, mycophenolate mofetil, and prednisone (16,17). The majority of transplant centers use some sort of antibody induction therapy (ALG, OKT3, or an anti-CD25 antibody), although recent reports have shown excellent results without antibody induction (18). Maintenance of adequate cyclosporine or tacrolimus levels seems important in reducing the rate of early rejection in the absence of an antibody protocol.

Rejection

The diagnosis of rejection is one of the most vexing problems in pancreas transplantation. The occurrence of hyperglycemia or hypoinsulinemia is a late sign of pancreatic dysfunction, implying the loss of 90% of islet function. Treatment of rejection at that late stage is often futile. For that reason, more sensitive methods of identifying pancreatic rejection have been sought. In the SPK setting, one frequently identifies renal rejection by a decrease in glomerular filtration rate (and a rise in creatinine) without any obvious sign of pancreatic dysfunction. The renal rejection, often confirmed by biopsy, is successfully treated, and the assumption is made that there must have been ongoing, unidentified, pancreatic rejection at the same time. It is primarily for this reason that pancreatic graft survival is better in the PSK group than with isolated pancreas transplants (see below).

Measures of exocrine function as an indicator of allograft rejection have been used with fair results, but are plagued by a lack of sensitivity and specificity. A rise in serum amylase is a very sensitive marker of rejection, but has little specificity for that diagnosis. Most commonly, urinary amylase has been followed, with a decrease in urinary amylase suggestive of rejection. Levels of urinary amylase vary depending on the dietary intake of the recipient and hydration status. As a result, urinary amylase levels must be measured at similar times of day, and either timed collections or amylase/creatinine ratios must be used to standardize results. In general, a decrease of 50% in urinary amylase is compatible with rejection.

More recently, in a number of centers the safety of percutaneous or transcystoscopic pancreatic needle biopsies in the diagnosis of rejection has been demonstrated (19). The percutaneous biopsies are either CT- or ultrasound-guided. Although this can allow for the accurate diagnosis of rejection, it is still necessary to have a clinical indication to perform the biopsy. Recent work in renal transplantation using molecular markers of cytotoxic T-lymphocyte activation for the diagnosis of rejection may also be applicable to pancreas transplantation as well (20,21).

Treatment of pancreatic rejection does not differ from that of renal allografts; generally, high-dose methylprednisolone or OKT3 is used, depending on center preference. Reversal of pancreatic rejection depends on early diagnosis; for that reason it is often more successful with SPK than isolated pancreatic grafts (22). Rarely, rejection of either the kidney or the pancreas may occur without loss of the other organ. In our experience, kidneys have been lost from chronic rejection, requiring a return to dialysis over several years, with preserved pancreatic function for many years following retransplantation of the kidney.

Results of Pancreatic Transplantation—Survival

Patient and graft survival rates have improved dramatically over the past decade of pancreatic transplantation. In the United States, current, 1-year graft survival is 81% with a 1-year patient survival of 94% (23). There is a significant difference in graft survival, depending on the presence or absence of a simultaneous kidney; 1-year survival for SPK is 83%, for PAK is 71%, and for solitary pancreas is 64%. This difference persists at 3 years with the results of 77%, 55%, and 50%, respectively. The poorer survival in the absence of a kidney from the same donor is attributed to the difficulty in identifying rejection. Many centers are reporting better results than the overall national data, with 1-year graft survivals of 90% to 100% (5,18).

Recent data have demonstrated a survival advantage for patients with type I diabetics who received a combined kidney-pancreas transplant compared with those who received a kidney transplant alone (24). In a 10-year study, Tyden et al reported a 20% mortality in the SPK group compared with 80% in the kidney alone group, and they speculated that this difference was the result of better glycemic control in the SPK patients. These data obviously have major implications regarding the beneficial effect of pancreas transplantation.

Results—Metabolic Effects

Patients with successful pancreas transplants maintain normal fasting-blood-glucose levels without exogenous insulin therapy. Glucose tolerance tests and 24-hour metabolic profiles are within normal range, and the HbA1c is also normal (25). Hyperglycemic glucose clamp studies (26,27) demonstrate high basal and stimulated insulin levels, presumably the result of the systemic drainage of the pancreas. This trended toward normal during 1 year of follow-up. Pancreas-kidney recipients had typical biphasic insulin release with normal hepatic glucose homeostasis.

In fact, pancreas-kidney recipients had more normal glucose homeostasis (as compared with normal controls) than did a control group of nondiabetic, steroid-treated kidney-transplant recipients. In our own experience, patients have not received any insulin from the time of their operation and have maintained normal HbA1c levels for over 11 years.

Because of concern over the possible deleterious effects of prologed hyperinsulinemia resulting from the systemic drainage of pancreatic venous blood, several groups led by Gaber et al (28,29) have championed the technique of portal venous drainage of the pancreas as a more physiologic method. At this time, there is not yet convincing evidence of the superiority of one technique over the other.

Results—Secondary Complications

The overall goal of pancreas transplantation is to prevent or halt the progression of typical, secondary complications in patients with diabetes: nephropathy, neuropathy, retinopathy, and cardiovascular disease. Preliminary data support the notion that, for some of these problems, transplantation of the pancreas is in fact helpful. For others, more data will be needed before definitive statements can be made. Recurrent diabetic nephropathy can be seen by biopsy in transplanted kidneys within 3 years after transplantation. This is manifest by increased glomerular basement membrane thickness and mesangial volume. Comparison of patients with diabetes receiving a pancreas-kidney transplant versus a kidney transplant alone shows progression of nephropathy in the kidney group but not in the group receiving a pancreas as well (30). More recently, the same investigators have demonstrated the reversal of typical diabetic glomerular lesions after 10 years in patients with diabetes who received isolated pancreas transplants (31). These data suggest that, if transplantation is performed early, those patients with diabetic nephropathy can have their disease arrested, preventing the progression to end-stage disease.

Improvement in motor and sensory nerve function has been reported comparing patients with pancreas transplants with those without (32). Additionally, those patients with neuropathy who retained a functioning pancreas transplant had better survival than those who did not (33). Preliminary data concerning retinopathy show no improvement in the early posttransplantation period, but they do suggest stabilization after 4 years (34).

There have been only anecdotal reports of improvement in cardiac or peripheral vascular disease at present. Morrissey et al (35) have raised the troubling possibility that peripheral vascular disease might actually be increased in patients receiving simultaneous pancreas/kidney transplants compared with patients with diabetes receiving kidney transplants alone. The study was non-randomized and retrospective, but again raises the possibility that systemic hyperinsulinemia might accelerate atherosclerosis. Alternatively, in this population with a great deal of pre-existing peripheral vascular disease, one may only be seeing the natural progression of advanced disease.

Conclusion

Pancreatic transplantation, in properly selected patients, can provide for insulin independence and normal glucose homeostasis with a high rate of success. Recent data suggest better patient survival for simultaneous pancreas-kidney transplants compared with kidney transplants alone in patients with diabetes who have end-stage nephropathy. Early pancreas transplantation may prevent progression of renal disease to end stage. Patients need careful preoperative evaluation, particularly looking for silent myocardial disease. Immunosuppression is similar to that used for renal transplantation, that is, triple or quadruple therapy based on cyclosporine. Most pancreas transplants are performed in concert with a kidney from the same cadaver donor, which permits better identification of early graft rejection.

References

1. Diabetes Control and Complications Trial Research Group. The effects of intensive treatment of diabetes on the development and progression of long-term complications in insulin-dependent diabetes mellitus. N Engl J Med 1993;329:977.
2. Boland EA, Grey M, Oesterle A, et al. Continuous subcutaneous insulin infusion: a new way to lower risk of severe hypoglycemia, improve metabolic control, and enhance coping in adolescents with type 1 diabetes. Diabetes Care 1999;22:1779.
3. Kelly WD, Lillehei RC, Merkel FK, et al. Allotransplantation of the pancreas and duodenum along with the kidney in diabetic nephropathy. Surgery 1967;61:827.
4. Sutherland DER, Dunn DL, Goetz FC, et al. A 10-year experience with 290 pancreas transplants at a single institution. Ann Surg 1989;210:274.
5. Sollinger HW, Odorico JS, Knechtle SJ, et al. Experience with 500 simultaneous pancreas-kidney transplants. Ann Surg 1998;228:284.
6. American Diabetes Association. Pancreas transplantation for patients with diabetes mellitus. Diabetes Care 1999;22:S82.
7. Port FK, Wolfe RA, Mauger EA, et al. Comparison of survival probabilities for dialysis patients vs cadaveric renal transplant recipients. JAMA 1993;270:1339.
8. Corry RJ, Nghiem DD. Evolution of technique and results of pancreas transplantation at the University of Iowa. Clin Transplantation 1987;1:52.
9. Nesto RW, Watson FS, Kowalchuk GJ, et al. Silent myocardial ischemia and infarction in diabetics with peripheral vascular disease: assessment by dipyridamole thallium-201 scintigraphy. Am Heart J 1990;120:1073.
10. Bates JR, Sawada SG, Segar DS, et al. Evaluation using dobutamine stress echocardiography in patients with insulin-dependent diabetes mellitus before kidney and/or pancreas transplantation. Am J Cardiol 1996;77:175.
11. D'Alessandro AM, Sollinger HW, Stratta RJ, et al. Comparison between duodenal button and duodenal segment in pancreas transplantation. Transplantation 1989;47:120.
12. Nghiem DD, Corry RJ. Technique of simultaneous renal pancreaticoduodenal transplantation with urinary drainage of pancreatic secretion. Am J Surg 1987;153:405.
13. West M, Gruessner AC, Metrakos P, et al. Conversion from bladder to enteric drainage after pancreaticoduodenal transplantations. Surgery 1998;124:883.
14. Groth CG, Tyden G, Lundgren G, et al. Segmental pancreatic transplantation with enteric exocrine diversion. World J Surg 1984;8:257.
15. Dubernard JM, Traeger J, Bosi E, et al. Transplantation for the treatment of insulin-dependent diabetes: clinical experience with polymer-obstructed pancreatic grafts using neoprene. World J Surg 1984;8:262.
16. Odorico JS, Pirsch JD, Knechtle SJ, et al. A study comparing mycophenolate mofetil to azathioprine in simultaneous pancreas-kidney transplantation. Transplantation 1998;66:1751.
17. Gruessner RW, Burke GW, Stratta R, et al. A multicenter analysis of the first experience with FK506 for induction and rescue therapy after pancreas transplantation. Transplantation 1996;61:261.
18. Shapiro ME, Abrams JM, Brown RS, et al. Successful pancreas-renal transplantation without anti-T cell antibody induction. Transplant Proc 1995;27:3087.
19. Kuo PC, Johnson LB, Schweitzer EJ, et al. Solitary pancreas allografts. The role of percutaneous biopsy and standardized histologic grading of rejection. Arch Surg 1997;132:52.
20. Strehlau J, Pavlakis M, Lipman M, et al. Quantitative detection of immune activation transcripts as a diagnostic tool in kidney transplantation. Proc Natl Acad Sci USA 1997;94:695.
21. Vasconcellos LM, Asher F, Schacter AD, et al. Cyctotoxic lymphocyte gene expression in peripheral blood leukocytes correlates with rejecting renal allografts. Transplantation 1998;66:562.
22. Stratta RJ, Sollinger HW, Perlman SB, et al. Early detection of rejection in pancreas transplantation. Diabetes 1989;38 (suppl 1):63.
23. Gruessner AC, Sutherland DER. Analysis of Untied States and non-US pancreas transplants as reported to the International Pancreas Transplant Registry and to the United Network for Organ Sharing. In: Cecka JM, Terasaki PI, eds. Clinical transplants. Los Angeles: UCLA Tissue Typing Laboratory, 1999.
24. Tyden G, Bolinder J, Solders G, et al. Improved survival in patients with insulin-dependent diabetes mellitus and end-stage diabetic nephropathy 10 years after combined pancreas and kidney transplantation. Transplantation 1999;67:645.
25. Robertson RP, Sutherland DE. Pancreas transplantation as therapy for diabetes mellitus. Annu Rev Med 1992;43:395.
26. Elahi D, Clark BA, McAloon-Dyke M, et al. Islet cell responses to glucose in human transplanted pancreas. Am J Physiol 1991;261:E800.
27. Elahi D, McAloon-Dyke M, Clark BA, et al. Sequential evaluation of islet cell responses to glucose in the transplanted pancreas in humans. Am J Surg 1993;165:15.
28. Gaber AO, Shokouh-Amiri MH, Hathaway DK, et al. Results of pancreas transplantation with portal venous and enteric drainage. Ann Surg 1995;221:613.
29. Hughes TA, Gaber AO, Amiri HS, et al. Kidney-pancreas transplantation. The effect of portal versus systemic venous drainage of the pancreas on the lipoprotein composition. Transplantation 1995;60:1406.
30. Bilous RW, Mauer SM, Sutherland DER, et al. The effects of pancreas transplantation on the glomerular structure of renal allografts in patients with insulin-dependent diabetes. N Engl J Med 1989;321:80.

31. Fioretto P, Steffes MW, Sutherland DE, et al. Reversal of lesions of diabetic nephropathy after pancreas transplantation. N Engl J Med 1998;339:69.
32. Kennedy WR, Navarro X, Goetz FC, et al. Effects of pancreatic transplantation on diabetic neuropathy. N Engl J Med 1990;322:1031.
33. Navarro X, Kennedy WR, Aeppli D, Sutherland DER. Neuropathy and mortality in diabetes: influence of pancreas transplantation. Muscle Nerve 1996;19:1009.
34. Ramsay RC, Goetz FC, Sutherland DER, et al. Progression of diabetic retinopathy after pancreas transplantation for insulin-dependent diabetes mellitus. N Engl J Med 1988;318:208.
35. Morrissey PE, Shaffer D, Monaco AP, et al. Peripheral vascular disease after kidney-pancreas transplantation in diabetic patients with end-stage renal disease. Arch Surg 1997;132:358.

Chapter 35

Cardiac Transplantation

Abdallah G. Kfoury
David O. Taylor
Dale G. Renlund

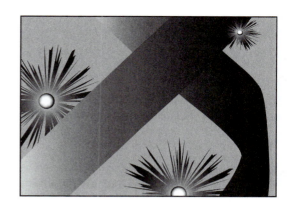

Survival and quality of life have improved after cardiac transplantation primarily because of advances in immunosuppression. However, over the past decade recipient selection and management (before and after transplantation) have also evolved, impacting the overall, long-term, medical management of the heart transplant recipient (1–3). The purpose of this chapter is to discuss various aspects of cardiac transplant recipient selection (4); some of the common non–infectious-related, non–rejection-related complications that occur after transplantation; and the development of coronary artery disease (5), the leading cause of morbidity and allograft loss late after transplantation. In addition, the clinical experience with some "newer" immunosuppressive therapies (in large trials) in heart transplantation will also be reviewed.

Recipient Selection

Recipient selection involves the selection of candidates who have a high mortality risk or severe functional incapacity without transplantation and who, after transplantation, are likely to survive with a meaningful quality of life (6). Only after excluding reversible or surgically amenable heart disease and optimizing medical therapy should cardiac transplantation be considered. Unfortunately, some patients undergo cardiac transplantation before optimal medical or surgical therapy is attempted, prompting ongoing efforts at standardization of candidacy criteria.

Although patients with intractable angina or life-threatening ventricular arrhythmias may infrequently warrant transplantation, candidates usually have heart failure with New York Heart Association (NYHA) class III to IV symptoms despite maximal medical therapy. Generally, patients have a low left ventricular ejection fraction (<20%), maximal oxygen consumption (Vo_2 < 14 mL/kg/minute or <50% of predicted), and cardiac index (<1.9 liter/m²). In these patients, one-year life expectancy is estimated to be less than 30% to 50% without heart transplantation. Patients with severe myocardial ischemia, not amenable to revascularization (by bypass surgery or angioplasty), may occasionally be considered if routine activity provokes significant symptoms or the coronary anatomy places them at especially high risk. Maximal antianginal therapy (including transmyocardial revascularization in selected patients) must clearly have been attempted and been demonstrated to have failed. Similarly,

patients with recurrent symptomatic and life-threatening ventricular arrhythmias, refractory to all accepted treatments, including automatic implantable cardioverter-defibrillator (AICD), may be evaluated.

Cardiac transplantation should not be considered when the only indication is a low, measured, left ventricular ejection fraction or simply because a history of NYHA class III or IV symptoms of heart failure is present. Furthermore, preclusion from coronary revascularization or valve replacement alone is also an inappropriate indication for cardiac transplantation. Most often, a Vo_2 of greater than 16 to 18 mL/kg/minute (or >60% of predicted) should delay consideration of transplantation.

Bearing these considerations in mind, once a decision to consider a patient for cardiac transplantation is made, a complete evaluation is performed. Psychosocial aspects, including motivation and coping abilities, are assessed, and past compliance with medical regimens is evaluated. Patients and their families must be well educated about transplantation to ensure that their expectations are realistic.

Table 35-1 indicates the studies usually performed to evaluate candidates for cardiac transplantation. Other studies may be considered if indicated as part of routine health maintenance (e.g., flexible sigmoidoscopy, mammography, Papanicolaou smear) or on the basis of the initial evaluation (e.g., carotid and peripheral Doppler testing, exercise test with peak oxygen consumption measurement, bone mineral density).

With a complete evaluation performed, the likelihood of successful transplantation can be determined. Table 35-2 lists several parameters to consider; however, recipient selection is made on an individual basis (6). Most "absolute" contraindications have, in fact, been successfully overcome in carefully selected, individual patients. Attempting to do so is not, however, necessarily advisable.

Pulmonary arterial hypertension documented on right-sided heart catheterization decreases the likelihood of successful transplantation (7,8) primarily because of the risk of right ventricular failure in the acute postoperative phase. If the pulmonary vascular resistance is greater than 8 Wood units (mean pulmonary artery pressure minus mean pulmonary capillary wedge pressure [millimeters of mercury] divided by cardiac output [liters per minute]) and is unresponsive to nitroprusside or other pulmonary vasodilator maneuvers, orthotopic cardiac transplantation is unlikely to be successful. Similarly, unresponsive pulmonary artery systolic pressures greater than 70 mm Hg and transpul-

Table 35-1. Candidate Evaluation

General Data	Cardiopulmonary Data	Immunologic Data	Serologies
Complete history and physical	Electrocardiogram	Blood type	Hepatitis screen
Blood chemistries	Chest x-ray film	Histocompatibility locus antigen typing	Herpes simplex
Thyroid function tests	Right-sided heart catheterization	Panel reactive antibodies screen	Human immunodeficiency virus
Complete blood cell count, differential, platelet count	Echocardiogram		Cytomegalovirus
Coagulation studies	Pulmonary function testing		Toxoplasmosis
Urinalysis			Epstein-Barr virus
Stool for occult blood			Venereal Disease Research Laboratory
Lipid profile			
Creatinine clearance			
Dental consultation			
Skin test for tuberculosis			

Table 35-2. Candidate Exclusion Criteria

Pulmonary hypertension (despite treatment)
  PVR 3 to 5 Wood units (mm Hg/liter/min)
  PAS > 70 mm Hg
  Mean PAP – PCW > 15 to 20 mm Hg
Infection
Irreversible hepatic disease
Irreversible renal disease
Irreversible pulmonary disease
Recent pulmonary infarction
Age greater than 65 years
Diabetes mellitus with significant end-organ damage
Cerebrovascular disease
Peripheral vascular disease
Peptic ulcer disease, active bleeding
Diverticulitis, recent
Chronic active hepatitis
HIV positive
Recent malignancy
Unresolved psychiatric disease
Substance abuse

PVR, pulmonary vascular resistance; PAS, pulmonary artery systolic pressure; HIV, human immunodeficiency virus; PAP, pulmonary artery pressure; PCWP, pulmonary capillary wedge pressure.

monary gradients (mean pulmonary artery pressure minus mean pulmonary capillary wedge pressure) of greater than 15 to 20 mm Hg likewise portend a poor outcome. In selected patients with significant and only partially reversible pulmonary arterial hypertension at initial pretransplant assessment, prolonged therapy with vasodilators and/or positive inotropes or mechanical circulatory support could allow successful transplantation after acceptable reversal of their pulmonary hypertension (9).

Clearly, in the setting of irreversible renal, hepatic, or pulmonary disease, multiorgan transplantation can be considered and may be performed with acceptable mortality. Age limitations are, of course, arbitrary. Older individuals can undergo successful transplantation if they are carefully selected to avoid concomitant diseases (10). Similarly, patients with diabetes mellitus (even insulin-dependent) can undergo successful transplantation. However, significant end-organ damage will generally lessen the quality of life after transplantation.

Patients with symptomatic, untreatable cerebrovascular or peripheral vascular disease are usually poor candidates, as are patients with chronic active hepatitis and human immunodeficiency virus carriers. A history of recent malignancy will generally exclude a patient from consideration, whereas a remote, "cured" malignancy will not necessarily preclude transplant consideration.

Management of the Recipient While Waiting for Heart Transplantation

Close follow-up and frequent reevaluation are required before transplantation to ensure that compensated heart failure is at least maintained. Electrolytes and liver and kidney function must be monitored frequently. Potassium and magnesium preparations should be supplemented to maintain normal or high normal levels. Warfarin use is desirable (though not routinely indicated) in patients with a low (<20%) left ventricular ejection fraction and normal sinus rhythm. Patients with a prior history of thromboembolism, intracardiac thrombus, or atrial fibrillation should receive warfarin chronically to minimize the risk of systemic thromboembolization. If significant azotemia, refractory salt and water overload, persistent hypotension, or altered mental status develops, hospitalization is warranted. Presyncope or syncope should be promptly and thoroughly investigated.

Table 35-3. Responses of the New Cardiac Allograft Compared with Normal

Unchanged Inotropic and Chronotropic Effect	Diminished Inotropic or Chronotropic Effect	Diminished or Absent Atrioventricular Nodal Effect
Isoproterenol	Dopamine	Atropine
Dobutamine	Ephedrine	Edrophonium
Epinephrine	Metaraminol	Digoxin
Norepinephrine	Mephentermine	Quinidine

Signs or symptoms of low cardiac output necessitate escalating treatment, beginning with intravenous diuretics followed by intravenous inotropic agents, intraaortic balloon counterpulsation, and mechanical circulatory support, as needed. Needless to say, potential recipients who develop irreversible end-organ failure (other than heart) or whose likelihood of survival after transplantation is poor should be withdrawn from the waiting list and not undergo transplantation.

All patients waiting for heart transplantation are routinely evaluated on an ongoing basis. For patients with prolonged waiting times, repeat right-sided catheterization should be performed every 3 to 6 months to ensure the continued presence of acceptable pulmonary pressures, and repeat panel reactive antibody (PRA) assays are performed. Additionally, because recovery of left ventricular function or exercise tolerance can occur in some patients (11), routine reevaluation of left ventricular function and functional capacity is advised if symptoms of left-sided failure abate. Recovery of function may obviate or defer the need for transplantation.

When a suitable cardiac donor becomes available and immediately before transplantation, the following steps are taken: The immunosupressive protocol of choice is begun; prophylactic antibiotics are ordered; the medical history and current medical regimen are reviewed; anticoagulation is discontinued and reversed; chemistries, hematology, and coagulation studies are evaluated; blood is obtained for final antidonor antibody crossmatching; a chest x-ray is obtained; and the anticipated blood products necessary for surgery are ordered.

Immediate Posttransplantation Care

After surgery, the hemodynamic management of the newly transplanted cardiac allograft is carefully monitored (12). The newly transplanted heart is totally denervated, and usually transiently dysfunctional because of the preceding ischemic insult. Adequate preload (right atrial pressure of 10 to 15 mm Hg or left atrial pressure of 15 to 20 mm Hg) is often required to avoid hemodynamic deterioration from decreased diastolic compliance. Even when adequately preloaded, inotropic and chronotropic support are necessary to obtain and maintain adequate cardiac output. Isoproterenol (0.25 to 5.00 µg/min) is infused to maintain the heart rate at 110 to 120 beats per minute and enhance diastolic relaxation. Isoproterenol should be continued even if the heart appears to contract well. Because sinus node dysfunction and

atrioventricular (AV) block can occur, AV pacing may be required through surgically installed leads. Sinus node dysfunction (usually sinus bradycardia) can especially occur in patients previously treated with the antiarrhythmic agent amiodarone. Theophylline has also been reported to be effective in the treatment of postoperative sinus bradycardia (13).

The response of the denervated heart to medication differs from that of the innervated heart in several important respects (Table 35-3), and knowledge of these alterations is particularly important in the early posttransplantation period. When inotropic support in addition to that provided by isoproterenol is required, dobutamine (5.0 to 20.0 µg/kg/min), epinephrine (1.0 to 5.0 µg/min), and/or milrinone (0.2 to 0.75 µcg/kg/min) may be used. The full β-adrenergic agonist epinephrine is an excellent inotropic agent in the denervated, transplanted heart because there is no neuronal uptake system to prevent access to myocardial β-adrenergic receptors. Although dopamine can reverse moderate systemic vasodilation, as seen rarely with disruption of central aortic reflexes or OKT3 first-dose reactions, severe vasodilation responds well to the pure ∂-adrenergic agonist phenylephrine. Inotropic support is usually maintained for 2 to 5 days.

Noninfectious, Noncardiac Complications after Transplantation

The immunosupressive agents used after heart transplantation contribute to an array of problems, some of which are noninfectious and noncardiac in nature. These complications, although not totally preventable, can be mitigated to some extent and ameliorated in part. Among the most common and serious are hypertension, hypercholesterolemia, osteoporosis, and malignancy (5,14,15).

Hypertension

Instead of relying completely on medical treatment for hypertension, limitation of salt intake, maintenance of ideal body weight, and moderate exercise should be stressed. Even if these steps are taken, most (>80%) cardiac transplant recipients require treatment. Blood pressures consistently greater than 140/90 mm Hg require treatment. Monotherapy may be attempted with either an angiotensin-converting enzyme (ACE) inhibitor (e.g., captopril, enalapril, lisinopril) or a calcium channel blocker (e.g., diltiazem, nifedipine, verapamil, amlodipine). In conventional doses, these agents can be effective as monotherapy. Care must be taken with ACE inhibitors in some patients because of potentially serious hyperkalemia resulting from the combined effect of cyclosporine and ACE inhibition on the kidney.

Care must also be taken when using diltiazem or verapamil because they decrease the metabolism of cyclosporine and could possibly cause serious toxicity. On the other hand, diltiazem can be used carefully to lower cyclosporine requirement and attendant costs. The extended-release preparations of calcium channel blockers are well tolerated and effective. Pedal edema can occur with calcium blocker use, but this side effect may be attenuated by the addition of an ACE inhibitor or low-dose diuretics. When monotherapy is unsuccessful, the use of both an ACE inhibitor and calcium channel blocker often proves effective. Diuretics are sometimes effective but seldom as effective as monotherapy. Dehydration should be avoided because the transplanted heart is more preload-dependent than the innervated heart.

When hypertension is inadequately controlled despite maximally tolerated doses of calcium channel blockers and ACE inhibitors, then ∂-blockers, clonidine, β-blockers (e.g., metoprolol, atenolol, propranolol, carvedilol), or hydralazine may sometimes be used with some success. Infrequently, reduction of the cyclosporine dose or conversion to tacrolimus may be required.

Hyperlipidemia

Hyperlipidemia is common after cardiac transplantation and requires treatment in more than 50% of recipients (16). This is most likely caused by corticosteroid and cyclosporine use and preexisting hyperlipidemia. Adequate control is important since it has been shown to be a predisposing factor for allograft coronary disease and coronary events after heart transplantation (17). As with hypertension, hyperlipidemia should be treated with rational health maintenance measures such as limitation of cholesterol and other fat intake, maintenance of ideal body weight, and moderate exercise. Minimization of cortecosteroid dose or avoidance, when possible, is helpful (18). Optimal control of blood sugar in diabetics is also important. Serum cholesterol greater than 240 mg/dL or low-density lipoprotein (LDL) cholesterol greater than 160 mg/dL, despite dietary or other behavior modification, should be treated. In recipients with known allograft coronary artery disease, target lipid levels are significantly lower (serum cholesterol <200 mg/dL and LDL <100 mg/dL).

Gemfibrozil (in doses up to 600 mg twice daily) can be effective in some patients with mild-to-moderate hyperlipidemia, especially in the setting of hypertriglyceridemia. Moderate-to-severe hypercholesterolemia usually requires the use of a 3-hydroxy-3-methylglutaryl coenzyme A (HMG-CoA) reductase inhibitor (e.g., lovastatin, simvastatin, pravastatin, fluvastatin, atorvastatin). The combination of any of the above lipid-lowering agents with cyclosporine increases the risk of rhabdomyolysis. Periodic creatine kinase and liver function tests should be performed. Prudence should especially be exerted if more than one agent is used with cyclosporine. As per routine recommendations, lipid-lowering agents should be started at a low dose and then gradually up-titrated as needed and tolerated. Nicotinic acid, bile acid sequestrants (e.g., cholestyramine, colestipol), probucol, and fish oil (omega-3 free fatty acids) are infrequently used because of intolerance or significant interactions with immunosuppressive agents. Other clinical benefits have also been reported with the use of selected lipid-lowering agents such as lower incidence of allograft rejection and better long-term outcome (16). As such (and because it is such a common problem), it is not surprising that a growing number of transplant centers now routinely use those agents on all their patients after transplantation.

Osteoporosis

Osteoporosis is a serious problem that often affects the quality of life after transplantation. Its true incidence is likely underestimated because of the lack of routine patient screening with bone densitometry.

Patients with end-stage heart failure who are undergoing transplantation are already at high risk of skeletal complications resulting from prolonged inactivity and, in some cases, long-term use of intravenous heparin (19). This risk of bone loss is further increased with the use of corticosteroids following transplantation. Bone loss is rapid in the first 6 months after transplantation and continues at a slower rate thereafter, despite continued use of moderate doses of corticosteroids. Bone loss is mostly marked in the lumbar spine. Clinically, vertebral compression fractures and aseptic necrosis of the femoral head are the most common skeletal complications. Pretransplantation prophylaxis in high-risk patients should be considered. In men, a serum testosterone level should be measured to rule out deficiency. Generally, postmenopausal women should be given estrogen replacement. All high-risk patients and those with pretransplantation osteoporosis should receive calcium salts (such as calcium carbonate up to 1500 mg daily in divided doses) and calcitriol (beginning at 0.25 μg every other day) indefinitely. More recently, the addition of biphosphonates such as alendronate (10 mg daily) has been shown to be safe and to effectively increase bone density (20). Other useful measures to minimize osteoporosis and its complications include exercise (21) and maintenance of ideal body weight. Surgical interventions (such as joint replacement) are usually successful and should be performed as indicated.

Malignancy

Malignancy is a serious complication after organ transplantation. In most instances, tumors develop de novo. Less commonly, tumors may preexist in the recipient or, rarely, be transplanted from the donor at the time of surgery (15). The causes of cancer are not fully understood, but impaired immunity and oncogenic viruses are believed to play a major additive role. While characteristics of prostate, colon, breast, and cervical cancers seem to be similar to those in the general population, skin cancer is especially common and mandates routine, periodic screening. When compared with the renal transplant patient, the cardiac recipient was found in one study to have a twofold greater increase in the incidence of all neoplasms, which was attributed to more intense immunosuppression (22). Another malignancy that deserves special attention in the transplant recipient is posttransplant lymphoproliferative disease (PTLD), including "frank" lymphomas. The incidence of lymphoma in heart recipients increased over eightfold when long courses of OKT3 were added to standard, triple-therapy, immunosuppressive regimens (23). The Epstein-Barr virus (EBV), a lymphotropic virus that infects over 90% of the population by adulthood, is thought to be responsible for the development of PTLD in immunocompromised patients. While rare in general, the incidence of PTLD can be as high as 50% in EBV-seronegative recipients that receive an EBV-seropositive organ (24). Presentation can be localized and benign or fulminant and fatal. Treatment usually involves reduction of immunosuppression, administration of high-dose acyclovir, and chemotherapy as needed for widespread disease.

Standard recommendations for cancer screening such as prostate-specific antigen level, mammography, lower gastrointestinal endoscopy, Papanicolaou smear, etcetera, should be applied to transplant recipients, especially since the latency period of some cancers seems to be shorter.

Allograft Coronary Artery Disease

Allograft coronary artery disease remains a major determinant of survival following the first year after transplantation (5,25). The prevalence of angiographically detectable disease is in the range of 10% to 20% at 1 year, 25% to 45% at 3 years, and 50% to 60% at 5 years. Yearly screening coronary angiography is recommended because of the high prevalence of disease and, usually, the lack of anginal symptoms. An effective prophylactic regimen to prevent allograft coronary artery disease is not currently available. Although the impact of risk-factor modification in allograft coronary artery disease remain unproven, avoidance or minimization of known risk factors for native coronary artery disease is advisable. In severe cases, retransplantation might be considered, but outcome results of retransplantation are far inferior to primary transplantation. Coronary revascularization with bypass surgery or various interventional catheterization procedures may be palliative in some patients. The impact of a growing number of such interventions on graft/patient survival remains to be reviewed on a large scale.

Clinical Use of Some "Newer" Immunosuppressive Agents in Heart Transplantation

For obvious reasons, major advances in immunosuppression in heart transplantation have emanated mostly from experience gained with other (especially kidneys) solid organ transplants. Indeed, it was not until recently that large prospective trials with immunosuppressive agents/protocols were carried out in the heart-transplant-recipient population. A brief review of some of this clinical experience follows, while omitting to comment on "standard" immunosuppressive practices using azathioprine, corticosteroids, and cyclosporine. More basic and pharmacologic characteristics of some of these agents are reviewed elsewhere in this book.

Mycophenolate Mofetil

Mycophenolate mofetil (MMF) is a potent, selective inhibitor of inosine monophosphate dehydrogenase, a key enzyme in the de novo purine biosynthesis (and thus DNA synthesis), in activated human lymphocytes (26). Cells capable of invoking the salvage pathway for purine biosynthesis such as erythrocytes and neutrophils are less adversely affected than lymphocytes (27), thus theoretically giving MMF a relative, selectivity advantage. Early dose-ranging and refractory-rejection studies in human cardiac transplant recipients suggested that MMF was safe to use and at least as effective as azathioprine in standard, triple-therapy, immunosuppressive regimens (28–31).

Recently, results of a large multicenter trial were reported (32); 650 patients, undergoing their first cardiac transplantation, were randomized in a double-blind, active-controlled trial to receive MMF or azathioprine, in addition to cyclosporine and corticosteroids. Rejection and survival data were collected for 6 and 12 months. Because of a large withdrawal rate (11%) before drug administration, data analyses were performed on both enrolled and treated patients. Survival and rejection were similar in enrolled patients. In treated patients, a 45% reduction in mortality at 12 months was observed in those on MMF versus azathioprine. A significant reduction in the need for rejection treatment (65.7% vs 73.7%) was also noted. Fewer MMF patients tended to have ≥IHSLT grade 3A rejections ($P = .055$) or required treatment with monoclonal or polyclonal antibodies (15.2% vs 21.1%). Opportunistic infections, mostly herpes simplex, were more common in the MMF group (53.3% vs 43.6%). Allograft coronary data at 1 year were, for the most part, similar in both MMF- and azathioprine-treated patients. Of note were large withdrawal rates in both groups (~40%). The survival benefit persisted at 36 months (35% mortality reduction) in MMF-treated patients (33). Coronary angiography data at 3 years await release.

Given the results of the multicenter MMF trial, what is the role of MMF in cardiac transplantation? Should MMF be given routinely to patients after cardiac transplantation? Extrapolating the results of any randomized, controlled trial to all future patients is always suspect. One must consider whether the patients randomized into the trial are truly representative of "all" future patients. In this particular trial, the patients randomized seemed quite representative of most cardiac transplant recipients based on baseline demographic data and the fact that there were few exclusion criteria. According to the intent-to-treat analysis, there were no significant differences in outcome measures, which was possibly because of the large withdrawal rate. When analyzed based only on patients who received at least one dose of the study drugs, there were at least strong trends toward benefit in almost all outcome measures in the MMF group. These results are only valid if this subgroup maintains the "randomization" effect for preexisting bias. The demographic analysis of this subgroup supports this contention. While these results cannot be considered conclusive, they certainly suggest that MMF is at least as effective as, and very possibly more effective than, azathioprine after cardiac transplantation. Even if one accepts the assertion that MMF is better, one must be cognizant of the large difference in cost and the facts that 25% of the azathioprine patients never had any treated rejection episodes and 47% never had a biopsy grade of 3A or greater. Thus, treating all patients with MMF would have subjected this subgroup to the excess costs without any presumed benefit. Therefore, a reasonable approach to the use of MMF after cardiac transplantation might be to individually tailor therapy based on the risk of rejection and/or prompt conversion of patients from azathioprine to MMF with their first, early or significant, rejection episode.

Tacrolimus

Tacrolimus (FK506, Prograf) is a macrolide antibiotic with immunosuppressive properties similar to those of cyclosporine. Though structurally different, they both inhibit the T-cell-receptor–mediated signal transduction pathway. In animal models, tacrolimus was found to prevent rejection of various solid-organ transplants. In humans, early clinical experience was limited to the use of tacrolimus for the treatment of refractory rejection in live transplant recipients (34). Other larger trials in liver and kidney transplantation followed. In cardiac transplantation, tacrolimus safety and efficacy were demonstrated for both primary and rescue immunosuppressive therapy in nonrandomized and small, single-center trials (35–38). More recently, results of the European Tacrolimus Multicenter Heart Study Group and the Tacrolimus US Heart Transplant Multicenter Study Group were revealed (39,40). Both trials randomized patients to receive tacrolimus or cyclosporine in an open-label fashion. At 12 months, no significant difference was found in patient or allograft survival nor in incidence of rejection between the two groups. In the European study, a subgroup analysis showed that early antibody therapy was associated with a reduced incidence of acute allograft rejection. However, the benefit was seen in both tacrolimus- and cyclosporine-treated groups, and the use of antibody therapy was not determined by randomization. The incidence of side effects such as infection, renal dysfunction, and glucose intolerance was similar in both groups. The European study showed that patients treated with tacrolimus had a reduced requirement for antihypertensive therapy. This finding was mirrored in the US multicenter trial. In addition, serum cholesterol and the need for lipid-lowering agents were lower in tacrolimus-treated patients. Thus, tacrolimus-based immunosuppression appears both effective and safe for early rejection prophylaxis in cardiac transplant recipients, with the added benefit of less incidence of hypertension and hyperlipidemia. While not conclusive, the combination of tacrolimus with antibody therapy early in the posttransplant period might provide an added efficacy in the prevention of acute allograft rejection.

Microemulsion Cyclosporine (Neoral)

Neoral is a microemulsion preparation of cyclosporine with superior pharmacokinetic properties such as improved absorption and bioavailability (41). In a large, multicenter, randomized, double-blind study, the safety, tolerability, and vascular effects of Neoral were compared with those of Sandimmune in heart transplant patients (42,43). Three hundred and eighty patients were randomized in a double-blind fashion to receive either Neoral or Sandimmune along with azathioprine and corticosteroids. Induction therapy with monoclonal or polyclonal antibodies was allowed as indicted by preoperative renal function. Primary end points included patient and/or graft survival and the incidence and severity of acute rejection episodes. Various safety variables were also monitored. Patient demographics showed a slightly higher percentage of pretransplant, idiopathic, dilated cardiomyopathy in the Sandimmune arm ($P = .031$). At 12 months, patient/graft survival and the incidence of rejections with any ISHLT biopsy score were similar. There were significantly less rejections requiring antibody therapy and lower cyclosporine dosages needed in the Neoral group. In addition, less cytomegalovirus infections were seen in the Neoral arm, possibly related to the decreased need for supplemental steroids (NS) and antilymphocyte antibodies ($P = .002$). With the exception of a slightly higher incidence of headache and nausea/vomiting in the Neoral group, there was no difference in the spectrum and incidence of cyclosporine-related side effects between the two groups. Quantitative coronary angiography, intravascular ultrasound, and echocardiographic data await review and release.

Photopheresis

Photopheresis is an immunomodulation technique during which white blood cells from a person are exposed to a photoactive compound and ultraviolet A light and then reinfused. Early experience in heart transplantation was limited to very few patients. Nonetheless, photopheresis was found to decrease levels of non–donor-specific anti-HLA antibodies and possibly the incidence of rejection (44), to reduce levels of panel-reactive antibodies early after transplantation, and to reduce coronary artery intimal thickness 1 and 2 years after transplantation (45). Furthermore, photopheresis was found to have moderate success in treating hemodynamically stable rejections and was associated with less infections when compared with high-dose corticosteroids (46). Recently, results of a small, multicenter, prospective trial were reported (47). Sixty patients were randomized to receive standard, triple, immunosuppressive therapy versus standard, triple therapy and prophylactic photopheresis. The primary end point of the study was the number and frequency of acute rejection episodes, and secondary end points included the incidence of clinically treated infections and survival without the need for retransplantation. Those end points were monitored for 6 months as part of the study, and then safety and survival follow-up was continued for an additional 6 months. At 6 months, the mean number of rejections per patient was less in the photopheresis group ($P = .04$). Fewer patients in the photopheresis group had two or more rejections. There was no significant difference in the time to a first rejection, the incidence of hemodynamically unstable rejections, or survival at 6 and 12 months between the two groups. The incidence of clinically relevant infections was similar, although cytomegalovirus DNA was detected significantly less in the photopheresis group ($P = .04$).

Other Immunosuppressive Agents

Another immunosuppressive agent that is currently being tested on a large scale in heart transplantation is a derivative of rapamycin designated as SDZ RAD.

Recently, the Food and Drug Administration approved a generic formulation of cyclosporine, SangCyA with bioequivalence to cyclosporine, for use in heart transplant recipients.

Outcomes

One-year and three-year survivals in the postcyclosporine era exceed 80% and 75%, respectively (48). Among the survivors, quality of life is excellent in approximately 50% to 60%. In 30% to 40% of transplanted patients, the quality of life is good but not excellent. In these patients, some aspect, usually a side effect of the medications, makes life less than excellent. This commonly involves nonspecific symptoms (e.g., fatigue or listlessness) or corticosteroid-related side effects (e.g., obesity, cushinoid habitus). Approximately 10% of survivors have side effects that cause excessive morbidity, making the quality of life poor. Generally, those in this latter category are older patients or those with musculoskeletal abnormalities. Clearly, quality of life for post-transplantation patients is not perfect (49). However, cardiac transplantation remains the treatment of choice for selected patients with refractory, end-stage heart failure.

References

1. Evans RW. Organ transplantation activity in the United States. In: Evans RW, Manninen DL, Dong FB, eds. The National Cooperative Transplantation Study: final report. Seattle: Battelle-Seattle Research Center, 1991.
2. Renlund DG, Bristow MR, Lee HR, O'Connell JB. Medical aspects of cardiac transplantation. J Cardiothoracic Anesth 1988;2:500–512.
3. Mudge GH, Goldstein S, Addonizio LJ, et al. Twenty-fourth Bethesda Conference: cardiac transplantation; Task Force 3: recipient guideline/prioritization. J Am Coll Cardiol 1993;22:21–31.
4. Francis GS. Determinants of prognosis in patients with heart failure. J Heart Lung Transplant 1994;13:S113–S116.
5. Miller LW, Schlant RC, Kobashigawa J, et al. Twenty-fourth Bethesda Conference: cardiac transplantation; Task Force 5: complications. J Am Coll Cardiol 1993;22:41–54.
6. Hastillo A, Hess ML. Selection of patients for cardiac transplantation. In: Thompson ME, ed. Cardiac transplantation. Philadelphia: FA Davis, 1990:107–120.
7. Kirklin JK, Naftel DC, Kirklin JW, et al. Pulmonary vascular resistance and the risk of heart transplantation. J Heart Transplant 1988;7:331–335.
8. Murali S, Kormos RL, Uretsky BF, et al. Preoperative pulmonary hemodynamics and early mortality after orthotopic cardiac transplantation: the Pittsburgh experience. Am Heart J 1993;126:896–904.
9. Farhoud H, Kfoury A, Renlund D, Taylor D. "Fixed" pulmonary hypertension in patients with end-stage heart failure considered for heart transplantation: how fixed is it? Circulation 1996;94(suppl 2):I-478. Abstract.
10. Renlund DG, Gilbert EM, O'Connell JB, et al. Age-associated decline in cardiac allograft rejection. Am J Med 1987;83:391–398.
11. Stevenson LW, Steimle AE, Fonarow G, et al. Improvement in exercise capacity of candidates awaiting heart transplantation. J Am Coll Cardiol 1995;25:163–170.
12. Young JB, Winters WL, Bourge R, Uretsky BF. Twenty-fourth Bethesda Conference: cardiac transplantation; Task Force 4: function of the heart transplant recipient. J Am Coll Cardiol 1993;22:31–41.
13. Bertolet BD, Eagle DA, Conti JB, et al. Bradycardia after heart transplantation: reversal with theophylline. J Am Coll Cardiol 1996;28:396–398.
14. Sambrook PN, Kelly PJ, Keogh AM, et al. Bone loss after heart transplantation: a prospective study. J Heart Lung Transplant 1994;13:116–121.
15. Penn I. Malignant neoplasia in the immunocompromised patient. In: The transplantation and replacement of thoracic organs. Kluwer Academic, 111–117.
16. Kobashigawa JA, Katznelson S, Laks H, et al. Effect of pravastatin on outcomes after cardiac transplantation. N Engl J Med 1995;333:621–627.
17. De Lorgeril M, Boissonat P, Mamelle N, et al. Platelet aggregation and HDL cholesterol are predictive of acute coronary events in heart transplant recipients. Circulation 1994;89:2590–2594.
18. Becker DM, Chamberlain B, Pearson TA, et al. Cumulative corticosteroids exposure and serum lipids in heart transplant recipients. Am J Med 1988;85:632–638.
19. Stein B, Takizawa M, Katz I, et al. Salmon calcitonin prevents cyclosporine A–induced high-turnover bone loss. Endocrinology 1991;299:92.
20. Van Cleemput J, Daenen W, Geusens P, et al. Prevention of bone loss in cardiac transplant recipients. A comparison of biphosphonates and vitamin D. Transplantation 1996;61:1495–1499.
21. Braith R, Mills R, Welsch M, et al. Resistance exercise training restores bone mineral density in heart transplant recipients. J Am Coll Cardiol 1996;28:1471–1477.
22. Lanza RP, Cooper DKC, Cassidy MJC, Barnard CN. Malignancy following cardiac transplantation. JAMA 1993;249:1746.
23. Swinnen LJ, Costanzo-Nordin MR, Fisher SG, et al. Increased incidence of lymphoproliferative disorder after immunosuppression with the monoclonal antibody OKT3 in cardiac transplant recipients. N Engl J Med 1990;323:1723–1728.
24. Walker RC, Paya CV, Marshall WF, et al. Pretransplantation seronegative Epstein-Barr virus status is the primary risk factor for posttransplantation lymphoproliferative disorder in adult heart, lung, and other solid organ transplantation. J Heart Lung Transplant 1995;14:214–221.
25. Schroeder JS, Gao S-Z, Hunt SA, Stinson EB. Accelerated graft coronary artery disease: diagnosis and prevention. J Heart Lung Transplant 1992;11:S258–S266.

26. Allison AC, Eugi EM. Immunosuppressive and other effects of mycophenolic acid and an ester prodrug, mycophenolate mofetil. Immunol Rev 1993;136:5.
27. Allison AC, Hovi T, Watts RWE, Webster ADB. The role of de novo purine synthesis lymphocyte transformation. Ciba Found Symp 1997;48:207.
28. Ensley RD, Bristow MR, Olsen SL, et al. The use of mycophenolate mofetil (RS-61443) in human heart transplant recipients. Transplantation 1993;56:75.
29. Kobashigawa JA, Renlund DG, Olsen SL, et al. Initial results of RS-61443 for refractory cardiac rejection. J Am Coll Cardiol 1992;19:203A. Abstract.
30. Kirklin JK, Deierhoi M, Naftel DC, et al. Treatment of recurrent cardiac rejection with RS-61443: initial clinical experience. J Heart Lung Transplant 1992;11:223. Abstract.
31. Taylor DO, Ensley RD, Olsen SL, et al. Mycophenolate mofetil (RS-61443): preclinical, clinical, and three year experience in heart transplantation. J Heart Lung Transplant 1994;13:571–582.
32. Kobashigawa JA, Miller LW, Renlund DG, et al. A randomized active-controlled trial of mycophenolate mofetil in heart transplant recipients. Transplantation 1998;66:507–515.
33. Keogh A, Bourge A, Costanzo M, et al. Three year results of the double-blind randomized multicenter trial of mycophenolate mofetil in heart transplant patients. J Heart Lung Transplant 1999;18:53. Abstract.
34. Fung JJ, Starzl TE. FK 506 in solid organ transplantation. Transplant Proc 1994;26:3017–3020.
35. Armitage JM, Kormos RL, Morita S, et al. Clinical trial of FK506 immunosuppression in adult cardiac transplantation. Ann Thorac Surg 1992;54:205–211.
36. Pham SM, Kormos RL, Hattler BG, et al. A prospective trial of tacrolimus (FK506) in clinical heart transplantation: intermediate-term results. J Thorac Cardiovasc Surg 1996;111:764–772.
37. Rinaldi M, Pellegrini C, Martinelli L, et al. FK506 effectiveness in reducing acute rejection after heart transplantation: a prospective randomized study. J Heart Lung Transplant 1997;16:1001–1010.
38. Meiser BM, Uberfuhr P, Fuchs A, et al. Single-center randomized trial comparing tacrolimus (FK506) and cyclosporine in the prevention of acute myocardial rejection. J Heart Lung Transplant 1998;17:782–788.
39. Reichart B, Meiser B, Vigano M, et al. European Tacrolimus Multicenter Heart Study Group. European multicenter tacrolimus (FK506) heart pilot study: one-year results. J Heart Lung Transplant 1998;17:775–781.
40. Taylor DO, Barr ML, Radovancevic B, et al. Decreased hypercholestrolemia and hypertension in heart transplant recipients receiving tacrolimus: a randomized, multicenter, cyclosporine-controlled trial. J Heart Lung Transplant 1999;18:336–345.
41. Mueller EA, Kovarik JM, van Bree JB, et al. Pharmacokinetics and tolerability of a microemulsion formulation of cyclosporine in renal allograft recipients—a concentration-controlled comparison with the commercial formulation. Transplantation 1994;57:1178–1182.
42. Eisen HJ, Hobbs RE, Davis SF, et al. Safety, tolerability and efficacy of cyclosporine microemulsion in heart transplant recipients: a randomized, multicenter, double-blind comparison with the oil-based formulations of cyclosporine—results at six months after transplantation. Transplantation 1999;68:663–671.
43. Eisen JH, Mueller EA, Turkin D, et al. The OLN351 Study Group. Multicenter, double-blind, randomized study of Neoral vs Sandimmune in heart transplantation: one year results. J Heart Lung Transplant 1999;18:93. Abstract.
44. Rose EA, Barr ML, Xu H, et al. Photochemotherapy in human heart transplant recipients at high risk for fatal rejection. J Heart Lung Transplant 1992;11:746–750.
45. Barr ML, McLaughlin SM, Murphy MP, et al. Prophylactic photopheresis and effect on graft atherosclerosis in cardiac transplantation. Transplant Proc 1995;27:1993–1994.
46. Costanzo-Nordin MR, Hubbell EA, O'Sullivan EJ, et al. Photopheresis versus corticosteroids in the therapy of heart transplant rejection: preliminary clinical report. Circulation 1992;86(suppl 2):II-242–II-250.
47. Barr ML, Meiser BM, Eisen HJ, et al. Photopheresis for the prevention of rejection in cardiac transplantation. N Engl J Med 1998;339:1744–1751.
48. Hosenpud JD, Bennett LE, Keck BM, et al. The registry of the International Society for Heart and Lung Transplantation: fifteenth official report—1998. J Heart Lung Transplant 1998;17:656–668.
49. Walden JA, Stevenson LW, Darcup K, et al. Extended comparison of quality of life between stable heart failure patients and heart transplant recipients. J Heart Lung Transplant 1994;13:1109–1118.

Chapter 36

Lung Transplantation

Steven J. Mentzer
Scott J. Swanson

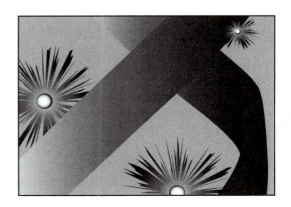

Overview

History

The first patient with end-stage lung disease treated by orthotopic human lung transplantation lived 8 days (1). The transplanted lung did not provide adequate gas exchange, and the patient remained ventilator dependent. Between the years of 1963 and 1980, approximately 40 additional lung transplant procedures were performed. The longest survival period was 10 months. The early failures in lung transplantation were mostly attributed to primary graft nonfunction, bronchial dehiscence, acute lung rejection, and pneumonia (2,3).

In 1983 the Toronto group succeeded in achieving long-term success with a single-lung transplant in a patient with idiopathic pulmonary fibrosis (IPF) (4–6). The problem of bronchial dehiscence was addressed by wrapping an omental pedicle around the bronchial anastomosis. The transplanted lung provided excellent gas exchange immediately after implantation. Because of the early functioning of the lung, prolonged mechanical ventilation and the associated infectious problems were avoided. The immunosuppressive regimen included cyclosporin A, azathioprine, and antilymphocyte globulin.

Results

Since the initial successful lung transplant, there has been a marked increase in the number of lung transplants performed worldwide. The number of single-lung transplants rose from one in 1984 to more than 700 in 1994 (Fig. 36-1) (7). Similarly, there was an increase in the total number of double-lung transplants in the late 1980s and early 1990s. The number of both single and double lung transplants plateaued in the late 1990s (see Fig. 36-1). In contrast, the frequency of heart-lung transplantation decreased in the late 1980s. An important reason for this decrease was the growing percentage of patients waiting for lung transplantation. Selective transplantation of the lung and the heart has increased the total number of potential transplant recipients. In addition, the timely transplantation of patients with primary lung disease has prevented the development of secondary cardiac failure.

The survival results of single-lung transplantation have demonstrated continuing improvement during the past decade. As the surgical technique and postoperative care have improved, perioperative mortality is less than 10% in most centers. The 1-year survival rate after single-lung transplantation is approximately 70% with 2-year survival rate greater than 60% (Fig. 36-2) (7). Double-lung transplantation has comparable survival rates.

Similar to other transplanted organs, a small percentage of grafts continue to be lost 2 and 3 years after transplantation. Because patient survival is dependent on graft function, survival also continues to decline. Infection is the most common cause of death within the first 2 years after transplantation (Fig. 36-3). Most of the late allograft losses are the result of chronic rejection manifested as obliterative bronchiolitis (OB). The gradual destruction of the small airways also leads to an increased susceptibility to infection.

Recipient Selection

Patients with a variety of pulmonary diseases are candidates for either single-lung or double-lung transplantation (Fig. 36-4). The most common indication for lung transplantation is emphysema, including chronic obstructive pulmonary disease (COPD) and alpha-1 antitrypsin deficiency. Other diseases that are common indications for lung transplantation include idiopathic pulmonary fibrosis (IPF), cystic fibrosis, and pulmonary hypertension.

Criteria

The selection criteria for lung transplantation continue to evolve as transplant risk factors are clarified (Table 36-1). In most transplant centers, a life expectancy of approximately 18 to 24 months is required for being placed on the transplant waiting list. An accurate assessment of life expectancy, however, can be difficult to establish in many diseases (8). The life expectancy of patients with cystic fibrosis, for example, can be unexpectedly shortened by severe infection (9). Similarly, patients with primary pulmonary hypertension (PPH) can experience sudden death or a rapidly progressive deterioration of right ventricular function.

Although the median recipient age range is 40 to 49 years (Fig. 36-5), most centers use 55 years as an age guideline for pretransplant evaluation. Although absolute age limits are unusual, most patients over 55 years have other systemic organ dysfunction that precludes transplantation. In appropriately selected patients over 50 years of age, lung transplant survival is comparable with that of younger recipients; their causes of death,

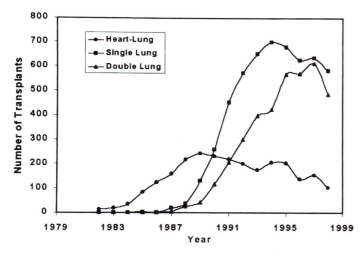

Figure 36-1. Number of lung transplants performed by year: single lung (*square*), double lung (*triangle*), and heart-lung (*circle*). (Source: International Society for Heart and Lung Transplantation Registry Report 1998.)

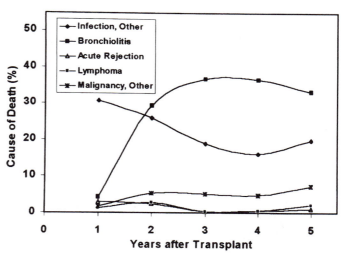

Figure 36-3. Causes of death of lung transplant recipients from 1 to 4 years after transplantation. (Source: International Society for Heart and Lung Transplantation Registry Report 1998.)

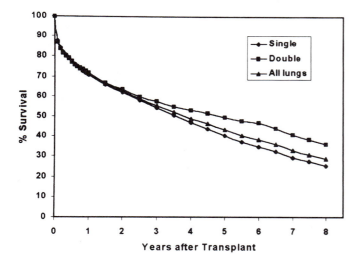

Figure 36-2. Survival of patients undergoing single (*diamond*) and double (*square*) transplantation. (Source: International Society for Heart and Lung Transplantation Registry Report 1998.)

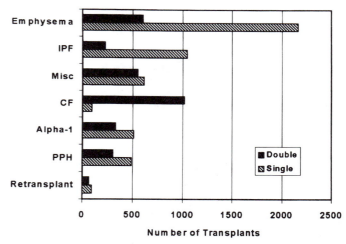

Figure 36-4. Indications for single (*diagonal*) and double (*solid*) lung transplantation. (Source: International Society for Heart and Lung Transplantation Registry Report 1998.)

however, are different from those of younger patients, suggesting a decrease in immunologic responsiveness with age (10). Despite the comparable survival, the restricted donor supply and the longer, average, waiting time on the transplant list have made 55 years a generally accepted age guideline.

The ideal lung transplant recipient has isolated pulmonary dysfunction (11). With a risk of transient graft dysfunction in the early postoperative period, cardiac reserve is important to maintain oxygen delivery to the peripheral tissues. With marginal oxygenation, prolonged tachycardia may be required to maintain tissue oxygen supply. Because of these demands, the pretransplant evaluation attempts to exclude coronary artery disease or right ventricular dysfunction. Patients with coronary artery disease sufficiently severe to limit oxygen delivery at near-anaerobic exercise levels are not appropriate for lung transplantation. Because of the technical limitations of noninvasive, cardiac-function measures, the assessment of right ventricular function can be problematic. In most centers, the clinical signs of right heart failure such as hepatomegaly or peripheral edema are contraindications to lung transplantation.

Table 36-1. Recipient Selection Guidelines

Irreversible pulmonary vascular disease
Isolated pulmonary disease; no other significant organ
  dysfunction
Substantial limitation in quality of life
Limited life expectancy
Participation in ambulatory rehabilitation
Acceptable nutritional status
Acceptable psychosocial profile and emotional support systems

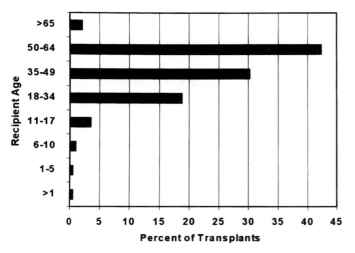

Figure 36-5. Age of lung transplant recipients. (Source: International Society for Heart and Lung Transplantation Registry Report 1998.)

Normal kidney function is particularly important for patients undergoing lung transplantation. In addition to the importance of maintaining fluid homeostasis, the kidneys must withstand several nephrotoxic insults in the posttransplant course. Most patients are maintained in negative fluid balance for the first several days after transplantation because of the transplanted lung's tendency to develop a capillary leak syndrome and increased lung water immediately after transplantation. The renal toxicity of commonly used drugs such as cyclosporin A and amphotericin B is amplified by the low circulating blood volumes. The transient hypoxemia, which is common after lung transplantation, also predisposes recipients to acute renal dysfunction.

Most lung transplant centers require potential recipients to actively participate in pulmonary rehabilitation programs (12). End-stage lung disease is associated with significant social and emotional disability. Continuous oxygen therapy, as well as the severe functional limitations of breathlessness, presents a major restriction in interactions with family and friends. Whereas pulmonary rehabilitation programs do not appear to improve gas exchange indices or spirometric measurements, they do contribute to improvements in muscle conditioning and social adaptation (13–15). Furthermore, the complete benefits of physical

rehabilitation and adequate muscle conditioning may not be realized until after the lung transplant when lung function is no longer limiting.

The psychologically adapted, medically compliant, and well-informed patient is critical to successful lung transplantation (16). An involved patient plays a particularly important role in maintaining the graft in the outpatient setting (17). The accurate interpretation of symptoms of breathlessness can be difficult even for experienced clinicians. Acute infection may not be associated with purulent sputum or fever. Similarly, acute rejection may only be manifested by a subtle change in lung compliance or drop in oxygen saturation. Patients who conscientiously monitor their lung function will detect these problems at an early and treatable stage.

Nutritional issues are important in recipient selection. Candidates for lung transplantation frequently have respiratory cachexia. In these patients the increased work of breathing can result in chronic, negative, nitrogen balance. Other patients may have central obesity and peripheral wasting from chronic steroid therapy and deconditioning. Both of these nutritional issues are associated with increased postoperative complications and should be addressed during the pretransplant evaluation process (8). Potential transplant recipients should maintain their weight within 20% of ideal body weight (8,18).

There are few absolute surgical contraindications to lung transplantation (Table 36-2). In our experience, the severely calcified hilum, with or without pulmonary artery aneurysms, is a contraindication to transplantation. The calcific hilum may be associated with life-threatening hemorrhage if the need for cardiopulmonary bypass (CPB) should arise. Mediastinal irradiation is a contraindication to lung transplantation primarily because of the adverse effects of radiation on bronchial healing. Mediastinal irradiation also implies previous malignancy. A history of malignancy is a contraindication to lung transplantation except in extraordinary circumstances. Finally, extensive pleural scarring has been associated with life-threatening hemorrhage in patients requiring CPB (19,20).

Single-Lung Transplants

Single-lung transplantation has been performed for a variety of benign lung diseases. The most common indication for single-lung transplant is emphysema (49%) from either chronic obstructive

Table 36-2. Contraindications for Lung Transplantation

Active extrapulmonary infection
Significant extrapulmonary organ dysfunction
Previous malignancy (rare exceptions)
Current cigarette smoking
Poor nutritional status
Poor rehabilitation potential
Significant psychosocial dysfunction (e.g., substance abuse,
  medical noncompliance)
Extensive pleural disease

pulmonary disease (COPD) (36%) or alpha-1-antitrypsin deficiency (13%). Fibrotic lung diseases, including IPF, are the next most common indication for transplantation (24%), followed by PPH (11%) (7).

The first successful lung transplant was performed in a patient with IPF (4). IPF was chosen because the disease is associated with progressive scarring of the lung and parallel decreases in both ventilation and perfusion. The relatively predictable course of the disease permits the listing of patients for transplant when the contralateral native lung function is sufficient to maintain the patient during the transplant procedure without CPB. The progression of the disease posttransplantation results in less blood flow to the native lung and more blood flow to the transplanted lung. This gradual shunt of pulmonary blood flow to the transplanted lung provides an opportunity to gradually adapt to the lung transplant.

In contrast to fibrotic lung disease, patients with emphysema have hyperexpanded and hypercompliant lungs (21,22). The physiology of emphysema has led to the theoretical concern that the enlarging native lung will compromise the ventilation of the transplanted lung (23). Although these theoretical concerns have not prevented successful, single-lung transplantation for emphysema, there are situations in which the hypercompliant native lung becomes a clinical problem. Immediately after lung transplantation, acute ventilation-perfusion mismatching in the transplanted lung may occur, requiring mechanical ventilation. Positive airway pressures can cause hyperexpansion of the emphysematous native lung with the consequence of compromised cardiac output and systemic oxygen delivery. In circumstances in which the transplanted lung requires high airway pressures, it is possible to differentially ventilate the native and transplanted lungs using a double-lumen endotracheal tube.

Chronic changes can also occur in the emphysematous native lung. Several years after transplantation, progression of emphysema in the native lung can eventually compromise ventilation of the transplanted lung. The hyperexpansion of the native lung appears to be exacerbated by a decrease in compliance of the transplanted lung caused by either chronic rejection or acute infections. These changes in the native lung have been used as a rationale for double-lung transplantation in emphysema (24).

The management of PPH is challenging both before and after transplantation (25,26). Patients diagnosed with PPH have a median survival of 2.8 years. The life expectancy for any individual patient, however, can be unpredictable (27). Patients may develop rapidly progressive right ventricular dysfunction or a sudden death syndrome (28,29). Careful monitoring of hemodynamic variables and physical limitations is important for the timely selection of patients for transplantation.

In the immediate posttransplant period, patients with PPH may develop pulmonary hypertensive crises. Although the etiology of these hypertensive episodes is unclear, the acute increase in pulmonary artery pressures can be sustained by the work-hypertrophied right ventricle. Because of the high resistance in the native hypertensive lung, most of the pulmonary perfusion is through the transplanted lung. Thus, any ventilation-perfusion

abnormalities in the transplanted lung are manifested by systemic hypoxemia (30). These observations have led the Washington University group to recommend sedation for a minimum of several days after lung transplantation (31).

Another solution to the problem of episodic pulmonary hypertension is double-lung transplantation. The presence of two transplanted lungs appears to avoid the hypertensive crises that occur after single-lung transplantation. Alternatively, the hyperreactive vasoconstriction in the transplanted lung may be addressed pharmacologically. The use of nitric oxide to improve ventilation-perfusion matching in the acute transplant setting has shown promising results. Organic nitrates, a precursor to nitric oxide, can also be given to improve the balance between pulmonary vasoconstrictors and vasodilators (32). Despite these advances, the management of PPH patients remains challenging.

Double-Lung Transplants

The dominant indication for double transplantation is septic lung disease (Table 36-3). Cystic fibrosis is the most common indication for double-lung transplantation (see Fig. 36-4). Fewer than 15% of the patients have undergone transplantation for bronchiectasis. Although patients have received double-lung transplants for emphysema and IPF, the potential for improved postoperative lung function is not an indication for double-lung transplantation. Exercise testing has shown no significant functional difference between patients receiving single-lung or double-lung transplants (33).

Lung transplantation for septic lung disease requires that both lungs be removed. Theoretically, there is the possibility that transplanting one lung would risk cross-contamination of the transplanted lung, as well as progression of the preexisting infection in the native lung. Alternatively, septic lung disease could be treated by the transplantation of one lung followed by removal of the contralateral lung. This approach has been used both experimentally and in isolated clinical cases. A practical problem is ensuring that the patient is sufficiently stable to permit resec-

Table 36-3. Recommended Procedures by Disease

Procedure	Disease state
Single-lung transplant	Fibrotic lung disease, emphysema, alpha-1 antitrypsin deficiency, primary pulmonary hypertension, Eisenmenger's complex with reparable heart anomaly
Double-lung transplant	Cystic fibrosis, bronchiectasis, rare patients with single-lung transplant indications
Heart-lung transplant	Eisenmenger's complex with irreparable heart defect, pulmonary hypertension with cor pulmonale, end-stage lung disease with secondary heart failure

tion of a septic native lung. In addition to removing functioning lung tissue, the pneumonectomy space poses its own risk of postoperative infection.

In recipients with cystic fibrosis, the indications for lung transplantation have continued to evolve (34–37). Many patients with cystic fibrosis have pancreatic failure and a gut malabsorption syndrome. Because of these problems, nutrition can be an important clinical issue both before and after transplantation. Pancreatic failure usually requires exogenous pancreatic enzymes and may require postoperative insulin. The poor absorption of oral medications, including cyclosporin A, is an important consideration in posttransplant immunosuppression.

Patients with cystic fibrosis are considered poor candidates for lung transplantation if they have significant hepatic or renal disease (38). Another relative contraindication for transplantation in cystic fibrosis is the presence of panresistant *Pseudomonas*. Although *Pseudomonas cepacia* has been implicated in poor outcomes, a variety of *Pseudomonas* species have been associated with multiple drug resistance and intractable postoperative pneumonias (37,39).

Despite the organ dysfunction and colonization with multiresistant bacteria, cystic fibrosis patients have a number of advantages for lung transplantation. The cystic fibrosis patients tend to be young patients with good cardiac and renal function. Perhaps most importantly, cystic fibrosis patients are highly motivated patients with experience in respiratory care and physical rehabilitation (40).

The other major septic lung disease, bronchiectasis, comprises only a small percentage of patients undergoing double-lung transplantation. Patients with bronchiectasis tend to be older with the comorbidity of chronic disability. The chronicity of pulmonary dysfunction can lead to pulmonary hypertension and an inflamed pleural space. The chronicity of their disease and the prolonged use of antibiotics are commonly associated with resistant *Pseudomonas* and colonization with *Aspergillus*. Both their chronic disability and fungal colonization are relative contraindications to transplantation.

Heart-Lung Transplants

The number of heart-lung transplants performed in the United States has gradually declined since 1988. The major practical limitation of heart-lung transplantation has been donor availability. Potential donors must have both heart and lungs suitable for transplantation. Less than 15% of heart donors also have lungs suitable for transplantation. Size matching of the heart-lung block can also complicate donor suitability.

The heart-lung donors are generally reserved for patients with combined heart and lung disease. As single-lung transplantation has been popularized, the number of patients with primary pulmonary disease and secondary cardiac failure has decreased. Single-lung transplantation associated with repair of congenital defects has also been reported (41). A remaining indication for heart-lung transplantation is the development of Eisenmenger's complex (see Table 36-3).

Donor Organs

The limited donor supply affects all organs, but it is a particular problem for lung transplantation. Only 5% to 15% of all organ donors have lung function suitable for transplantation. The low percentage of suitable donors reflects the premorbid condition of the lungs, the mechanism of death, and prolonged attempts of life support prior to the declaration of brain death. The most common mechanism of death leading to lung donation in the United States is a gunshot wound. The second most frequent cause of donor death is a neurologic event, including isolated head trauma or spontaneous intracranial hemorrhage. The criteria for acceptable donor lungs are generally conservative and reflect the importance of early graft function. With the discouraging results from extracorporeal life support, early acceptable graft function appears to be essential for recipient survival. In addition to selecting suitable organs, the potential lung donor must be carefully managed prior to donation (42). Finally, the donor lungs must be procured with a technique that promotes early graft function.

Donor Criteria

The premorbid condition of the lungs becomes an important issue with donors of advancing age, smoking histories, or occupational exposure (Table 36-4). As the average age for the donor population increases, most transplant centers have attempted to increase the age of acceptable donors. This strategy is limited by the predictable decline in lung function with age, and most centers prefer donors less than 60 years old. In addition, the donor should not have a physician's diagnosis of respiratory disease or a smoking history of more than 20 to 30 pack years. Other medical contraindications to lung donation include any history of extracranial malignancy.

The mechanism of donor death is frequently associated with pulmonary complications. Aspiration pneumonia is a common consequence of a loss of consciousness in an unintubated patient. Motor vehicle trauma is often associated with severe chest trauma that may result in traumatic or neurogenic pulmonary edema. Finally, life-ending penetrating trauma frequently involves injury to intrathoracic organs.

Many potential donors have been exposed to prolonged resuscitation attempts. Intensive care unit ventilatory support of more than 1 week is associated with a high incidence of bacter-

Table 36-4. Donor Selection Guidelines

Age <65 years
No severe infection
Chest radiograph without infectious infiltrate
Minimal purulent secretions
Negative HIV serology
Match for hepatitis B and C
Lung size match within 10%
ABO compatibility

ial or fungal pneumonitides. Established pneumonias can rapidly progress with posttransplant immunosuppression. Most centers have avoided transplanting lungs with established pneumonias.

The functional assessment of the potential donor lung is primarily based on gas exchange indices. Arterial blood gases obtained on optimal ventilatory settings and a 100% FIO_2 should have a PO_2 of 250 to 300 torr. The chest radiograph should show no significant infiltrates or evidence of pneumonia. The most common finding on chest radiograph is basilar atelectasis caused by hypoventilation. These radiographic findings typically resolve with increased tidal volumes (10cc/kg) and positive end-expiratory airway pressures (10cm H_2O).

Lung donors are matched for ABO compatibility. HLA matching is not routinely performed because of the time constraints for lung donation and the practical limitations of a small donor supply. Cytomegalovirus (CMV) matching has been attempted in some centers; however, the limited donor supply has made CMV matching largely impractical as well. All potential lung donors have negative serologies for HIV. Hepatitis B– or C–positive donor organs are usually reserved for seropositive recipients.

Donor-recipient size matching is an important consideration in lung transplantation (43). Lungs that are too large for the recipient are insufficiently expanded resulting in alveolar hypoventilation and intrapulmonary shunting. Undersized lungs may oxygenate adequately, but may also suffer from suboptimal ventilation. Although the mechanical requirements for optimal ventilation are not yet defined, the size of the donor lung should be within 10% of the size of the recipient lung. An adequate size match is more important in double-lung transplants than in single-lung transplants. In addition to compromised ventilation, oversized lungs can result in cardiac compression.

Lung Preservation

The delicate alveolar-capillary membrane network in the lung is extraordinarily sensitive to mechanical, chemical, and ischemic injury (44). Damage to the donor lung during the ischemic period and immediately after transplantation most likely reflects a variety of injuries. These injury mechanisms appear to include leukocyte activation, complement activation, oxygen-free radical formation, and the generation of inflammatory mediators and arachidonic acid metabolites (44). The current procurement techniques have resulted in a significant drop in the percentage of recipients with early graft failure.

The central goal in lung procurement is to preserve gas-exchange function after ischemic storage for 4 to 6 hours. The original technique of lung procurement used topical cooling of the lung after absorption atelectasis (5). The most widely used technique today is single-flush perfusion of the lung followed by static cold storage. With some variation, the technique of lung procurement involves the flush of the donor lungs with 1000cc to 2000cc of cold Euro-Collins solution. Prior to the flush, donors are generally pretreated with prostaglandins (prostaglandin E_1 or prostacyclin), corticosteroids, and calcium channel blockers.

During the flush, the lungs are inflated close to total lung capacity to ensure vascular recruitment. The lungs are oxygenated with 100% FIO_2 in most centers to provide an increase in alveolar oxygen concentration during transport in cold storage. After the lung flush, the airway is stapled closed to preserve lung inflation during transportation.

A range of transport times has been associated with successful lung transplantation. In most cases an ex vivo transport time of less than 6 hours is desirable. Despite careful preservation and short transport times, there continues to be a risk of a "reimplantation response." The reimplantation response is a capillary leak syndrome that is associated with acute graft dysfunction (45). This capillary leak syndrome is thought to be an ischemia and reperfusion event; however, the mechanism is likely to be multifactorial. The syndrome is characterized radiographically by patchy infiltrates in the transplanted lung (Fig. 36-6). Infiltrates attributable to the reimplantation response should resolve within the first 3 to 5 days. If the infiltrates do not resolve within this period, alternative explanations for the radiographic abnormality should be considered (46).

Surgical Procedure

Intraoperative Management

The intraoperative challenge in lung transplantation is the support of gas exchange and oxygen delivery during the transplant procedure. Patients with end-stage lung disease can become unstable with the simple induction of general anesthesia. This challenge is amplified during the extraction and implantation of the replacement lung. In most cases the patient's cardiac function is adequate, and oxygen delivery depends on adequate gas exchange. The impairment of gas exchange reflects the underlying disease process, but can include both hypercarbia and hypoxemia.

The anesthetic management of a lung transplant recipient is tailored to the primary disease process. For example, patients with septic lung disease often have thick and tenacious airway secretions (47). These secretions can result in relative airway obstruction and alveolar hypoventilation. Mucolytics such as the recently developed DNAase have proved to be effective in liquefying airway secretions and preventing airway obstruction.

In contrast, lung transplant recipients with emphysema generally do not have anatomic airway obstruction, but rather extraordinary sensitivity to positive pressure ventilation. The poor elastic recoil of the emphysematous lung results in hyperinflation and "gas trapping." The stacking of sequential positive pressure breaths can result in increased mean intrathoracic pressure and life-threatening hypotension.

Cardiopulmonary bypass (CPB) may be required in 10% to 30% of adults while undergoing lung transplantation. Because most lung transplant recipients have adequate cardiac reserve, CPB is used primarily for the support of gas exchange. CPB

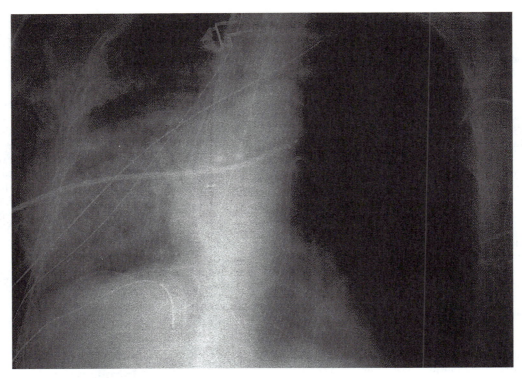

Figure 36-6. Chest radiograph of a patient 3 days after single-lung transplantation demonstrating a severe reimplantation response.

can be associated with a significant increase in lung water and impaired ventilation-perfusion matching. Postoperative bleeding has also been associated with the heparinization required for conventional CPB. Patients with pulmonary hypertension such as those with PPH require early CPB to support oxygen delivery during both the extraction and the implantation of the transplanted lung. Similarly, all patients receiving heart-lung transplants require prolonged CPB support during the transplant procedure.

In single-lung transplant recipients, the decision to transplant the left or right lung is usually dictated by the availability of donor organs. On occasion, the potential recipient will be listed with the organ procurement organization for only the left or right lung because of technical considerations. If all the surgical variables are equal, most transplant centers would prefer to transplant the most abnormal lung. This maximizes the opportunity to avoid CPB during extraction and implantation. A functioning native lung can also be useful postoperatively should the transplanted lung develop a reimplantation response or transient posttransplant dysfunction.

Surgical Technique

The surgical technique of lung transplantation involves the anastomosis of the airway, pulmonary artery, left atrium, and pulmonary veins (48) (Fig. 36-7). The anastomosis can be performed using a variety of approaches and surgical techniques. For maximal exposure during implantation, the bronchial anastomosis is usually constructed first followed by the pulmonary artery and atrial anastomoses.

Prior to the first successful transplant in 1983, bronchial dehiscence was a major cause of early transplant mortality (Fig. 36-8). The reasons for bronchial dehiscence appear to be related to the bronchial blood supply (49,50). In the usual circumstance, the bronchial blood flow is antegrade through systemic bronchial arteries. These bronchial arteries are disrupted in both single- and sequential single-lung transplantation. Because there is no antegrade blood flow, the blood supply to the mainstem bronchus depends on retrograde perfusion from the pulmonary circulation. This anatomic arrangement results in an ischemic watershed at the level of the mainstem bronchial anastomosis.

The first successful solution to this problem was proposed by the Toronto lung transplant group. Cooper et al used abdominal omentum to buttress the anastomosis and facilitate bronchial healing (5). The omental pedicle was brought through a substernal tunnel and wrapped around the bronchial anastomosis. The omental pedicle prevented dehiscence in the event of anastomotic separation and largely prevented the life-threatening septic complications (51). Experimental studies also suggested that the omental pedicle facilitated revascularization of the bronchial anastomosis.

More recently, a successful approach to bronchial anastomosis has relied on shortening the bronchial anastomosis and minimizing the extent of the ischemic watershed (51). The

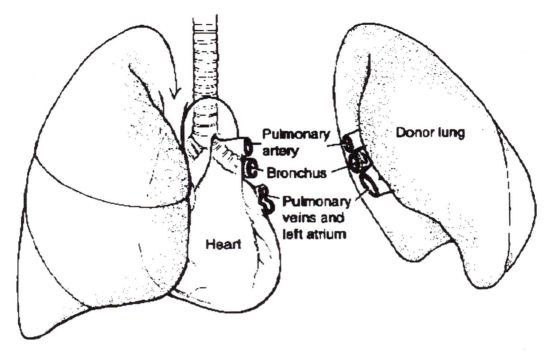

Figure 36-7. Schematic of the surgical anastomoses performed during single-lung transplantation.

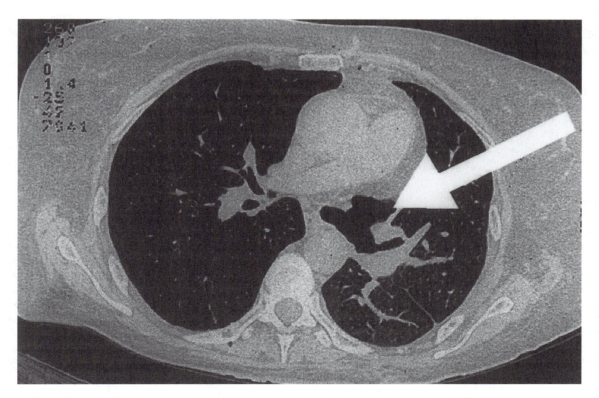

Figure 36-8. Chest CT scan of a bronchial dehiscence 3 weeks after single-lung transplantation. The arrow indicates the extraluminal air at the site of dehiscence.

bronchus is further protected by "telescoping" of the donor bronchus one to two cartilaginous rings inside the recipient bronchus (52). Although a limited ischemic watershed still exists, the ischemic donor airway is reinforced by the surrounding recipient bronchus. This "telescoping" technique generally permits healing of the bronchus without dehiscence or stricture (52).

An alternative to the telescoping anastomosis is the use of bronchial artery revascularization (53). Bronchial artery revascularization uses a variety of techniques to reestablish airway blood supply through the small bronchial arteries. Reestablishing bronchial blood flow appears to decrease the incidence of airway dehiscence. The limitation of these procedures is the additional surgical time that is required. The theoretical possibility that bronchial artery revascularization decreases the incidence of chronic rejection has not been demonstrated in early studies.

The original double-lung transplant technique was developed by Patterson and colleagues of the Toronto group (54). This technique involved CPB during the implantation of a double-lung block. The original en bloc implantation was performed using a single tracheal, arterial, and atrial anastomosis. The early failures of this procedure were related to the dehiscence of the single tracheal anastomosis. The dehiscence of the tracheal anastomosis suggested that the retrograde blood flow from the lung parenchyma was insufficient to maintain viability of the distal trachea. In contrast to heart-lung transplantation, there were no heart collaterals to augment airway circulation.

The problems with tracheal healing have led to the development of sequential lung transplantation for most patients requiring two lungs (55). This technique involves bilateral airway, pulmonary artery, and atrial anastomoses. An advantage of the sequential single-lung transplantation technique is that it can be performed without CPB and systemic heparinization. This advantage has been particularly useful in patients with extensive pleural disease who were previously considered inoperable because of the risk of life-threatening hemorrhage associated with CPB (19,20).

Rejection

In the past, the failure of the graft to support gas exchange was frequently ascribed to immunologic mechanisms. As experience with lung transplantation grows, early graft dysfunction has become less common. The reasons for the improvement in early graft function are probably related to improved graft preservation rather than changes in immunosuppression. Because the lung inflammation, regardless of the etiology, results in increased capillary permeability and an impairment in gas exchange, the potential role of hyperacute rejection in graft non-function is difficult to evaluate. In contrast, acute rejection usually does not occur within 2 weeks of transplantation. As more aggressive early immunosuppression has evolved, the first episode of acute rejection is typically seen more than 3 weeks after transplantation.

Clinical Manifestation

The clinical presentation of acute lung rejection is similar to that of other solid-organ transplants. Patients typically manifest a mild fever and leukocytosis. Patients may complain of breathlessness related to measurable ventilation-perfusion mismatching and systemic hypoxemia. Acute rejection can also cause a decrease in lung compliance. Increased stiffness of the lung causes increased work of breathing. The clinical consequence is an increase in respiratory rate and the use of accessory muscles. Spirometry demonstrates a drop in expiratory flow rates such as FEV_1 and FVC (56). The radiographic presentation of acute rejection can be variable. In most cases, lung rejection can be seen as a patchy infiltrate (57).

The primary differential diagnosis of acute lung rejection is lung infection. Early after the lung transplant, donor-related bacterial infections are common. Donor aspiration is a frequent cause of graft infection in the early posttransplantation period. Infections with cytomegalovirus, caused by either endogenous or donor-derived virus, may stimulate a rejection episode. Fungal infections are also common in patients exposed to prolonged courses of broad-spectrum antibiotics. The incidence of cytomegalovirus and fungal infections increases 4 to 6 weeks after transplantation (58).

Diagnosis

The diagnosis of acute rejection is typically based on the findings from fiberoptic bronchoscopy (11). The presence of sputum in the airways can confirm the diagnosis of a bacterial pneumonia. Bronchoalveolar lavage has also been used to confirm the presence of neutrophils and bacterial organisms (59). In patients with aspiration pneumonitis, lavage cultures will only reveal oral flora. Because it can be difficult to exclude oral contamination from aspiration of mouth organisms, we prefer to use protected-brush cultures of the distal airway. The protective sheath on the culture brush prevents contamination by oral flora in the mouth. Protected-brush specimens demonstrating oral flora in the distal airways are diagnostic of aspiration.

In the absence of purulent sputum, tissue biopsies are usually required to differentiate viral infection from acute rejection (60). Transbronchial biopsies can be performed using the fiberoptic bronchoscope (59). In most patients, these biopsies can be performed as an outpatient. The average transbronchial biopsy can yield a lung tissue specimen consisting of 300 or more alveoli. These biopsies usually contain both the small vessels and airways associated with acute rejection. Although the number of biopsies required to document acute rejection is varied, experimental studies have shown that five transbronchial biopsies in the involved lobes yield a sensitivity to mild rejection in excess of 90% (60).

The earliest pathologic abnormality in acute lung rejection is the infiltration of small vessels by mononuclear cells. These infiltrates are often sparse and require adequate tissue for diagnosis. In some cases, mononuclear infiltrates will also be seen in the small airways. With increasing severity, the infiltrates become more cellular. The inflammation associated with acute rejection may extend into the alveolar walls and airspaces. In the most severe cases, the small-airway inflammation progresses to alveolar damage with diffuse tissue necrosis.

This progression of acute rejection has been incorporated into a working formulation for the classification of pulmonary rejection (61). The main features of the grading system include a measure of severity, as well as anatomic localization. Grade 1 shows infrequent infiltrates that may or may not be associated with bronchiolar inflammation. Grade 2 inflammation demonstrates endotheleitis, as well as endothelial inflammation with accompanying lymphocytic bronchiolitis. Grade 3 shows extension of the infiltrate into the small airways and alveoli. Grade 4 is diffuse inflammation that may be associated with parenchymal necrosis. A potentially important pathologic observation is that lymphocytic bronchiolitis can be seen in the absence of perivascular mononuclear infiltrates. It is likely that these early airway inflammatory cells represent the precursor to the development of small-airway scarring and obliterative bronchiolitis (62).

Immunosuppression

The standard immunosuppression of lung transplant recipients is similar to that for other solid organs. The unique aspect of lung transplantation is the aggressive level of immunosuppression. The significant morbidity associated with acute rejection in the first several weeks after transplant has led to aggressive therapy with cyclosporin A, steroids, and azathioprine. In addition, the prominence of lung-associated lymphoid tissue and the role of the lung as an immunologic tissue have led to the theoretic argument that aggressive early immunosuppression may facilitate lung mononuclear cell turnover and graft adaptation (62).

Also unique to lung transplantation is the toxicity of conventional immunosuppression. In the early transplant period, recipients are maintained in negative fluid balance because of the susceptibility of the graft to increase lung water. The diminished extracellular fluid volume in lung transplant recipients potentiates renal toxicity of cyclosporin A. Other problems with immunosuppression are related to the primary disease process. For example, the transition of intravenous to oral cyclosporin A can be unpredictable in patients with the gut malabsorption syndrome associated with cystic fibrosis. The high incidence of cytomegalovirus infections and the increased use of prophylactic ganciclovir have led to an increased incidence of bone marrow toxicity and a more cautious use of azathioprine in lung transplant recipients.

Another unique aspect of lung transplant immunosuppression is the toxicity of antilymphocyte immunoglobulin such as OKT3 or antithymocyte globulin. The use of OKT3, in particular, has been associated with an increased incidence of pulmonary edema (63). A reasonable speculation is that the known ability of anti-CD3 antibodies such as OKT3 to stimulate lymphocyte cytokines can produce a capillary leak syndrome in the lung. This observation is unpredictable, and in many cases the OKT3 can be given with minimal side effects and no pulmonary edema.

Infection

Bacterial

Early after lung implantation the risk of infection is related to donor-derived organisms. Cultures are routinely obtained of the donor airways prior to organ procurement. These cultures are usually repeated at the time of the operation. In our center, we routinely use a second-generation cephalosporin until those culture results are obtained. If the donor lungs have had prolonged mechanical ventilation, broader antibiotic coverage may be required.

The most frequent source of recipient-derived infection in the early transplant period is aspiration. The use of protected-brush specimens has documented the significant incidence of oral flora in the distal airways. This observation is consistent with other work in patients who have undergone pneumonectomies for other indications. Although the mechanism of aspiration is unclear, the changes in intrathoracic pressure after pneumonectomy or transplantation may contribute to an increased incidence of clinically significant aspiration pneumonia.

In patients with cystic fibrosis, chronic colonization of their sinuses with both fungus and *Pseudomonas* has been associated with complications after transplantation. In high-risk patients, prophylactic antibiotics are routinely used for 1 to 2 weeks after lung transplantation. Drainage of the nasal sinuses is performed prior to lung transplantation to decrease "seeding" of the transplanted airway. Nasal irrigation and inhaled aminoglycosides have also been used to effectively decrease colonization of resistant *Pseudomonas*.

Viral

Cytomegalovirus (CMV) is an increasingly troublesome infection in lung transplant recipients. The typical CMV infection presents 3 to 9 weeks after lung transplantation. Although CMV infection is rare in seronegative recipients receiving a seronegative donor lung, pretransplant CMV matching has become impractical given the limited donor supply and constraints on size matching. Patients with a CMV serologic mismatch develop a clinical CMV infection in 20% to 90% of lung transplants (58,64). Thus, CMV is second only to bacterial pneumonias as the most common cause of lung infection.

The clinical presentation of CMV is varied (65). Some patients may manifest fever, cough, hypoxemia, and a chest radiograph infiltrate. These pulmonary symptoms are suggestive of rejection and require bronchoscopy to exclude this possibility. In other lung transplant recipients, cytomegalovirus may result in other organ dysfunction such as bone marrow suppression and hepatic dysfunction.

The diagnosis of CMV can be made by bronchoscopic lavage culture or by tissue biopsy (66). Although bronchoscopy can usually obtain culture evidence of CMV infection, the delay in culture results can be impractical in a patient with increasing hypoxemia. Alternatively, transbronchial biopsy can provide

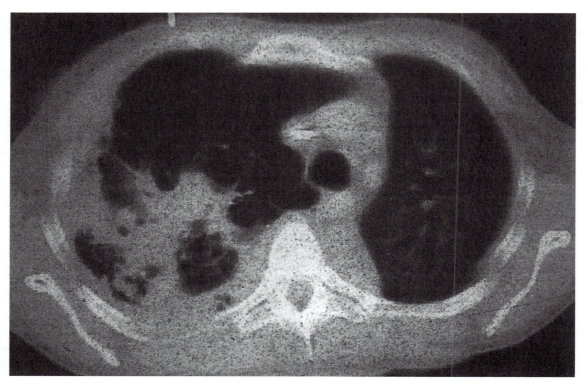

Figure 36-9. Chest radiograph of a patient after left, single-lung transplantation with a lobar aspergillus pneumonia in the native lung.

sufficient tissue for an accurate cytologic diagnosis (67). The typical cytopathic changes with characteristic CMV inclusion bodies are considered diagnostic in the lung transplant recipient.

Patients with clinical CMV disease are generally treated with extended courses of antiviral therapy. Because of the potential life-threatening risk of outpatient CMV pneumonitides, CMV mismatch may require ganciclovir therapy for 6 to 12 months after transplantation (68). The prolonged course of antiviral therapy permits a tapering of the immunosuppression and allows time for adequate pulmonary rehabilitation.

Fungal

Fungal infections also present significant morbidity and mortality after lung transplantation (69,70). Fungal infections can develop from weeks to years after the lung transplant. The most common organism identified is *Candida albicans. Candida* can be cultured from the airway in most donors who have had prolonged mechanical ventilation. Although the demonstration of invasive *Candida* may be difficult, the presence of *Candida* in lung cultures is sufficient to encourage preemptive therapy with amphotericin B.

Similarly, the presence of *Aspergillus* in the airways may represent colonization and not invasive disease. Because of the current lack of effective antifungal therapy in lung transplant recipients, patients with positive *Aspergillus* cultures require aggressive preemptive therapy. In most cases, antifungal therapy with amphotericin B should be instituted before the documentation of fungal disease. In patients with chronic obstructive pulmonary disease, fungal infections of the native lung may also occur (Fig. 36-9).

Obliterative Bronchiolitis

Solid-organ transplantation is associated with characteristic manifestations of chronic rejection. In the lung, chronic rejection is found in 20% to 30% of long-term survivors. The histologic finding and clinical symptoms are referred to as obliterative bronchiolitis (OB). Although OB can be associated with environmental exposure and autoimmune diseases, the most devastating clinical consequence of OB is observed in lung transplant recipients. Obliterative bronchiolitis is a major cause of death in patients 2 or more years after transplantation (see Fig. 36-3).

Obliterative bronchiolitis is an inflammatory process that primarily affects small conducting airways of the lung. The pathologic finding in obliterative bronchiolitis is the submucosal scarring of respiratory bronchioles. The airway scarring may be variable, and it may be associated with a destruction of the smooth muscle. In active bronchiolitis the scarring can be associated with the mononuclear infiltrates. Obliterative bronchiolitis has been associated with a variety of etiologies, including chronic lung transplant rejection. Although the immunologic triggers may be varied, the final common pathway is an inflammation that results in damage and fibrosis of the bronchiolar epithelium.

In some patients without obliterative bronchiolitis, the scarring of the small airways may spare a significant amount of interstitium. The spirometry and radiographic presentations of these patients may mimic chronic obstructive pulmonary disease. Alternatively, the scarring of the small airways may lead to a mixed restrictive and obstructive ventilatory defect (71). These patients may present with a clinical picture similar to that of patients with other fibrotic lung diseases (72).

The clinical presentation of bronchiolitis is rarely evident within the first year after transplantation. As has been suggested in other organ transplants, obliterative bronchiolitis is associated with a high incidence of acute rejection episodes (62,73,74) unless these episodes are treated aggressively. The first symptom of OB is usually an increase in dyspnea. Spirometry typically demonstrates a fall in the midportion of the expiratory flow. This obstructive defect is typically progressive over the course of months. This process ultimately results in a decrease in all expiratory flow indices.

The chest radiograph in a patient with OB can demonstrate peribronchial and interstitial infiltrates. More commonly, the chest radiograph is relatively normal. The chest radiograph may show a decrease in vascular markings and apparent hyperinflation; however, the radiograph belies the clinical course of progressive respiratory insufficiency.

The functional consequences of OB are a decrease in small airway flow and impaired mucociliary clearance. This results in an increased incidence of pneumonia. The coexistence of OB and chronic infection can lead to diagnostic uncertainty regarding the underlying pathophysiology of patients with progressive pulmonary failure.

The diagnosis of obliterative bronchiolitis is controversial. For many clinicians, the progressive decline in pulmonary function in the face of a characteristic chest radiograph is diagnostic of OB. Others have relied on transbronchial biopsy or open-lung biopsy to document the presence of bronchiolar inflammation and scarring (74). Localized lymphocyte bronchitis/bronchiolitis may respond to increased immunosuppression (73), but established scarring of the conducting airways is a poor prognostic sign.

The treatment of bronchiolitis obliterans continues to be unrewarding. Similar to other solid organs developing chronic rejection, there has been little success with an increase in immunosuppression. The predisposition of the lung to infection further complicates aggressive immunosuppressive therapy. A variety of aggressive therapies, including total lymphoid irradiation, OKT3, increased steroids, and antilymphocyte globulin, have been used with little demonstrable benefit.

References

1. Raju S, Heath BJ, Warren ET, Hardy JD. Single- and double-lung transplantation. Problems and possible solutions. Ann Surg 1990;211:681–691.
2. Dark J, Corris PA. The current state of lung transplantation. Thorax 1989;44:689–692.
3. Kaiser LR, Cooper JD. The current status of lung transplantation. Adv Surg 1992;25:259–307.
4. Toronto Lung Transplant Group. Unilateral lung transplantation for pulmonary fibrosis. N Engl J Med 1986;314:1140–1145.
5. Cooper JD, Pearson FG, Patterson GA, et al. Technique of successful lung transplantation in humans. J Thorac Cardiovasc Surg 1987;93:173–181.
6. Grossman RF, Frost A, Zamel N, et al. The Toronto Lung Transplant Group. Results of single-lung transplantation for bilateral pulmonary fibrosis. N Engl J Med 1990;322:727–733.
7. Annual ISHLT Heart/Lung Registry Data Report. International Society for Heart and Lung Transplantation, 1999.
8. Onofrio JM, Emory WB. Selection of patients for lung transplantation. Med Clin North Am 1992;76:1207–1219.
9. Kerem E, Reisman J, Corey M, et al. Prediction of mortality in patients with cystic fibrosis. N Engl J Med 1992;326:1187–1191.
10. Snell GI, De Hoyos A, Winton T, Maurer JR. Lung transplantation in patients over the age of 50. Transplantation 1993;55:562–566.
11. Heritier F, Madden B, Hodson ME, Yacoub M. Lung allograft transplantation: indications, preoperative assessment and postoperative management. Eur Respir J 1992;5:1262–1278.
12. McGregor CG, Daly RC, Peters SG, et al. Evolving strategies in lung transplantation for emphysema. Ann Thorac Surg 1994;57:1513–1520.
13. Curtis JR, Deyo RA, Hudson LD. Pulmonary rehabilitation in chronic respiratory insufficiency. VII. Health-related quality of life among patients with chronic obstructive pulmonary disease. Thorax 1994;49:162–170.
14. Olopade CO, Beck KC, Viggiano RW, Staats BA. Exercise limitation and pulmonary rehabilitation in chronic obstructive pulmonary disease. Mayo Clin Proc 1992;67:144–157.
15. Niederman MS, Clemente PH, Fein AM, et al. Benefits of a multidisciplinary pulmonary rehabilitation program. Improvements are independent of lung function [see comments]. Chest 1991;99:798–804.
16. Bright MJ, Craven JL, Kelly PJ. Toronto Lung Transplant Group. Assessment and management of psychosocial stress in lung transplant candidates. Health Soc Work 1990;15:125–132.
17. Craven JL, Bright J, Dear CL. Psychiatric, psychosocial, and rehabilitative aspects of lung transplantation. Clin Chest Med 1990;11:247–257.
18. Morrison DL, Maurer JR, Grossman RF. Preoperative assessment for lung transplantation. Clin Chest Med 1990;11:207–215.
19. Noirclerc MJ, Metras D, Vaillant A, et al. Bilateral bronchial anastomosis in double lung and heart-lung transplantations. Eur J Cardiothorac Surg 1990;4:314–317.
20. Pasque MK, Cooper JD, Kaiser LR, et al. Improved technique for bilateral lung transplantation: rationale and initial clinical experience. Ann Thorac Surg 1990;49:785–791.
21. Mal H, Andreassian B, Pariente R. Single-lung transplantation in hyperinflated patients. Chest 1990;97:110S–111S.
22. Kaiser LR, Cooper JD, Trulock EP, et al. The Washington University Lung Transplant Group. The evolution of single

lung transplantation for emphysema. J Thorac Cardiovasc Surg 1991;102:333–339.

23. Trulock EP, Egan TM, Kouchoukos NT, et al. Washington University Lung Transplant Group. Single lung transplantation for severe chronic obstructive pulmonary disease. Chest 1989;96:738–742.

24. Emery RW, Graif JL, Hale K, et al. Treatment of end-stage chronic obstructive pulmonary disease with double lung transplantation. Chest 1991;99:533–537.

25. Pasque MK, Kaiser LR, Dresler CM, et al. Single lung transplantation for pulmonary hypertension. Technical aspects and immediate hemodynamic results. J Thorac Cardiovasc Surg 1992;103:475–481.

26. Levine SM, Gibbons WJ, Bryan CL, et al. Single lung transplantation for primary pulmonary hypertension. Chest 1990;98:1107–1115.

27. Glanville AR, Burke CM, Theodore J, Robin ED. Primary pulmonary hypertension. Length of survival in patients referred for heart-lung transplantation. Chest 1987;91: 675–681.

28. Dinh Xuan AT, Higenbottam TW, Scott JP, Wallwork J. Primary pulmonary hypertension: diagnosis, medical and surgical treatment. Respir Med 1990;84:189–197.

29. Palevsky HI, Fishman AP. The management of primary pulmonary hypertension. JAMA 1991;265:1014–1020.

30. Levine SM, Jenkinson SG, Bryan CL, et al. Ventilation-perfusion inequalities during graft rejection in patients undergoing single lung transplantation for primary pulmonary hypertension. Chest 1992;101:401–405.

31. Pasque MK, Trulock EP, Kaiser LR, Cooper JD. Single-lung transplantation for pulmonary hypertension. Three-month hemodynamic follow-up. Circulation 1991;84:2275–2279.

32. Mentzer SJ, Reilly JJ, DeCamp M, et al. Potential mechanism of vasomotor dysregulation after lung transplantation for primary pulmonary hypertension. J Heart Lung Transplant 1995;14(2):387–393.

33. Miyoshi S, Trulock EP, Schaefers HJ, et al. Cardiopulmonary exercise testing after single and double lung transplantation. Chest 1990;97:1130–1136.

34. Egan TM. Lung transplantation in cystic fibrosis. Semin Respir Infect 1992;7:227–239.

35. Shennib H, Adoumie R, Noirclerc M. Current status of lung transplantation for cystic fibrosis. Arch Intern Med 1992;152:1585–1588.

36. Starnes VA, Lewiston N, Theodore J, et al. Cystic fibrosis: target population for lung transplantation in North America in the 1990s. J Thorac Cardiovasc Surg 1992;103:1008–1014.

37. Snell GI, De Hoyos A, Krajden M, et al. *Pseudomonas cepacia* in lung transplant recipients with cystic fibrosis. Chest 1993;103:466–471.

38. Shennib H, Noirclerc M, Ernst P, et al. Double-lung transplantation for cystic fibrosis. Ann Thorac Surg 1992;54: 27–32.

39. Flume PA, Egan TM, Paradowski LJ, et al. Infectious complications of lung transplantation: impact of cystic fibrosis. Am J Respir Crit Care Med 1994;149:1601–1607.

40. Bartholomew LK, Parcel GS, Swank PR, Czyzewski DI. Measuring self-efficacy expectations for the self-management of cystic fibrosis. Chest 1993;103:1524–1530.

41. Fremes SE, Patterson GA, Williams WG, et al. Toronto Lung Transplant Group. Single lung transplantation and closure of patent ductus arteriosus for Eisenmenger's syndrome. J Thorac Cardiovasc Surg 1990;100:1–5.

42. Griffith BP, Zenati M. The pulmonary donor. Clin Chest Med 1990;11:217–226.

43. Lloyd KS, Barnard PA, Holland VA, et al. Lung transplantation for end-stage pulmonary disease. Effects of donor lung size on pulmonary function. Chest 1990;97:110S.

44. Novick RJ, Gehman KE, Ali IS, Lee J. Lung preservation: the importance of endothelial and alveolar type II cell integrity. Ann Thorac Surg 1996;62:302–314.

45. Corris PA, Odom NJ, Jackson G, McGregor CG. Reimplantation injury after lung transplantation in a rat model. J Heart Transplant 1987;6:234–237.

46. Herman SJ, Rappaport DC, Weisbrod GL, et al. Single-lung transplantation: imaging features. Radiology 1989;170:89–93.

47. Soberman MS, Kraenzler EJ, Licina M, et al. Airway management during bilateral sequential lung transplantation for cystic fibrosis. Ann Thorac Surg 1994;58:892–894.

48. Egan TM, Cooper JD. Surgical aspects of single lung transplantation. Clin Chest Med 1990;11:195–205.

49. Schafers HJ, Haydock DA, Cooper JD. The prevalence and management of bronchial anastomotic complications in lung transplantation. J Thorac Cardiovasc Surg 1991;101:1044–1052.

50. Patterson GA, Todd TR, Cooper JD, et al. Toronto Lung Transplant Group. Airway complications after double lung transplantation. J Thorac Cardiovasc Surg 1990;99: 14–20.

51. Miller JD, DeHoyos A. An evaluation of the role of omentopexy and of early perioperative corticosteroid administration in clinical lung transplantation. J Thorac Cardiovasc Surg 1993;105:247–252.

52. Calhoon JH, Grover FL, Gibbons WJ, et al. Single lung transplantation. Alternative indications and technique. J Thorac Cardiovasc Surg 1991;101:816–824.

53. Schreinemakers HH, Weder W, Miyoshi S, et al. Direct revascularization of bronchial arteries for lung transplantation: an anatomical study. Ann Thorac Surg 1990;49:44–53.

54. Patterson GA. Double lung transplantation. Clin Chest Med 1990;11:227–233.

55. Kaiser LR, Pasque MK, Trulock EP, et al. Bilateral sequential lung transplantation: the procedure of choice for double-lung replacement. Ann Thorac Surg 1991;52:438–445.

56. Becker FS, Martinez FJ, Brunsting LA, et al. Limitations of spirometry in detecting rejection after single-lung transplantation. Am J Respir Crit Care Med 1994;150:159–166.

57. Herman SJ. Radiologic assessment after lung transplantation. Radiol Clin North Am 1994;32:663–678.

58. Wreghitt TG, Hakim M, Gray JJ, et al. A detailed study of cytomegalovirus infections in the first 160 heart and heart/lung transplant recipients at Papworth Hospital, Cambridge, England. Transplant Proc 1987;19:2495–2496.

59. Shennib H, Nguyen D. Bronchoalveolar lavage in lung transplantation. Ann Thorac Surg 1991;51:335–340.

60. Tazelaar HD, Nilsson FN, Rinaldi M, et al. The sensitivity of transbronchial biopsy for the diagnosis of acute lung rejection. J Thorac Cardiovasc Surg 1993;105:674–678.

61. Randhawa P, Yousem SA. The pathology of lung transplantation. Pathol Annu 1992;27:247–279.

62. Yousem SA, Dauber JA, Keenan R, et al. Does histologic acute rejection in lung allografts predict the development of bronchiolitis obliterans? Transplantation 1991;52:306–309.
63. Shennib H, Massard G, Reynaud M, Noirclerc M. Efficacy of OKT3 therapy for acute rejection in isolated lung transplantation. J Heart Lung Transplant 1994;13:514–519.
64. Ettinger NA, Bailey TC, Trulock EP, et al. Cytomegalovirus infection and pneumonitis: impact after isolated lung transplantation. Am Rev Respir Dis 1993;147:1017–1023.
65. Duncan AJ, Dummer JS, Paradis IL, et al. Cytomegalovirus infection and survival in lung transplant recipients. J Heart Lung Transplant 1991;10:638–644.
66. Paradis IL, Duncan SR, Dauber JH, et al. Distinguishing between infection, rejection, and the adult respiratory distress syndrome after human lung transplantation. J Heart Lung Transplant 1992;11:S232–S236.
67. Nakhleh RE, Bolman RM, Henke CA, Hertz MI. Lung transplant pathology. A comparative study of pulmonary acute rejection and cytomegaloviral infection. Am J Surg Pathol 1991;15:1197–1201.
68. Merigan TC, Renlund DG, Keay S, et al. A controlled trial of ganciclovir to prevent cytomegalovirus disease after heart transplantation. N Engl J Med 1992;326:1182–1186.
69. Dauber JH, Paradis IL, Dummer JS. Infectious complications in pulmonary allograft recipients. Clin Chest Med 1990;11: 291–308.
70. Laghi F, Yeldandi V, McCabe M, Garrity ER Jr. Common infections complicating lung transplantation. N Engl J Med 1993;90:317–319.
71. King TE Jr. Bronchiolitis obliterans. Lung 1989;167:69–93.
72. Morrish WF, Herman SJ, Weisbrod GL, Chamberlain DW. The Toronto Lung Transplant Group. Bronchiolitis obliterans after lung transplantation: findings at chest radiography and high-resolution CT. Radiology 1991;179:487–490.
73. Yousem SA. Lymphocytic bronchitis/bronchiolitis in lung allograft recipients. Am J Surg Pathol 1993;17:491–496.
74. Paradis I, Yousem S, Griffith B. Airway obstruction and bronchiolitis obliterans after lung transplantation. Clin Chest Med 1993;14:751–763.

Chapter 37

Hemopoietic Stem Cell Transplantation

Voravit Ratanatharathorn
James L. M. Ferrara

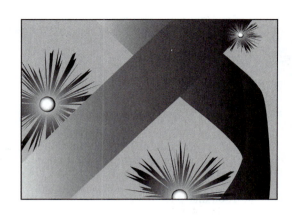

The landmark experiment of Lorenz in 1950 demonstrated the capability of marrow injection to rescue mice from a lethal dose of radiation (1). This observation sparked the imaginations of many investigators and led them to explore the use of high-dose therapy for treating refractory malignancies and to exploit the ability of marrow infusion to rescue patients from lethal toxicity of chemoradiotherapy in both autologous and allogeneic settings. In the mid-1950s, patients with advanced malignancies were first treated with high-dose therapy and marrow rescue, but none of these patients attained durable remission; all patients died from regimen-related toxicity, relapse of their malignancies, or "secondary disease," which is now known as "graft-versus-host disease" (GVHD)(2). The discovery of histocompatibility antigens a decade later established the foundation for transplantation biology. Using these new immunogenetic principles, the first success of allogeneic stem cell transplantation from a human leukocyte antigen (HLA)–matched sibling was reported in 1969 (3). Over the years, many advances in the management of immunocompromised hosts, in antibiotic regimens, and in blood component therapy have dramatically improved the outcome of this procedure. Presently, stem cell transplantation is the treatment of choice for many nonmalignant and malignant disorders (Table 37-1) (4).

Hemopoietic Stem Cells

Despite the widespread use of hemopoietic stem cell transplantation, our knowledge of the precise identity and biology of the hemopoietic stem cell remains incomplete. The spleen colony assay in lethally irradiated animals provided us with the first glimpse into the biologic characteristics of pleuripotential hemopoietic stem cells (5). The advents of in vitro culture (6), hybridoma technology (7), and fluorescent cytometry and cell sorting (8) all represent successive milestones in hemopoietic stem cell research.

In the early 1980s, a monoclonal antibody raised against a human myeloid cell line, anti-My-10, was found to bind to a cell surface glycophosphoprotein on early lymphohematopoietic stem and progenitor cells called "CD34" (9). As a marker for hemopoietic stem/progenitor cells, CD34 identified only 1.5% of the nucleated cells in the marrow and less than 0.5% of the peripheral blood mononuclear cells. Early multipotential progenitor cells—CFU-blast and long-term culture initiating cells (LT-CICs)—were enriched in the CD34^{bright} population. Eventually, enumeration of CD34^{bright} cells was used to quantitate the content of stem/progenitor cells in the stem cell graft. In murine studies, true stem cells seem to represent 1 in 10^4 to 1 in 10^5 cells; thus the CD34^{bright} population contains many early progenitors as well as stem cells. In order to ensure engraftment, the optimal dose of CD34^{bright} cells is estimated to be at the minimum of 2×10^6/kg of recipient body weight (10,11).

Hemopoietic stem cells used in clinical transplantation can be harvested from bone marrow, peripheral blood, fetal liver, and cord blood. For several decades, bone marrow has been the predominant source of stem cells. Recently, the use of cytokine-mobilized peripheral blood stem cells for transplantation has increased rapidly. In autotransplantation, mobilized peripheral blood has been the main source of stem cells since 1993, and its use in allotransplantation is on the rise (11). Initially, there was concern about using peripheral blood stem cells for allogeneic transplantation because of concern over the increased risk of GVHD owing to a high content of T cells in the stem cell graft (see below). However, the shorter time to engraftment associated with peripheral blood stem cell transplantation and the faster tempo of immunologic reconstitution, owing to large numbers of progenitor cells in the mobilized apheresis products, are beneficial.

Other sources of stem cells, such as fetal liver cells, have been rarely used for transplantation because of ethical concerns and the quality control of the tissues obtained from aborted fetuses. Of the several reports of fetal liver transplantation, many patients did not show convincing evidence of stable engraftment (12–14). The low yield of progenitor/stem cells from fetal hemopoietic tissues (fetal liver or cord blood) limits their use to recipients of small body size. The major advantage of using fetal hemopoietic stem cells is the low incidence of GVHD, probably owing to a high concentration of primitive stem cells and a low frequency of mature T cells compared with stem cell grafts obtained from marrow or mobilized peripheral blood (15).

The feasibility of using cryopreserved cord blood as a source of unrelated hemopoietic stem cells has renewed interest in the use of fetal hemopoietic tissue for transplantation. Patients who receive cord blood transplantation from unrelated donors appear to have an early mortality rate similar to that of patients who receive unrelated marrow transplantation, but the rate of acute GVHD is apparently lower, despite the higher degree of HLA

Table 37-1. Diseases Treated with Hemopoietic Stem Cell Transplantation

Acquired		Congenital	
Malignant	**Nonmalignant**		
Acute myeloid leukemia	Aplastic anemia	Immunodeficiencies: Severe combined immunodeficiencies Combined immunodeficiencies Leukocyte adhesion defects Actin deficiency Chronic mucocutaneous candidiasis Others	Mucopolysaccharidoses: Hurler's syndrome Hunter's syndrome Maroteaux-Lamy syndrome Others
Acute lymphoid leukemia	Paroxysmal nocturnal hemoglobinuria		
Chronic myeloid leukemia	Acquired immunodeficiency syndrome		Mucolipidoses: Metachromatic leukodystrophy Adrenoleukodystrophy Other lipidoses
Chronic lymphoid leukemia		Hematologic defects: Wiskott-Aldrich syndrome Fanconi's anemia Blackfan-Diamond anemia Thalassemia Sickle cell disease Glanzmann's thrombasthenia Gaucher's disease Chronic granulomatous disease Congenital neutropenia Chédiak-Higashi syndrome Langerhan's cell histiocytosis Dyskeratosis congenita Congenital amegakaryocytosis Thrombocytopenia–absent radius syndrome Familial erythrophagocytic lymphohistiocytosis Others	
Non-Hodgkin's lymphoma			Other lysosomal diseases: Lesch-Nyhan syndrome Type IIA glycogen storage disease
Hodgkin's disease			
Multiple myeloma			
Myelodysplastic syndromes			
Neuroblastoma			
Breast cancer			
Germ cell tumors			
Other selected solid tumors		Osteopetrosis	

disparity in the recipients of cord blood stem cells (16,17). The lower rate of acute GVHD in cord blood stem cell recipients may be attributable to the low numbers of mature T cells in the grafts and the younger age of both cord blood donors and recipients. With greater age disparity between donors and recipients in unrelated donor transplantation, it has been shown that donor age is an important predictor of acute and chronic GVHD (16,18). Therefore, it is conceivable that the lower rate of acute GVHD associated with cord blood transplantation is associated with hemopoietic stem cell donation from the youngest possible living donor.

Rationale for Hemopoietic Stem Cell Transplantation

The purpose of hemopoietic stem cell transplantation is to provide the host with hemopoietic tissue with the capacity for self-renewal and repopulation. The underlying pathologic states for which hemopoietic stem cell transplantation are performed can be categorized as follows.

Malignancies That Require High-Dose Therapy Resulting in Prolonged Marrow Aplasia

Many malignancies cannot be cured with conventional doses of therapy. The dose-response relationship of several chemotherapeutic agents and radiation has been shown in experimental models as well as in clinical trials (19,20). In order to overcome the resistance of tumor cells to conventional doses of therapy, the antitumor regimen is often escalated beyond the dose that would completely ablate the bone marrow. In this situation, hemopoietic stem cell transplantation functions as a biologic rescue after myeloablative therapy.

Nonmalignant, Acquired Disorders of Lymphohemopoietic Stem Cells

Bone marrow failure syndromes comprise a relatively rare category of diseases in which autoimmune mechanisms may damage lymphohemopoietic cells. Autoimmune destruction of erythroid, granulocytic, and megakaryocytic progenitors may result in aplastic anemia (21). Somatic mutation of the hemopoietic stem cells can also result in clonal disorders such as paroxysmal nocturnal hemoglobinuria (PNH) (22). Allogeneic transplantation is often necessary to correct the aplasia that accompanies PNH (23).

Congenital Defects of Lymphohemopoietic Stem Cells

This category consists of a variety of rare congenital disorders ranging from the developmental absence of a specific lineage of cells derived from lymphohemopoietic stem cells (e.g., severe combined immune deficiency, osteopetrosis, and amegakaryocytosis) to abnormalities in the synthesis of hematologic proteins (e.g., sickle cell anemia, thalassemia, and Glanzmann's thrombasthenia). Myeloablative therapy is needed to eliminate the defective hemopoietic clones, and allogeneic transplantation is used to reconstitute normal hemopoiesis.

Congenital Deficiencies of Enzymes Not Limited to Lymphohemopoietic Tissues

This diverse group of diseases is caused by deficiencies of enzymes that are not limited to the lymphohemopoietic system, commonly referred to as "storage diseases." The dominant manifestations of these disorders include degenerative changes in the CNS, hepatosplenomegaly, myocardial dysfunction, and dysmorphia. The goal of hemopoietic stem cell transplantation is to provide normal, self-renewing hemopoietic cells as an indefinite source for replenishment of the deficient enzymes (24). Progression of CNS manifestations of these diseases sometimes can be prevented following successful stem cell transplantation, but preexisting disease is often not reversible. Microglial and astroglial cells derived from transplanted stem cells are the likely sources of enzyme replacement in the CNS (25).

Donor Selection

The underlying disease of a patient is the most important determining factor in the choice of the source of hemopoietic stem cells. Autologous stem cell transplantation clearly is not an option for patients with aplastic anemia and congenital diseases. Autologous transplantation for malignancies of the marrow is unsuccessful if tumor cells cannot be completely removed from the stem cell graft (26,27). Autologous transplantation can be curative in patients with Hodgkin's disease and lymphomas without history of marrow involvement. For allogeneic transplantation, the most desirable sources of stem cells are human leukocyte antigen (HLA)–identical siblings and sometimes other close blood relatives. Since 1986, the National Marrow Donor Registry has facilitated searches for unrelated donors. There are more than 3 million volunteer donors in the registry worldwide typed for major histocompatibility complex (MHC) class I antigens (A and B loci), and many have been typed for MHC class II loci (DR loci). The chance of finding a closely matched donor is increas-

ing, especially among patients of northern European extraction (16). Another source that should be considered is cord blood stem cells—especially in pediatric patients (17). The strategy of selecting an appropriate source of allogeneic stem cells is often complex. Factors to be considered in the selection include urgency of transplantation, risk of GVHD, graft failure, cytomegalovirus (CMV) infection/disease, and minimization of risk for a child donor. Preferences for donor selection are as follows:

1. HLA-phenotypically identical family member (i.e., syngeneic donor and sibling donor where family analysis permits identification as genotypically identical; for certain malignancies genotypically matched sibling donor preferable over syngeneic donor)
2. HLA-phenotypically identical family member (first-degree relative preferred—e.g., sibling, parent, or child is preferable over any other blood relative)
3. Single-antigen mismatched family member (graft rejection direction)
4. Single-antigen mismatched family member (GVHD or bidirectional direction)
5. Fully matched (6/6) unrelated donor compared to 5/6 or 6/6 matched unrelated cord blood
   a. Unrelated donor preferred if recipient has malignant condition
   b. Cord blood preferred in nonmalignant conditions if cell dose is no less than 3×10^7 mononuclear cells/kg body weight of recipient
6. Single-antigen mismatched unrelated donor compared to 4/6 (or 3/6 in some cases) matched unrelated cord blood
   a. Unrelated donor preferred if recipient has malignant condition
   b. Cord blood preferred in nonmalignant conditions if cell dose is no less than 3×10^7 mononuclear cells/kg body weight of recipient
7. If a fully matched or single-antigen mismatched unrelated donor is not available, a zero-to-three-antigen mismatched cord blood may be used provided the cell dose is no less than 2×10^7 mononuclear cells/kg body weight of recipient (i.e., patients with malignant or nonmalignant conditions with no suitable unrelated donor can still come to transplant if a cord blood that meets minimum cell dose requirements is available).

When more than one donor is available, the following order of preference is followed:

1. CMV-negative donor if recipient is CMV-negative
2. Larger donor (if recipient is significantly larger than donor)
3. ABO-compatible donor
4. Male or nulliparous female over parous female

Obviously, the order of preference for donor selection outlined above will need frequent revision, because new technologies (e.g., ex vivo expansion of stem cells, genomic typing, and GVHD prophylaxis) may alter the risks of a particular group of donors so as to render that group more favorable than others.

Preparative Regimens for Hemopoietic Stem Cell Transplantation

For most patients, a preparative regimen is needed to ensure stable engraftment. The preparative regimen has two main biologic components:

1. *Immunosuppression.* This component is essential to prevent rejection of allogeneic hemopoietic stem cells. Rejection mechanisms include inherent immunity, allosensitization, and an autoimmune response against the host tissue microenvironment (e.g., aplastic anemia and various autoimmune diseases) (21).
2. *Cytoreduction.* This component is crucial for patients with malignancies regardless of hematologic or nonhematologic origins. Selection of agents for a preparative regimen is largely empirical. Agents with broad antitumor activity (e.g., alkylating agents and total body irradiation) are the most commonly used.

The proportional effects of these two components depend on the source of the donor stem cells (syngeneic, autologous, or allogeneic) and on the underlying disorder. Eradication of the tumor cells should be the primary goal of conditioning in autologous and syngeneic transplantation, because there is no graft-versus-tumor effect (see below) or graft rejection. Syngeneic transplantation for patients with aplastic anemia is an exception; immunosuppression is needed because the pathogenesis of the disease is mediated by immune mechanisms (28).

Agents used in the preparative regimen can be categorized as follows:

1. *Antineoplastic agents with low immunosuppressive activity.* The prototype for this group of agents is busulfan. This agent is highly toxic against myeloid stem cells and precursors but exhibits little immunosuppressive activity.
2. *Immunosuppressive agents.* Cyclosporine, tacrolimus, and sirolimus are immunosuppressive agents used in solid organ transplantation and stem cell transplantation. These agents act by inhibiting interleukin-2 (IL-2) gene transcription. Antithymocyte globulin (ATG) and monoclonal antibodies against T cells (anti-CD3, anti-CD2, anti-CD6, anti-CD5, anti-Tac) selectively bind to the T cells or their subsets (29). Corticosteroids and mycophenolic acid exhibit preferential cytotoxicity against lymphoid cells (30,31).
3. *Agents exhibiting both antineoplastic and immunosuppressive activities.* Cyclophosphamide and total body irradiation (TBI) are typical examples of this category of agents. Total lymphoid irradiation (TLI) is considered predominantly immunosuppressive because the exposure is limited to axial lymphoid tissue (32).

Because the intensity of the regimen contributes significantly to the morbidity and mortality of hemopoietic stem cell transplantation, attempts have been made to attenuate the antineoplastic component of the preparative regimen while maintaining high levels of immunosuppression. This strategy attempts to exploit the graft-versus-leukemia (or graft-versus-tumor) effect of such "adoptive immunotherapy," which is partly responsible for cures in allograft recipients (33,34). The scope of application is currently the subject of active clinical investigation.

Procurement and Preparation of Stem Cell Graft

Harvesting of bone marrow stem cells is performed under sterile conditions in the operating room. The primary harvest site is the posterior iliac crests. In situations where higher cell dose is critical to achieve engraftment, additional marrow can be obtained from anterior iliac crests and, rarely, from the sternum. In general, 10 to 15 mL/kg of marrow can be safely harvested. The marrow is pooled in a sterile container mixed with 10% media and anticoagulant and then passed through filters of graduated sizes to remove bone particles and form a mononuclear suspension. In a donor-recipient pair with a major ABO incompatibility, depletion of RBC from the marrow graft by centrifugation is necessary to avoid serious hemolytic transfusion reactions. The final product after RBC depletion usually contains 15 to 50 mL of packed RBC. Plasma exchange, plasma immunoadsorption, or whole-blood immunoadsorption should be performed prior to marrow infusion into patients with very high titer of isoantibodies against the donor red cells to reduce potential intravascular hemolysis. During infusion of an ABO-incompatible marrow graft, the patient should be closely observed and treated prophylactically for a transfusion reaction with hydration, diphenhydramine, and glucocorticoids. In a donor-recipient pair with minor ABO incompatibility, plasma depletion alone is adequate.

Harvesting of peripheral blood stem cells (PBSCs) requires mobilization with chemotherapy, growth factors, or a combination of growth factors and chemotherapy (11). Sequential administration of chemotherapy and granulocyte colony-stimulating factor (G-CSF) or granulocyte-macrophage colony-stimulating factor (GM-CSF) produces a better yield than G-CSF or GM-CSF alone. In patients in whom chemotherapy is used for stem cell mobilization, the dose of chemotherapy should be sufficiently myelosuppressive to obtain a good yield. The chemotherapeutic agent most commonly used in stem cell mobilizing protocols is cyclophosphamide. Other agents used less frequently, such as etoposide, ara-C, thio-TEPA, ifosphamide, and anthracycline, are usually administered in combination with cyclophosphamide and given as an induction regimen preceding stem cell harvesting. The major drawback of chemotherapy-mobilizing regimens is the accompanying neutropenic sepsis. Favorable indicators that predict the yield of stem cell harvesting are the absence of marrow disease, little prior chemotherapy, and absence of radiation treatment to the marrow-containing areas (35). Prior treatment with chemotherapy that is toxic for stem cells such as carmustine (BCNU) and melphalan predicts a poor yield. The quality of the stem cell graft is reflected in the tempo of hemopoietic recovery and is predicted by the number of CD34[bright] cells in the graft.

In recent years, several new hemopoietic cytokines have been introduced in clinical trials. G-CSF is currently used most frequently to mobilize stem cells. Neither PIXY321 (a GM-CSF/IL-3 fusion molecule) given as a single agent nor IL-3 given sequentially with GM-CSF has been shown to have any advantage over G-CSF alone (11). Additionally, side effects of these two molecules (fever and bone pain) appear to limit their clinical use as stem cell mobilizing agents. Early trials of stem cell factor (SCF) enhanced the yield of CD34^{bright} cells in PBSC grafts when compared with G-CSF alone, but it is not yet in wide clinical use (36).

For allogeneic transplantation, the large majority of normal donors who receive G-CSF as a mobilizing agent require only one or two leukaphereses to achieve a cell dose of 2×10^8 cells/kg. At least in the short term, administration of G-CSF and PBSC harvest appear to be safe. Although there is no identifiable contraindication to PBSC mobilization in hematologically normal donors, current practice is to exclude donors who have a potential for complication of mobilization—i.e., individuals with autoimmune inflammatory disease and atherosclerotic disease of the heart or CNS (37).

Posttransplantation Care

The care of patients after transplantation involves a broad range of clinical problems that encompass several medical disciplines. Toxicities from preparative regimens are primarily apparent during the first 30 days of transplantation (38). In addition to severe pancytopenia, patients may suffer toxicity of the kidney (caused by platinum, nephrotoxic antimicrobials, cyclosporine, or tacrolimus); liver (veno-occlusive disease, caused by chemoradiotherapy and preexisting liver diseases); heart (caused by prior anthracycline therapy and cyclophosphamide); and lung (caused by chemoradiotherapy). Multisystem organ failure is a major cause of morbidity and mortality after stem cell transplantation (39). Aggressive supportive care is crucial for a good long-term outcome, because many of these organ toxicities are reversible. During aplasia shortly after conditioning, almost all patients require transfusion support, especially RBC and platelets. Posttransplantation administration of hemopoietic growth factors can enhance the recovery of hemopoiesis in patients who have received marrow transplantation. Moreover, administration of hemopoietic growth factors may be beneficial in patients with poor graft function by accelerating neutrophil recovery (40). The use of growth factors after transplantation is not universal, however. In one study, a combination of GM-CSF/G-CSF or IL-3/GM-CSF did not improve the recovery of neutrophil over G-CSF or GM-CSF alone (11,41). The benefit of hemopoietic growth factors administered after PBSC transplantation is less apparent than after marrow transplantation because the cytopenic phase is shorter than after marrow transplantation. Some investigators have attempted to eliminate the granulocytopenic phase altogether through transfusion of G-CSF mobilized granulocytes. The overall benefit and practicality of this approach remain to be determined (42).

Most patients develop fever during the neutropenic phase and require empiric antibiotic therapy. Prophylactic antibiotics have been used to reduce the incidence of bacterial infection (43). With modern antibiotic therapy, mortality resulting from infectious complications during the neutropenic phase is low; however, opportunistic infections—particularly in the setting of GVHD—are frequently fatal. Therefore, routine infectious prophylaxis against opportunistic infections is an important part of posttransplantation care and is begun within the first month after transplantation. The drugs of choice for prophylaxis against *Pneumocystis carinii* and CMV are trimethoprim/sulfamethoxazole and ganciclovir, respectively. The latter is indicated only in patients who have positive serology for CMV or who are recipients of stem cells from donors with positive CMV serology. In patients who are positive for herpes simplex virus (HSV) serology, the risk of reactivation of HSV is very high, and therefore acyclovir is routinely used in this group. Fluconazole is also used as antifungal prophylaxis in most centers. Occasionally, superinfection with a fluconazole-resistant organism (e.g., *Candida kruzei*) may become problematic. Nevertheless, prophylaxis with fluconazole has been shown to improve survival in the recipients of unrelated marrow transplantation (44).

Clinical Results

Congenital Disorders

Immunodeficiency Syndromes

Allogeneic stem cell transplantation is the treatment of choice for severe combined immune deficiency (SCID) (45,46). With few exceptions [e.g., some patients with adenosine deaminase (ADA) deficiency, patients with Wiskott-Aldrich syndrome, and recipients of unrelated cord blood], engraftment can be achieved without an intensive preparative regimen. A unique aspect of allogeneic transplantation in SCID is the high success rate experienced using T-depleted grafts from a parent (i.e., a haploidentical graft). The reasons for such a high success rate include a low incidence of GVHD and low-intensity preparative conditioning, which minimizes tissue injury. Mixed lymphoid chimerism usually occurs and is sufficient to achieve long-term reconstitution of lymphoid function. While T-cell function reconstitutes completely in most patients, B-cell function remains abnormal in the recipients of T-depleted haploidentical marrow. More than half of these patients continue to require immunoglobulin replacement.

For patients with ADA deficiency, experimental therapeutic options other than allogeneic stem cell transplantation are currently available—for example, polyethylene glycol–adenosine deaminase (PEG-ADA) (47), infusions of autologous T cells genetically corrected by insertion of a normal ADA gene and expanded ex vivo (48), and infusion of autologous umbilical cord blood CD34$^+$ cells transduced with the ADA gene (49). Nontransplant treatment options also exist for other congenital diseases, such as Kostmann's syndrome (G-CSF) (50) and chronic granulomatous disease [interferon-γ (IFN-γ) (51)]. These options are not uniformly successful in all stages of the disease, and allogeneic transplantation remains the treatment of choice for patients with advanced or accelerated disease. The cost of replacement therapy and the risks of organ damage are crucial factors in considering the timing and feasibility of the transplant option.

Thalassemia and Sickle Cell Disease

Cures of thalassemia and sickle cell disease with allogeneic transplantation are well documented (52–54). Preparative regimens containing busulfan and cyclophosphamide are the ones used most frequently. An intensive (myeloablative) preparative regimen is required to eliminate preexisting abnormal hemopoiesis. Allosensitization from transfusion predisposes patients to graft rejection, and toxicity from preparative regimens can potentially exacerbate organ dysfunction from iron overload, resulting in significant peritransplant morbidity. Therefore, the selection of a candidate for an allograft and the timing of the transplant procedure are crucial for an optimal outcome.

Storage Disease

As detailed above, storage diseases comprise a heterogeneous group of disorders with variable outcomes after allogeneic transplantation. Stabilization or improvement of clinical signs and symptoms is often observed in patients with adrenoleukodystrophy (55), globoid cell leukodystrophy (56), and Hurler's syndrome (57). Clinical benefit is less apparent in metachromatic leukodystrophy (58) and Hunter's syndrome whereas for others, such as Sanfilippo's syndrome, allogeneic transplantation may be contraindicated. Gaucher's disease can be cured with allogeneic transplantation, but replacement therapy is now also an option (59).

Aplastic Anemia

Allogeneic transplantation is the treatment of choice for patients with aplastic anemia who have HLA-matched sibling donors (60). For patients who do not have HLA-identical siblings, immunosuppressive therapy is the best alternative therapy, with consideration of allogeneic transplantation from unrelated donors in patients for whom this therapy has been unsuccessful (16). Allosensitization (through transfusion) should be avoided if possible in patients who have HLA-identical sibling donors because of an increased risk of graft rejection after allosensitization (61). Although graft rejection can be overcome with donor lymphocyte infusions, the risk of chronic GVHD is increased by this maneuver (62). In allosensitized patients, the addition of TBI or TLI to cyclophosphamide (50 mg/kg/day for 4 days) can significantly reduce the risk of graft rejection (32,63). Nonetheless, the risk of secondary malignancies increases with inclusion of radiation in the preparative regimen (64,65). Alternatively, ATG can be used to improve engraftment (66). Nearly 90% survival with sustained engraftment can be expected in patients who receive ATG and cyclophosphamide as a preparative regimen.

Lymphohemopoietic Malignancies

Acute Lymphocytic Leukemia

The majority of children and approximately 30% to 70% of adult patients with acute lymphocytic leukemia (ALL) can be cured with chemotherapy (67). Allogeneic transplantation of ALL in first remission does not improve long-term leukemia-free survival and is not currently recommended for most adult patients (68). However, allogeneic transplantation is the treatment of choice for patients who are in first remission with high-risk features such as the presence of chromosomal abnormalities [e.g., Ph^1 chromosome, 11q23 abnormalities, or t(1;19) translocation] and for patients who have relapses or induction failures (69–71). Autologous transplantation with a purged stem cell graft and allogeneic transplantation from an unrelated donor are reasonable options for patients in relapse or in later remission who have no matched sibling donors (72).

Chronic Lymphocytic Leukemia

Both autologous and allogeneic transplantation have been used in patients with chronic lymphocytic leukemia (73). Complete remissions have been documented in these patients, but long-term follow-up is limited and additional information is needed to assess the efficacy of stem cell transplantation in this disease.

Acute Myeloid Leukemia

Several large cooperative groups have conducted prospective studies to evaluate the role of transplantation in postremission therapy for patients in first remission (74,75). In these studies, allogeneic transplantation has a marginal advantage over autologous transplantation and chemotherapy intensification. The outcomes of these trials are not surprising given the heterogeneity of the prognostic variables not included in the initial analysis. Allogeneic transplantation is not recommended for patients with "core-binding" karyotypes [e.g., t(8;21), inv(16), t(16;16), and del(16)], because long-term survival can be achieved in 78% of these patients with high-dose cytarabine (76). Additionally, patients with acute promyelocytic leukemia treated with all-*trans*-retinoic acid now experience excellent survival and should not receive allogeneic transplantation in remission (77). On the other hand, patients with unfavorable karyotypes are unlikely to benefit from high-dose cytarabine and therefore allogeneic transplantation in first remission should be considered in these patients. The role of autologous transplantation as postremission intensification is still a subject of controversy (78). Allogeneic transplantation from an HLA sibling matched donor is the treatment of choice for all patients not in first remission, although autologous transplantation and allogeneic transplantation from an unrelated donor are viable options (79).

Chronic Myeloid Leukemia

Presently, allogeneic stem cell transplantation is the only curative therapy for this disease. Allogeneic transplantation from a sibling donor and from an unrelated donor should be offered to all patients age 55 years and younger (80,81). Interferon (with or without cytarabine or hydroxyurea) therapy should be considered in older patients, because improvement of survival with disappearance of Ph^1 chromosome has been shown in several studies (82,83). Patients who do not respond to interferon can be considered for allogeneic transplantation. However, pretransplant treatment with interferon for 6 months or longer increases the risk of severe acute GVHD and mortality in recipients of unrelated donor marrow (84). Treatment options with interferon and allogeneic transplantation should be considered in the context of all of a patient's risk factors (85,86). Autologous transplantation using breakpoint cluster region–abelson (bcr-abl)-negative CD34^{bright} cells is under investigation (87).

Myelodysplastic Syndromes

The natural history of this group of disorders varies according to the histologic subtypes defined by the French-American-British (FAB) Classification. Assignment of a prognostic group according to the scoring system has been developed to aid therapeutic decisions (88). Histologic subtypes of chronic myelomonocytic leukemia and refractory anemia with excess blasts (with or without transformation) carry ominous prognoses, and allogeneic transplantation from a sibling or an unrelated donor should be offered as soon as possible. Depending on the risk category, disease-free survival rates of 30% to 70% can be expected (89,90).

Non-Hodgkin's Lymphoma

Non-Hodgkin's lymphoma comprises a heterogeneous group of diseases with several different histologic features and variable natural histories (91). Conventional chemotherapy can result in a cure for 30% to 50% of patients with diffuse aggressive histology. Autologous stem cell transplantation can be curative in patients with relapse or with disease resistant to conventional chemotherapy, and is the optimal salvage therapy in patients with chemotherapy-sensitive disease. It is not yet clear whether patients with slow responses to conventional chemotherapy can benefit from autologous transplantation (92). The main cause of treatment failure after autotransplantation is relapse, possibly related to marrow contamination with lymphoma cells. There is some evidence that marrow purging may reduce the relapse rate after autografting because patients who receive marrow that is effectively purged of lymphoma cells have a significantly higher disease-free survival rate (93). It is not clear whether successful purging of the marrow is simply an association with a lower tumor burden or represents better responsiveness to cytoreductive regimen. Other strategies to improve the outcome of autografting have focused on tumor-targeted therapy with radiolabeled monoclonal antibodies (94). An alternative approach to lowering the relapse rate is allogenic transplantation, which provides a tumor-free source of stem cells and may confer a graft-versus-lymphoma effect. One prospective study comparing autologous with allogeneic transplantation has been reported (95). Patients receiving allografts had a significantly lower relapse rate (20% for allograft compared with 69% for autograft), but the progression-free survival rate was not significantly different

(47% for allograft compared with 24% for autograft). The role of allogeneic transplantation has now been expanded to other histologic subtypes of lymphoma including low-grade lymphoma (96,97). Some investigators have employed T-depleted allografts to reduce GVHD-related complications, but long-term outcomes of this approach are unknown.

Hodgkin's Disease

Autologous transplantation represents the best salvage therapy for patients with refractory or relapsed Hodgkin's disease (98). Poor prognostic factors include "B" symptoms at relapse, extranodal disease at relapse, and initial remission duration of less than 1 year (99). Patients with no more than one risk factor have a probability of disease-free survival of more than 80%. The results of allogeneic transplantation in this disease have been disappointing, probably as a result of excessive toxicity from preparative regimen and complications from GVHD (100).

Solid Tumors

Hemopoietic stem cell transplantation has been used with increasing frequency in patients with solid tumors. Since 1995, the number of autologous transplants for breast cancer has exceeded the number of transplants for lymphoma (101). A high rate of complete remission in patients with metastatic disease after autotransplantation is encouraging, although long-term follow-up is limited and it is not clear whether the high response rate translates into a survival advantage. Promising results have also been reported in groups of patients with inflammatory and stage II disease for whom autotransplantation was used as neoadjuvant or adjuvant therapy (102). Several large randomized trials for these earlier stages are ongoing. Allogeneic transplantation has been reported in a patient with breast cancer in whom MHC class I antigen–restricted cytotoxic T lymphocytes specific for breast carcinoma target cells were isolated from the peripheral blood, indicating a possible graft-versus-tumor effect (103). Induction of autologous GVHD using low-dose cyclosporine has also been attempted, but its biologic impact on the tumoricidal effect is not known (104).

Autotransplantation is also in the early stages of clinical testing for patients with ovarian cancer (105) and brain tumors (106). Long-term outcome for these patients and for selected subsets of patients who might derive benefit from this therapy will not be known for several years.

The role of autotransplantation in solid tumors has been most clearly established for testicular cancer (107) and neuroblastoma (108). Approximately 50% of patients with testicular cancer who are refractory to chemotherapy or in relapse now exhibit long-term survival with this treatment. Both high-dose chemotherapy and I^{131} metaiodobenzylguantidine (MIBG) have been used for cytoreduction of neuroblastoma (109). Patients with stage IV disease are likely to benefit from high-dose therapy and autotransplantation (110). Comparative analysis of allogeneic and autologous transplantation does not show statistical differences for either survival or relapse (111). With the poor prognosis of patients with bone and marrow involvement at diagnosis, allogeneic transplantation in these subsets of patients may be preferable (112).

Pathophysiology of Acute Graft-versus-Host Disease

The major complication of allogeneic hemopoietic stem cell transplantation remains graft-versus-host disease (GVHD). Our understanding of the pathophysiology of GVHD has dramatically improved with recent advances in our knowledge of the cellular and humoral interactions that are intrinsic to all inflammatory processes. It is important to remember that in hemopoietic stem cell transplantation, donor lymphocytes are infused into a host that has been profoundly damaged. The effects of the underlying disease, prior infection, and the conditioning regimen may result in substantial proinflammatory changes in endothelial and epithelial cells. Donor cells rapidly encounter not only a foreign environment, but also one that has been altered to promote the activation and proliferation of inflammatory cells by the increased expression of adhesion molecules, cytokines, and cell surface recognition molecules. The donor lymphocytes respond in turn by reacting in a fashion that would foster the control or resolution of infection under ordinary circumstances. Thus, the pathophysiology of GVHD may be considered a distortion of the cellular response to viral and gram-negative bacterial infection.

The target organs of GVHD support the close relationship between GVHD and infection. The skin, gut, and liver all share an extensive exposure to endotoxins and other bacterial products that can trigger and amplify local inflammation. This exposure distinguishes them from organs, such as the heart and kidneys, that are not GVHD targets. The lung is an organ of controversy in this regard. While the lungs are not classic GVHD targets, accumulating evidence suggests that they share some degree of GVHD susceptibility with the skin, gut, and liver (113,114). Because of their roles as primary barriers to infection, these target organs have large populations of professional antigen-presenting cells (APCs), such as macrophages and dendritic cells, that may enhance the graft-versus-host (GVH) reaction.

Recent findings have implicated the inappropriate production of cytokines, which are the central regulatory molecules of the immune system, as a primary cause of the induction and maintenance of experimental and clinical GVHD (115,116). Dysregulation of complex cytokine networks occurring in three sequential phases can be considered a framework for the pathophysiology of acute GVHD (115–117).

Phase One: Conditioning Regimen

The earliest phase of acute GVHD starts before the donor cells are infused (Fig. 37-1). The transplant conditioning regimen is an important variable in the pathogenesis of acute GVHD because it damages and activates host tissues, including the intestinal mucosa, liver, and other tissues. Activated host cells secrete inflammatory cytokines such as tumor necrosis factor-α (TNF-α) and IL-1 (118), growth factors such as GM-CSF (119,120), and many others (121). The presence of inflammatory cytokines

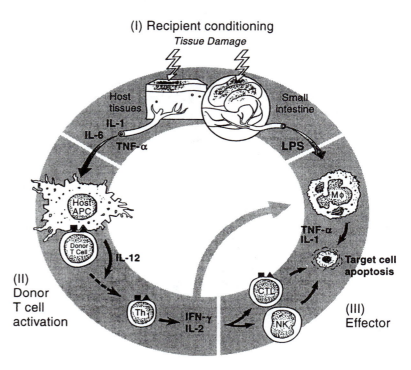

Figure 37-1. Inflammatory cytokine cascades during acute GVHD. The pathophysiology of acute GVHD can be conceptualized from the perspective of cytokines as a three-step process. After allogeneic BMT, T cells and mononuclear phagocytes interact both at the initiation of a GVHD reaction and in the subsequent injury to host tissues; during these interactions, cytokines play critical roles. The first step emphasizes the importance of the transplant conditioning regimen in the damage and activation of host tissues, including intestinal mucosa, liver, and other tissues. Activated host cells then secrete inflammatory cytokines (e.g., TNF-α and IL-1) (118). The consequences of the action of this cytokine release are the expression of adhesion molecules (e.g., ICAM-1 and VCAM-1) (119–121) and of MHC class II antigens (122,123). These events enhance the recognition of host MHC antigens and/or mHAs by mature donor T cells after allogeneic BMT.

during this phase may up-regulate adhesion molecules (122) and MHC antigens (123–125), thereby enhancing the recognition of host MHC or minor histocompatibility antigens by mature donor T cells after the cellular component of the transplantation has been infused. This process is in accordance with the observation that an enhanced risk of GVHD after clinical bone marrow transplantation (BMT) is associated with intensive preparative regimens that cause extensive injury to epithelial and endothelial surfaces with a subsequent release of inflammatory cytokines and increases in expression of cell surface adhesion molecules (126–128). The relationship among intensity of the preparative regimen, inflammatory cytokines, and GVHD severity was recently further supported in animal models (129). Moreover, the risk of inducing severe acute GVHD appears to be less if the lymphocytes are infused well after the primary tissue injury has resolved (130,131).

Phase Two: Donor T-Cell Activation

The second phase of acute GVHD consists of donor T-cell activation, and it includes antigen presentation, activation of individual T cells, and proliferation and differentiation of activated T cells (see Fig. 37-1). During antigen presentation, large proteins are digested by APCs into smaller fragments; these antigenic peptides bind to HLA (class I or class II) molecules and are displayed on the surfaces of the APCs as peptide-HLA complexes. T cells recognize this complex through antigen-specific T-cell receptors (TCRs). In allogeneic interactions such as GVHD, mature donor T cells recognize recipient peptide-HLA complexes (alloantigens) in which both the HLA molecules and the bound peptides are foreign. These peptides represent minor histocompatibility antigens (mHAs), some of which have been recently identified (132,133).

Efforts to identify and understand target-effector interactions have also led to interesting observations of the TCR repertoire in the blood and in the organs involved in GVHD. After transplantation, there may be oligoclonal reconstitution of T cells (134,135). In mice, there is the additional observation that the vertical transmission of retroviruses results in the thymic deletion of T cells with specific Vβ subfamily specificities, which occurs because some retroviral proteins function as superantigens (i.e., they bind to portions of the TCR that are not antigen specific). These superantigens are then interpreted as "self" in the thymus, and reactive cells are eliminated. Because mouse strains vary in Vβ deletions, transplantation between strains allows the role of Vβ specificity to be determined in GVHD. It is clear that, in mice, T cells do not expand all TCR families equally, and that the superantigens identified by transplanted T cells in an H2-compatible strain result in interferon secretion and GVHD (136,137). In both experimental and clinical BMT, there appear to be oligoclonal populations of T cells in target organs that preferentially utilize specific Vβ segments (135,138,139). Furthermore, analysis of T cells in target organs affected by GVHD is more likely to show specific Vβ usage compared with blood, supporting the idea of local expansion of T-cell clones reactive to host alloantigens (134,140).

Recently, the role of CD40-CD40 ligand (CD40L) interactions in T-cell activation has been defined (141–143). Alloantigen composition of the host determines which T-cell subset proliferates and differentiates. MHC class II (HLA-DR, -DR, and -DQ) differences stimulate CD4+ T cells; MHC class I (HLA-A, -B, and -C) differences stimulate CD8+ T cells. In mouse models of GVHD, where genetic differences between multiple strain combinations can be controlled, CD4+ cells induce GVHD to MHC class II differences, and CD8+ cells induce GVHD to MHC class I differences (144). Thus, both CD4+ and CD8+ T-cell subsets can initiate the afferent phase of GVHD. In the majority of clinical HLA-identical marrow transplant recipients, GVHD may be induced by either subset or simultaneously by both.

Host APCs provide costimulatory activation signals by B7-CD28 interaction and IL-1 (145). In addition to the TCR, accessory molecules such as CD4, CD8, leukocyte function-associated antigen (LFA)-1, LFA-2, and CD44 participate in effector-target cell interactions by intensifying cellular contact and communication (146). Antigen presentation induces the activation of individual T cells, initiating the transcription of the genes for cytokines, such as IL-2, IL-12, and IFN-γ, and their receptors. Cytokines produced in response to alloantigens are predominantly secreted by the T-helper 1 (Th1) subset of T cells (147,148). Both IL-2 and IFN-γ have long been implicated in the pathophysiology of acute GVHD (see below), and they play central roles in further T-cell activation, induction of cytotoxic T lymphocytes (CTLs) and natural killer (NK) cell responses, and the priming of additional donor and residual host mononuclear phagocytes to produce IL-1 and TNF-α. The T-cell activation phase is followed by clonal expansion and differentiation. DNA synthesis commences within 24 hours of antigen recognition and is maximal 3 to 5 days later. Functional differentiation then occurs as cells produce proteins required for specific effector functions, such as the protein esterases that are required for CTLs (149). The expression of many cell surface molecules is altered; receptors for lymphocyte homing and migration may be down-regulated; and other adhesion molecules (e.g., LFA-1) may be up-regulated, thus altering the T cells' ability to traffic in vivo (150).

While inflammatory effector functions of mononuclear phagocytes are stimulated by IL-2 and IFN-γ, which are secreted by activated Th1 T-cell subsets, these effector functions are inhibited by IL-4 and IL-10, cytokines that are produced by activated Th2 T cells. There is now considerable evidence that the preferential expansion of Th2 T cells after allogeneic transplantation is associated with the development of a GVHD syndrome that is similar to chronic GVHD and is associated with less lethality and antibody formation in murine systems (151–155).

The preincubation of donor T cells in the presence of murine recombinant IL-4 ex vivo during a primary mixed lymphocyte culture (MLC) to alloantigens was sufficient to polarize these T cells toward a Th2 cytokine phenotype (156). Transplantation of these polarized Th2 T-cell populations failed to induce acute GVHD to MHC class I or class II antigens. These experiments strongly supported the concept that the balance in Th1 and Th2 cytokines is critical for the development (or prevention) of acute GVHD. Further issues that need to be addressed include the preservation of a graft-versus-leukemia effect after transplantation of polarized Th2 cells (157,158). and whether they can support lymphohematopoietic engraftment. Peripheral blood hematopoietic cells collected after mobilization with G-CSF suggests that Th1 → Th2 polarization may be underway, albeit indirectly, resulting in less GVHD compared with saline-treated controls (159–161). This effect also changes the production of other inflammatory cytokines such as TNF-α (162).

Phase Three: Inflammatory Effectors

The third phase of acute GVHD is complex and has only recently been appreciated. The initial hypothesis that the cytolytic function of CTLs directly causes the majority of tissue damage and necrosis in GVHD targets is too limited (163). Large granular lymphocytes (LGLs) or NK cells appear to be prominent in the effector arm of GVHD in several animal models, and they may contribute to the pathologic damage—that is, induce the changes of GVHD following the T-cell–mediated GVH reaction (163,164). LGLs do not recognize HLA proteins as targets, but they can be recruited by cytokines released by T cells. The precise relationship between cytokines induced during the second phase and mediators of tissue damage during this phase is an area of active investigation.

Mononuclear phagocytes, which have been primed with Th1 cytokines during phase two, receive a second, triggering signal to increase the secretion of the inflammatory cytokines TNF-α and IL-1. This stimulus may be provided by lipopolysaccharide (endotoxin, LPS), which can leak through the intestinal mucosa damaged by the conditioning regimen. LPS subsequently may stimulate gut-associated lymphocytes and macrophages (165). LPS reaching skin tissues may also stimulate keratinocytes, dermal fibroblasts, and macrophages to produce similar cytokines in the dermis and epidermis (119–121). TNF-α can cause direct tissue damage by inducing necrosis of target cells, or it may induce tissue destruction during GVHD through apoptosis, or programmed cell death. The induction of apoptosis commonly occurs after activation of the TNF-α-Fas antigen pathway (166). Apoptosis is probably critical to GVHD in the large intestine (167), skin (168,169), and possibly endothelial cells (170). In addition to these proinflammatory cytokines, excess nitric oxide (NO) produced by activated macrophages may contribute to the deleterious effects on GVHD target tissues, particularly immunosuppression (171–173). Thus, the induction of inflammatory cytokines may synergize with the cellular damage caused by CTLs and NK cells (163,174), resulting in the amplification of local tissue injury and further promotion of an inflammatory response, which ultimately lead to the observed target tissue destruction in the BMT host.

Phase Three: Cytolytic Effectors

Although cytokines clearly play important roles in the morbidity and mortality of systemic GVHD, their relative importance as mediators of damage in GVHD target organs is less well established. The unusual cluster of GVHD target organs (skin, gut, and liver) is not adequately explained by the systemic release of cytokines. For example, intravenous infusion of TNF-α and IL-1 does not cause the lymphomononuclear cell infiltration of liver and skin observed in GVHD. Furthermore, the absence of GVHD toxicity in other visceral organs, such as the kidneys, argues against circulating cytokines as the sole causation of tissue-specific damage. The infiltrates observed in GVHD target organs are generally thought to contain T cells responding to alloantigens on host tissues. As mentioned earlier, LPS leakage through the skin or mucosa may act as an adjuvant to the antigens expressed in these tissues, attracting and activating alloreactive donor T cells. A second possibility is that tissue-specific neoantigens are expressed at these sites as the result of ongoing inflammation. Such inflammation may alter the ligands for homing receptors on T cells (e.g., selectins) that enable them to traffic into specific tissues.

It is clear in murine systems that cellular effectors contribute to GVHD (Table 37-2). The application of knockout technology and the identification of pertinent mutant mice have provided important tools for dissection of effector mechanisms. Three pathways that have been identified need to be considered as GVHD effectors—the perforin–granzyme B pathway, the Fas–Fas ligand (FasL) pathway, and direct cytokine-mediated injury.

Clearly, additional overlapping but as yet unidentified mechanisms may be present as well. Direct cellular cytotoxicity through the perforin–granzyme B pathway contributes to target

Table 37-2. Mechanisms of Graft-versus-Host Disease

Effector	Target Damage*	Systemic Toxicity*
CD4+ T cells	±	++
Secreted cytokine		
CD8+ T cells		
Fas–Fas ligand system	+	±
Perforin–granzyme B pathway	++	−
Monocytes, granulocytes	+	±
Nitric oxide, others	+	±

*− negative; ± minimal; + moderate; ++ severe.

cell injury in GVHD. Perforin causes membrane pore formation, but it is not adequate to initiate apoptosis on its own (175). Granzyme B enters the cell through the perforin-derived pore and causes apoptosis. Granzyme B appears to be most effective in MHC class I mismatches and is less critical in GVHD resulting from MHC class II mismatches (176). Donor cells from both perforin-deficient and granzyme B–deficient knockout mice can mediate GVHD, but the onset of clinical manifestations is significantly delayed compared with control animals. This suggests that the perforin–granzyme B pathway is an early-acting mechanism, but that an additional late mechanism of cytotoxicity exists (177,178). One candidate for the late-acting mechanism is the Fas-FasL interaction (179–181). Fas is a member of the TNF receptor family that is expressed on numerous cell types (182), while FasL is expressed on activated T cells. Interactions between a Fas-bearing target and a FasL-bearing T cell result in apoptosis of the target cell. Thus, a setting in which FasL molecules are up-regulated by cytokines is likely to result in destruction of both specific targets and nonspecific, innocent bystanders that express Fas. When mutant mice that are deficient in FasL (*gld* mice) are used as transplant donors, GVHD occurs in an attenuated fashion. While FasL-deficient donors can mediate hepatic and cutaneous GVHD, the mice do not develop cachexis (178), supporting the concept of yet a third pathway. When Fas-deficient mice are crossed with those having perforin or granzyme B knockouts, the use of lymphocytes from these donors further diminishes but does not abrogate GVHD. Thus, neither FasL nor perforin is necessary for GVHD and, in the absence of both cellular effectors, GVHD can still occur (183). Cytokines such as TNF-α may also contribute to cytotoxicity (177,184); TNF may be either circulating or membrane bound. Interestingly, in a murine model of acute GVHD, the infusion of metalloproteinase inhibitors reduced the shedding of both TNF-α and FasL by effector cells and reduced both clinical GVHD manifestations and mortality (185). A recent detailed analysis of a patient with transfusion-associated GVHD supports this notion of multiple effectors in human GVHD (186).

This conceptual framework of these sequential steps helps to explain a variety of unique and seemingly unrelated aspects of GVHD. For example, several analyses of clinical transplants noted increased risks of GVHD associated with advanced-stage leukemia, certain intensive conditioning regimens, and viral infections (126–128). Similarly, the reduction in GVHD seen in gnotobiotic mice (187,188) and in patients with aplastic anemia undergoing transplantation in laminar airflow environments with gut decontamination (189) may be explained by the reduction of bacterial LPS on the skin and gut. The LPS may leak through damaged intestinal mucosal surfaces and stimulate the numerous gut-associated lymphocytes and macrophages to produce inflammatory cytokines. The beneficial effects of protective environments may be less apparent in patients receiving transplants for malignancies, because prior therapy and associated infections may have resulted in an environment that facilitates GVHD. Viral infections are commonly associated with GVHD. They are more frequent in patients with GVHD, and a viral illness may cause the initiation of GVHD or worsening of established GVHD. Cytomegalovirus (CMV) has a particularly close relationship with GVHD (190,191), as does herpes simplex virus (HSV) (192,193), and possibly human herpesvirus 6 (HHV-6) (194). The precise pathophysiology of this connection remains uncertain. While it has been hypothesized that viral antigen expression on target cells might function as an mHA, direct evidence proving this association is lacking. Certainly, cellular damage to the intestine or liver may increase the permeability of those organs, resulting in increased absorption of bacterial products such as LPS. Alternatively, GVHD targets could be innocent bystanders of either an NK-cell attack a virus-induced activated T-cell attack. (195,196).

Clinical Manifestations and Management of Graft-versus-Host Disease

GVHD comprises two clinical syndromes with distinctly different manifestations. Acute GVHD with its onset during the first 100 days posttransplantation involves skin, liver, and GI tract. GVHD that persists or manifests its onset more than 100 days after transplantation is called chronic GVHD.

Acute GVHD

"Satellitosis" is a pathologic description of eosinophilic cytoplasmic degeneration and necrosis in acute GVHD, which is a characteristic feature observed on the epithelium of target organs (197). Skin involvement often precedes visceral manifestations, but isolated involvement of the liver or the GI tract is occasionally observed. The severity of each organ may vary. Clinical staging of the severity of the involved organs depends on the surface area of skin involvement, the level of total bilirubin, and the volume of diarrhea. Several grading systems based on the composite stages of the target organs have been proposed (198–200). The fundamental problem with any of these grading systems is the difficulty in ascertaining the cause of a particular organ dysfunction, because tissue biopsy is either not feasible or nondiagnostic. Thus, the diagnosis, staging, and grading of acute GVHD rely on careful analysis of the physical signs and symptoms, laboratory data, and the clinical course of the patient. Despite these difficulties, recognition and grading of acute GVHD is one of the most important parts of daily management of patients undergoing allogeneic transplantation.

Factors associated with increased risk of acute GVHD in sibling-donor allograft recipients include transplant from an HLA-disparate donor (201), older recipient age (202), and sex mismatch of donor and recipient (127). In unrelated allogeneic transplantation where potential histocompatibility is more pronounced, genomic typing of class I and class II alleles is becoming an important element for donor selection (203,204). Additionally, older donor age has been shown to increase the risk of acute GVHD in unrelated donor transplantation (18).

Table 37-3. Graft-versus-Host Disease Prophylaxis

T-lymphocyte depletion of donor marrow in vitro:
    Complete
    Selective (CD5, CD8)
    With partial add-back
In vivo treatment of patient:
    Tacrolimus, cyclosporine, methotrexate, and others
    Polyclonal anti–T-cell antibodies
    Monoclonal anti–T-cell antibodies
        Murine
        Humanized
Gnotobiosis

Prophylaxis of Acute GVHD

Without posttransplant immunosuppressive therapy, significant acute GVHD invariably develops in all patients after allotransplantation (205). Therefore, all allograft recipients require prophylactic treatment for GVHD (Table 37-3). The main agent in GVHD prophylaxis is either cyclosporine or tacrolimus. These agents are commonly used in combination with methotrexate and/or steroids (206–208). Despite drug prophylaxis, acute GVHD still occurs in approximately 30% to 40% of allograft recipients. Promising new agents (e.g., mycophenolate and sirolimus) are currently in the early stages of preclinical and clinical trials (209–211). Mycophenolic acid, an active hydrolyzed metabolite of mycophenolate mofetil, is a potent noncompetitive inhibitor of inosine monophosphate dehydrogenase (IMPDH) that leads to inhibition of the de novo pathway of guanosine nucleotide synthesis, which is critical for T and B lymphocytes.

An approach to reduction or elimination of GVHD is to deplete T cells from the graft. T-cell depletion can be accomplished by incubation with monoclonal antibody against T cells and complement, elutriation, CD34-positive selection, and soybean agglutination. The major drawbacks of using T-depleted grafts are higher rates of leukemia relapse and graft failure (212–214). Moreover, patients receiving T-depleted grafts without developing GVHD have a higher relapse rate than patients who receive non-T-depleted allografts and do not develop GVHD. These findings underscore the importance of the graft-versus-leukemia (GVL) effect in allogeneic stem cell transplantation. Dissociation of GVHD, facilitation of engraftment, and graft-versus-tumor effects has been difficult. Adoptive transfer of a specific CD8 cytotoxic T-lymphocyte clone recognizing host alloantigen or donor T cells expressing disparate MHC class I molecules has been shown to facilitate engraftment without causing GVHD (215,216). Furthermore, adoptive transfer of selective donor CD8 subsets generated by in vitro culture can facilitate engraftment without GVHD while preserving the GVL effect in leukemia-bearing animals (156,217).

Treatment of Acute GVHD

Corticosteroid treatment is the most commonly used initial therapy for acute GVHD. Responses usually occur in 35% to 50% of patients in at least one organ, with an overall partial and complete response rate of 44% (218). It is not uncommon to observe exacerbation of acute GVHD during the tapering phase of corticosteroid treatment. The results of acute GVHD therapy with other agents have been unsatisfactory (219). One clinical trial of mycophenolate mofetil in 17 patients with acute GVHD showed a 65% response rate (209). Further study of this drug is warranted.

Chronic GVHD

Chronic GVHD occurs in approximately 50% of the long-term survivors among HLA-identical marrow recipients, and the risk increases with the use of peripheral blood stem cell transplantation (220). Clinical manifestations of chronic GVHD are similar to those of autoimmune collagen vascular diseases, which include oral ulceration (lichen planus), keratoconjunctivitis sicca, xerostomia, polyserositis, esophagitis and esophageal stricture, vaginal ulceration and stricture, intrahepatic obstructive liver disease, obstructive pulmonary disease, scleroderma, morphea, fasciitis, and myositis (221). In contrast to those of acute GVHD, the clinical manifestations of chronic GVHD are unique and less likely to be confounded by other complications, leading to a high diagnostic concordance rate among physicians (222). The classification of chronic GVHD proposed by Sullivan et al (221) is based on the extent of organ involvement as well as the presence of pathologic features that are known to be associated with poor prognosis, such as bridging necrosis or cirrhosis on liver biopsy. Unfortunately, the current classification does not fully address the significance of other organ involvement (e.g., lung involvement, hematologic abnormalities, and immune deficiencies).

Although there is no specific prophylactic therapy for chronic GVHD, the most important risk factor for the development of chronic GVHD is a prior diagnosis of acute GVHD. The probability of chronic GVHD ranges from 59% to 85% among those who have had grade II to grade IV acute GVHD, and from 28% for those who have not had acute GVHD to 49% for those who have had grade I acute GVHD (223). Other prognostic factors associated with higher risk of chronic GVHD are recipient age greater than 20 years, use of non-T-cell–depleted bone marrow, and alloimmune female donors for male recipients. In one study, chronic GVHD developed de novo in 62% of patients who had all three of these adverse prognostic factors (223). Pharmacologic approaches to the prevention of chronic GVHD have been disappointing. One recent prospective, randomized, double-blind study using thalidomide, an agent known to exhibit activity in the treatment of chronic GVHD, resulted in a paradoxical outcome with a higher incidence of chronic GVHD and a lower overall survival rate in patients who received thalidomide (224).

The diversity of organ involvement, the chronicity of the illness, and hematologic and immunologic dysfunctions contribute to the difficulties of treating and evaluating chronic GVHD. The success of treatment is related to risk factors associated with chronic GVHD. Three features of chronic GVHD are associated with poor survival: the "progressive" form of chronic

GVHD, lichenoid changes in the skin histology, and elevated bilirubin. In one study, the actuarial survival at 6 years was 70% in patients with none of these risk factors, 43% in patients with one of these risk factors, and 20% in patients with any combination of two or more of these factors (225). The "progressive" form of chronic GVHD is the type that evolves without a hiatus from active acute GVHD. Patients with progressive chronic GVHD are likely to receive corticosteroids and tacrolimus or cyclosporine at its onset, but it is less responsive to other types of immunosuppressive therapy (221). By contrast, patients who develop chronic GVHD after an interval of response to treatment for acute GVHD (quiescent form) and patients who have never had acute GVHD (de novo form) are more responsive to therapy. In these latter situations, reinstitution of primary prophylactic regimen for GVHD, such as tacrolimus or cyclosporine in combination with glucocorticoids, is often effective. In patients with extensive chronic GVHD and platelet counts of 100,000/μL or higher, addition of azathioprine to prednisone actually resulted in a poorer survival than that of patients treated with prednisone alone (5-year survival rates of 47% and 61%, respectively) (226). Patients with extensive chronic GVHD who had platelet counts of 100,000/μL or higher, most of whom had "progressive" chronic GVHD, had the poorest survival (5-year survival rate of 26%). A subsequent trial using alternate-day cyclosporine and prednisone has shown improvement of this subset of patients with extensive chronic GVHD with thrombocytopenia (227).

Another agent that has been reported to have efficacy in chronic GVHD is thalidomide. Thalidomide (N-phthalimidoglutarimide), a sedative with teratogenic effects that was withdrawn from the market 30 years ago, has found a new role in the treatment of chronic GVHD. Although its precise immunomodulatory mechanisms are not known, thalidomide had been shown to decrease the number of CD4 cells and the CD4/CD8 ratio and to prolong cardiac graft survival in animals (228,229). It has also been shown to prevent as well as treat established acute GVHD in rats transplanted with MHC-incompatible marrow (230). The experience with thalidomide for treatment of acute GVHD in humans is limited (231,232), but the efficacy of thalidomide in chronic GVHD is well established in both adults and children. The response rate in patients with steroid-resistant chronic GVHD ranges from 20% to 76% (233–235), and 48% with high-risk chronic GVHD (mostly the "progressive" form) responded. Responses of patients with chronic pulmonary GVHD have also been reported (236). Common side effects of thalidomide are somnolence, constipation, neuritis, rashes, and neutropenia. These side effects may limit widespread application of this drug (233).

Immunologic Reconstitution after Hemopoietic Stem Cell Transplantation

Immunologic reconstitution after hemopoietic transplantation is determined both by host factors (e.g., HLA disparity from donor, presence of GVHD, degree of posttransplant immunosuppression, and age) and by donor factors (e.g., T-cell depletion of graft

and source of stem cells: peripheral blood versus marrow). The most important inherent host factor in immunologic reconstitution is the thymic function, which declines at an early age. Studies in thymic-deficient mice show that T-cell regeneration occurs primarily through antigen-driven expansion of mature peripheral T cells. This mechanism of T-cell regeneration limits the recovery of immune competence because of the quantitative deficiencies in T-cell number and the restricted diversity of the regenerated T-cell receptor (TCR) repertoire (237). Because the recovery of the T-cell function is primarily an antigen-driven process, it may be possible to skew the T-cell repertoire toward a specific antigenic target using vaccine strategy during immune reconstitution in stem cell transplant recipients. It should be noted that acute and chronic GVHD are inherently immunosuppressive, and their treatment with additional immunosuppressive agents causes further delay of recovery of T-cell function (238).

Given the restrictions of T-cell reconstitution noted above, it is not surprising that recipients of T-depleted grafts exhibit a sustained period of immunodeficiency. The tempo of immune reconstitution is probably related to the level of T-cell depletion. These patients show early appearance of NK cells, whose numbers remain constant, while T- and B-cell functions may take 2 to 3 years to return to normal (238,239). Addition of posttransplant immunosuppression to prevent graft failure in these T-depleted stem cell recipients further delays immune reconstitution, resulting in prolonged inversion of the CD4/CD8 ratio, increased numbers of activated CD8⁺ T cells, and delayed recovery of T-cell mitogen responses (240). These patients have depressed levels of CD4⁺ T cells, with associated increased risks of Epstein-Barr virus–associated lymphoproliferative disorders, opportunistic infections, and relapse of malignancy (240,241). Similarly, autologous transplantation with autologous CD34^bright cells (a process resulting in profound T-cell depletion) is associated with serious opportunistic infections, characteristic of delayed immune reconstitution (242).

Recently, studies comparing immune reconstitution in recipients of peripheral blood stem cell transplantation (PBSCT) and bone marrow transplantation (BMT) from both autologous and allogeneic donors have been reported (243,244). After autologous transplantation, PBSCT recipients had significantly faster recovery of circulating monocytes (CD14⁺ cells), NK (CD56⁺) cells, T helper (CD4⁺) cells, TCR gamma/delta cells, and naive T lymphocytes (CD45RA⁺), compared with recipients of BMT; by contrast, BMT recipients had more rapid increases in the frequency of T suppressor/effector (CD8⁺) cells, B (CD19⁺) cells, CD34⁺ cells, polymorphonuclear (PMN) leukocytes, and memory T lymphocytes (CD45RO⁺). The CD4:CD8 and CD45RA: CD45RO ratios were consistently higher in the PBSCT recipients, resulting in a greater response to mitogen (243). In the case of allogeneic donors, PBSCT recipients exhibited significantly faster recovery of naive (CD4⁺CD45RA⁺) helper T cells, memory (CD4⁺CD45RO⁺) helper T cells, B (CD19⁺) cells, and proliferative responses to mitogen (244). Longer follow-up studies of immune reconstitution in PBSCT recipients will be needed before we can determine its potential advantage over BMT recipients.

Delayed Complications of Stem Cell Transplantation

Stem cell transplantation represents an extremely aggressive form of therapy. Survival and quality of life after transplantation often depend on the careful management of delayed complications. Acute toxicity to various organs, such as heart and lungs, are common after administration of preparative regimens, but these effects are usually reversible. A minority of patients continue to manifest clinical organ dysfunction on long-term follow-up. Routine pretransplant evaluations of organ functions in asymptomatic patients without specific risk factors usually do not predict the occurrence of delayed organ dysfunction. While organ toxicities from preparative regimens are the main causes of morbidity and mortality in the early course of transplantation, delayed complications, such as sicca syndrome, scleroderma, and cataracts, are most often related to chronic GVHD. Post-transplant lymphoproliferative diseases (PTLDs) after allogeneic transplantation have histologic features that resemble diffuse large cell lymphoma and are usually of donor origin. The majority of cases occur within 6 months after transplantation, although some patients develop PTLDs more than a year after the procedure. The risk of PTLD increases with the use of unrelated or HLA-disparate grafts, the use of anti–T-cell antibody, and T-cell depletion (16). T-cell depletion or CD34[bright] selection of hemopoietic graft is the most important risk factor for the development of PTLD in autologous transplantation (245,246). Treatment of PTLD with IFN-α, donor lymphocyte infusion, or Epstein-Barr virus–specific donor T cells is usually effective (247,248). Other malignant complications of stem cell transplantation are myelodysplastic syndrome or acute myeloblastic leukemia which occur in up to 18% of patients who receive autologous transplantation (249,250). The duration of cytotoxic therapy prior to autologous transplantation appears to be the major risk factor for the development of these complications. The risks of solid tumors also increase in both autologous and allogeneic transplant recipients; risk factors are chronic GVHD, irradiation, T-depleted graft, and male gender (251,252). The strategies for decreasing the risks of secondary malignancies include development of less toxic preparative regimens, improvement of immune reconstitution, and prevention of chronic GVHD.

Future Directions

Although the role of hemopoietic stem cell transplantation for curative therapy of many diseases is well recognized, the risks associated with this procedure have limited its potential application to incurable diseases. The critical areas of research that should improve the safety of this procedure include new strategies for prevention of GVHD (through cytokine modulation or new immunosuppressive agents), blockade of costimulatory molecules with novel reagents such as CTLA1-Ig (253), and enhancement of immune reactivity against tumor cells and viruses (through adoptive cellular therapy and/or cytokines). The possibility of engraftment of allogeneic stem cells in recipients conditioned with nonmyeloablative regimens (which is associated with minimal morbidity and mortality) will permit innovative approaches for many patients who would not currently be eligible for BMT (254,255) or patients with severe autoimmune disorders such as multiple sclerosis, myasthenia gravis, and systemic lupus erythematosus. Similar strategies can also be employed to create mixed chimerism with donor-specific tolerance to solid organ grafts (256). The potential application of this therapy is being aggressively pursued in many diseases, and its role is expected to expand significantly over the next few years.

References

1. Lorenz E, Uphoff D, Reid TR, Shelton E. Modification of radiation injury in mice and guinea pigs by bone marrow injections. J Natl Cancer Inst 1951;12:197–201.
2. Bortin MM. A compendium of reported human bone marrow transplants. Transplantation 1970;9(6):571–587.
3. Meuwissen HJ, Gatti RA, Terasaki PI, et al. Treatment of lymphopenic hypogammaglobulinemia and bone-marrow aplasia by transplantation of allogeneic marrow. Crucial role of histocompatibility matching. N Engl J Med 1969; 281(13):691–697.
4. Appelbaum FR. The use of bone marrow and peripheral blood stem cell transplantation in the treatment of cancer [see comments]. CA Cancer J Clin 1996;46(3):142–164.
5. Till JE, McCulloch EA. A direct measurement of the radiation sensitivity of normal mouse bone marrow cells. Radiat Res 1961;14:213–222.
6. Bradley TR, Metcalf D. The growth of mouse bone marrow cells in vitro. Aus J Exp Biol Med Sci 1966;44:287–300.
7. Kohler G, Milstein C. Continuous cultures of fused cells secreting antibody of predefined specificity. Nature 1975; 256(5517):495–497.
8. Civin CI, Banquerigo ML, Strauss LC, Loken MR. Antigenic analysis of hematopoiesis. VI. Flow cytometric characterization of My-10-positive progenitor cells in normal human bone marrow. Exp Hematol 1987;15(1):10–17.
9. Krause DS, Fackler MJ, Civin CI, May WS. CD34: structure, biology, and clinical utility [see comments]. Blood 1996;87(1):1–13.
10. Korbling M, Huh YO, Durett A, et al. Allogeneic blood cell transplantation: peripheralization and yield of donor-derived primitive hematopoietic progenitor cells (CD34+ Thy-1dim) and lymphoid subsets, and possible predictors of engraftment and graft-versus-host disease. Blood 1995; 86(7):2842–2848.
11. To LB, Haylock DN, Simmons PJ, Juttner CA. The biology and clinical uses of blood stem cells. Blood 1997;89(7): 2233–2258.
12. Morrison SJ, Hemmati HD, Wandycz AM, Weissman IL. The purification and characterization of fetal liver hematopoietic stem cells. Proc Natl Acad Sci USA 1995;92(22): 10302–10306.
13. Lucarelli G, Izzi T, Porcellini A, et al. Fetal liver transplantation in 2 patients with acute leukaemia after total body irradiation. Scand J Haematol 1982;28(1):65–71.

14. Kochupillai V, Sharma S, Francis S, et al. Fetal liver infusion in aplastic anaemia. Thymus 1987;10(1–2):95–102.

15. Broxmeyer HE, Douglas GW, Hangoc G, et al. Human umbilical cord blood as a potential source of transplantable hematopoietic stem/progenitor cells. Proc Natl Acad Sci USA 1989;86(10):3828–3832.

16. Kernan NA, Bartsch G, Ash RC, et al. Analysis of 462 transplantations from unrelated donors facilitated by the National Marrow Donor Program [see comments]. N Engl J Med 1993;328(9):593–602.

17. Rubinstein P, Carrier C, Scaradavou A, et al. Outcomes among 562 recipients of placental-blood transplants from unrelated donors processing and cryopreservation of placental/umbilical cord blood for unrelated bone marrow reconstitution. N Engl J Med 1995;92(22):10119–10122.

18. Kollman C, Confer D, Matlack M, et al. The effect of donor age on recipient outcome following unrelated donor bone marrow transplant. Blood 1998;92:686a.

19. Hryniuk W, Levine MN. Analysis of dose intensity for adjuvant chemotherapy trials in stage II breast cancer. J Clin Oncol 1986;4(8):1162–1170.

20. Kwak LW, Halpern J, Olshen RA, Horning SJ. Prognostic significance of actual dose intensity in diffuse large-cell lymphoma: results of a tree-structured survival analysis [see comments]. J Clin Oncol 1990;8(6):963–977.

21. Young NS, Maciejewski J. The pathophysiology of acquired aplastic anemia. N Engl J Med 1997;336(19):1365–1372.

22. Hillmen P, Lewis SM, Bessler M, et al. Natural history of paroxysmal nocturnal hemoglobinuria. N Engl J Med 1995;333(19):1253–1258.

23. Szer J, Deeg HJ, Witherspoon RP, et al. Long-term survival after marrow transplantation for paroxysmal nocturnal hemoglobinuria with aplastic anemia. Ann Intern Med 1984;101(2):193–195.

24. Krivit W, Sung JH, Shapiro EG, Lockman LA. Microglia: the effector cell for reconstitution of the central nervous system following bone marrow transplantation for lysosomal and peroxisomal storage diseases. Cell Transplant 1995;4(4):385–392.

25. Eglitis MA, Mezey E. Hematopoietic cells differentiate into both microglia and macroglia in the brains of adult mice. Proc Natl Acad Sci USA 1997;94(8):4080–4085.

26. Brenner MK, Rill DR, Moen RC, et al. Gene-marking to trace origin of relapse after autologous bone-marrow transplantation. Lancet 1993;341(8837):85–86.

27. Rill DR, Santana VM, Roberts WM, et al. Direct demonstration that autologous bone marrow transplantation for solid tumors can return a multiplicity of tumorigenic cells. Blood 1994;84(2):380–383.

28. Hinterberger W, Rowlings PA, Hinterberger-Fischer M, et al. Results of transplanting bone marrow from genetically identical twins into patients with aplastic anemia [see comments]. Ann Intern Med 1997;126(2):116–122.

29. Przepiorka D, Chan KW, Champlin RE, et al. Prevention of graft-versus-host disease with anti-CD5 ricin A chain immunotoxin after CD3-depleted HLA-nonidentical marrow transplantation in pediatric leukemia patients. Bone Marrow Transplant 1995;16(6):737–741.

30. Langhoff E, Ladefoged J, Dickmeiss E. The immunosuppressive potency of various steroids on peripheral blood lymphocytes, T cells, NK and K cells. Int J Immunopharmacol 1985;7(4):483–489.

31. Hood KA, Zarembski DG. Mycophenolate mofetil: a unique immunosuppressive agent. Am J Health Syst Pharm 1997;54(3):285–294.

32. Ramsay NK, Kim TH, McGlave P, et al. Total lymphoid irradiation and cyclophosphamide conditioning prior to bone marrow transplantation for patients with severe aplastic anemia. Blood 1983;62(3):622–626.

33. Sullivan KM, Storb R, Buckner CD, et al. Graft-versus-host disease as adoptive immunotherapy in patients with advanced hematologic neoplasms. N Engl J Med 1989;320(13):828–834.

34. Horowitz MM, Gale RP, Sondel PM, et al. Graft-versus-leukemia reactions after bone marrow transplantation. Blood 1990;75(3):555–562.

35. Bensinger W, Appelbaum F, Rowley S, et al. Factors that influence collection and engraftment of autologous peripheral-blood stem cells. J Clin Oncol 1995;13(10):2547–2555.

36. Moskowitz CH, Stiff P, Gordon MS, et al. Recombinant methionyl human stem cell factor and filgrastim for peripheral blood progenitor cell mobilization and transplantation in non-Hodgkin's lymphoma patients—results of a phase I/II trial. Blood 1997;89(9):3136–3147.

37. Anderlini P, Korbling M, Dale D, et al. Allogeneic blood stem cell transplantation: considerations for donors [editorial]. Blood 1997;90(3):903–908.

38. Bearman SI, Appelbaum FR, Buckner CD, et al. Regimen-related toxicity in patients undergoing bone marrow transplantation. J Clin Oncol 1988;6(10):1562–1568.

39. Bearman SI, Appelbaum FR, Back A, et al. Regimen-related toxicity and early posttransplant survival in patients undergoing marrow transplantation for lymphoma. J Clin Oncol 1989;7(9):1288–1294.

40. Weisdorf DJ, Verfaillie, CM, Davies SM, et al. Hematopoietic growth factors for graft failure after bone marrow transplantation: a randomized trial of granulocyte-macrophage colony-stimulating factor (GM-CSF) versus sequential GM-CSF plus granulocyte-CSF. Blood 1995;85(12):3452–3456.

41. Crump M, Couture F, Kovacs M, et al. Interleukin-3 followed by GM-CSF for delayed engraftment after autologous bone marrow transplantation. Exp Hematol 1993;21(3):405–410.

42. Adkins D, Spitzer G, Johnston M, et al. Transfusions of granulocyte-colony-stimulating factor-mobilized granulocyte components to allogeneic transplant recipients: analysis of kinetics and factors determining posttransfusion neutrophil and platelet counts. Transfusion 1997;37(7):737–748.

43. Momin F, Chandrasekar PH. Antimicrobial prophylaxis in bone marrow transplantation. Ann Intern Med 1995;123(3):205–215.

44. Hansen JA, Gooley TA, Martin PJ, et al. Bone marrow transplants from unrelated donors for patients with chronic myeloid leukemia [see comments]. N Engl J Med 1998;338(14):962–968.

45. Parkman R. The biology of bone marrow transplantation for severe combined immune deficiency. Adv Immunol 1991;49:381–410.

46. Buckley RH, Schiff SE, Schiff RI, et al. Hematopoietic stem-cell transplantation for the treatment of severe combined immunodeficiency. N Engl J Med 1999;340(7):508–516.

47. Hershfield MS. PEG-ADA: an alternative to haploidentical bone marrow transplantation and an adjunct to gene therapy for adenosine deaminase deficiency. Hum Mutat 1995;5(2):107–112.

48. Blaese RM. Development of gene therapy for immunodeficiency: adenosine deaminase deficiency. Pediatr Res 1993;33(1 suppl):S49–S53; discussion S53–S55.

49. Kohn DB, Weinberg KI, Nolta JA, et al. Engraftment of gene-modified umbilical cord blood cells in neonates with adenosine deaminase deficiency. Nat Med 1995;1(10):1017–1023.

50. Boxer LA, Hutchinson R, Emerson S. Recombinant human granulocyte-colony-stimulating factor in the treatment of patients with neutropenia. Clin Immunol Immunopathol 1992;62(1 Pt 2):S39–S46.

51. Gallin JI. Interferon-gamma in the treatment of the chronic granulomatous diseases of childhood. Clin Immunol Immunopathol 1991;61(2 Pt 2):S100–S105.

52. Lucarelli G, Galimberti M, Polchi P, et al. Bone marrow transplantation in patients with thalassemia. N Engl J Med 1990;322(7):417–421.

53. Lucarelli G, Galimberti M, Polchi P, et al. Marrow transplantation in patients with thalassemia responsive to iron chelation therapy [see comments]. N Engl J Med 1993;329(12):840–844.

54. Walters MC, Patience M, Leisenring W, et al. Bone marrow transplantation for sickle cell disease [see comments]. N Engl J Med 1996;335(6):369–376.

55. Moser HW, Moser AB, Smith KD, et al. Adrenoleukodystrophy: phenotypic variability and implications for therapy [published erratum appears in J Inherit Metab Dis 1992;15(6):918]. J Inherit Metab Dis 1992;15(4):645–664.

56. Krivit W, Shapiro EG, Peters C, et al. Hematopoietic stem-cell transplantation in globoid-cell leukodystrophy. N Engl J Med 1998;338(16):1119–1126.

57. Peters C, Shapiro EG, Anderson J, et al. Hurler syndrome: II. Outcome of HLA-genotypically identical sibling and HLA-haploidentical related donor bone marrow transplantation in fifty-four children. The Storage Disease Collaborative Study Group. Blood 1998;91(7):2601–2608.

58. Dhuna A, Toro C, Torres F, et al. Longitudinal neurophysiologic studies in a patient with metachromatic leukodystrophy following bone marrow transplantation. Arch Neurol 1992;49(10):1088–1092.

59. Zimran A, Elstein D, Kannai R, et al. Low-dose enzyme replacement therapy for Gaucher's disease: effects of age, sex, genotype, and clinical features on response to treatment [see comments]. Am J Med 1994;97(1):3–13.

60. Storb R, Leisenring W, Anasetti C, et al. Long-term follow-up of allogeneic marrow transplants in patients with aplastic anemia conditioned by cyclophosphamide combined with antithymocyte globulin [letter]. Blood 1997;89(10):3890–3891.

61. Storb R, Prentice RL, Thomas ED. Marrow transplantation for treatment of aplastic anemia. An analysis of factors associated with graft rejection. N Engl J Med 1977;296(2):61–66.

62. Storb R, Prentice RL, Sullivan KM, et al. Predictive factors in chronic graft-versus-host disease in patients with aplastic anemia treated by marrow transplantation from HLA-identical siblings. Ann Intern Med 1983;98(4):461–466.

63. Gordon BG, Strandjord SE, Warkentin PI, et al. Successful treatment of severe aplastic anemia by bone marrow transplantation from HLA nonidentical family members: preliminary results utilizing cyclophosphamide and 600 cGY fractionated total body irradiation [see comments]. Am J Pediatr Hematol Oncol 1991;13(1):29–33.

64. Deeg HJ, Socie G, Schoch G, et al. Malignancies after marrow transplantation for aplastic anemia and Fanconi anemia: a joint Seattle and Paris analysis of results in 700 patients. Blood 1996;87(1):386–392.

65. Deeg HJ, Socie G. Malignancies after hematopoietic stem cell transplantation: many questions, some answers. Blood 1998;91(6):1833–1844.

66. Storb R, Etzioni R, Anasetti C, et al. Cyclophosphamide combined with antithymocyte globulin in preparation for allogeneic marrow transplants in patients with aplastic anemia. Blood 1994;84(3):941–949.

67. Pui CH, Evans WE. Acute lymphoblastic leukemia. N Engl J Med 1998;339(9):605–615.

68. Zhang MJ, Hoelzer D, Horowitz, MM, et al. Long-term follow-up of adults with acute lymphoblastic leukemia in first remission treated with chemotherapy or bone marrow transplantation. The Acute Lymphoblastic Leukemia Working Committee. Ann Intern Med 1995;123(6):428–431.

69. Chao NJ, Forman SJ, Schmidt GM, et al. Allogeneic bone marrow transplantation for high-risk acute lymphoblastic leukemia during first complete remission. Blood 1991;78(8):1923–1927.

70. Faderl S, Kantarjian HM, Talpaz M, Estrov Z. Clinical significance of cytogenetic abnormalities in adult acute lymphoblastic leukemia. Blood 1998;91(11):3995–4019.

71. Forman SJ, Schmidt GM, Nademanee AP, et al. Allogeneic bone marrow transplantation as therapy for primary induction failure for patients with acute leukemia. J Clin Oncol 1991;9(9):1570–1574.

72. Weisdorf DJ, Billett AL, Hannan P, et al. Autologous versus unrelated donor allogeneic marrow transplantation for acute lymphoblastic leukemia. Blood 1997;90(8):2962–2968.

73. Michallet M, Archimbaud E, Bandini, G, et al. HLA-identical sibling bone marrow transplantation in younger patients with chronic lymphocytic leukemia. European Group for Blood and Marrow Transplantation and the International Bone Marrow Transplant Registry. Ann Intern Med 1996;124(3):311–315.

74. Ravindranath Y, Yeager AM, Change MN, et al. Autologous bone marrow transplantation versus intensive consolidation chemotherapy for acute myeloid leukemia in childhood. Pediatric Oncology Group. N Engl J Med 1996;334(22):1428–1434.

75. Zittoun RA, Mandelli F, Willemze R, et al. Autologous or allogeneic bone marrow transplantation compared with intensive chemotherapy in acute myelogenous leukemia. European Organization for Research and Treatment of Cancer (EORTC) and the Gruppo Italiano Malattie Ematologiche Maligne dell'Adulto (GIMEMA) Leukemia Cooperative Groups [see comments]. N Engl J Med 1995;332(4):217–223.

76. Bloomfield CD, Lawrence D, Byrd JC, et al. Frequency of prolonged remission duration after high-dose cytarabine intensification in acute myeloid leukemia varies by cytogenetic subtype. Cancer Res 1998;58(18):4173–4179.

77. Tallman MS, Andersen JW, Schiffer CA, et al. All-trans-retinoic acid in acute promyelocytic leukemia [see comments] [published erratum appears in N Engl J Med 1997 Nov 27;337(22):1639]. N Engl J Med 1997;337(15):1021–1028.

78. Gorin NC. Autologous stem cell transplantation in acute myelocytic leukemia. Blood 1998;92(4):1073–1090.

79. Busca A, Anasetti C, Anderson G, et al. Unrelated donor or autologous marrow transplantation for treatment of acute leukemia. Blood 1994;83(10):3077–3084.

80. Appelbaum FR, Clift R, Radich J, et al. Bone marrow transplantation for chronic myelogenous leukemia. Semin Oncol 1995;22(4):405–411.

81. McGlave P. Unrelated donor transplant therapy for chronic myelogenous leukemia. Hematol Oncol Clin North Am 1998;12(1):93–105.

82. Kantarjian HM, Giles FJ, O'Brien SM, Talpaz M. Clinical course and therapy of chronic myelogenous leukemia with interferon-alpha and chemotherapy. Hematol Oncol Clin North Am 1998;12(1):31–80.

83. Guilhot F, Chastang C, Michallet M, et al. Interferon alfa-2b combined with cytarabine versus interferon alone in chronic myelogenous leukemia. French Chronic Myeloid Leukemia Study Group [see comments]. N Engl J Med 1997;337(4):223–229.

84. Morton AJ, Gooley T, Hansen JA, et al. Association between pretransplant interferon-alpha and outcome after unrelated donor marrow transplantation for chronic myelogenous leukemia in chronic phase. Blood 1998;92(2):394–401.

85. Gale RP, Hehlmann R, Zhang MJ, et al. Survival with bone marrow transplantation versus hydroxyurea or interferon for chronic myelogenous leukemia. The German CML Study Group. Blood 1998;91(5):1810–1819.

86. Lee SJ, Kuntz KM, Horowitz MM, et al. Unrelated donor bone marrow transplantation for chronic myelogenous leukemia: a decision analysis. Ann Intern Med 1997;127(12):1080–1088.

87. Verfaillie CM, Bhatia R, Steinbuch M, et al. Comparative analysis of autografting in chronic myelogenous leukemia: effects of priming regimen and marrow or blood origin of stem cells. Blood 1998;92(5):1820–1831.

88. Greenberg P, Cox C, LeBeau MM, et al. International scoring system for evaluating prognosis in myelodysplastic syndromes [see comments] [published erratum appears in Blood 1998 Feb 1;91(3):1100]. Blood 1997;89(6):2079–2088.

89. Ratanatharathorn V, Karanes C, Uberti J, et al. Busulfan-based regimens and allogeneic bone marrow transplantation in patients with myelodysplastic syndromes. Blood 1993;81(8):2194–2199.

90. Anderson JE, Appelbaum FR, Schoch G, et al. Allogeneic marrow transplantation for myelodysplastic syndrome with advanced disease morphology: a phase II study of busulfan, cyclophosphamide, and total-body irradiation and analysis of prognostic factors [see comments]. J Clin Oncol 1996;14(1):220–226.

91. Armitage JO. Treatment of non-Hodgkin's lymphoma. N Engl J Med 1993;328(14):1023–1030.

92. Verdonck LF, van Putten WL, Hagenbeek A, et al. Comparison of CHOP chemotherapy with autologous bone marrow transplantation for slowly responding patients with aggressive non-Hodgkin's lymphoma [see comments]. N Engl J Med 1995;332(16):1045–1051.

93. Gribben JG, Freedman AS, Neuberg D, et al. Immunologic purging of marrow assessed by PCR before autologous bone marrow transplantation for B-cell lymphoma [see comments]. N Engl J Med 1991;325(22):1525–1533.

94. Press OW, Eary JF, Appelbaum FR, et al. Radiolabeled-antibody therapy of B-cell lymphoma with autologous bone marrow support [see comments]. N Engl J Med 1993;329(17):1219–1224.

95. Ratanatharathorn V, Uberti J, Karanes C, et al. Prospective comparative trial of autologous versus allogeneic bone marrow transplantation in patients with non-Hodgkin's lymphoma. Blood 1994;84(4):1050–1055.

96. Adkins D, Brown R, Goodnough LT, et al. Treatment of resistant mantle cell lymphoma with allogeneic bone marrow transplantation. Bone Marrow Transplant 1998;21(1):97–99.

97. van Besien K, Sobocinski KA, Rowlings PA, et al. Allogeneic bone marrow transplantation for low-grade lymphoma. Blood 1998;92(5):1832–1836.

98. Horning SJ, Chao NJ, Negrin RS, et al. High-dose therapy and autologous hematopoietic progenitor cell transplantation for recurrent or refractory Hodgkin's disease: analysis of the Stanford University results and prognostic indices. Blood 1997;89(3):801–813.

99. Reece DE, Connors JM, Spinelli JJ, et al. Intensive therapy with cyclophosphamide, carmustine, etoposide +/– cisplatin, and autologous bone marrow transplantation for Hodgkin's disease in first relapse after combination chemotherapy [see comments]. Blood 1994;83(5):1193–1199.

100. Gajewski JL, Phillips GL, Sobocinski KA, et al. Bone marrow transplants from HLA-identical siblings in advanced Hodgkin's disease. J Clin Oncol 1996;14(2):572–578.

101. Antman KH, Rowlings PA, Vaughan WP, et al. High-dose chemotherapy with autologous hematopoietic stem-cell support for breast cancer in North America [see comments]. J Clin Oncol 1997;15(5):1870–1879.

102. Cagnoni PJ, Shpall EJ. High-dose chemotherapy for the treatment of breast and ovarian cancer [see comments]. Curr Opin Oncol 1997;9(2):122–125.

103. Eibl B, Schwaighofer H, Nachbaur D, et al. Evidence for a graft-versus-tumor effect in a patient treated with marrow ablative chemotherapy and allogeneic bone marrow transplantation for breast cancer. Blood 1996;88(4):1501–1508.

104. Kennedy MJ, Beveridge R, Vogelsang G, et al. Phase I study of cyclosporin A (CSA) to induce graft-versus-host disease (GVHD) following high-dose chemotherapy (HDC) with autologous marrow reinfusion (AMR) for metastatic breast cancer (MBC). Proc Annu Meet Am Soc Clin Oncol 1991;10:A48. Meeting abstract.

105. Stiff PJ, Bayer R, Kerger C, et al. High-dose chemotherapy with autologous transplantation for persistent/relapsed ovarian cancer: a multivariate analysis of survival for 100 consecutively treated patients [see comments]. J Clin Oncol 1997;15(4):1309–1317.

106. Mason WP, Grovas A, Halpern S, et al. Intensive chemotherapy and bone marrow rescue for young children with newly diagnosed malignant brain tumors. J Clin Oncol 1998;16(1):210–221.

107. Broun ER, Nichols CR, Gize G, et al. Tandem high dose chemotherapy with autologous bone marrow transplantation for initial relapse of testicular germ cell cancer. Cancer 1997;79(8):1605–1610.

108. Johnson FL, Goldman S. Role of autotransplantation in neuroblastoma. Hematol Oncol Clin North Am 1993; 7(3):647–662.

109. Goldberg SS, Desantes K, Huberty JP, et al. Engraftment after myeloablative doses of 131I-metaiodobenzylguanidine followed by autologous bone marrow transplantation for treatment of refractory neuroblastoma. Med Pediatr Oncol 1998;30(6):339–346.

110. Stram DO, Matthay KK, O'Leary M, et al. Consolidation chemoradiotherapy and autologous bone marrow transplantation versus continued chemotherapy for metastatic neuroblastoma: a report of two concurrent Children's Cancer Group studies [see comments]. J Clin Oncol 1996;14(9):2417–2426.

111. Matthay KK, Seeger RC, Reynolds CP, et al. Allogeneic versus autologous purged bone marrow transplantation for neuroblastoma: a report from the Childrens Cancer Group. J Clin Oncol 1994;12(11):2382–2389.

112. Matthay KK, Atkinson JB, Stram DO, et al. Patterns of relapse after autologous purged bone marrow transplantation for neuroblastoma: a Childrens Cancer Group pilot study. J Clin Oncol 1993;11(11):2226–2233.

113. Drize NJ, Keller JR, Chertkov JL. Local clonal analysis of the hematopoietic system shows that multiple small short-living clones maintain life-long hematopoiesis in reconstituted mice. Blood 1996;88(8):2927–2938.

114. Cooke KR. TNF alpha production to LPS stimulation by donor cells predicts the severity of experimental acute graft-versus-host disease. J Clin Invest 1999 (in press).

115. Antin JH, Ferrara JL. Cytokine dysregulation and acute graft-versus-host disease. Blood 1992;80(12):2964–2968.

116. Krenger W, Ferrara JL. Dysregulation of cytokines during graft-versus-host disease. J Hematother 1996;5(1):3–14.

117. Jadus MR, Wepsic HT. The role of cytokines in graft-versus-host reactions and disease [published erratum appears in Bone Marrow Transplant 1993 Jan;11(1):89]. Bone Marrow Transplant 1992;10(1):1–14.

118. Xun CQ, Thompson JS, Jennings CD, et al. Effect of total body irradiation, busulfan-cyclophosphamide, or cyclophosphamide conditioning on inflammatory cytokine release and development of acute and chronic graft-versus-host disease in H-2-incompatible transplanted SCID mice. Blood 1994;83(8):2360–2367.

119. Luger TA, Schwarz T. Evidence for an epidermal cytokine network. J Invest Dermatol 1990;95(6 suppl):100S–104S.

120. McKenzie RC, Sauder DN. The role of keratinocyte cytokines in inflammation and immunity. J Invest Dermatol 1990;95(6 suppl):105S–107S.

121. Kupper TS. Immune and inflammatory processes in cutaneous tissues. Mechanisms and speculations [published erratum appears in J Clin Invest 1991 Feb;87(2):753]. J Clin Invest 1990;86(6):1783–1789.

122. Norton J, Sloane JP. ICAM-1 expression on epidermal keratinocytes in cutaneous graft-versus-host disease. Transplantation 1991;51(6):1203–1206.

123. Cavender DE, Haskard DO, Joseph B, Ziff M. Interleukin 1 increases the binding of human B and T lymphocytes to endothelial cell monolayers. J Immunol 1986;136(1): 203–207.

124. Chang RJ, Lee SH. Effects of interferon-gamma and tumor necrosis factor-alpha on the expression of an Ia antigen on a murine macrophage cell line. J Immunol 1986;137(9): 2853–2856.

125. Thornhill MH, Wellicome SM, Mahiouz DL, et al. Tumor necrosis factor combines with IL-4 or IFN-gamma to selectively enhance endothelial cell adhesiveness for T cells. The contribution of vascular cell adhesion molecule-1-dependent and -independent binding mechanisms. J Immunol 1991;146(2):592–598.

126. Clift RA, Buckner CD, Appelbaum FR, et al. Allogeneic marrow transplantation in patients with acute myeloid leukemia in first remission: a randomized trial of two irradiation regimens [see comments]. Blood 1990;76(9):1867–1871.

127. Gale RP, Bortin MM, van Bekkum DW, et al. Risk factors for acute graft-versus-host disease. Br J Haematol 1987;67 (4):397–406.

128. Ringden O. Viral infection and graft-versus-host disease. In: Burakoff SJ, Deeg HJ, Ferrara J, Atkinson K, eds. Graft-versus-host disease. New York: Marcel Dekker, 1990:467.

129. Hill GR, Crawford JM, Cooke KR, et al. Total body irradiation and acute graft-versus-host disease: the role of gastrointestinal damage and inflammatory cytokines. Blood 1997;90(8):3204–3213.

130. Johnson BD, Drobyski WR, Truitt RL. Delayed infusion of normal donor cells after MHC-matched bone marrow transplantation provides an antileukemia reaction without graft-versus-host disease. Bone Marrow Transplant 1993;11(4): 329–336.

131. Johnson BD, Truitt RL. Delayed infusion of immunocompetent donor cells after bone marrow transplantation breaks graft-host tolerance allows for persistent antileukemic reactivity without severe graft-versus-host disease. Blood 1995;85(11):3302–3312.

132. Goulmy E, Schipper R, Pool J, et al. Mismatches of minor histocompatibility antigens between HLA-identical donors and recipients and the development of graft-versus-host disease after bone marrow transplantation [see comments]. N Engl J Med 1996;334(5):281–285.

133. den Haan JM, Sherman NE, Blokland E, et al. Identification of a graft versus host disease-associated human minor histocompatibility antigen. Science 1995;268(5216):1476–1480.

134. Liu X, Chesnokova V, Forman SJ, Diamond DJ. Molecular analysis of T-cell receptor repertoire in bone marrow transplant recipients: evidence for oligoclonal T-cell expansion in graft-versus-host disease lesions. Blood 1996;87(7):3032–3044.

135. Gaschet J, Trevino MA, Cherel M, et al. HLA-target antigens and T-cell receptor diversity of activated T cells invading the skin during acute graft-versus-host disease. Blood 1996;87(6):2345–2353.

136. Jones MS, Riley R, Hamilton BL, et al. Endogenous superantigens in allogeneic bone marrow transplant recipients rapidly and selectively expand donor T cells which can produce IFN-gamma. Bone Marrow Transplant 1994;14(5): 725–735.

137. Miconnet I, Roger T, Seman M, Bruley-Rosset M. Critical role of endogenous Mtv in acute lethal graft-versus-host disease. Eur J Immunol 1995;25(2):364–368.

138. Goulmy E, Pool J, van den Elsen PJ. Interindividual conservation of T-cell receptor beta chain variable regions by minor histocompatibility antigen-specific HLA-A→1-restricted cytotoxic T-cell clones. Blood 1995;85(9):2478–2481.

139. Kubo K, Yamanaka K, Kiyoi H, et al. Different T-cell receptor repertoires between lesions and peripheral blood in acute graft-versus-host disease after allogeneic bone marrow transplantation. Blood 1996;87(7):3019–3026.

140. Howell CD, Li J, Roper E, Kotzin BL. Biased liver T cell receptor V beta repertoire in a murine graft-versus-host disease model. J Immunol 1995;155(5):2350–2358.

141. Blazar BR, Taylor PA, Panoskaltsis-Mortari A, et al. Blockade of CD40 ligand-CD40 interaction impairs CD4+ T cell-mediated alloreactivity by inhibiting mature donor T cell expansion and function after bone marrow transplantation. J Immunol 1997;158(1):29–39.

142. Buhlmann JE, Noelle RJ. Therapeutic potential for blockade of the CD40 ligand, gp39. J Clin Immunol 1996;16(2):83–89.

143. Durie FH, Aruffo A, Ledbetter J, et al. Antibody to the ligand of CD40, gp39, blocks the occurrence of the acute and chronic forms of graft-vs-host disease. J Clin Invest 1994;94(3):1333–1338.

144. Korngold R, Sprent J. T cell subsets in graft-versus-host disease. In: Burakoff SJ, Deeg HJ, Ferrara J, Atkinson K, eds. Graft-versus-host disease: immunology, pathophysiology and treatment. New York: Marcel Dekker, 1990:31–50.

145. Unanue ER, Allen PM. The basis for the immunoregulatory role of macrophages and other accessory cells. Science 1987;236(4801):551–557.

146. Weiss A, Imboden JB. Cell surface molecules and early events involved in human T lymphocyte activation. Adv Immunol 1987;41:1–38.

147. Mosmann TR, Cherwinski H, Bond MW, et al. Two types of murine helper T cell clone. I. Definition according to profiles of lymphokine activities and secreted proteins. J Immunol 1986;136(7):2348–2357.

148. Sad S, Marcotte R, Mosmann TR. Cytokine-induced differentiation of precursor mouse CD8+ T cells into cytotoxic CD8+ T cells secreting Th1 or Th2 cytokines. Immunity 1995;2(3):271–279.

149. Weiss A. T lymphocyte activation. In: Paul WE, ed. Fundamental immunology. New York: Raven, 1989:359–384.

150. Hemler ME. Adhesive protein receptors on hematopoietic cells. Immunol Today 1988;9(4):109–113.

151. Allen RD, Staley TA, Sidman CL. Differential cytokine expression in acute and chronic murine graft-versus-host-disease. Eur J Immunol 1993;23(2):333–337.

152. Garlisi CG, Pennline KJ, Smith SR, et al. Cytokine gene expression in mice undergoing chronic graft-versus-host disease. Mol Immunol 1993;30(7):669–677.

153. Umland SP, Razac S, Nahrebne DK, Seymour BW. Effects of in vivo administration of interferon (IFN)-gamma, anti-IFN-gamma, or anti-interleukin-4 monoclonal antibodies in chronic autoimmune graft-versus-host disease. Clin Immunol Immunopathol 1992;63(1):66–73.

154. Doutrelepont JM, Moser M, Leo O, et al. Hyper IgE in stimulatory graft-versus-host disease: role of interleukin-4. Clin Exp Immunol 1991;83(1):133–136.

155. De Wit D, Van Mechelen M, Zanin C, et al. Preferential activation of Th2 cells in chronic graft-versus-host reaction. J Immunol 1993;150(2):361–366.

156. Krenger W, Snyder KM, Byon JC, et al. Polarized type 2 alloreactive CD4+ and CD8+ donor T cells fail to induce experimental acute graft-versus-host disease. J Immunol 1995;155(2):585–593.

157. Fowler DH, Kurasawa K, Husebekk A, et al. Cells of Th2 cytokine phenotype prevent LPS-induced lethality during murine graft-versus-host reaction. Regulation of cytokines and CD8+ lymphoid engraftment. J Immunol 1994;152(3):1004–1013.

158. Fowler DH, Kurasawa K, Smith R, et al. Donor CD4-enriched cells of Th2 cytokine phenotype regulate graft-versus-host disease without impairing allogeneic engraftment in sublethally irradiated mice. Blood 1994;84(10):3540–3549.

159. Pan L, Delmonte J Jr, Jalonen CK, Ferrara JL. Pretreatment of donor mice with granulocyte colony-stimulating factor polarizes donor T lymphocytes toward type-2 cytokine production and reduces severity of experimental graft-versus-host disease. Blood 1995;86(12):4422–4429.

160. Pan L, Bressler S, Cooke KR, et al. Long-term engraftment, graft-vs.-host disease, and immunologic reconstitution after experimental transplantation of allogeneic peripheral blood cells from G-CSF-treated donors [see comments]. Biol Blood Marrow Transplant 1996;2(3):126–133.

161. Zeng D, Dejbakhsh-Jones S, Strober S. Granulocyte colony-stimulating factor reduces the capacity of blood mononuclear cells to induce graft-versus-host disease: impact on blood progenitor cell transplantation. Blood 1997;90(1):453–463.

162. Kitabayashi A, Hirokawa M, Hatano Y, et al. Granulocyte colony-stimulating factor downregulates allogeneic immune responses by posttranscriptional inhibition of tumor necrosis factor-alpha production. Blood 1995;86(6):2220–2227.

163. Ghayur T, Seemayer TA, Kongshavn PA, et al. Graft-versus-host reactions in the beige mouse. An investigation of the role of host and donor natural killer cells in the pathogenesis of graft-versus-host disease. Transplantation 1987;44(2):261–267.

164. Ferrara JL, Guillen FJ, van Dijken PJ, et al. Evidence that large granular lymphocytes of donor origin mediate acute graft-versus-host disease. Transplantation 1989;47(1):50–54.

165. Nestel FP, Price KS, Seemayer TA, Lapp WS. Macrophage priming and lipopolysaccharide-triggered release of tumor necrosis factor alpha during graft-versus-host disease. J Exp Med 1992;175(2):405–413.

166. Laster SM, Wood JG, Gooding LR. Tumor necrosis factor can induce both apoptic and necrotic forms of cell lysis. J Immunol 1988;141(8):2629–2634.

167. Suzuki M, Suzuki Y, Ikeda H, et al. Apoptosis of murine large intestine in acute graft-versus-host disease after allogeneic bone marrow transplantation across minor histocompatibility barriers. Transplantation 1994;57(8):1284–1287.

168. Langley RG, Walsh N, Nevill T, et al. Apoptosis is the mode of keratinocyte death in cutaneous graft-versus-host disease. J Am Acad Dermatol 1996;35(2 Pt 1):187–190.

169. Gilliam AC, Whitaker-Menezes D, Korngold R, Murphy GF. Apoptosis is the predominant form of epithelial target cell injury in acute experimental graft-versus-host disease. J Invest Dermatol 1996;107(3):377–383.

170. Lindner H, Holler E, Ertl B, et al. Peripheral blood mononuclear cells induce programmed cell death in human endothelial cells and may prevent repair: role of cytokines. Blood 1997;89(6):1931–1938.

171. Langrehr JM, Murase N, Markus PM, et al. Nitric oxide production in host-versus-graft and graft-versus-host reactions in the rat. J Clin Invest 1992;90(2):679–683.

172. Falzarano G, Krenger W, Snyder KM, et al. Suppression of B-cell proliferation to lipopolysaccharide is mediated through induction of the nitric oxide pathway by tumor necrosis factor-alpha in mice with acute graft-versus-host disease. Blood 1996;87(7):2853–2860.

173. Krenger W, Falzarano G, Delmonte J Jr, et al. Interferon-gamma suppresses T-cell proliferation to mitogen via the nitric oxide pathway during experimental acute graft-versus-host disease. Blood 1996;88(3):1113–1121.

174. Hakim FT, Sharrow SO, Payne S, Shearer GM. Repopulation of host lymphohematopoietic systems by donor cells during graft-versus-host reaction in unirradiated adult F1 mice injected with parental lymphocytes. J Immunol 1991;146(7):2108–2115.

175. Duke RC, Persechini PM, Chang S, et al. Purified perforin induces target cell lysis but not DNA fragmentation. J Exp Med 1989;170(4):1451–1456.

176. Graubert TA, Russell JH, Ley TJ. The role of granzyme B in murine models of acute graft-versus-host disease and graft rejection. Blood 1996;87(4):1232–1237.

177. Braun MY, Lowin B, French L, et al. Cytotoxic T cells deficient in both functional fas ligand and perforin show residual cytolytic activity yet lose their capacity to induce lethal acute graft-versus-host disease. J Exp Med 1996;183(2):657–661.

178. Baker MB, Altman NH, Podack ER, Levy RB. The role of cell-mediated cytotoxicity in acute GVHD after MHC-matched allogeneic bone marrow transplantation in mice. J Exp Med 1996;183(6):2645–2656.

179. Chu JL, Ramos P, Rosendorff A, et al. Massive upregulation of the Fas ligand in lpr and gld mice: implications for Fas regulation and the graft-versus-host disease-like wasting syndrome. J Exp Med 1995;181(1):393–398.

180. Shresta S, Russell JH, Ley TJ. Mechanisms responsible for granzyme B-independent cytotoxicity. Blood 1997;89(11):4085–4091.

181. Via CS, Nguyen P, Shustov A, et al. A major role for the Fas pathway in acute graft-versus-host disease. J Immunol 1996;157(12):5387–5393.

182. Leithauser F, Dhein J, Mechtersheimer G, et al. Constitutive and induced expression of APO-1, a new member of the nerve growth factor/tumor necrosis factor receptor superfamily, in normal and neoplastic cells. Lab Invest 1993;69(4):415–429.

183. Baker MB, Podack ER, Levy RB. Perforin- and Fas-mediated cytotoxic pathways are not required for allogeneic resistance to bone marrow grafts in mice. Biol Blood Marrow Transplant 1995;1(2):69–73.

184. Lee RK, Spielman J, Zhao DY, et al. Perforin, Fas ligand, and tumor necrosis factor are the major cytotoxic molecules used by lymphokine-activated killer cells. J Immunol 1996;157(5):1919–1925.

185. Hattori K, Hirano T, Ushiyama C, et al. A metalloproteinase inhibitor prevents lethal acute graft-versus-host disease in mice. Blood 1997;90(2):542–548.

186. Nishimura M, Uchida S, Mitsunaga S, et al. Characterization of T-cell clones derived from peripheral blood lymphocytes of a patient with transfusion-associated graft-versus-host disease: Fas-mediated killing by CD4+ and CD8+ cytotoxic T-cell clones and tumor necrosis factor beta production by CD4+ T-cell clones. Blood 1997;89(4):1440–1445.

187. Jones JM, Wilson R, Bealmear PM. Mortality and gross pathology of secondary disease in germfree mouse radiation chimeras. Radiat Res 1971;45(3):577–588.

188. Bekkum DW, van Roodenburg J, Heidt PJ, der Waaij DV. Mitigation of secondary disease of allogeneic mouse radiation chimeras by modification of the intestinal microflora. J Natl Cancer Inst 1974;52(2):401–404.

189. Storb R, Prentice RL, Buckner CD, et al. Graft-versus-host disease and survival in patients with aplastic anemia treated by marrow grafts from HLA-identical siblings. Beneficial effect of a protective environment. N Engl J Med 1983;308(6):302–307.

190. Miller W, Flynn P, McCullough J, et al. Cytomegalovirus infection after bone marrow transplantation: an association with acute graft-v-host disease. Blood 1986;67(4):1162–1167.

191. Einsele H, Ehninger G, Hebart H, et al. Incidence of local CMV infection and acute intestinal GVHD in marrow transplant recipients with severe diarrhoea. Bone Marrow Transplant 1994;14(6):955–963.

192. Gratama JW, Sinnige LG, Weijers TF, et al. Marrow donor immunity to herpes simplex virus: association with acute graft-versus-host disease. Exp Hematol 1987;15(7):735–740.

193. Gratama JW, Zwaan FE, Stijnen T, et al. Herpes-virus immunity and acute graft-versus-host disease. Lancet 1987;1(8531):471–474.

194. Appleton AL, Sviland L, Peiris JS, et al. Human herpes virus-6 infection in marrow graft recipients: role in pathogenesis of graft-versus-host disease. Newcastle upon Tyne Bone Marrow Transport Group. Bone Marrow Transplant 1995;16(6):777–782.

195. Matzinger P. Tolerance, danger, and the extended family. Annu Rev Immunol 1994;12:991–1045.

196. Fuchs EJ, Matzinger P. Is cancer dangerous to the immune system? Semin Immunol 1996;8(5):271–280.

197. Sale GE, Buckner CD. Pathology of bone marrow in transplant recipients. Hematol Oncol Clin North Am 1988;2(4):735–756.

198. Glucksberg H, Storb R, Fefer A, et al. Clinical manifestations of graft-versus-host disease in human recipients of marrow from HL-A-matched sibling donors. Transplantation 1974;18(4):295–304.

199. Przepiorka D, Weisdorf D, Martin P, et al. 1994 Consensus Conference on Acute GVHD Grading. Bone Marrow Transplant 1995;15(6):825–828.

200. Rowlings PA, Przepiorka D, Klein JP, et al. IBMTR Severity Index for grading acute graft-versus-host disease: retrospective comparison with Glucksberg grade. Br J Haematol 1997;97(4):855–864.

201. Beatty PG, Clift RA, Mickelson EM, et al. Marrow transplantation from related donors other than HLA-identical siblings. N Engl J Med 1985;313(13):765–771.

202. Ringden O, Nilsson B. Death by graft-versus-host disease associated with HLA mismatch, high recipient age, low marrow cell dose, and splenectomy. Transplantation 1985;40(1):39–44.

203. Sasazuki T, Juji T, Morishima Y, et al. Effect of matching of class I HLA alleles on clinical outcome after transplantation of hematopoietic stem cells from an unrelated donor. Japan Marrow Donor Program [see comments]. N Engl J Med 1998;339(17):1177–1185.

204. Petersdorf EW, Gooley TA, Anasetti C, et al. Optimizing outcome after unrelated marrow transplantation by comprehensive matching of HLA class I and II alleles in the donor and recipient [In Process Citation]. Blood 1998; 92(10):3515–3520.

205. Sullivan KM, Deeg HJ, Sanders J, et al. Hyperacute graft-v-host disease in patients not given immunosuppression after allogeneic marrow transplantation. Blood 1986;67(4): 1172–1175.

206. Storb R, Deeg HJ, Whitehead J, et al. Methotrexate and cyclosporine compared with cyclosporine alone for prophylaxis of acute graft versus host disease after marrow transplantation for leukemia. N Engl J Med 1986;314(12):729–735.

207. Storb R, Pepe M, Deeg HJ, et al. Long-term follow-up of a controlled trial comparing a combination of methotrexate plus cyclosporine with cyclosporine alone for prophylaxis of graft-versus-host disease in patients administered HLA-identical marrow grafts for leukemia [letter]. Blood 1992;80(2):560–561.

208. Jacobson P, Uberti J, Davis W, Ratanatharathorn V. Tacrolimus: a new agent for the prevention of graft-versus-host disease in hematopoietic stem cell transplantation. Bone Marrow Transplant 1998;22(3):217–225.

209. Basara N, Blau WI, Romer E, et al. Mycophenolate mofetil for the treatment of acute and chronic GVHD in bone marrow transplant patients. Bone Marrow Transplant 1998; 22(1):61–65.

210. Yu C, Seidel K, Nash RA, et al. Synergism between mycophenolate mofetil and cyclosporine in preventing graft-versus-host disease among lethally irradiated dogs given DLA-nonidentical unrelated marrow grafts. Blood 1998;91(7):2581–2587.

211. Hale DA, Gottschalk R, Maki T, Monaco AP. Determination of an improved sirolimus (rapamycin)-based regimen for induction of allograft tolerance in mice treated with anti-lymphocyte serum and donor-specific bone marrow. Transplantation 1998;65(4):473–479.

212. Marmont AM, Horowitz MM, Gale RP, et al. T-cell depletion of HLA-identical transplants in leukemia. Blood 1991;78(8):2120–2130.

213. Drobyski WR, Ash RC, Casper JT, et al. Effect of T-cell depletion as graft-versus-host disease prophylaxis on engraftment, relapse, and disease-free survival in unrelated marrow transplantation for chronic myelogenous leukemia. Blood 1994;83(7):1980–1987.

214. Champlin RE, Horowitz MM, van Bekkum DW, et al. Graft failure following bone marrow transplantation for severe aplastic anemia: risk factors and treatment results. Blood 1989;73(2):606–613.

215. Kusunoki Y, Chen W, Martin PJ. Prevention of marrow graft rejection without induction of graft-versus-host disease by a cytotoxic T-cell clone that recognizes recipient alloantigens. Blood 1998;91(11):4038–4044.

216. Martin PJ. Prevention of allogeneic marrow graft rejection by donor T cells that do not recognize recipient alloantigens: potential role of a veto mechanism. Blood 1996;88(3): 962–969.

217. Fowler DH, Whitfield B, Livingston M, et al. Non-host-reactive donor CD8+ T cells of Tc2 phenotype potently inhibit marrow graft rejection. Blood 1998;91(11):4045–4050.

218. Martin PJ, Schoch G, Fisher L, et al. A retrospective analysis of therapy for acute graft-versus-host disease: initial treatment. Blood 1990;76(8):1464–1472.

219. Martin PJ, Schoch G, Fisher L, et al. A retrospective analysis of therapy for acute graft-versus-host disease: secondary treatment. Blood 1991;77(8):1821–1828.

220. Storek J, Gooley T, Siadak M, et al. Allogeneic peripheral blood stem cell transplantation may be associated with a high risk of chronic graft-versus-host disease. Blood 1997;90 (12):4705–4709.

221. Sullivan KM, Shulman HM, Storb R, et al. Chronic graft-versus-host disease in 52 patients: adverse natural course and successful treatment with combination immunosuppression. Blood 1981;57(2):267–276.

222. Atkinson K, Horowitz MM, Gale RP, et al. Consensus among bone marrow transplanters for diagnosis, grading and treatment of chronic graft-versus-host disease. Committee of the International Bone Marrow Transplant Registry. Bone Marrow Transplant 1989;4(3):247–254.

223. Atkinson K, Horowitz MM, Gale RP, et al. Risk factors for chronic graft-versus-host disease after HLA-identical sibling bone marrow transplantation. Blood 1990;75(12): 2459–2464.

224. Chao NJ, Parker PM, Niland JC, et al. Paradoxical effect of thalidomide prophylaxis on chronic graft-vs.-host disease. Biol Blood Marrow Transplant 1996;2(2):86–92.

225. Wingard JR, Piantadosi S, Vogelsang GB, et al. Predictors of death from chronic graft-versus-host disease after bone marrow transplantation. Blood 1989;74(4):1428–1435.

226. Sullivan KM, Witherspoon RP, Storb R, et al. Prednisone and azathioprine compared with prednisone and placebo for treatment of chronic graft-v-host disease: prognostic influence of prolonged thrombocytopenia after allogeneic marrow transplantation. Blood 1988;72(2):546–554.

227. Sullivan KM, Witherspoon RP, Storb R, et al. Alternating-day cyclosporine and prednisone for treatment of high-risk chronic graft-v-host disease. Blood 1988;72(2):555–561.

228. Keenan RJ, Eiras G, Burckart GJ, et al. Immunosuppressive properties of thalidomide. Inhibition of in vitro lymphocyte proliferation alone and in combination with cyclosporine or FK506. Transplantation 1991;52(5):908–910.

229. Ostraat O, Riesbeck K, Qi Z, et al. Thalidomide prolonged graft survival in a rat cardiac transplant model but had no inhibitory effect on lymphocyte function in vitro. Transpl Immunol 1996;4(2):117–125.

230. Vogelsang GB, Hess AD, Gordon G, Santos GW. Treatment and prevention of acute graft-versus-host disease with thalidomide in a rat model. Transplantation 1986;41(5): 644–647.

231. Lim SH, McWhannell A, Vora AJ, Boughton BJ. Successful treatment with thalidomide of acute graft-versus-host disease after bone-marrow transplantation [letter]. Lancet 1988;1(8577):117.

232. Ringden O, Aschan J, Westerberg L. Thalidomide for severe acute graft-versus-host disease [letter]. Lancet 1988;2 (8610):568.

233. Parker PM, Chao N, Nademanee A, et al. Thalidomide as salvage therapy for chronic graft-versus-host disease. Blood 1995;86(9):3604–3609.
234. Heney D, Norfolk DR, Wheeldon J, et al. Thalidomide treatment for chronic graft-versus-host disease. Br J Haematol 1991;78(1):23–27.
235. Rovelli A, Arrigo C, Nesi F, et al. The role of thalidomide in the treatment of refractory chronic graft-versus-host disease following bone marrow transplantation in children. Bone Marrow Transplant 1998;21(6):577–581.
236. Forsyth CJ, Cremer PD, Torzillo P, et al. Thalidomide responsive chronic pulmonary GVHD [see comments]. Bone Marrow Transplant 1996;17(2):291–293.
237. Mackall CL, Gress RE. Pathways of T-cell regeneration in mice and humans: implications for bone marrow transplantation and immunotherapy. Immunol Rev 1997;157: 61–72.
238. Kook H, Goldman F, Padley D, et al. Reconstruction of the immune system after unrelated or partially matched T-cell-depleted bone marrow transplantation in children: immunophenotypic analysis and factors affecting the speed of recovery. Blood 1996;88(3):1089–1097.
239. Lamb LS Jr, Gee AP, Henslee-Downey PJ, et al. Phenotypic and functional reconstitution of peripheral blood lymphocytes following T cell-depleted bone marrow transplantation from partially mismatched related donors. Bone Marrow Transplant 1998;21(5):461–471.
240. Small TN, Avigan D, Dupont B, et al. Immune reconstitution follwing T-cell depleted bone marrow transplantation: effect of age and posttransplant graft rejection prophylaxis. Biol Blood Marrow Transplant 1997;3(2):65–75.
241. Cavazzana-Calvo M, Bordigoni P, Michel G, et al. A phase II trial of partially incompatible bone marrow transplantation for high-risk acute lymphoblastic leukaemia in children: prevention of graft rejection with anti-LFA-1 and anti-CD2 antibodies. Societe Francaise de Greffe de Moelle Osseuse. Br J Haematol 1996;93(1):131–138.
242. Nachbaur D, Fink FM, Nussbaumer W, et al. CD34+-selected autologous peripheral blood stem cell transplantation (PBSCT) in patients with poor-risk hematological malignancies and solid tumors. A single-centre experience. Bone Marrow Transplant 1997;20(10):827–834.
243. Talmadge JE, Reed E, Ino K, et al. Rapid immunologic reconstitution following transplantation with mobilized peripheral blood stem cells as compared to bone marrow. Bone Marrow Transplant 1997;19(2):161–172.
244. Ottinger HD, Beelen DW, Scheulen B, et al. Improved immune reconstitution after allotransplantation of peripheral blood stem cells instead of bone marrow. Blood 1996;88(7):2775–2779.
245. Anderson KC, Soiffer R, DeLage R, et al. T-cell-depleted autologous bone marrow transplantation therapy: analysis of immune deficiency and late complications. Blood 1990;76(1):235–244.
246. Chao NJ, Berry GJ, Advani R, et al. Epstein-Barr virus-associated lymphoproliferative disorder following autologous bone marrow transplantation for non-Hodgkin's lymphoma. Transplantation 1993;55(6):1425–1428.
247. O'Reilly RJ, Small TN, Papadopoulos E, et al. Biology and adoptive cell therapy of Epstein-Barr virus-associated lymphoproliferative disorders in recipients of marrow allografts. Immunol Rev 1997;157:195–216.
248. Gross TG, Steinbuch M, DeFor T, et al. B cell lymphoproliferative disorders following hematopoietic stem cell transplantation: risk facors, treatment and outcome. Bone Marrow Transplant 1999;23:251–258.
249. Miller JS, Arthur DC, Litz CE, et al. Myelodysplastic syndrome after autologous bone marrow transplantation: an additional late complication of curative cancer therapy [see comments]. Blood 1994;83(12):3780–3786.
250. Kollmannsberger C, Beyer J, Droz JP, et al. Secondary leukemia following high cumulative doses of etoposide in patients treated for advanced germ cell tumors. J Clin Oncol 1998;16(10):3386–3391.
251. Deeg HJ, Socie G. Malignancies after hematopoietic stem cell transplantation: many questions, some answers. Blood 1999;91(6):1833–1844.
252. Curtis RE, Rowlings PA, Deeg HJ, et al. Solid cancers after bone marrow transplantation [see comments]. N Engl J Med 1997;336(13):897–904.
253. Guinan EC. Boussiotis VA, Neuberg D, et al. Transplantation of anergic histoincompatible bone marrow allografts. N Engl J Med 1999;340:1704–1714.
254. McSweeney PA, Storb R. Mixed chimerism: preclinical studies and clinical applications. Biol Blood Marrow Transplant 1999;5:192–203.
255. Sykes M, Preffer F, McAfee S, et al. Mixed lymphohaemopoietic chimerism and graft-versus-lymphoma effects after non-myeloablative therapy and HLA-mismatched bone-marrow transplantation. Lancet 1999;353:1755–1759.
256. Starzl TE, Demetris AJ, Murase N, et al. The lost chord: microchimerism and allograft survival. Immunol Today 1996;17(12):577–584; discussion 588.

Chapter 38

Cell Transplantation

Luca Inverardi
Alberto Pugliese
Camillo Ricordi

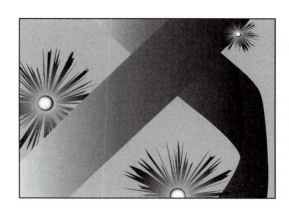

History

The long history of cell transplantation begins in the 15th century, when the very first blood transfusions were attempted in humans. This form of transplantation preceded by 2 centuries the first morphologic description of a cell as a definite biologic unit (1) that followed the invention of the microscope. At the beginning of this century, after the discovery of enzymes capable of cell separation with the preservation of cell viability, scientists understood the striking potentials of cell transplantation and began to develop procedures for cell isolation from solid organs for transplantation of the purified cell suspension (2,3). Their efforts have led to the substantial progress that we have witnessed in the last 2 decades.

Today a wide variety of cell types are used for clinical transplantation, and even more models are currently being tested for future clinical applications. One of the greatest advantages of most cell-transplantation approaches is that the transplantation can be generally performed through relatively safe and noninvasive procedures, which do not require general anesthesia or major surgery.

Isolation Procedures

Most types of cell transplants share common problems related to their retrieval from the original tissue or organ (i.e., cell separation and purification), and there is significant technical overlap for many procedures that facilitates the sharing of experience and progress in different fields.

Excluding harvesting of peripheral blood and bone marrow, where cells are already physically separated, obtaining isolated cell preparations often requires some degree of processing of the native solid organ or tissue. Separation is accomplished by a variety of mechanical, chemical, and/or enzymatic techniques. This is an important stage because the traumatic stress induced by these procedures can affect the yield and quality of the recovered cells (4). During the last decade, improved procedures for the separation of cell clusters from tissues and organs have been developed to minimize mechanical stress (5–8). Collagenase is presently the most commonly used and effective enzyme in tissue digestion. On the other hand, because of its poor characterization and significant variability in enzymatic activity, even the most standardized isolation procedure may yield variable amounts of viable cells, depending on the batch of the enzyme used. To minimize this variability, new classes of collagenase with more defined chemical and catalytic properties are being developed (9–11).

In some instances, cell separation results in a mixture of cell types, and only further purification allows the isolation of the desired cell population. This can be achieved in several ways, including isopicnic or isokinetic centrifugation on density gradients (12). Other means of purification are based on the different functional properties of each cell type (e.g., adhesion to plastic or substrate-coated surfaces) or on the presence of different antigens on the cell surface (i.e., techniques of panning or adhesion to magnetic beads coated with specific antibodies). Antigenic differences can also be used to select the desired cell type with a fluorescence-activated cell sorter (FACS) after labeling the cells with specific fluorochrome-conjugated antibodies (13,14).

Major Factors Affecting Cell Engraftment

One of the key elements for the success of a cell transplant is the adequate engraftment of the transplanted cells. Engraftment probably depends on the availability of oxygen and nutrients, initially by diffusion and subsequently by neovascularization (15–18).

It still remains controversial whether reinnervation is crucial to the long-term survival and optimal function of the graft (19–21). Other factors that might affect the outcome of a cellular transplant are the local availability of relevant growth factors or immunoregulatory proteins (22).

The nonspecific inflammatory reaction commonly observed at the transplant site may adversely affect cell engraftment, as a result of the release by immune cells of soluble inflammatory mediators, including selected cytokines and nitric oxide, which are potentially cytotoxic to the transplanted cells (23–28).

New observations have recently emerged that expand our knowledge of the obstacles to successful engraftment, including anoikis and local activation of coagulation and complement. Anoikis (homelessness) defines the occurrence of apoptosis of isolated cells that is initiated by their loss of interaction with extracellular matrix proteins. This indeed might represent one of the concurrent causes of poor cell engraftment, since extracellular matrix proteins are largely removed by commonly used isolation procedures. Islets of Langerhans, among other cells, have been shown to be susceptible to anoikis after isolation (29). Lastly, implanting cellular grafts in the blood stream might pose an additional hurdle to successful engraftment, since the procedure has been shown to efficiently initiate coagulation and complement activation in a model where islets were implanted in the portal vein (30).

Our growing understanding of these mechanisms will lead to efficient strategies to improve cell survival and engraftment that will contribute to a better overall outcome of cell transplantation.

Immune Recognition of Transplanted Cells

A second major element affecting the outcome of a cell graft is the immune response of the host. The basic mechanism of rejection is the recognition by the recipient immune system of foreign cell surface antigens on the membrane of the transplanted cells. Although still controversial, it appears that the enzymatic digestion or other procedures such as cryopreservation that are performed during or after the separation and purification procedures of different cell types may modify the expression of relevant cell-surface antigens (31,32).

Separation, purification, and preservation procedures could also render isolated cells more susceptible to immune recognition compared with the whole native organ. Furthermore, non-specific inflammation occurring at the site of cell implant might amplify subsequent, specific, immune recognition. This could partly explain measurable differences in the fate of cell transplants versus whole-organ transplants for selected diseases such as diabetes mellitus, where islet transplants have a lower rate of success than pancreas transplants.

Because of the poor availability of markers allowing early recognition of an imminent rejection, rescue attempts with immunosuppressive drugs are not always possible. This problem becomes even more prevalent when transplanting immature tissues (i.e., fetal cells), since transplanted cells need to become mature and fully competent before their functional activity can be monitored, thus making it difficult, if not impossible, to diagnose rejection episodes early.

Two strategies, which are not mutually exclusive, have been utilized with the aim of preventing immune recognition and rejection. The first is based on immunosuppression of the recipient (which will be extensively covered in other chapters of this text). The second approach relies on strategies aimed at rendering transplanted cells "less immunogenic." This can be achieved by manipulations of the cells prior to grafting, by the use of physical barriers (bioartificial membranes), or by implantation into immunoprivileged sites such as the thymus, the testis, and the anterior chamber of the eye (33–36).

Cell graft manipulation prior to transplantation includes elimination of highly immunogenic ("antigen presenting") cells from tissue grafts by selected in vitro culture conditions (low temperature, high oxygen concentration, hyperbaric storage), by monoclonal antibodies or UV-radiation–based purging, and by FACS-based mechanical separation (37–40). Similar techniques might also result in the modulation or alteration of the pattern of cell-membrane antigen expression, namely MHC molecules. Some of these approaches have proven to significantly increase graft survival in a variety of experimental models (37–41).

In recent years, following the development of new biocompatible and long-lasting artificial interfaces, there has been increasing attention toward the possible use of membranes or capsules to isolate cellular grafts from the host environment. Once encapsulated, transplanted cells are surrounded by a physical barrier that prevents interactions between the immune system of the host and the graft, but does not compromise oxygen and nutrient exchanges (42–52).

There are two main types of encapsulation: 1) microencapsulation refers to the inclusion of single or few islets or other cell clusters into a matrix coated by a semipermeable outer layer; 2) macroencapsulation aims to comprise larger amounts of cells within single devices such as hollow fibers, vascular prostheses, or diffusion chambers.

Cell Preservation

Another important issue in cell transplantation is the preservation of cells. In fact, at least for some cell-transplant applications, a significant delay between the time of cell preparation and the actual transplant time might occur. For instance, a combination of cells from more than one donor may be needed to obtain enough tissue for adequate graft function, requiring the development of efficient strategies for the preservation of viable cells. While most cell lineages are amenable to short-term culture, longer preservation times are often a necessity such as in the case of human-cell harvesting with the obvious unpredictability of donor availability. Cells can be frozen in the presence of cryoprotective agents, thus allowing long-term storage without the formation of ice crystals that disrupt the cell membrane and structure with consequent cell death (53,54). Cells are stored at very low temperatures (in liquid nitrogen at 196°C below zero), which decreases the metabolic rate to near nil and allows indefinite preservation of viability and function, once thawed and transplanted. New cryoprotective agents and methods of cryopreservation are being developed to further improve quantitative and qualitative recovery of cell preparations (55–57).

Current and Potential Clinical Applications of Cell Transplantation

Significant progress has been achieved in the last 10 years in cell transplantation–related technology and immunosuppressive strategies, and several clinical trials for the treatment by cellular transplantation of many human diseases have begun. Table 38-1 lists current applications of cell transplantation, procedures from

Table 38-1. Cell Transplantation Models in Clinical Practice and Research Development

Bone-marrow and stem-cell transplantation	**Chondrocyte transplantation**

Bone-marrow and stem-cell transplantation

Hematopoietic malignancies
   Acute leukemia
   Chronic myeloid leukemia
   Lymphoma
   Myelodysplastic syndromes
Bone-marrow depression from chemotherapy of
   Breast carcinoma
   Neuroblastoma
   Germ-line-cell tumors
Nonmalignant diseases and metabolic diseases
   Aplastic anemia
   Sickle cell anemia
   Immunologic dysfunctions
   Severe, combined, immunodeficiency syndrome
   Wiskott-Aldrich syndrome
   Chediak-Higashi syndrome
   Thalassemia
   Gaucher's disease
Tolerance induction to other organ or cellular grafts
Therapy of autoimmune diseases
   Lupus
   Reumathoid arthritis
   Multiple sclerosis
   Diabetes
Treatment of nonhematologic, nonautoimmune diseases
   Muscular dystrophy
   Liver diseases

Transplantation of islets of Langerhans

Treatment of insulin-dependent (type I) diabetes mellitus
Treatment of type II diabetes mellitus

Chondrocyte transplantation

Articular cartilage defects

Epidermal-cell transplantation

Extensive wounds
Burns

Hepatocyte transplantation

Enzymatic defects
   Bilirubin UDP-glucuronil transferase
   Albumin synthase
   Mucopolysaccaridosis
Liver failure

Myoblast and myocyte transplantation

Muscular dystrophy (Duchenne)
Myocardial infarction

Neural-cell transplantation

Spinal cord injury
Parkinson's disease
Huntington's disease
Hypothalamus deficiencies in production of releasing hormones
Retinal lesions
Alleviation of acute/chronic pain

Vascular endothelial-cell transplantation

Internal lining of vascular prosthetic devices
Prevention of postangioplasty restenosis

---

already established models (i.e., bone-marrow transplantation), and experimental protocols.

Transplantation of Bone Marrow and Stem Cells

Bone-marrow transplantation is a well-established model of cell transplantation, dating back more than 60 years (58,59). The aim of bone-marrow transplantation is to provide the patient with a multipotent stem-cell population capable of self-renovation and differentiation into mature blood cells to replace deficient or pathologic cells of the host (60,61). Some of the major indications for bone-marrow transplantation are aplastic anemia, acute and chronic leukemia, and selected types of lymphoma. One of the most exciting potential applications of bone-marrow transplantation is presently being tested, which consists of the administration of donor bone marrow to induce donor-specific hyporesponsiveness to either solid organs or tissues transplanted concurrently (62). Although graft-versus-host disease (GVHD) is still a feared complication, it has been possible to drastically

reduce its incidence by depleting the donor bone marrow of those T cells responsible for the development of GVHD (63,64). However, T-cell–depleted bone-marrow preparations have reduced engraftment ability with the potential of leading to graft failure and, in the case of hemopoietic malignancies, to the relapse of the original disease (65).

Stem-cell isolation from the peripheral blood could be an alternative to bone-marrow transplantation when a contraindication to the latter procedure exists (e.g., aplastic syndrome or bone-marrow contamination by malignant cells [66,67]).

Recent exciting data have been obtained on the potential therapeutic role of bone-marrow transplantation in diseases of nonhematologic origin. A beneficial role of allogeneic or autologous bone-marrow transplantation has been reported in selected autoimmune diseases refractory to conventional therapy (68–75), and clinical trials to confirm and extend this preliminary observation are being planned. Also, data are accumulating that indicate the unexpected multipotency of bone-marrow–derived stem cells (including mesenchymal stem cells) in giving rise to a remarkably diverse progeny, which includes myocytes, chondrocytes, osteoblasts, and hepatocytes (76–78), thus opening up exciting possibilities of new therapeutic approaches for numerous diseases.

Transplantation of Islets of Langerhans

Administration of exogenous insulin is still the therapy of choice for insulin-dependent diabetes mellitus. Although insulin therapy allows patients to live an almost normal life, it has been associated with the development of long-term vascular complications. Moreover, even multiple blood-glucose measurements, repeated daily injections, strict dietary habits, and constant exercise do not always prevent the onset of late complications, and these measures significantly decrease patients' quality of life. The ideal solution to overcome these problems is represented by successful biologic replacement of insulin-producing tissue and, in particular, by pancreatic islet transplantation. After the first unsuccessful attempts of the 1970s and 1980s, newer isolation techniques with higher purification, greater yield of islets, and better immunosuppressive strategies have renewed the interest in clinical islet transplantation. Between 1974 and 1996, a total of 305 islet transplants were performed worldwide in 35 institutions; 215 of these transplants were performed between 1990 and 1996. Insulin independence for more than 1 week was documented in 33 of 305 patients, and 30 of these patients were among the 215 transplanted between 1990 and 1996. Partial graft function persisted for longer than 1 year in 33% of the 167 patients with negative C-peptide before transplantation (79,80).

Several ongoing trials are evaluating the key issues for islet functional survival such as the influence of the transplant microenvironment, the role of novel immunosuppression regimens, HLA matching procedures, immunoalteration of islets prior to transplantation, and cotransplantation of donor bone-marrow cells for the induction of immune hyporesponsiveness.

Transplantation of Epidermal Cells

There are patients in whom the skin has suffered such extensive damage that it does not allow conventional full-thickness replacement (81,82). Autologous epidermal cells can be cultured and expanded for the treatment of such extensive burns or wounds. While the first clinical trials have shown only limited proliferation and differentiation of epidermal cells in culture toward full functional epidermis (83–85), new data suggest that the improvement of in vitro culture conditions might indeed result in dramatic progress in keratinocyte transplantation success (86). Although allogeneic skin grafts seem to be successful in animal models (87), the survival of allotransplanted epidermal cells in clinical trials was only temporary, but it accelerated wound healing (88). Cotransplantation of as little as 5% of autologous keratinocytes in an allogeneic graft results in a better take and a reduced allospecific immune response, potentially broadening the indication for epidermal-cell transplantation in patients considered ineligible (89).

Transplantation of Hepatocytes

Rodent experimental models have proven that hepatocyte transplantation can correct several congenital enzyme deficiencies (90–92). Moreover, the development of bioartificial devices (93) used as storage chambers for hepatocytes has been shown to reverse congenital enzyme deficiencies and to restore lost hepatic function (94–96). A similar approach was partially successful in a monkey model system where hepatic-cell autografts were performed (97). The safety of this procedure has been confirmed also in human studies. However, sustained graft function has not yet been achieved (98). Liver assist devices, on the other hand, have been utilized in clinical pilot trials in patients with fulminant hepatic failure to bridge them to a liver transplant. This has been made possible by recent improvements in hepatocyte isolation and culture and by the availability of new biocompatible materials (99). One of the key issues in the field of hepatocyte transplantation is the characterization of those stimulators and hepatotrophic factors that are present in the portal vein blood and that derive at least in part from the pancreas (100–105). Further investigations are needed to determine the relative importance of these factors and their minimal requirement to warrant functional survival of hepatocellular tissue transplanted in ectopic sites.

Transplantation of Chondrocytes

There have been reports of chondrocyte transplantation in animal models to correct articular cartilage defects either after traumatic lesions or during the course of chronic inflammatory disease. The current direction of research is to explore the origin and functional properties of chondrocytes in an allogeneic environment (106–108).

Transplantation of Myoblasts and Myocytes

Myoblasts have recently been used in a variety of promising applications. For instance, some forms of hereditary muscular dystrophy have been ameliorated in experimental animal models by transplanting functionally preserved myoblasts (109–111). The first clinical trials were attempted in patients suffering from Duchenne's muscular dystrophy in whom allogeneic myoblasts were transplanted intramuscularly (112,113). It was clear, however, that in these cases there was an absolute requirement for immunosuppression even to obtain a short-term survival of the graft. Further studies are ongoing to determine whether the increased muscular strength noted in these first transplanted patients is caused by the transplant itself or by other external factors. Recent applications of myocyte transplantation include the use of autologous cells to improve functional performance of the heart after experimental scarring or induced infarction. Autologous cardiomyocytes were also shown to prevent scar thinning in both small and large animals (114,115).

Transplantation of Neural Tissue

Increasing attention is focused on the progress made in the field of neural-tissue transplantation. Cell transplantation could be used to replace those neuronal populations lost in Parkinson's or Huntington's diseases and, in turn, would restore endogenous production of those neurotransmitters whose deficiency is responsible for the clinical signs and symptoms of these diseases. Different potential sources have been described such as the adrenal medulla, fetal mesencephalic tissue, cells derived from the substantia nigra (dopaminergic replacement), or cholinergic brain cells (for the treatment of Huntington's disease) (116).

Other clinical settings in which neuronal-cell transplantation could be useful include chronic pain, epilepsy, and schizophrenia. Moreover, cells derived from the hypothalamus could be used to correct deficiencies in the production of hypothalamic hormone–releasing factors (e.g., gonadotropins), and the use of retinal-cell grafting could prove useful to replace damaged cells in the host retina (117,118).

Recent observations have further extended the potential of neural-cell transplantation by suggesting the feasibility of global cell replacement by administration of neural stem cells in a murine system of diffuse demyelination of the CNS (119).

Also, alternative approaches are being explored in which lost functions of the CNS could be assumed by engineered cells of a different origin, as in a recent report (120) where L-DOPA–producing marrow stromal cells were impanted in Parkinson rats.

Another area of intensive studies in this field implements transplantation of parts of the peripheral nervous system to restore the vital functions after spinal-cord injuries (121–123). For instance, these procedures have been tried to up-regulate alternative neural pathways, rather than replacing the lost main tract, or to transplant peripheral nerves into the gap created in spinal cord transaction to promote growth of neural tissue (124,125). Recently, hollow-fiber implants containing Schwann's-cell strings have been tested as a potential means of nerve regeneration after spinal-cord transection.

Transplantation of Vascular Endothelial Cells

The internal lining of endothelial cells in vascular prostheses has been proposed in vascular reconstructive surgery to prevent or decrease the incidence of thrombosis. The patency of dog artificial vascular devices was improved by internally coating such devices with a layer of fibronectin and endothelial cells. With these devices no immunologic acute response was detected even in an allogeneic model (126). The first clinical trials have applied this technology to tibial and coronary arterial grafts and to venous replacement grafts (127).

Endothelial-cell grafts have also been shown to hold promise for preventing restenosis after angioplasy in a porcine, large-animal model (128). The potential clinical implications of this approach, if its efficacy is confirmed, are obvious.

Future Perspectives in Cell Transplantation

Cell-transplant procedures have been traditionally intended to restore lost functional tissue following infection, trauma, toxicity, or autoimmune disease and to replace genetically dysfunctional/deficient cell populations (i.e., inherited metabolic diseases). However, the potential of many new and exciting applications has yet to be tested. For instance, the use of cell-transplant techniques to induce tolerance of donor cells, tissues, or solid organs or the use of genetically engineered autologous cells to restore a lost function (i.e., insulin secretion, growth hormone synthesis) has enormous clinical potential.

The infusion of donor bone marrow in combination with other organ or tissue/cell grafts is believed to enhance a state of posttransplantation chimerism in which immunocompetent cells from both the donor and the recipient coexist in the same individual. The interaction between the host and recipient immune systems might lead to a state of unresponsiveness or even donor-specific tolerance (129,130). This crucial observation was first described in animal models where the hypothesis was raised that the cell type responsible for the induction of the tolerant state could be an antigen-presenting cell, in particular, the dendritic cell (62). This hypothesis was later supported by circumstantial evidence in patients who stopped immunosuppressive therapy after liver transplantation. In these patients, cell migration from the graft into most of the recipient's tissues was clearly documented, and the migrating cells appeared to be similar to dendritic cells (62,131–133). Further experimental studies are currently evaluating the significance and characteristics of these cells, which seem capable of modulating the host immune system toward unresponsiveness and tolerance. Meanwhile, clinical trials have started to evaluate the relationships between the chimeric state that follows bone-marrow infusion and solid-organ graft acceptance with encouraging preliminary data (134–136).

Genetic Engineering of Cells

Transfection of cells with functional genes may lead to a new era for cell transplantation, even though targeted gene therapy may eventually make cells obsolete as a vehicle of gene products (137,138). For the time being, however, transplanting cells that carry a functional gene into patients specifically lacking a gene product could be instrumental in restoring production of the missing hormones, proteins, and other molecules that are fundamental for the function of the human body. Several viral vectors are presently available for gene transfer, with different vectors being suitable for different applications, depending on their properties and limitations. Among these, retroviruses pose problems connected with the possible random integration of the viral genes into the cells' genome, with a significant potential for the unwanted disruption of genes and even tumorigenesis. Moreover, even if retroviruses are able to infect a large variety of cells, they predominantly penetrate into dividing cells, and this limits the number of cell types that they can successfully transduce (139). Research is now focusing on the use of retroviral strains capable of infecting nondividing cells and of other viral vectors such as herpes viruses, adenoviruses, adenoassociated viruses, and lentiviruses (140–144).

Several techniques have been tested for gene delivery into cells in addition to viral vectors. These include microinjection, electroporation, lipofection, or precipitation with calcium phosphate or diethylaminoethyl (DEAE) dextran.

Several clinical trials have recently started following the encouraging results obtained in experimental studies (138,145, 146). Disease states in which gene therapy could be beneficial include genetically transmitted enzyme deficiencies (adenosine deaminase, alpha-1-antitrypsin, phenylalanine hydroxylase, purine-nucleoside phosphorilase, glucocerebrosidase in Gaucher's disease, and factor VIII in hemophilia) or genetic diseases in which the translation of the mutated gene product leads to a dysfunctional form of protein or enzyme (thalassemia, sickle cell anemia, cystic fibrosis [147], altered low-density lipoprotein [LDL], and thyroid-stimulating-hormone [TSH] receptors).

Concluding Remarks

In conclusion, the field of cell transplantation is rapidly evolving. The latest advances deriving from research and experimental models await further testing in clinical trials, which will allow an increasing number of cell-transplant applications to be developed. The transition from research to clinical practice will be subject to ethical and scientific regulations, but that hopefully will not block or delay the implementation of research breakthroughs in the clinical setting at qualified academic institutions.

References

1. Hooke K. Micrographia or some physiological descriptions of minute bodies made by magnifying glasses with observation and inquires thereupon. London: Martyn and Allestry, 1665:112.
2. Rous P, Jones FS. A method for obtaining suspensions of living cells from fixed tissues and for the plating out of individual cells. J Exp Med 1916;23:549.
3. Oakley CL, Warrack GH, Van Hevningen WE. The collagenase (k toxin) of *Clostridium welchii* type A. J Pathol Bacteriol 1946;58:229.
4. Waymouth C. To disaggregate or not to disaggregate. Injury and cell disaggregation, transient or permanent. In Vitro 1974;10:97.
5. Ricordi C, Lacy PE, Finke EH, et al. Automated method for isolation of human pancreatic islets. Diabetes 1988;37: 413–420.
6. Ricordi C, Socci C, Davalli A, et al. Isolation of elusive pig islet. Surgery 1990;107:688–694.
7. Ricordi C, Tzakis AG, Carroll PB, et al. Human islet isolation and allotransplantation in 22 consecutive cases. Transplantation 1992;53:407–414.
8. Lakey JRT, Warnock GL, Brierton M, et al. Development of an automated computer controlled islet isolation system. Cell Transplant 1997;6:47–57.
9. Linetsky E, Bottino R, Lehmann R, et al. Improved human islet isolation using a new enzyme blend, Liberase™. Diabetes 1997;46:1120–1123.
10. Lakey JR, Cavanagh TJ, Zieger MA, Wright M. Evaluation of a purified enzyme blend for the recovery and function of canine pancreatic islets. Cell Transplant 1998;7:365.
11. Klock G, Kowalski MB, Hering BJ, et al. Fractions from commercial collagenase preparations: use in enzymic isolation of the islets of Langerhans from porcine pancreas. Cell Transplant 1996;5:543.
12. London NJM, Robertson GSM, Chadwick DR, et al. Adult islet purification. In: Ricordi C, ed. Methods in cell transplantation. Austin, Texas: RG Landes, 1995:439–454.
13. Davies JE, James RF, London NJ, Robertson GS. Optimization of the magnetic field used for immunomagnetic islet purification. Transplantation 1995;59:767.
14. Lilja H, Arkadopoulos N, Blanc P, et al. Fetal rat hepatocytes: isolation, characterization, and transplantation in the Nagase analbuminemic rats. Transplantation 1997;64:1240.
15. Davalli AM, Scaglia L, Brevi M, et al. Pituitary cotransplantation significantly improves the performance, insulin content, and vascularization of renal subcapsular islet grafts. Diabetes 1999;48:59.
16. Beger C, Cirulli V, Vajkoczy P, et al. Vascularization of purified pancreatic islet-like cell aggregates (pseudoislets) after syngeneic transplantation. Diabetes 1998;47:559.
17. Ajioka I, Akaike T, Watanabe Y. Expression of vascular endothelial growth factor promotes colonization, vascularization, and growth of transplanted hepatic tissues in the mouse. Hepatology 1999;29:396.
18. Schrezenmeir J, Gero L, Laue C, et al. The role of oxygen supply in islet transplantation. Transplant Proc 1992;24: 2925.
19. Rosenberg L. Clinical islet cell transplantation. Are we there yet? Int J Pancreatol 1998;24:145.
20. Korsgren O, Jansson L, Sundler F. Reinnervation of transplanted fetal porcine endocrine pancreas. Evidence for initial growth and subsequent degeneration of nerve fibers in the islet grafts. Transplantation 1996;62:352.
21. Pundt LL, Kondoh T, Conrad JA, Low WC. Transplantation of human striatal tissue into a rodent model of Huntington's disease: phenotypic expression of transplanted neurons and host-to-graft innervation. Brain Res Bull 1996;39:23.
22. Danova M, Aglietta M. Cytokine receptors, growth factors and cell cycle in human bone marrow and peripheral blood hematopoietic progenitors. Haematologica 1997;82:622.
23. Nagata M, Mullen Y, Matsuo S. The impact of T cells in nonspecific destruction of β cells in mice. Transplant Proc 1992;24:988.
24. Kaufman DB, Platt JL, Rabe FL, et al. Differential roles of Mac-1+ cells, and CD4+ and CD8+ T lymphocytes in primary nonfunction and classic rejection of islet allografts. J Exp Med 1990;172:291.
25. London NJM, Robertson GSM, Chadwick DR, et al. Human pancreatic islet isolation and transplantation. Clin Transplant 1994;8:421.
26. Stevens RB, Lokeh A, Ansite JD, et al. Role of nitric oxide in the pathogenesis of early pancreatic islet dysfunction during rat and human intraportal islet transplantation. Transplant Proc 1994;26:692.

27. Nussler AK, Ricordi C, Carroll PB, et al. Hepatic nitric oxide generation as a putative mechanism for failure of intrahepatic cell grafts. Transplant Proc 1992;24:2997.

28. Simeonovic CJ. Xenogeneic islet transplantation. Xenotransplantation 1999;6:1.

29. Wang RN, Rosenberg L. Maintenance of beta cell function and survival following islet isolation requires reestablishment of the islet-matrix interaction. J Endocrinol 1999;163:181.

30. Bennet W, Sundberg B, Groth C-G, et al. Incompatibility between human blood and isolated islets of Langerhans. A finding with implication for clinical intraportal islet transplantation? Diabetes 1999;48:1907.

31. Iwasa K, Izumi R, Shimizu K, et al. Effect of cryopreservation on the immunogenicity of pancreatic islets in xenotransplantation. Transplant Proc 1994;26:2439.

32. Gramberg D, Ernst E, Liu X, et al. Isokinetic gradients decrease islet graft immunogenicity. Transplant Proc 1994;26:753.

33. Okamoto S, Hara Y, Streilein JW. Induction of anterior chamber-associated immune deviation with lymphoreticular allogeneic cells. Transplantation 1995;59:377.

34. Ar'Rajab A, Dawidson IJ, Harris RB, Sentementes JT. Immune privilege of the testis for islet xenotransplantation (rat to mouse). Transplant Proc 1994;26:3446.

35. Turvey SE, Hara M, Morris PJ, Wood KJ. Mechanisms of tolerance induction after intrathymic islet injection: determination of the fate of alloreactive thymocytes. Transplantation 1999;68:30.

36. Moulian N, Berrih-Aknin S. Fas/APO-1/CD95 in health and autoimmune disease: thymic and peripheral aspects. Semin Immunol 1998;10:449.

37. Scharp DW, Lacy PE. Islet transplantation: a review of the objective, the concepts, the problems, the progress, and the future. In: Dubemard JM, Sutherland DER, eds. International handbook of pancreas transplantation. Dordrecht, The Netherlands: Kluwer, 1989:455.

38. Lafferty KJ, Prowse SJ, Simeonovic C. Immunobiology of tissue transplantation: a return of the passenger leukocyte concept. Annu Rev Immunol 1987;1:143.

39. Lau H, Reemstma K, Hardy MA. Prolongation of rat islet allograft survival by direct ultraviolet irradiation of the graft. Science 1984;223:607.

40. Alejandro R, Latif Z, Noel J, et al. Effect of anti Ia antibodies, culture and cyclosporine on prolongation of canine islet allograft survival. Diabetes 1987;36:269.

41. Kenyon NS, Strasser S, Alejandro R. Ultraviolet light immunomodulation of canine islets for prolongation of allograft survival. Diabetes 1990;39:305.

42. Morris PJ. Immunoprotection of therapeutic cell transplants by encapsulation. Trends Biotechnol 1996;14:163.

43. Cotton CK. Engineering challenges in cell-encapsulation technology. Trends Biotechnol 1996;14:158.

44. Zekorn TD, Horcher A, Mellert J, et al. Biocompatibility and immunology in the encapsulation of islets of Langerhans (bioartificial pancreas). Int J Artif Organs 1996;19:251.

45. Davis MW, Vacanti JP. Toward development of an implantable tissue engineered liver. Biomaterials 1996;17:365.

46. Lanza RP, Hayes JL, Chick WL. Encapsulated cell technology. Nat Biotechnol 1996;14:1107.

47. Lanza RP, Chick WL. Transplantation of pancreatic islets. Ann N Y Acad Sci 1997;831:323.

48. Lanza RP, Chick WL. Immunoisolation: at a turning point. Immunol Today 1997;18:135.

49. Lanza RP, Chick WL. Transplantation of encapsulated cells and tissues. Surgery 1997;121:1.

50. Hottinger AF, Aebischer P. Treatment of diseases of the central nervous system using encapsulated cells. Adv Tech Stand Neurosurg 1999;25:3.

51. Davis MW, Vacanti JP. Toward development of an implantable tissue engineered liver. Biomaterials 1996;17:365.

52. Stange J, Mitzner S. Hepatocyte encapsulation—initial intentions and new aspects for its use in bioartificial liver support. Int J Artif Organs 1996;19:45.

53. Rajotte RV, Warnock GL, Kneteman NM. Cryopreservation of insulin producing tissue in rats and dogs. World J Surg 1984;8:179.

54. Ricordi C, Kneteman NM, Scharp DW, et al. Transplantation of insulin producing tissue in rats and dogs. World J Surgery 1988;12:861.

55. Beattie GM, Crowe JH, Lopez AD, et al. Trehalose: a cryoprotectant that enhances recovery and preserves function of human pancreatic islets after long-term storage. Diabetes 1997;46:519.

56. Rajotte RV. Islet cryopreservation protocols. Ann N Y Acad Sci 1999;18:875.

57. Arita S, Kasraie A, Une S, et al. Improved recovery of cryopreserved canine islets by use of beraprost sodium. Pancreas 1999;19:289.

58. Osgood EE, Riddle MC, Matthews TJ. Aplastic anemia treated with diilv transfusions and intravenous marrow: a case report. Ann Intern Med 1939;13:357.

59. Thomas ED, Lochte HL, Lu WC, et al. Intravenous infusion of bone marrow in patients receiving radiation and chemotherapy. N Engl J Med 1957;257:491.

60. Hardy RE, Ikpeazu EV. Bone marrow transplantation: a review. J Nat Med Assoc 1989;81:518.

61. DeMagalhaes-Silverinan M, Donnenberg AD, Pincus SM, et al. Bone marrow transplantation: a reivew. Cell Transplant 1993;2:75.

62. Starzl TE, Demetris AJ, Murase N, et al. Donor cell chimerism permitted by immunosuppressive drugs: a new view of organ transplantation. Immunol Today 1993;14:326.

63. Butturini A, Gale P. T-cell depletion in bone marrow transplantation for leukemia. Br J Hematol 1989;72:1.

64. Ramsay N, Kersey J. Indications for marrow transplantation in acute lymphoblastic leukemia. Blood 1990;75:815.

65. Patterson J, Prentice HG, Brenner MK, et al. Graft rejection following HLA matched T lymphocyte depleted bone marrow transplantation. Br J Haematol 1986;63:221.

66. Lasky LC. Hematopoietic reconstitution using progenitors recovered from blood. Transfusion 1989;29:552.

67. Broxmeyer HE, Gluckman E, Auerbach A, et al. Human umbilical cord blood: a clinically useful source of transplantable hematopoietic stem/progenitor cells. Int J Cell Cloning 1990;8:76.

68. Martini A, Maccario R, Ravelli A, et al. Marked and sustained improvement two years after autologous stem cell transplantation in a girl with systemic sclerosis. Arthritis Rheum 1999;42:807.

69. Olalla JI, Ortin M, Hermida G, et al. Disappearance of lupus anticoagulants after allogeneic bone marrow transplantation. Bone Marrow Transplant 1999;23:83.
70. Brodsky RA, Smith BD. Bone marrow transplantation for autoimmune diseases. Curr Opin Oncol 1999;11:83.
71. Marmont AM. Stem cell transplantation for severe autoimmune diseases: progress and problems. Haematologica 1998;83:733.
72. Wang B, Yamamoto Y, El-Badri NS, Good RA. Effective treatment of autoimmune disease and progressive renal disease by mixed bone marrow transplantation that establishes a stable mixed chimerism in BXSB recipient mice. Proc Natl Acad Sci USA 1999;96:3012.
73. Sherer Y, Shoenfeld Y. Autoimmune diseases and autoimmunity post bone marrow transplantation. Bone Marrow Transplant 1998;22:873.
74. Ikehara S. Autoimmune diseases as stem cell disorders: normal stem cell transplant for their treatment. Int J Mol Med 1998;1:5.
75. Tyndall A. Hematopoietic stem cell transplantation in rheumatic diseases other than systemic sclerosis and systemic lupus erythematosus. J Rheumatol Suppl 1997;48:94.
76. Pittenger MF, Mackay AM, Beck SC, et al. Multilineage potential of adult human mesenchymal stem cells. Science 1999;284:143.
77. Prockop DJ. Marrow stromal cells as stem cells for non-hematopoietic tissues. Science 1997;276:71.
78. Petersen BE, Bowen WC, Patrene KD, et al. Bone marrow as a potential source of hepatic oval cells. Science 1999;284:1168.
79. Hering BJ, Ricordi C. Islet transplantation for patients with type I diabetes: results, research priorities and reasons for optimism. Graft 1999;2:12.
80. Hering BJ, Brendel MD, Schultz AO, et al. Int Islet Transpl Reg Newslett 1996;6:1.
81. Green H, Kehinde O, Thomas J. Growth of cultured human epidermal cells into multiple epithelia suitable for grafting. Proc Natl Acad Sci USA 1979;76:5665.
82. Rheinwald JG, Green H. Serial cultivation of strains of human epidermal keratinocytes: the formation of keratinizing colonies from single cells. Cell 1975;6:331.
83. O'Connor NE, Mulliken JB, Banks-Schlegel S, et al. Grafting of burns with cultured epithelium prepared from autologous epidermal cells. Lancet 1981;1:75.
84. O'Connor NE, Gallico GG, Compton CC, et al. Grafting of burns with cultured epithelium prepared from autologous epidermal cells. II. Intermediate term results on three pediatric patients. In: Hunt TK, Heppenstall KB, Pines E, et al, eds. Soft and hard tissue repair—biological and clinical aspects. Vol. 2. New York: Praeger Scientific, 1984: 283.
85. Gallico GG III, O'Connor NE, Compton CC, et al. Permanent coverage of large burn wounds with autologous cultured human epithelium. N Engl J Med 1984;311:448.
86. Pellegrini G, Ranno R, Stracuzzi G, et al. The control of epidermal stem cells (holoclones) in the treatment of massive full-thickness burns with autologous keratinocytes cultured on fibrin. Transplantation 1999;68:868.
87. Demidem A, Chiller JM, Kanagawa O. Dissociation of antigenicity and immunogenicity of neonatal epidermal allografts in the mouse. Transplantation 1990;49:966.
88. Philips TJ, Provan A, Colbert D, et al. A randomized single-blind controlled study of cultured epidermal allografts in the treatment of split-thickness skin graft donor sites. Arch Dermatol 1993;129:879.
89. Larochelle F, Ross G, Rouabhia M. Permanent skin replacement using engineered epidermis containing fewer than 5% syngeneic keratinocytes. Lab Invest 1998;78: 1089.
90. Matas AJ, Sutherland DER, Steffes MW, et al. Hepatocellular transplantation for metabolic deficiencies: decrease of plasma bilirubin in gunn rats. Science 1976;192:892.
91. Groth CG, Arborgh B, Bjorken C, et al. Correction of hyperbilirubinemia in the glucuronyltransferase-deficient rat by intraportal hepatocyte transplantation. Transplant Proc 1977;19:313.
92. Vroemer JPAM, Buurman WA, Heirweg KPM, et al. Hepatocyte transplantation for enzyme deficiency disease in congeneic rats. Transplantation 1984;38:23.
93. Fremond B, Malandain C, Guyomard C, et al. Correction of bilirubin conjugation in the gunn rat using hepatocytes immobilized in alginate gel beads as an extracorporeal bioartificial liver. Cell Transplant 1993;2:453.
94. Nyberg SL, Shirabe K, Madhusudan VP, et al. Extracorporeal application of a gel-entrapment, bioartificial liver: demonstration of drug metabolism and other biochemical functions. Cell Transplant 1993;2:441.
95. Ribeiro J, Nordlinger B, Ballet F, et al. Intrasplenic hepatocellular transplantation corrects hepatic encephalopathy in portocaval shunt rats. Hepatology 1992;15:12.
96. Tompkins RG, Yarmush ML. Prospects for an artificial liver. Transplant Rev 1993;7:191.
97. Kasai S, Sawa M, Mito M, et al. Evaluation of an artificial liver support device using isolated hepatocytes. Prog Artif Organs 1983;2:734.
98. Mito M, Kusano M. Hepatocyte transplantation in man. Cell Transplant 1993;2:65.
99. Kamohara Y, Rozga J, Demetriou AA. Artificial liver: review and Cedars Sinai experience. J Hepatobiliary Pancreatic Surg 1998;5:273.
100. Starzl TE, Porter KA, Putnam CW. Intraportal insulin protects from the liver injury of portocaval shunt in dogs. Lancet 1975;2:1241.
101. Starzl TE, Terblanche J. Hepatotrophic substances. Prog Liver Dis 1979;6:135.
102. Starzl TE, Porter KA, Francavilla A, et al. 100 years of hepatotrophic controversy. In: Porter R, Whelan J, eds. Hepatotrophic factors. Ciba Foundation Symposium No. 55. Amsterdam, The Netherlands: Excerpta Medica (Elsevier), 1978:111.
103. Starzl TE, Porter KA, Watanabe K, et al. The effect of insulin, glucagon and insulin/glucagon infusion upon liver morphology and cell division after complete portocaval shunt in dogs. Lancet 1976;6:821.
104. Ricordi C, Lacy PE, Callery MP, et al. Trophic factors from pancreatic islet in combined hepatocyte-islet allografts enhance hepatocellular survival. Surgery 1989;105:218.
105. Ricordi C, Zeng Y, Tzakis A, et al. Evidence that canine pancreatic islets promote the survival of human hepatocytes in nude mice. Transplantation 1991;52:749.
106. Brittberg M. Autologous chondrocyte transplantation. Clin Orthop 1999;367(suppl):S147.

107. Frenkel SR, Di Cesare PE. Degradation and repair of articular cartilage. Front Biosci 1999;4:D671.

108. Chen FS, Frenkel SR, Di Cesare PE. Chondrocyte transplantation and experimental treatment options for articular cartilage defects. Am J Orthop 1997;26:396.

109. Morgan JE, Hoffman EP, Partridge TA. Normal myogenic cells from newborn mice restore normal histology to degenerating muscles of the mdx mouse. J Cell Biol 1990; 111:2437.

110. Partridge TA, Morgan JE, Coulton GR, et al. Conversion of mdx myofibers from dystrophin-negative to dystrophin-positive by injection of normal myoblasts. Nature 1989;337: 176.

111. Partridge TA. Myoblast transfer. A possible therapy for inherited myopathies? Muscle Nerve 1991;14:197.

112. Tremblay JP, Malouin F, Roy R, et al. Results of a triple blind clinical study of myoblast transplantations without immunosuppressive treatment in young boys with Duchenne muscular dystrophy. Cell Transplant 1993;2: 99.

113. Law PK, Goodwin TG, Fang Q. Cell transplantation as an experimental treatment for Duchenne muscular dystrophy. Cell Transplant 1993;2:485.

114. Sakai T, Li RK, Weisel RD, et al. Autologous heart cell transplantation improves cardiac function after myocardial injury. Ann Thorac Surg 1999;68:2074.

115. Li RK, Weisel RD, Mickle DA, et al. Autologous porcine heart cell transplantation improved heart function after a myocardial infarction. J Thorac Cardiovasc Surg 2000;119: 62.

116. Freed WJ. Neural transplantation: prospects for clinical use. Cell Transplant 1993;2:13.

117. Fine A. Cell transplantation: report of a conference held at the Royal College of Physicians. JR Coll Physicians Lond 1988;22:188.

118. Kohen S, Kohen L, Gabrielian K, et al. Influence of anti-CD4 (W3/23) therapy on the prevention of rejection of transplanted retinal pigment epithelia in a rat model. Invest Ophthalmol Vis Sci 1993;34:1095.

119. Yandava BD, Billinghurst LL, Snyder EY. "Global" cell replacement is feasible via neural stem cell transplantation: evidence from the dysmyelinated shiverer mouse brain. Proc Natl Acad Sci USA 1999;96:7029.

120. Schwarz EJ, Alexander GM, Prockop DJ, Azizi SA. Multi-potential marrow stromal cells transduced to produce L-DOPA: engraftment in a rat model of Parkinson disease. Hum Gene Ther 1999;10:2539.

121. Notias F, Horvat JC, Nfira JC, et al. Double step neural transplants to replace degenerated motoneurons. In: Dunnet SB, Richards SJ, eds. Neural transplantation: from molecular basis to clinical applications. Amsterdam, The Netherlands: Elsevier, 1990:239.

122. Reier PJ, Houle JD, Jakeman L, et al. Transplantation of fetal spinal cord tissue into acute and chronic hemisection and contusion lesions of the adult rat spinal cord. In: Gash DM, Sladek JR, eds. Transplantation in the mammalian CNS. Amsterdam, The Netherlands: Elsevier, 1988:173.

123. Tesler A. Intraspinal transplants. Ann Neurol 1991;29: 115.

124. Bray GM, Villegas-Perez MP, Vidal-Sanz, et al. The use of peripheral nerve grafts to enhance neuronal survival, promote growth and permit terminal reconnections in the central nervous system of adult rats. J Exp Biol 1987; 132:5.

125. Paino CL, Bunge MB. Induction of axon growth into Schwann cells implants grafted into lesioned adult rat spinal cord. Exp Neurol 1991;14:254.

126. Hess F, Steeghs S, Jerusalem R, et al. Patency and morphology of fibrous polyurethane vascular prostheses implanted in the femoral artery of dogs after seeding with subcultivated endothelial cells. Eur J Vasc Surg 1993;7:402.

127. Herring MB. The use of the endothelial seeding of prosthetic arterial bypass grafts. Surg Ann 1991;23:157.

128. Nugent HM, Rogers C, Edelman ER. Endothelial implants inhibit intimal hyperplasia after porcine angioplasty. Circ Res 1999;84:384.

129. Ildstadt ST, Starzl TRE, Ricordi C. Bone marrow chimerism and pancreatic islet grafts. In: Ricordi C, ed. Pancreatic islet transplantation. Austin, TX: Landes, 1992:168.

130. Zeng Y, Ricordi C, Tzakis AG, et al. Long-term survival of donor-specific pancreatic islet xenografts in fully xenogeneic chimeras (WF rat → B 10 mouse). Transplantation 1992;53:277.

131. Ricordi C, Ildstadt ST, Demetris AJ, et al. Host dendritic cells are replaced ubiquitously with those of the donor following rat to mouse transplantation. Lancet 1992;339: 1610.

132. Starzl TE, Demetris AJ, Trucco M, et al. Chimerism and donor specific nonreactivity 27 to 29 years after kidney allotransplantation. Transplantation 1993;55:1272.

133. Starzl TE, Demetris AJ, Trucco M, et al. Systemic chimerism in human female recipients of male livers. Lancet 1992; 340:876.

134. Fontes P, Rao A, Demetris AJ, et al. Augmentation with bone marrow of donor leukocyte migration for kidney, liver, heart, and pancreas islet transplantation. Lancet 1994;344:151.

135. Ricordi C, Karatzas T, Nery J, et al. High-dose donor bone marrow infusion to enhance allograft survival: the effect of timing. Transplantation 1997;63:7.

136. Garcia-Morales R, Carreno M, Mathew J, et al. The effects of chimeric cells following donor bone marrow infusions as detected by PCR-flow assays in kidney transplant recipients. J Clin Invest 1997;99:1118.

137. Anderson WF. Prospects for human gene therapy. Science 1984;226:401.

138. Anderson WF. Human gene therapy. Science 1992;256: 808.

139. Roe T, Reynolds TC, Yu G, et al. Integration of murine leukemia virus DNA depends on mitosis. EMBO J 1993;12:2099.

140. Kochanek S. High-capacity adenoviral vectors for gene transfer and somatic gene therapy. Hum Gene Ther 1999; 19:2451.

141. Grimm D, Kleinschmidt JA. Progress in adeno-associated virus type 2 vector production: promises and prospects for clinical use. Hum Gene Ther 1999;10:2445.

142. Salmons B, Gunzburg WH. Targeting of retroviral vectors for gene therapy. Hum Gene Ther 1993;4:129.

143. Klimatcheva E, Rosenblatt JD, Planelles V. Lentiviral vectors and gene therapy. Front Biosci 1999;4:D481.
144. Haggerty S, Dempsey MP, Stevenson K. Retroviral sequences to allow infection of non-dividing cells. In: Whelan WJ, Ahmad F, Baumbach L, et al, eds. Advances in gene technology: molecular biology and human disease. Miami Short Reports. Vol. 4. Oxford: IRL Press, 1994:95.
145. Parkman R. The application of bone marrow transplantation to the treatment of genetic disease. Science 1986;32:1373.
146. Culver KW, Anderson WF, Bleise RM. Lymphocyte gene therapy. Hum Gene Ther 1991;2:17.
147. Hyde SC, Gill DR, Higgins CF, et al. Correction of the ion transport defect in cystic fibrosis transgenic mice by gene therapy. Nature 1993;362:250.

Chapter 39

Liver Transplantation

Roberto Gedaly

James J. Pomposelli

Roger L. Jenkins

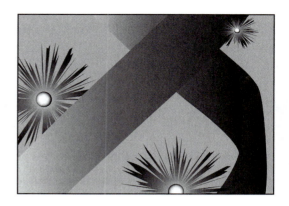

Recipient Selection

Liver transplantation has become the treatment of choice for end-stage liver disease. With improvements in patient selection, organ preservation, surgical technique, and perioperative care, combined with safer and more efficacious immunosuppressive agents, patients now enjoy survival rates that exceed 85% at 1 year and 70% at 5 years after liver transplantation (1,2). Although the number of patients waiting for liver transplantation increases each year (approximately 16,000 currently), the number of available donors has remained relatively stable over the past 10 years (approximately 4000) (3). The disparity between the number of individuals waiting and the number of available organs has resulted in a waiting-list mortality of approximately 25%. The shortage of available organs has put a premium on maximizing the use of every potential donor while efforts are continuing to increase cadaver-organ donation. Novel surgical techniques such as split-liver and living-donor liver transplantation provide an opportunity to expand the donor pool and to significantly reduce waiting-list mortality (4,5).

In this chapter we will provide an overview of liver transplantation with emphasis on surgical indications and new techniques to expand the donor pool. The clinical application of immunosuppressive agents and complications commonly encountered in the postoperative period will be explored.

Recipient Selection

The success of liver transplantation is closely related to the rational selection of patients most likely to benefit from surgery. To obtain maximal benefit from every available organ, there has been increasing emphasis on careful patient selection to improve overall survival. Previously, many organs were lost in futile attempts to save patients in unsalvageable states.

Perhaps the greatest challenge facing transplant physicians and surgeons in the era of donor-organ shortage is accurate timing of liver replacement. Ideally, patients should be identified and referred for evaluation early so that sufficient time can be accrued on the transplant waiting list before complications develop. Unfortunately, many patients are referred for transplantation after significant complications of cirrhosis and portal hypertension have already developed (1,6).

The indications for liver transplantation include the following (7):

1. Nonalcoholic cirrhosis (primary biliary cirrhosis, cryptogenic cirrhosis, primary sclerosing cholangitis)
2. Alcoholic cirrhosis (patients should have documented abstinence for a period of 6 months with a reform program in place)
3. Acute and chronic viral hepatitis (fulminate hepatitis A, B, and/or C)
4. Vascular disorders (Budd-Chiari syndrome)
5. Metabolic disorders (alpha-1 antitrypsin deficiency, Wilson's disease, hemochromatosis, galactosemia, tyrosinemia, glycogen storage disease, familial amyloidotic polyneuropathy)
6. Congenital biliary disorders (biliary atresia, Byler's disease, hepatic fibrosis)
7. Nonmetastatic primary hepatobiliary tumors
8. Selective metastatic liver neoplasms

Patients who are appropriate to undergo liver-transplant evaluation should have abnormalities in at least two parameters listed in the Child's Turcott Pugh (CTP) scoring system (Table 39-1) (7). The system is based on five parameters: two clinical parameters and three laboratory tests. Each parameter is assigned 1 (normal), 2 (abnormal), or 3 (severe abnormality) points depending on disease severity. Therefore, the CTP score ranges between 5 to 15 points. The clinical parameters include the presence or absence of ascites and/or hepatic encephalopathy. For example, a patient without ascites would be given 1 CTP point. A patient with controlled ascites with diuretic therapy would be given 2 points. Intractable ascites despite aggressive medical therapy is assigned 3 points. Laboratory tests include serum albumin, total bilirubin, and prothrombin time. A score of 7 points is the minimal amount required for transplant evaluation (Table 39-2).

Patients listed with the United Network of Organ Sharing (UNOS) with a CTP score between 7 and 9 points are considered status-3 patients. Patients with a CTP score of 10 or more points are qualified for urgency status upgrade to status 2B. Chronically ill patients who have life-threatening decompensation may be upgraded to status 2A. Acutely ill patients with fulminate hepatic failure and a life expectancy of less than 1 week receive the highest priority at status 1. Status 1 and 2A patients are considered "high urgency" and should obtain the next available liver in the region with the appropriate blood type. In addition to disease severity, overall time on the transplant waiting list is another parameter used to stratify patients with similar disease severity.

Table 39-1. Child's Turcott Pugh Scoring System

Parameter	1	2	3
Ascites	None	Easily controlled	Intractable
Encephalopathy	None	Easily controlled	Coma
Albumin	>3.5 mg/dL	2.8–3.5 mg/dL	<2.8 mg/dL
Prothrombin time (INR)	<15 (1.7) sec	15–17 (1.7–2.1) sec	>17 (2.1) sec
Total bilirubin	<2 mg/dL	2–3 mg/dL	>3 mg/dL
for cholestatic disease	<4 mg/dL	4–10 mg/dL	>10 mg/dL

Table 39-2. United Network for Organ Sharing (UNOS) Listing Status

- **Status 1**—Fulminant liver failure with a life expectancy of less than 7 days. Included in this group are those with fulminant liver failure as traditionally defined, primary graft nonfunction, or hepatic artery thrombosis within 7 days of transplantation.
- **Status 2A**—Adults with chronic liver disease in the ICU with a life expectancy of less than 7 days.
- **Status 2B**—Adults with chronic liver disease who have a Child-Pugh score >10, or >7 and meet one of four criteria: persistent variceal hemorrhage despite treatment, hepatorenal syndrome, refractory ascites or hepatohydrothorax, or stage 3 or 4 encephalopathy.
- **Status 3**—Requires continuous medical care; hospitalized or at home, but not meeting status 2B criteria.

Table 39-3. Absolute, Relative Contraindications and Patients at High Risk

Absolute Contraindications

HIV positivity
Extrahepatic malignancy
Active sepsis
Advanced cardiopulmonary disease
Inability to comply with an immunosuppression protocol

Patients at High Risk

Renal insufficiency
Obesity (body mass index ≥35)
Retransplantation
Advanced liver disease
Multiorgan transplants

Relative Contraindications

Active alcohol or drug abuse
Intrahepatic tumor >5 cm or multicentric hepatoma
Cholangiocarcinoma
Hepatitis B, HbeAg (+), hepatitis B virus-DNA (+)

Potential donors are matched by ABO blood group compatibility. Cross matching is not performed as is done in renal transplantation.

Because of organ shortages, an increasing number of patients are transplanted at higher urgency status. Not surprisingly, patients who received liver transplantation early in their disease course had improved overall survival rate and lower hospital costs compared with patients who were transplanted after complications developed (8,9).

Contraindications

The list of absolute and relative contraindications to liver transplantation is shown in Table 39-3. Recent myocardial infarction, advanced cardiopulmonary disease, uncontrolled bacterial or fungal infection, HIV positivity, and extrahepatic malignancy are considered absolute contraindications in most centers (10).

Relative contraindications to liver transplantation include age over 65 years (older patients in relatively good health can be considered), acute or chronic renal failure (not hepatorenal syndrome), recurrent biliary sepsis, severe hypoxemia resulting from right to left shunts, uncontrolled underlying psychiatric disorder, active alcohol or drug abuse, intrahepatic tumor >5 cm or multicentric hepatoma, spontaneous bacterial peritonitis (treated for less than 5 days), systemic bacterial infection, cholangiocarcinoma, and hepatitis E antigen or hepatitis B virus-DNA positivity. Inadequate social or family support and inability to maintain the medical regimen can also exclude a patient (6,10,11).

Pretransplant Evaluation

Before patients can be listed for transplant, an extensive medical, social, and psychiatric evaluation is performed. Complete history and physical exam, laboratory studies, viral serologys, and organ-specific evaluations are carried out (8,12).

Measurement of the serum alpha-fetoprotein concentration and liver imaging using MRI, CT scan, and ultrasound are essential to identify possible hepatocellular carcinoma and to define the vascular anatomy. Cardiopulmonary evaluation includes electrocardiogram and echocardiography. Patients with hypoxemia should undergo careful evaluation to determine the etiologic factor. Particular attention should be directed toward ruling out the presence of pulmonary hypertension, which significantly increases operative mortality. Chest radiography and pulmonary function testing are performed in all cases (8).

Evaluation by a social worker and a psychiatrist should be included to establish social and psychiatric stability of the patient and family (13). Patients need significant support during the long waiting time prior to liver transplantation and during the follow-up period, which requires frequent follow-up visits and obtaining proper medications.

Evaluation by infectious-disease specialists is an important part of the evaluation process to screen for underlying infectious disease and to establish a baseline. Immunizations against pneumococcus and hepatitis A and B viruses are also part of the pretransplant evaluation in most centers.

Immunologic Considerations

ABO blood compatibility between donor and recipient is preferred in liver transplantation. However, ABO-incompatible liver transplants have been performed in urgent settings with 1-year survival rates approximately one-half those observed inpatients without an ABO discrepancy (14).

Unlike renal transplantation, hyperacute rejection is rare after liver transplantation; therefore, T-cell cross matching is not routinely performed preoperatively. In addition, a positive cross-match does not reliably predict hyperacute rejection after liver transplantation as it does after kidney transplantation. HLA typing is not performed preoperatively because of relatively short preservation times, but may be of some advantage in patients requiring a second transplant (15).

Cadaveric Donors

Suitable cadaveric donors must meet strict brain-death criteria as promulgated by law. Usually, each hospital has its own mechanism for declaring legal death. The declaration of brain death is never made by any personnel associated with UNOS, the regional organ bank, or the organ recovery teams. Suitable donors must demonstrate biochemical evidence of acceptable hepatic function, be free of transmissible disease (HIV negative, HBsAg negative), and have no underlying malignancy (some brain tumors are the exception). Other important factors used to evaluate the donor status are age, hemodynamic stability, mechanism of donor's death, and the level of hepatic or intraabdominal trauma. Donor features that have been associated with poor initial graft function include fat infiltration of more than 30%, cold preservation time greater than 12 hours, and donor age greater than 60 years (16,17). Because of the severe organ shortage, many centers are using these "marginal donors" to expand the donor pool (16).

The use of grafts obtained from patients who demonstrate hepatitis B core antibody (HbcAb), but are surface antigen (HbsAg) and surface antibody (HbsAb) negative, is controver-

sial. A study reviewing 25 donors who were HBcAb positive but negative to HBsAg and HBsAb demonstrated a hepatitis B transmission rate of 50% to the liver recipients (10). A similar study showed that the risk of transmission was much lower for grafts that were from donors who were B core antibody positive (8.2%) than those that were from donors who were surface antibody positive (12.5%) (18).

Recipients transplanted with grafts infected with hepatitis C test positive for HCV RNA in up to 97% of the cases 1 to 4 years after follow-up (19,20). With such a high transmission rate, many authors believe the use of HCV-infected organs should be restricted to life-saving organs only (liver, heart, lung). Currently, we restrict the use of HCV-positive livers to HCV-positive recipients or to a critically ill patient in need of urgent transplantation.

Orthotopic Liver Transplantation

Successful liver transplantation requires the management of severe coagulopathy, metabolic derangement, massive fluid shifts and blood loss, temperature derangement, hemodynamic instability, and renal dysfunction. Full, invasive monitoring is mandatory with direct arterial, central venous, and pulmonary artery pressure sensors so that hemodynamic profiles can be calculated and appropriately managed. Adequate venous access is necessary to permit rapid, massive transfusions if required. Fluid and external warmers are used to avoid hypothermia.

The surgical procedure can be described in three distinct sequential phases: 1) hepatectomy of the recipient, 2) anhepatic phase and revascularization of the graft, and 3) biliary reconstruction.

Hepatectomy of the Recipient

This phase is characterized by meticulous dissection of the liver and porta hepatis. Portal hypertension, prior abdominal surgery, and severe coagulopathy can make the procedure extremely difficult. To decrease portal pressures during hepatectomy, many centers resort to venovenous bypass (21). This involves placing catheters in the femoral and portal veins to decompress the systemic circulation during vena cava cross-clamping and returning the blood volume to the heart by means of an external pump and a third catheter placed in the subclavian vein. The theoretic advantages of venovenous bypass are the reduction of portal hypertension and improved hemodynamic stability during inferior vena cava cross-clamping. The disadvantages of venovenous bypass include the necessity of placing large-bore cannulas in the femoral, subclavian, and portal veins; additional operative time; and the potential for wound complications. The potential for cytokine release from activated white cells induced by the plastic tubing in the circuit and agitation from the external pump can also lead to increased fluid requirement and complications (21,22).

Selective use of venovenous bypass is becoming more widespread. The "piggyback" technique of inferior vena cava preservation during recipient hepatectomy is quickly becoming the standard procedure. During this procedure, the liver is resected off the vena cava by systematically ligating and dividing all of the small hepatic vein branches to the right, left, and caudate lobes. Eventually, the liver is only attached by the vasculature in the porta hepatis and the three main hepatic veins (right, middle, and left). The major advantage of the "piggyback" technique is that venovenous bypass can be avoided since the liver can be removed simply by clamping the inflow and outflow vessels directly without cross-clamping the vena cava. Using this technique, the patient remains relatively hemodynamically stable during the anhepatic phase.

Anhepatic Phase and Revascularization of the Graft

Once the recipient liver has been resected, the rapid development of progressive coagulopathy and fibrinolysis characterizes the anhepatic phase. Infusion of fresh-frozen plasma, cryoprecipitate, and platelets helps maintain some level of hemostasis. Routine uses of antifibrinolitic agents such as aminocaproic may contribute to the reestablishment of hemostasis, but can also be associated with graft thrombosis.

During the "piggyback" technique, the suprahepatic vena cava of the graft is sutured to the confluence of the middle and left hepatic veins. The right hepatic vein is then oversewn. The portal vein is anastomosed next, and the graft is revascularized after a blood flush to remove preservation fluid. The graft hepatic artery is anastomosed directly to the recipient's hepatic artery. When the recipient artery is inadequate, a "jump" graft from the aorta using donor iliac vessels is required.

Biliary Reconstruction

Direct end-to-end bile duct anastomosis (choledococholedocostomy) is the reconstruction of choice in most cases. Occasionally, reconstruction of the biliary tree using Roux-en-Y hepaticojejunostomy is performed. Common indications for this type of reconstruction include primary sclerosing cholangitis, biliary atresia, or other technical factors such as extreme size mismatch.

Living-Donor Liver Transplantation

The severe organ shortage has lead to the surgical innovation of living-donor liver transplantation. The problem has been exacerbated in the pediatric population where appropriate size–matched grafts are uncommon. The procedure was first performed in 1987 between a mother and a child in Brazil, but was unsuccessful. The first successful series of pediatric living-donor liver transplantation was reported by Broelsch et al from the University of Chicago in 1989 (23,24). In these cases, the left lateral segment of the donor (20% of donor liver volume) is resected without compromising blood flow to the graft and transplanted into the recipient. Because of the regenerative properties of the liver, both the resected lobe in the donor and the liver graft in the recipient grow to the appropriate size for the host.

To date, over 1500 pediatric living-donor liver transplants have been performed worldwide. Outcomes now exceed those observed with cadaveric transplants with patients enjoying 90% 1-year survival. The obvious disadvantage to living-donor liver transplantation is the risk of morbidity and mortality for the donor. In the worldwide literature, two donor deaths have been reported to date. In both cases, the complication leading to death (pulmonary embolus, drug reaction) occurred during the postoperative period.

As a result of the success in living-donor liver transplantation in children, several groups have begun adult-to-adult living-donor liver transplantation. Since the left lateral segment does not provide enough liver volume to sustain the recipient, either the right lobe (60% donor liver volume) or left lobe (40% donor liver volume) is used. Currently, approximately 350 adult-to-adult living-donor liver transplant procedures have been performed worldwide. Because of cultural beliefs, the majority of these have been performed in Asia where brain death criteria have not been established.

In December of 1998 our group initiated an adult-to-adult living-donor liver transplant program to help solve the problem of organ shortages. In our own experience, approximately 25% of our patients waiting for liver transplant die from complications of their liver disease prior to transplantation.

To date, the outcome with adult-to-adult living-donor liver transplantation has not been equivalent to cadaveric transplantation. The major difference has been the increased bile-duct complications observed after living donation. Whereas 10% of cadaveric liver transplant recipients experience a bile-duct complication (leak or stricture), approximately 20% of patients receiving a live-donor liver transplant experience biliary complications (25). The results of large patient series will determine if adult-to-adult living-donor liver transplantation can provide outcomes similar to cadaveric transplantation.

Immunosupression

Most liver transplant centers use double-drug therapy (prednisone plus either cyclosporine or tacrolimus) or triple-drug (prednisone plus either cyclosporine or tacrolimus plus azathioprine) immunosuppression regimens. Some groups have replaced azathioprine with mycophenolate mofetil (MMF) (26). Several preliminary studies suggest that mycophenolate mofetil used as a primary agent in combination with tacrolimus or cyclosporine reduces the incidence of rejection and allows steroid withdrawal (27).

It has been our practice to use double-drug therapy with gradual withdrawal of steroids after 1 to 2 years, providing there is stable graft function. Both cyclosporine and tacrolimus are used in our armamentarium and have provided equally excellent results. Often, patient tolerance will dictate which regimen they are prescribed.

Table 39-4. Cause of Allograft Dysfunction After Orthotopic Liver Transplantation

1 to 7 Days After Transplantation

Hepatic artery thrombosis
Primary graft nonfunction
Hyperacute rejection
Functional cholestasis
Bile leaks
Acute cellular rejection

7 to 30 Days After Transplantation

Acute cellular rejection
Bile leaks
Drug toxicity
Hepatic artery thrombosis

More Than 30 Days After Transplantation

CMV infection
Acute cellular rejection
Biliary complications
Ductopenic rejection
Hepatitis C
Hepatitis B
Recurrent PBC or PSC
Portal vein thrombosis
Drug toxicity

There have been two large trials, one conducted in United States and the other in Europe, comparing immunosuppression regimens based on either cyclosporine or tacrolimus (28–30). Retransplantation rate and patient and graft survivals were similar in both groups. Steroid-resistant rejection was significantly higher in the cyclosporine-treated patients.

As mentioned previously, steroids may be withdrawn safely from stable patients after liver transplantation to reduce the risk of posttransplant obesity, hyperlipidemia, diabetes mellitus, hypertension, and metabolic bone disease.

Hyperacute Rejection

Hyperacute rejection is characterized by the rapid destruction of the graft, usually within hours of reperfusion. Preformed IgG antibodies within recipient serum mediate this dramatic immunologic response. Fortunately, this is a rare complication of liver transplantation.

Acute Cellular Rejection

Despite recent improvements in immunosuppressive therapy, acute cellular rejection remains a major cause of morbidity and late graft loss in patients undergoing liver transplantation (31).

Acute cellular rejection is defined as an acute deterioration in allograft function that is associated with specific histologic changes in the graft, including mixed, inflammatory-cell infiltrates involving portal tracts (lymphocytes, monocytes, eosinophils, and neutrophils) and disruption of biliary and vascular endothelium by lymphocytes (endotheliitis).

Acute cellular rejection develops in approximately 70% of liver transplant recipients treated with cyclosporine-or tacrolimus-based immunosuppression regimens (32). Although, cellular rejection usually occurs within the first 3 weeks after transplantation, late cellular rejection episodes are now being reported. These episodes are often associated with low blood cyclosporine or tacrolimus concentrations. Approximately 5% to 10% of liver transplant recipients who develop acute cellular rejection progress to severe ductopenic rejection that may require retransplantation. In the early stage of acute rejection most patients are asymptomatic. Clinical manifestations can be subtle and include fever, abdominal pain, malaise, fatigue, and poor appetite.

Laboratory indicators of acute rejection most commonly include a rise in serum bilirubin level, with more modest elevations in alkaline phosphatase and aminotransferases. Prothrombin time and albumin are usually unaffected. However, these biochemical parameters are neither sensitive nor specific for distinguishing acute cellular rejection from other causes of hepatic allograft dysfunction and do not correlate with the severity of the rejection episode. Routine and liberal use of percutaneous liver biopsy is the best means to diagnose acute cellular rejection.

The differential diagnosis of graft dysfunction depends on when it occurs after surgery (Table 39-4). For example, graft dysfunction within the first few days after transplantation may reflect technical or functional problems such as hepatic artery thrombosis, preservation injury, biliary anastomosis leakage or stenosis, primary graft nonfunction, or infection. Other causes of liver allograft dysfunction include cytomegalovirus (CMV), Epstein-Barr virus infections, recurrent hepatitis B virus or hepatitis C virus infection (HCV), functional cholestasis, or tacrolimus or cyclosporine toxicity.

The distinction between HCV and allograft rejection may be difficult because of the overlap in the histologic features. Bile-duct injury and portal lymphocytic infiltration are features of both conditions. The biopsy findings of lobular hepatitis plus immunohistochemical staining for HCV may be helpful. In patients with recurrent hepatitis B the presence of the HBsAg in the serum, high titers of HBV-DNA, and histologic findings confirm the diagnosis.

Functional cholestasis is a unique entity, which typically occurs in the early posttransplant period. This form of cholestasis is independent of rejection, parenteral nutrition, or the use of specific drugs. Liver histology shows cholestasis in zones 2 and 3 and may be associated with ballooning of the hepatocytes in these areas. Cyclosporine or tacrolimus toxicity should be suspected when abnormal liver tests are seen in conjunction with otherwise unexplained elevations in serum creatinine.

Once hepatic allograft dysfunction has been detected, abdominal ultrasound should be used to assess hepatic artery and portal venous blood flow. The possibility of intraabdominal collection and infection should also be evaluated. Blood tests for CMV antigen, HBsAg, HBV DNA, HCV DNA, and drug concentration should be obtained. A cholangiogram should be obtained to rule out biliary leak of stricture. Finally, percutaneous liver biopsy should be performed to help established a definitive diagnosis.

Treatment of Acute Cellular Rejection

First-line therapy for acute cellular rejection generally consists of high-dose corticosteroids. Approximately 70% of episodes of acute cellular rejection resolve after a course of high-dose corticosteroids. Different schemes have been utilized. In our institution, 1000 mg of methylprednisolone is administered daily for 3 days. Biochemical and histologic improvement is generally observed within 3 to 5 days when high-dose corticosteroid therapy is successful. Approximately 80% to 90% of rejection episodes respond to bolus doses of methylprednisolone. When biochemical improvement is not seen within 72 hours, a repeat liver biopsy is performed to diagnose ongoing rejection. In these cases, monoclonal antibody therapy is added using OKT3 (33). OKT3 is generally given to the approximately 20% of patients in whom acute cellular rejection is not reversed by high-dose corticosteroid therapy. OKT3 is a murine monoclonal antibody to the CD3 antigen-receptor complex present on mature T lymphocytes. Binding of OKT3 to the CD3 complex leads to clearance of circulating T lymphocytes by the reticuloendothelial system and interferes both with antigen recognition by the T-cell receptor and with T-cell activation (34).

OKT3 is administered daily as a 5-mg intravenous bolus for 10 to 14 days. Fever, rigors, nausea, vomiting and diarrhea, hypotension, chest pain, dyspnea, or wheezing may develop within 30 to 60 minutes of the first few doses. Premedications include diphenhydramine, acetaminophen, and corticosteroids to minimize the common first-dose reactions. OKT3 therapy is successful in treating most of those patients who develop steroid-resistant rejection. A small percentage of patients will be refractory to therapy for acute cellular rejection and progress to severe ductopenic rejection necessitating retransplantation.

The major risks posed by treatment for acute cellular rejection include increased susceptibility to infection and the development of posttransplantation lymphoproliferative disease (PTLD) (35). PTLD has been associated with the use of monoclonal antibody, which is used either for induction therapy or for the treatment of steroid-resistant rejection and Epstein-Barr virus infection. Therapy usually consists of reducing immunosuppression to minimal levels. Patients with monoclonal PTLD usually fail to respond to immunosuppression withdrawal and require chemotherapy. Prognosis is poor in these situations.

The cumulative immunosuppressive effect of high-dose corticosteroid or OKT3 therapy to treat rejection also increases the susceptibility to oral candidiasis, cytomegalovirus (CMV) infection, *Aspergillus*, *Pneumocystis carinii*, and bacterial pathogens.

Other potential side effects include hyperglycemia, gastrointestinal hemorrhage, and mood changes. The administration of OKT3 for steroid-resistant, liver-transplant rejection has been associated with rapid progression of recurrent hepatitis C to liver failure in patients with preexisting HCV infection (36).

Chronic Ductopenic Rejection: "Vanishing Bile-Duct Syndrome"

Ductopenic rejection affects approximately 10% of liver transplant patients. It rarely occurs during the first 2 months after OLT, and, like acute cellular rejection, the diagnosis is based in histologic criteria. Ductopenic rejection is defined as the histologic loss of bile ducts in over 50% or more of portal tracts when 20 or more portal tracts are available for evaluation. A sclerosing arteriopathy affecting large- and medium-size arteries characterized by intima foam-cell infiltration has also been described (37).

No treatment can reverse the progression of bile-duct loss. When the diagnosis is confirmed, patients should be relisted for liver transplantation even if graft function is adequate. This is especially important in the setting of organ shortages where UNOS waiting times around the country exceed 1 year in most areas and approach 3 years in others.

Summary

Liver transplantation is the procedure of choice for treatment of end-stage liver diseases. Improved survival in patients undergoing OLT has been associated with better selection criteria, improved surgical technique, and immunosuppression regimens.

The use of newly developed artificial-support devices such as the bioartificial liver may serve as an adequate bridge to transplantation. The bioartificial liver, an ex vivo apparatus for hepatic support consisting of porcine hepatocytes attached to a hollow-fiber dialysis cassette, has shown promise in reducing cerebral edema and has shown mild improvement in biochemical parameters.

A critical shortage of suitable donor organs remains the single most important barrier to transplantation. Surgical innovations such as living-donor and split-liver transplantation have helped to increase the pool of suitable organs and may contribute to reducing waiting-list mortality. As these technologies develop, early referral of the patient with end-stage liver disease to a center with an active transplant program affords the patient the best chance at successful outcome.

References
1. Rosen HR, Shackleton CR, Martin P. Indications for and timing of liver transplantation. Med Clin North Am 1996;80:1069–1102.
2. Ghobrial RM, Farmer DG, Baquerizo A, et al. Orthotopic liver transplantation for hepatitis C: outcome, effect of immunosuppression, and causes of retransplantation during

an 8-year single-center experience. Ann Surg 1999;229: 824–833.

3. Kauffman HM, McBride MA, Rosendale JD, et al. Trends in organ donation, recovery and disposition: UNOS data for 1988–1996. Transplant Proc 1997;29:3303–3304.

4. Malago M, Rogiers X, Hertl M, et al. Optimization of the use of the cadaveric liver. Transplant Proc 1998;30:3902–3903.

5. Rogiers X, Malago M, Gawad K, et al. In situ splitting of cadaveric livers. The ultimate expansion of a limited donor pool. Ann Surg 1996;224:331–341.

6. Lake JR. Changing indications for liver transplantation. Gastroenterol Clin North Am 1993;22:213–229.

7. Lucey MR, Brown KA, Everson GT, et al. Minimal criteria for placement of adults on the liver transplant waiting list: a report of a national conference organized by the American Society of Transplant Physicians and the American Association for the Study of Liver Diseases [see comments]. Liver Transpl Surg 1997;3:628–637.

8. Chung SW, Greig PD, Ca Hral MS, et al. Evaluation of liver transplantation for high-risk indications. Br J Surg 1997;84:189–195.

9. Yoong KF, Gunson BK, Buckels JA, et al. Repeat orthotopic liver transplantation in the 1990s: is it justified? Transpl Int 1998;11(suppl 1):S221–S223.

10. Everson GT, Kam I. Liver transplantation: current status and unresolved controversies. Adv Inter Med 1997;42:505–553.

11. Consensus statement on indications for liver transplantation: Paris, June 22–23, 1993. Hepatology 1994;20:63S–68S.

12. O'Brien JD, Ettinger NA. Pulmonary complications of liver transplantation. Clin Chest Med 1996;17:99–114.

13. Surman OS, Cosimi AB. Ethical dichotomies in organ transplantation. A time for bridge building. Gen Hosp Psychiatry 1996;18(suppl 6):13S–19S.

14. Reding R, Veyckemans F, de ville de Goyet J, et al. ABO-incompatible orthotopic liver allografting in urgent indications. Surg Gynecol Obstet 1992;174:59–64.

15. Wong T, Donaldson P, Devlin J, Williams R. Repeat HLA-B and -DR loci mismatching at second liver transplantation improves patient survival. Transplantation 1996;61:440–444.

16. Fishbein TM, Feil MI, Emre S, et al. Use of livers with microvesicular fat safely expands the donor pool. Transplantation 1997;64:248–251.

17. Deschenes M, Forbes C, Tchervenkov J, et al. Use of older donor livers is associated with more extensive ischemic damage on intraoperative biopsies during liver transplantation [see comments]. Liver Transpl Surg 1999;5:357–361.

18. Van Thiel DH, De Maria N, Colantoni A, Friedlander L. Can hepatitis B core antibody positive livers be used safely for transplantation: hepatitis B virus detection in the liver of individuals who are hepatitis B core antibody positive. Transplantation 1999;68:519–522.

19. Pereira BJ, Levey AS. Hepatitis C infection in cadaver organ donors: strategies to reduce transmission of infection and prevent organ waste. Pediatr Nephrol 1995;9(suppl): S23–S28.

20. Chazouilleres O, Wright TL. Hepatitis C and liver transplantation. J Gastroenterol Hepatol 1995;10:471–480.

21. Chari RS, Gan TJ, Robertson KM, et al. Venovenous bypass in adult orthotopic liver transplantation: routine or selective use? J Am Coll Surg 1998;186:683–690.

22. Johnson SR, Marterre WF, Alonso MH, Hanto DW. A percutaneous technique for venovenous bypass in orthotopic cadaver liver transplantation and comparison with the open technique. Liver Transpl Surg 1996;2:354–361.

23. Broelsch CE, Whitington PF, Emond JC, et al. Liver transplantation in children from living related donors. Surgical techniques and results. Ann Surg 1991;214:428–439.

24. Malago M, Rogiers X, Broelsch CE. Liver splitting and living donor techniques. Br Med Bull 1997;53:860–867.

25. Chen CL, Chen YS, Liu PP, et al. Living related donor liver transplantation. J Gastroenterol Hepatol 1997;12:S342–S345.

26. McDiarmid SV. Mycophenolate mofetil as induction therapy after liver transplantation. Liver Transpl Surg 1999;5(suppl 1):S85–S89.

27. Trouillot TE, Shrestha R, Kam I, et al. Successful withdrawal of prednisone after adult liver transplantation for autoimmune hepatitis [see comments]. Liver Transpl Surg 1999;5:375–380.

28. The U.S. Multicenter FK 506 Liver Study Group. A comparison of tacrolimus (FK 506) and cyclosporine for immunosuppression in liver transplantation [see comments]. N Engl J Med 1994;331:1110–1115.

29. Klintmalm GB, Goldstein R, Gonwa T, et al. The U.S. Multicenter FK 506 Liver Study Group. Use of Prograf (FK 506) as rescue therapy for refractory rejection after liver transplantation. Transplant Proc 1993;25:679–688.

30. European FK 506 Multicentre Liver Study Group. Randomised trial comparing tacrolimus (FK 506) and cyclosporin in prevention of liver allograft rejection [see comments]. Lancet 1994;344:423–428.

31. Nicolette LA, Reichard KW, Falkenstein K, et al. Results of transplantation for acute and chronic hepatic allograft rejection. J Pediatr Surg 1998;33:909–912.

32. Neuberger J. Incidence, timing, and risk factors for acute and chronic rejection. Liver Transpl Surg 1999;5(suppl 1):S30–S36.

33. Wall WJ, Ghent CN, Roy A, et al. Use of OKT3 monoclonal antibody as induction therapy for control of rejection in liver transplantation. Dig Dis Sci 1995;40:52–57.

34. Alegre ML, Lenschow DJ, Bluestone JA. Immunomodulation of transplant rejection using monoclonal antibodies and soluble receptors. Dig Dis Sci 1995;40:58–64.

35. Ben-Ari Z, Amlot P, Lachmanan SR, et al. Posttransplantation lymphoproliferative disorder in liver recipients: characteristics, management, and outcome. Liver Transpl Surg 1999;5:184–191.

36. Rosen HR, Shackelton CR, Higa L, et al. Use of OKT3 is associated with early and severe recurrence of hepatitis C after liver transplantation [see comments]. Am J Gastroenterol 1997;92:1453–1457.

37. van Hoek B, Wiesner RH, Krom RA, et al. Severe ductopenic rejection following liver transplantation: incidence, time of onset, risk factors, treatment, and outcome. Semin Liver Dis 1992;12:41–50.

Chapter 40

Xenotransplantation

Tomasz Sablinski
David K. C. Cooper
David H. Sachs

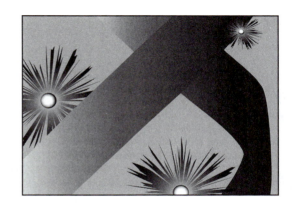

The enormous success that we have witnessed in clinical allotransplantation over the past 2 decades has paradoxically led to a new limitation to further progress in this field by causing a shortage of available donor organs. The consequent necessity of finding another source of organs has evoked a worldwide resurgence of interest in xenotransplantation, that is, the replacement of human organs or tissues with those from a "donor" of a different species. Although routine clinical application of this therapeutic modality remains in the future, recent progress offers cause for optimism (1–4). Many efforts in the field of transplantation immunobiology are currently concentrated on xenotransplantation, suggesting that we can expect exciting new developments in the near future.

Here, we shall briefly review the need for an alternative source of organs for humans, the clinical experience with xenotransplants, and the current research efforts in this field, with emphasis on studies directed toward understanding the mechanisms of xenotransplant rejection and developing new methods for prolongation of xenograft survival.

The Need

The insufficient supply of donor organs is a critical problem facing the field of transplantation. The discrepancy between the number of patients waiting for an organ transplant and the number of organs that become available each year is steadily increasing (5). In the United States alone over 70,000 patients await an organ transplant, and yet in the current year less than one-third of these will undergo a transplant procedure. More than ten people die every day while waiting for an organ. In addition, because of the severe shortage of organs, the criteria for receiving a transplant are restrictive, so there are many patients who could be saved by a transplant who are denied placement on the waiting list. To many clinicians and scientists, xenotransplantation seems to be the only plausible choice for meeting this increasing need. Nevertheless, for reasons mainly related to the potential for transfer of infection from the transplanted animal organ to the recipient and possibly into the community, there is not universal agreement on the prudence of xenotransplantation. The field must also contend with the voices of organizations that traditionally oppose any kind of animal research, even if it would save human lives.

The Choice of Animal as an Organ Source for Humans

On the basis of the phylogenetic distance between the species combination, the rapidity of the rejection process, and the levels of detectable preformed antibodies, xenotransplants have been classified into two groups. As proposed by Calne (6), mammals that belong to evolutionarily distant species and that reject organs in a hyperacute manner are termed "discordant." In contrast, if an animal rejects a xenograft at a rate similar to that observed in allotransplantation, the relationship between the species is called "concordant." Although this terminology has shortcomings, it is widely accepted in the transplantation literature and will be used in this chapter.

Understandably, early efforts to apply xenotransplantation to clinical practice concentrated on nonhuman primates as donors. Clearly, from a phylogenetic point of view, nonhuman primates are closest to humans (Table 40-1). The nearest primates are the great apes; however, as members of endangered species, these primates can be ruled out as a future source of organs. The most available nonhuman primate is the baboon. However, transmission of infectious agents from nonhuman primates to humans, particularly viruses, is of great concern (7,8). There are also potential problems of size and availability, and there are, of course, ethical considerations associated with the use of any nonhuman primate donor (Table 40-2). The FDA has issued guidelines regarding the use of nonhuman primates as a source of organs for clinical transplantation (9), which indicate growing concern over the use of nonhuman, primate-derived tissues for transplantation and make concordant xenotransplantation unlikely to take place.

The Pig As a Source Of Organs and Tissues in Humans

Most investigators now believe that discordant species will provide the ultimate solution, and many have chosen the pig as a suitable xenograft donor, largely because of its unlimited availability, its favorable breeding characteristics, and the similarity of many of its organ systems to those of humans (see Table 40-2) (10,11). In the authors' laboratory, work has focused on miniature swine as potential donors. Partially inbred miniature swine have been produced

Table 40-1. Comparison of the Evolutionary Relationship Between Certain Primate and Nonprimate Species

Species	Index of Dissimilarity*
Primates	
Humans and apes	
Human	1.0
Chimpanzee	1.14
Gorilla	1.09
Orangutan	1.22
Gibbon	1.28–1.30
Old World monkeys	2.23–2.65
New World monkeys	2.7–5.0
Prosimians, e.g., lemur	8.6–18
Nonprimates	
Bull	32
Pig	>35

*Based on reactivity in the microcomplement fixation test to human serum albumin. The greater the discrepancy from 1.0, the more distant is the evolutionary relationship with humans.
Source: Adapted from Sarich VM. In: Washburn SL, Jay PC, eds. Perspectives on human evolution. New York: Holt, Rhinehart and Winston, 1968.

by a selective breeding program over the past 25 years (12) and have a variety of advantages as potential xenograft donors:

1. Size: Miniature swine achieve adult weights of approximately 120 to 140 kg, making it possible to obtain a miniature swine of appropriate size as an organ donor for any potential human recipient, from a newborn baby to a large adult. In contrast, domestic swine reach mature weights of over 450 kg, clearly larger than necessary for organ donation and difficult to handle as a laboratory animal.
2. Physiology: Many organ systems of swine have been shown to be similar physiologically to their human counterparts, including the cardiovascular (Table 40-3), renal (Table 40-4), pulmonary, and digestive systems.
3. Breeding characteristics: Like other breeds of swine, miniature swine have favorable breeding characteristics for the production of organ-source animals. Swine are one of the few large animal species in which it is possible to carry out a breeding program to establish genetic characteristics. Swine have large litter sizes (five to ten offspring), early sexual maturity (5 months), short gestation time (114 days), and frequent estrus cycles (every 3 weeks). It is for these reasons that we have been able to produce animals homozygous for the major histocompatibility complex (MHC) in a relatively short time, and we currently have one inbred line that has reached a greater than 70% coefficient of inbreeding.
4. Genetic engineering: It is theoretically possible to incorporate any number of transgenes into a line of miniature swine to modify the animal to make it more appropriate as a donor species, for example, by the introduction of a gene for a human complement-regulatory protein. There might be great benefit if all groups interested in producing transgenic pigs for xeno-

transplantation used the same inbred recipient herd. This would permit crossbreeding and selection of inbred donors carrying the new genes in a much shorter time than would be possible if different breeding stock were used.
5. Blood type: Swine can be typed for ABO blood type. All are A or H (O). For the purposes of organ transplantation, group H (O) swine have been selectively bred to ensure no immune response directed against AB antigens.
6. Tissue type: If knowledge of the tissue type of the potential donor pig herd is available, genetic engineering of the *recipient's* tissues is also feasible. For example, by using gene therapy techniques, it may be possible to induce tolerance to the products of some of the most important xenogeneic antigens by introducing the corresponding swine genes into the bone-marrow stem cells of the recipient. After a gene ubiquitous in the herd has been introduced into the potential recipient, a subsequent organ transplant can be carried out using an organ from any member of the herd. This procedure, which has been termed "molecular chimerism," has been shown to be effective for prolonging the survival of allotransplants (13,14). Preliminary studies have been carried out in the pig-to-nonhuman primate model (15).

Concerns have been expressed that transplantation of porcine organs into humans may result in a public health risk (16). This concern was triggered largely by data demonstrating the in vitro transmission of porcine endogenous retroviruses from pig cells to human cells (17). It is feared that porcine endogenous retroviruses might be transferred to the human recipient with a transplanted organ and that these retroviruses then may be spread to other members of the community by contact with the recipient. To date, however, more than 100 patients have been exposed to living porcine tissue in various forms (liver perfusion, splenic perfusion, islet xenotransplantation, etc.) with no definite evidence of cross-species infection with porcine endogenous retroviruses (18). Thus, despite some concerns, the overall climate for pig-to-human transplantation remains favorable, and many scientists, including ourselves, urge that the field should proceed actively but with caution (19).

Clinical Experience of Xenotransplantation

Early in the development of clinical organ transplantation, several investigators experimented with the use of xenografts to treat terminally ill patients (20). Reemtsma (21) and subsequently Starzl (22) and others performed a limited number of clinical xenogeneic transplants using kidneys and hearts from chimpanzees and baboons. Even though the immunosuppressive regimens were far more primitive than those used today, one of Reemtsma's patients survived for 9 months with a functioning chimpanzee kidney transplant, which remains the longest survival ever achieved in clinical xenotransplantation. Twenty years later, using immunosuppression with cyclosporine, one baboon-to-human cardiac xenotransplant was performed (23). The recipient

Table 40-2. Relative Advantages and Disadvantages of Baboons and Pigs As Potential Donors of Organs and Tissues for Humans

	Baboon	Pig
Availability	Limited	Unlimited
Breeding potential	Poor	Good
Period to reproductive maturity	3–5 years	4–8 months
Length of pregnancy	173–193 days	114 ± 2 days
Number of offspring	1–2	5–12
Growth	Slow (9 years to reach maximum size)	Rapid (adult human size within 6 months)[a]
Size of adult organs	Inadequate*	Adequate
Cost of maintenance	High	Significantly lower
Anatomic similarity to humans	Close	Moderately close
Physiologic similarity to humans	Close	Moderately close
Relationship of immune system to humans	Close	Distant
Knowledge of tissue typing	Limited	Considerable (in selected herds)
Necessity for blood type compatibility with humans	Important	Probably unimportant
Experience with genetic engineering	None	Considerable
Risk of transfer of infection (xenozoonosis)	High	Low
Availability of specific pathogen-free animals	No	Yes
Public opinion	Mixed	More in favor

*The size of certain organs, e.g., the heart, would be inadequate for transplantation into adult humans.
[a] Breeds of miniature swine are approximately 50% of the weight of domestic pigs at birth and sexual maturity, and they reach a maximum weight of approximately 30% of standard breeds.
Source: Cooper DKC, Lanza RP, XENO—the promise of transplanting animal organs into humans. New York: Oxford University Press, 2000.

(Baby Fae), an infant with hypoplastic left heart syndrome, survived for 20 days before antibody-mediated rejection led to her death. More recently, there have been two attempts to achieve long-term survival of baboon livers in humans (24). Although at the time of the patients' deaths (at 28 and 70 days after transplantation, respectively) neither transplanted liver showed signs of rejection, this may have been the result of overimmunosuppression. Unsuccessful attempts to achieve survival of pig livers and hearts have been undertaken by other investigators (20,25,26). Despite these disappointments, an important conclusion from this limited clinical experience is that animal kidneys and hearts can support the vital functions of humans.

Immunologic Hurdles

Hyperacute Rejection

Experimental data from a variety of animal models have demonstrated that transplantation of primarily vascularized organs across a discordant barrier leads to hyperacute rejection (HAR) (4,27–29). As its name implies, this is a rapid process, leading to loss of the organ by interstitial hemorrhage and vascular thrombosis in minutes or hours after transplantation. In some species combinations, for example, pig-to-primate, HAR is initiated by preformed natural antibodies, that is, antibodies that are directed against target antigens and that are present before exposure to the donor tissues (30). Antibody-antigen binding results in complement activation and in activation/injury of the vascular endothelium of the transplanted organ. Much attention has been focused on this problem during the past decade, and a variety of encouraging approaches to its solution have been explored (28,31–36). These approaches relate largely to depletion of antibody and/or complement in the recipient and to modification of antigen expression and/or of complement-regulatory proteins in the donor organ. The results have been significant prolongation of survival of porcine organs in nonhuman primates, with survival now measured in weeks, rather than in minutes or hours (37,38).

Preformed Natural Antibodies

The dramatic response initiated by preformed natural antibodies (nAb) is comparable with the anti-HLA antibody-mediated HAR seen in allografts in presensitized recipients (39). By definition, nAb are those that are circulating in an individual in the absence of obvious immunization (40). Our current understanding is that these nAb develop in infancy as a response to the presence of common, gastrointestinal, environmental antigens and that they cross-react with carbohydrate antigens on the surface of the pig vascular endothelium (41) (Table 40-5). Germ-free rodents have been shown to have very low titers of nAb, substantiating such correlation (42). However, other physiologic reasons for the presence of nAb have been proposed, including

Table 40-3. Comparative Hemodynamic Measurements in Humans and Pigs

Parameter	Human	Pig*
Heart rate (bpm)	60–100	95–115
Stroke index[a]	32–58 mL/m^2	0.43–1.92 mL/kg[a]
Ejection fraction	0.59–0.75	0.40–0.44
Cardiac output (1/min.)	4–6	8–10
Cardiac output index[a]	2.6–4.2 L/min/m^2	45–240 mL/min/kg[a]
Blood pressures (mm Hg)		
Right atrium	0–8	2–10
Right ventricle	15–30/0–8	22–31/1–6
Pulmonary artery	15–30/3–12	14–22
Left atrium and PCWP	1–10	10–14
Left ventricle	100–140/3–12	56–120/2–8
Mean arterial pressure	70–105	45–89
Systemic vascular resistance (dynes-sec-cm^{-5})	700–1600	2540–2850
Pulmonary vascular resistance (dynes-sec-cm^{-5})	20–130	350–420

* Cardiovascular parameters in swine vary with weight and breed. Range of some data is wide as they were selected from studies using pigs of appropriate weight but of several breeds.
[a] Estimation of body surface area has proved difficult in pigs, necessitating the use of inconsistent units for these measurements.
PCWP, Pulmonary capillary wedge pressure.
Source: Modified from Appel JZ, Buhler L, Cooper DKC. The pig as a source of cardiac xenografts. J Cardiac Surg (in press).

Table 40-4. Comparative Measurements of Renal Function in Humans and Pigs

Parameter	Human	Pig
Maximal concentration (mOsm/L)	1160	1080
Maximal urine/plasma osmol. ratio	4.0	3.3
Glomerular filtration rate (mL/min/70 kg)	130	126–175
Total renal blood flow (mL/min/g)	4	3.0–4.4

Source: Modified from Kirkman RL. Of swine and men: organ physiology in different species. In: Hardy MA, ed. Xenograft 25. Amsterdam: Excerpta Medica, 1989:125–132.

Table 40-5. Structure of the Main Carbohydrate Epitopes Exposed at the Surface of Human and Porcine Vascular Endothelia

Human	Pig
Galβ1-4GlcNAcβ1-R*	Galβ1-4GlcNAcβ1-R*
ABH-Galβ1-4GlcNAcβ1-R[a]	**Galα1-3**Galβ1-4GLcNAcβ1-R[b]
NeuAcα2-3Galβ1-4GlcNAcβ1-R[c]	NeuAcα2-3Galβ1-4GlcNAcβ1-R[c]
	NeuGcα2-3Galβ1-4GlcNAcβ1-R[d]

Only the epitopes shown in bold type and underlined are different between the two species. R are glycolipid or glycoprotein carrier molecules anchored in the cell membrane.
* N-acetyllactosamine.
[a] The A, B, H, or AB blood group antigen.
[b] The α-galactosyl antigen.
[c] N-acetylneuraminic acid.
[d] N-glycolylneuraminic acid.
Source: Cooper DKC. Xenoantigens and xenoantibodies. Xenotransplantation 1998;5:6–17.

surveillance against neoplastic cells (43) or cytokine regulation (44). Using sensitive techniques, low levels of nAb can be detected in concordant species combinations, as in the detection of mouse nAb targeted to rat bone marrow cells (45,46), but these are generally insufficient to cause HAR.

The role of nAb in rejection of a discordant xenograft remains the best-studied component of the xenogeneic response. The binding of nAb to antigens on the surface of the donor vascular endothelium activates the complement cascade, which causes rapid destruction of the xenograft (30). In some species combinations, removal of nAb from the recipients' blood effectively prolongs survival of xenografts (28,31,32), adoptive transfer of sera with high titers of nAb accelerates

rejection of the xenograft (47), and deposits of immunoglobulin on the tissues of the transplanted organ are a feature of discordant xenogeneic rejection (28,29,48). The majority of nAb are IgM. Thus, effective removal of IgM antibodies, with adequate blocking of both an induced humoral and a cellular response (or induction of tolerance—see below), may facilitate xenotransplantation.

Determination of the targets of nAb remains an active area of investigation. From the point of view of potential clinical application, the most relevant studies are those involving human antiporcine responses (Table 40-6) (49). Studies by Platt et al demonstrated that human sera contain antibodies against a triad of glycoproteins of molecular weights 115, 125, and 135 kDa, which appear to be major targets on the surface of pig endothelial cells (50). These results probably reflected the presence of the Galα1-3Gal (αGal) epitope on these abundant glycoproteins (34,51,52). Normal human serum contains both IgM and IgG antibodies reactive with this epitope, which is found as the terminal sugar residue of many glycoproteins and glycolipids on the surface of many cells of all mammals, except those of humans, apes, and Old World monkeys (53–55). The majority of human antipig nAb are directed toward this αGal epitope, which is formed by a single glycosyltransferase. This finding raises the possibility of producing genetically engineered pigs lacking the epitope following targeted destruction of the relevant α1, 3galactosyltransferase (αGT) gene (51), and studies in this direction are under way at several centers. An alternative approach is to down-regulate expression of the oligosaccharide by introducing a gene for an enzyme that produces another sugar and that competes with the αGT for a common substrate (51,56). Both of these possibilities are described below.

Table 40-6. Known Non-αGal Carbohydrate Antigens Against Which Humans Can Have Naturally Occurring Antibodies

1. A: GalNAcα1-3 (Fucα1-2) Galβ1-4GlcNAcβ-R
2. B: Galα1-3 (Fucα1-2) Galβ1-4GlcNAcβ-R
3. Thomsen-Friedenreich (T or TF) Galβ1-3GalNAcα1-R
4. Tn (TF precursor) GalNAcα-R
5. Sialosyl-Tn: NeuAcα2-6GalNAcα1-R
6. p^K: Galα1-4Galβ1-4Glcβ1-R
7. Other P antigens
8. Sulfatide I: SO$_4$-3Gal-R
9. Forssman: GalNAcα1-3GalNAcβ1-3Galα1-4Galβ1-4Glcβ1-R
10. i: Galβ1-4GlcNAcβ1-3Galβ1-4GlcNAcβ-R*
11. I: Galβ1-4GlcNAcβ1-3 (Galβ1-4Glcβ1-6) Galβ1-4GlcNAcβ-R*
12. αRhamnose-containing oligosaccharides
    L-Rhm-α-Rhm
    L-Rhm-α1-3GlcNAcβ1-2L-Rhm-α-R
13. βGlcNAc-containing oligosaccharides
    GlcNAcβ-R
    GlcNAcβ1-4GlcNAcβ-R

R are glycolipid or glycoprotein carrier molecules anchored in the cell membrane.
*The core structures of the ABH antigen system, which are fucosylated by H transferase to generate H substance.
Source: Cooper DKC. Xenoantigens and xenoantibodies, Xenotransplantation 1998;5:6–17.

The prerequisite condition for prolongation of discordant xenograft survival is avoidance of the effects of these nAb. This can be achieved by the removal and/or blocking of nAb or by the circumvention of the subsequent mechanisms that lead to injury of the vascular endothelium such as complement-mediated cytotoxicity. Several approaches are being used to achieve this goal.

Modification of the Recipient's Immune Response

Removal of Antipig Antibodies

Plasmapheresis. Based on earlier successful experience in recipients of allogeneic kidneys from ABO blood group—incompatible donors (57), plasmapheresis (or plasma exchange) has been used to remove nAb from nonhuman primates prior to xenotransplantation of pig organs (31,58). Plasmapheresis can effectively remove IgM antibodies and, when combined with other therapy (e.g., splenectomy, T-cell depletion, pharmacologic immunosuppression), has resulted in prolonged (<23 days) survival of renal or heterotopic pig cardiac grafts in baboons. Because of the lack of specificity in the removal of immunoglobulins by plasmapheresis, a more specific method is needed.

Extracorporeal Organ Perfusion. One of the most specific methods of nAb removal is perfusion of the recipient's blood through an organ from the donor, which leads to prolonged survival of a subsequently transplanted organ from the same donor (28). Perfusion of a pig kidney or liver with baboon or monkey blood successfully removes nAb from the circulation and is relatively well tolerated (28,59,60). Additional support for the safety of this approach comes from limited but well-documented clinical applications in which pig livers have been used ex vivo for detoxification of patients in hepatic coma, without profound adverse effects (61,62).

Specific Immunoadsorption of Anti-αGal Antibodies. The perfusion of recipient plasma through immunoaffinity columns of synthetic αGal epitopes, which bind anti-αGal antibodies specifically, has proved successful (63–66). Over 99% of anti-αGal IgM and 97% of anti-Gal IgG can be depleted by this technique (67). In a variant of this procedure, the same synthetic αGal sugars have been infused intravenously into baboons with the intent of binding the circulating anti-αGal antibody and thus inhibiting it from binding to a subsequently transplanted pig organ. Although success has been reported using a similar technique in preventing HAR of allografts transplanted across the ABO blood group barrier (34), this method has proved less successful in discordant xenogeneic systems (68,69).

Anti-IgM Antibodies. The use of anti-IgM antibodies to inactivate circulating IgM has been reported to be effective for this purpose in a rodent model (70) and is currently being tested in primates (71).

Splenectomy

Splenectomy results in decreased levels of circulating IgM (72), and in quantitative assays a reduction in preformed nAb levels of up to 40% has been observed. Splenectomy is believed to disturb the proliferative response of circulating B lymphocytes (73) and is widely used in experimental models of xenotransplantation (4,74). It has been demonstrated to prolong survival of pig organs in nonhuman primates (74). Additional support for the effectiveness of splenectomy in diminishing the humoral response comes from its use in ABO-incompatible kidney transplants (57), but few controlled data are available.

Suppression of Antibody Production

Several pharmacologic agents are reported to be effective in suppressing B-cell function and subsequently in decreasing the level of nAb in the circulation, particularly when used in combination with well-established T-cell immunosuppressants such as cyclosporine or tacrolimus. Cyclophosphamide, rapamycin (and its analog RAD), brequinar, 15-deoxyspergualin, mycophenolate mofetil, and several other agents have been used with varying degrees of success to maintain low nAb levels (75–80), although total suppression of anti-αGal production has yet to be achieved.

B cells can be targeted with monoclonal antibodies directed against B-cell–specific surface antigens. For example, CD20 is targeted by the human-mouse chimeric monoclonal antibody IDEC-C2B8. In our laboratory, baboons have been treated with a 4-week course after which no B cells could be detected in the blood or bone marrow for up to 3 months (79). Lymph nodes showed an 80% decrease in B cells, which was extended to 100% reduction after treatment with 150 cGy of whole-body irradiation. Despite the absence of B cells, anti-Gal antibody production was only modestly reduced. The use of immunotoxins also directed against B-cell surface antigens has been similarly disappointing.

Immunologic Tolerance

Studies in rodents have indicated that the induction of mixed hematopoietic cell chimerism (81,82) or of molecular chimerism (83) results in B-cell tolerance and leads to a cessation of specific anti-αGal production (discussed below). This state has not yet been achieved in the pig-to-nonhuman primate model.

Down-regulation of αGal Expression on the Donor Vascular Endothelium

The ideal approach might be to breed a pig in which the αGal epitopes have been "knocked out" by disruption of the αGT gene by homologous recombination. As pig embryonic stem cells are not yet available, it is currently not possible to create such an αGal-knockout pig. αGal-knockout mice, however, have been bred (84,85), and, although hearts from these mice are less susceptible than those from αGal-positive mice to the cytotoxic effects of human serum, they still undergo injury, suggesting the presence of other targets against which human antibodies may be directed.

Alternative approaches have been proposed (56) (Fig. 40-1). The introduction of a gene that would compete with αGT for its substrate, N-acetyllactosamine, is one such approach and has been termed "competitive glycosylation" (86). In vitro studies by Sandrin et al in COS cells have demonstrated that competition for this substrate takes place between αGT and α1, 2 fucosyltransferase (αFT), the enzyme that makes the H (O) blood group antigen, in the Golgi apparatus (86). As αFT takes precedence, this results in the cell expressing more H (O) antigen than αGal. Mice transgenic for αFT demonstrate a major decrease in αGal expression, and their cells show increased resistance to human serum cytotoxicity (87). However, not all of the αGal epitopes are replaced by the H (O) epitopes, and therefore the organ is still susceptible to antibody-mediated rejection. The addition of a second transgene, that for αgalactosidase, which removes terminal αGal epitopes, results in cells where there is a complete absence of αGal expression (88). No work in pigs has yet been carried out to indicate the success of this approach in this species.

Although our inability to isolate pig embryonic stem cells has prevented the knockout of the αGT gene, this can be achieved in single cells, for example, pig fibroblasts. If this modified nuclear material is then transferred into embryonic cells from which the nucleus has been removed and these cells are then implanted into surrogate sows, the resulting genetically modified piglet should express no αGal. Although not yet accomplished in the pig, this technique of nuclear transfer and cloning (89) may allow progress in this area.

Depletion or Inhibition of Complement

Activation of the complement system is believed to be of crucial importance in the HAR of xenotransplants (90). The relative role of the classic and alternative pathways in the pathogenesis of HAR varies with the species combination. In nonhuman primates, following binding of nAb to the vascular endothelium of the donor organ, complement is activated directly by the classic pathway (90). However, activation of complement by the alternative pathway has been shown to contribute to rejection in some species combinations (91,92). Complement can be depleted or its action inhibited by a number of agents.

Exogenous Molecules. Soluble complement receptor 1, a protein that blocks C3, thereby inhibiting both classic and alternative pathways of complement activation, has been reported to prevent or delay HAR in both rodents and primates

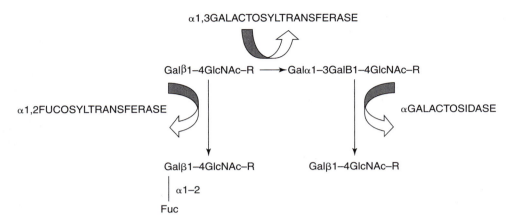

Figure 40-1. Biosynthetic pathway for synthesis of Galα1-3Gal. The α1,3 galactosyltransferase enzyme adds galactose to N-acetyllactosamine (Galβ1-4GlcNAc) to generate Galα1-3Gal. The same substrate can be utilized by transgenically introduced α1,2 fucosyltransferase to produce the H(O) histo-blood group epitope. Galα1-3Gal can also be eliminated by the introduction of α-galactosidase, which enables the N-acetyllactosamine substrate to be available again for further fucosylation. (Modified from Sandrin MS, Cohney S, Osman N, McKenzie IFC. Overcoming the anti–Galα1-3Gal reaction to avoid hyperacute rejection: molecular genetic approaches. In: Cooper DKC, Kemp E, Platt JL, White DJG, eds. Xenotransplantation. 2nd ed. Heidelberg: Springer, 1997:683–700.)

(93). Cobra venom factor, a potent deactivator of complement, also prolongs xenograft survival in some species combinations (94–96).

Membrane-Bound Molecules. Studies of membrane-bound, complement-regulatory proteins such as membrane cofactor protein (MCP, CD46), decay accelerating factor (DAF, CD55), and CD59 have led to an increased interest in their potential use in prevention of complement activation in xenotransplantation. These proteins are believed to decrease the activation of complement by antibodies of the same, but not of discordant, species (97), although recent work suggests that species specificity may not be as important as an overall increase in the expression of these molecules (98). Genes for MCP, DAF, and CD59 have each been introduced into cultured cells to test for their effect on complement-mediated damage (99–101), and they have demonstrated inhibition of cytotoxity. Several groups are now producing transgenic pigs expressing one or more human genes for these complement-regulatory proteins to produce organ donors that will take advantage of this decreased capacity to activate human complement. Of particular interest is the work of the Cambridge, UK, group (Imutran/Novartis), which has produced pigs transgenic for human DAF (102). These pigs are now well characterized and express human DAF in levels sufficient to avoid HAR (103). Indeed, it is the use of organs from this herd of pigs that has resulted in the longest survival (99 days) of non–life-supporting, pig-to-primate organs to date (104). Pig kidney transplantation has supported life in cynomolgus monkeys for up to 73 days with a median of 33 days (38,105). Pig orthotopic heart

transplantation has maintained baboons for up 39 days, with a median of 14 days (37,106).

Suppression of Endothelial Cell Activation

There is evidence suggesting that hemorrhage, edema, and thrombosis in HAR result from activation and/or injury to endothelial cells, which in turn lead to loss of the anticoagulant properties of the endothelium (107–109). Antibody and complement binding may indeed exert some of their effects as a result of such activation. In addition, nonimmunologic factors such as molecular incompatibilities may contribute to this effect. Activated endothelium is permeable to plasma proteins and stimulates thrombin generation.

Acute Vascular Rejection—the Induced Antibody and Cellular Responses

If the problems caused by nAb could be resolved, the induced antibody and cellular responses to the discordant xenograft will then have to be overcome. Most recent evidence indicates that, in the case of in vitro pig-to-primate responses, the T-cell response is as great as, or greater than, that toward an allotransplant (110–112) and that, in addition, other cellular populations such as NK cells and macrophages may play a role (113). It is also clear that there is a potent, induced antibody response to xenografts that is dependent on T-cell help and that may therefore also be avoided by suppression of the cellular immune response.

Acute Vascular Rejection

A step in this direction has been taken by administration of an anti-CD40L monoclonal antibody that, when combined with other therapeutic modalities, has prevented sensitization in the pig-to-baboon model (79,114) (Fig. 40-2). However, despite prevention of an induced antibody response, baseline nAb production continues. As costimulatory blockade directly affects only T-cell function, thus inhibiting T-cell help to B cells, this observation lends support to the long-held opinion that nAb production is T-cell independent.

Investigation of the mechanisms involved in the development of acute vascular rejection, which is less well understood than HAR, has shown it to be a complex process in which antibody and various cell types play roles. Activation of the vascular endothelium, probably by antibody, may accentuate the molecular incompatibilities known to exist between pig and human and may result in disorders of coagulation. For example, disseminated

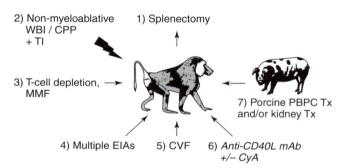

Figure 40-2. Schematic representation of our immunomodulation regimen (aimed at obtaining mixed hematopoietic chimerism and inducing tolerance) in baboons. (**1**) A splenectomy is performed, followed by (**2**) 300cGy whole body (WBI) and thymic (TI) irradiation or induction therapy with cyclophosphamide (CPP). (**3**) T-cell depletion is with antithymocyte globulin. A continuous intravenous infusion of mycophenolate mofetil (MMF) is commenced and continued for 30 days. (**4**) The baboon undergoes three extracorporeal immunoadsorptions (EIAs) using immunoaffinity columns of synthetic αGal oligosaccharide. (**5**) Anticomplement therapy is initiated with cobra venom factor, dosed according to the results of the measurement of CH50 and continued for 30 days. (**6**) Anti-CD40L mAb therapy (20 mg/kg) is initiated prior to the first infusion of porcine mobilized peripheral blood progenitor cells (PBPC) and continued on alternate days for 14 days (total 8 doses). In some cases, cyclosporine (CYA) and/or macrophage blockade with medronate liposomes have been added to the protocol. (**7**) A total of 3×10^{10} PBPCs/kg is infused over 3 days and porcine hematopoietic growth factors (cytokines) are administered to help engraftment. A pig organ transplant may also be transplanted at this time. (Modified from Alwayn IPJ, Buhler L, Basker M, Cooper DKC. Immunomodulation strategies in xenotransplantation. In: Sayegh M, Remuzzi G, eds. Current and future immunosuppressive therapies following transplantation. Dordrecht, The Netherlands: Kluwer [in Press].)

intravascular coagulation has been reported in some baboons undergoing pig-organ transplants (108,109). This complication is manifest by a steady reduction in fibrinogen level with a late, dramatic increase in prothrombin time. If the xenograft is not excised as an emergency, a bleeding diathesis can be fatal.

Work by Bach et al suggests that activation of the vascular endothelium is associated with the up-regulation of certain detrimental genes, whereas accommodation (in which the antibody does not cause injury despite the presence of the specific antigen—see below) is associated with the up-regulation of "protective" genes (115). This opens the possibility of the insertion into the donor animal of one or more protective genes, though this approach has not yet been attempted. The concept of accommodation derives largely from observations made in patients undergoing ABO-incompatible allografts and, to a lesser extent, in HLA-sensitized patients receiving allografts (57,116). This phenomenon can be summarized as the absence of antibody-mediated rejection of a vascularized organ despite the presence of circulating antibodies that are potentially reactive with antigens on the vascular endothelium of the graft (117). It has not been conclusively documented in αGal-incompatible, large animal models. Possible explanations have been proposed and include changes in the isotype, affinity, and/or specificity of the antibodies or subtle changes in the surface antigens or endothelial cells (117).

Cellular Rejection

In vitro testing of cellular immunity to xenogeneic antigens has sometimes shown lower reactivity than the comparable alloresponses (118,119). However, most of these data were obtained in rodent systems and involved weak or absent direct recognition of xenoantigens (120). Direct recognition, which is the main factor thought to be responsible for the strength of alloresponses, apparently does not occur in the mouse antihuman response, possibly because of the failure of effective function of accessory and surface adhesion molecules such as LFA-1 and ICAM-1. However, more recent testing of human T-cell responses to xenogeneic stimulator cells has shown direct recognition comparable with that observed for alloreactions (111,120). In the human, antipig, mixed lymphocyte reaction, for example, peak reactivity occurred with similar kinetics, and secondary responses are comparable (111,112). Data also indicate that cultured, porcine endothelial cells are capable of directly presenting xenogeneic MHC molecules to human T cells and elicit a response that appears markedly stronger than the allogeneic anti-endothelial response (110).

Immunosuppressive Therapy

Numerous immunosuppressive agents have been developed to suppress cellular immunity to allografts. However, it seems likely that the intensity of immunosuppression that will be required to avoid rejection of a discordant xenograft will be greater than that required for control of allograft rejection. Indeed, in long-surviving pig-to-primate xenografts, the high level of immunosuppression required has been responsible for the loss of several recipients from infection or other drug-related complications (37,38,104–106).

The Induction of Tolerance to Xenografts

Mixed Hematopoietic Cell Chimerism

Since the level of immunosuppression needed for allografts already causes the transplant recipient to be susceptible to infectious complications and to the development of neoplasia, it would be highly desirable to eliminate the cellular response to a xenograft through specific immune modulation, that is, through the induction of tolerance. Our laboratory has therefore concentrated on adapting a successful methodology for inducing allogeneic transplantation tolerance to the discordant xenograft combination of pig-to-nonhuman primate. This approach involves the induction of mixed hematopoietic chimerism as a means of specifically eliminating the immune response to the transplanted organ without diminishing the immune response to other antigens.

Bone marrow transplantation (BMTx) is usually carried out clinically as a treatment for hematologic malignancy. In this case it is usually essential that all host hematopoietic elements be ablated to ensure that the malignant condition is eliminated. An additional consequence of BMTx is that tolerance is induced to the bone marrow donor, and that tolerance extends to any organ or tissue from that donor. Tolerance has been demonstrated following BMTx in numerous animal systems, as well as in clinical practice when a BMTx recipient has subsequently received a kidney transplant from the same donor (121–123). Recently, a further step was taken when a kidney allotransplant was performed successfully at the same time as BMTx from the same donor (124).

However, when BMTx is used for the induction of transplantation tolerance, rather than for treatment of a hematologic malignancy, it is neither necessary nor desirable to completely ablate the recipient's hematopoietic system. On the contrary, it is advantageous to leave the host's hematopoietic system as intact as possible, but to ensure that sufficient bone marrow elements from the donor survive in the reconstituted recipient to allow tolerance to be maintained. This is especially true when the transplant is carried out across MHC barriers, since the presence of host antigen-presenting cells is essential to ensure immunocompetence in the recipient (125,126). Certain cells from the donor marrow inoculum must survive to induce and maintain transplantation tolerance (127), although the level of chimerism can be very low and still be sufficient for this purpose. It is not yet clear exactly which cells must survive nor where they must reside, although likely contenders are dendritic cells in the thymus, a combination known to be capable of negative selection for newly developing T cells (128,129).

Our laboratory has previously demonstrated that mixed hematopoietic chimerism provides an effective means of inducing long-term tolerance to skin allografts across full MHC barriers in mice (130,131) and, more recently, to kidney allografts in cynomolgus monkeys (132). The most effective procedure for inducing mixed chimerism for this purpose involves T-cell depletion in vivo with anti–T-cell antibodies, low-dose whole-body irradiation, and administration of allogeneic bone marrow prior to, or at the same time as, the organ allograft. The addition of costimulatory blockade is currently being explored. We have also demonstrated that a similar protocol is effective in producing long-term specific hyporesponsiveness to xenogeneic grafts in the concordant species combinations of rat-to-mouse (133) and baboon-to-monkey (134).

Mixed Chimerism and Swine-to-Nonhuman Primate Renal Transplantation

On the basis of previous success in allogeneic and concordant xenogeneic systems, we have established a program of discordant renal xenotransplantation using the principle of mixed xenogeneic chimerism. One protocol aimed at inducing tolerance is illustrated schematically in Figure 40-2. This protocol parallels very closely that which we have previously demonstrated to be effective for inducing long-term renal allograft acceptance in fully MHC-mismatched cynomolgus monkeys (132). The main difference from the allograft protocol involves the need to remove nAb from the recipient's circulation to avoid HAR. This has been accomplished by the intraoperative perfusion of the primate's blood through an isolated pig liver (35,60,63) or by the pretransplant perfusion of plasma through a synthetic α1-3Gal immunoadsorption column (63,64,66,109). This procedure has been successful in consistently avoiding HAR. The induced IgG response to the graft can be successfully prevented by costimulatory blockade with an anti-CD40L monoclonal antibody (79,114).

Pig kidney xenografts have functioned for up to 29 days, achieving normal BUN and creatinine levels for most of that period (Buhler L et al, unpublished data). However, the kidney eventually succumbs to a vascular form of rejection, often associated with the development of a state of disseminated intravascular coagulation (109). There has been evidence of pig cell microchimerism in the blood for up to 1 month. At the time of rejection, IgM (and sometimes IgG) antibodies have been detected by immunofluorescence in the vessels of the graft.

Our studies in allogeneic systems have demonstrated that at least transient chimerism is a requirement for achieving lasting transplantation tolerance. Our current efforts are therefore focusing on means for increasing the engraftment of pig bone marrow cells in nonhuman primate recipients, for example, by the administration of pig, recombinant, hematopoietic growth factors (135).

Molecular Chimerism

A second approach to the induction of tolerance is by gene therapy in an attempt to induce what has been termed molecular chimerism. For example, B-cell tolerance might be achieved if the primate recipient could be induced to express the Gal epitope on its tissues, which might lead to the suppression of production of anti-Gal antibody. Autologous transplantation of bone marrow from αGal-knockout mice transduced ex vivo with the gene αGT, the enzyme that leads to the production of the Gal epitopes, resulted in suppression of production of anti-αGal and the achievement of B-cell tolerance to αGal (83). Preliminary studies in baboons, however, demonstrated only transient expression of αGal following the infusion of transduced, autologous, bone marrow cells. The transduction efficiency of baboon bone marrow cells is currently being optimized with the use of improved vectors and culture parameters.

T-cell tolerance might be achieved by the introduction into the recipient of a gene encoding a swine MHC (SLA) class II antigen. The presence of a donor-specific class II antigen in the recipient (following gene transduction of bone marrow cells) has been demonstrated to lead to tolerance to a kidney allograft in miniature swine (14), and its importance has been tested in the pig-to-baboon model (15). Ex vivo transduction of baboon bone marrow cells with an SLA class II gene of a specific, MHC-inbred, miniature-swine genotype was performed. Autologous transplantation of these transduced cells led to detection of the transgene in blood and bone marrow, but the transcription was transient. Subsequent pig skin or organ grafts (from a pig matched to the transgene) were rejected within 8 to 22 days from an antibody-mediated mechanism. In contrast to control baboons, however, the induction of IgG against non-αGal antigens was prevented, suggesting prevention of a T-cell response.

Discordant Thymic Xenotransplantation

Our center is also involved with the induction of T-cell tolerance by the transplantation of a thymic graft from the donor. The transplantation of fetal pig thymic tissue has been shown in a mouse model to be capable of inducing discordant xenograft tolerance (136). Initial data from Wu et al (137) indicate that porcine thymic tissue transplanted into thymectomized, T-cell–depleted, nonhuman primates permits the development of immunocompetence and induces long-term, in vitro hyporesponsiveness to pig antigens. Yamada et al (138,139) have demonstrated in our MHC-inbred herd of pigs that autologous thymic tissue, when transplanted under the renal capsule, becomes vascularized, regenerates, and functions normally. When these "thymokidney" composite grafts are transplanted across a fully mismatched allogeneic barrier, in a T-cell–depleted and thymectomized recipient, they are able to induce T-cell tolerance (Yamada K et al, manuscript in preparation). If anti-αGal could be successfully depleted for a limited period, the transplantation of a pig thymokidney could potentially induce T-cell tolerance in the pig-to-primate model. The problem of providing an anti-αGal-free environment that would allow T-cell tolerance to develop, however, remains unresolved at the present time.

It is our hope that by combining approaches directed toward the humoral xenograft response with tolerance at the cellular level, long-term acceptance of discordant xenografts in the pig-to-primate combination will be achieved.

Nonimmunologic Considerations in Discordant Xenotransplantation

There are a number of anatomic and physiologic similarities between swine and humans with respect to parameters of importance to transplantation (10,140), which have been discussed by Hammer (141). Many functional parameters of the cardiovascular and renal systems are essentially identical in the two species. Indeed, the reported greater-than-2-month survival of life-supporting pig kidneys in cynomolgus monkeys, with essentially normal parameters of renal function, provides evidence for physiologic compatibility (38,105). Nevertheless, it seems almost certain that not all of the metabolic and hormonal functions of pig organs will be adequate after transplantation into the human host (141). The liver, for example, produces so many proteins and metabolites that it would be surprising if all of the porcine products were compatible in primates. However, it is possible that transgenic technology may permit the introduction of human genes that enable production of the desired product.

Comment

Although we are still far from a solution to all of the problems associated with xenografting, none of the obstacles appear to us to be insurmountable. Recent consistent success in overcoming HAR gives hope for further progress and makes it feasible to plan for a cautious, stepwise approach to clinical trials. Given the recent advances and the enormous motivation imposed by clinical necessity, it seems likely that xenotransplantation will eventually become a therapeutic modality.

Acknowledgements
The authors thank Mrs. Lisa A. Bernardo for expert secretarial assistance. The work in our laboratory was supported in part by NIH Grant 1R01 AI37692 and in part by a Sponsored Research Agreement between the Massachusetts General Hospital and BioTransplant, Inc.

References
1. Auchincloss H Jr, Sachs DH. Transplantation and graft rejection. In: Paul WE, ed. Fundamental immunology. New York: Raven, 1993:1099–1142.
2. Cooper DKC, Kemp E, Platt JL, White DJG, eds. Xeno-transplantation. 2nd ed. Heidelberg: Springer, 1997:1–854.
3. Buhler L, Friedman T, Iacomini J, Cooper DKC. Xeno-transplantation—state of the art: update 1999. Front Biosci 1999;4:416–432.
4. Lambrigts D, Sachs DH, Cooper DKC. Discordant organ xenotransplantation in primates: world experience and current status. Transplantation 1998;66:547–561.
5. United Network for Organ Sharing. 1997 Annual Report.
6. Calne RY. Organ transplantation between widely disparate species. Transplant Proc 1970;2:550–556.

7. Michaels MG, Simmons RL. Xenotransplant-associated zoonoses. Strategies for prevention. Transplantation 1994; 57:1–7.

8. Koralnik IJ, Boeri E, Saxinger WC, et al. Phylogenetic associations of human and simian T-cell leukemia/lymphotropic virus type I strains: evidence for interspecies transmission. J Virol 1994;68:2693–2707.

9. US Department of Health and Human Services Public Health Service. Guidance for industry: public health issues posed by the use of nonhuman primate xenografts in humans. Fed Reg 1999;64:16743–16744.

10. Cooper DKC, Ye Y, Rolf LL, Zuhdi N. The pig as potential organ donor for man. In: Cooper DKC, Kemp E, Reemtsma K, White DJG, eds. Xenotransplantation. 1st ed. Heidelberg: Springer, 1991:481–500.

11. Sachs DH. The pig as a potential xenograft donor. Vet Immunol Immunopathol 1994;43:185–191.

12. Sachs DH. MHC homozygous miniature swine. In: Swindle MM, Moody DC, Phillips LD, eds. Swine as models in biomedical research. Ames, Iowa: Iowa State University Press, 1992:3–15.

13. Sykes M, Sachs DH, Nienhuis AW, et al. Specific prolongation of skin graft survival following retroviral transduction of bone marrow with an allogeneic major histocompatibility complex gene. Transplantation 1993;55:197–202.

14. Emery DW, Sablinski T, Shimada H, et al. Expression of an allogeneic MHC DRB transgene, through retroviral transduction of bone marrow, induces specific reduction of alloreactivity. Transplantation 1997;64:1414–1423.

15. Ierino FL, Gojo S, Banerjee PI, et al. Transfer of swine MHC class I genes into autologous bone marrow cells of baboons for the induction of tolerance across xenogeneic barriers. Transplantation 1999;67:1119–1128.

16. Bach FH, Fishman JA, Daniels N, et al. Uncertainty in xenotransplantation: individual benefit versus collective risk. Nat Med 1998;4:141–144.

17. Patience C, Takeuchi Y, Weiss RA. Infection of human cells by an endogenous retrovirus of pigs. Nat Med 1997;3: 282–286.

18. Paradis K, Langford G, Long Z, et al. Search for cross-species transmission of porcine endogenous retrovirus in patients treated with living pig tissue. Science 1999;285: 1236–1241.

19. Sachs DH, Colvin RB, Cosimi AB, et al. Xenotransplantation—caution, but no moratorium. Nat Med 1998;4:372. Letter.

20. Taniguchi S, Cooper DKC. Clinical xenotransplantation—past, present and future. Ann R Coll Surg Engl 1997;79: 13–19.

21. Reemtsma K, McCracken BH, Schlegel JU, et al. Renal heterotransplantation in man. Ann Surg 1964;160:384–410.

22. Starzl TE, Marchioro TL, Peters GN. Renal heterotransplantation from baboon to man: experience with six cases. Transplantation 1964;2:752–776.

23. Bailey LL, Nehlsen-Cannarella SL, Concepcion W, Jolley WB. Baboon-to-human cardiac xenotransplantation in a neonate. J Am Med Assoc 1985;254:223.

24. Starzl TE, Fung J, Tzakis A, et al. Baboon-to-human liver transplantation. Lancet 1993;341:65–71.

25. Makowka L, Cramer DV, Hoffman A, et al. Pig liver xenografts as a temporary bridge for human allografting. Xeno 1993;1:27–29.

26. Czaplicki J, Blonska B, Religa Z. The lack of hyperacute xenogeneic heart transplant rejection in a human. J Heart Lung Transplant 1992;11:393–397. Letter.

27. Busch GJ, Martins ACP, Hollenberg NK, et al. A primate model of hyperacute renal allograft rejection. Am J Pathol 1975;79:31–36.

28. Cooper DKC, Human PA, Lexer G, et al. Effects of cyclosporine and antibody adsorption on pig cardiac xenograft survival in the baboon. J Heart Lung Transplant 1988;7:238–246.

29. Platt JL, Fischel RJ, Matas AJ, et al. Immunopathology of hyperacute xenograft rejection in a swine-to-primate model. Transplantation 1991;52:214–220.

30. Perper RJ, Najarian JS. Experimental renal heterotransplantation. I. In widely divergent species. Transplantation 1966;4:377–388.

31. Alexandre GPJ, Gianello P, Latinne D, et al. Plasmapheresis and splenectomy in experimental renal xenotransplantation. In: Hardy MA, ed. Xenograft 25. New York: Excerpta Medica, 1989:259–266.

32. Fischel RJ, Bolman RM III, Platt JL, et al. Removal of IgM anti-endothelial antibodies results in prolonged cardiac xenograft survival. Transplant Proc 1990;22:1077–1078.

33. Dalmasso AP, Vercellotti GM, Platt JL, Bach FH. Inhibition of complement-mediated endothelial cell cytotoxicity by decay-accelerating factor. Potential for prevention of xenograft hyperacute rejection. Transplantation 1991;52: 530–533.

34. Cooper DKC. Depletion of natural antibodies in nonhuman primates—a step towards successful discordant xenografting in humans. Clin Transpl 1992;6:178–183.

35. Latinne D, Gianello P, Smith CV, et al. Xenotransplantation from pig to cynomolgus monkey: approach toward tolerance induction. Transplant Proc 1993;25:336–338.

36. Langford GA, Yannoutsos N, Cozzi E, et al. Production of pigs transgenic for human decay accelerating factor. Transplant Proc 1994;26:1400–1401.

37. Schmoeckel M, Bhatti FN, Zaidi A, et al. Orthotopic heart transplantation in a transgenic pig-to-primate model. Transplantation 1998;65:1570–1577.

38. Zaidi A, Schmoeckel M, Bhatti FN, et al. Life-supporting pig-to-primate renal xenotransplantation using genetically modified donors. Transplantation 1998;65:1584–1590.

39. Kissmeyer-Nielsen F, Olsen S, Petersen VP, Fjeldborg O. Hyperacute rejection of kidney allografts, associated with pre-existing humoral antibodies against donor cells. Lancet 1966;2:662–665.

40. Hammer C. Preformed natural antibodies (PNAB) and possibilities of modulation of hyperacute xenogeneic rejection (HXAR). Transplant Proc 1989;21:522–523.

41. Galili U, Mandrell RE, Hamadeh RM, et al. Interaction between human natural anti-αgalactosyl immunoglobulin G and bacteria of the human flora. Infect Immunol 1988;56: 1730–1737.

42. Hammer C. Isohemagglutinins and preformed natural antibodies in xenogeneic organ transplantation. Transplant Proc 1987;19:4443–4447.

43. Galili U, Flechner I, Knyszynski A, et al. The natural anti-alpha-galactosyl IgG on human normal senescent red blood cells. Br J Haematol 1986;62:317–324.

44. Bendtzen K, Svenson M, Jonsson V, Hippe E. Autoantibodies to cytokines—friends or foes. Immunol Today 1990;11: 167–169.

45. Aksentijevich I, Sachs DH, Sykes M. Natural antibodies against bone marrow cells of a concordant xenogeneic species. J Immunol 1991;147:79–85.

46. Sablinski T, Hancock WW, Wasowska BA, et al. Modulation of acute and hyperacute rejection of xenografts in concordant hamster to rat combination. Transplant Rev 1993;25: 432–434.

47. Perper RJ, Najarian JS. Experimental renal heterotransplantation. III. Passive transfer of transplantation immunity. Transplantation 1967;5:514–533.

48. Geller RL, Bach FH, Turman MA, et al. Evidence that polyreactive antibodies are deposited in rejected discordant xenografts. Transplantation 1993;55:168–172.

49. Cooper DKC. Xenoantigens and xenoantibodies. Xenotransplantation 1998;5:6–17.

50. Platt JL, Lindman BJ, Hen H, et al. Endothelial cell antigens recognized by xenoreactive human natural antibodies. Transplantation 1990;50:817–822.

51. Cooper DKC, Koren E, Oriol R. Oligosaccharides and discordant xenotransplantation. Immunol Rev 1994;141:31–58.

52. Sandrin MS, Vaughan HA, Dabkowski PL, McKenzie IFC. Anti-pig IgM antibodies in human serum react predominantly with Gal (alpha 1–3) Gal epitopes. Proc Natl Acad Sci USA 1993;90:11391–11395.

53. Galili U, Clark MR, Shohet SB, et al. Evolutionary relationship between the natural anti-Gal antibody and the alpha 1–3 Gal epitope in primates. Proc Natl Acad Sci USA 1987;84:1369–1373.

54. Oriol R, Ye Y, Koren E, Cooper DKC. Carbohydrate antigens of pig tissues reacting with human natural antibodies as potential targets for hyperacute rejection in pig-to-man organ transplantation. Transplantation 1993;56: 1433–1442.

55. Oriol R, Candelier J-J, Taniguchi S, et al. Major carbohydrate epitopes in tissues of domestic and African wild animals of potential interest for xenotransplantation research. Xenotransplantation 1999;6:79–89.

56. Cooper DKC, Koren E, Oriol R. Genetically engineered pigs. Lancet 1993;342:682–683. Letter.

57. Alexandre GPJ, Squifflet JP, De Bruyere M, et al. Present experiences in a series of 26 ABO-incompatible living donor renal allografts. Transplant Proc 1987;19:4538–4542.

58. Leventhal JR, Sakilayak P, Witson J, et al. The synergistic effect of combined antibody and complement depletion on discordant cardiac xenograft survival in nonhuman primates. Transplantation 1994;57:974–978.

59. Tanaka M, Latinne D, Gianello P, et al. Xenotransplantation from pig to cynomolgus monkey: the potential for overcoming xenograft rejection through induction of chimerism. Transplant Proc 1994;26:1326–1327.

60. Sablinski T, Gianello PR, Bailin M, et al. Pig to monkey bone marrow and kidney xenotransplantation. Surgery 1997;121:381–391.

61. Norman JC, Brown ME, Saravis CA, et al. Perfusion techniques in temporary human-isolated ex vivo porcine liver cross circulation. Possible adjunct in the treatment of hepatic failure. Surgery 1996;6:121–125.

62. Collins BH, Chari RS, Magee JC, et al. Mechanisms of injury in porcine livers perfused with blood of patients with fulminant hepatic failure. Transplantation 1994;58:1162–1171.

63. Sablinski T, Latinne D, Gianello P, et al. Xenotransplantation of pig kidneys to nonhuman primates. I. Development of the model. Xenotransplantation 1995;2:264–270.

64. Xu Y, Lorf T, Sablinski T, et al. Removal of anti-porcine natural antibodies from human and nonhuman primate plasma in vitro and in vivo by a Galalpha1-3Galbeta1-4betaGlc-X immunoaffinity column. Transplantation 1998;65:172–179.

65. Taniguchi S, Neethling FA, Korchagina EY, et al. *In vivo* immunoadsorption of anti-pig antibodies in baboons using a specific Galα1-3Gal column. Transplantation 1996;10: 1379–1384.

66. Kozlowski T, Ierino FL, Lambrigts D, et al. Depletion of anti-αGal1-3Gal antibodies in baboons by specific immunoaffinity columns. Xenotransplantation 1998;5:122–131.

67. Watts A, Foley A, Awwad M, et al. Plasma perfusion by apheresis through a Gal immunoaffinity column successfully depletes anti-Gal antibody: experience with 280 aphereses in baboons. Presentation at the Fifth Congress of the International Xenotransplantation Association, 1999, Nagoya, Japan. Abstract 0099.

68. Simon PM, Neethling FA, Taniguchi S, et al. Intravenous infusion of Galalpha1-3Gal oligosaccharides in baboons delays hyperacute rejection of porcine heart xenografts. Transplantation 1998;65:346–353.

69. Romano E, Neethling FA, Nilsson K, et al. Intravenous synthetic αGal saccharides delay hyperacute rejection following pig-to-baboon heart transplantation. Xenotransplantation 1999;6:36–42.

70. Soares MP, Latinne D, Elsen M, et al. *In vivo* depletion of xenoreactive natural antibodies with an anti-mu monoclonal antibody. Transplantation 1993;56:1427–1433.

71. Dehoux J-P, Horri S, Talpe S, et al. In baboon, the complete elimination of circulating IgM by anti-μ monoclonal antibody allows a pig kidney xenograft to survive up to 6 days. Presentation at the Fifth Congress of the International Xenotransplantation Association, 1999, Nagoya, Japan. Abstract 0189.

72. Westerhausen M, Worsdorfer O, Gessner U, et al. Immunological changes following posttraumatic splenectomy. Blood 1981;43:345–353.

73. Foster PN, Trejdosiewicz LK. Impaired proliferative response of peripheral blood B cells from splenectomized subjects to phorbol esther and ionophore. Clin Exp Immunol 1992;89:369–373.

74. Schmoeckel M, Bhatti FN, Zaidi A, et al. Splenectomy improves survival of hDAF transgenic pig kidneys in primates. Transplant Proc 1999;31:961.

75. Murase N, Starzl TE, Demetris AJ, et al. Hamster to rat heart and liver xenotransplantation with FK506 plus antiproliferative drugs. Transplantation 1993;55:701–708.

76. Cosenza A, Tuso PJ, Chapman FA, et al. Prolonged survival following combination therapy with brequinar sodium and cyclosporine. Transplant Proc 1993;25:59–61.

77. Leventhal JR, Flores HC, Gruber SA, et al. Evidence that 15-deoxyspergualin inhibits natural antibody production but fails to prevent hyperacute rejection in a discordant xenograft model. Transplantation 1992;54:26–31.

78. Lambrigts D, Van Calster, Xu Y, et al. Pharmacologic immunosuppressive therapy and extracorporeal immunoadsorption in the suppression of anti-alpha Gal antibody in the baboon. Xenotransplantation 1998;5:274–283.

79. Alwayn IPJ, Buhler L, Basker M, Cooper DKC. The problem of anti-pig antibodies in pig-to-primate xenografting: current and novel methods of depletion and/or suppression of production of anti-pig antibodies. Xenotransplantation 1999;6:157–168.

80. Alwayn IPJ, Buhler L, Basker M, Cooper DKC. Immunomodulation strategies in xenotransplantation. In: Sayegh M, Remuzzi G, eds. Current and future immunosuppressive therapies following transplantation. Dordrecht. The Netherlands: Kluwer, (in Press).

81. Aksentijevich I, Sachs DH, Sykes M. Humoral tolerance in xenogeneic bone marrow transplant recipients conditioned with a non-myeloablative regimen. Transplantation 1992;53:1108–1114.

82. Yang Y-G, DeGoma E, Ohdan H, et al. Tolerization of anti-Galα1-3Gal natural antibody-forming B cells by induction of mixed chimerism. J Exp Med 1998;187:1335–1342.

83. Bracy JL, Sachs DH, Iacomini J. Inhibition of xenoreactive natural antibody production by retroviral gene therapy. Science 1998;281:1845–1847.

84. Thall AD, Maly P, Lowe JB. Oocyte Galα1, 3Gal epitopes implicated in sperm adhesions to the zona pelucida glycoprotein ZP3 are not required for fertilization in the mouse. J Biol Chem 1995;270:21437–21440.

85. Tearle RG, Tange MJ, Zannettino ZL, et al. The α-1,3-galactosyltransferase knockout mouse. Implications for xenotransplantation. Transplantation 1996;61:13–19.

86. Sandrin MS, Fodor WL, Mouhtouris E, et al. Enzymatic remodelling of the carbohydrate surface of a xenogenic cell substantially reduces human antibody binding and complement-mediated cytolysis. Nat Med 1995;1:1266–1267.

87. Shinkel TA, Chen G-C, Salvaris E, et al. Changes in cell surface glycosylation in α1,3 galactosyltransferase knockout and α1,2 fucosyltransferase transgenic mice. Transplantation 1997;63:197–204.

88. Osman N, McKenzie IF, Ostenried K, et al. Combined transgenic expression of alpha-galactosidase and alpha 1,2-fucosyltransferase leads to optimal reduction in the major xenoepitope Galalpha(1,3). Proc Natl Acad Sci USA 1997;94:14677–14682.

89. Wilmut I, Schnieke AE, McWhir J, et al. Viable offspring derived from fetal and adult mammalian cells. Nature 1997;385:810–813.

90. Dalmasso AP. The complement system in xenotransplantation. Immunopharmacology 1992;24:149–160.

91. Johnston PS, Lim SML, Wang MW, et al. Hyperacute rejection of xenografts in the complete absence of antibody. Transplant Proc 1991;23:877–879.

92. Miyagawa S, Hirose H, Shirakura R, et al. The mechanism of discordant xenograft rejection. Transplantation 1988;46:825–830.

93. Pruitt SK, Baldwin WM III, Marsh HC Jr, et al. The effect of soluble complement receptor type 1 on hyperacute xenograft rejection. Transplantation 1991;52: 868–873.

94. Gewurz H, Clark DS, Cooper MD, et al. Effect of cobra venom induced inhibition of complement activity on allograft and xenograft rejection reactions. Transplantation 1967;5:1296–1303.

95. Leventhal JR, Dalmasso AP, Cromwell JW, et al. Prolongation of cardiac xenograft survival by depletion of complement. Transplantation 1993;55:857–866.

96. Kobayashi T, Taniguchi S, Neethling FA, et al. Delayed xenograft rejection of pig-to-baboon cardiac transplants after cobra venom factor therapy. Transplantation 1997;64:1255–1261.

97. Ansch G, Hammer CH, Vangory P, Shin ML. Homologous species restriction in lysis of erythrocytes by terminal complement proteins. Proc Natl Acad Sci USA 1981;78: 5118–5121.

98. Hinchliffe SJ, Rushmere NK, Hanna SM, Morgan BP. Molecular cloning and functional characterization of the pig analogue of CD59: relevance to xenotransplantation. J Immunol 1998;160:3924–3932.

99. Oglesby TJ, Allen CJ, Liszewski MK, et al. Membrane cofactor protein (CD46) protects cells from complement mediated attack by an intrinsic mechanism. J Exp Med 1992;175:1547–1551.

100. Lublin DM, Coyne KE. Phospholipid-anchored and transmembrane versions of either decay-accelerating factor or membrane cofactor protein show equal efficiency in protection from complement-mediated damage. J Exp Med 1991;174:35–44.

101. Walsh JA, Tone M, Waldmann H. Transfection of human CD59 complementary DNA into rat cells confers resistance to human complement. Eur J Immunol 1992;21:847–850.

102. Cozzi E, Tucker AW, Langford GA, et al. Characterization of pigs transgenic for human decay-accelerating factor. Transplantation 1997;64:1383–1392.

103. Rosengard AM, Cary NR, Langford GA, et al. Tissue expression of human complement inhibitor, decay-accelerating factor, in transgenic pigs. A potential approach for preventing xenograft rejection. Transplantation 1995;59: 1325–1333.

104. Bhatti FN, Schmoeckel M, Zaidi A, et al. Three-month survival of hDAF transgenic pig hearts transplanted into primates. Transplant Proc 1999;31:958.

105. Ostlie DJ, Cozzi E, Vial CM, et al. SDZ RAD permits prolonged life-supporting function in HDAF pig-to-primate renal transplantation. Presentation at the Fifth Congress of the International Xenotransplantation Association, 1999, Nagoya, Japan. Abstract 0813A.

106. Vial CM, Bhatti FNK, Ostlie DJ, et al. Enhanced survival of orthotopic cardiac xenografts in an HDAF transgenic pig-to-baboon model. Presentation at the Fifth Congress of the International Xenotransplantation Association, 1999, Nagoya, Japan. Abstract 0134.

107. Platt JL, Vercellotti GM, Dalmasso AP, et al. Transplantation of discordant xenografts: a review of progress. Immunol Today 1990;11:450–456.

108. Ierino FL, Kozlowski T, Siegel JB, et al. Disseminated intravascular coagulation in association with the delayed

rejection of pig-to-baboon renal xenografts. Transplantation 1998;66:1439–1450.

109. Kozlowski T, Shimizu A, Lambrigts D, et al. Porcine kidney and heart transplantation in baboons undergoing a tolerance induction regimen and antibody adsorption. Transplantation 1999;67:18–30.

110. Murray AG, Khodadoust MM, Pober JS, Bothwell AL. Porcine aortic endothelial cells activate human T cells: direct presentation of MHC antigens and costimulation by ligands for human CD2 and CD28. Immunity 1994;1:57–63.

111. Kumagai-Braesch M, Satake M, Korsgren O, et al. Characterization of cellular human anti-porcine xenoreactivity. Clin Transpl 1993;7:273–280.

112. Yamada K, Sachs DH, DerSimonian H. Human anti-porcine xenogeneic T-cell response. Evidence for allelic specificity of mixed leukocyte reaction and for both direct and indirect pathways of recognition. J Immunol 1995;155: 5249–5256.

113. Blakely ML, Van der Werf WJ, Berndt MC, et al. Activation of intragraft endothelial and mononuclear cells during discordant xenograft rejection. Transplantation 1994;58: 1059–1066.

114. Buhler L, Awwad M, Basker M, et al. A nonmyeloablative regimen with CD40L blockade leads to humoral/cellular hyporesponsiveness to pig hematopoietic cells in baboons. Presentation at the Fifth Congress of the International Xenotransplantation Association, 1999, Nagoya, Japan. Abstract 0139.

115. Bach FH, Ferran C, Hechenleitner P, et al. Accommodation of vascularized xenografts: expression of "protective genes" by donor endothelial cells in a host Th2 cytokine environment. Nat Med 1997;3:196–204.

116. Palmer A, Taube D, Welsh K, et al. Removal of HLA antibodies by extracorporeal immunoadsorption to enable renal transplantation. Lancet 1989;1:10–12.

117. Bach FH, Platt JL, Cooper DKC. Accommodation—the role of natural antibody and complement in discordant xenograft rejection. In: Cooper DKC, Kemp E, Reemtsma K, White DJG, eds. Xenotransplantation. 1st ed. Heidelberg: Springer, 1991:81–105.

118. Widmer MB, Bach FH. Allogeneic and xenogeneic response in mixed leukocyte cultures. J Exp Med 1972;135:1204–1208.

119. Moses RD, Pierson RN III, Winn HJ, Auchincloss H Jr. Xenogeneic proliferation and lymphokine production are dependent on CD4+ helper T cells and self antigen-presenting cells in the mouse. J Exp Med 1990;172:567–575.

120. Auchincloss H Jr. Cell-mediated xenoresponses: strong or weak? Clin Transpl 1994;8:155–159.

121. Helg C, Chapuis B, Bolle JF, et al. Renal transplantation without immunosuppression in a host with tolerance induced by allogeneic bone marrow transplantation. Transplantation 1994;58:1420–1422.

122. Jacobsen N, Taaning E, Ladefoged J, et al. Tolerance to an HLA-B, DR disparate kidney allograft after bone-marrow transplantation from same donor. Lancet 1994;343:800. Letter.

123. Sayegh MH, Fine NA, Smith JL, et al. Immunologic toler-ance to renal allografts after bone marrow transplants from the same donors. Ann Inter Med 1991;114:954–955.

124. Spitzer TR, Delmonico F, Tolkoff-Rubin N, et al. Combined histocompatibility leukocyte antigen–matched donor bone marrow and renal transplantation for multiple myeloma with end-stage renal diseases: the induction of allograft tolerance through mixed lymphohematopoietic chimerism. Transplantation 1999;68:480–484.

125. Zinkernagel RM, Althage A, Callahan G, Welsh RM Jr. On the immunocompetence of H-2 incompatible irradiation bone marrow chimeras. J Immunol 1980;124:2356–2365.

126. Singer A, Hathcock KS, Hodes RJ. Self-recognition in allogeneic radiation bone marrow chimeras. J Exp Med 1981;153:1286–1301.

127. Sharabi Y, Abraham VS, Sykes M, Sachs DH. Mixed allogeneic chimeras prepared by a non-myeloablative regimen: requirement for chimerism to maintain tolerance. Bone Marrow Transplant 1992;9:191–197.

128. Blackman M, Kappler J, Marrack P. The role of the T-cell receptor in positive and negative selection of developing T cells. Science 1990;248:1335–1341.

129. Inaba M, Inaba K, Hosono M, et al. Distinct mechanisms of neonatal tolerance induced by dendritic cells and thymic B cells. J Exp Med 1991;173:549–559.

130. Ildstad ST, Sachs DH. Reconstitution with syngeneic plus allogeneic or xenogeneic bone marrow leads to specific acceptance of allografts or xenografts. Nature 1984;307: 168–170.

131. Sharabi Y, Sachs DH. Mixed chimerism and permanent specific transplantation tolerance induced by a nonlethal preparative regimen. J Exp Med 1989;169:493–502.

132. Kawai T, Cosimi AB, Colvin RB, et al. Mixed allogeneic chimerism and renal allograft tolerance in cynomolgus monkeys. Transplantation 1995;59:256–262.

133. Sharabi Y, Aksentijevich I, Sundt TM III, et al. Specific tolerance induction across a xenogeneic barrier: production of mixed rat/mouse lymphohematopoietic chimeras using a nonlethal preparative regimen. J Exp Med 1990;172: 195–202.

134. Ko DSC, Kawai T, Sogawa H, et al. Efficacy of mycophenolate mofetil induction in prolongation of kidney xenograft survival in a nonhuman concordant primate model. Presentation at the Fifth Congress of the International Xenotransplantation Association, Nagoya, Japan, 1999. Abstract 0073.

135. Sablinski T, Emery DW, Monroy R, et al. Long-term discordant xenogeneic (porcine-to-primate) bone marrow engraftment in a monkey treated with porcine-specific growth factors. Transplantation 1999;67:972–977.

136. Lee LA, Gritsch HA, Sergio JJ, et al. Specific tolerance across a discordant xenogeneic transplantation barrier. Proc Natl Acad Sci USA 1994;91:10864–10867.

137. Wu A, Esnaola NF, Yamada K, et al. Xenogeneic thymic transplantation in a pig-to-nonhuman primate model. Transplant Proc 1999;31:957.

138. Yamada K, Shimizu A, Ierino FL, et al. Thymic transplantation in miniature swine: I. Development and function of the "thymokidney." Transplantation 1999;68:1684–1692.

139. Yamada K, Shimizu A, Ierino FL, et al. Allogeneic

thymokidney transplants induce stable tolerance in miniature swine. Transplant Proc 1999;31:1199.

140. Kirkman RL. Of swine and men: organ physiology in different species. In: Hardy MA, ed. Xenograft 25. Amsterdam: Excerpta Medica, 1989:125–132.

141. Hammer C. Evolutionary obstacles to xenotransplantation. In: Cooper DKC, Kemp E, Platt JL, White DJG, eds. Xenotransplantation. 2nd. ed. Heidelberg: Springer, 1997: 716–735.

Chapter 41

Cellular Therapy

Philip D. Greenberg
Stanley R. Riddell

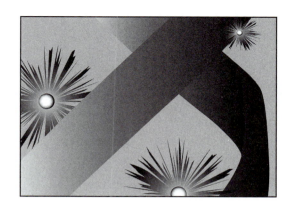

Adoptive cellular immunotherapy, in which large numbers of effector cells are administered to reconstitute or establish an immune response, is emerging as a modality for the treatment of infections and malignant diseases. Studies in animal models have defined many of the principles for effective cellular therapy and have provided valuable insights for application of this approach to the treatment of humans. Advances in cellular and molecular immunology have made it possible to overcome or circumvent many of the obstacles to effective immunotherapy and have fostered the design of clinical trials of adoptive cellular therapy, in particular specific T-cell therapy, for human disease. This chapter briefly reviews the preclinical studies that provide the foundations of adoptive T-cell therapy, describes the recent clinical studies, and discusses future prospects for cellular therapy of human virus infections and tumors.

Adoptive Cellular Therapy of Viral Diseases

The design of successful immunologic strategies to treat human viral infections requires an understanding of the effector responses that participate in control of infection and of the mechanisms by which viruses evade such responses. The cellular immune response to viruses includes nonspecific effector cells such as natural killer (NK) cells and macrophages, $\gamma\delta^+$ T cells with limited diversity for antigen recognition, and specific $\alpha\beta^+$ T cells and antibody-producing B cells with enormous diversity for antigen recognition. Studies in animal models have demonstrated that the predominant role of nonspecific effectors is during the initial phase of infection to limit viral replication and tissue injury while the T-cell response is developing, although observations in several inherited human immunodeficiency syndromes have suggested that a functional NK-cell compartment, as well as T-cell immunity, is required for successful resolution of particular viral infections (1,2). However, for most viruses, CD4$^+$ T helper (Th) and CD8$^+$ cytolytic (Tc) $\alpha\beta^+$ T-cell responses can mediate or induce the effector mechanisms necessary and sufficient to resolve acute infection (3,4) and they can provide the protective memory responses responsible for resistance to reexposure and for controlling reactivation of latent infections. In the struggle to survive and assure transmission, viruses have evolved diverse

strategies to evade these $\alpha\beta^+$ T-cell responses (5–8), but in the majority of clinical settings the host immune response ultimately prevails and controls the infection. Vaccination with viral proteins or attenuated viruses provides an effective means to further tip the balance in favor of the immune system, facilitating more rapid clearance of virus and mitigating disease. Thus, adoptive therapy with virus-specific effector T cells does not need to be considered for the treatment of most viral infections. However, there are identifiable clinical situations in which people frequently fail to mount effective responses to either a prophylactic vaccine or the infectious virus, placing them at high risk of severe or fatal disease.

Adoptive cellular therapy is currently being pursued in settings in which the host has a known immunodeficiency. Recipients of solid organ or hematopoietic stem cell transplants are rendered less immunocompetent because of the administration of immunosuppressive drugs to prevent graft rejection and to facilitate graft tolerance. The result is an increased incidence of life-threatening viral infections, including acute infections with viruses such as respiratory syncitial virus (RSV) and reactivation of persistent viruses such as cytomegalovirus (CMV), Epstein-Barr virus (EBV), and herpes zoster. The use of peptide-MHC tetramers has made it possible to quantitate T cells reactive with specific viral epitopes and has revealed that control of virus infection is associated with the generation of a very expanded virus-specific CD8$^+$ T-cell response (9–12), which is not possible in the presence of immunosuppressive drugs. Studies with viruses in immunosuppressed mice have suggested that administration of virus-specific T cells might overcome this defect and restore protective immunity (13–15). Another form of immunodeficiency occurs in individuals infected with human immunodeficiency virus (HIV-1). The continuous viral replication associated with interference and escape from immune responses ultimately results in progressive destruction of the host immune system and an immunodeficient state (16,17). Studies in HIV-infected individuals and primate models suggest that the dramatic reduction of HIV-1 viral burden following acute infection and the containment of viral replication during the asymptomatic phase of infection are mediated by CD8$^+$ HIV-1–specific T cells (18–23), and that loss of the CD8$^+$ response results in disease progression (24–27). Thus, augmentation of this HIV-1–specific T-cell response has the potential to selectively enhance resistance to viral spread and control of virus.

The principles for adoptive T-cell therapy of virus infections elucidated in animal models and preclinical studies have led to clinical trials using transfer of αβ⁺ T cells for treatment of human viral diseases. Although settings in which a selected cell subset is missing or deleted suggest that other cell populations have antiviral activities, preclinical and animal model studies have not provided enough evidence suggesting that augmenting these effector responses will substantially improve control of virus to warrant advancing to clinical trials of adoptive cell transfer. Nonspecific effector cells such as activated NK cells would likely have only limited efficacy in the treatment of infection, since the major antiviral activity mediated by this population appears to be transient control of virus during the early phases of infection prior to T-cell immunity (1,28). Thus, not only would the administration of large numbers of NK cells have the potential for significant toxicities as a result of binding to many uninfected normal cells such as endothelial cells (29), but would likely be ineffective in the absence of T-cell immunity. Although γδ⁺ T cells with reactivity to virally infected cells have been isolated and could potentially be transferred, the role γδ⁺ T cells play in resolving viral infection is still unclear (3,30). The bulk of evidence would suggest that these cells play an immunoregulatory role and link innate immunity with the adaptive response and may contribute to the resolution of inflammation (31–33), but this evidence does not suggest a critical role in the presence of a response by αβ⁺ T cells. Thus, at the present time, adoptive therapy with virus-specific αβ⁺ T cells provides the greatest promise for a cell therapy strategy with the goals of maximal therapeutic efficacy and minimal toxicity.

Effector T Cells: Role of CD4+ and CD8+ T Cells in Controlling Viral Infections

Studies in animal models have provided evidence that, under appropriate experimental circumstances, either CD4⁺ or CD8⁺ T cells individually can be sufficient to provide protective immunity to challenge with viruses such as influenza, parainfluenza, and herpes simplex virus (13,34–37). However, for viruses such as lymphocytic choriomeningitis virus (LCMV), murine cytomegalovirus, and a murine gamma herpes virus, CD4⁺ T cells cannot adequately control infection, and CD8⁺ Tc appear to be the essential effector cells required (14,38,39). Indeed, following acute infection with LCMV or gamma herpes virus, an enormous expansion of virus-specific CD8⁺ CTL occurs (40–42), but a CD4⁺ Th response is required to sustain this CTL response and clear chronic infection (39,43,44). Cumulatively, these studies have highlighted the significant antiviral activities of both CD4⁺ and CD8⁺ T cells, but do not clearly define how best to proceed from experimental animal models to protocols for adoptive therapy of naturally occurring human viral disease.

The generation of mice lacking potential contributions by CD8⁺ T cells, because of lack of expression of class I molecules by targeted disruption of the β-2 microglobulin gene, or by CD4⁺ T cells, because of disruption of a class II structural gene or the CD4 gene, has provided an opportunity to more clearly evaluate the roles of CD4⁺ and CD8⁺ T cells in viral immunity (45,46). β-

2m−/− mice are severely deficient in CD8⁺ T cells, which is caused by the absence of positive selection during thymic ontogeny (47,48). These mice have significantly impaired resistance to LCMV and Theiler's virus, consistent with the critical role of CD8⁺ Tc previously observed in these infections, but only subtle defects in clearance of influenza, vaccinia, and Sendai virus (49–54). However, a more extensive analysis with influenza demonstrated that, while β-2m−/− mice clear virus of low virulence, challenge with strains of higher virulence results in delayed clearance and increased morbidity and mortality in comparison with β-2m+/+ mice (54). Thus, CD8⁺ Tc appear to have a major role in the host response to most viruses, while for selected exposures to low doses of virus and/or to strains of low virulence, the plasticity of the immune system, presumably reflecting induction of CD4⁺ Th responses and recruitment of NK cells, γδ⁺ T cells, and/or antibody-secreting B cells, may be sufficient to compensate for selective deficiencies in CD8⁺ Tc responses (39).

Experiments in mice with deficient CD4⁺ responses have supported and extended these conclusions. Class II −/− mice, despite the absence of CD4⁺ Th, have the ability to generate CD8⁺ Tc and resist challenge with LCMV or influenza virus (55,56). However, further studies in mice with a disrupted CD4 or class II gene have demonstrated that maintenance of the CD8⁺ Tc effector response requires CD4⁺ Th (43,57), and that the outcome of challenge in CD4-deficient mice depended on the dose and virulence of the virus. Similarly, following vaccinia infection of CD4-deficient mice, sufficient IL-2 was produced by the initially responding CD8⁺ T cells to generate a functional response independent of CD4⁺ Th cells, but maintenance of this response shortly became dependent on exogenous IL-2 or a CD4⁺ Th response (58). Thus, the importance of CD4⁺ Th, particularly in the context of adoptive therapy with CD8⁺ effector Tc, is most likely to become evident in chronic infections characterized by viral persistence and reactivation or in the setting of a high viral load.

Effector T Cells: Mechanisms by Which CD4+ and CD8+ T Cells Mediate Antiviral Responses

Adoptive therapy with T-cell populations is predicated on the assumption that the transferred cells can mediate the desired antiviral effect. Defining the specific effector functions used by each subset and the potential limitations of such activity has become increasingly important, because recent technical advances have made it possible to overcome some of the qualitative and quantitative obstacles to efficacy of cellular therapy by concurrently administering recombinant cytokines or by genetically modifying the T cells prior to transfer. The majority of insights regarding the effector mechanisms operative in elimination of viruses have been derived from animal studies.

CD4⁺ T cells can only recognize the limited range of target cells that present peptide antigens in association with class II heterodimers. Although class II⁺ cells infected with some viruses such as measles, HSV-1, and HIV-1 can be lysed by CD4[+] effector cells (59–61), the CD4[+] response is commonly limited to recognizing antigen-presenting cells (APC) that present endocytosed viral antigens rather than infected cells actively synthesizing viral proteins. Thus, the major antiviral effects of CD4[+] T cells usually result from secretion of cytokines that activate other effector responses. Differentiated CD4[+] T cells can be separated into two major subsets based on the profile of secreted cytokines (62). Th1 cells produce IL-2, IFNγ, and TNF, thereby promoting cell-mediated immune responses, including activation of CD8[+] Tc, NK cells, and macrophages, and enhancing the resistance of uninfected cells to virus (63–66). Th2 cells, by contrast, produce IL-4, IL-5, and IL-10, and predominantly promote humoral immune responses and the activation of eosinophils and mast cells (62,67–70). For intracellular pathogens such as viruses, Th1 responses and the associated cell-mediated immunity and local inflammatory reactions appear to be the most important, although promoting antibody responses can clearly facilitate early containment and clearance of virus. The importance of Th1 responses is supported both by adoptive-transfer experiments and by detection of IL-2 and IFNγ as the predominant cytokines being produced in lymphocytes that are present in draining lymph nodes and bronchoalveolar lavage fluid after acute, nonfatal infection of mice (71,72). Adoptive therapy studies in mice infected with influenza demonstrated that influenza-specific CD4[+] Th1 clones were protective, whereas Th2 clones were not (73). Studies in mice challenged with RSV revealed an additional and potentially important consideration for human studies—the transfer of RSV-specific CD4[+] Th2 cells induced an eosinophil-rich inflammatory response with hemorrhage and neutrophils in the lung and increased host morbidity/mortality (74).

CD8[+] T cells, in distinction to CD4[+] T cells, recognize viral peptides in association with class I molecules—thus, virtually all cells infected by a virus can be recognized by this effector population. CD8[+] Tc have also been divided into two major subsets based on cytokine secretion. The Tc1 subset produces Th1-type cytokines, and the Tc2 subset produces Th2-type cytokines (75). These cytokines may contribute to clearance of virus by engaging distinct, auxilliary, effector mechanisms (76,77). CD8[+] T cells can also secrete other molecules that have antiviral activity (78,79). However, the cytolytic function of CD8[+] T cells is the distinguishing and likely critical contribution of this population of effector cells. This conclusion is supported by studies in mice lacking perforin or Fas expression, thereby preventing cytolysis by CD8[+] T cells, which cannot efficiently clear viral infections such as LCMV and influenza (80,81).

IL-2 and IFNγ appear to be the cytokines produced by CD4[+] and CD8[+] T cells that most significantly contribute to the antiviral effects of the cellular immune response. Deficiencies of IL-2 would be predicted to severely impair the host response to viral pathogens by virtue of its role as the principle growth factor for T cells. Although IL-2 –/– knockout mice can generate initial CD8[+] Tc responses to viruses such as LCMV and vaccinia, these mice are deficient in secondary responses to viruses unless IL-2 is provided (82,83). This is most problematic for chronic, persis-

tent viral infections such as LCMV in which IL-2 or CD4[+] Th activity is required for maintenance of a functional, protective CD8[+] response (44,84,85). As predicted by these studies, humans with congenital defects in IL-2 production have exhibited increased susceptibility to viral infections (86,87). In adoptive therapy studies in settings in which a prolonged immune response is required, IL-2 is critical to support the in vivo persistence and proliferation of transferred CD8[+] T cells (88,89). These results have important implications for the design of adoptive therapy protocols for human viral diseases. Since human effector CD8[+] Tc that have been expanded in vitro do not produce significant amounts of IL-2 following antigen stimulation, long-term maintenance and in vivo expansion of adoptively transferred CD8[+] Tc responses will likely require the provision of exogenous IL-2 or concurrent administration of CD4[+] Th cells.

IFNγ has many activities that enhance the efficacy of cellular antiviral responses, including direct inhibition of viral replication, activation of nonspecific effector cells such as NK cells and macrophages, and up-regulation of cellular genes involved in the presentation of viral antigens for recognition by CD8[+] Tc, including TAP, LMP, and class I genes (1,90–95). Several experimental strategies to abrogate IFNγ activity in vivo have been used to define the requirement for IFNγ in host resistance to virus, including administering anti-IFNγ neutralizing monoclonal antibodies and constructing knockout mice that are either IFNγ –/– or IFNγ receptor –/–. These studies have suggested that IFNγ enhances the ability of the host to limit viral replication, but that, in general, even in the absence of IFNγ activity, the host can generate CD4[+] Th and CD8[+] Tc responses and resolve viral infections (96–98). Studies in humans found to have inherited abnormalities resulting in disruptions of the IFNγ signaling pathway have revealed a unique increase in susceptibility to intracellular bacteria, especially mycobacteria, with little increase in viral infections (99,100). Thus, these analyses in murine models and man, which highlight the principle that the effector responses to most viruses are sufficiently plastic and redundant to potentially overcome the loss of an individual component, suggest that the concurrent administration of IFNγ would not be expected to significantly enhance the therapeutic efficacy of transferred effector T cells.

Adoptive Therapy of Viral Diseases: Potential Obstacles to Efficacy

Viruses have evolved many diverse strategies to evade recognition and elimination by the host cellular immune response (Table 41-1). These mechanisms, by promoting prolongation of acute infection and/or facilitating establishment of persistent infection, provide the virus with adequate time to be transmitted to a new host. Defining the viral evasion strategies operative during particular viral infections is of practical importance for the design of adoptive-immunotherapy regimens, since it may influence the specificity, phenotype, or amount of T cells required to achieve therapeutic efficacy.

Table 41-1. Mechanisms by Which Viruses Evade T-Cell Responses

- Mutations in epitopes recognized by CD8$^+$ Tc
- Interference with antigen processing and presentation
- Secretion of proteins that block cytokine or chemokine activity
- Production of proteins that subvert effector responses
- Production of proteins that inhibit apoptosis of infected cells
- Establishment of latent infection with episodes of reactivation
- Elimination of virus-reactive T cells
- Inactivation of virus-reactive CD8$^+$ Tc effector functions

Mutational events in viruses that occur either within the coding region of an MHC binding peptide or in flanking sequences that affect antigen processing can interfere with T-cell elimination of the virus (101–105). Although this could occur with any virus, it is most likely to be biologically relevant for viruses that have high error rates during replication and/or that induce a highly focused, immunodominant, host T-cell response. Mutations resulting in changes in the epitopes recognized by T cells have been shown not only to provide a means to escape recognition, but also potentially to antagonize recognition of wild-type epitopes binding to the same MHC molecule, perhaps by inducing an anergic signal (106–108). Mutation as a viral evasion strategy has been demonstrated with LCMV and Gross virus in murine models (109,110), with EBV in human population studies (111), and with HIV-1 in studies of infected patients (8,112–114). In situations in which virus mutational escape is commonly observed, adoptive cellular therapy protocols will likely need to include transfer of T cells specific for multiple epitopes to minimize the risk of outgrowth of variant viruses.

The multistep process involved in the processing and presentation of viral antigens affords many distinct cellular sites at which viruses have been shown to interfere with recognition and elimination by CD8$^+$ Tc. For example, adenoviruses and herpes viruses encode proteins that decrease the amount of antigen presented on a target cell by down-regulating expression of class I genes, promoting degradation of class I molecules, retaining peptide-loaded class I molecules in the endoplasmic reticulum (ER) to prevent transport to the cell surface, blocking the transport of peptides into the ER to bind with class I molecules, and interfering with peptide loading of class I in the ER (6,115–117). Effective adoptive therapy in these settings will require the transfer of CD8$^+$ T cells that recognize viral antigens presented by infected cells prior to interference with the processing machinery, the transfer of CD8$^+$ Tc of high affinity that require expression of fewer peptide-MHC complexes by the target, and/or the administration of cytokines such as IFNγ that increase the activity of the antigen-processing machinery, as well as for some viruses the transfer of CD4$^+$ rather than CD8$^+$ effector T cells. However, viruses can also potentially disrupt the class II processing pathway or interfere with APC function, thereby interfering with the generation of a CD4$^+$ T-cell response (6,118,119). Fortunately, most of these evasion strategies are incomplete and

represent a means by which the virus normally prolongs its life span in the host but one that can be overcome with an appropriately targeted T-cell response.

The secretion of cytokines by cells participating in the immune response to virus often significantly augments the generation and recruitment of an effective response and enhances the effector activity of the response. However, viruses can produce proteins that interfere with these functions (7). For example, EBV produces BCRF1, a protein homologous to IL-10 that promotes skewing of the CD4$^+$ T-cell response toward the Th2 phenotype (120–122), and vaccinia viruses produce an IL-1 binding protein that inhibits IL-1 initiation of the CD4$^+$ T-cell response (123,124). IFNα/β produced by inflammatory cells can inhibit viral replication in infected cells, but adenovirus, EBV, and HIV produce RNA molecules that block this cytokine's intracellular activity (5). TNF and IFNγ are effector cytokines with antiviral activity, but Shope fibroma virus and myxoma virus secrete soluble proteins that bind and neutralize these cytokines (5,125,126). Adenoviruses produce proteins that render infected cells resistant to the cytolytic effects of TNF (5,116). Finally, the secretion of chemokines at sites of infection recruit the cell populations necessary for establishing an effective response, and some viruses secrete molecules that can neutralize chemokines (124,127). Such viral evasion strategies could be particularly problematic for adoptive therapy in the setting of an overwhelming infection and might be addressed with direct countermeasures such as administration of a specific cytokine, if providing large numbers of effector T cells proves insufficient to circumvent the blockade.

The establishment of viral latency, as observed with HSV, VZV, CMV, EBV, and HIV-1 infections, in which some infected cells containing the viral genome do not express any immunogenic viral proteins, makes it possible for the virus to persist during the height of the immune response but subsequently to replicate and spread after it has declined (128–133). Although episodes of viral reactivation are usually efficiently controlled by rapid host memory T-cell responses to the virus, individuals with iatrogenic or other acquired immunodeficiency states associated with impaired T-cell responses may succumb to progressive and life-threatening infections from viruses that had formerly been effectively contained. Adoptive T-cell transfer in immunocompromised hosts for treatment of viruses with latent phases may need to provide not only adequate effector cells for the immediate control of virus but also, depending on the duration of the immunocompromised state, cells capable of persisting to provide long-term immunity.

Rapidly replicating viruses can mediate unique escape mechanisms in that the large number of infected targets may eventually overwhelm the effector T-cell response and lead to deletion or dysfunction of the reactive T cells. For example, mice infected with a virulent strain of LCMV initially exhibit an expanding CD8$^+$ Tc response, but, with persistent viral replication, the LCMV-reactive CD8$^+$ Tc can become undetectable (134). Similarly, CD8$^+$ Tc transferred into these mice can mediate a transient antiviral effect, but subsequently are deleted (135). Evaluation of the loss of CD8$^+$ effector-cell activity in this setting has revealed not only deletion of reactive T cells but also the persistence of virus-specific CD8⁺ T cells that can no longer mediate antiviral activities such as cytolysis or cytokine production (84). Although the mechanisms by which these deletional events and functional defects occur in CD8⁺ T cells have not been fully defined, the outcomes are similar to those observed in mice rendered deficient in CD4⁺ helper T cells and infected with LCMV (44,84). Thus, the loss of CD8⁺ Tc function and viability may be a consequence of incomplete signaling following activation through the TCR, with the T cells failing, following repetitive target recognition, to receive growth and survival signals normally provided by concurrently responding CD4⁺ T cells. Indeed, a similar loss of CD8⁺ Tc is observed in HIV-infected individuals in whom the initially strong CD8⁺ Tc response contributes to control of disease but subsequently declines in association with persistent viral replication and the failure to sustain an HIV-specific CD4⁺ T-cell response (85,136,137). Although studies have not yet adequately addressed the issue of the presence of non-functional HIV-specific CD8⁺ T cells in HIV-infected individuals, data are accumulating to suggest this population is indeed dysfunctional (138–140). Thus, effective adoptive therapy of replicating persistent viruses with CD8⁺ Tc may require that concurrent CD4⁺ helper T cells, factors, or signals be provided, and that the function of the transferred CD8⁺ Tc be monitored to ascertain that the persistent T cells retain the capacity to function.

Adoptive Transfer of Virus-Specific T Cells As Treatment of Human Viral Diseases

Clinical trials have begun to evaluate T-cell transfer as a strategy for restoring protective immunity to persistent CMV and EBV infection in immunocompromised, hematopoietic stem cell transplant (HCT) recipients and for augmenting T-cell responses to HIV in HIV-infected individuals. These studies, as reviewed below, have demonstrated that the adoptive transfer of virus-specific T cells can safely augment virus-specific T-cell immunity and restore protective responses in immunocompromised patients. These studies also provided direction for efforts to broadly apply this approach to immunocompromised patients at risk for viral infection.

T-Cell Therapy of CMV

The design of human trials of T-cell therapy for CMV has been facilitated by studies in a murine model of CMV disease. Infection of normal mice with murine CMV (MCMV) results in a limited, acute infection followed by a persistent, latent infection. Immunosuppression of such chronically infected mice leads to a progressive fatal infection characterized by pneumonia and hematopoietic failure (14,141,142). Encouragingly, adoptive transfer of MCMV-specific CD8⁺ Tc into MCMV-infected, immunosuppressed mice can provide protection from this fatal CMV disease (14,143). Human CMV poses similar problems, and more than 70% of the individuals who harbor latent CMV infection and receive the intense immunosuppressive regimen associ-

ated with allogeneic HCT exhibit reactivation of CMV. In the absence of antiviral drug therapy, approximately 50% of patients reactivating CMV will develop CMV pneumonia or enteritis (144). Analysis of immunologic reconstitution during the first 100 days post-BMT has demonstrated that CMV disease occurs exclusively in the subset of patients that lack CD8⁺ T-cell responses, suggesting that this effector cell is also essential for resistance to human CMV disease (145). Thus, the animal model studies and correlative clinical data have made CMV disease in HCT patients an attractive setting to pursue the first trial for treating human disease by the adoptive transfer of CD8⁺ virus-specific T-cell clones.

The biology of CMV has suggested that only particular viral proteins may be appropriate targets for T-cell therapy. Cells replicating CMV do not efficiently present newly synthesized viral proteins to CD8⁺ T cells because of the down-regulation of class I MHC molecules mediated by the products of CMV genes (6,146–148). However, structural viral proteins such as the CMV matrix protein pp65 that enter the cell following virus penetration and uncoating are presented to CD8⁺ Tc before modulation of class I MHC expression. CD8⁺ Tc specific for such viral antigens are maintained at high levels in immunocompetent hosts and are presumed to represent the protective host response (149,150). Therefore, a protocol was designed to treat allogeneic HCT patients by the infusion of CD8⁺ T-cell clones that were derived from the HLA-identical, sibling donor; that were selected for recognition of structural CMV proteins; and that expanded to large numbers in vitro. Such donor T cells should theoretically be capable of only recognizing CMV-infected targets and unable to cause GVHD.

In the initial study of T-cell therapy for CMV, 14 patients received four weekly infusions of escalating doses of CD8⁺ CMV-specific T-cell clones after transplant. The patients were monitored for reconstitution of CMV-specific T-cell immunity, toxicity, and antiviral effects. Transfer of CMV-specific T-cell immunity was detected following infusion of even the lowest cell dose, and the level of reactivity achieved after the fourth infusion was equivalent to the protective responses detected in immunocompetent donors (151,152). Long-term (>12 weeks) persistence of the transferred Tc was documented in this study by monitoring for the presence in CMV-specific CD8⁺ T cells in the peripheral blood using the DNA sequence derived from the rearranged TCR Vβ genes of the infused clones as a marker for transferred T cells (152). As predicted from murine models, in which maintenance of CD8⁺ T-cell immunity to chronic viral infections requires a concurrent CD4⁺ Th response (44,84), the subset of HCT recipients on this study who did not recover endogenous CMV-specific CD4⁺ Th responses demonstrated a continuous decline in the magnitude of CMV-specific CD8⁺ Tc responses over the 12-week monitoring period. By contrast, recipients who recovered CD4⁺ Th responses to CMV maintained CD8⁺ Tc responses at levels equivalent to the normal donors. A transient fever after a single infusion was the only toxicity observed, and none of the 14 patients developed CMV viremia or disease. These results demonstrated that CD8⁺ T-cell immunity to CMV could be safely and effectively restored by the transfer of T-cell clones, but they also suggested that the cotransfer of CD4⁺ Th may be necessary for long-term persistence of transferred CD8⁺ Tc responses (152).

A larger, ongoing study in which both CMV-specific CD8⁺ Tc and CD4⁺ Th are being adoptively transferred to allogeneic HCT recipients has confirmed both the safety of this approach and the effective augmentation or restoration of deficient T-cell responses to CMV. However, it has also identified a subset of patients who pose an additional obstacle to successful immunologic reconstitution by adoptive T-cell therapy. A proportion of HCT recipients who develop severe graft-versus-host disease (GVHD) from the alloreactive T cells infused with the stem cell-inoculum require additional intensive immunosuppression with prednisone. Preliminary analysis of the function and persistence of adoptively transferred CMV-specific T cells in HCT recipients receiving high-dose prednisone suggests that the transferred cells fail to function normally, persist for a shorter duration, and are less effective in limiting virus replication (153).

T-Cell Therapy of EBV-induced Lymphoproliferative Disease

Epstein-Barr virus (EBV) is a ubiquitous herpes virus that infects approximately 95% of adults and persists in immunocompetent hosts in a latent form in B cells. The reservoir of latently infected B cells maintains the EBV genome as an episome, but expresses only the EBNA-1 gene (154–157). These cells escape immunologic detection because of the poor antigen-presenting capacity of resting B cells and the presence of unique, glycine-alanine repeat sequences in the EBNA-1 protein, which serve to abrogate processing of this protein and presentation by class I MHC molecules (158,159). Activation of latently infected B cells or de novo infection of B cells in vitro can lead to the lytic phase of the viral life cycle with expression of the full array of viral genes and production of new virions. However, this activation more commonly results in the expression of only a limited subset of viral latency genes, including those encoding the nuclear antigens EBNA-1,-2,-3A,-3B,-3C, and LP, and the latent membrane proteins LMP 1 and 2. These latent proteins do not cause cell lysis or death, but rather function to induce and maintain a transformed state (160). In response to chronic EBV infection, immunocompetent hosts develop high levels of CD8⁺ Tc usually specific for one or more of the EBNA-3A,-3B, or -3C proteins and minor responses to EBNA-2, LP, LMP-1, or LMP-2, which are thought to prevent the outgrowth of transformed B cells (10,161,162). In fact, EBV-transformed B cells expressing these eight EBV latent proteins will grow out of in vitro cultures of B lymphocytes from EBV⁺ individuals providing the T cells are removed from the cultures or suppressed with cyclosporin (163).

In chronically immunosuppressed EBV⁺ solid-organ-transplant recipients, especially those who receive anti-CD3 mAb to deplete T cells in vivo to prevent or treat rejection, as well as in allogeneic HCT recipients who receive a T-cell–depleted HCT or

are administered anti-CD3 mAb in vivo to prevent or treat GVHD (164–169), B-cell lymphoproliferative disease caused by EBV is a significant clinical problem. The proliferative B cells, which phenotypically represent EBV-infected B cells expressing the limited set of viral latency genes, may be polyclonal in the initial phases, but often become monoclonal with selection of more malignant cells as the disease progresses. These patients have a grave prognosis, responding poorly to antiviral drug therapy, as well as to conventional chemotherapy or radiotherapy (170,171).

The association of EBV-LPD with immunosuppressive regimens that specifically eliminate T cells, the correlation between the temporal occurrence of EBV-LPD after HCT and the period of deficient cytotoxic T-cell responses, and the expression of EBV proteins in the proliferating cells that are recognized by Tc suggested not only that the loss of virus-specific T cells may play a critical role in the pathogenesis of EBV-LPD, but that this disease may be amenable to cellular immunotherapy (171–173). The initial study of cellular therapy for EBV-LPD was performed in patients who developed EBV-LPD following T-cell–depleted allogeneic HCT and attempted to correct the deficiency of EBV-reactive T cells by infusing polyclonal lymphocytes obtained from the allogeneic donor. This therapy led to expansion of EBV-reactive Tc in vivo and the sustained resolution of EBV LPD in most patients. However, two patients with advanced LPD involving the lungs suffered fatal respiratory complications, and the majority of responding patients developed graft-versus-host disease because of the presence of alloreactive T cells in the infused population (171,174). Subsequently, donor T cells containing both CD4⁺ and CD8⁺ T cells highly enriched for EBV reactivity by prior in vitro culture with irradiated EBV-LCL stimulators were used to successfully treat EBV-LPD after allogeneic HCT, and these donor T cells did not cause significant GVHD (175,176). In these latter studies, a marker gene was introduced into the transferred T cells by retrovirus-mediated gene transfer, and T cells containing the marker gene were detected infiltrating the sites of EBV-LPD and could be isolated from the blood up to 18 months after the infusions (176). Recently, prophylactic infusions by EBV-reactive T cells generated from the donor PBL have been used to prevent the development of EBV-LPD in immunodeficient recipients of T-cell–depleted HCT (177).

The studies of cellular immunotherapy for EBV-LPD in HCT recipients have established the therapeutic benefits of this approach, but several issues have limited the efforts to extend the use of T-cell therapy to the solid-organ-transplant recipients at highest risk, individuals who are EBV seronegative at the time of transplant and receive a transplanted organ from an EBV⁺ donor. These issues include the difficulty of isolating EBV-reactive T cells from the EBV-negative recipient for use in therapy and the necessity for these patients to continue immunosuppressive drug therapy to prevent or treat T-cell–mediated rejection of the transplanted organ. However, as discussed later in this chapter, the ability to introduce TCR genes into T cells that confer a desired antigen specificity and/or genes that confer resistance to immunosuppressive drugs may overcome these obstacles.

T-Cell Therapy of HIV Infection

Several observations support a role for HIV-specific CD8[+] Tc and/or CD4[+] Th responses in controlling virus replication. These include the findings that clearance of viremia and recovery of CD4[+] T-cell counts following primary HIV-1 infection is associated with the development of HIV-specific CD8[+] Tc responses (19,23); that individuals who maintain strong CD8[+] Tc responses exhibit lower viral loads, longer asymptomatic periods, and slower declines in CD4[+] T-cell counts (21,22,25); and that a decline in recoverable CD8[+] Tc responses is associated with disease progression and increasing viremia (178). A characteristic of most HIV-infected individuals is a lack of CD4[+] HIV-specific Th (179,180). However, rare patients with strong CD4[+] Th responses to HIV have been identified, and these patients typically exhibit a nonprogressive infection characterized by low levels of plasma viremia and normal CD4[+] T-cell numbers (136). These correlative data have led to the development of clinical trials to determine if more effective control of HIV infection in individuals with progressive infection can be achieved by augmenting CD8[+] and CD4[+] T-cell responses to HIV-1.

Our laboratory has examined the adoptive transfer of autologous CD8[+] HIV-specific T-cell clones isolated from HIV-infected patients, selected for recognition of epitopes that are conserved in the patient's virus, and expanded to large numbers in vitro prior to infusion. To facilitate analysis of in vivo persistence and migration, the CD8[+] Tc were modified by retrovirus-mediated gene transfer to contain a neomycin phosphotransferase marker gene, which permitted the detection of transferred cells in vivo by flow cytometry using in situ PCR and hybridization for *neo* sequences. CD8[+] Tc were administered to patients in doses of $1 \times 10^8/m^2$ to $3.3 \times 10^9/m^2$. The cell infusions were well tolerated, although a mild flulike illness lasting up to 2 days was observed in patients with a high viral load, potentially reflecting activation and cytokine release by transferred Tc following recognition of infected cells in vivo. One day following the infusion of 3.3×10^9 CTL/m^2, 1.5% to 3.7% of CD8[+] T cells in the peripheral blood contained the marker gene, which was associated with a significant increase in the HIV-specific cytolytic activity of freshly isolated peripheral blood lymphocytes (181). Over the ensuing 4 days, the gene-marked T cells trafficked to and accumulated in lymph nodes at sites adjacent to cells actively replicating HIV and caused a reduction in the numbers of circulating HIV-infected cells in the blood (181). However, in these hosts with decreased CD4 counts and absent CD4[+] T-cell responses to HIV, the transferred Tc persisted for only several days and virus replication subsequently rebounded to pretreatment levels.

The adoptive transfer of large numbers of CD8[+] HIV-specific T-cell clones has provided direct evidence for the antiviral activities of CD8[+] Tc in HIV infection and insight into factors that may limit the efficacy of both the transferred endogenous CD8[+] Tc responses. A deficiency of IL-2–producing CD4[+] HIV-specific Th cells is characteristic of the majority of HIV-1–infected individuals, and, as observed in mice with LCMV infection, this lack of CD4[+] Th may result in dysfunction, short-

ened survival, and eventual deletion of virus-specific CD8[+] Tc (44,84). Therefore, strategies to potentially circumvent the CD4 deficiency and to prolong CD8[+] Tc survival and antiviral activity are being developed for second-generation studies. One approach is to develop helper-independent CD8[+] T cells by introducing a modified cytokine receptor that can deliver an autocrine IL-2 growth signal in response to a cytokine such as GM-CSF that is produced in a regulated fashion by the CD8[+] T cell in response to target recognition. High-affinity binding of IL-2 by the natural IL-2R requires the three α, β, and γ IL-2 receptor (IL-2R) chains, but the intracellular signaling is mediated entirely as a result of the dimerization of the cytoplasmic domains of the β and γ chains (182,183). Chimeric receptors that are composed of the extracellular, ligand-binding domains of the α and β chains of the two-chain GM-CSF receptor that are fused respectively to the cytoplasmic signaling domains of the IL-2R γ and β chains have been constructed and introduced into T cells. These receptor chains dimerize on binding GM-CSF and signal downstream biochemical events and proliferation identical to those induced by the authentic IL-2R (182). Recent studies demonstrate that the introduction of these GM-CSF/IL-2R chimeric receptors into virus-specific CD8[+] Tc clones will result in autocrine proliferation following target recognition (184). Further studies in vitro and in animal models are required to determine if providing a regulated growth signal will also overcome some of the functional abnormalities observed in HIV-specific CD8[+] Tc in infected individuals, but the engineering of bifunctional CD8[+] Tc by genetic modification offers the potential to overcome one of the obstacles to therapy with CD8[+] Tc in CD4-deficient hosts.

In many HIV[+] patients, rare CD4[+] HIV-specific Th can be detected and isolated in vitro. Therefore an alternative approach to provide HIV-specific Th function is to confer an HIV-resistant phenotype to CD4[+] HIV-specific Th by the introduction of genes that interfere with critical steps in the virus life cycle such as binding, entry, and replication. These HIV-resistant CD4[+] Th could then be expanded in vitro and adoptively transferred to the patient. Both RNA- and protein-based strategies have been developed for inhibiting HIV replication. RNA-based inhibitors include transactivation response (TAR) element decoys and Rev response element (RRE) decoys that sequester Tat or Rev and ribozymes engineered to cleave specific HIV sequences (185–187). Protein-based inhibitors include a dominant negative Rev protein, intracellular antibodies that bind and inhibit the function of HIV proteins required for virus replication, and modified chemokine ligands that bind and retain in the ER HIV coreceptors required for virus entry (188–192). Early clinical trials, in which polyclonal autologous CD4[+] T cells were modified to express a dominant negative Rev protein (RevM10) and were infused into HIV[+] patients, have provided evidence that survival of CD4[+] T cells can be improved by expression of genes that inhibit HIV replication (193,194). Thus, it may be possible to establish an effective CD4[+] Th response by the transfer of expanded numbers of CD4[+] HIV-specific Th clones rendered genetically resistant to HIV.

The difficulty isolating and expanding HIV-specific T cells from patients with advanced disease has led to the development of approaches to engineer HIV reactivity in nonspecifically expanded cells by the introduction of chimeric receptors that can recognize infected targets. Receptors containing extracellular domains composed of either the variable region of an envelope-specific antibody or the CD4 molecule fused to the cytoplasmic signaling domain of the TCR zeta chain have been expressed in T cells and shown to bind and kill HIV-infected targets in vitro (195,196). Adoptive transfer of these genetically modified cytolytic cells may need to overcome the problem posed by the large, cell-free HIV burden in some patients that may occupy the receptor, and it is unclear if repetitive triggering through these chimeric receptors in vivo will be sufficient to result in retention of cytolytic activity or permit cell survival. Clinical trials are being conducted in HIV-infected patients to assess these issues and should provide directions for developing this cellular therapy regimen.

Adoptive T-Cell Therapy of Viral Diseases: Future Potential

The adoptive transfer of virus-specific T cells is emerging as a useful approach for the prophylaxis or treatment of CMV and EBV infections in immunodeficient recipients of allogeneic HCT. Several limitations of this approach have been identified and will need to be addressed in future studies. One is the susceptibility of transferred T cells to the inhibitory effects of the intensive immunosuppressive drug therapy that is often being concurrently administered to these patients. This could potentially be overcome by genetically modifying the transferred T cells to be resistant to one or more of the immunosuppressive drugs. Strategies for rendering cells resistant to cyclosporin by expressing a mutant calcineurin protein have been described (197), and similar approaches are being pursued for other commonly used agents. A second issue, related to the use of T-cell therapy for CMV and EBV in solid-organ transplant patients who develop a primary infection from the transplanted organ, is the difficulty isolating T cells from the recipient for use in therapy. This obstacle could potentially be resolved by introducing the TCR α and β genes derived from a T-cell clone of known antigen specificity and MHC restriction into T cells from the recipient to confer the desired reactivity (198).

Reservoirs of replicating and latent HIV persist in infected individuals despite combination antiretroviral drug therapy, and maintaining HIV-specific T-cell responses by adoptive transfer could assist in reducing these viral reservoirs. However, as discussed above, it may be necessary to genetically modify CD8+ T cells to overcome limitations imposed by the CD4+ Th deficiency in these individuals, and it will be essential to ensure that T cells can traffic to the tissue sites containing reservoirs of HIV.

Viruses such as EBV, HPV, and KSHV have been associated with the development of malignancies in humans, and an emerging area of interest is to augment T-cell responses to viral proteins expressed in tumor cells by vaccination or T-cell therapy. This issue will be discussed more extensively in the next section. However, a more complete understanding of the mechanisms these tumors use to evade recognition, despite the expression of immunogenic proteins, is likely to be necessary to design appropriate therapeutic strategies.

Adoptive Cellular Therapy of Tumors

Cellular therapy has been more extensively pursued for the treatment of human malignancy than for human viral diseases. This has in part reflected the intense need to develop new treatment strategies for cancer and has resulted in testing not only specific T cells but the more readily generated nonspecific effector-cell populations that can lyse tumor cells in vitro and that also have in vivo activity in animal tumor models. However, the initial human clinical trials, particularly with nonspecific effector cells, have had limited success, and the substantial obstacles to effectively and broadly translating this strategy to human tumor therapy must be resolved before the potential demonstrated in murine models can be realized. These obstacles appear more profound than those previously described for developing therapy for viral infections, as a result of both the failure of most tumors to encode readily characterizable novel antigens that induce strong T-cell responses and the more complex biology of tumors as compared with viruses. However, recent advances in cellular and molecular immunology have provided approaches for identifying target antigens at which to direct an immunologic attack, as well as insights into the underlying biology. Thus, it can be expected that cellular therapy using specific tumor-reactive T cells will become increasingly available and hopefully effective for the treatment of a wide range of malignancies.

Effector Cells Capable of Mediating Antitumor Responses

Adoptive transfer studies in mice have been informative for examining the operative in vivo effector mechanisms and contributions to tumor eradication of cell populations that exhibit antitumor activity in vitro. Several cell types with distinct modes of tumor cell recognition have been shown to promote the regression of established tumors in syngeneic hosts, including nonspecific effector cells (such as NK cells, lymphokine-activated killer (LAK) cells, and activated monocytes) and MHC-restricted CD4+ and CD8+ tumor-reactive T cells (88,199–203). Although the relative ease with which nonspecific effectors can be generated makes such cells attractive for use in adoptive therapy, even in animal models the in vivo activity of these cell populations has been limited and often restricted to localized tumors. The clinical trials performed in human cancer patients with nonspecific effector cells have provided provocative but ultimately largely disappointing results (204–206), and no clear strategies are available to overcome the lack of tumor specificity and inability to selectively localize at sites of tumor. Thus, since CD4+ and CD8+ tumor-reactive T cells exhibit specificity for target antigens expressed by tumor cells, homing to sites of antigen expression and the most significant and reproducible in vivo antitumor activity in murine models, this chapter will focus on the development of cellular therapy with $\alpha\beta^+$ T cells. Although most of these T cells recognize proteins in the context of classic MHC antigens, reports of T cells recognizing tumors by non-classic MHC molecules are appearing (207,208).

Class I–restricted CD8$^+$ tumor-specific CTL directly lyse class I–positive tumor cells in vitro, and adoptively transferred CD8$^+$ CTL mediate regression of a wide range of experimental tumors in vivo (88,209–211). The effector mechanisms employed by CD8$^+$ T cells extend beyond direct cytolysis and include the antitumor activities of secreted cytokines (212). Since the majority of tumors express or can be induced to express class I molecules, CD8$^+$ CTL represent the effector cell of choice for adoptive transfer in most therapy settings. However, as the elimination of established tumors generally requires a prolonged in vivo antitumor response (213), the therapeutic efficacy of transferred CD8$^+$ CTL is influenced by the availability of cytokines normally provided in an immune response by CD4$^+$ T cells such as IL-2, which is required to promote proliferation and survival of these effector cells. Thus, it has generally been necessary in murine models either to administer IL-2 or to concurrently transfer tumor-reactive CD4$^+$ T cells to achieve tumor eradication (88,209,211,214,215). As an exception, CD8$^+$ CTL that produce IL-2 in response to tumor recognition can be occasionally isolated from mice. The improved in vivo efficacy observed in tumor therapy with such bifunctional, helper-independent CD8$^+$ CTL has also provided direct support for the critical need to provide IL-2 in tumor therapy, if the more classic IL-2–dependent CD8$^+$ CTL are being administered alone (216).

Class II–restricted CD4$^+$ T cells, in addition to providing helper function for CD8$^+$ T cells by providing IL-2 and/or by activating professional antigen-presenting cells to effectively stimulate CD8$^+$ cells (217–219), can independently mediate antitumor effects (220,221). For class II$^+$ tumors such as B-cell lymphomas, CD4$^+$ T cells may directly lyse the target cells (222,223). Moreover, studies in murine models with a wide range of histologic tumor types have demonstrated that noncytolytic CD4$^+$ T cells can also mediate rejection of class II$^-$ tumors in the absence of participation by CD8$^+$ T cells (201,202,224). This presumably requires class II$^+$ APC to present tumor antigens to stimulate the CD4$^+$ T cells to secrete cytokines that are directly tumoricidal; to recruit and activate tumoricidal effector cells such as NK cells, macrophages, and eosinophils; and/or to interfere with tumor angiogenesis (225). Unfortunately, these studies in animal models have not identified the settings in which CD4$^+$ T cells that recognize a tumor antigen can be predicted to be effective in the absence of CD8$^+$ T cells, or in which the effector responses promoted by CD4$^+$ T cells provide an obligate contribution to the efficacy of CD8$^+$ Tc. Until such principles are defined, some human tumor therapy trials using only tumor-reactive CD4$^+$ T cells or only CD8$^+$ T cells may be unsuccessful and may underestimate the potential antitumor activity of the infused T-cell population.

Molecular strategies have now provided the means to generate a new population of hybrid effector cells—cytolytic effector T cells into which have been inserted, by gene transfer with retroviruses or alternative vectors, a chimeric receptor with an extracellular binding domain derived from a tumor-reactive antibody and a cytoplasmic signaling domain derived from the zeta chain (or a functional surrogate) of the T-cell receptor (226). By molecular engineering, it is possible to construct this entire receptor from one gene encoding a single chain containing the antibody V_H and V_L regions separated by a flexible linker that permits formation of the high-affinity antibody-binding site fused inframe to the signaling tail. Effector CD8$^+$ cells expressing these "T-body" receptors have been shown to recognize and lyse tumor cells and to eradicate tumors in in vivo animal models (226–228). This approach has the obvious advantages of greatly broadening the range of antigens that can serve as targets for therapy and of circumventing some of the immune evasion strategies employed by tumors, while still utilizing the effector mechanisms mediated by T cells. However, there are several limitations that must be addressed. Firstly, the receptor could potentially be occupied/triggered by soluble antigen, which would prevent therapeutic efficacy. Secondly, the receptor affinities and target interactions may preclude the necessary kinetics of binding and release required for normal, T-cell function and survival. Thirdly, the inability of these receptors to assemble a complete TCR complex and to engage all the appropriate accessory molecules on target recognition could attenuate T-cell function. Because of these differences between the T-body receptor and a normal TCR, there is only limited evidence to suggest that these effector cells can mediate serial engagement and killing of targets and antigen-induced proliferation (229), which is required to sustain a prolonged in vivo response. Ongoing, basic, preclinical and clinical investigations to improve receptor functioning and signaling offer significant promise (230,231), however, and may provide substantial benefit in the future.

Identification of Tumor Antigens Recognized by T Cells

In contrast to viral diseases and experimental murine tumors that express novel antigens and readily elicit T-cell responses that can be examined for therapeutic efficacy, initial studies with human tumors failed to detect T-cell responses in the majority of tumor-bearing hosts. Thus, a major obstacle to developing T-cell therapy for human malignancy has been the absence of defined antigens expressed by tumors to be appropriate targets for an immunologic attack. In the past decade, considerable effort has been devoted to the identification of human tumor antigens, and the success of these efforts has now provided the foundation for developing cellular therapy of human malignancy using T cells specific for defined tumor antigens.

Three strategies, initially used to identify proteins in murine tumor cells that give rise to antigenic peptides recognized by CD8$^+$ or CD4$^+$ T cells, are now being used to study human tumors. The first approach, pioneered by Thierry Boon et al, has used tumor-reactive Tc as the reagents to identify immunogenic proteins. Pools of DNA from an immunogenic murine P815 tumor cell were transfected into target cells, and the targets screened for recognition by tumor-reactive Tc clones (232). Using this strategy, two antigens, P91A and P198, were identified to be encoded by mutated genes. Peptides encompassing the amino acid substitutions encoded by the mutations were demonstrated to contain the epitopes recognized by P815-specific Tc (233,234). A third antigen recognized by the antitumor Tc response—designated P1A—was identified and surprisingly found to be encoded by a normal, nonmutated gene (235).

The use of tumor-reactive T cells isolated from cancer patients as reagents to screen expression libraries from human tumors for the genes encoding human tumor antigens has been most productive in malignant melanoma. This is primarily because investigators have had the greatest success isolating tumor-reactive T cells from patients with this malignancy. Several genes expressed in human tumors that encode antigens recognized by CD8$^+$ Tc have been characterized. These genes include the RAGE, MAGE, BAGE, GAGE, and NY-ESO families of proteins, which are normal proteins that in adults are expressed only in the testes and some tumors, and tyrosinase, TRP-1, TRP-2, melan A, and gp100, which are expressed both in normal melanocytes and in melanoma cells (236–248). The finding that normal proteins present in tumor cells from many patients may be targets for immunologic therapy was greeted with considerable enthusiasm because this simplifies the design and interpretation of cellular therapy studies for a large population.

Tumor antigens recognized by either CD8$^+$ Tc or CD4$^+$ Th and encoded by mutated gene products have also been identified by screening expression libraries. These include epitopes resulting from point mutations in the MUM-1, CDK-4 and β-catenin, and triosephosphate isomerase genes, and from the fusion site of a chimeric protein expressed as a result of chromosomal rearrangement in the tumor (249–253). Mutated antigens may have potential advantages over normal proteins as therapeutic targets, including reduced toxicity to normal tissues and an increased likelihood that T cells with high avidity for the antigen will not have been deleted in the host (254). However, these antigens have not yet been pursued aggressively as therapeutic targets since the mutations are typically not shared by tumor cells from other patients.

The second strategy for identifying tumor antigens has also used tumor-reactive T cells as the reagents to probe for the immunogen. This involves eluting peptides bound by the class I MHC molecules on the tumor cell, separating the peptide peaks by HPLC fractionation, identifying the peaks that contain peptides recognized by tumor reactive Tc, and sequencing the relevant peptide peaks by tandem mass spectrometry (255,256). Using this approach, peptides encoded by genes expressed in murine lung carcinoma, melanoma, and human lung carcinoma have been identified (255,257). The peptide-elution approach requires large numbers of tumor cells and is technically complex, but has the advantage of identifying epitopes that have undergone posttranslational modifications of peptide epitopes that may alter MHC binding or T-cell recognition (258,259).

In a third approach to antigen identification, a protein or peptide known to be expressed in the tumor cell is presumed to be potentially immunogenic and is used to elicit T-cell responses by in vitro stimulation or in vivo immunization. This has been most extensively studied in murine tumors induced by oncogenic viruses and resulted in the identification of viral proteins such as the SV40 T antigen, adenovirus type 5 E1A antigen, and F-MuLV gag antigen that can be targets of an effective antitumor immune response (209,260,261). These results have encouraged the development of studies evaluating viral proteins as targets for human virus-associated cancers such as Hodgkin's disease with EBV and cervical cancer with HPV. However, this approach is also being applied to human tumors that are not virus-associated but are known to express novel genes. These include B-cell lymphomas that express a unique immunoglobulin molecule arising from gene rearrangement and somatic mutation (262,263); leukemias such as CML and APL that have chromosomal translocations that give rise to the chimeric BCR/ABL and PML/RARα proteins, respectively (264,265); and tumors that express mutated ras and p53 (266,267). The strategy has also been applied to tumors that are known to selectively express or overexpress normal proteins that are involved in maintaining the malignant phenotype such as the catalytic subunit of telomerase and Her2/neu (268–270). To evaluate immunogenicity, typically, either the proteins are introduced into APC using recombinant vectors, or MHC binding peptides derived from the protein are cultured with APC, and the APC are then used in vitro to stimulate reactive T cells. Using the latter approach, CD4$^+$ and/or CD8$^+$ MHC-restricted T cells reactive with epitopes derived from mutated ras, mutated p53, BCR/ABL, PML/RARα, telomerase, Her2/neu, and EBV-encoded proteins have been identified (264–271). Unfortunately, many of the T cells isolated with this approach failed to recognize tumor cells. This likely reflects in part the elimination of high-avidity Tc from the cultures by activation-induced cell death following restimulation with high concentrations of peptide and the resulting selective outgrowth of T cells with low avidity for the peptide/MHC complex (272,273), coupled with the relatively lower density of antigen being presented by the tumor cell. However, Tc that recognize tumor cells have been occasionally isolated with this strategy, including T cells reactive with epitopes derived from telomerase, which is expressed in >85% of human tumors (270). Recent studies, using soluble, class I MHC molecules complexed to the relevant peptide to stain and sort high-avidity cells by flow cytometry early in the culture process, suggest that this general approach can be made more efficient for isolating potentially therapeutic tumor-reactive T cells (274–277).

A unique situation in which T-cell responses to antigens expressed by tumor cells may be manipulated for therapeutic benefit is following allogeneic HCT. In this setting, T cells reactive with minor histocompatibility (H) antigens that are encoded by polymorphic genes that differ between the donor and the recipient can be isolated from patients after transplant. Such T cells are presumed to be involved in both GVHD and graft-versus-leukemia (GVL) reactions (278,279). In fact, minor H antigen–specific Tc have been directly shown to lyse leukemic blasts, to inhibit leukemic colony formation in vitro, and to prevent the engraftment of human AML in immunodeficient mice, suggesting they may exert antileukemic activity in patients (280–282). Since some minor H antigens appear to exhibit expression restricted to hematopoietic cells, these antigens may be appropriate targets for directing a selective GVL response that will not be complicated by the toxicity of GVHD.

Both the expression-library cloning strategy and the peptide-elution approach are now being used to identify the genes encoding human minor H antigens that can then be used for molecular screening of tissue expression. CD8+ Tc clones isolated from HCT patients have been used to define seven minor H antigens encoded by autosomal genes and designated HA-1 to HA-7 (279). By in vitro cytotoxicity assays, HA-3, -4, -5, -6, and -7 are expressed by hematopoietic cells, endothelial cells, epithelial cells, and fibroblasts, suggesting derivation from a ubiquitously expressed gene, and would not likely be suitable targets for inducing a selective GVL effect (283). However, HA-1– and HA-2–specific Tc do not lyse nonhematopoietic cells such as keratinocytes, fibroblasts, and renal epithelial cells in vitro (283). Using the peptide-elution approach, the HA-1 peptide was found to be encoded by a polymorphic gene KIAA0223 of unknown function, and the HA-2 peptide closely matches that of a class I myosin gene (284,285). Detailed molecular studies analyzing the expression of HA-1 in tissues that are targets of GVHD have not yet been reported. However, studies evaluating the association of donor/recipient mismatching for HA-1 with the development of GVHD after BMT and a study using class I MHC tetramers to detect HA-1–specific Tc have suggested that mismatching of HA-1 and expansion of HA-1–specific Tc are associated with the development of grade 2 to 4 GVHD, thus engendering skepticism regarding its potential as a target to induce a selective GVL response (286,287). These findings are consistent with a much broader expression of HA-1 in vivo than predicted by prior in vitro studies using cultured cells and suggest that HA-1 may not be a suitable target for GVL therapy.

The expression-library screening approach has been used to define a gene encoding a minor H antigen denoted HB-1, which is presented to CD8+ Tc by HLA B44 and is expressed in EBV-transformed B cells and B-ALL cells but not skin fibroblasts, T cells, or monocytes (288). Molecular analysis has confirmed the selective expression of HB-1 in transformed B cells, suggesting it may be an appropriate target for adoptive immunotherapy of B-ALL after allogeneic BMT (289).

Minor H antigens encoded by the Y chromosome have also been identified and may be relevant for inducing GVL responses in male recipients of female HCT. The peptide-elution approach was used to identify epitopes recognized by HLA A2– and HLA B7–restricted, H-Y–specific T–cell clones, and both epitopes were found to be encoded by the SMCY gene (259,290). However, SMCY is transcribed in all tissues, and cells of both hematopoietic and nonhematopoietic derivation are recognized by the T-cell clones specific for SMCY (283). Thus, SMCY is a potential target for T cells mediating GVHD (291), but is unlikely to be a suitable target for T-cell therapy to induce a selective GVL response. Recently, CD8+ T-cell clones specific for a novel H-Y antigen presented by HLA B8 have been isolated in our lab. These H-Y–specific Tc lyse hematopoietic cells, including AML blasts but not skin fibroblasts obtained from male donors (292). Despite the development of a Tc response against this H-Y

antigen, the transplant recipient did not develop GVHD, suggesting that this antigen may be a good candidate to pursue as a target for GVL activity. These studies of allogeneic HCT recipients suggest that additional specificities relevant for inducing GVL responses will be identified in the future.

The discovery of what is now a large number of antigens expressed by human tumors has dispelled the notion that malignancies are inherently nonimmunogenic, and distinct classes of antigens that might be capable of inducing therapeutic T-cell responses have been identified. These antigens include proteins encoded by viruses, proteins encoded by mutated genes, normal proteins that exhibit selective or relatively selective expression or are overexpressed in tumor cells, and minor histocompatibility antigens (Table 41-2). The opportunity now exists to design clinical trials to define the potential therapeutic benefits and/or limitations of cellular therapy or vaccination to augment T-cell responses to selected tumor-associated antigens.

Obstacles to Adoptive T-Cell Therapy of Tumors

Studies of tumor immunobiology in murine models, and more recently in humans, have helped identify many of the issues that must be addressed to facilitate effective T-cell therapy of tumors. Historically, the most substantial obstacle has been the difficulty in identifying tumor antigens that can be used to detect/generate tumor-reactive T cells. Improvements in T-cell cloning technology, optimization of antigen presentation by the selec-

Table 41-2. Categories of Potential Antigens Expressed by Human Tumors

- Viral gene products in virus-associated malignancies (e.g., HPV E6 and E7 proteins [cervical cancer]; EBV LMP-1 and EBNA-1 proteins [Hodgkin's disease, nasopharyngeal carcinoma])
- Proteins encoded by mutated genes or chromosomal rearrangements (e.g., p21 ras [~10% of tumors]; BCR/ABL [chronic myelogenous leukemia]; PML/RARα [acute promyelocytic leukemia]; β catenin, MUM-1, triosephosphate isomerase [melanoma])
- Normal gene products that are selectively expressed or overexpressed in the tumor (e.g., telomerase [~85% of tumors]; Her-2/neu [breast and ovarian cancer])
- Normal gene products that are tissue-specific and expressed by the tumor (e.g., tyrosinase, melan A, gp100, TRP-1, TRP-2 [melanoma])
- Normal gene products not expressed or minimally expressed in adult tissues (e.g., MAGE, BAGE, GAGE, RAGE, and NY/ESO proteins [melanoma and other tumors])
- Idiotypic proteins (e.g., immunoglobulin molecules [B-cell lymphoma])
- Minor histocompatibility antigens expressed selectively by hematopoietic cells in allogeneic HCT recipients

tion of potentially immunodominant epitopes and by the use of activated dendritic cells as stimulator cells, and the development of in vivo immunization strategies that maximize costimulatory signals and/or that use tumor cells genetically modified to increase immunogenicity have now made it increasingly possible to isolate tumor-reactive T cells. However, it is unlikely that all such T cells will be useful in therapy, and defining the conditions necessary for success and designing the strategies to overcome the obstacles represent major challenges for the next decade.

There are many reasons why potentially tumor-reactive T cells may fail to be effective in therapy (Table 41-3). The nature of many of the target tumor antigens, which represent normal cellular proteins also expressed in healthy tissues, may preclude isolation of T cells with a high-affinity TCR because of the mechanisms operative in vivo for deletion of self-reactive T cells. Thus, only T cells with a low affinity for the antigen may be obtainable (293,294), and the efficacy of such cells in therapy will obviously depend on the density of antigen and accessory adhesion molecules expressed by the tumor cells. Achieving therapeutic benefit will likely be enhanced if the effector T cells can be screened for the ability to recognize fresh tumor cells and/or can be selected with tetramer-binding assays for high TCR affinity (276,277).

Therapy may be ineffective as a result of the presence of variant tumor cells that have lost expression of the target antigen, which is expected in malignant cells that exhibit genomic instability. However, it may be particularly problematic for target antigens such as the normal melanosomal proteins expressed by melanoma cells that are characteristic of the tissue of origin but not related to the malignant phenotype, since loss of expression should not result in a growth disadvantage for the cell. Alternatively, tumors may escape recognition by mutations in the epitope or a region adjacent to the epitope that affects processing of the protein (295). Overcoming these obstacles may require targeting several distinct proteins simultaneously. Another means of acquiring an antigen-loss phenotype is by decreasing epitope presentation such as by down-regulating expression of HLA class I antigens, β-2 microglobulin, or components of the antigen-processing machinery. These obstacles may be partially corrected

Table 41-3. Mechanisms by Which Tumors Evade T-Cell Responses to Tumor Antigens

- Deletion of T cells expressing high-affinity TCR
- Limited expression of the tumor antigen
- Antigen loss by mutations or deletions in tumor variants
- Interference with antigen processing and presentation
- Secretion of proteins that subvert responses
- Expression of molecules that directly interfere with effector mechanisms
- Elimination of tumor-reactive T cells
- Induction of anergy in tumor-reactive T cells
- Modulation of tumor vasculature to prevent access

in a subset of tumors by the administration of cytokines such as IFN-α or IFN-γ that enhance the functioning of the antigen-processing machinery, although some tumor cells have been shown to evade immune responses by acquiring unresponsiveness to IFN-γ (296,297).

Tumor cells may directly interfere with T-cell function by targeting distinct phases required for tumor eradication. Complete tumor elimination generally requires a prolonged response, and tumors can secrete cytokines such as IL-10, TGF-β, or prostaglandins that interfere with activation of reactive T cells (298–300). Alternatively, tumors may express FasL, which can bind to Fas molecules expressed by activated T cells and induce apoptosis of the effector populations (301,302). Such FasL expression has been shown to be at least in part responsible for the immunologic privilege afforded certain tissue sites such as the eye and the testes, but the role of FasL in protecting tumor cells by eliminating T cells remains controversial (302–304). Theoretically, this evasion activity by the tumor might be circumvented by introducing genes that block Fas signaling into the T cells being transferred such as FLIP (305,306). Indeed, some tumors have been shown to overexpress FLIPs, presumably because of the selective benefit of attenuating death signals mediated by FasL (307,308). Tumors can also express molecules such as RCAS1 or DF3/MUC1 that bind to molecules on T cells, inducing a signal that interferes with cell-cycle progression following activation and resulting in apoptosis of the activated T cells (309–311). Overcoming this escape mechanism might be accomplished by the administration of antibodies that block the interaction of these inhibitory molecules with the T cells. Finally, growing tumor cells can induce anergy in potentially reactive CD4+ and CD8+ T cells (312,313), a finding recently confirmed in humans by direct analysis of melanoma-reactive CD8+ T cells isolated from the peripheral blood of patients (314). Although the precise mechanisms are unclear, biochemical changes that interfere with the ability of the TCR or IL-2R to deliver competent signals have been identified (315–317). Overcoming this problem will require more complete analysis of the abnormalities present in anergic T cells and elucidation of the signaling events responsible for inducing this state and/or required to prevent it.

Tumor eradication requires that the infused T cells exit the vascular tree and enter the tumor site. However, studies have suggested that the tumor microvasculature may be qualitatively abnormal (318–321). The extravasation of T cells into a tumor requires a multistep process mediated by several families of cell adhesion molecules, including integrins, selectins, and members of the Ig superfamily, as well as chemokine receptors. Leukocytes, which stick to normal capillary endothelium, stick poorly to some intratumoral capillaries (318,322). This likely reflects several abnormalities, including the failure of tumor endothelium to respond to inflammatory cytokines such as TNFα or IL-2 by up-regulating expression of adhesion molecules such as VCAM-1 (321,323), and ultimately results in poor lymphocyte infiltration into the tumor mass (324). An improved understanding of the biology of the tumor vasculature and how the tumor microenvironment regulates expression of adhesion molecules will be required to design strategies to facilitate T-cell entry into tumors.

Despite all these potential obstacles, T-cell therapy will likely be successful in the treatment of some tumors. However, in settings in which T-cell therapy is unsuccessful, it will be imperative to evaluate the basis for failure so that rational approaches can be designed and tested to overcome the relevant obstacle(s).

Human Trials of Cellular Immunotherapy for Malignant Diseases

Adoptive Transfer of MHC-Restricted, Tumor-Specific T Cells to Patients with Malignancy

Prior to the identification of antigens expressed by tumor cells that were recognized by MHC-restricted T cells, the adoptive transfer of lymphocytes activated to a nonspecific cytolytic state with high concentrations of IL-2 was evaluated in patients with advanced malignancy, but did not provide antitumor effects beyond those observed with high-dose IL-2 alone. Studies in tumor-bearing mice demonstrated that lymphocytes infiltrating tumor sites were more likely to exhibit MHC-restricted, tumor-specific reactivity than lymphocytes obtained from the peripheral blood and were more potent than LAK cells in adoptive-therapy models (325). Thus, it was anticipated that isolating and culturing lymphocytes infiltrating human tumors might facilitate the identification of tumor-specific T cells that could be expanded for use in therapy.

Lymphocytes have been obtained from biopsies of tumors of several histologies and cultured in high concentrations of IL-2. In the majority of tumor types, tumor-infiltrating lymphocyte (TIL) cultures contained both CD8$^+$ and CD4$^+$ T cells, but mediated only non–MHC-restricted cytolytic activity for tumor targets, consistent with the induction of promiscuous cytolytic activity by high-dose IL-2 rather than the selective expansion of tumor-specific T cells (326–328). However, a proportion of TIL cultures from patients with melanoma and with squamous-cell carcinoma of the head and neck exhibited class I MHC–restricted lysis of autologous tumor (326–329).

The functional and phenotypic heterogeneity of TIL cultures has posed a problem for the design and interpretation of clinical trials of cellular therapy because of the difficulty in defining effector mechanisms responsible for toxicity and/or efficacy. However, trials evaluating the adoptive transfer of TIL cells cultured with IL-2 have proceeded in patients with a variety of advanced malignancies for which alternative therapies were limited. With the exception of patients with advanced melanoma in whom an improved response rate was observed in comparison with historic results in patients treated with IL-2 alone or with IL-2 combined with nonspecific cytolytic cells derived from the blood and activated in culture with high concentrations of IL-2 (330), the results of therapy with TIL have been disappointing.

The observation that higher response rates were observed in patients with melanoma (the tumor for which MHC-restricted, tumor-specific T cells were most frequently detected in TIL cul-

tures) focused attention on the development of more sophisticated techniques for selectively isolating and manipulating tumor-specific T cells in vitro. A major advance has been the development of soluble class I MHC tetramers, which can be used to isolate T cells reactive with tumor-derived peptides from blood, lymph node mononuclear cell suspensions, and in vitro cultures (276,277). Many of the T cells selected in this fashion exhibit cytolytic activity for the tumor and can be propagated in vitro for use in adoptive transfer. Class I MHC tetramers are being used in our lab to select T cells specific for the melanocyte differentiation antigens gp100, MART-1, or tyrosinase for adoptive therapy of melanoma. Several issues are being addressed in this initial trial, including the potential for toxicity to normal melanocytes, the ability of transferred T cells to migrate to tumor sites and eliminate tumor cells bearing the antigen, the selection of escape variants that lack the target antigen or components of the antigen-processing machinery, and the long-term persistence and function of transferred T cells. It is anticipated the results of this trial and others using T cells specific for defined antigens expressed in melanoma will assist in identifying the potential limitations of cellular therapy and in designing future studies to improve the efficacy of this approach for melanoma and other malignancies.

Cellular Immunotherapy of Leukemia After Allogeneic HCT

Allogeneic HCT is curative for some malignancies in part as a result of a graft-versus-tumor effect mediated by donor T cells specific for minor H antigens. The potency of the GVL effect is best illustrated by studies in which patients who relapse after allogeneic HCT are induced into a complete remission by the infusion of additional lymphocytes from the HCT donor. In HCT patients with relapse of chronic-phase chronic myeloid leukemia, 50% to 70% can be subsequently induced into a complete remission with this approach (331,332). Unfortunately, only a minority of patients who relapse with blast crisis of CML or with acute leukemia respond to donor lymphocyte infusions, potentially reflecting the difficulty treating a rapidly expanding tumor burden with only T-cell therapy. An additional problem with this therapy is that the majority of the responding patients also develop GVHD. However, recent studies using donor lymphocytes modified to express the HSV-TK gene to permit their in vivo ablation provide a potential approach to reversing this toxicity (333).

In an attempt to improve efficacy and reduce the occurrence of GVHD associated with unselected donor lymphocyte infusions, efforts are in progress to use T-cell clones specific for minor H antigens for adoptive therapy. The high relapse rate in patients who receive an allogeneic HCT for advanced AML or ALL makes it feasible to prospectively isolate and characterize T-cell clones specific for recipient minor H antigens. This process would involve selecting those clones with in vitro reactivity for recipient leukemic cells, but not for nonhematopoietic cells, and storing those clones for potential use in adoptive immunotherapy if the patient relapses. Under ideal circumstances, T-cell clones specific for minor H antigens encoded by defined genes known to be expressed only in hematopoietic cells would be used in therapy to minimize the potential for causing GVHD, but a complete molecular analysis of the target antigen will not always be available at the time some patients require treatment. Recent developments in gene therapy may provide strategies for safely evaluating therapy with T-cell clones specific for minor H antigens that have not yet been characterized at the molecular level. For example, the HSV-TK gene could be introduced into minor H antigen–specific T-cell clones to permit their ablation in vivo (333). A clinical trial of this approach is now in progress and should assist in defining the potential to safely augment GVL activity after allogeneic HCT by the adoptive transfer of T-cell clones specific for recipient minor H antigens.

Adoptive T-Cell Therapy of Malignancy: Future Potential

Advances in basic immunology, insights derived from animal-model studies of cellular therapy for malignancy, and the identification of tumor antigens that elicit CD8[+] and CD4[+] T-cell responses have provided new opportunities to pursue a rigorous evaluation of adoptive T-cell therapy for human malignancy with purified T cells specific for defined tumor-associated antigens. However, as discussed earlier in this chapter, the identification of a plethora of strategies that tumors may use to evade detection and elimination by host immune responses suggests that there will be formidable obstacles to the development of effective cellular therapy for cancer. The task for the next generation of clinical studies will be to provide an improved understanding of the reasons for both the failures and the successes of T-cell therapy so that strategies for improving efficacy can be developed for subsequent studies. This will require carefully designed clinical trials and the use of sophisticated immunologic, molecular, and histologic techniques for analysis of treated patients. As discussed earlier in this chapter, it may be necessary to concurrently administer cytokines or to use T cells that are genetically modified to overcome defined obstacles and improve efficacy. Advances in gene therapy have made it possible to modify antigen-specific T cells to express novel functions. Such functions include the expression of cytokine receptors that might improve T-cell survival (184,334), cytokines that have direct antitumor activity or counteract immunosuppressive factors produced by the tumor (335), receptors that might improve migration and localization at tumor sites, and receptors that impart specificity such as T-cell receptors or chimeric single-chain Fv receptors (336,337). Future studies incorporating the insights derived from clinical trials and the evolving cellular and molecular strategies to modify and improve T-cell function should make it possible to begin realizing the therapeutic potential of T-cell therapy in cancer.

References

1. Biron CA, Nguyen KB, Pien GC, et al. Natural killer cells in antiviral defense: function and regulation by innate cytokines. Annu Rev Immunol 1999;17:189–220.

2. Biron CA, Byron KS, Sullivan JL. Severe herpesvirus infections in an adolescent without natural killer cells. N Engl J Med 1989;320:1731–1735.

3. Doherty PC, Allan W, Eichelberger M, Carding SR. Roles of alpha beta and gamma delta T-cell subsets in viral immunity. Annu Rev Immunol 1992;10:123–151.

4. Koszinowski UH, Reddehase MJ, Jonjic S. The role of CD4 and CD8 T cells in viral infections. Curr Opin Immunol 1991;3:471–475.

5. Gooding LR. Virus proteins that counteract host immune defenses. Cell 1992;71:5–7.

6. Ploegh HL. Viral strategies of immune evasion. Science 1998;280:248–253.

7. Spriggs MK. One step ahead of the game: viral immunomodulatory molecules. Annu Rev Immunol 1996;14:101–130.

8. McMichael A. T-cell responses and viral escape. Cell 1998;93:673–676.

9. Callan MF, Tan L, Annels N, et al. Direct visualization of antigen-specific CD8+ T cells during the primary immune response to Epstein-Barr virus in vivo. J Exp Med 1998;187:1395–1402.

10. Tan LC, Gudgeon N, Annels NE, et al. A re-evaluation of the frequency of CD8+ T cells specific for EBV in healthy virus carriers. J Immunol 1999;162:1827–1835.

11. He XS, Rehermann B, Lopez-Labrador FX, et al. Quantitative analysis of hepatitis C virus-specific CD8(+) T cells in peripheral blood and liver using peptide-MHC tetramers. Proc Natl Acad Sci USA 1999;96:5692–5697.

12. Kuroda MJ, Schmitz JE, Charini WA, et al. Emergence of CTL coincides with clearance of virus during primary simian immunodeficiency virus infection in rhesus monkeys. J Immunol 1999;162:5127–5133.

13. Ada GL, Jones PD. The immune response to influenza infection. Curr Top Microbiol Immunol 1986;128:1–54.

14. Reddehase MJ, Weiland F, Munch K, et al. Interstitial murine cytomegalovirus pneumonia after irradiation: characterization of cells that limit viral replication during established infection of the lungs. J Virol 1985;55:264–273.

15. Dharakul T, Rott L, Greenberg HB. Recovery from chronic rotavirus infection in mice with severe combined immunodeficiency: virus clearance mediated by adoptive transfer of immune CD8+ T lymphocytes. J Virol 1990;64:4375–4382.

16. Pantaleo G, Fauci AS. New concepts in the immunopathogenesis of HIV infection. Annu Rev Immunol 1995; 13:487–512.

17. Shearer GM. HIV-induced immunopathogenesis. Immunity 1998;9:587–593.

18. Pantaleo G, Demarest JF, Soudeyns H, et al. Major expansion of CD8+ T cells with a predominant V beta usage during the primary immune response to HIV. Nature 1994;370:463–467.

19. Koup RA, Safrit JT, Cao Y, et al. Temporal association of cellular immune responses with the initial control of viremia in primary human immunodeficiency virus type 1 syndrome. J Virol 1994;68:4650–4655.

20. Chen ZW, Kou ZC, Lekutis C, et al. T-cell receptor V beta repertoire in an acute infection of rhesus monkeys with simian immunodeficiency viruses and a chimeric simian-human immunodeficiency virus. J Exp Med 1995; 182:21–31.

21. Musey L, Hughes J, Schacker T, et al. Cytotoxic-T-cell responses, viral load, and disease progression in early human immunodeficiency virus type 1 infection. N Engl J Med 1997;337:1267–1274.

22. Ogg GS, Jin X, Bonhoeffer S, et al. Quantitation of HIV-1–specific cytotoxic T lymphocytes and plasma load of viral RNA. Science 1998;279:2103–2106.

23. Borrow P, Lewicki H, Hahn BH, et al. Virus-specific CD8+ cytotoxic T-lymphocyte activity associated with control of viremia in primary human immunodeficiency virus type 1 infection. J Virol 1994;68:6103–6110.

24. Klein MR, van Baalen CA, Holwerda AM, et al. Kinetics of Gag-specific cytotoxic T-lymphocyte responses during the clinical course of HIV-1 infection: a longitudinal analysis of rapid progressors and long-term asymptomatics. J Exp Med 1995;181:1365–1372.

25. Carmichael A, Jin X, Sissons P, Borysiewicz L. Quantitative analysis of the human immunodeficiency virus type 1 (HIV-1)–specific cytotoxic T-lymphocyte (CTL) response at different stages of HIV-1 infection: differential CTL responses to HIV-1 and Epstein-Barr virus in late disease. J Exp Med 1993;177:249–256.

26. Schmitz JE, Kuroda MJ, Santra S, et al. Control of viremia in simian immunodeficiency virus infection by CD8+ lymphocytes. Science 1999;283:857–860.

27. Ogg GS, Kostense S, Klein MR, et al. Longitudinal phenotypic analysis of human immunodeficiency virus type 1–specific cytotoxic T lymphocytes: correlation with disease progression. J Virol 1999;73:9153–9160.

28. Welsh RM, Vargas-Cortes M. Natural killer cells in viral infection. In: Lewis CE, McGee JOD, eds. The natural killer cell. Oxford: IRL Press, 1992:108–150.

29. Fujita S, Puri RK, Yu ZX, et al. An ultrastructural study of in vivo interactions between lymphocytes and endothelial cells in the pathogenesis of the vascular leak syndrome induced by interleukin-2. Cancer 1991;68:2169–2174.

30. Sciammas R, Johnson RM, Sperling AI, et al. Unique antigen recognition by a herpesvirus-specific TCR-gamma delta cell. J Immunol 1994;152:5392–5397.

31. Welsh RM, Lin MY, Lohman BL, et al. Alpha beta and gamma delta T-cell networks and their roles in natural resistance to viral infections. Immunol Rev 1997;159:79–93.

32. Boismenu R, Havran WL. An innate view of gamma delta T cells. Curr Opin Immunol 1997;9:57–63.

33. Born W, Cady C, Jones-Carson J, et al. Immunoregulatory functions of gamma delta T cells. Adv Immunol 1999; 71:77–144.

34. Kast WM, Bronkhorst AM, de-Waal LP, Melief CJ. Cooperation between cytotoxic and helper T lymphocytes in protection against lethal Sendai virus infection. Protection by T cells is MHC-restricted and MHC-regulated: a model for MHC-disease associations. J Exp Med 1986;164:723–738.

35. Lightman S, Cobbold S, Waldmann H, Askonas BA. Do L3T4+ T cells act as effector cells in protection against influenza virus infection? Immunology 1987;62:139–144.

36. Mackenzie CD, Taylor PM, Askonas BA. Rapid recovery of lung histology correlates with clearance of influenza virus by specific CD8+ cytotoxic T cells. Immunology 1989;67:375–381.

37. Nash AA, Jayasuriya A, Phelan J, et al. Different roles for L3T4+ and Lyt 2+ T-cell subsets in the control of an acute herpes simplex virus infection of the skin and nervous system. J Gen Virol 1987;68:825–833.

38. Byrne JA, Oldstone MB. Biology of cloned cytotoxic T lymphocytes specific for lymphocytic choriomeningitis virus. VI. Migration and activity in vivo in acute and persistent infection. J Immunol 1986;136:698–704.

39. Doherty PC, Topham DJ, Tripp RA, et al. Effector CD4+ and CD8+ T-cell mechanisms in the control of respiratory virus infections. Immunol Rev 1997;159:105–117.

40. Murali-Krishna K, Altman JD, Suresh M, et al. Counting antigen-specific CD8 T cells: a reevaluation of bystander activation during viral infection. Immunity 1998;8:177–187.

41. Butz EA, Bevan MJ. Massive expansion of antigen-specific CD8+ T cells during an acute virus infection. Immunity 1998;8:167–175.

42. Stevenson PG, Belz GT, Altman JD, Doherty PC. Changing patterns of dominance in the CD8+ T-cell response during acute and persistent murine gamma-herpesvirus infection. Eur J Immunol 1999;29:1059–1067.

43. Cardin RD, Brooks JW, Sarawar SR, Doherty PC. Progressive loss of CD8+ T cell–mediated control of a gamma-herpesvirus in the absence of CD4+ T cells. J Exp Med 1996;184:863–871.

44. Matloubian M, Concepcion RJ, Ahmed R. CD4+ T cells are required to sustain CD8+ cytotoxic T-cell responses during chronic viral infection. J Virol 1994;68:8056–8063.

45. Raulet DH. MHC class I–deficient mice. Adv Immunol 1994;55:381–421.

46. Cosgrove D, Gray D, Dierich A, et al. Mice lacking MHC class II molecules. Cell 1991;66:1051–1066.

47. Koller BH, Marrack P, Kappler JW, Smithies O. Normal development of mice deficient in beta 2M, MHC class I proteins, and CD8+ T cells. Science 1990;248:1227–1230.

48. Zijlstra M, Bix M, Simister NE, et al. Beta 2-microglobulin–deficient mice lack CD4–8+ cytolytic T cells. Nature 1990;344:742–746.

49. Eichelberger M, Allan W, Zijlstra M, et al. Clearance of influenza virus respiratory infection in mice lacking class I major histocompatibility complex–restricted CD8+ T cells. J Exp Med 1991;174:875–880.

50. Hou S, Doherty PC, Zijlstra M, et al. Delayed clearance of Sendai virus in mice lacking class I MHC–restricted CD8+ T cells. J Immunol 1992;149:1319–1325.

51. Spriggs MK, Koller BH, Sato T, et al. Beta 2-microglobulin, CD8+ T-cell–deficient mice survive inoculation with high doses of vaccinia virus and exhibit altered IgG responses. Proc Natl Acad Sci USA 1992;89:6070–6074.

52. Fiette L, Aubert C, Brahic M, Rossi CP. Theiler's virus infection of beta 2-microglobulin–deficient mice. J Virol 1993;67:589–592.

53. Muller D, Koller BH, Whitton JL, et al. LCMV-specific, class II–restricted cytotoxic T cells in beta 2-microglobulin–deficient mice. Science 1992;255:1576–1578.

54. Bender BS, Croghan T, Zhang L, Small PA Jr. Transgenic mice lacking class I major histocompatibility complex–restricted T cells have delayed viral clearance and increased mortality after influenza virus challenge. J Exp Med 1992;175:1143–1145.

55. Bodmer H, Obert G, Chan S, et al. Environmental modulation of the autonomy of cytotoxic T lymphocytes. Eur J Immunol 1993;23:1649–1654.

56. Laufer TM, von-Herrath MG, Grusby MJ, et al. Autoimmune diabetes can be induced in transgenic major histocompatibility complex class II–deficient mice. J Exp Med 1993;178:589–596.

57. Battegay M, Moskophidis D, Rahemtulla A, et al. Enhanced establishment of a virus carrier state in adult CD4+ T-cell–deficient mice. J Virol 1994;68:4700–4704.

58. Mizuochi T, Hugin AW, Morse HCI, et al. Role of lymphokine-secreting CD8+ T cells in cytotoxic T-lymphocyte responses against vaccinia virus. J Immunol 1989;142:270–273.

59. Malnati MS, Marti M, LaVaute T, et al. Processing pathways for presentation of cytosolic antigen to MHC class II–restricted T cells. Nature 1992;357:702–704.

60. Koelle DM, Corey L, Burke RL, et al. Antigenic specificities of human CD4+ T-cell clones recovered from recurrent genital herpes simplex virus type 2 lesions. J Virol 1994;68:2803–2810.

61. Miskovsky EP, Liu AY, Pavlat W, et al. Studies of the mechanism of cytolysis by HIV-1–specific CD4+ human CTL clones induced by candidate AIDS vaccines. J Immunol 1994;153:2787–2799.

62. Mosmann TR, Cherwinski H, Bond MW, et al. Two types of murine helper T-cell clone. I. Definition according to profiles of lymphokine activities and secreted proteins. J Immunol 1986;136:2348–2357.

63. Farrar JJ, Benjamin WR, Hilfiker ML, et al. The biochemistry, biology, and role of interleukin-2 in the induction of cytotoxic T-cell and antibody-forming B-cell responses. Immunol Rev 1982;63:129–166.

64. Biron CA, Young HA, Kasaian MT. Interleukin 2–induced proliferation of murine natural killer cells in vivo. J Exp Med 1990;171:173–188.

65. Staeheli P. Interferon-induced proteins and the antiviral state. Adv Virus Res 1990;38:147–200.

66. Wong GH, Goeddel DV. Tumour necrosis factors alpha and beta inhibit virus replication and synergize with interferons. Nature 1986;323:819–822.

67. Chen WF, Zlotnik A. IL-10: a novel cytotoxic T-cell differentiation factor. J Immunol 1991;147:528–534.

68. Paul WE. Interleukin-4: a prototypic immunoregulatory lymphokine. Blood 1991;77:1859–1870.

69. Lopez AF, Sanderson CJ, Gamble JR, et al. Recombinant human interleukin-5 is a selective activator of human eosinophil function. J Exp Med 1988;167:219–224.

70. Coffman RL, Seymour BW, Lebman DA, et al. The role of helper T-cell products in mouse B-cell differentiation and isotype regulation. Immunol Rev 1988;102:5–28.

71. Carding SR, Allan W, McMickle A, Doherty PC. Activation of cytokine genes in T cells during primary and secondary murine influenza pneumonia. J Exp Med 1993;177:475–482.

72. Sarawar SR, Doherty PC. Concurrent production of interleukin-2, interleukin-10, and gamma interferon in the regional lymph nodes of mice with influenza pneumonia. J Virol 1994;68:3112–3119.

73. Graham MB, Braciale VL, Braciale TJ. Influenza virus–specific CD4+ T helper type 2 lymphocytes do not promote recovery from experimental virus infection. J Exp Med 1994;180:1273–1282.

74. Alwan WH, Kozlowska WJ, Openshaw PJ. Distinct types of lung disease caused by functional subsets of antiviral T cells. J Exp Med 1994;179:81–89.

75. Mosmann TR, Li L, Sad S. Functions of CD8 T-cell subsets secreting different cytokine patterns. Semin Immunol 1997;9:87–92.

76. Li L, Sad S, Kagi D, Mosmann TR. CD8Tc1 and Tc2 cells secrete distinct cytokine patterns in vitro and in vivo but induce similar inflammatory reactions. J Immunol 1997;158:4152–4161.

77. Cerwenka A, Morgan TM, Harmsen AG, Dutton RW. Migration kinetics and final destination of type 1 and type 2 CD8 effector cells predict protection against pulmonary virus infection. J Exp Med 1999;189:423–434.

78. Levy JA, Mackewicz CE, Barker E. Controlling HIV pathogenesis: the role of the noncytotoxic anti-HIV response of CD8+ T cells. Immunol Today 1996;17:217–224.

79. Yang OO, Kalams SA, Trocha A, et al. Suppression of human immunodeficiency virus type 1 replication by CD8+ cells: evidence for HLA class I–restricted triggering of cytolytic and noncytolytic mechanisms. J Virol 1997;71:3120–3128.

80. Kagi D, Ledermann B, Burki K, et al. Cytotoxicity mediated by T cells and natural killer cells is greatly impaired in perforin-deficient mice. Nature 1994;369:31–37.

81. Topham DJ, Tripp RA, Doherty PC. CD8+ T cells clear influenza virus by perforin or Fas-dependent processes. J Immunol 1997;159:5197–5200.

82. Schorle H, Holtschke T, Hunig T, et al. Development and function of T cells in mice rendered interleukin-2 deficient by gene targeting. Nature 1991;352:621–624.

83. Kundig TM, Schorle H, Bachmann MF, et al. Immune responses in interleukin-2–deficient mice. Science 1993;262:1059–1061.

84. Zajac AJ, Blattman JN, Murali-Krishna K, et al. Viral immune evasion due to persistence of activated T cells without effector function. J Exp Med 1998;188:2205–2213.

85. Kalams SA, Walker BD. The critical need for CD4 help in maintaining effective cytotoxic T-lymphocyte responses. J Exp Med 1998;188:2199–2204.

86. Weinberg K, Parkman R. Severe combined immune deficiency due to a specific defect in interleukin-2 production. N Engl J Med 1990;322:1718–1723.

87. DiSanto JP, Keever CA, Small TN, et al. Absence of interleukin-2 production in a severe combined immunodeficiency disease syndrome with T cells. J Exp Med 1990;171:1697–1704.

88. Greenberg PD. Adoptive T-cell therapy of tumors: mechanisms operative in the recognition and elimination of tumor cells. Adv Immunol 1991;49:281–355.

89. Reddehase MJ, Mutter W, Koszinowski UH. In vivo application of recombinant interleukin-2 in the immunotherapy of established cytomegalovirus infection. J Exp Med 1987;165:650–656.

90. Boehm U, Klamp T, Groot M, Howard JC. Cellular responses to interferon-gamma. Annu Rev Immunol 1997;15:749–795.

91. Fruh K, Yang Y. Antigen presentation by MHC class I and its regulation by interferon gamma. Curr Opin Immunol 1999;11:76–81.

92. Young HA, Hardy KJ. Role of interferon-gamma in immune cell regulation. J Leukoc Biol 1995;58:373–381.

93. Biron CA. Cytokines in the generation of immune responses to, and resolution of, virus infection. Curr Opin Immunol 1994;6:530–538.

94. Billiau A, Heremans H, Vermeire K, Matthys P. Immunomodulatory properties of interferon-gamma. An update. Ann N Y Acad Sci 1998;856:22–32.

95. Farrar MA, Schreiber RD. The molecular cell biology of interferon-gamma and its receptor. Annu Rev Immunol 1993;11:571–611.

96. Wille A, Gessner A, Lother H, Lehmann-Grube F. Mechanism of recovery from acute virus infection. VIII. Treatment of lymphocytic choriomeningitis virus–infected mice with anti-interferon-gamma monoclonal antibody blocks generation of virus-specific cytotoxic T lymphocytes and virus elimination. Eur J Immunol 1989;19:1283–1288.

97. Huang S, Hendriks W, Althage A, et al. Immune response in mice that lack the interferon-gamma receptor. Science 1993;259:1742–1745.

98. Graham MB, Dalton DK, Giltinan D, et al. Response to influenza infection in mice with a targeted disruption in the interferon gamma gene. J Exp Med 1993;178:1725–1732.

99. Newport MJ, Huxley CM, Huston S, et al. A mutation in the interferon-gamma-receptor gene and susceptibility to mycobacterial infection. N Engl J Med 1996;335:1941–1949.

100. Jouanguy E, Lamhamedi-Cherradi S, Lammas D, et al. A human IFNGR1 small deletion hotspot associated with dominant susceptibility to mycobacterial infection. Nat Genet 1999;21:370–378.

101. Bergmann CC, Yao Q, Ho CK, Buckwold SL. Flanking residues alter antigenicity and immunogenicity of multi-unit CTL epitopes. J Immunol 1996;157:3242–3249.

102. Yellen-Shaw AJ, Wherry EJ, Dubois GC, Eisenlohr LC. Point mutation flanking a CTL epitope ablates in vitro and in vivo recognition of a full-length viral protein. J Immunol 1997;158:3227–3234.

103. Moudgil KD, Sercarz EE, Grewal IS. Modulation of the immunogenicity of antigenic determinants by their flanking residues. Immunol Today 1998;19:217–220.

104. Mylin LM. Context-dependent immunogenicity of an S206G-substituted H-2Db-restricted simian virus 40 large T antigen epitope I variant. J Immunol 1999;162:2171–2179.

105. Yewdell JW, Bennink JR. Immunodominance in major histocompatibility complex class I–restricted T-lymphocyte responses. Annu Rev Immunol 1999;17:51–88.

106. Bertoletti A, Sette A, Chisari FV, et al. Natural variants of cytotoxic epitopes are T-cell receptor antagonists for antiviral cytotoxic T cells. Nature 1994;369:407–410.

107. Klenerman P, Rowland-Jones S, McAdam S, et al. Cytotoxic T-cell activity antagonized by naturally occurring HIV-1 Gag variants. Nature 1994;369:403–407.

108. Sloan-Lancaster J, Shaw AS, Rothbard JB, Allen PM. Partial T-cell signaling: altered phospho-zeta and lack of zap70 recruitment in APL-induced T-cell anergy. Cell 1994;79:913–922.

109. Pircher H, Moskophidis D, Rohrer U, et al. Viral escape by selection of cytotoxic T cell–resistant virus variants in vivo. Nature 1990;346:629–633.

110. Green WR. Cytotoxic T lymphocytes to endogenous mouse retroviruses and mechanisms of retroviral escape. Immunol Rev 1999;168:271–286.

111. de Campos Lima PO, Gavioli R, Zhang QJ, et al. HLA-A11 epitope loss isolates of Epstein-Barr virus from a highly A11+ population. Science 1993;260:98–100.

112. Borrow P, Lewicki H, Wei X, et al. Antiviral pressure exerted by HIV-1–specific cytotoxic T lymphocytes (CTLs) during primary infection demonstrated by rapid selection of CTL escape virus. Nat Med 1997;3:205–211.

113. Goulder PJ, Phillips RE, Colbert RA, et al. Late escape from an immunodominant cytotoxic T-lymphocyte response associated with progression to AIDS. Nat Med 1997;3:212–217.

114. McMichael AJ, Phillips RE. Escape of human immunodeficiency virus from immune control. Annu Rev Immunol 1997;15:271–296.

115. Pamer E, Cresswell P. Mechanisms of MHC class I–restricted antigen processing. Annu Rev Immunol 1998;16:323–358.

116. Mahr JA, Gooding LR. Immune evasion by adenoviruses. Immunol Rev 1999;168:121–130.

117. Bennett EM, Bennink JR, Yewdell JW, Brodsky FM. Cutting edge: adenovirus E19 has two mechanisms for affecting class I MHC expression. J Immunol 1999;162:5049–5052.

118. Tomazin R, Boname J, Hegde NR, et al. Cytomegalovirus US2 destroys two components of the MHC class II pathway, preventing recognition by CD4+ T cells. Nat Med 1999;5:1039–1043.

119. Abendroth A, Arvin A. Varicella-zoster virus immune evasion. Immunol Rev 1999;168:143–156.

120. Moore KW, Vieira P, Fiorentino DF, et al. Homology of cytokine synthesis inhibitory factory (IL-10) to the Epstein-Barr virus gene BCRFI. Science 1990;248:1230–1234.

121. Hsu DH, de Waal Malefyt R, Fiorentino DF, et al. Expression of interleukin-10 activity by Epstein-Barr virus protein BCRF1. Science 1990;250:830–832.

122. Moore KW, O'Garra A, de-Waal-Malefyt R, et al. Interleukin-10. Annu Rev Immunol 1993;11:165–190.

123. Alcami A, Smith GL. A soluble receptor for interleukin-1 beta encoded by vaccinia virus: a novel mechanism of virus modulation of the host response to infection. Cell 1992;71:153–167.

124. Smith GL, Symons JA, Khanna A, et al. Vaccinia virus immune evasion. Immunol Rev 1997;159:137–154.

125. Upton C, Mossman K, McFadden G. Encoding of a homolog of the IFN-gamma receptor by myxoma virus. Science 1992;258:1369–1372.

126. Nash P, Barrett J, Cao JX, et al. Immunomodulation by viruses: the myxoma virus story. Immunol Rev 1999;168:103–120.

127. Bodaghi B, Jones TR, Zipeto D, et al. Chemokine sequestration by viral chemoreceptors as a novel viral escape strategy: withdrawal of chemokines from the environment of cytomegalovirus-infected cells. J Exp Med 1998;188:855–866.

128. Daheshia M, Feldman LT, Rouse BT. Herpes simplex virus latency and the immune response. Curr Opin Microbiol 1998;1:430–435.

129. Kinchington PR. Latency of varicella zoster virus: a persistently perplexing state. Front Biosci 1999;15:D200–211.

130. Sinclair J, Sissons P. Latent and persistent infections of monocytes and macrophages. Intervirology 1996;39:293–301.

131. Cohen JI. The biology of Epstein-Barr virus: lessons learned from the virus and the host. Curr Opin Immunol 1999;11:365–370.

132. McCune JM. Viral latency in HIV disease. Cell 1995;82:183–188.

133. Finzi D, Blankson J, Siliciano JD, et al. Latent infection of CD4+ T cells provides a mechanism for lifelong persistence of HIV-1, even in patients on effective combination therapy. Nat Med 1999;5:512–517.

134. Moskophidis D, Lechner F, Pircher H, Zinkernagel RM. Virus persistence in acutely infected immunocompetent mice by exhaustion of antiviral cytotoxic effector T cells. Nature 1993;362:758–761.

135. Moskophidis D, Laine E, Zinkernagel RM. Peripheral clonal deletion of antiviral memory CD8+ T cells. Eur J Immunol 1993;23:3306–3311.

136. Rosenberg ES, Billingsley JM, Caliendo AM, et al. Vigorous HIV-1–specific CD4+ T-cell responses associated with control of viremia. Science 1997;278:1447–1450.

137. Kalams SA, Buchbinder SP, Rosenberg ES, et al. Association between virus-specific cytotoxic T-lymphocyte and helper responses in human immunodeficiency virus type 1 infection. J Virol 1999;73:6715–6720.

138. Trimble LA, Lieberman J. Circulating CD8 T lymphocytes in human immunodeficiency virus–infected individuals have impaired function and downmodulate CD3 zeta, the signaling chain of the T-cell receptor complex. Blood 1998;91:585–594.

139. Brander C, Walker BD. T-lymphocyte responses in HIV-1 infection: implications for vaccine development. Curr Opin Immunol 1999;11:451–459.

140. Andersson J, Behbahani H, Lieberman J, et al. Perforin is not co-expressed with granzyme A within cytotoxic granules in CD8 T lymphocytes present in lymphoid tissue during chronic HIV infection. AIDS 1999;13:1295–1303.

141. Shanley JD, Jordan MC, Cook ML, Stevens JG. Pathogenesis of reactivated latent murine cytomegalovirus infection. Am J Pathol 1979;95:67–80.

142. Mutter W, Reddehase MJ, Busch FW, et al. Failure in generating hemopoietic stem cells is the primary cause of death from cytomegalovirus disease in the immunocompromised host. J Exp Med 1988;167:1645–1658.

143. Jonjic S, del Val M, Keil GM, et al. A nonstructural viral protein expressed by a recombinant vaccinia virus protects against lethal cytomegalovirus infection. J Virol 1988;62:1653–1658.

144. Meyers JD, Flournoy N, Thomas ED. Risk factors for cytomegalovirus infection after human marrow transplantation. J Infect Dis 1986;153:478–488.

145. Reusser P, Riddell SR, Meyers JD, Greenberg PD. Cytotoxic T-lymphocyte response to cytomegalovirus after human allogeneic bone marrow transplantation: pattern of recovery and correlation with cytomegalovirus infection and disease. Blood 1991;78:1373–1380.

146. Riddell SR, Rabin M, Geballe AP, et al. Class I MHC–restricted cytotoxic T-lymphocyte recognition of cells infected with human cytomegalovirus does not require endogenous viral gene expression. J Immunol 1991;146:2795–2804.

147. Gilbert MJ, Riddell SR, Li CR, Greenberg PD. Selective interference with class I major histocompatibility complex presentation of the major immediate-early protein following infection with human cytomegalovirus. J Virol 1993;67:3461–3469.

148. Jones TR, Hanson LK, Sun L, et al. Multiple independent loci within the human cytomegalovirus unique short region down-regulate expression of major histocompatibility complex class I heavy chains. J Virol 1995;69:4830–4841.

149. McLaughlin-Taylor E, Pande H, Forman S, et al. Identification of the major late human cytomegalovirus matrix protein pp65 as a target antigen for CD8+ virus-specific cytotoxic T lymphocytes. J Med Virol 1994;43:103–110.

150. Wills MR, Carmichael AJ, Mynard K, et al. The human cytotoxic T-lymphocyte (CTL) response to cytomegalovirus is dominated by structural protein pp65: frequency, specificity, and T-cell receptor usage of pp65-specific CTL. J Virol 1996;70:7569–7579.

151. Riddell SR, Watanabe KS, Goodrich JM, et al. Restoration of viral immunity in immunodeficient humans by the adoptive transfer of T-cell clones. Science 1992;257:238–241.

152. Walter EA, Greenberg PD, Gilbert MJ, et al. Reconstitution of cellular immunity against cytomegalovirus in recipients of allogeneic bone marrow by transfer of T-cell clones from the donor. N Engl J Med 1995;333:1038–1044.

153. Riddell SR, Greenberg PD. Unpublished data.

154. Miyashita EM, Yang B, Babcock GJ, Thorley-Lawson DA. Identification of the site of Epstein-Barr virus persistence in vivo as a resting B cell. J Virol 1997;71:4882–4891.

155. Decker LL, Klaman LD, Thorley-Lawson DA. Detection of the latent form of Epstein-Barr virus DNA in the peripheral blood of healthy individuals. J Virol 1996;70:3286–3289.

156. Chen F, Zou JZ, di Renzo L, et al. A subpopulation of normal B cells latently infected with Epstein-Barr virus resembles Burkitt lymphoma cells in expressing EBNA-1 but not EBNA-2 or LMP1. J Virol 1995;69:3752–3758.

157. Miyashita EM, Yang B, Lam KM, et al. A novel form of Epstein-Barr virus latency in normal B cells in vivo. Cell 1995;80:593–601.

158. Levitskaya J, Coram M, Levitsky V, et al. Inhibition of antigen processing by the internal repeat region of the Epstein-Barr virus nuclear antigen-1. Nature 1995;375:685–688.

159. Levitskaya J, Sharipo A, Leonchiks A, et al. Inhibition of ubiquitin/proteasome-dependent protein degradation by the Gly-Ala repeat domain of the Epstein-Barr virus nuclear antigen 1. Proc Natl Acad Sci USA 1997;94:12616–12621.

160. Kieff E. Epstein-Barr Virus and its replication. In: Fields BN, Knipe DM, Howley PM, eds. Fields' virology. Philadelphia: Raven, 1996:2343–2396.

161. Murray RJ, Kurilla MG, Brooks JM, et al. Identification of target antigens for the human cytotoxic T-cell response to Epstein-Barr virus (EBV): implications for the immune control of EBV-positive malignancies. J Exp Med 1992;176:157–168.

162. Khanna R, Burrows SR, Kurilla MG, et al. Localization of Epstein-Barr virus cytotoxic T-cell epitopes using

recombinant vaccinia: implications for vaccine development. J Exp Med 1992;176:169–176.

163. Moss DJ, Rickinson AB, Pope JH. Long-term T-cell–mediated immunity to Epstein-Barr virus in man. I. Complete regression of virus-induced transformation in cultures of seropositive donor leukocytes. Int J Cancer 1978;22:662–668.

164. Nalesnik MA. Lymphoproliferative disease in organ transplant recipients. Springer Semin Immunopathol 1991;13:199–216.

165. Shapiro RS, McClain K, Frizzera G, et al. Epstein-Barr virus–associated B-cell lymphoproliferative disorders following bone marrow transplantation. Blood 1988;71:1234–1243.

166. Zutter MM, Martin PJ, Sale GE, et al. Epstein-Barr virus lymphoproliferation after bone marrow transplantation. Blood 1988;72:520–529.

167. Swinnen LJ, Costanzo-Nordin MR, Fisher SG, et al. Increased incidence of lymphoproliferative disorder after immunosuppression with the monoclonal antibody OKT3 in cardiac-transplant recipients. N Engl J Med 1990;323:1723–1728.

168. Morrison VA, Dunn DL, Manivel JC, et al. Clinical characteristics of post-transplant lymphoproliferative disorders. Am J Med 1994;97:14–24.

169. Curtis RE, Travis LB, Rowlings PA, et al. Risk of lymphoproliferative disorders after bone marrow transplantation: a multi-institutional study. Blood 1999;94:2208–2216.

170. Fischer A, Blanche S, Le Bidois J, et al. Anti–B-cell monoclonal antibodies in the treatment of severe B-cell lymphoproliferative syndrome following bone marrow and organ transplantation. N Engl J Med 1991;324:1451–1456.

171. O'Reilly RJ, Small TN, Papadopoulos E, et al. Biology and adoptive cell therapy of Epstein-Barr virus–associated lymphoproliferative disorders in recipients of marrow allografts. Immunol Rev 1997;157:195–216.

172. Heslop HE, Rooney CM. Adoptive cellular immunotherapy for EBV lymphoproliferative disease. Immunol Rev 1997;157:217–222.

173. Lucas KG, Small TN, Heller G, et al. The development of cellular immunity to Epstein-Barr virus after allogeneic bone marrow transplantation. Blood 1996;87:2594–2603.

174. Papadopoulos EB, Ladanyi M, Emanuel D, et al. Infusions of donor leukocytes to treat Epstein-Barr virus–associated lymphoproliferative disorders after allogeneic bone marrow transplantation. N Engl J Med 1994;330:1185–1191.

175. Rooney CM, Smith CA, Ng CY, et al. Use of gene-modified virus-specific T lymphocytes to control Epstein-Barr-virus–related lymphoproliferation. Lancet 1995;345:9–13.

176. Heslop HE, Ng CY, Li C, et al. Long-term restoration of immunity against Epstein-Barr virus infection by adoptive transfer of gene-modified virus-specific T lymphocytes. Nat Med 1996;2:551–555.

177. Rooney CM, Smith CA, Ng CY, et al. Infusion of cytotoxic T cells for the prevention and treatment of Epstein-Barr virus-induced lymphoma in allogeneic transplant recipients. Blood 1998;92:1549–1555.

178. Safrit JT, Koup RA. The immunology of primary HIV infection: which immune responses control HIV replication? Curr Opin Immunol 1995;7:456–461.

179. Wahren B, Morfeldt-Mansson L, Biberfeld G, et al. Characteristics of the specific cell-mediated immune response in human immunodeficiency virus infection. J Virol 1987;61:2017–2023.

180. Rosenberg ES, Walker BD. HIV type 1–specific helper T cells: a critical host defense. AIDS Res Hum Retroviruses 1998;14:S143–147.

181. Brodie SJ, Lewinsohn DA, Patterson BK, et al. In vivo migration and function of transferred HIV-1–specific cytotoxic T cells. Nat Med 1999;5:34–41.

182. Nelson BH, Lord JD, Greenberg PD. Cytoplasmic domains of the interleukin-2 receptor beta and gamma chains mediate the signal for T-cell proliferation. Nature 1994;369:333–336.

183. Nakamura Y, Russell SM, Mess SA, et al. Heterodimerization of the IL-2 receptor beta- and gamma-chain cytoplasmic domains is required for signalling. Nature 1994;369:330–333.

184. Evans LS, Wittee PR, Feldhaus AL, et al. Expression of chimeric granulocyte-macrophage colony–stimulating factor/interleukin-2 receptors in human cytotoxic T-lymphocyte clones results in granulocyte-macrophage colony–stimulating factor-dependent growth. Hum Gene Ther 1999;10:1941–1951.

185. Lisziewicz J, Sun D, Smythe J, et al. Inhibition of human immunodeficiency virus type 1 replication by regulated expression of a polymeric Tat activation response RNA decoy as a strategy for gene therapy in AIDS. Proc Natl Acad Sci USA 1993;90:8000–8004.

186. Sarver N, Cantin EM, Chang PS, et al. Ribozymes as potential anti–HIV-1 therapeutic agents. Science 1990;247:1222–1225.

187. Bahner I, Kearns K, Hao QL, et al. Transduction of human CD34+ hematopoietic progenitor cells by a retroviral vector expressing an RRE decoy inhibits human immunodeficiency virus type 1 replication in myelomonocytic cells produced in long-term culture. J Virol 1996;70:4352–4360.

188. Fox BA, Woffendin C, Yang ZY, et al. Genetic modification of human peripheral blood lymphocytes with a transdominant negative form of Rev: safety and toxicity. Hum Gene Ther 1995;6:997–1004.

189. Marasco WA, Haseltine WA, Chen SY. Design, intracellular expression, and activity of a human anti–human immunodeficiency virus type 1 gp120 single-chain antibody. Proc Natl Acad Sci USA 1993;90:7889–7893.

190. Levy-Mintz, P, Duan L, Zhang H, et al. Intracellular expression of single-chain variable fragments to inhibit early stages of the viral life cycle by targeting human immunodeficiency virus type 1 integrase. J Virol 1996;70:8821–8832.

191. Chen JD, Bai X, Yang AG, et al. Inactivation of HIV-1 chemokine co-receptor CXCR-4 by a novel intrakine strategy. Nat Med 1997;3:1110–1116.

192. Bai X, Chen JD, Yang AG, et al. Genetic co-inactivation of macrophage- and T-tropic HIV-1 chemokine coreceptors CCR-5 and CXCR-4 by intrakines. Gene Ther 1998;5:984–994.

193. Ranga U, Woffendin C, Verma S, et al. Enhanced T-cell engraftment after retroviral delivery of an antiviral gene in HIV-infected individuals. Proc Natl Acad Sci USA 1998;95:1201–1206.

194. Woffendin C, Ranga U, Yang Z, et al. Expression of a protective gene prolongs survival of T cells in human immunodeficiency virus–infected patients. Proc Natl Acad Sci USA 1996;93:2889–2894.

195. Roberts MR, Qin L, Zhang D, et al. Targeting of human immunodeficiency virus–infected cells by CD8+ T lymphocytes armed with universal T-cell receptors. Blood 1994;84:2878–2889.

196. Yang OO, Tran AC, Kalams SA, et al. Lysis of HIV-1–infected cells and inhibition of viral replication by universal receptor T cells. Proc Natl Acad Sci USA 1997;94:11478–11483.

197. Zhu D, Cardenas ME, Heitman J. Calcineurin mutants render T lymphocytes resistant to cyclosporin A. Mol Pharmacol 1996;50:506–511.

198. Clay TM, Custer MC, Sachs J, et al. Efficient transfer of a tumor antigen–reactive TCR to human peripheral blood lymphocytes confers anti-tumor reactivity. J Immunol 1999;163:507–513.

199. Mule JJ, Shu S, Rosenberg SA. The anti-tumor efficacy of lymphokine-activated killer cells and recombinant interleukin-2 in vivo. J Immunol 1985;135:646–652.

200. Greenberg PD. Therapy of murine leukemia with cyclophosphamide and immune Lyt-2+ cells: cytolytic T cells can mediate eradication of disseminated leukemia. J Immunol 1986;136:1917–1922.

201. Greenberg PD, Kern DE, Cheever MA. Therapy of disseminated murine leukemia with cyclophosphamide and immune Lyt-1+,2- T cells. Tumor eradication does not require participation of cytotoxic T cells. J Exp Med 1985;161:1122–1134.

202. Fujiwara H, Fukuzawa M, Yoshioka T, et al. The role of tumor-specific Lyt-1+2- T cells in eradicating tumor cells in vivo. I. Lyt-1+2- T cells do not necessarily require recruitment of host's cytotoxic T-cell precursors for implementation of in vivo immunity. J Immunol 1984;133:1671–1676.

203. Levitsky HI, Lazenby A, Hayashi RJ, Pardoll DM. In vivo priming of two distinct antitumor effector populations: the role of MHC class I expression. J Exp Med 1994;179:1215–1224.

204. Thompson JA, Shulman KL, Benyunes MC, et al. Prolonged continuous intravenous infusion interleukin-2 and lymphokine-activated killer-cell therapy for metastatic renal cell carcinoma. J Clin Oncol 1992;10:960–968.

205. Paciucci PA, Holland JF, Glidewell O, Odchimar R. Recombinant interleukin-2 by continuous infusion and adoptive transfer of recombinant interleukin-2–activated cells in patients with advanced cancer. J Clin Oncol 1989;7:869–878.

206. Rosenberg SA, Lotze MT, Yang JC, et al. Prospective randomized trial of high-dose interleukin-2 alone or in conjunction with lymphokine-activated killed cells for the treatment of patients with advanced cancer. J Natl Cancer Inst 1993;85:622–632.

207. Griffiths E, Ong H, Soloski MJ, et al. Tumor defense by murine cytotoxic T cells specific for peptide bound to nonclassical MHC class I. Cancer Res 1998;58:4682–4687.

208. Housseau F, Bright R, Simonis T, et al. Recognition of a shared human prostate cancer–associated antigen by nonclassical MHC-restricted CD8+ T cells. J Immunol 1999;163:6330–6337.

209. Kast WM, Offringa R, Peters PJ, et al. Eradication of adenovirus E1–induced tumors by E1A-specific cytotoxic T lymphocytes. Cell 1989;59:603–614.

210. Barker E, Mokyr MB. Importance of Lyt-2+ T cells in the resistance of melphalan-cured MOPC-315 tumor bearers to a challenge with MOPC-315 tumor cells. Cancer Res 1988;48:4834–4842.

211. Melief CJ. Tumor eradication by adoptive transfer of cytotoxic T lymphocytes. Adv Cancer Res 1992;58:143–175.

212. Dobrzanski MJ, Reome JB, Dutton RW. Therapeutic effects of tumor-reactive type 1 and type 2 CD8+ T-cell subpopulations in established pulmonary metastases. J Immunol 1999;162:6671–6680.

213. Greenberg PD, Cheever MA, Fefer A. Detection of early and delayed antitumor effects following curative adoptive chemoimmunotherapy of established leukemia. Cancer Res 1980;40:4428–4432.

214. Cheever MA, Greenberg PD, Fefer A, Gillis S. Augmentation of the anti-tumor therapeutic efficacy of long-term cultured T lymphocytes by in vivo administration of purified interleukin-2. J Exp Med 1982;155:968–980.

215. Bear HD, Susskind BM, Close KA, Barrett SK. Phenotype of syngeneic tumor–specific cytotoxic T-lymphocytes and requirements for their in vivo generation from tumor-bearing host and immune spleens. Cancer Res 1988;48:1422–1427.

216. Klarnet JP, Matis LA, Kern DE, et al. Antigen-driven T-cell clones can proliferate in vivo, eradicate disseminated leukemia, and provide specific immunologic memory. J Immunol 1987;138:4012–4017.

217. Schoenberger SP, Toes RE, van de Voort EI, et al. T-cell help for cytotoxic T lymphocytes is mediated by CD40-CD40L interactions. Nature 1998;393:480–483.

218. Bennett SR, Carbone FR, Karamalis F, et al. Help for cytotoxic-T-cell responses is mediated by CD40 signalling. Nature 1998;393:478–480.

219. Ridge JP, Di Rosa F, Matzinger P. A conditioned dendritic cell can be a temporal bridge between a CD4+ T- helper and a T-killer cell. Nature 1998;393:474–478.

220. Toes RE, Ossendorp F, Offringa R, Melief CJ. CD4 T cells and their role in antitumor immune responses. J Exp Med 1999;189:753–756.

221. Pardoll DM, Topalian SL. The role of CD4+ T-cell responses in antitumor immunity. Curr Opin Immunol 1998;10:588–594.

222. Weiss S, Bogen B. MHC class II–restricted presentation of intracellular antigen. Cell 1991;64:767–776.

223. Wen YJ, Lim SH. T cells recognize the VH complementarity-determining region 3 of the idiotypic protein of B-cell non-Hodgkin's lymphoma. Eur J Immunol 1997;27:1043–1047.

224. Mumberg D, Monach PA, Wanderling S, et al. CD4(+) T cells eliminate MHC class II–negative cancer cells in vivo by indirect effects of IFN-gamma. Proc Natl Acad Sci USA 1999;96:8633–8638.

225. Hung K, Hayashi R, Lafond-Walker A, et al. The central role of CD4(+) T cells in the antitumor immune response. J Exp Med 1998;188:2357–2368.

226. Eshhar Z, Bach N, Fitzer-Attas CJ, et al. The T-body approach: potential for cancer immunotherapy. Springer Semin Immunopathol 1996;18:199–209.

227. Hwu P, Yang JC, Cowherd R, et al. In vivo antitumor activity of T cells redirected with chimeric antibody/T-cell receptor genes. Cancer Res 1995;55:3369–3373.

228. Altenschmidt U, Klundt E, Groner B. Adoptive transfer of in vitro–targeted, activated T lymphocytes results in total tumor regression. J Immunol 1997;159:5509–5515.

229. Weijtens ME, Willemsen RA, Valerio D, et al. Single-chain Ig/gamma gene-redirected human T lymphocytes produce cytokines, specifically lyse tumor cells, and recycle lytic capacity. J Immunol 1996;157:836–843.

230. Patel SD, Moskalenko M, Smith D, et al. Impact of chimeric immune receptor extracellular protein domains on T-cell function. Gene Ther 1999;6:412–419.

231. Finney HM, Lawson AD, Bebbington CR, Weir AN. Chimeric receptors providing both primary and costimulatory signaling in T cells from a single gene product. J Immunol 1998;161:2791–2797.

232. Boon T, Cerottini JC, Van-den-Eynde B, et al. Tumor antigens recognized by T lymphocytes. Annu Rev Immunol 1994;12:337–365.

233. Lurquin C, Van-Pel A, Mariam'e B, et al. Structure of the gene of tum- transplantation antigen P91A: the mutated exon encodes a peptide recognized with Ld by cytolytic T cells. Cell 1989;58:293–303.

234. Sibille C, Chomez P, Wildmann C, et al. Structure of the gene of tum- transplantation antigen P198: a point mutation generates a new antigenic peptide. J Exp Med 1990;172:35–45.

235. Van den Eynde B, Lethe B, Van Pel A, et al. The gene coding for a major tumor rejection antigen of tumor P815 is identical to the normal gene of syngeneic DBA/2 mice. J Exp Med 1991;173:1373–1384.

236. van der Bruggen P, Traversari C, Chomez P, et al. A gene encoding an antigen recognized by cytolytic T lymphocytes on a human melanoma. Science 1991;254:1643–1647.

237. Brichard V, Van-Pel A, Wolfel T, et al. The tyrosinase gene codes for an antigen recognized by autologous cytolytic T lymphocytes on HLA-A2 melanomas. J Exp Med 1993;178:489–495.

238. van der Bruggen P, Szikora JP, Boel P, et al. Autologous cytolytic T lymphocytes recognize a MAGE-1 nonapeptide on melanomas expressing HLA-Cw*1601. Eur J Immunol 1994;24:2134–2140.

239. Kawakami Y, Eliyahu S, Delgado CH, et al. Cloning of the gene coding for a shared human melanoma antigen recognized by autologous T cells infiltrating into tumor. Proc Natl Acad Sci USA 1994;91:3515–3519.

240. Kawakami Y, Eliyahu S, Delgado CH, et al. Identification of a human melanoma antigen recognized by tumor-infiltrating lymphocytes associated with in vivo tumor rejection. Proc Natl Acad Sci USA 1994;91:6458–6462.

241. Boel P, Wildmann C, Sensi ML, et al. BAGE: a new gene encoding an antigen recognized on human melanomas by cytolytic T lymphocytes. Immunity 1995;2:167–175.

242. Gaugler B, Van den Eynde B, van der Bruggen P, et al. Human gene MAGE-3 codes for an antigen recognized on a melanoma by autologous cytolytic T lymphocytes. J Exp Med 1994;179:921–930.

243. Jager E, Chen YT, Drijfhout JW, et al. Simultaneous humoral and cellular immune response against cancer-testis antigen NY-ESO-1: definition of human histocompatibility leukocyte antigen (HLA)-A2–binding peptide epitopes. J Exp Med 1998;187:265–270.

244. Van den Eynde B, Peeters O, De Backer O, et al. A new family of genes coding for an antigen recognized by autologous cytolytic T lymphocytes on a human melanoma. J Exp Med 1995;182:689–698.

245. Boon T, van der Bruggen P. Human tumor antigens recognized by T lymphocytes. J Exp Med 1996;183:725–729.

246. Wang RF, Robbins PF, Kawakami Y, et al. Identification of a gene encoding a melanoma tumor antigen recognized by HLA-A31–restricted tumor-infiltrating lymphocytes. J Exp Med 1995;181:799–804.

247. Wang RF, Parkhurst MR, Kawakami Y, et al. Utilization of an alternative open reading frame of a normal gene in generating a novel human cancer antigen. J Exp Med 1996;183:1131–1140.

248. Wang RF, Johnston SL, Southwood S, et al. Recognition of an antigenic peptide derived from tyrosinase-related protein-2 by CTL in the context of HLA-A31 and -A33. J Immunol 1998;160:890–897.

249. Coulie PG, Lehmann F, Lethe B, et al. A mutated intron sequence codes for an antigenic peptide recognized by cytolytic T lymphocytes on a human melanoma. Proc Natl Acad Sci USA 1995;92:7976–7980.

250. Wolfel T, Hauer M, Schneider J, et al. A p16INK4a-insensitive CDK4 mutant targeted by cytolytic T lymphocytes in a human melanoma. Science 1995;269:1281–1284.

251. Robbins PF, El-Gamil M, Li YF, et al. A mutated beta-catenin gene encodes a melanoma-specific antigen recognized by tumor infiltrating lymphocytes. J Exp Med 1996;183:1185–1192.

252. Wang RF, Wang X, Atwood AC, et al. Cloning genes encoding MHC class II–restricted antigens: mutated CDC27 as a tumor antigen. Science 1999;284:1351–1354.

253. Wang RF, Wang X, Rosenberg SA. Identification of a novel major histocompatibility complex class II-restricted tumor antigen resulting from a chromosomal rearrangement recognized by CD4(+) T cells. J Exp Med 1999;189:1659–1668.

254. Gilboa E. The makings of a tumor rejection antigen. Immunity 1999;11:263–270.

255. Mandelboim O, Berke G, Fridkin M, et al. CTL induction by a tumour-associated antigen octapeptide derived from a murine lung carcinoma. Nature 1994;369:67–71.

256. Hunt DF, Henderson RA, Shabanowitz J, et al. Characterization of peptides bound to the class I MHC molecule HLA-A2.1 by mass spectrometry. Science 1992;255:1261–1263.

257. Hogan KT, Eisinger DP, Cupp SR, et al. The peptide recognized by HLA-A68.2–restricted, squamous cell carcinoma of the lung-specific cytotoxic T lymphocytes is derived from a mutated elongation factor 2 gene. Cancer Res 1998; 58:5144–5150.

258. Skipper JC, Hendrickson RC, Gulden PH, et al. An HLA-A2–restricted tyrosinase antigen on melanoma cells results from posttranslational modification and suggests a novel pathway for processing of membrane proteins. J Exp Med 1996;183:527–534.

259. Meadows L, Wang W, den Haan JM, et al. The HLA-A*0201–restricted H-Y antigen contains a posttranslationally modified cysteine that significantly affects T-cell recognition. Immunity 1997;6:273–281.

260. Klarnet JP, Kern DE, Okuno K, et al. FBL-reactive CD8+ cytotoxic and CD4+ helper T lymphocytes recognize distinct Friend murine leukemia virus–encoded antigens. J Exp Med 1989;169:457–467.

261. Tanaka Y, Tevethia MJ, Kalderon D, et al. Clustering of antigenic sites recognized by cytotoxic T-lymphocyte clones in the amino-terminal half of SV40 T antigen. Virology 1988;162:427–436.

262. Hsu FJ, Caspar CB, Czerwinski D, et al. Tumor-specific idiotype vaccines in the treatment of patients with B-cell lymphoma—long-term results of a clinical trial. Blood 1997;89:3129–3135.

263. Kwak LW, Campbell MJ, Czerwinski DK, et al. Induction of immune responses in patients with B-cell lymphoma against the surface-immunoglobulin idiotype expressed by their tumors. N Engl J Med 1992;327:1209–1215.

264. Yotnda P, Firat H, Garcia-Pons F, et al. Cytotoxic T-cell response against the chimeric p210 BCR-ABL protein in patients with chronic myelogenous leukemia. J Clin Invest 1998;101:2290–2296.

265. Gambacorti-Passerini C, Grignani F, Arienti F, et al. Human CD4 lymphocytes specifically recognize a peptide representing the fusion region of the hybrid protein pml/RAR alpha present in acute promyelocytic leukemia cells. Blood 1993;81:1369–1375.

266. Jung S, Schluesener HJ. Human T lymphocytes recognize a peptide of single point–mutated, oncogenic ras proteins. J Exp Med 1991;173:273–276.

267. Houbiers JG, Nijman HW, van-der-Burg SH, et al. In vitro induction of human cytotoxic T lymphocyte responses against peptides of mutant and wild-type p53. Eur J Immunol 1993;23:2072–2077.

268. Yoshino I, Goedegebuure PS, Peoples GE, et al. HER2/neu-derived peptides are shared antigens among human non–small cell lung cancer and ovarian cancer. Cancer Res 1994;54:3387–3390.

269. Fisk B, Chesak B, Pollack MS, et al. Oligopeptide induction of a cytotoxic T-lymphocyte response to HER-2/neu proto-oncogene in vitro. Cell Immunol 1994;157:415–427.

270. Vonderheide RH, Hahn WC, Schultze JL, Nadler LM. The telomerase catalytic subunit is a widely expressed tumor-associated antigen recognized by cytotoxic T lymphocytes. Immunity 1999;10:673–679.

271. Redchenko IV, Rickinson AB. Accessing Epstein-Barr virus–specific T-cell memory with peptide-loaded dendritic cells. J Virol 1999;73:334–342.

272. Alexander-Miller MA, Leggatt GR, Berzofsky JA. Selective expansion of high- or low-avidity cytotoxic T lymphocytes and efficacy for adoptive immunotherapy. Proc Natl Acad Sci USA 1996;93:4102–4107.

273. Alexander-Miller MA, Leggatt GR, Sarin A, Berzofsky JA. Role of antigen, CD8, and cytotoxic T-lymphocyte (CTL) avidity in high-dose antigen induction of apoptosis of effector CTL. J Exp Med 1996;184:485–492.

274. Valmori D, Pittet MJ, Rimoldi D, et al. An antigen-targeted approach to adoptive transfer therapy of cancer. Cancer Res 1999;59:2167–2173.

275. Luxembourg AT, Borrow P, Teyton L, et al. Biomagnetic isolation of antigen-specific CD8+ T cells usable in immunotherapy. Nat Biotechnol 1998;16:281–285.

276. Yee C, Savage PA, Lee PP, et al. Isolation of high-avidity melanoma-reactive CTL from heterogeneous populations using peptide-MHC tetramers. J Immunol 1999;162:2227–2234.

277. Dunbar PR, Chen JL, Chao D, et al. Cutting edge: rapid cloning of tumor-specific CTL suitable for adoptive immunotherapy of melanoma. J Immunol 1999;162:6959–6962.

278. Warren EH, Gavin M, Greenberg PD, Riddell SR. Minor histocompatibility antigens as targets for T-cell therapy after bone marrow transplantation. Curr Opin Hematol 1998;5:429–433.

279. Goulmy E. Human minor histocompatibility antigens: new concepts for marrow transplantation and adoptive immunotherapy. Immunol Rev 1997;157:125–140.

280. van der Harst D, Goulmy E, Falkenburg JH, et al. Recognition of minor histocompatibility antigens on lymphocytic and myeloid leukemic cells by cytotoxic T-cell clones. Blood 1994;83:1060–1066.

281. Falkenburg JH, Goselink HM, van der Harst D, et al. Growth inhibition of clonogenic leukemic precursor cells by minor histocompatibility antigen–specific cytotoxic T lymphocytes. J Exp Med 1991;174:27–33.

282. Bonnet D, Warren EH, Greenberg PD, et al. CD8(+) minor histocompatibility antigen–specific cytotoxic T-lymphocyte clones eliminate human acute myeloid leukemia stem cells. Proc Natl Acad Sci USA 1999;96:8639–8644.

283. de Bueger M, Bakker A, Van Rood JJ, et al. Tissue distribution of human minor histocompatibility antigens. Ubiquitous versus restricted tissue distribution indicates heterogeneity among human cytotoxic T-lymphocyte–defined non-MHC antigens. J Immunol 1992;149:1788–1794.

284. den Haan JM, Meadows LM, Wang W, et al. The minor histocompatibility antigen HA-I: a diallelic gene with a single amino acid polymorphism. Science 1998;279:1054–1057.

285. den Haan JM, Sherman NE, Blokland E, et al. Identification of a graft-versus-host disease–associated human minor histocompatibility antigen. Science 1995;268:1476–1480.

286. Goulmy E, Schipper R, Pool J, et al. Mismatches of minor histocompatibility antigens between HLA-identical donors and recipients and the development of graft-versus-host disease after bone marrow transplantation. N Engl J Med 1996;334:281–285.

287. Tseng LH, Lin MT, Hansen JA, et al. Correlation between disparity for the minor histocompatibility antigen HA-1 and the development of acute graft-versus-host disease after allogeneic marrow transplantation. Blood 1999;94:2911–2914.

288. Dolstra H, Fredrix H, Preijers F, et al. Recognition of a B-cell leukemia–associated minor histocompatibility antigen by CTL. J Immunol 1997;158:560–565.

289. Dolstra H, Fredrix H, Maas F, et al. A human minor histocompatibility antigen specific for B-cell acute lymphoblastic leukemia. J Exp Med 1999;189:301–308.

290. Wang W, Meadows LR, den Haan JM, et al. Human H-Y: a male-specific histocompatibility antigen derived from the SMCY protein. Science 1995;269:1588–1590.

291. Mutis T, Gillespie G, Schrama E, et al. Tetrameric HLA class I minor histocompatibility antigen peptide complexes demonstrate minor histocompatibility antigen–specific

cytotoxic T lymphocytes in patients with graft-versus-host disease. Nat Med 1999;5:839–842.

292. Warren EH, Greenberg PD, Riddell SR. Cytotoxic T-lymphocyte–defined human minor histocompatibility antigens with a restricted tissue distribution. Blood 1998;91: 2197–2207.

293. Morgan DJ, Kreuwel HT, Fleck S, et al. Activation of low-avidity CTL specific for a self-epitope results in tumor rejection but not autoimmunity. J Immunol 1998;160:643–651.

294. Sherman LA, Theobald M, Morgan D, et al. Strategies for tumor elimination by cytotoxic T lymphocytes. Crit Rev Immunol 1998;18:47–54.

295. Theobald M, Ruppert T, Kuckelkorn U, et al. The sequence alteration associated with a mutational hotspot in p53 protects cells from lysis by cytotoxic T lymphocytes specific for a flanking peptide epitope. J Exp Med 1998;188:1017–1028.

296. Dighe AS, Richards E, Old LJ, Schreiber RD. Enhanced in vivo growth and resistance to rejection of tumor cells expressing dominant negative IFN gamma receptors. Immunity 1994;1:447–456.

297. Kaplan DH, Shankaran V, Dighe AS, et al. Demonstration of an interferon gamma–dependent tumor surveillance system in immunocompetent mice. Proc Natl Acad Sci USA 1998;95:7556–7561.

298. Musiani P, Modesti A, Giovarelli M, et al. Cytokines, tumour-cell death and immunogenicity: a question of choice. Immunol Today 1997;18:32–36.

299. Levy LS, Bost KL. Mechanisms that contribute to the development of lymphoid malignancies: roles for genetic alterations and cytokine production. Crit Rev Immunol 1996;16:31–57.

300. Chen Q, Daniel V, Maher DW, Hersey P. Production of IL-10 by melanoma cells: examination of its role in immunosuppression mediated by melanoma. Int J Cancer 1994;56:755–760.

301. Hahne M, Rimoldi D, Schroter M, et al. Melanoma cell expression of Fas(Apo-1/CD95) ligand: implications for tumor immune escape. Science 1996;274:1363–1366.

302. Walker PR, Saas P, Dietrich PY. Role of Fas ligand (CD95L) in immune escape: the tumor cell strikes back. J Immunol 1997;158:4521–4524.

303. Walker PR, Saas P, Dietrich PY. Tumor expression of Fas ligand (CD95L) and the consequences. Curr Opin Immunol 1998;10:564–572.

304. Chappell DB, Restifo NP. T cell-tumor cell: a fatal interaction? Cancer Immunol Immunother 1998;47:65–71.

305. Kataoka T, Schroter M, Hahne M, et al. FLIP prevents apoptosis induced by death receptors but not by perforin/granzyme B, chemotherapeutic drugs, and gamma irradiation. J Immunol 1998;161:3936–3942.

306. Zaks TZ, Chappell DB, Rosenberg SA, Restifo NP. Fas-mediated suicide of tumor-reactive T cells following activation by specific tumor: selective rescue by caspase inhibition. J Immunol 1999;162:3273–3279.

307. Irmler M, Thome M, Hahne M, et al. Inhibition of death receptor signals by cellular FLIP. Nature 1997;388:190–195.

308. Tschopp J, Irmler M, Thome M. Inhibition of fas death signals by FLIPs. Curr Opin Immunol 1998;10:552–558.

309. Gimmi CD, Morrison BW, Mainprice BA, et al. Breast cancer–associated antigen, DF3/MUC1, induces apoptosis of activated human T cells. Nat Med 1996;2:1367–1370.

310. Nakashima M, Sonoda K, Watanabe T. Inhibition of cell growth and induction of apoptotic cell death by the human tumor-associated antigen RCAS1. Nat Med 1999;5:938–942.

311. Villunger A, Strasser A. The great escape: is immune evasion required for tumor progression? Nat Med 1999;5:874–875.

312. Staveley-O'Carroll K, Sotomayor E, Montgomery J, et al. Induction of antigen-specific T-cell anergy: an early event in the course of tumor progression. Proc Natl Acad Sci USA 1998;95:1178–1183.

313. Shrikant P, Mescher MF. Control of syngeneic tumor growth by activation of CD8+ T cells: efficacy is limited by migration away from the site and induction of nonresponsiveness. J Immunol 1999;162:2858–2866.

314. Lee PP, Yee C, Savage PA, et al. Characterization of circulating T cells specific for tumor-associated antigens in melanoma patients. Nat Med 1999;5:677–685.

315. Mizoguchi H, O'Shea JJ, Longo DL, et al. Alterations in signal transduction molecules in T lymphocytes from tumor-bearing mice. Science 1992;258:1795–1798.

316. Kolenko V, Wang Q, Riedy MC, et al. Tumor-induced suppression of T-lymphocyte proliferation coincides with inhibition of Jak3 expression and IL-2 receptor signaling: role of soluble products from human renal cell carcinomas. J Immunol 1997;159:3057–3067.

317. Correa MR, Ochoa AC, Ghosh P, et al. Sequential development of structural and functional alterations in T cells from tumor-bearing mice. J Immunol 1997;158:5292–5296.

318. Wu NZ, Klitzman B, Dodge R, Dewhirst MW. Diminished leukocyte-endothelium interaction in tumor microvessels. Cancer Res 1992;52:4265–4268.

319. Jain RK, Koenig GC, Dellian M, et al. Leukocyte-endothelial adhesion and angiogenesis in tumors. Cancer Metastasis Rev 1996;15:195–204.

320. Ellem KA, Schmidt CW, Li CL, et al. The labyrinthine ways of cancer immunotherapy—T cell, tumor cell encounter: "how do I lose thee? Let me count the ways." Adv Cancer Res 1998;75:203–249.

321. Piali L, Fichtel A, Terpe HJ, et al. Endothelial vascular cell adhesion molecule 1 expression is suppressed by melanoma and carcinoma. J Exp Med 1995;181:811–816.

322. Brown NJ, Ali S, Reed MW, et al. Trafficking of activated lymphocytes into the RENCA tumour microcirculation in vivo in mice. Br J Cancer 1997;76:1572–1578.

323. Ogawa M, Umehara K, Yu WG, et al. A critical role for a peritumoral stromal reaction in the induction of T-cell migration responsible for interleukin-12–induced tumor regression. Cancer Res 1999;59:1531–1538.

324. Ganss R, Hanahan D. Tumor microenvironment can restrict the effectiveness of activated antitumor lymphocytes. Cancer Res 1998;58:4673–4681.

325. Rosenberg SA, Spiess P, Lafreniere R. A new approach to the adoptive immunotherapy of cancer with tumor-infiltrating lymphocytes. Science 1986;233:1318–1321.

326. Topalian SL, Muul LM, Solomon D, Rosenberg SA. Expansion of human tumor–infiltrating lymphocytes for use in immunotherapy trials. J Immunol Methods 1987;102:127–141.

327. Topalian SL, Solomon D, Rosenberg SA. Tumor-specific cytolysis by lymphocytes infiltrating human melanomas. J Immunol 1989;142:3714–3725.

328. Aebersold P, Hyatt C, Johnson S, et al. Lysis of autologous melanoma cells by tumor-infiltrating lymphocytes: association with clinical response. J Natl Cancer Inst 1991;83:932–937.

329. Yasumura S, Hirabayashi H, Schwartz DR, et al. Human cytotoxic T-cell lines with restricted specificity for squamous cell carcinoma of the head and neck. Cancer Res 1993;53:1461–1468.

330. Rosenberg SA, Packard BS, Aebersold PM, et al. Use of tumor-infiltrating lymphocytes and interleukin-2 in the immunotherapy of patients with metastatic melanoma. A preliminary report. N Engl J Med 1988;319:1676–1680.

331. Kolb HJ, Schattenberg A, Goldman JM, et al. European Group for Blood and Marrow Transplantation Working Party Chronic Leukemia. Graft-versus-leukemia effect of donor lymphocyte transfusions in marrow grafted patients. Blood 1995;86:2041–2050.

332. Collins R Jr, Shpilberg O, Drobyski WR, et al. Donor leukocyte infusions in 140 patients with relapsed malignancy after allogeneic bone marrow transplantation. J Clin Oncol 1997;15:433–444.

333. Bonini C, Ferrari G, Verzeletti S, et al. HSV-TK gene transfer into donor lymphocytes for control of allogeneic graft-versus-leukemia. Science 1997;276:1719–1724.

334. Nagoya S, Greenberg PD, Yee C, et al. Helper T-cell–independent proliferation of CD8+ cytotoxic T lymphocytes transduced with an IL-1 receptor retrovirus. J Immunol 1994;153:1527–1535.

335. Marincola FM, Ettinghausen S, Cohen PA, et al. Treatment of established lung metastases with tumor-infiltrating lymphocytes derived from a poorly immunogenic tumor engineered to secrete human TNF-alpha. J Immunol 1994;152:3500–3513.

336. Jensen M, Tan G, Forman S, et al. CD20 is a molecular target for scFvFc:zeta receptor redirected T cells: implications for cellular immunotherapy of CD20+ malignancy. Biol Blood Marrow Transplant 1998;4:75–83.

337. Eshhar Z, Waks T, Gross G, Schindler DG. Specific activation and targeting of cytotoxic lymphocytes through chimeric single chains consisting of antibody-binding domains and the gamma or zeta subunits of the immunoglobulin and T-cell receptors. Proc Natl Acad Sci USA 1993;90:720–724.

Chapter 42

Genetically Engineered Cancer Vaccines

Glenn Dranoff

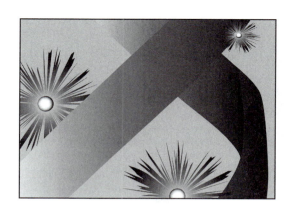

Tumor immunology appears to be on the verge of achieving some well-deserved respectability. The field at last seems to have emerged from the sortie of impassioned criticisms launched its way over the course of many decades. Despite Dr. Coley's demonstration, nearly 100 years ago, that the administration of bacterial toxins to patients with cancer could result in clinically meaningful tumor destruction (1), the low frequency of tumor response together with the troublesome systemic toxicities rendered his findings, in the eyes of many, a curiosity devoid of general applicability. The experimental models underlying this field similarly were viewed with a large dose of skepticism. While admittedly the preliminary findings of antitumor immunity in murine systems were revealed to reflect unrecognized major histocompatibility complex (MHC) disparities (2), convincing evidence for antitumor immunity in the autochthonous host (3) was answered with the retort that carcinogen-induced tumors bore little resemblance to the cancers plaguing humans (4). Even after spontaneous murine tumors were shown to be immunogenic by virtue of chemical mutagenesis techniques (5), some still maintained that human tumors simply were nonimmunogenic (6).

The combination of improved insights into the host-tumor relationship and informed empiricism in the design of clinical trials may finally have effectively silenced this rhetoric. The application of contemporary genetic, biochemical, and cellular methodologies to the experimental problems of tumor immunology has resulted in an impressive body of data that demonstrates that cancer patients can develop productive antitumor immune responses (7). A substantial number of tumor antigens that evoke humoral and/or cellular reactions have been defined at the molecular level (8). Importantly, some of these antigens have been incorporated into vaccination strategies that efficiently result in tumor destruction in both patients with advanced cancer (9–11) and murine models (12,13).

These critical findings highlight the inherent value of rodent tumor systems and the power of contemporary approaches to translate into patient benefits. Indeed, the first convincing demonstration that tumor vaccination can modulate the natural history of human cancer has now been presented. Dr. Pinedo and colleagues established through a large randomized clinical trial that patients with early stage colorectal carcinoma experience a 61% reduction in the risk for recurrent disease if they are immunized with autologous, irradiated tumor cells admixed with Bacille Calmette-Guérin (BCG) (14). This landmark study reflects the tenacity of clinical investigators who steadfastly sought to delineate the therapeutic potential of BCG, which was first suggested in murine tumor models 40 years ago (15). In a similar spirit, large-scale testing of other classic immunization schemes is also under way in patients with metastatic melanoma who harbor minimal residual disease following surgical intervention (16).

It is clear that a new and exciting era in tumor immunology has been ushered in. Gene transfer technologies have contributed in important ways to the achievement of this long-awaited beginning. In this chapter I will review the accumulating pre-clinical and clinical data that indicate that gene transfer is likely to maintain a prominent position in the quest to develop efficacious immunotherapy for many forms of cancer.

Experimental Foundations

One of the cornerstones of contemporary tumor immunology is the crafting of several strategies to identify tumor antigens. A key insight underlying this work is the recognition that T lymphocytes respond to target antigens as processed peptides, derived from cellular proteins, inserted into the grooves of MHC molecules (17). Based on this understanding, Boon and colleagues devised the first informative approach to this problem in which tumor-specific cytolytic T-cell clones were used to screen cDNA expression libraries, derived from tumor samples, transfected into recipient cells expressing the appropriate MHC class I molecules (8). This powerful approach recently was validated through the demonstration in murine models that vaccination with P1A or mutated, mitogen-activated protein kinase (genes identified by this scheme) efficiently protected against challenges with the appropriate parental tumors (12,13); further, immunization of patients with metastatic melanoma with peptides derived from the MAGE-3 and gp100 gene products resulted in tumor regression in some cases as well (9–11). A related approach, pioneered by Hunt and collaborators, uses tumor-specific T cells to screen candidate peptides that are acid-eluted from MHC molecules and sequenced using reverse-phase, high-performance liquid chromatography or mass spectrometry (18).

A third informative strategy, developed by Pfreundschuh and colleagues, employs antibodies to screen cDNA expression libraries prepared from tumor cell–derived mRNA (19). This scheme is grounded in the hypothesis that at least some tumor antigens recognized by high-titer IgG antibodies are also targets for CD4- and CD8-positive T lymphocytes. Indeed, the development of significant IgG titers implies, at a minimum, that CD4-positive T cells have been stimulated to provide signals necessary for isotype switching. In support of this hypothesis, serologic techniques have been used to identify the MAGE-1 and tyrosinase gene products, antigens initially discovered by T-cell cloning methods (19). Perhaps more noteworthy, however, is the finding that NY-ESO-1, a protein of unknown function first discovered through antibody-based cloning, subsequently was shown to be recognized by MHC class I–restricted cytotoxic T lymphocytes as well (20,21). These results suggest that serology-based methods may ultimately prove to be the most informative of all, since patient tumors and sera are widely available and, in contrast to the stringent requirement for generating T-cell clones for the first two approaches, limited manipulations of antibodies are necessary for library screening. It seems likely that serology-based methods will yield many novel targets in a variety of cancers; a recent detailed study of patients with colorectal carcinoma revealed the provocative finding that nuclear proteins may be an especially rich source of antigens (22).

The cumulative efforts of the three tumor-antigen-discovery strategies have provided insights into the range of cancer-associated molecules that can become targets for immune responses. Four major classes of antigens have emerged thus far (7,8). One group, represented by the MAGE, BAGE, and GAGE gene families, consists of oncofetal antigens that are widely expressed during fetal development, but restricted to the testis and placenta in the adult; these characteristics have inspired the term "cancer-testis" antigens. A second group of targets, surprisingly, consists of normal differentiation proteins; these have been delineated most thoroughly in malignant melanomas where they function as key components of the melanin biosynthetic pathway. They include tyrosinase, Melan A/MART-1, gp75 (tyrosinase related protein-1, TRP-1), TRP-2, and gp100/Pmel 17. The potential of nonmutated cellular proteins to serve as tumor antigens highlights the connections between antitumor immunity and autoimmunity; studies further exploring this interaction are likely to reveal important mechanisms underlying the maintenance of peripheral tolerance (23). A third group of antigens is composed of mutated cellular proteins, some of which may contribute to the transformed phenotype such as cyclin-dependent protein kinase 4, β-catenin, and caspase 8. A final group consists of short peptides encoded by intronic sequences that are aberrantly expressed in cancer cells; examples of this class include MUM-1, p15, *N*-acetylglucosaminyltransferase V, and a novel form of TRP-2.

Naturally Occurring Antitumor Immunity

The plethora of tumor antigens revealed by genetic and biochemical techniques indicates that tumors frequently evoke immune responses. At first blush, since these observations were made in tumor-bearing hosts, it would seem prudent to conclude that such reactions typically are ineffective in controlling tumor progression. However, a more detailed examination uncovers a striking correlation between long-term patient survival and specific patterns of host antitumor immunity. The landmark investigations of Clark and Mihm in maligant melanoma are especially provocative in this context (24–27). These pathologists discovered that, although the vertical-growth phase of primary melanoma is infiltrated diffusely with T lymphocytes only infrequently, this response nonetheless is tightly correlated with prolonged survival and a low incidence of recurrent disease. The development of brisk T-cell infiltrates in melanomas that already have metastasized to regional lymph nodes similarly predicts improved survival when compared with tumors that fail to evoke this host response.

These correlations now have been extended to early-stage colon carcinoma, where the presence of CD8-positive T lymphocytes within nests of the primary tumor proves to be as strong a prognostic indicator for survival as the widely used Duke's staging system (28). Lymphocytic infiltrates are associated with many other tumors to a variable degree, suggesting that additional clinicopathologic analyses should be performed to clarify the generality of these findings. Finally, although the increased incidence of viral-associated neoplasms in immunocompromised patients is well documented (29), the studies of Clark and Mihm strongly indicate that the issue of immunosurveillance in normal hosts should be revisited.

The Failure of Antitumor Immunity

Naturally occurring, antitumor immunity ultimately fails to restrain cancer growth in most patients. The means by which tumors escape remain to be fully delineated, but evidence for several possibilities already has been marshalled. One pathway of resistance involves the selection of antigen-loss variants or clones with defects in the antigen-presentation machinery (30–32). These lesions can include the loss of MHC molecules, $\beta 2$-microglobulin, or TAP gene products and mutations in the T-cell epitope that alter the binding affinity for the MHC groove; mutations flanking the epitope may also compromise the efficiency at which the proteasome processes the native protein.

A second mechanism underlying cancer progression involves the finding that tumor cells frequently do not stimulate maximal immune responses. Increasing evidence suggests that dendritic cells are specialized to initiate immunity because of their abilities to process antigens efficiently into both MHC class I and II pathways and their high-level expression of costimulatory molecules (33). Tumor cells, in contrast to dendritic cells, are less endowed with the capacity for antigen processing and usually do not express the full complement of costimulatory molecules (34). Tumor cells generally also fail to incite the local recruitment and activation of professional antigen-presenting cells. Together, these considerations render it unlikely for T and B lymphocytes to be exposed to tumor antigens in an optimal immunologic environment; reactive cells may be driven to abortive responses or become dysfunctional. It is worth highlighting in this regard that mouse models of chronic viral infection reveal that if CD8-positive T-cell responses are generated in the absence of CD4-positive T-cell help, the CD8 population is compromised in antigen-specific cytotoxicity and cytokine production (35).

Another crucial factor determining the outcome of the host antitumor response is the mixture of cytokines produced in the tumor microenvironment. Forni et al first established the importance of this factor through their studies involving the injection of recombinant cytokines into the sites of growing tumors (36). Their work demonstrated that specific molecules, especially interleukin-2 (IL-2), could alter the host-tumor balance and elicit tumor destruction through the local activation of neutrophils, eosinophils, macrophages, natural killer cells, and lymphocytes. Tumor destruction endowed the mice with protective immunity against wild-type tumor challenge. These important experiments suggested the potential of therapeutic strategies aimed at altering the cytokine profiles found in the tumor milieu.

A final item in the accounting of tumor escape relates to the ability of cancer cells to undergo apoptosis in response to immune effector mechanisms. Although mutations in p53 and other key gene products have been most thoroughly explored in the context of resistance to chemotherapy and radiation therapy (37), it is possible that these defects may be relevant to immunotherapy as well. Indeed, a mutant caspase 8 molecule, identified as a potential T-cell target in a patient with squamous cell carcinoma of the head and neck, proved to be defective in initiating the proteolytic cascade that culminates in cell death (38). Additional studies will be required to delineate whether alterations in apoptotic pathways can undermine immunotherapy in the same way as has been observed with conventional cancer treatments.

Genetically Modified Tumor Cells Enhance Antitumor Immunity

The discovery of Forni et al that the intratumoral injection of recombinant cytokines stimulated the host antitumor response (36) spearheaded a large number of experiments investigating the antitumor activities of various immunostimulatory molecules. These efforts were advanced substantially through the introduction of gene-transfer techniques, which afforded in vivo gene expression superior to that achieved with inoculation of recombinant proteins. This advantage uncovered novel properties of gene products that otherwise were not detectable with conventional modes of drug delivery.

Retroviral vectors were used most frequently in these studies because of their versatility in achieving stable, high-level gene expression without the concomitant production of replication competent virus (39). An impressive number of molecules with diverse immunologic functions were evaluated for the ability to abrogate tumorigenicity following transduction into tumor

cells (40). While several gene products manifested antitumor activities in different models, IL-12 and IL-2 emerged as the most potent molecules across the entire range of studies (41–43). The repertoire of antitumor effector cells generated in the various experiments depended on the cytokine introduced and the characteristics of the model system, which, unfortunately, still remain poorly defined. Nonetheless, CD4- and CD8-positive T lymphocytes, natural killer cells, macrophages, neutrophils, and eosinophils were all stimulated, suggesting that multiple immunologic pathways could mediate tumor inhibition. An intriguing finding, still not satisfactorily understood, was that the abrogation of tumorigenicity could be dissociated from the development of protective immunity against subsequent wild-type tumor challenge.

This puzzling observation motivated a second series of experiments testing the relative activities of engineered tumor cells to stimulate systemic antitumor immunity. To circumvent the confounding variable that many gene products failed to abrogate tumorigenicity, these studies used growth-arrested tumor cells for vaccination. Irradiation was used most frequently for this purpose; while this treatment results in G_2-cell-cycle arrest, it does not significantly inhibit transgene expression, likely because the transfected vectors are much smaller than the typical targets for double-stranded DNA breaks (44). Our own group performed a comprehensive analysis of more than thirty different gene products in this way. We found that immunization with irradiated tumor cells engineered to secrete granulocyte-macrophage colony-stimulating factor (GM-CSF) proved to be the most effective for augmenting potent, specific, and long-lasting antitumor immunity in multiple murine tumor models (45). GM-CSF based vaccinations require both CD4- and CD8-positive T lymphocyes and likely involve the improved uptake and processing of irradiated tumor cells by activated dendritic cells and macrophages recruited to the immunization site.

Two points of controversy have not yet been fully resolved in this field. The first relates to the use of live versus irradiated tumor cells for vaccination. In some model systems, live tumor cells lead to higher levels of systemic immunity than irradiated tumor cells (46). These observations are complicated, however, by Schirrmacher's finding that some live, genetically altered tumor cells are never rejected by the host following inoculation; rather, these cells enter a poorly understood state of dormancy that is tightly associated with the maintenance of long-lasting systemic immunity (47). The persistence of live tumor cells underscores a potential safety concern for application in clinical trials, but also poses an intriguing issue for further study.

A second unresolved issue involves the differences between using vaccination to treat preexisiting tumors versus to prophylax against subsequent tumor challenges. A widely held view is that preexisting treatment models more closely resemble the clinical context in which tumor vaccinations will be employed (48). In the treatment assay, IL-12 administered by a variety of techniques convincingly emerges as the most potent cytokine identified to date, eliciting substantial antitumor effects particularly in immunogenic systems (49). Investigation into the mechanisms underlying this activity thus far has delineated a complicated cascade of events; an initial inhibition of angiogenesis combined with the destruction of nascent tumor blood vessels gradually evolves into a typical Th-1 delayed-type hypersensitivity reaction (50). The early vascular targeting appears critical, as the ability of specific T-cell responses to be generated in the short interval prior to the establishment of a large tumor is limited.

Immunization with irradiated tumor cells engineered to secrete GM-CSF, in contrast to IL-12, elicits destruction of only small burdens of established tumors (45). However, as discussed below, clinical testing of vaccination with lethally irradiated, autologous, melanoma cells engineered to secrete GM-CSF surprisingly demonstrated substantial antitumor effects in patients with advanced disease (51). Extensive tumor necrosis was induced, even against large metastases, in direct contrast to the results predicted by the treatment assays in the mouse model. These findings raise the possibility that murine treatment models overestimate the kinetics of angiogenesis and have less predictive value for the clinic than generally believed.

Clinical Investigations

Several phase I clinical studies of vaccination with genetically modified tumor cells have been initiated (44). These trials involve patients with advanced disease, since the primary aim of these trials is establishing safety and toxicity. At this stage of the illness, clonal evolution operating within an environment of immunologic selection likely has given rise to the most resistant and diverse malignant cells. The immune system has been damaged as a consequence of prior treatments and heavy tumor burdens. The prospects for clinical activity in these settings are small, although it should be possible to delineate preliminary evidence of biologic activity.

One set of investigations is defining the effects of immunization with established human tumor cell lines engineered to express immunostimulatory molecules. This approach enjoys the practical advantage of ease in manufacturing and the suitability for large numbers of patients. The rationale underlying this strategy is that shared tumor antigens are attractive targets (8). Nonetheless, the potency of these targets for vaccination remains to be defined, and thus it is currently unclear whether generic cell lines will possess sufficient antigenic relevance to tumors originating de novo in patients. A pilot study of immunization with IL-2 secreting, allogeneic melanoma cells demonstrated that inflammation could be provoked at sites of distant metastases, although this did not result in tumor regression (52). Studies exploring the activities of GM-CSF and B7-1 transfected cells are under way, but have not yet been published.

A second, more demanding approach involves autologous tumor cells. The therapeutic efficacy of vaccination with irradiated colorectal cells admixed with BCG in early-stage patients (14) provides a strong foundation for testing potential improvements on this approach. In this strategy, tumor cells from individual patients are processed to single-cell suspension, introduced into short-term culture, and then genetically engineered with a variety of vectors to secrete immunostimulatory molecules.

Two small trials of vaccination with lethally irradiated, autologous melanoma cells engineered to secrete gamma-interferon have been published (53,54). Convincing evidence for the enhancement of humoral antimelanoma immunity was obtained through these studies. ELISA and RIA analyses demonstrated greater increases in the levels of IgG2a antibodies directed against melanoma cells than had been observed when BCG was used as the adjuvant. A few minor clinical responses were noted in this small group of patients.

Initial experience with immunization using irradiated, GM-CSF secreting, autologous renal-cell carcinoma cells has been presented (55). Vaccination sites revealed an influx of macrophages, dendritic cells, eosinophils, and lymphocytes, analogous to that observed in the murine systems. Following, but not before vaccination, injections of nontransfected tumor cells stimulated reactions composed of lymphocytes, eosinophils, and macrophages. One partial response of almost a year's duration was observed in a group of three patients receiving an active biologic dose of cells.

We have recently published the results of a phase I trial of 21 metastatic melanoma patients who were vaccinated with irradiated, autologous melanoma cells engineered to secrete GM-CSF (51). All patients developed impressive admixtures of dendritic cells, macrophages, eosinophils, and T lymphocytes at vaccination sites. This constellation of cells is consistent with the idea that GM-CSF functions to enhance antitumor immunity by increasing the numbers and activities of host, professional, antigen-presenting cells. Each patient also developed, as a consequence of immunization, intense infiltrates of T lymphocytes and eosinophils in response to injections of irradiated, nontransfected melanoma cells. This type of reaction could be readily distinguished from those previously observed in vaccination trials using BCG as an adjuvant (56); the quality of these reactions, moreover, suggested striking parallels to the immune responses characteristic of allergic disease or parasitic infection (57). The similarities to these conditions also extended to the development of peripheral eosinophilia, which likely reflected the induction of IL-3, IL-5, and GM-CSF by tumor-reactive T cells (51).

The most important finding of our study was that distant metastases, in 11 of 16 cases examined, were diffusely infiltrated following, but not before, vaccination with large numbers of T lymphocytes and plasma cells (51). Immunohistochemical studies showed that both CD4- and CD8-positive T cells formed rosettes around dying melanoma cells. The coordinated activation of T lymphocytes and plasma cells led to the destruction of at least 80% of the tumor cells in the infiltrated metastases. Intriguingly, the host reactions in most cases did not produce clinical regressions; rather, the tumor masses became replaced with inflammatory cells, edema, and fibrosis. In contrast to the results in the murine tumor models (45), these impressive reactions were found in well-established metastases in a variety of locations.

Several potential antitumor mechanisms were suggested through both pathologic and laboratory analysis (51). Studies of the tumor-infiltrating T lymphocytes and plasma cells indicated that lymphocyte-mediated cytotoxicity, cytokine production, and antibody formation could mediate tumor destruction. A provocative finding, not predicted by the murine studies, was the targeted destruction of the tumor vasculature; damaged endothelium was infiltrated with lymphocytes admixed with degranulating eosinophils and neutrophils. It is possible that tumor-reactive T cells initially recognize tumor antigens presented by endothelial cells and then secrete cytokines, which leads to the secondary recruitment and activation of eosinophils.

Conclusions

The landmark study of Pinedo and colleagues has established that autologous tumor cell–based vaccines can lead to important improvements in clinical outcome (14). This finding provides a strong rationale for evaluating many other cancer-vaccination schemes. Since most new therapies will initially be evaluated in the patient population with advanced disease, investigators will need to provide convincing evidence of biologic activity in these early studies to identify those strategies most appropriate for further clinical development within large, randomized trials. A combination of pathologic analysis and in vitro antitumor T-cell and humoral assays should render it possible to discriminate among the myriad approaches entering the clinic that include, in addition to genetically modified tumor cells, peptide immunizations, dendritic cell–based schemes, and naked DNA injections. Few vaccination strategies will overcome all of the substantive obstacles confronting large-scale clinical testing. It seems likely, however, that the next generation of cancer therapeutics will prominently showcase cancer vaccines.

References

1. Nauts H, Fowler G, Bogatko F. A review of the influence of bacterial infection and of bacterial products (Coley's toxins) on malignant tumors in man. Acta Med Scand 1953:5–103.
2. Gorer PA. The antigenic basis of tumor transplantation. J Pathol Bacteriol 1938;47:231–252.
3. Klein G, Sjogren HO, Klein E, Hellstrom KE. Demonstration of resistance against methylcholanthrene-induced sarcomas in the primary autochthonous host. Cancer Res 1960; 20:1561–1572.
4. Hewitt HB, Blake ER, Walder AS. A critique of the evidence for active host defense against cancer based on personal studies of 27 murine tumors of spontaneous origin. Br J Cancer 1976;33:241–259.
5. Van Pel A, Vessiere F, Boon T. Protection against two spontaneous mouse leukemias conferred by immunogenic variants obtained by mutagenesis. J Exp Med 1983;157:1992 –2001.
6. Scott O. Tumor transplantation and tumor immunity: a personal view. Cancer Res 1991;51:757–763.
7. Old L, Chen Y-T. New paths in human cancer serology. J Exp Med 1998;187:1163–1167.
8. Boon T, van der Bruggen P. Human tumor antigens recognized by T lymphocytes. J Exp Med 1996;183:725–729.

9. Marchand M, Weynants P, Rankin E, et al. Tumor regression responses in melanoma patients treated with a peptide encoded by gene MAGE-3. Int J Cancer 1995;63:883–885.
10. Marchand M, van Baren N, Weynants P, et al. Tumor regressions observed in patients with metastatic melanoma treated with an antigenic peptide encoded by gene MAGE-3 and presented by HLA-A1. Int J Cancer 1999;80:219–230.
11. Rosenberg S, Yang J, Schwartzentruber D, et al. Immunologic and therapeutic evaluation of a synthetic peptide vaccine for the treatment of patients with metastatic melanoma. Nat Med 1998;4:321–327.
12. Brandle D, Bilsborough J, Rulicke T, et al. The shared tumor-specific antigen encoded by mouse gene P1A is a target not only for cytolytic T lymphocytes but also for tumor rejection. Eur J Immunol 1998;28:4010–4019.
13. Ikeda H, Ohta N, Furukawa K, et al. Mutated mitogen-activated protein kinase: a tumor rejection antigen of mouse sarcoma. Proc Natl Acad Sci USA 1997;94:6375–6379.
14. Vermorken J, Claessen A, van Tinteren H, et al. Active specific immunotherapy for stage II and stage III human colon cancer: a randomised trial. Lancet 1999;353:345–350.
15. Old L, Clarke D, Benacerraf B. Effect of bacillus Calmette-Guerin (BCG) infection on transplanted tumors in the mouse. Nature 1959;184:291–292.
16. Livingston P, Wong G, Adluri S, et al. Improved survival in stage III melanoma patients with GM2 antibodies: a randomized trial of adjuvant vaccination with GM2 ganglioside. J Clin Oncol 1994;12:1036–1044.
17. Townsend A, Bodmer H. Antigen recognition by class I–restricted T-lymphocytes. Annu Rev Immunol 1989; 7:601–624.
18. Cox A, Skipper J, Chen Y, et al. Identification of a peptide recognized by five melanoma-specific human cytotoxic T-cell lines. Science 1994;264:716–719.
19. Sahin U, Tureci O, Schmitt H, et al. Human neoplasms elicit multiple specific immune responses in the autologous host. Proc Natl Acad Sci USA 1995;92:11810–11813.
20. Chen Y-T, Scanlan M, Sahin U, et al. A testicular antigen aberrantly expressed in human cancers detected by autologous antibody screening. Proc Natl Acad Sci USA 1997;94:1914–1918.
21. Jager E, Chen Y-T, Drijfhout J, et al. Simultaneous humoral and cellular immune response against cancer-testis antigen NY-ESO-1: definition of human histocompatibility leukocyte antigen (HLA)-A2–binding peptide epitopes. J Exp Med 1998;187:265–270.
22. Scanlan M, Chen Y-T, Williamson B, et al. Characterization of human colon cancer antigens recognized by autologous antibodies. Int J Cancer 1998;76:652–658.
23. Houghton A. Cancer antigens: immune recognition of self and altered self. J Exp Med 1994;180:1–4.
24. Clark W, From L, Bernardino E, Mihm M. The histogenesis and biologic behavior of primary human malignant melanomas of the skin. Cancer Res 1969;29:705–726.
25. Clark W, Elder D, Guerry D, et al. Model predicting survival in stage I melanoma based on tumor progression. J Natl Cancer Inst 1989;81:1893–1904.
26. Clemente C, Mihm M, Bufalino R, et al. Prognostic value of tumor infiltrating lymphocytes in the vertical growth phase of primary cutaneous melanoma. Cancer 1996;77: 1303–1310.

27. Mihm M, Clemente C, Cascinelli N. Tumor infiltrating lymphocytes in lymph node melanoma metastases—a histopathologic prognostic indicator and an expression of local immune response. Lab Invest 1996;74:43–47.
28. Naito Y, Saito K, Shiiba K, et al. CD8+ T cells infiltrated within cancer cell nests as a prognostic factor in human colorectal cancer. Cancer Res 1998;58:3491–3494.
29. Papadopoulos EB, Ladanyi M, Emanuel D, et al. Infusions of donor leukocytes to treat Epstein-Barr virus–associated lymphoproliferative disorders after allogeneic bone marrow transplantation. N Engl J Med 1994;330:1185–1191.
30. Hicklin D, Wang Z, Arienti F, et al. Beta2-microglobulin mutations, HLA class I antigen loss, and tumor progression in melanoma. J Clin Invest 1998;101:2720–2729.
31. Jager E, Ringhoffer M, Altmannsberger M, et al. Immuno-selection in vivo: independent loss of MHC class I and melanocyte differentiation antigen expression in metastatic melanoma. Int J Cancer 1997;71:142–147.
32. Theobald M, Ruppert T, Kuckelkorn U, et al. The sequence alteration associated with a mutational hotspot in p53 protects cells from lysis by cytotoxic T lymphocytes specific for a flanking peptide epitope. J Exp Med 1998;188:1017–1028.
33. Bancereau J, Steinman R. Dendritic cells and the control of immunity. Nature 1998;392:245–252.
34. Guinan E, Gribben J, Boussiotis V, et al. Pivotal role of the B7:CD28 pathway in transplantation tolerance and tumor immunity. Blood 1994;84:3261–3282.
35. Zajac A, Blattman J, Murali-Krishna K, et al. Viral immune evasion due to persistence of activated T cells without effector function. J Exp Med 1998;188:2205–2213.
36. Forni G, Fujiwara H, Martino F, et al. Helper strategy in tumor immunology: expansion of helper lymphocytes and utilization of helper lymphokines for experimental and clinical immunotherapy. Cancer Metastasis Rev 1988;7:289–309.
37. Lowe SW, Ruley HE, Jacks T, Housman DE. p53-dependent apoptosis modulates the cytotoxicity of anticancer agents. Cell 1993;74:957–967.
38. Mandruzzato S, Brasseur F, Andry G, et al. A CASP-8 mutation recognized by cytolytic T lymphocytes on a human head and neck carcinoma. J Exp Med 1997;186:785–793.
39. Mulligan RC. The basic science of gene therapy. Science 1993;260:926–932.
40. Dranoff G, Mulligan RC. Gene transfer as cancer therapy. Adv Immunol 1995;58:417–454.
41. Fearon ER, Pardoll DM, Itaya T, et al. Interleukin-2 production by tumor cells bypasses T helper function in the generation of an antitumor response. Cell 1990;60:397–403.
42. Gansbacher B, Zier K, Daniels B, et al. Interleukin-2 gene transfer into tumor cells abrogates tumorigenicity and induces protective immunity. J Exp Med 1990;172:1217–1224.
43. Tahara H, Zeh HJ, Storkus WJ, et al. Fibroblasts genetically engineered to secrete interleukin-12 can suppress tumor growth and induce antitumor immunity to a murine melanoma in vivo. Cancer Res 1994;54:182–189.
44. Dranoff G. Cancer gene therapy: connecting basic research with clinical inquiry. J Clin Oncol 1998;16:2548–2556.
45. Dranoff G, Jaffee E, Lazenby A, et al. Vaccination with irradiated tumor cells engineered to secrete murine granulocyte-macrophage colony-stimulating factor stimulates potent, specific, and long-lasting anti-tumor immunity. Proc Natl Acad Sci USA 1993;90:3539–3543.
46. Allione A, Consalvo M, Nanni P, et al. Immunizing and curative potential of replicating and nonreplicating murine mammary adenocarcinoma cells engineered with interleukin (IL)-2, IL-4, IL-6, IL-7, IL-10, tumor necrosis factor α, granulocyte-macrophage colony-stimulating factor, and γ-interferon gene or admixed with conventional adjuvants. Cancer Res 1994;54:6022–6026.
47. Khazaie K, Prifti S, Beckhove P, et al. Persistence of dormant tumor cells in the bone marrow of tumor cell–vaccinated mice correlates with long-term immunological protection. Proc Natl Acad Sci USA 1994;91:7430–7434.
48. Tepper RI, Mule JJ. Experimental and clinical studies of cytokine gene-modified tumor cells. Hum Gene Ther 1994;5:153–164.
49. Brunda MJ, Luistro L, Warrier RR, et al. Antitumor and antimetastatic activity of interleukin-12 against murine tumors. J Exp Med 1993;178:1223–1230.
50. Cavallo F, Di Carlo E, Butera M, et al. Immune events associated with the cure of established tumors and spontaneous metastases by local and systemic interleukin-12. Cancer Res 1999;59:414–421.
51. Soiffer R, Lynch T, Mihm M, et al. Vaccination with irradiated, autologous melanoma cells engineered to secrete human granulocyte-macrophage colony stimulating factor generates potent anti-tumor immunity in patients with metastatic melanoma. Proc Natl Acad Sci USA 1998;95:13141–13146.
52. Belli F, Arienti F, Sule-Suso J, et al. Active immunization of metastatic melanoma patients with interleukin-2–transduced allogeneic melanoma cells: evaluation of efficacy and tolerability. Cancer Immunol Immunother 1997;44:197–203.
53. Abdel-Wahab Z, Weltz C, Hester D, et al. A phase I clinical trial of immunotherapy with interferon-γ gene-modified autologous melanoma cells. Cancer 1997;80:401–412.
54. Nemunaitis J, Bohart C, Fing T, et al. Phase I trial of retroviral vector-mediated interferon (IFN)-gamma gene transfer into autologous tumor cells in patients with metastatic melanoma. Cancer Gene Ther 1998;5:292–300.
55. Simons JW, Jaffee EM, Weber CE, et al. Bioactivity of autologous irradiated renal cell carcinoma vaccines generated by ex vivo granulocyte-macrophage colony-stimulating factor gene transfer. Cancer Res 1997;57:1537–1546.
56. Barth A, Hoon DSB, Foshag LJ, et al. Polyvalent melanoma cell vaccine induces delayed-type hypersensitivity and in vitro cellular immune response. Cancer Res 1994;54:3342–3345.
57. Gleich GJ, Adolphson CR. The eosinophilic leukocyte: structure and function. Adv Immunol 1986;39:177–253.

Chapter 43

Gene Therapy for Inherited Immunodeficiencies

Fabio Candotti
R. Michael Blaese

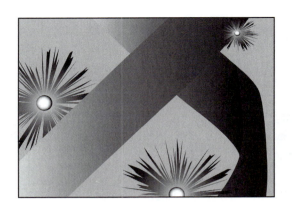

The idea of correcting human diseases at the molecular level, as opposed to merely treating the clinical manifestations originating from genetic aberrations, is extremely attractive for obvious reasons. Genetic correction of somatic cells is therefore often considered the ultimate form of therapy. In the last 10 to 15 years we have witnessed the evolution of gene therapy from its theoretic inception to early clinical trials. During this period the potential applications of this new branch of medicine have broadened. Besides representing a revolutionary new form of treatment for inherited disorders, clinical gene transfer is now commonly exploited for therapeutic approaches to a variety of non-inherited diseases such as cancer and HIV infection.

In September 1990 a clinical gene-therapy protocol based on the repeated infusions of gene-corrected, autologous T lymphocytes (1) was launched at the National Institutes of Health for the treatment of children affected by severe combined immunodeficiency (SCID) caused by deficit of adenosine deaminase (ADA). The two children affected with ADA-SCID in this protocol were the first to be treated by gene therapy, just as a patient with X-linked SCID was the first to be successfully treated by allogeneic bone-marrow transplantation 2 decades earlier (2).

In the last decade, progress in molecular medicine has led to the identification of molecular defects underlying a wide variety of inherited immunodeficiency diseases (IDDs), thus opening the way to new possibilities for genetic intervention. Since most IDDs that are curable by allogeneic bone-marrow transplantation (BMT) are also good candidates for gene therapy, several investigators have become attracted by the possibility of developing corrective gene-transfer approaches as potential alternative therapies for these disorders.

Although this wide interest has generated important preclinical data, the current clinical experience with gene therapy for IDDs is certainly limited. As of June 1999, almost 300 clinical gene-transfer protocols were approved in the United States, Europe, China, and Japan, and several hundred individuals have received genetically modified cells (3). These numbers clearly show the logarithmic growth and the evolution of the gene-therapy field since 1990. However, as few as 10 of these clinical protocols involve strategies for gene therapy of IDDs, and data on only 11 ADA-SCID patients (4–9) and eight subjects affected with chronic granulomatous disease (10,11) treated by gene therapy have been published to date (Table 43-1).

As is the case with other genetic diseases, developing gene-therapy strategies for IDDs involves a series of critical considerations (Table 43-2). Extensive knowledge of the genomic characteristics, physiologic regulation, and pattern of expression of the gene of interest is of central importance. Several genes identified as responsible for IDDs have expression restricted to specific lymphoid or hematopoietic elements or particular stages of cell differentiation (e.g., BTK, CD40L, and RAG1-2). The use of first-generation gene transfer vectors carrying transgenes under the transcriptional control of strong viral promoters routinely results in unregulated expression of the transferred gene in the transduced cells and their progeny. Unregulated transgene expression means that, if a multipotent stem cell were successfully gene modified, transgene expression might be expected in all lineages derived from such stem cell. Such constitutive "ectopic" expression of the transgene could have undesirable or detrimental consequences on the differentiation and/or function of targeted populations. Theoretically, the use of gene-specific promoter and/or enhancer elements could be exploited to obtain regulated expression of the therapeutic gene, or, alternatively, inducible or repressible systems could also be used to achieve some control of transgene expression.

The possibility of adverse effects resulting from the gene-transfer procedure must be seriously considered and tested for in laboratory and animal models. Unfortunately, animal models are not always adequate for many important human diseases, including IDDs, and often results obtained in animals are not indicative of responses in human applications. Nevertheless, the study of safety and efficacy of gene-therapy strategies in animal models of human disease remains of critical importance. It is also critical to verify that transfer and expression of the gene of interest can result in adequate correction of the biologic defects characteristic of the disease. This is especially important in those cases where the mutations do not result in complete lack of the encoded proteins ("null" mutations) but where residual levels of mutated gene products can be detected. In these situations, the mutated molecules can potentially manifest dominant-negative effects against the transduced, normal proteins, and it is important to establish what levels of expression of the transgene need to be achieved to obtain phenotypic correction. Finally and importantly, the possibilities of success of experimental gene-therapy approaches for any specific IDDs should be always weighed

Table 43-1. Gene Therapy Clinical Trials for Inherited Immune Disorders

Disease	Investigators	Vector	Target Cells	No. Patients	References
ADA-SCID	R.M. Blaese	LASN	T lymphocytes	2	(6)
ADA-SCID	C. Bordignon	DCA*l* DCA*m*	T lymphocytes BM cells	2*	(5)
ADA-SCID	D.B. Kohn	LASN	CB CD34+ cells	3	(4, 9)
ADA-SCID	A. Fischer R.J. Lewinsky D. Valerio	LgAL(Δmo + PyF101)	BM cells	3	(7)
ADA-SCID	Y. Sakiyama	LASN	T lymphocytes	1	(8, 57)
CGD (p47phox)	H.M. Malech	MFGS p47phox	PB CD34+ cells	5	(10)
X-CGD (gp91phox)	H.M. Malech	MFGS gp91phox	PB CD34+ cells	3	(11)

*Three additional patients have been treated for whom no data are yet available.
BM, bone marrow; PB, peripheral blood.

Table 43-2. Issues for Gene Therapy of Inherited Immune Disorders

- Knowledge of molecular and functional characteristics of the gene of interest
- Efficacy of gene transfer to reverse aberrant phenotype
- Long-term gene expression
- Effective gene transfer into hematopoietic stem cell
- Effects of constitutive/unregulated gene expression
- Safety and efficacy studies in animal models
- Efficacy of established therapies

against the record of success and efficacy of established alternative therapies.

Methods and Tools for Gene Therapy of Immunodeficiency Diseases

In general, current gene therapy strategies for the treatment of genetic diseases are based on the reconstitution of the function(s) of the mutated gene by providing the patient's cells or tissues with a copy of the normal gene. Such "gene addition" strategies are technically much easier than other possible approaches aiming at the substitution of the defective gene with a functional one ("gene replacement"). The very low efficiency with which homologous recombination would occur between the mutated gene and the normal sequence has been thus far the major obstacle to the development and clinical application of gene-replacement strategies. In the case of IDDs, integrating gene-transfer systems are probably indispensable for efficient gene therapy since, by promoting stable integration of the exogenous genetic material into the host cell genome, they ensure transmission of the transferred gene to the progeny of that cell during normal cell division. Cells of the immune system are often very actively replicating, and, in the absence of integration, the transferred gene may be diluted out as the cell divides and the therapeutic effects would consequently be lost. Moreover, for efficient gene therapy of the immune system, the ultimate goal is the integration of the therapeutic gene of interest into the self-renewing, hematopoietic stem cell (HSC). This would provide a limitless supply of genetically corrected cells capable of continually replacing senescent or dying "affected" populations.

Among the variety of systems developed for gene transfer into mammalian cells, vectors based on retroviruses and adeno-associated viruses (AAV) allow stable integration of the transduced gene and have now been tested in clinical applications. Recently, great interest has been devoted to a new generation of gene transfer vectors based on lentiviruses, largely because of their ability to integrate into quiescent cells. Finally, hybrid viral systems have recently been developed that combine advantages of different vectors and try to eliminate the respective pitfalls. Among those worth mentioning are AAV-HSV vector system based on AAV- and herpes simplex virus–derived components (12) and a more recent "adeno-retro" gene-transfer strategy using adenoviral constructs able to convert transduced cells in retroviral producer cells in vivo (13).

Regardless the gene transfer system used to obtain integration of the therapeutic gene of interest, "gene addition" strategies are far from perfect, as the random integration of the transduced gene and the control of its expression by constitutive viral or mammalian promoters make the therapeutic gene totally evicted from physiologic cellular control.

Very recently, a novel technique has been developed that could be of great importance for the direct correction of genetic defects ("gene repair") without the need for substituting the whole mutated gene. By using chimeric oligonucleotides composed of DNA and modified RNA residues, Allyson Cole-Strauss and coworkers were able to correct with high efficiency the specific mutation in the hemoglobin β_s allele of EBV-immortalized B-cell lines, thus providing the basis for gene correction of sickle cell anemia (14). The results of this first report were confirmed by other studies describing the efficient introduction of single-nucleotide mutation in the alkaline phosphatase gene of human hepatoma cells "in vitro" (15) and in the factor IX gene of intact liver tissue in an "in vivo" rat model (16). The use of DNA-RNA chimeric oligonucleotides for gene therapy would have the disadvantage of requiring the construction of chimeric molecules specific for each patient's mutation, but would also grant the extraordinary advantage of providing the correction of the mutated gene "in situ" and therefore within physiologic transcriptional control. Furthermore, it is possible that such a strategy would allow the initiation of gene therapy studies for disorders where the mutated gene has been identified, but its specific function(s) and the mechanisms controlling its expression are still unclear (e.g., X-linked agammaglobulinemia and Wiskott-Aldrich syndrome).

Retroviral Vectors

Reproducing the replication and integration mechanisms of retroviruses, retroviral vectors (Fig. 43-1) are the most commonly used gene transfer system in human gene therapy (3). Most of these vectors are based on the genome structure of murine retroviruses such as the Moloney murine leukemia virus (MoMLV). These retroviruses are rendered incapable of replicating by deleting the genes encoding for critical viral proteins (reverse transcriptase, integrase, structural proteins of the capsid and the envelope) and by replacing them with selectable markers and/or cloning sites for the insertion of therapeutic genes. The expression of the gene of interest may be driven by the MoMLV long terminal repeat (LTR) promoter or other murine retroviral LTRs such as those from the myeloproliferative sarcoma virus (MPSV) or the murine stem-cell virus (MSCV) LTRs. Other strong viral (e.g., cytomegalovirus) or mammalian (e.g., phosphoglycerate kinase) promoters are also often used.

"Packaging" cell lines that express the retroviral *gag*, *pol*, and *env* genes products are then used to obtain preparations of these "crippled" viral particles to be used to infect (or "transduce") target-cell populations. The ability of a retroviral vector to infect a specific target cell depends on the characteristics of the envelope protein. Ecotropic retroviruses are only able to infect mouse- and rat-derived cells, whereas amphotropic vectors can transduce a broader range of cell types, including monkey and human (17). Furthermore, retroviral particles can be obtained that contain the gibbon-ape leukemia virus (GALV) envelope protein (18), thus allowing their binding to the GALV receptor, Pit-1, on the cell membrane. The levels of expression of Pit-1 are higher in some cell types such as hematopoietic cells and progenitors than the amphotropic receptor Pit-2 and can be metabolically up-regulated (19), making GALV-expressing packaging cells an attractive tool for gene transfer into hematopoietic elements or stem cells. Envelopes derived from the cat endogenous virus have also been shown to target hematopoietic cells. In addition, retroviral particles resistant to the lytic effects of human serum can be obtained by using packaging lines derived from human rather than murine cells (20).

Retroviral vectors with a broad host range have also been obtained by incorporating of the vesicular-stomatitis virus envelope G-protein (VSV-G) into the virions of MoMLV-derived vectors. The viral particles containing the VSV-G have the advantage of withstanding centrifugation procedures that permit the concentration of the viral supernatants and obtain higher-titer retroviral preparations.

Recently, retroviral vectors have been successfully directed to specific cell targets by incorporating into the viral envelope moieties able to specifically recognize certain membrane receptors. The first example demonstrating that such specific targeting was possible came from the elegant experiments of Kasahara et al who, using retroviral vectors engineered to express the polypeptide hormone erythropoietin as part of their envelope, were able to efficiently and specifically transduce cells expressing the erythropoietin receptor (21). The ability to specifically direct gene transfer vectors to the appropriate target cells could find several applications in treating disorders of the immune system.

The major advantage of using retroviral vectors for gene therapy is that these vectors promise efficient and stable integration of the transgene in the target-cell population, an essential feature for long-term correction of genetic defects. However, this class of vectors will only deliver genes to cells that are actively dividing. This is the major limitation of using retroviral vectors for stem cell gene therapy of IDDs since the "true" hematopoietic progenitor is mostly in the quiescent G0/G1 phase of the cellular cycle, thus being refractory to integration of the proviral genome. Extensive experience in murine models has clearly shown that retrovirus-mediated gene transfer into marrow stem cells is achievable. However, data from experiments conducted in dogs and nonhuman primates and the early protocols in humans (4,5,7,9,10,22) have shown that retrovirus-mediated gene transfer into the HSC is still inefficient and must clearly be improved before gene therapy involving these cells will be routinely successful.

Other disadvantages of the retrovirus-based technology include the following: 1) the limited amount of genetic material that they can accommodate (only ~8 Kb), which prevents the transfer of large genomic sequences; 2) the problem of the random integration of the proviral genome that, on the one hand, is responsible for the high variability of gene expression often observed in different cell clones and that, on the other, may theoretically lead to insertional mutagenesis; and 3) the high cost of production of clinical-grade retroviral supernatants. It is, however, worth noting that cDNAs encoding for most genes can be easily inserted in retroviral vector cassettes and that the "position effect" may not constitute a problem for those genes that operate without tightly regulated ranges of expression. Finally, the use of replication incompetent vectors minimizes the potential risk of oncogenesis resulting from the use of these vectors.

Adeno-Associated Viral Vectors

Genetic vectors based on adeno-associated virus (AAV) have become appealing tools for gene transfer mostly because of the

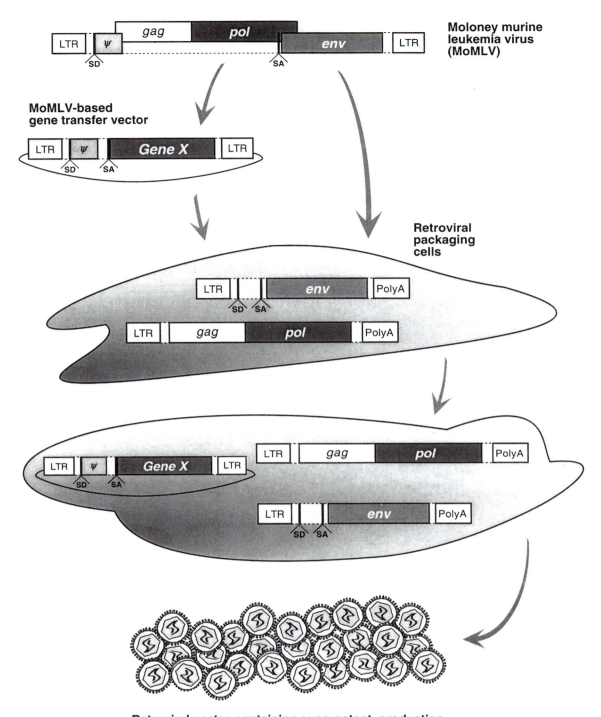

Retroviral vector-containing supernatant production

Figure 43-1. Generation of recombinant retroviral vectors. Retroviral vector cassettes are generated by removing the *gag, pol,* and *env* coding regions from the retroviral genome and replacing them with the gene of interest. In simple constructs, the viral long-terminal repeat (LTR) drives expression of a single transgene. The packaging signal sequence (ψ) is necessary to allow encapsidation of the recombinant genome into complete virions. Splice donor (SD) and acceptor (SA) sites may also be conserved to mimic the wild-type virus transcriptional mechanisms and improve gene expression. Portions of the murine retroviral genome are used to produce "packaging" cell lines, stably expressing the viral *gag, pol,* and *env* genes and thus providing the necessary structural proteins and enzymes to produce complete, infectious viral particles. Retroviral constructs are then transfected into packaging cells and are packaged into complete virions that can be collected with the culture supernatants.

nonpathogenic nature of the wild-type AAVs (23) and their ability to transfer and express genes in nondividing cells (24). This last characteristic makes them particularly attractive for gene transfer into the HSC (25,26).

AAV-based vectors (Fig. 43-2) are produced by deleting the *rep* and *cap* genes from the human AAV serotype 2 DNA and replacing them with the transcriptional unit (promoter + experimental gene) of interest (27). The production of complete recombinant AAV particles is then obtained by cotransfection of cells infected with a helper virus (adenovirus or herpes simplex virus), with the cassette containing the therapeutic gene ("vector") and a "helper" plasmid providing in *trans* the expression of *rep* and *cap* genes, which encode for a series of peptides necessary for viral DNA replication and AAV encapsidation. This transient expression system does not allow a long-term production of recombinant AAV vectors, nor the generation of viral stocks with standardized, reproducible characteristics and makes scale-up procedures cumbersome. In addition, AAV-vector stocks produced by this cotransfection strategy are contaminated with helper virus and often also with wild-type AAV generated by recombination between the "vector" and "helper" plasmids. A series of modifications are being developed to address these problems, which include the construction of replication-deficient "helper" viruses (28) and the generation of AAV vector packaging cell lines, stably expressing the *rep* and *cap* genes and thus reducing the risk of recombination events arising during the transfection procedures (29–33).

In infected cells, AAV vectors may either persist in an episomal stage or integrate in the host-cell genome. In contrast with the characteristics of wild-type AAV infections, integration of AAV-based vectors seems to take place only at very high multiplicities of infection and is not specifically directed to chromosome 19. Among the disadvantages of using AAV-based vectors is their limited capacity for foreign DNA, since they cannot accommodate segments above 4.7 kb in length.

AAV vectors have been demonstrated to infect hematopoietic tissues and have been tested in preclinical studies for the treatment of hemoglobinopathies. In addition, preliminary results on the use of AAV-based vectors for the treatment of congenital hematologic defects such as chronic granulomatous disease and Fanconi's anemia have shown that the expression of the genes responsible for these diseases can be successfully restored in B-cell lines and CD34+ progenitors (34–36). AAV vector–mediated gene expression, however, can occur in the absence of integration (37), and further studies demonstrating the persistence of gene expression obtained in these trials will be important to determine the real potential of AAV-based gene transfer into the HSC.

Similar to retroviral vectors, AAV vectors capable of targeting specific cell types have been generated. Of particular interest for the potential application to the field of gene therapy for IDDs is the recent work by Yang et al who have included chimeric anti-CD34, single-chain, antibody-AAV capsid proteins within an AAV virion. The use of this engineered vector significantly increased infectivity of the CD34+ cell, which is normally refractory to AAV transduction (38).

Lentiviral Vectors

As already mentioned, one of the central obstacles to effective gene transfer into the HSCs is the quiescent G0/G1 status of these cells that makes them refractory to integrating gene-transfer systems like retroviral vectors. For integrating of retroviral sequences in the genome of the host cell, dissolution of the nuclear envelope that occurs during mitosis appears to be necessary. The replicative cycle of lentiviruses, on the other hand, is independent of cell division, and for this reason gene transfer vectors based on this distinct group of retroviruses have recently attracted the interest of investigators in the field of gene therapy (Fig. 43-3).

The genome of human immunodeficiency virus type 1 (HIV-1) is more complex than that of other retroviruses in that, in addition of the structural *gag*, *pol*, and *env* genes, it also contains two regulatory genes (*tat* and *rev*) and four additional transcripts (*vif*, *vpr*, *vpu*, and *nef*) that encode for accessory proteins critical for viral replication and pathogenesis. The HIV-1 LTR contains *cis*-acting sequences necessary for transcription, polyadenylation, and integration. A major splice donor site is located downstream of the 5' LTR and is followed by a not yet fully characterized packaging signal sequence (ψ) that, similar to other retroviruses, extends into the *gag* coding region. The core proteins are encoded by this gene, whereas virion-associated enzymes (such as reverse transcriptase and integrase) originate from transcription of the *pol* region. Finally, the *env* gene encodes for the envelope glycoprotein. On infection, Nef is required for viral capsid disassembly, whereas the *gag*-encoded protein MA, the integrase, and Vpr (all containing nuclear localization signals) form a stable preintegration complex and mediate its transport through the intact nuclear membrane. After reverse transcription and integration, the HIV-1 LTR has only weak basal transcription activity that results in accumulation of small quantities of Tat, Rev, and Nef proteins. Tat is a strong transcriptional *trans*-activator of HIV gene expression that operates by binding to the TAR (Tat activation response) element localized downstream of the transcription initiation site of the viral mRNA. The increase in transcription mediated by Tat leads to amplification of Rev expression, which promotes transport of unspliced viral mRNAs from the nucleus to the cytoplasm by binding to a Rev response element (RRE) found in the *env* gene. This is a critical step for the HIV replication cycle as it allows production of viral structural and late proteins and generation of new viral particles. Vif is important during virion assembly to promote infectivity of viral particles in subsequent early steps of viral infection, while Vpu has been shown to enhance the release of budding viral particles from infected cells.

A number of gene-transfer systems based on HIV-1, HIV-2, and other lentiviruses (equine infectious anemia virus—EIAV, feline immunodeficiency virus—FIV) have been described (39–45). Naldini et al were the first to describe an HIV-1–based gene transfer system where replication defective viral particles were pseudotyped by the use of heterologous envelope proteins such as the Moloney leukemia virus amphotropic envelope or the vesicular-stomatitis virus G-protein (39), thus broadening the

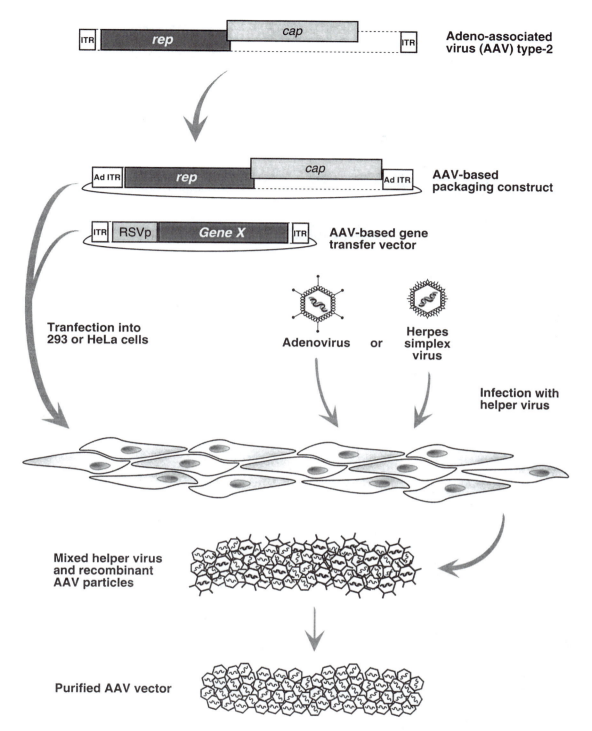

Figure 43-2. Generation of recombinant AAV vectors. The two-plasmid, "helper-vector" system for generation of an AAV-based, gene transfer vector uses a "helper" construct containing the viral *rep* and *cap* genes inserted between two copies of the adenoviral inverted-terminal repeats (Ad ITR) and a gene transfer "vector" where the AAV encoding sequences have been replaced by a transcriptional unit (in this case driven by the respiratory sincytial virus promoter [RSVp]) expressing the gene of interest. These two constructs are transfected into human cells (usually embryonic kidney 293 cells or cervical carcinoma HeLa cells). To obtain productive AAV replication, cells are then infected with adenovirus or herpes simplex virus. A progeny of recombinant AAV vectors is thus produced and can be purified from cell lysates. The original system depicted here is difficult to scale up for clinical use and leads to viral stocks contaminated with adenovirus (or herpes virus), as well as wild-type AAV deriving from recombination between the "helper" and "vector" constructs. More recent systems use "packaging" cells carrying the *rep* and *cap* genes that are stably integrated (and thus less prone to recombination) and modified adenoviral or herpes constructs that are able to provide the necessary function for productive AAV replication, but are unable to produce infectious viral particles. These improved systems are more adaptable to scale-up procedures and should provide better-defined viral stocks suitable for clinical use.

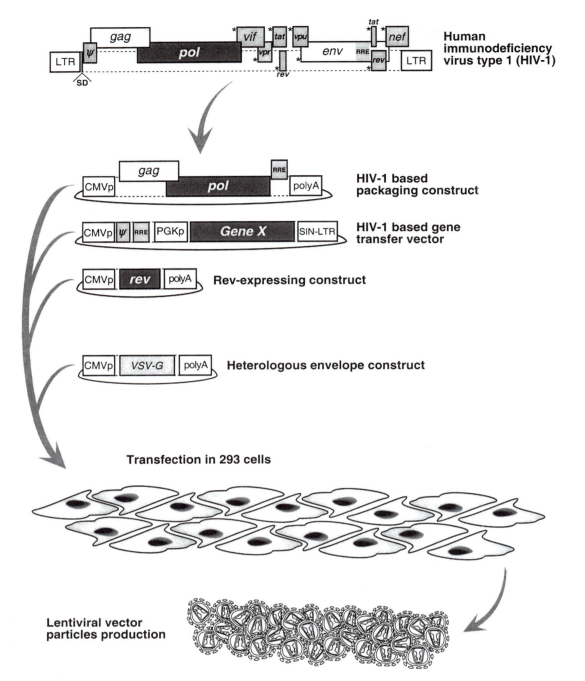

Figure 43-3. Generation of recombinant lentiviral vectors. Several systems are being used to produce HIV-based vectors for preclinical studies. The majority of them use transfection of the different lentiviral components into embryonic kidney 293 cells. The schematic representation reported here has been modified from Dull et al (53). Driven by a strong viral promoter (i.e., cytomegalovirus promoter [CMVp]), the *gag* and *pol* genes are expressed by using a construct that also contains the *rev*-responsive element (RRE), which allows *rev*-mediated transport of the respective transcripts from the nucleus to the cytoplasm. The use of the CMVp instead of the HIV LTR eliminates the need for the presence of *tat*. Preliminary experiments indicate that the accessory genes can also be omitted without severely affecting the transduction capabilities of lentiviral vectors. The HIV-based gene transfer vector also carries the RRE, in addition to the trancriptional unit expressing the gene of interest under the control of an internal promoter such as the phosphoglycerate kinase promoter (PGKp). A series of modifications are exploited in this system to reduce the possibility that, by recombination between the packaging construct and the gene-transfer vector, replication competent viruses can be generated during the transfection procedures. First, the 3′ HIV LTR can be inactivated by deletions in the U3 region (52,54). During retrotranscription and integration events, the inactivating deletion LTR is copied at the 5′ of the integrated proviral genome, which now lacks functioning terminal repeats. Constructs using these modified LTRs are called self-inactivating (SIN). In addition, the *rev* sequence can be expressed by an independent plasmid, thus introducing the need for a further recombination event to provide the originating virus with this critical gene. Finally, the HIV envelope is substituted with a heterologous, and independently expressed, envelope protein (i.e., vesicular stomatitis virus G-protein [VSV-G]), which broadens the host range of the recombinant vector particles, making the HIV-based vector usable for gene transfer into a wide variety of target cells. Similarly to retroviral vectors, recombinant lentiviral particles can be collected with the culture supernatant. When VSV-G is used as the envelope protein, supernatants can then be concentrated by centrifugation.

tropism of the vector and opening the way to a wide variety of different applications. In recent years, several groups have demonstrated that lentiviral vectors can efficiently transduce nondividing cells (41,43,45–51). These lentiviral vectors therefore could represent very useful tools for gene therapy of diseases affecting tissues and/or organs composed of quiescent or post-mitotic cells such as the central nervous system, liver, muscle, and lymphohematopoietic system. The application of lentiviral vectors in clinical practice, however, raises relevant biosafety concerns, especially in the case of the HIV-1–based constructs that are derived from a highly pathogenic human virus. The major issue resides with the possibility that recombinants could be generated during the vector production step with the consequent exposure of the recipient to the risk of infection by an "HIV-like" agent. In addition, in patients treated with HIV-1–based vectors, the possibility exists that, on subsequent exposure to wild-type HIV-1 and recombination events, the vector and the therapeutic gene could be "mobilized" and spread to unwanted targets. Through the generation of systems using nonoverlapping, split-genome, packaging constructs and self-inactivating vector cassettes, these risks have been greatly reduced (52–54). The lack of suitable animal models for HIV-1 infection, however, makes it difficult to test these improved systems in laboratory animals before their application in clinical trials. For these reasons, vectors based on HIV-2 (41,42), testable in nonhuman primates, or nonhuman pathogenic lentiviruses such as EIAV (44) or FIV (43) may provide a more acceptable alternative. However, our knowledge of the biology of these viruses is definitely less extensive than that of HIV-1, and the potential effects of the introduction in the human species of recombinant viruses arising from HIV-2 or nonprimate lentiviruses remain unpredictable.

Early and Current Clinical Trials

Adenosine Deaminase Deficiency

Adenosine deaminase (ADA) deficiency leads to one of most severe disorders of immunity characterized by virtual absence of circulating T and B lymphocytes and consequent lack of both cellular and humoral responses. Similar to what is observed in other forms of severe combined immunodeficiency (SCID), this disease results in extreme susceptibility to recurrent and life-threatening infections, failure to thrive, and death early in life. ADA deficiency accounts for 25% to 30% of all SCIDs and can be cured by allogeneic bone-marrow transplantation (BMT). In the absence of suitable bone-marrow donors, enzyme replacement therapy with bovine ADA conjugated to polyethylene glycol (PEG-ADA) (55) represents a life-saving treatment and has provided immunologic and clinical improvement for many patients. PEG-ADA administration, however, is costly ($250,000 to $400,000/year), and in some cases its efficacy has faded with time. Alternative forms of therapy are therefore needed for this disease.

Several characteristics make ADA-SCID an ideal candidate disease to be treated with gene therapy, and they explain why in the mid 1980s it was selected for pioneer experimental testing of clinical gene transfer. These attributes include a good understanding of ADA gene structure and function, the wide range of ADA enzyme concentrations compatible with normal immune function, and the demonstrated selective advantage of ADA-expressing cells over the enzyme-deficient ones. In terms of corrective gene transfer strategies, this translates into the significant advantage that tight regulation of gene expression was not required and that relatively low transduction efficiency could still produce therapeutic effects.

A variety of approaches have been undertaken by different research groups to attempt genetic correction of ADA-SCID patients by targeting both peripheral lymphocytes and hematopoietic progenitors from various sources. In 1990, Blaese and collaborators launched the first gene therapy protocol for the treatment of ADA-SCID at the National Institutes of Health (1). The strategy of targeting autologous T lymphocytes was chosen because of the disappointing early results of gene transfer into the hematopoietic stem cell of large experimental animals. This approach was conceptually supported by the finding that some ADA-SCID patients treated by BMT, but engrafted with only donor T cells, had shown full reconstitution of their immune responses, thus suggesting that the genetic correction of the patients' own lymphocytes could provide clinical benefit.

Over a 2-year period, two ADA deficient girls received 11 and 12 infusions of autologous T lymphocytes transduced with the LASN vector (56). The patients subsequently were shown to have reconstituted several immune responses that were absent or barely detectable before gene therapy. These included restoration of normal T-cell counts, development of cutaneous delayed-type hypersensitivity to various antigens, normalization of isohemoagglutinins titers, and antibody responses to vaccines (6). Both patients showed similar improvements; however, a marked difference with respect to the levels of gene transfer and of ADA enzyme expression achieved in the patients' T cells was noted. While in Patient 1 it could be demonstrated that more than 50% of circulating peripheral blood lymphocytes carried the retroviral ADA gene and that cellular ADA enzyme activity reached levels of half the amount found in heterozygous patients, analysis of Patient 2 showed only a small fraction (0.1% to 1%) of circulating T cells containing the inserted ADA gene (6). Further studies have shown that immune-mediated elimination of gene-transduced cells in Patient 2 could provide an explanation for these differences, as both cytotoxic T lymphocytes against the neomycin resistance gene product and precipitating antibodies to a cell-associated fetal calf serum protein have been demonstrated in this patient (R.M. Blaese, personal communication).

Following protocol and vector preparations identical to those used in the NIH trial, Sakiyama and colleagues from the Department of Pediatrics of the Hokkaido University, School of Medicine in Sapporo treated a Japanese ADA-SCID patient with 11 infusions of genetically modified, autologous T lymphocytes transduced with the human ADA cDNA over 20 months. This clinical trial started in August 1995, and periodic analysis of peripheral blood lymphocytes has shown transduction frequencies of 10% to 20% (8,57), accompanied by gradual increase of ADA enzyme activity in the patient's circulating T cells to levels comparable with those of a heterozygous carrier individual. Evidence of improvement of the patient's immune function after gene therapy included increased T-lymphocyte counts and DTH responses, appearance of isohemagglutinins, increase in serum immune globulin, and specific antibody production (8,57). Taken together with the results of the NIH trial, these findings indicate the effectiveness of T lymphocyte–directed gene transfer as a viable treatment option for ADA-SCID.

From the pioneer experiments of T lymphocyte–directed gene therapy, it can be concluded that the introduction of foreign genetic material did not alter the biology of mature T lymphocytes, some of which are still present in the circulation of the first patient treated more than 8 years after the last infusion. Although T lymphocytes can clearly be long-lived, their life span cannot be assumed unlimited and gene-corrected T cells are therefore destined to disappear. Further, when T-cell clones with new immune specificities develop in response to environmental stimuli, they will not have been "gene-corrected" by the previous therapy and thus will be unable to persist. For this reason, self-renewing hematopoietic progenitor cells have been the logical targets of three additional gene therapy protocols for ADA-SCID.

In 1992 in Italy, Bordignon and coworkers enrolled two ADA-SCID patients in a clinical protocol involving separate transductions of lymphocytes and bone-marrow progenitors using two distinguishable forms of the same DCA retroviral vector (58). After nine and five administrations of gene-modified cells, respectively, Patient 1 and Patient 2 showed normalization of lymphocyte counts and mitogen- and antigen-specific T-cell proliferative responses. Improvement of isohemoagglutinin titers and restoration of antigen-specific antibody production were also observed (5). More importantly, the integrated provirus was detectable in the DNA obtained from both patients' BFU-E, CFU-GM, and CFU-GEMM colonies, and ADA enzyme activity was demonstrated also in mature granulocytes and erythrocytes, thus indicating some degree of genetic correction of bone-marrow progenitors (5).

In the spring of 1993, Kohn and collaborators opted for umbilical-cord blood as a source of CD34+ hematopoietic progenitors to be used as the target for gene correction. Cord blood was collected at birth from three ADA-SCID newborns, and repeated retroviral transductions of CD34+ progenitors were performed before cells were infused in the newborns on their fourth day of life. Serial molecular studies demonstrated that integrated vector sequences were detectable in bone marrow–derived CD34+ cells, CFU-GM colonies, and in both the mononuclear and polymorphonuclear leukocyte populations of all three infants (4). Four years after the infusion of gene-corrected cells, 1% to 10% of circulating T lymphocytes contained the transduced gene, whereas only 0.01% to 0.1% of other hematopoietic elements were vector-positive.

PEG-ADA treatment was stopped in the patient carrying the highest percentage of gene-corrected T lymphocytes (~10%). As a result, proliferative response to tetanus toxoid was lost, as well as most of the circulating B and NK cells. Reduction of the total number of CD3+ and CD4+ T lymphocytes was also observed; however, the percentage of circulating T cells containing the transduced ADA gene increased to 30% to 100%, and the lymphocyte proliferation response to PHA was retained. These findings and the development of an upper respiratory tract infection induced the investigators to reinstate PEG-ADA therapy that resulted in the restoration of clinical and laboratory findings to prewithdrawal levels (9). On the one hand, these observations established that ADA gene–corrected T cells do have a selective survival advantage over unmodified lymphocytes, but, on the other, also demonstrated that the level of transduced progenitors (particularly for B and NK cells) was not sufficiently high to guarantee adequate immune function in the absence of enzyme replacement. Confirmation of the validity of the selective-advantage postulate is of significant importance as improved gene-therapy techniques are developed for this and other disorders (i.e., X-SCID, JAK3-SCID, XLA) where accumulation of gene-corrected cells could help overcome the limitations of low transduction efficiency.

Also in 1993, Valerio, Fischer, and Levinsky headed a multi-center gene-therapy protocol for ADA-SCID patients based on the retroviral transduction of hematopoietic stem cells isolated from bone marrow. Two French and one British ADA-deficient children were enrolled in the study. The results obtained were disappointing, since vector-containing cells were detectable by PCR 6 months after the treatment in the bone marrow of only one patient and no signal was detected in the peripheral blood of any of the three children. No clinical improvement could be observed in these patients (7). The reasons for the different responses observed in this trial are unknown and could be related to the different vector design, different transduction procedures, and/or different nature of target cells.

Chronic Granulomatous Disease

Chronic granulomatous disease (CGD) is an immune deficiency affecting the phagocyte system and is inherited as an X-linked or autosomal-recessive trait. Mutations of any of four different genes encoding for subunits of the NAPDH oxidase (gp91phox, p22phox, p47phox, p67phox) have been found to be responsible for this disease. As a consequence of the impairment of phagocytic-cell functions, CGD is characterized by recurrent bacterial and fungal infections that induce formation of granuloma and threaten the life of the affected individuals. Current management of CGD patients includes antibiotic prophylaxis, administration of interferon-γ (γ-IFN), and allogeneic BMT. For several patients, however, available therapeutic options remain unsatisfactory, making the development of new strategies based on gene transfer highly desirable.

Mature phagocytes are characterized by a very limited life span and attempts to achieve genetic corrections of these labile elements would not lead to long-term beneficial effects. For these reasons, the ultimate target for gene therapy of CGD is the hematopoietic stem cell. In vitro preclinical studies have demonstrated that CD34+ hematopoietic progenitors derived from G-

CSF mobilized peripheral blood and genetically corrected by retrovirus-mediated gene transfer showed restoration of superoxide production when induced to differentiate into mature monocytes and neutrophils (59–63). In addition, in vivo restoration of respiratory burst in p47phox and gp91phox "knock-out" mice has been demonstrated, following gene correction of bone-marrow cells with retroviral vectors (64,65). On the basis of these encouraging results, Malech and coworkers at the National Institutes of Health initiated a phase I clinical study for gene therapy of the autosomal-recessive form of CGD, caused by defective expression of the NAPDH complex p47phox subunit. Five CGD patients were subjected to pharmacologic mobilization of CD34+ hematopoietic progenitors that were then collected from the peripheral blood by apheresis. Enriched CD34+ cells were transduced "in vitro" using a retroviral vector expressing the p47phox cDNA and then reinfused into the patients. Appearance of NAPDH oxidase activity in PMA-stimulated peripheral blood granulocytes was followed in each subject over time. At variable intervals between 15 and 32 days after infusion of transduced progenitors, all patients showed the presence of oxidase-positive granulocytes, with maximum percentages ranging between 0.004% and 0.05%. The presence of the transduced gene in the DNA of peripheral blood lymphocytes was confirmed by PCR detection. Oxydase-positive cells were detected for a minimum of 79 and a maximum of 172 days (66). Although silencing of the transduced gene has not been excluded, these findings are consistent with the loss of the transduced cells and with the pos-sibility that more differentiated progenitors, rather than true self-renewing hematopoietic stem cells, were targeted in this study.

More recently, the same research group has started a second clinical trial aimed at the genetic correction of the more-common X-linked form of CGD (X-CGD), caused by mutation of the gp91phox subunit of NAPDH oxidase. Using a high-titer retroviral vector and improved transduction procedures, three X-CGD patients each received two infusions of gp91phox- transduced CD34+ cells. Preliminary results reported in abstract form indicated that levels of NAPDH-positive neutrophils were markedly higher than those observed in the previous trial and ranged from 0.2% to 0.06% at 3 to 4 weeks after treatment (11).

Contrary to ADA-SCID, no selective advantage of gene-corrected populations is expected in this disease, and significant levels of HSCs transduction will probably be needed to obtain a clear clinical benefit.

X-Linked, Severe, Combined Immune Deficiency

Accounting for approximately 50% of all forms, X-linked, severe, combined immune deficiency (X-SCID) is the most commonly diagnosed variant of SCID. X-SCID is caused by mutations of the common gamma chain (γ_c) of the receptors for interleukin (IL)-2, IL-4, IL-7, IL-9, and IL-15 (85) that profoundly impair lymphoid development and lead to virtual lack of circulating T and NK cells in affected patients. B lymphocytes are usually present in normal or even elevated numbers. Clinically, affected boys present with severe, recurrent infections, leading to failure to thrive and early

death unless their immune function is reconstituted by allogeneic bone marrow transplantation (BMT). Both HLA-identical BMTs from related donors (generally a sibling), or from unrelated volunteers, and partially matched, T-cell–depleted transplants from parents have been performed on a relatively large number of X-SCID patients with good success (86,87). Transplantation procedures, however, are not available for all patients and can be associated with serious complications such as graft-versus-host disease (GvHD). In addition, transplanted patients often achieve little or no reconstitution of B-lymphocyte function and continue to have defective, humoral, immune responses that require the institution of continuous replacement therapy with intravenous immune globulins. Genetic correction and reinfusion of autologous hematopoietic stem cells (HSCs) would represent a better therapeutic alternative, one that is free from the threat of GvDH and available to all patients.

Retrovirus-mediated transfer of the γ_c into B lymphoblastoid cell lines derived from X-SCID patients has shown that several cellular defects could be corrected by gene transfer, including γ_c membrane expression, IL-2 high-affinity binding and internalization, and ligand binding–mediated phosphorylation of JAK1 and JAK3 tyrosine kinases, as well as IL-2–induced cell proliferation (68–70). Subsequent studies have focused on genetic correction of X-SCID HSCs, the logical target for clinical applications, and have demonstrated that γ_c gene transfer into X-SCID bone-marrow cells restores the ability of X-SCID HSCs to mature into T lymphocytes (72) and NK cells (71) in vitro. Animal experiments aimed at restoring immune function in γ_c "knockout" mice have demonstrated the safety and efficacy of γ_c gene transfer in vivo (113–115).

Based on the preclinical results, a clinical trial of gene therapy for X-SCID has been recently started by Cavazzana-Calvo and colleagues at the Necker Hospital in Paris, France. The results published on the first two treated patients show good reconstitution of T-cell numbers and both humoral and cellular immune function, up to 9 months after infusion of gene-corrected CD34+ autologous cells (116).

Preclinical Studies for Future Applications

A number of IDDs of known genetic origin appear as good candidates for gene therapy and include those diseases caused by genes whose expression is not strictly regulated or confined to a particular cell type, cell cycle phase, or differentiation stage. A large body of literature is available describing in vitro and in vivo preclinical studies aimed at assessing the safety and feasibility of gene-based strategies as alternative therapy for these diseases, and both encouraging and cautionary notes have emerged (67–82).

Purine Nucleoside Phosphorylase Deficiency

Purine nucleoside phosphorylase (PNP) deficiency is a rare disorder of the same purine salvage pathway affected in ADA-SCID. Lack of PNP activity leads to failure of the cell-mediated arm of the immune system and consequent complete defeat of the natural defenses in affected patients, who usually die in their first decade of overwhelming infections (83). Allogeneic HLA-matched bone marrow transplantation is the current therapy of choice, although reports indicating its success in PNP-deficient patients are limited (84). Because PNP deficiency and ADA-SCID are caused by similar biochemical aberrations, it also seems likely that genetic correction of PNP deficiency could lead to potential benefits. In preclinical studies using retrovirus-mediated gene transfer, "in vitro" reconstitution of PNP activity in T lymphocytes derived from PNP-deficient subjects has been described (67). These results suggest that T cells could potentially be used as vehicles for therapeutic PHP gene expression, and a clinical protocol testing this hypothesis has been proposed. PNP-deficient patients are usually lymphopenic and, contrary to ADA-SCID, no enzyme replacement treatment is available for this disease. For this reason the possibility remains that PNP-deficient patients will not have a sufficiently developed peripheral T-cell repertoire to achieve meaningful immune reconstitution with T-lymphocyte–directed gene therapy, and correction of the gene defect at the level of the hematopoietic stem cells seems the best strategy for this disease.

JAK3-Deficient SCID

Genetic lesions impairing expression and/or function of JAK3, a member of the Janus family of tyrosine kinases, result in a variant of SCID phenotypically identical to X-SCID, but inherited as an autosomal-recessive trait. JAK3 intimately interacts with γ_c in all γ_c-containing receptors (88), and such an association explains the equivalent effects of the lack of JAK3 on the development of the immune system. JAK3-SCID is a good candidate disease for stem-cell gene therapy because it can also be cured by allogeneic BMT. Also analogous to X-SCID, BMT in JAK3-SCID patients may cause GvHD and result in continuous B-cell impairment. Gene transfer with retroviral vectors has been demonstrated to correct JAK3 expression and signal transduction in lymphoblastoid B cells obtained from JAK3-SCID patients (73). More importantly, retrovirus-mediated gene correction of bone marrow–derived progenitors has been shown to result in restoration of cellular and humoral immune responses in JAK-3 "knock-out" mice (75,76), thus indicating that a similar strategy could be successful in humans.

ZAP-70 Deficiency

The tyrosine kinase ZAP-70 is expressed in T and natural killer (NK) cells and associates with the ζ chain of the T-cell receptor (TcR) complex after TcR engagement (89–91). Mutations in the ZAP-70 coding sequence result in a rare form of autosomal-recessive profound IDD characterized by absence of mature circulating CD8+ T lymphocytes and TcR signal transduction defects in peripheral CD4+ T cells. Normal levels of B lymphocytes and serum immunoglobulins, as well as adequate "in vitro" NK activity, can be detected (92–94).

Preliminary studies of corrective gene transfer have been performed using HTLV-1–transformed T-cell lines and have shown that retrovirus-mediated gene transduction of the normal ZAP-70 cDNA resulted in production of ZAP-70 kinase that was appropriately tyrosine phosphorylated upon TcR engagement. In addition, in vitro ZAP-70 kinase activity was also restored, as was calcium mobilization on TcR stimulation in the gene-corrected cells (77).

Clinical application of gene therapy for ZAP-70 deficiency will probably require gene correction at the level of the hematopoietic stem cell. Also, because of the characteristic restricted expression of the ZAP-70 protein in specific lymphoid lineages, the development of gene-transfer systems allowing tight gene regulation will probably be necessary to avoid potential deleterious effects of the "ectopic" expression of ZAP-70 in cell types normally not expressing this protein. Preclinical experiments in ZAP-70 "knockout" mice will be necessary to address this issue.

Deficiency of Expression of MHC Class II Molecules

This disorder is caused by genetic defects affecting the expression of the *trans*-activating regulatory factor CIITA (class II *trans*-activator) (95), the RFX5 binding protein (96), and the RFXAP protein (97) and, as opposed to ZAP-70 deficiency, is characterized by low numbers of CD4+ lymphocytes. Reduced T-cell responses to antigens and the absence of specific antibody production in response to vaccines are also found in patients affected with this severe IDD, who usually present with failure to thrive, multiple infections, and death in the first or second decade of life (98). Allogeneic BMT is potentially curative, but its success rate for this disease is very low (99,100). Alternative forms of therapy are therefore needed, and HSCs-directed gene therapy could be beneficial for these patients. Exploring this possibility, Bradley et al have shown that retrovirus-mediated gene transfer of the CIITA factor could restore expression of MHC class II in B lymphoblastoid lines and peripheral blood cells from an MHC class II–deficient patient (78).

A cautionary note comes from the reports indicating that ectopic expression of MHC class II genes can result in pathologic hyperactivity of CD4+ lymphocytes (101). Since expression of MHC class II molecules is regulated in important cell types such as T lymphocytes, fibroblasts, and endothelial cells, it will be important to determine if tissue-specific expression of the therapeutic gene will be needed for clinical applications.

Leukocyte Adhesion Deficiency Type I (LAD I)

Absence or reduced levels of expression of the common β_2-integrin subunit (CD18) are at the basis of this syndrome, which is clinically characterized by retarded separation of the umbilical cord and recurrent, severe bacterial and fungal infections characterized by high leukocyte counts, impaired pus formation, and delayed wound healing. These clinical findings are explained by the impairment of LAD 1 granulocyte motion (adhesion to endothelial cells and transmigration) and the failure of these granulocytes to migrate into inflamed tissues and exert their phagocytic functions. Bone marrow transplantation is curative, and it is therefore probable that stem cell gene correction may lead to a cure for this disease. Preclinical experiments in murine BMT models have shown that retroviral transduction of hematopoietic progenitors resulted in successful expression of the human CD18 in circulating granulocytes (79,80,102). In further studies, LAD 1 CD34+ peripheral blood stem cells were transduced with a retroviral vector expressing CD18 and induced to differentiate in vitro with granulocyte colony-stimulating factor (G-CSF) and granulocyte-macrophage CSF (GM-CSF). Normal CD18 surface expression and CD18-mediated adhesion were demonstrated (81), indicating that ex vivo gene transfer of CD18 and reinfusion of autologous CD34+ cells may restore granulocyte functions in LAD1 patients. Based on these encouraging studies, a clinical protocol for gene therapy of LAD 1 was recently opened at the Department of Pediatrics of the University of Washington in Seattle, WA. The expression of CD18 is limited to myeloid cells and lymphocytes; however, functional adhesion molecules require dimerization of CD18 with the CD11a, CD11b, or CD11c subunits also expressed only in the same cells. For this reason, it seems reasonable to assume that expression of CD18 in other types deriving from transduced HSCs and normally not expressing CD18 should not result in unregulated and potentially dangerous expression of complete adhesion molecules.

Similar to CGD, no selective advantage of cells deriving from transduced HSCs is expected, and the success of gene therapy for LAD 1 will probably depend on the achievement of high transduction efficiency of target cells.

Wiskott-Aldrich Syndrome (WAS)

Boys affected with WAS present with thrombocytopenia with small-sized platelets variably associated with eczema and immunodeficiency, leading to increased susceptibility to infection from all classes of pathogens. Sepsis and severe intracerebral hemorrhages represent frequent causes of death among WAS patients who also have a higher risk of lymphoid cancer than the normal population. All clinical aspects of the disease are curable by allogeneic bone marrow transplantation (BMT) with high success when histocompatible sibling donors are available. Good success has also been reported when matched, unrelated (MUD) transplants are performed in the first years of life. Unfortunately, MUD BMTs in older WAS patients and T cell–depleted, haploidentical transplants carry a much higher incidence of BMT-related severe complications (103,104). Therefore, patients lacking suitable BMT donors could benefit from the development of gene-based therapeutic strategies. However, our understanding of the regulation and function of the Wiskott-Aldrich syndrome protein (WASP) is still to incomplete to comfortably propose gene therapy for this disease. Several lines of evidence have linked this protein to mechanisms of cytoskeleton organization in hematopoietic cells (105), but information on its role in HSCs differentiation is still undefined.

Preliminary studies assessing the feasibility of genetic correction of WAS cells by retrovirus-mediated gene transfer have demonstrated that constitutive expression of WASP in lymphoblastoid B cells is not toxic and leads to correction of actin polymerization defects observed in WAS lines (74). However, because WAS affects multiple hematopoietic cell types, the hematopoietic stem cell is the ultimate target for corrective gene transfer. Because myeloablation is a necessary prerequisite to successful engraftment of normal allogeneic, WASP-expressing, hematopoietic stem cells (104,106), it is reasonable to conclude that gene-corrected hematopoietic progenitors would not have selective advantage over residual, unmodified stem cells. Myeloblation would probably still be required before the reinfusion of genetically engineered cells to achieve clinical benefit. Alternatively, "in vivo" positive selection of transduced progenitors could represent a way of increasing the efficacy of gene-transfer procedures and could be achieved by adding in vivo selectable drug-resistance genes (e.g., DHFR, MGMT) to the retroviral vector cassette.

X-Linked Immunodeficiency with Hyper-IgM (X-HIGM)

Mutations affecting the expression of the CD40 ligand molecule (CD40L) are responsible for faulty T-cell-B-cell cooperation resulting in the defective humoral and cellular immunity found in the X-linked hyper-IgM syndrome. X-HIGM patients are unable to produce IgG, IgA, and IgE, while IgM levels are normal or even elevated. B lymphocytes are detected in normal numbers. Impairment of antigen-specific T-cell responses is also often reported. Pyogenic and opportunistic agents (*Pneumocystis carinii, Cryptosporidium*) are common causes of acute and chronic infections. In addition, neutropenia, lymphoproliferative complications, and autoimmune disorders are also commonly reported. Despite antibiotic and IVIg prophylaxis, X-HIGM patients show a severely reduced survival (107), and allogeneic BMT is being evaluated as potential definitive therapy. Gene therapy could provide clinical benefit for X-HIGM patients, and both peripheral T lymphocytes and hematopoietic stem cells are conceivable targets for corrective gene transfer. Unfortunately, CD40L expression is highly regulated and restricted to "activated" CD4+ lymphocytes, thus introducing the need for regulated gene-transfer systems. The necessity of strictly regulating the expression of CD40L on gene-corrected cells has been recently stressed by the results obtained by Brown et al, who performed transplantation of retrovirally gene-corrected bone-marrow or thymic cells in CD40L "knockout" mice. Humoral and cellular immune responses of treated mice to influenza virus were partially or fully restored; however, more than 60% of these mice developed lymphoproliferative disease in the form of prelymphoma of T-lymphoblastic lymphoma, likely the result of enhanced positive selection driven by the constitutive expression of CD40L on developing thymocytes (82). Gene transfer systems allowing effective regulation of CD40L therefore will have to be developed before similar gene correction approaches can be proposed for the treatment of X-HIGM.

Soluble CD40L is available and could represent an alternative form of therapy for X-HIGM patients. If proven beneficial, the administration of autologous cells or "pseudo-organs" that are engineered to produce CD40L and that are easily removable could be attempted as a more economic option.

Prospects of Gene Therapy for Other Immunodeficiencies

Many other IDDs exist for which gene therapy could represent an advantageous form of treatment. For example, the recent identification of the recombination activating genes 1 and 2 (RAG-1 and RAG-2) as genetic causes of autosomal-recessive SCID (108) and Omenn's syndrome (109) has opened the way for possible attempts of hematopoietic stem cell gene correction as treatment for those patients lacking suitable bone marrow donors. However, the regulation of RAG gene expression in humans is poorly understood. RAG-1 and RAG-2 are expressed in immature lymphocytes in bone marrow and thymus and are downregulated in mature T- and B-lymphocyte populations. Interestingly, activated, mature B cells reexpress the RAG gene products in the context of germinal centers. The mechanisms controlling RAG activation are therefore complex, and the development of gene-therapy approaches for RAG-1/RAG-2 deficiencies must await further investigations.

Similar considerations are valid for other IDDs of known genetic origin such as Chediak-Higashi syndrome and X-linked lymphoproliferative syndrome. These syndromes are curable by allogeneic bone marrow transplantation, and therefore corrective gene transfer at the level of the hematopoietic stem cell could be equally effective. However, the available information relative to the function and regulation of the causative gene is still too limited to predict the effects of constitutive gene expression. Further studies and preclinical models are therefore warranted to explore safety and feasibility of therapeutic gene transfer for these diseases.

The potential role of gene therapy is currently unclear for those IDDs that are usually characterized by less overwhelming clinical presentations and generally considered not severe enough to expose affected patients to the risks of bone marrow transplantation. Both cellular immunity defects (such as MHC class I deficiency, CD3ε or CD3γ deficiency, autoimmune lymphoproliferative syndrome) and antibody deficiencies (i.e., X-linked agammaglobulinemia) can be included in this group of diseases for which, in addition to more information on the biology of the causative genes, the demonstration that gene correction could lead to efficient restoration of the missing function(s) still needs to be obtained.

At its current stage of development, gene therapy cannot offer solutions for syndromes such as ataxia telangiectasia (AT) and Bloom's syndrome (BS), where the immune system is only one of the multiple systems affected by the disease. The great difficulty posed by delivering genes to a multiplicity of different tissues and organs, including the central nervous system in the case of AT, represents a major barrier to gene therapy for these syndromes. One potential approach for genetic correction of AT and BS could be fetal gene therapy. The advantages of gene delivery in the early stages of fetal development would include the theoretic feasibility of exposing most tissues to gene transfer using a relatively low amount of vector and the possibility of restoring normal gene function before the potential establishment of irreversible negative effects (i.e., genomic instability) caused by lack of expression of the mutated gene.

The recently described family of IDDs characterized by the inability to produce or respond to interferon γ (IFN-γ) (110) may benefit from gene therapy approaches. It is conceivable that the defective expression of IL-12, IL-12 receptor β1 chain (IL12Rβ1), and IFN-γ receptor chains 1 and 2 (IFN-γR1, IFN-γR2) can be restored by corrective stem cell gene transfer. Preclinical experiments in animal models will determine whether regulated gene expression will be needed for gene therapy of these disorders. In particular, IL12Rβ1 deficiency seems eligible for T-lymphocyte–directed gene-therapy approaches, which would avoid the difficulties of gene transfer into the hematopoietic stem cell.

Concluding Remarks

Inherited immune deficiencies have played a major role in the development and early clinical applications of gene therapy, and the results of the numerous gene transfer experiments involving genes responsible for IDDs have taught us invaluable lessons. In particular, the pioneer clinical trials have begun addressing the primary concern of safety. The first human subject to be treated with a therapeutic gene has now been followed for more than 8 years with no signs of adverse effects, although the transduced gene is detectable in as many as ~50% of the circulating lymphocytes. Because of the limited number of patients treated in the early trials, the efficacy issue has been more difficult to address. Although a series of immune functions that were absent before gene therapy in ADA-SCID patients were clearly detectable after treatment (5,6), a major criticism in the interpretation of these findings has been that PEG-ADA enzyme replacement therapy was continued in all cases, thus making the clinical benefit deriving uniquely from gene correction difficult to assess.

The first gene therapy trials aiming at genetic correction of hematopoietic stem cells have shown low efficiency and limited or no clinical benefits (7,9,10), indicating that improvements in gene transfer procedures are needed for future applications. Current gene transfer systems have shown clear improvement over the first generation of vectors used and hold promise for improved transduction in future clinical studies. In addition, continuing studies have shed more light on the biology of the hematopoietic stem cell and will have a major impact on gene-therapy approaches for IDDs. The very promising results obtained in France with gene therapy of X-SCID are based on these incremental improvements and will hopefully withstand the test of time.

The necessity for tissue-specific and/or precise regulation of transgene expression represents a formidable challenge for the development of gene therapies for IDDs and for genetic diseases in general. Pharmacologic activation/suppression of gene expression has been obtained in mice (111) and nonhuman primates (112), and these results will hopefully open the way for application in humans. In addition, the use of fail-safe, "suicide" mechanisms is also envisionable for eliminating engineered cells and thus for controlling the effects of gene transfer.

Ethical issues will have to be resolved as gene therapy approaches are developed for those IDDs that are successfully curable with traditional forms of therapy. Solid preclinical data will have to be produced before established and life-saving treatment could comfortably be postponed or withheld to allow testing of experimental gene therapies. However, if gene therapy approaches are designed such that potential failures will not preclude or alter the success of traditional treatment, clinical scenarios can be envisioned where the ethical concern may be relieved. Clinical settings where gene therapy can be delivered concurrently with traditional therapy (i.e., together with PEG-ADA for ADA-SCID or with allogeneic BMT for other forms of SCID) or after failure of prior therapeutic approaches (after unsuccessful or only partially successful BMT) may raise less ethical issues, but may also result in clinical outcomes that are difficult to interpret.

In summary, gene therapy holds the promise to cure many forms of IDDs; the pioneer human experiments have exposed the crucial problems and issues to be solved to allow the successful development and general application of this novel and modern branch of medicine.

References

1. Blaese RM. The ADA human gene therapy clinical protocol. Hum Gene Ther 1990;1:327–362.
2. Gatti RA, Meuwissen HJ, Allen HD, et al. Immunological reconstitution of sex-linked lymphopenic immunological deficiency. Lancet 1968;2:1366–1369.
3. Human Gene Marker/Therapy Protocols. Hum Gene Ther 1998;9:2805–2852.
4. Kohn DB, Weinberg KI, Nolta JA, et al. Engraftment of gene-modified umbilical cord blood cells in neonates with adenosine deaminase deficiency. Nat Med 1995;1:1017–1023.
5. Bordignon C, Notarangelo LD, Nobili N, et al. Gene therapy in peripheral blood lymphocytes and bone marrow for ADA-immunodeficient patients. Science 1995;270:470–475.
6. Blaese RM, Culver KW, Miller AD, et al. T lymphocyte–directed gene therapy for ADA-SCID: initial trial results after 4 years. Science 1995;270:475–480.
7. Hoogerbrugge PM, van Beusechem VW, Fischer A, et al.

8. Onodera M, Ariga T, Kawamura N, et al. Successful peripheral T lymphocyte–directed gene transfer for a patient with severe combined immune deficiency due to adenosine deaminase deficiency. Blood 1998;91:30–36.
9. Kohn DB, Hershfield MS, Carbonaro D, et al. T lymphocytes with a normal ADA gene accumulate after transplantation of transduced autologous umbilical cord blood CD34+ cells in ADA-deficient SCID neonates. Nat Med 1998;4:775–780.
10. Malech HL, Maples PB, Whiting-Theobald N, et al. Prolonged production of NADPH oxidase-corrected granulocytes after gene therapy of chronic granulomatous disease. Proc Natl Acad Sci USA 1997;94:12133–12138.
11. Malech HL, Horwitz ME, Linton GF, et al. Extended production of oxidase normal neutrophils in X-linked chronic granulomatous disease (CGD) following gene therapy with gp91(phox) transduced CD34+ cells. Blood 1998;92:690A.
12. Johnston KM, Jacoby D, Pechan PA, et al. HSV/AAV hybrid amplicon vectors extend transgene expression in human glioma cells. Hum Gene Ther 1997;8:359–370.
13. Ramsey WJ, Caplen NJ, Li Q, et al. Adenovirus vectors as transcomplementing templates for the production of replication defective retroviral vectors. Biochem Biophys Res Commun 1998;246:912–919.
14. Cole-Strauss A, Yoon K, Xiang Y, et al. Correction of the mutation responsible for sickle cell anemia by an RNA-DNA oligonucleotide. Science 1996;273:1386–1389.
15. Kren BT, Cole-Strauss A, Kmiec EB, Steer CJ. Targeted nucleotide exchange in the alkaline phosphatase gene of HuH-7 cells mediated by a chimeric RNA/DNA oligonucleotide. Hepatology 1997;25:1462–1468.
16. Kren BT, Bandyopadhyay P, Steer CJ. In vivo site-directed mutagenesis of the factor IX gene by chimeric RNA/DNA oligonucleotides. Nat Med 1998;4:285–290.
17. Miller AD. Retrovirus packaging cells. Hum Gene Ther 1990;1:5–14.
18. Miller AD, Garcia JV, von Suhr N, et al. Construction and properties of retrovirus packaging cells based on gibbon ape leukemia virus. J Virol 1991;65:2220–2224.
19. Bunnell BA, Muul LM, Donahue RE, et al. High-efficiency retroviral-mediated gene transfer into human and non-human primate peripheral blood lymphocytes. Proc Natl Acad Sci USA 1995;92:7739–7743.
20. Cosset FL, Takeuchi Y, Battini JL, et al. High-titer packaging cells producing recombinant retroviruses resistant to human serum. J Virol 1995;69:7430–7436.
21. Kasahara N, Dozy AM, Kan YW. Tissue-specific targeting of retroviral vectors through ligand-receptor interactions. Science 1994;266:1373–1376.
22. Brenner MK. The contribution of marker gene studies to hemopoietic stem cell therapies. Stem Cells 1995;13:453–461.
23. Berns KI. Parvoviridae: the viruses and their replication. In: Fields BN, Knipe DM, Howley PM, eds. Virology. Philadelphia, PA: Lippincott-Raven, 1995:2173–2197.
24. Podsakoff G, Wong KK Jr, Chatterjee S. Efficient gene transfer into nondividing cells by adeno-associated virus-based vectors. J Virol 1994;68:5656–5666.
25. Broxmeyer HE, Cooper S, Etienne-Julan M, et al. Cord blood transplantation and the potential for gene therapy.

Gene transduction using a recombinant adeno-associated viral vector. Ann NY Acad Sci 1995;770:105–115.

26. Lubovy M, McCune S, Dong JY, et al. Stable transduction of recombinant adeno-associated virus into hematopoietic stem cells from normal and sickle cell patients. Biol Blood Marrow Transplant 1996;2:24–30.

27. Samulski RJ, Chang LS, Shenk T. Helper-free stocks of recombinant adeno-associated viruses: normal integration does not require viral gene expression. J Virol 1989;63:3822–3828.

28. Gao GP, Qu G, Faust LZ, et al. High-titer adeno-associated viral vectors from a *rep/cap* cell line and hybrid shuttle virus. Hum Gene Ther 1998;9:2353–2362.

29. Flotte TR, Barraza-Ortiz X, Solow R, et al. An improved system for packaging recombinant adeno-associated virus vectors capable of in vivo transduction. Gene Ther 1995;2:29–37.

30. Clark KR, Voulgaropoulou F, Fraley DM, Johnson PR. Cell lines for the production of recombinant adeno-associated virus. Hum Gene Ther 1995;6:1329–1341.

31. Clark KR, Voulgaropoulou F, Johnson PR. A stable cell line carrying adenovirus-inducible *rep* and *cap* genes allows for infectivity titration of adeno-associated virus vectors. Gene Ther 1996;3:1124–1132.

32. Tamayose K, Hirai Y, Shimada T. A new strategy for large-scale preparation of high-titer recombinant adeno-associated virus vectors by using packaging cell lines and sulfonated cellulose column chromatography. Hum Gene Ther 1996;7:507–513.

33. Inoue N, Russell DW. Packaging cells based on inducible gene amplification for the production of adeno-associated virus vectors. J Virol 1998;72:7024–7031.

34. Thrasher AJ, de Alwis M, Casimir CM, et al. Functional reconstitution of the NADPH-oxidase by adeno-associated virus gene transfer. Blood 1995;86:761–765.

35. Walsh CE, Nienhuis AW, Samulski RJ, et al. Phenotypic correction of Fanconi anemia in human hematopoietic cells with a recombinant adeno-associated virus vector. J Clin Invest 1994;94:1440–1448.

36. Frisch VL, Wang S, Malech HL, Walsh CE. Phenotypic correction of human hematopoietic progenitor cells from a patient with X-linked chronic granulomatous disease using a recombinant adeno-associated virus vector. Blood 1995;86:242a.

37. Flotte TR, Afione SA, Zeitlin PL. Adeno-associated virus vector gene expression occurs in nondividing cells in the absence of vector DNA integration. Am J Respir Cell Mol Biol 1994;11:517–521.

38. Yang Q, Mamounas M, Yu G, et al. Development of novel cell surface CD34-targeted recombinant adenoassociated virus vectors for gene therapy. Hum Gene Ther 1998;9:1929–1937.

39. Naldini L, Blomer P, Gallay P, et al. In vivo gene delivery and stable transduction of nondividing cells by a lentiviral vector. Science 1996;273:263–267.

40. Reiser J, Harmison G, Kluepfel-Stahl S, et al. Transduction of nondividing cells using pseudotyped defective high-titer HIV type 1 particles. Proc Natl Acad Sci USA 1996;93:15266–15271.

41. Poeschla E, Gilbert J, Li X, et al. Identification of a human immunodeficiency virus type 2 (HIV-2) encapsidation deter-

minant and transduction of nondividing human cells by HIV-2–based lentivirus vectors. J Virol 1998;72:6527–6536.

42. Arya SK, Zamani M, Kundra P. Human immunodeficiency virus type 2 lentivirus vectors for gene transfer: expression and potential for helper virus–free packaging. Hum Gene Ther 1998;9:1371–1380.

43. Poeschla EM, Wong-Staal F, Looney DJ. Efficient transduction of nondividing human cells by feline immunodeficiency virus lentiviral vectors. Natl Med 1998;4:354–357.

44. Olsen JC. Gene transfer vectors derived from equine infectious anemia virus. Gene Ther 1998;5:1481–1487.

45. Uchida N, Sutton RE, Friera AM, et al. HIV, but not murine leukemia virus, vectors mediate high efficiency gene transfer into freshly isolated G0/G1 human hematopoietic stem cells. Proc Natl Acad Sci USA 1998;95:11939–11944.

46. Naldini L, Blomer U, Gage FH, et al. Efficient transfer, integration, and sustained long-term expression of the transgene in adult rat brains injected with a lentiviral vector. Proc Natl Acad Sci USA 1996;93:11382–11388.

47. Miyoshi H, Takahashi M, Gage FH, Verma IM. Stable and efficient gene transfer into the retina using an HIV-based lentiviral vector. Proc Natl Acad Sci USA 1997;94:10319–10323.

48. Zufferey R, Nagy D, Mandel RJ, et al. Multiply attenuated lentiviral vector achieves efficient gene delivery in vivo. Natl Biotechnol 1997;15:871–875.

49. Kafri T, Blomer U, Peterson DA, et al. Sustained expression of genes delivered directly into liver and muscle by lentiviral vectors. Natl Genet 1997;17:314–317.

50. Miyoshi H, Smith KA, Mosier DE, et al. Transduction of human CD34+ cells that mediate long-term engraftment of NOD/SCID mice by HIV vectors. Science 1999;283:682–686.

51. Case SS, Price MA, Jordan CT, et al. Stable transduction of quiescent CD34(+)CD38(–) human hematopoietic cells by HIV-1–based lentiviral vectors. Proc Natl Acad Sci USA 1999;96:2988–2993.

52. Miyoshi H, Blomer U, Takahashi M, et al. Development of a self-inactivating lentivirus vector. J Virol 1998;72:8150–8157.

53. Dull T, Zufferey R, Kelly M, et al. A third-generation lentivirus vector with a conditional packaging system. J Virol 1998;72:8463–8471.

54. Zufferey R, Dull T, Mandel RJ, et al. Self-inactivating lentivirus vector for safe and efficient in vivo gene delivery. J Virol 1998;72:9873–9880.

55. Hershfield MS, Buckley RH, Greenberg ML, et al. Treatment of adenosine deaminase deficiency with polyethylene glycol-modified adenosine deaminase. N Engl J Med 1987;316:589–596.

56. Hock RA, Miller AD, Osborne WR. Expression of human adenosine deaminase from various strong promoters after gene transfer into human hematopoietic cell lines. Blood 1989;74:876–881.

57. Egashira M, Ariga T, Kawamura N, et al. Visible integration of the adenosine deaminase (ADA) gene into the recipient genome after gene therapy. Am J Med Genet 1998;75:314–317.

58. Hantzopoulos PA, Sullenger BA, Ungers G, Gilboa E. Improved gene expression upon transfer of the adenosine deaminase minigene outside the transcriptional unit of a

retroviral vector. Proc Natl Acad Sci USA 1989;86:3519–3523.

59. Sekhsaria S, Gallin JI, Linton GF, et al. Peripheral blood progenitors as a target for genetic correction of p47phox-deficient chronic granulomatous disease. Proc Natl Acad Sci USA 1993;90:7446–7450.
60. Li F, Linton GF, Sekhsaria S, et al. CD34+ peripheral blood progenitors as a target for genetic correction of the two flavocytochrome b558 defective forms of chronic granulomatous disease. Blood 1994;84:53–58.
61. Porter CD, Parkar MH, Collins MK, et al. Efficient retroviral transduction of human bone marrow progenitor and long-term culture-initiating cells: partial reconstitution of cells from patients with X-linked chronic granulomatous disease by gp91-phox expression. Blood 1996;87:3722–3730.
62. Weil WM, Linton GF, Whiting-Theobald N, et al. Genetic correction of p67phox-deficient chronic granulomatous disease using peripheral blood progenitor cells as a target for retrovirus mediated gene transfer. Blood 1997;89:1754–1761.
63. Becker S, Wasser S, Hauses M, et al. Correction of respiratory burst activity in X-linked chronic granulomatous cells to therapeutically relevant levels after gene transfer into bone marrow CD34+ cells. Hum Gene Ther 1998;9:1561–1570.
64. Mardiney MR, Jackson SH, Spratt SK, et al. Enhanced host defense after gene transfer in the murine p47phox-deficient model of chronic granulomatous disease. Blood 1997;89:2268–2275.
65. Bjorgvinsdottir H, Ding C, Pech N, et al. Retroviral-mediated gene transfer of gp91phox into bone marrow cells rescues defect in host defense against *Aspergillus fumigatus* in murine X-linked chronic granulomatous disease. Blood 1997;89:41–48.
66. Malech HL, Sekhsaria S, Whiting-Theobald N, et al. Prolonged detection of oxidase-positive neutrophils in the peripheral blood of five patients following a single cycle of gene therapy for chronic granulomatous disease. Blood 1996;88(suppl 1):486a.
67. Nelson DM, Butters KA, Markert ML, et al. Correction of proliferative responses in purine nucleoside phosphorylase (PNP)–deficient T lymphocytes by retroviral-mediated PNP gene transfer and expression. J Immunol 1995;154:3006–3014.
68. Candotti F, Johnston JA, Puck JM, et al. Retroviral-mediated gene correction for X-linked severe combined immunodeficiency. Blood 1996;87:3097–3102.
69. Taylor N, Uribe L, Smith S, et al. Correction of interleukin-2 receptor function in X-SCID lymphoblastoid cells by retrovirally mediated transfer of the gamma-c gene. Blood 1996;87:3103–3107.
70. Hacein-Bey S, Cavazzana-Calvo M, Le Deist F, et al. Gamma-c gene transfer into SCID X1 patients' B-cell lines restores normal high-affinity interleukin-2 receptor expression and function. Blood 1996;87:3108–3116.
71. Cavazzana-Calvo M, Hacein-Bay S, de Saint Basile G, et al. Role of interleukin-2 (IL-2), IL-7, and IL-15 in natural killer cell differentiation from cord blood hematopoietic progenitor cells and from gc transduced severe combined immunodeficiency X1 bone marrow cells. Blood 1996;88:3901–3909.

72. Hacein-Bey S, Basile GD, Lemerle J, et al. Gamma-c gene transfer in the presence of stem cell factor, FLT-3L, interleukin-7 (IL-7), IL-1, and IL-15 cytokines restores T-cell differentiation from gamma-c(–) X-linked severe combined immunodeficiency hematopoietic progenitor cells in murine fetal thymic organ cultures. Blood 1998;92:4090–4097.
73. Candotti F, Oakes S, Johnston JA, et al. In vitro correction of JAK3-deficient severe combined immunodeficiency by retroviral-mediated gene transduction. J Exp Med 1996;183:2687–2692.
74. Candotti F, Facchetti F, Blanzuoli L, et al. Retroviral-mediated WASP gene transfer corrects defective actin polymerization in B-cell lines from Wiskott-Aldrich syndrome patients carrying "null" mutations. Gene Ther 1999;6:1170–1174.
75. Bunting KD, Sangster MY, Ihle JN, Sorrentino BP. Restoration of lymphocyte function in Janus kinase 3–deficient mice by retroviral-mediated gene transfer. Nat Med 1998;4:58–64.
76. Bunting KD, Flynn KJ, Riberdy JM, et al. Virus-specific immunity after gene therapy in a murine model of severe combined immunodeficiency. Proc Natl Acad Sci USA 1999;96:232–237.
77. Taylor N, Bacon KB, Smith S, et al. Reconstitution of T-cell receptor signaling in AZP-70–deficient cells by retroviral transduction of the ZAP-70 gene. J Exp Med 1996;184:2031–2036.
78. Bradley MB, Fernandez JM, Ungers G, et al. Correction of defective expression in MHC class II deficiency (bare lymphocyte syndrome) cells by retroviral transduction of CIITA. J Immunol 1997;159:1086–1095.
79. Krauss JC, Bond LM, Todd RFD, Wilson JM. Expression of retroviral transduced human CD18 in murine cells: an in vitro model of gene therapy for leukocyte adhesion deficiency. Hum Gene Ther 1991;2:221–228.
80. Wilson RW, Yorifuji T, Lorenzo I, et al. Expression of human CD18 in murine granulocytes and improved efficiency for infection of deficient human lymphoblasts. Hum Gene Ther 1993;4:25–34.
81. Bauer TR, Schwartz BR, Conrad Liles W, et al. Retroviral-mediated gene transfer of the leukocyte integrin CD18 into peripheral blood CD34+ cells derived from a patient with leukocyte adhesion deficiency type 1. Blood 1998;91:1520–1526.
82. Brown MP, Topham DJ, Sangster MY, et al. Thymic lymphoproliferative disease after successful correction of CD40 ligand deficiency by gene transfer in mice. Nat Med 1998;4:1253–1260.
83. Markert ML. Purine nucleoside phosphorylase deficiency. Immunodefic Rev 1991;3:45–81.
84. Buckley RH, Schiff SE, Sampson HA, et al. Development of immunity in human severe primary T-cell deficiency following haploidentical bone marrow stem cell transplantation. J Immunol 1986;136:2398–2407.
85. Leonard WJ, Noguchi M, Russell SM, McBride OW. The molecular basis of X-linked severe combined immunodeficiency: the role of the interleukin-2 receptor gamma chain as a common gamma chain, gamma c. Immunol Rev 1994;138:61–86.
86. Haddad E, Landais P, Friedrich W, et al. Long-term immune reconstitution and outcome after HLA-nonidentical

T-cell–depleted bone marrow transplantation for severe combined immunodeficiency: a European retrospective study of 116 patients. Blood 1998;91:3646–3653.

87. Buckley RH, Schiff SE, Schiff RI, et al. Hematopoietic stem-cell transplantation for the treatment of severe combined immunodeficiency. N Engl J Med 1999;340:508–516.

88. O'Shea JJ. Jaks, STATs, cytokine signal transduction, and immunoregulation: are we there yet? Immunity 1997;7:1–11.

89. Chan AC, Iwashima M, Turck CW, Weiss A. ZAP-70: a 70-kd protein-tyrosine kinase that associates with the TCR zeta chain. Cell 1992;71(4):649–662.

90. Irving BA, Chan AC, Weiss A. Functional characterization of a signal transducing motif present in the T-cell antigen receptor zeta chain. J Exp Med 1993;177:1093–1103.

91. Chan AC, van Oers NS, Tran A, et al. Differential expression of AZP-70 and Syk protein tyrosine kinases, and the role of this family of protein tyrosine kinases in TCR signaling. J Immunol 1994;152:4758–4766.

92. Arpaia E, Shahar M, Dadi H, et al. Defective T-cell receptor signaling and CD8+ thymic selection in humans lacking zap-70 kinase. Cell 1994;76:947–958.

93. Chan AC, Kadlecek TA, Elder ME, et al. AZP-70 deficiency in an autosomal recessive form of severe combined immunodeficiency. Science 1994;264:1599–1601.

94. Elder ME, Lin D, Clever J, et al. Human severe combined immunodeficiency due to a defect in ZAP-70, a T-cell tyrosine kinase. Science 1994;264:1596–1599.

95. Steimle V, Otten LA, Zufferey M, Mach B. Complementation cloning of an MHC class II transactivator mutated in hereditary MHC class II deficiency (or bare lymphocyte syndrome). Cell 1993;75:135–146.

96. Steimle V, Durand B, Barras E, et al. A novel DNA-binding regulatory factor is mutated in primary MHC class II deficiency (bare lymphocyte syndrome). Genes Dev 1995;9:1021–1032.

97. Durand B, Sperisen P, Emery P, et al. RFXAP, a novel subunit of the RFX DNA binding complex is mutated in MHC class II deficiency. EMBO J 1997;16:1045–1055.

98. Griscelli C, Lisowska-Grospierre B, Mach B. Combined immunodeficiencies with defective expression in MHC class II genes. In: Rosen FS, Seligman M, eds. Immunodeficiencies. Philadelphia, PA: Harwood Academic, 1993:141–154.

99. Klein C, Cavazzana-Calvo M, Le Deist F, et al. Bone marrow transplantation in major histocompatibility complex class II deficiency: a single-center study of 19 patients. Blood 1995;85:580–587.

100. Huss R, Nepom GT, Deeg HJ. Defective CD4+ T-lymphocyte reconstitution in major histocompatibility complex class II–deficient transplant models. Blood 1995;85:3354–3356.

101. Bottazzo GF, Todd I, Mirakian R, et al. Organ-specific autoimmunity: a 1986 overview. Immunol Rev 1986;94:137–169.

102. Krauss JC, Mayo-Bond LA, Rogers CE, et al. An in vivo animal model of gene therapy for leukocyte adhesion deficiency. J Clin Invest 1991;88:1412–1417.

103. Brochstein JA, Gillio AP, Ruggiero M, et al. Marrow transplantation from human leukocyte antigen-identical or haploidentical donors for correction of Wiskott-Aldrich syndrome. J Pediatr 1991;119:907–912.

104. Filipovich A. Stem cell transplantation from unrelated donors for correction of primary immunodeficiencies. Immunol Allerg Clin North Am 1996;16(2):377–392.

105. Ochs HD. The Wiskott-Aldrich syndrome. Springer Semin Immunopathol 1998;19:435–458.

106. Fischer A, Landais P, Friedrich W, et al. Bone marrow transplantation (BMT) in Europe for primary immunodeficiencies other than severe combined immunodeficiency: a report from the European Group for BMT and the European Group for Immunodeficiency. Blood 1994;83:1149–1154.

107. Levy J, Espanol-Boren T, Thomas C, et al. The clinical spectrum of X-linked hyper IgM syndrome. J Pediatr 1997;131:47–54.

108. Schwarz K, Gauss GH, Ludwig L, et al. RAG mutations in human B-cell–negative SCID. Science 1996;274:97–99.

109. Villa A, Santagata S, Bozzi F, et al. Partial V(D)J recombination activity leads to Omenn syndrome. Cell 1998;93:885–896.

110. Ottenhoff TH, Kumararatne D, Casanova JL. Novel human immunodeficiencies reveal the essential role of type-I cytokines in immunity to intracellular bacteria. Immunol Today 1998;19:491–494.

111. Kistner A, Gossen M, Zimmermann F, et al. Doxycycline-mediated quantitative and tissue-specific control of gene expression in transgenic mice. Proc Natl Acad Sci USA 1996;93:10933–10938.

112. Ye X, Rivera VM, Zoltick P, et al. Regulated delivery of therapeutic proteins after in vivo somatic cell gene transfer. Science 1999;283:88–91.

113. Lo M, Bloom ML, Imada K, et al. Restoration of lymphoid populations in a murine model of X-linked severe combined immunodeficiency by a gene-therapy approach. Blood 1999;94:3027–3036.

114. Otsu M, Anderson SM, Bodine DM, et al. Lymphoid development and function in X-linked severe combined immunodeficiency mice after stem cell gene therapy. Mol Ther 2000;1:145–153.

115. Soudais C, Shiho T, Sharara Li, et al. Stable and functional lymphoid reconstitution of common cytokine receptor gamma chain deficient mice by retroviral-mediated gene transfer. Blood 2000;95:3071–3077.

116. Cavazzana-Calvo M, Hacein-Bey S, de Saint Basile G, et al. Gene therapy of human severe combined immunodeficiency (SCID)-X1 disease. Science 2000;288:669–672.

Chapter 44

Plasmapheresis and Immunoadsorption

Siân Griffin
C. Martin Lockwood
Charles D. Pusey

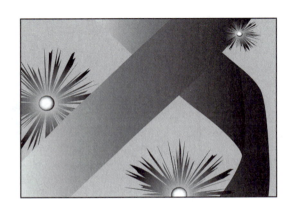

Plasmapheresis, with the removal of plasma and fluid replacement, has been employed extensively for a range of diverse indications. The effectiveness of this technique in the treatment of the autoantibody-mediated diseases, Goodpasture's syndrome, and myasthenia gravis was demonstrated in the 1970s and was followed by widespread enthusiasm for the use of plasmapheresis in a range of other conditions with a recognized immunologic component. Variable benefit was reported, usually on the basis of case reports or uncontrolled trials. More recently, rigorous analysis has been made of the benefits of plasmapheresis, especially in the context of modern immunosuppressive drug regimens and novel immunotherapeutic interventions. In a small number of diseases, a clear benefit has been borne out, and therapeutic plasmapheresis, with the replacement of removed plasma by colloid, is a valuable intervention. In other cases, it remains an adjuvant therapy, with its use indicated for patients resistant to, or intolerant of, other forms of therapy.

The feasibility of plasmapheresis was first demonstrated in an experimental (canine) model by Abel et al in 1914 (1). This involved the removal of whole blood, separation into cells and plasma, and then subsequent return of the cells to the animal. The technique was refined and used to collect plasma from humans during World War II. The benefit to patients was subsequently demonstrated with the amelioration of the symptoms of hyperviscosity associated with multiple myeloma and Waldenstrom's macroglobulinemia (2,3). It was the successful treatment of anti–glomerular basement membrane (GBM) disease in 1975 (4) that led to the full therapeutic potential of plasmapheresis being realized and thereafter its application to a wide range of diseases. Although many medical specialties now have experience with this therapy, there remains a degree of variability in the success claimed.

Extracorporeal immunoadsorption (IA) is a technique in which immunologic interactions are used to selectively remove pathogenic molecules from the plasma. In current practice this generally involves a modification of plasmapheresis, in which the separated plasma is passed through a column containing a ligand with affinity for the component concerned. Although IA could theoretically be used to treat whole blood, major problems with biocompatibility remain to be overcome.

In immunotherapy IA is most often used to remove alloantibodies or autoantibodies. Although this is the aim of plasmapheresis in many disorders, it should be remembered that the two processes differ in some aspects and cannot be regarded as equivalent. In particular, plasmapheresis also removes other plasma proteins, including complement components and coagulation factors, that may be involved in inflammation (5). In addition, the nature of the replacement fluid used for plasmapheresis, for example, fresh frozen plasma (FFP) in thrombotic thrombocytopenic purpura (TTP), may contribute to the biologic effect (6). Thus, the demonstration of benefit from plasmapheresis (PE) cannot necessarily be extrapolated to IA.

Techniques for Plasmapheresis

Cells are separated from plasma by either membrane filtration or centrifugation. Membrane filtration may be carried out using a hemodialysis system and thus has historically been the mode of plasmapheresis preferred by nephrologists (7). For patients with acute renal failure requiring dialysis, additional plasmapheresis may be carried out using the same dialysis machine. Filtration is achieved by pumping blood through microporous membranes, arranged either as hollow fibres or as a parallel plate. The pore diameter is usually $0.2\,\mu m$ to $0.5\,\mu m$, allowing the removal of immunoglobulins (Ig) and most immune complexes, with the cells passing through the separator and returning to the patient with the replacement fluid. The rate of fluid replacement is adjusted according to the rate of plasma separation, with maintenance of a constant circulating volume. Large immune complexes and IgM may not be removed as effectively as IgG, which should be remembered in the treatment of diseases where these molecules are implicated in pathogenesis. The extracorporeal gelling of cryoglobulins in the cooler environment will also impair the efficiency of their clearance.

The separated plasma may be further treated using membranes of different pore size. The aim here is to improve the selectivity of removal, for example, of cryoglobulins or immune complexes; to avoid depletion of other essential molecules, for example, clotting factors; or to reduce the requirement for replacement colloid. This "cascade filtration" has been found useful for the selective removal of IgM; however, a membrane to give adequate separation of IgG and albumin does not yet exist. The technique is not widely used.

Cell separators involve the centrifugal removal of plasma, by either a continuous or discontinuous flow system. Blood is pumped into the centrifuge bowl, and, in the continuous-flow technique, cells and plasma are separately removed from different ports on the bowl. In the discontinuous system, following the separation and removal of the plasma, centrifugation is stopped to allow reinfusion of the cells to the patient. Approximately 500 mL of blood are processed with each cycle. The discontinuous system has the disadvantages of being slower and requiring a larger extracorporeal volume than the continuous.

The vascular access required and complications of the procedure are similar for both methods, although the precise biologic effects may differ. For example, exposure to an artificial surface, as occurs during membrane filtration, may lead to complement activation and cell damage. The replacement colloid currently preferred is 5% human albumin solution, as the risk of associated complications is low, although the possibility of hemorrhage is an indication for the use of FFP. The short intravascular half-life of synthetic plasma expanders precludes their use as the main fluid replacement in intensive treatment courses of plasmapheresis.

The rate of clearance of individual molecules varies and is determined not only by their intravascular and extravascular distributions but also by their rates of synthesis and breakdown (8). These factors will therefore dictate the efficiency of the procedure and the frequency at which it is required. For example, one 4-litre plasma exchange will cause a 60% reduction in serum IgG and will deplete body stores by 20% (9). The autoantibody synthesis rate is variable between patients, even in the absence of immunosuppressive modulation, so that accurate measurement of levels (where possible) may be invaluable for planning frequency of plasmapheresis therapy.

Systems for Immunoadsorption

The system using protein A as an immunoadsorbent (Excorim) will be discussed as the prototype (10). In this technique plasma is first separated from other components of blood by plasma filtration and then pumped sequentially over one of two protein A columns in parallel. Each column has a volume of 62.5 mL and a capacity to bind approximately 1.5 g of antibody. They are perfused alternately and regenerated during their resting phase using a pH gradient. This alternating system theoretically allows antibody to be removed indefinitely, and it eliminates the need for a column of sufficient size to deplete the plasma of a significant proportion of Ig. Anticoagulation is maintained by low-dose heparin (for the plasma filter) and acid citrate dextrose (for the IA columns). The treated plasma is returned to the patient with the separated blood cells, so no plasma substitute is required. In a typical treatment session, two to three plasma volumes (5 to 7 litres) are processed, and this procedure takes 4 to 6 hours. The incidence of side effects using this system is extremely low, probably because of the negligible release of protein A from the columns. A variety of adverse effects have, however, been reported using different systems (11).

Mechanisms of Action

Plasmapheresis

Several explanations may account for the beneficial effects of plasmapheresis.

1. Removal of pathogenic autoantibodies has been suggested as a main mechanism of action, and this is a compelling explanation for the improvement seen in diseases such as anti-GBM disease, myasthenia gravis, and Eaton-Lambert syndrome (4,12,13). Improvement is not inevitable in autoantibody-associated diseases, which may reflect either the transient, and possibly ineffectual, lowering of antibody levels; the presence of these antibodies as epiphenomena rather than as pathogenic molecules; or the late institution of this therapy after tissue damage has already become established. Removal of antibody may stimulate B-cell proliferation and hence further antibody production (14). These stimulated cells will be sensitized to the effects of cytotoxic drugs, which may have implications for the optimal timing of immunosuppressive drugs used in conjunction with plasmapheresis (15).
2. Circulating immune complexes may be found in many diseases such as systemic lupus erythematosus (SLE) and mixed essential cryoglobulinemia (MEC). Although their pathogenicity has not been proved, their detection prompted the use of plasmapheresis in these conditions. It is now believed that tissue immune complexes usually arise from in situ formation; therefore removal of circulating complexes is probably less relevant than that of autoantibodies.
3. Impairment of the function of the reticuloendothelial system (RES) may be demonstrated in patients with vasculitis, SLE, and MEC, as evidenced by clearance of isotope-labelled, antibody-coated, senescent red blood cells (16–18). This clearance improves following plasmapheresis, and levels of immune complexes may continue to fall further thereafter, indicating that the beneficial effect on clearance may be maintained for some time. Clearance of microaggregated albumin has also been shown to improve following plasmapheresis in SLE (19).

Other theories have been suggested, generally with little substantiating evidence. No reproducible alterations in lymphocyte populations have been observed. The depletion of complement components or cytokines may explain therapeutic efficacy and remains an attractive, yet unproven, hypothesis. However, removal of other immunologically active compounds may also contribute to the therapeutic efficacy of plasmapheresis.

Immunoadsorption

Three different approaches have been taken to IA (20).

1. The chemical interactions between immunoglobulins and amino acids such as tryptophan and phenylalanine have been used. This binding process may depend on charge, as well as noncovalent hydrophobic interactions, which are semiselective for Ig but not specific. A relatively greater removal of

certain autoantibodies, for example, anti–acetyl choline receptor antibodies, than of total Ig has been reported using such devices, although this is difficult to explain.

2. In widest clinical use at present, the interaction between staphylococcal protein A and the Fc portion of Ig has been utilized (10,21). Protein A is a cell wall component of staphylococci that has particular affinity for IgG subclasses 1, 2, and 4, but will also bind IgG$_3$, IgA, and IgM. This approach allows selective, but again not specific, antibody removal.

3. The covalent binding between a specific antigen and the F(ab)$_2$ portion of Ig has been used. Although there are few clinical studies in this area, the specificity of the interaction offers considerable therapeutic advantages, and this is the approach that seems likely to be pursued in the future. Since there are practical difficulties and potential hazards in using naturally occurring antigens, further development of this approach depends on the production of synthetic or recombinant antigens in the correct conformation.

There are several advantages to IA over plasmapheresis in situations where antibody removal itself is the important factor in treatment (10). Since clotting components are not removed, there is less risk of bleeding and less need for the potentially hazardous FFP, the use of which has been associated with the most serious reactions to plasmapheresis. Avoidance of a plasma substitute also reduces the risk of transmission of infectious agents, particularly viruses. Hemodynamic disturbances are less common, particularly when compared with intermittent flow cell centrifugation. IA also has theoretic advantages in terms of the efficiency of removal of antibodies when large volumes of plasma are treated (20). When specific as opposed to selective IA is used, then there is the additional advantage of removing only the pathogenic antibody, while leaving those of other specificities that are perhaps essential to the host's repertoire of defense against infection.

Disease Applications

Ideally, plasmapheresis and, more particularly, IA should be considered for disorders in which circulating factors such as antibodies have been clearly shown to contribute significantly to disease pathogenesis. Assays for these should be available to guide treatment, and their removal should lead to improvement. In most cases long-term IA is not feasible, so the disease should be self-limiting or be amenable to control by other therapeutic agents, at least in the longer term. An important prerequisite is that it should be possible to purify or synthesize the ligand for IA in sufficient quantities, and it should be conformationally stable on the column. In practice, both procedures have often been introduced empirically, rarely justifiable except in uncommon, severe diseases or in the context of a controlled trial.

This section will only consider the use of IA and plasmapheresis in immune-mediated diseases, although immunologic interactions could also be used to remove other pathogenic molecules. For example, lipoproteins can be removed by the use of columns carrying antilipoprotein antibodies.

Renal Diseases

Anti–Glomerular Basement Membrane Disease

In anti-GBM disease an autoimmune response is mounted to the noncollagenous domain of the α3 chian of type IV collagen present in the alveolar and glomerular basement membranes (22). The prognosis of the disease if untreated is dismal, with mortality approaching 90% (23,24). Following the demonstration of the pathogenicity of the autoantibody (25), the aim of treatment has become the removal of this antibody from the circulation, together with immunosuppression by cytotoxic drugs to prevent further synthesis. Lockwood et al in 1975 (4) first described the resultant striking clinical improvement in predialysis patients, compared with historic controls. An aggressive regimen of plasmapheresis was used—daily 4-litre exchanges for 14 days. Antibody titres fell rapidly, there was improvement in the serum creatinine levels of the predialysis patients, and pulmonary hemorrhage was controlled in the majority of patients. Plasmapheresis, in combination with immunosuppression, is now established as the treatment of choice in patients with independent renal function, although success depends on prompt, early use (26–28). With the evolution of more selective immunotherapy, a few cases have now been successfully treated using protein A IA (29).

A retrospective analysis of 29 patients treated with immunosuppression and plasma exchange revealed that 41% of patients showed improved renal function, and this proportion rose to 66% when patients with initial oligoanuria were excluded (30). Effective anti-GBM antibody removal is well documented, most notably with the intensive regimen as described above (31).

Although widely accepted, there has been a lack of controlled evidence supporting the use of plasmapheresis in anti-GBM disease. Johnson et al (32) described benefit in a small series of 17 patients, with improvement in 1 of 9 patients randomized to receive immunosuppressive treatment only, compared with 4 of 8 who additionally received plasmapheresis. This trial used a nonintensive regimen, with 4-litre exchanges every 3 days. Generally, daily 4-litre exchanges for 14 days are considered necessary to achieve optimal lowering of antibody levels, with continuation to 30 days if autoantibody levels remain elevated or there is persistent pulmonary hemorrhage (30,33).

Patients who are oligoanuric at presentation tend to respond less well, and, in the absence of lung hemorrhage, plasmapheresis is not usually indicated (31,34–36). The exceptions are those who on renal biopsy have favorable features such as evidence of superimposed vasculitis or a relatively low proportion of either crescents or sclerosed glomeruli (28), or those in whom from a clinical viewpoint there is reason to believe that acute tubular necrosis may be a contributory factor. An additional indication would be prior to renal transplantation, in the unusual patient in whom antibody levels persist (37). Recurrence of anti-GBM disease is unusual, and successfully treated patients have a good long-term prognosis.

Renal Vasculitis: Focal Necrotizing Glomerulonephritis

Rapidly progressive glomerulonephritis (RPGN) associated with crescent formation may develop during the course of several renal diseases, and this section will consider that associated with the small vessel vasculitides, Wegener's granulomatosis (WG), and microscopic polyangiitis. A renal limited form of vasculitis is also seen, referred to as idiopathic RPGN. These conditions are characterized histologically by a pauci-immune, focal necrotizing glomerulonephritis and the presence of circulating autoantibodies to monocyte and neutrophil cytoplasm, the antineutrophil cytoplasm antibodies (ANCA) (38,39). Although their role in pathogenesis remains controversial (40), several lines of evidence implicate ANCA in the development of vasculitic injury (41). The development of specific immunoaffinity depletion may be an alternative, future treatment possibility since recombinant forms of both the major ANCA autoantigens proteinase 3 (Pr3) and myeloperoxidase (MPO) have been produced.

Systemic vasculitis with RPGN usually responds well to immunosuppressive drug regimens, particularly when cyclophosphamide is used early in the course of the disease, and 80% of patients may be expected to show at least an initial improvement (42). The role for plasmapheresis remains controversial and is not yet clearly established, as demonstration of any additional benefit requires the study of large numbers of patients. Early, uncontrolled trials suggested improved outcome (43–49); however, later, more rigorous, randomized trials have often failed to demonstrate benefit. The determination of the benefit of plasmapheresis has been clouded by several confounding factors. The studies have frequently included patients with other causes of RPGN such as Henoch-Schönlein purpura, lupus nephritis, and infection-related glomerulonephritis. Also patients are not consistently stratified for degree of renal injury at entry, and plasmapheresis may not be carried out at the optimal frequency with sufficient volume removal.

Glöckner et al (50) reported the results of a multicentre, randomized, prospective trial of intensive plasmapheresis and immunosuppression versus immunosuppression alone in the treatment of necrotizing, crescentic glomerulonephritis. Twenty-six patients were enrolled, of whom 21 had idiopathic RPGN; the remainder had WG, IgA nephropathy, lupus nephritis, polyarteritis nodosa, or scleroderma. All renal biopsies showed crescent formation in greater than 70% glomeruli, with a creatinine clearance of less than 50 mL/minute. Twelve patients were dialysis dependent at the time of presentation. Immunosuppression consisted initially of oral methylprednisolone (1.5 mg/kg/day) with oral cyclophosphamide (3 mg/kg/day) and oral azathioprine (1 mg/kg/day). Plasmapheresis was carried out three times a week.

After 4 weeks, nonresponders in the immunosuppression-only group were offered plasmapheresis. Plasmapheresis was discontinued after 4 weeks in the nonresponders in the plasmapheresis-plus-immunosuppression group. Eight of 11 patients (73%) receiving immunosuppressive therapy alone and monitored for at least 8 weeks were considered responders on the basis of improved serum creatinine levels, including three of

the four patients initially requiring dialysis. After 6 months, the average serum creatinine had fallen from 619 μmol/L (pretreatment) to 221 μmol/L. Nine of 13 patients (69%) who additionally received plasmapheresis were improved at 8 weeks, including five of the eight who were dialysis dependent initially. At 6 months, the average serum creatinine had fallen from 548 μmol/L (pretreatment) to 248 μmol/L.

Although the eventual extent of recovery was similar in both groups, the speed of response was more rapid in those receiving additional plasmapheresis (50% response rate at 4 weeks, compared with 33% in the immunosuppression-alone group). The extent of improvement of the dialysis-dependent patients was also greater in those receiving plasmapheresis (average serum creatinine at 6 months 150 μmol/L versus 486 μmol/L), but the number of patients (12) was too small to draw any definite conclusions. Similar good response rates to immunosuppressive therapy alone have been reported by others using a variety of regimens (51–53).

The benefit to patients who are dialysis dependent at presentation was also demonstrated by Pusey et al (54) who in 1991 reported the results of a randomized, prospective trial in which patients with vasculitis or idiopathic RPGN received either prednisolone and cytotoxic drugs alone or additional plasmapheresis. The only statistically significant benefit was seen in the group requiring dialysis, in which 10 of 11 plasmapheresis patients, compared with 3 of 8 control patients, had recovered renal function after 4 weeks of treatment (P = .041). Long-term prognosis was difficult to assess because of the small numbers and the death of several patients; however, those who did survive maintained independent renal function.

Cole et al (55) published the results of a study involving similar treatment regimens in a similar patient population, although the immunosuppressive therapy consisted of pulse intravenous methylprednisolone with azathioprine as the sole cytotoxic agent. Eleven of 32 patients enrolled were dialysis dependent, and 3 of 4 of the plasmapheresis group subsequently recovered independent renal function, compared with 2 of 7 receiving immunosuppression alone. Of the nondialyzed patients, similar improvements were seen in each treatment group (7 of 9 receiving immunosuppression alone; 8 of 12 receiving additional plasmapheresis). These improvement rates were comparable with the previous trials, despite the differences in immunosuppressive drugs used.

Pooling the results of these three trials, 26 of 31 patients (84%) who did not require dialysis responded to an immunosuppressive regimen alone. Of the dialysis-dependent patients, 77% of those treated with additional plasmapheresis improved, compared with 42% of those who received immunosuppression alone. Therefore, in contrast to anti-GBM disease, patients with systemic vasculitis or idiopathic RPGN who are dialysis dependent at presentation are the group most likely to benefit from intensive plasmapheresis. There have also been encouraging reports of the use of protein A IA in these patients (56,57), suggesting that more specific forms of IA using immobilized recombinant autoantigen might be advantageous. A comparable benefit has been described for the initial use of methylprednisolone (52), and a direct comparison of the two treatment options is currently under way (58).

Plasmapheresis may also be helpful in the management of patients with intractable disease, refractory to conventional immunosuppressive drugs, and for those in whom these drugs have produced intolerable side effects such as profound myelotoxicity.

Systemic Lupus Erythematosus

Systemic lupus erythematosus (SLE) is a multisystem autoimmune disorder characterized by the presence of a polyclonal, multispecific, autoantibody response with related immune complexes, which follows a remitting and relapsing clinical course. Renal biopsies from patients with lupus nephritis show a wide variety of appearances, ranging from minimal histologic changes visible only by electron microscopy, to a fulminant, rapidly progressive glomerulonephritis with severe proliferative changes. The World Health Organization (WHO) classification is now widely accepted and provides a reproducible basis for the rationalization of treatment protocols. Additionally, this classification is strongly predictive of the ultimate outcome of renal function (59). The direct involvement of the autoantibodies in pathogenesis has not been demonstrated. Nevertheless, the active humoral immune response seen in these patients makes plasmapheresis theoretically an attractive therapeutic approach.

The use of plasmapheresis in SLE was first reported by Verrier-Jones et al (60), and following this many uncontrolled studies described benefit (61–66). Plasmapheresis acutely reduces levels of autoantibodies and immune complexes (67,68) and improves RES function with a sustained fall in immune complexes (16,18), but these serologic markers have not always correlated with a clinical improvement.

The Lupus Nephritis Study Group reported the results of a controlled trial of plasmapheresis therapy in severe lupus nephritis in 1992 (69). Patients with lesser degrees of glomerular involvement were excluded, as their prognosis is much more favorable irrespective of the type of therapy given. Eighty-six patients were recruited between April 1981 and September 1986, with renal biopsy changes of WHO type III (severe segmental and proliferative lupus nephritis with active or necrotizing lesions in less than 50% of the glomeruli), type IV (diffuse proliferative nephritis), or type V (membranous nephritis with superimposed severe segmental or diffuse proliferative changes). All were dialysis independent at enrollment, with a serum creatinine less than 530 μmol/L. Patients were randomized to receive standard immunosuppression with prednisolone and cyclophosphamide, or similar immunosuppression with additional plasmapheresis, three times a week for 4 weeks. The trial was terminated after the results of studies in these 86 patients failed to show any additional benefit in the plasmapheresis-treated group. There were similar rates of death (6 of 46 in the conventional-therapy group versus 8 of 40 in the plasmapheresis group), progression to end-stage renal failure (8 of 46 versus 10 of 40), and disease remission (19 of 46 versus 16 of 40). Disease remission was considered to be a serum creatinine of less than 124 μmol/L and a 24-hour urinary

protein excretion of less than 0.3 g/day. Extended follow-up of these patients was continued until the spring of 1990, and again no differences in outcome were identified between the two treatment groups (69).

Although the clinical responses were similar in both groups, there was a marked difference in the serologic indices, with a more rapid and more profound decrease in serum concentrations of anti-dsDNA antibodies, cryoglobulins, and complement components C3 and C4 during the first 2 weeks of treatment with plasmapheresis. These results confirmed that the therapeutic aim to remove circulating, potentially pathogenic molecules had been achieved. It was subsequently argued that perhaps synchronized, high-dose pulse cyclophosphamide might have been more effective in preventing rebound B-cell proliferation and thereby would have allowed benefit from plasmapheresis to have been seen (70,71). The results of such a trial are still awaited. However, the rapid and sustained lowering of the serologic indices of lupus seen in the Lupus Nephritis Study Group trial suggests that adequate immunosuppression had occurred.

Despite these negative findings, plasmapheresis may still have a role to play in those patients with cerebral lupus or lung hemorrhage (72) and in those who prove refractory to, or intolerant of, standard immunosuppressive regimes. Small numbers of patients have been treated by IA, using protein A or dextran sulphate (57,73,74). Effective removal of anti-DNA antibodies has also been achieved using a column bearing salmon DNA (75). However, as with plasmapheresis, there have been no convincing clinical consequences of such treatment.

Focal Segmental Glomerulosclerosis

Hoyer et al (76) first described the recurrence of focal segmental glomerulosclerosis (FSGS) following renal transplantation, and since then the search for the putative circulating factor implicated in pathogenesis has continued. Plasmapheresis and IA have been used by several groups in an attempt to remove this serum factor, with varying degrees of success (77–81). The recurrence rate in grafts following transplantation is approximately 30% (82), and it is in the treatment of this group that most experience has accumulated. The inclusion of cyclosporin in the immunosuppressive regimen has modified the course of recurrent disease, but has not reduced its incidence (83,84). Indeed, these patients may be more susceptible to cyclosporin nephrotoxicity (85).

Encouraging results were recently reported by Artero et al (86). A group of nine patients was studied, all of whom had biopsy-proven FSGS as their primary diagnosis. Recurrent proteinuria greater than 3 g/24 hours had developed in all nine at an average of 28 days posttransplantation (range 9 to 91 days), and recurrent FSGS was confirmed by renal transplant biopsy. Plasmapheresis was carried out on 3 consecutive days and then alternate days for a total of nine sessions. Six of nine patients in whom the diagnosis of recurrent FSGS was made and in whom plasmapheresis was initiated within 1 week of the onset of proteinuria achieved clinical remissions, with proteinuria decreasing in these patients from a mean of 11 g/24 hours of 2 g/24 hours.

Three of the nine patients did not respond to plasmapheresis; of these, one had had proteinuria for 12 weeks before commencing plasmapheresis and two had evidence of established hyalinosis on renal biopsy. Two patients subsequently relapsed and a repeat course of plasmapheresis was successful in inducing remission. The conclusions of this study were that plasmapheresis is effective in reducing the proteinuria of recurrent FSGS following transplantation, provided it is instituted early and before the development of glomerular scarring.

Patients treated with IA by protein A columns have also shown improvement (87). In these studies, eight patients with recurrent proteinuria following transplantation received one to three cycles of two to seven sessions of protein adsorption. The results in individual patients were variable, but the average reduction in proteinuria following a treatment cycle was 82%. Proteinuria subsequently returned to pretreatment levels in all but one patient over the next 2 months. Compared with the study by Artero et al, immunotherapy was initiated much later, usually several weeks after the onset of proteinuria, which may explain the variability of the results. Both groups confirmed the removal of an abnormal plasma constituent capable of inducing proteinuria. Artero et al (86) demonstrated the presence of a factor capable of increasing permeability to albumin in isolated rat glomeruli, and Dantal et al (87) provoked proteinuria in rats by injecting the eluate from the protein A columns used in treatment.

Plasmapheresis has also been used together with oral prednisolone and intravenous cyclophosphamide in the treatment of native kidney FSGS (88). Eleven patients with persistent proteinuria despite prolonged treatment with oral prednisolone (initially 1 to 2 mg/kg, tapering after 3 to 4 months to 10 mg daily) and subsequent cyclophosphamide (5 to 10 mg/kg monthly for three doses, then alternate months to a total of 10 doses) received additional plasmapheresis (17 sessions of 2-litre exchanges over 6 months). One month after the last plasmapheresis session, eight of eleven patients were in clinical remission, which was maintained at 6 months in six of eleven.

Although results increasingly suggest benefit for plasmapheresis and IA in the treatment of recurrent FSGS, a prospective controlled trial is needed to confirm efficacy.

Renal Transplantation

Pretransplantation.   Plasmapheresis has been used successfully to treat highly sensitized recipients prior to renal transplantation. Such patients now constitute approximately 20% of the dialysis population, and transplantation has previously been considered contraindicated, as the presence of the antibodies can be responsible for hyperacute rejection. High panel reactivity frequently correlates with antibodies that recognize a restricted number of human leukocyte antigens (HLA), which are present in high titres and give a high incidence of positive cross matches. Taube et al (89) reported the successful transplantation of four of five highly sensitized patients treated with intensive PE, together with prednisolone and cyclophosphamide, to prevent resynthesis of

anti-HLA antibodies. Their success has subsequently been repeated by other groups (90).

The use of IA columns has had variable success (91–94). Initial results with the use of protein A columns were promising (95), with seven of eight transplanted patients in this study having functioning allografts at 12 to 18 months. Experience elsewhere has shown a similar favorable outcome (96). However, Esnault et al (97) treated six hyperimmunized patients with protein A IA and immunosuppression with prednisolone and cyclophosphamide, but were unable to transplant four patients because of the persistence of the anti-HLA antibodies. Of the two patients transplanted, one developed early vascular rejection and died of infection on day 40. The other returned to hemodialysis on day 285, with graft failure resulting from transplant glomerulopathy.

Modified pretransplantation IA has also been carried out using a tryptophan column (98), together with immunosuppression as above. Five of eight patients were successfully transplanted, and, of the three grafts lost, only one was the result of rejection. Similarly, because in some instances organ transplantation is precluded by blood group (ABO) incompatibility, protein A IA has been used to remove anti-A or anti-B alloantibodies. A more specific approach has used A or B antigens (99,100). In one series, using A or B antigens bound to a silicon column, 60 patients were treated of whom 47 received a transplant, and for 37 this produced a good outcome (99).

Posttransplantation.   After transplantation, the development of anti-HLA antibodies against mismatched antigens has been associated with vascular rejection, as has the finding of antiendothelial antibodies (101). In a nonrandomized study, Vangelista et al (102) demonstrated that plasmapheresis and cyclophosphamide reduced anti-HLA antibodies to undetectable levels after two to five exchanges; this reduction was maintained after cessation of plasmapheresis. Titres were unchanged by pulse methylprednisolone or cyclophosphamide alone, and removal of the antibodies was associated with an improvement in renal function. A more recent study supported these findings (103), although this remains controversial (104,105). Gurland et al (106) presented a review of the literature concerning the use of plasmapheresis for both acute and chronic rejection. No benefit was found, possibly a reflection of the heterogeneity of the patient population.

Two controlled trials (107,108) have shown improved graft survival following the treatment of acute-rejection episodes with plasmapheresis. However, in the Bonomini trial the rejection episodes occurred unusually late following transplantation, at a mean of 10 months; in the Cardella trial there was no significant difference in graft survival when only patients given blood transfusions prior to transplantation were considered. The effective application of plasmapheresis for rejection following transplantation will probably be limited to those patients with high titres of anti-HLA antibodies, although there are as yet no studies comparing plasmapheresis with other second-line treatment strategies for rejection such as antilymphocyte globulin and monoclonal antibodies.

Alport's disease is most commonly inherited as an X-linked recessive disorder, although both autosomal dominant and recessive inheritance has been described (109). The X-linked disease is caused by the abnormal expression of the gene for the noncollagenous domain of the α5 chain of type IV collagen (110). Following transplantation, recipients may uncommonly develop anti-GBM antibodies directed to the α5 chain, to which they are not immunologically tolerant. Rarely, this may result in frank nephritis and graft loss (111,112): in these unusual patients plasmapheresis may be effective treatment, as it is in primary anti-GBM disease.

Other Renal Diseases

Although immunologic mechanisms are implicated in the development of many other types of glomerular injury, there is no conclusive evidence supporting a role for the use of plasmapheresis in the treatment of other forms of glomerulonephritis. Anecdotally, benefit has been reported in mesangial IgA disease with crescent formation (113,114), mesangiocapillary glomerulonephritis (115–117), and membranous nephropathy; however, these results have not been substantiated by larger, controlled, randomized trials (118–120).

Neurologic Disease

Myasthenia Gravis

The autoantibodies to the acetyl choline receptor (AChR) present in myasthenia gravis are known to be pathogenic, and early reports of the benefit of plasmapheresis have been widely confirmed (12,121). A clinical response is generally seen after about 2 days, but electrophysiologic improvement can be detected earlier (122,123). Rebound of antibody synthesis can be prevented by concomitant treatment with immunosuppressive drugs. Plasmapheresis has a clear role in the short-term improvement of acute severe myasthenia, especially to relieve the weakness of respiration or swallowing. It may also be used to control symptoms pending the effects of thymectomy or drug therapy. However, on the basis of uncontrolled studies, there is probably no role for plasmapheresis in long-term management (124). The Lambert Eaton syndrome, cased by autoantibodies to the calcium channel on the presynaptic nerve terminal, also responds to plasmapheresis, although more slowly than myasthenia gravis (13).

Considerable experience has now accumulated in the treatment of myasthenia gravis by IA. The anti-AChR antibodies can be removed, with increasing specificity, by using tryptophan, protein A, or synthetic AChR (125–127).

Inflammatory Polyneuropathy

There were several reports of the benefit of plasmapheresis in acute, inflammatory, demyelinating polyneuropathy (Guillain-Barré syndrome). These are now supported by the results from two large controlled trials. Both the Guillain-Barré Study Group (245 patients) (128) and the French randomized trial (188 patients) (129) demonstrated benefit from plasmapheresis in the short term and at 6 months. Patients treated within 1 week of onset, or if ventilator dependent, improved if given five 50 mL/kg exchanges within the first 7 to 14 days. Similar results have been achieved using protein A IA (130). A comparable response may be seen with intravenous immunoglobulin (IVIg), which has the advantage of ease of administration (85,131).

There are several anecdotal reports of benefit with plasmapheresis in chronic, inflammatory, demyelinating polyneuropathy, which runs a slowly progressive or relapsing course. One small controlled trial in patients with severe disease supported these reports; however, larger trials with longer follow-up are required (132).

Multiple Sclerosis

Evidence is increasing that multiple sclerosis (MS) is an autoimmune disease, although cellular rather than humoral mechanisms are receiving most attention. However, recent work suggests that antimyelin oligodendrocyte glycoprotein (MOG) antibodies may be important in pathogenesis. Plasmapheresis has been studied in several uncontrolled series and controlled trials; however, these are difficult to interpret because of the tendency of symptoms in MS to undergo remission and exacerbation over long periods (5). On balance, there is insufficient evidence to recommend plasmapheresis widely. It may be helpful to patients with severe acute attacks or those with frequently relapsing disease (133). Successful results have also been achieved using protein A IA (134).

Hematologic Disease

Myeloma and Cryoglobulinemia

In myeloma or macroglobulinemia associated with hyperviscosity syndrome, plasmapheresis is the logical choice for short-term treatment. In acute renal failure related to myeloma, possibly caused by obstruction of, or toxicity to, the renal tubules by myeloma protein, the role of plasmapheresis is unclear. Several uncontrolled studies suggest that plasmapheresis is of benefit in recovery of renal function (135). One controlled trial (29 patients) concluded that renal function was more likely to recover in patients given at least five exchanges in addition to chemotherapy (136). However, a more recent trial (21 patients) failed to show any benefit from plasmapheresis (137).

In type I cryoglobulinemia, characterized by a monoclonal cryoglobulin of unknown specificity, symptoms related to hyperviscosity or peripheral cryoprecipitation generally respond well to plasmapheresis (138). In type II cryoglobulinemia, characterized by a monoclonal rheumatoid factor (usually IgM) complexed with polyclonal IgG, symptoms are more often related to deposition of immune complexes. These are efficiently removed by plasmapheresis, but tend to rebound rapidly in the absence of immunosuppression. Many clinical features, especially of skin and joints, improve promptly following plasmapheresis. Renal disease, usually in the form of mesangiocapillary glomerulonephritis, may also respond, but evidence for long-term benefit is unclear (139,140). The close association of type II cryoglobulins with hepatitis C virus is promoting a reexamination of treatment approaches; however, plasmapheresis still has a role in severe, acute disease. Type III cryoglobulinemia, characterized by polyclonal rheumatoid factors complexed with polyclonal IgG, is usually secondary to a wide range of infective, inflammatory, or neoplastic disease. Treatment is directed at the underlying disease, but plasmapheresis may be of short-term benefit for cryoglobulin-related symptoms.

Thrombotic Thrombocytopenic Purpura

Plasmapheresis is widely reported to be effective in thrombotic thrombocytopenic purpura (TTP), recently reported to develop in association with an autoantibody directed against von Willebrand factor–cleaving protease (141,142). A similar beneficial effect has been observed by some following infusion of FFP or cryosupernatant alone (143,144). A recent trial of 102 patients showed that plasmapheresis for TTP led to an improved outcome, both short term and at six months, compared with controls given FFP infusions only (6). However, the plasmapheresis groups received more FFP, and whether the effect of plasmapheresis relates to the more intensive replacement of deficient factors or to removal of pathogenic factors remains unclear. Nonetheless, plasmapheresis remains the most effective treatment available for TTP. The effectiveness of plasmapheresis in the management of the hemolytic uraemic syndrome (HUS) has been studied less intensively. The clinical presentation may be similar to that of TTP, and in such cases plasmapheresis may be warranted. Postdiarrheal HUS in children usually resolves spontaneously, but plasmapheresis may be considered in adults with severe or persistent disease.

Idiopathic Thrombocytopenia Purpura

Immune thrombocytopenia purpura (ITP) is associated with antiplatelet antibodies which lead to the splenic destruction of platelets. There are several anecdotal reports and two uncontrolled studies suggesting benefit from plasmapheresis (145,146). ITP usually responds to splenectomy, to treatment with immunosuppressive drugs, or to IVIg, and the future role of plasmapheresis is likely to remain limited to refractory cases.

Alloantibodies in Hematologic Disease

Alloantibodies to factor VIII and factor IX can limit effective treatment for hemophiliacs, and PE has been used together with the appropriate factor infusion in the management of severe hemorrhage (147). Protein A IA has been described to reduce the alloantibody titres and to allow a better response to clotting factors (148). Plasmapheresis is the treatment of choice for severe, posttransfusion purpura, associated with antiplatelet antibodies (149).

Rheumatologic Disease

Plasmapheresis has been widely used in the treatment of severe rheumatoid arthritis, associated with rheumatoid factor, either alone or as part of a lymphoplasmapheresis procedure. Unfortunately, a review of the literature does not provide support for benefit in the majority of patients (5). Most trials have given unconvincing results or shown only short-term improvement. For example, one controlled crossover trial of plasmapheresis in 26 patients who had failed to respond to drug therapy, showed no significant clinical change despite improvement in several laboratory parameters. More convincingly, success has been claimed in patients with rheumatoid vasculitis, and further controlled studies are needed in this subset of patients (150).

There are also claims of benefit, on the basis of small series or case reports, in the early stages of scleroderma, dermatomyositis, polymyositis, Sjogren's syndrome, and Behçet's disease. However, as with rheumatoid arthritis, a controlled trial of plasmapheresis in 39 patients with dermatomyositis or polymyositis failed to confirm advantage (151). There is insufficient evidence to recommend plasmapheresis in these disorders.

Several studies, including one small controlled trial, have suggested amelioration of severe Raynaud's phenomenon following plasmapheresis (152). It will clearly reduce plasma viscosity in these patients, which may account for the effect, and would seem a reasonable approach in those with severe digital ischemia unresponsive to other therapy.

Dermatologic Disease

Pemphigus vulgaris is associated with antibodies to the squamous epithelium, and there are many reports of the use of plasmapheresis for severe disease. However, not all studies support a role for plasmapheresis, and its use should perhaps be restricted to severe, steroid-resistant cases (153–155). Similarly, bullous pemphigoid, associated with antibodies to the dermal basement membrane, has been reported to respond to plasmapheresis (156).

Numerous other skin diseases, in which immune mechanisms are less clear, have also been treated by plasmapheresis (157). A subgroup of patients with severe, drug-resistant cutaneous vasculitis have been reported to improve following long-term intermittent plasmapheresis (158). Other disorders treated include pyoderma gangrenosum, dermatitis herpetiformis, herpes gestationis, and acquired bullous epidermolysis, but the evidence for benefit is generally lacking.

Complications

Plasmapheresis is generally a safe procedure when possible complications are anticipated and corrective steps taken. A recent study evaluated all plasmapheresis procedures carried out at the University of Connecticut over a period of 30 months, comprising 699 treatments (159). Their incidence of complications (9.7%) was compared with a review of the literature, giving a total of 15,658 treatments. A similar rate of side effects was seen with both the centrifugal and membrane systems, and the majority were described as mild/moderate. However, eight of the 15,658 patients died at a time when plasmapheresis was felt to be contributory. Because of the different techniques involved, the incidence of complications related to IA is even lower.

Wide-bore vascular access is prone to the same complications as when inserted for other procedures such as hemodialysis, namely, pneumothorax at the time of insertion, catheter related thrombosis and infection, and bleeding at the time of removal. Episodes of hypovolemia may occur, particularly when using the discontinuous flow system and when fluids hypo-oncotic to plasma are used. Hypocalcemia is reported to occur in 1.5% to 9% of treatments (160,161) and is a result of citrate infusion, either as an anticoagulant for the procedure or in FFP, which contains approximately 14% citrate by volume. Hypocalcemia is detected more frequently when FFP rather than albumin is used as the replacement fluid (162). Although usually manifest as only perioral or distal extremity parasthesias, there is often also lengthening of the QT interval on the electrocardiogram, thus predisposing to cardiac arrhythmias (163). In patients receiving repeated treatments over a prolonged period, significant loss of calcium may occur. These complications are readily prevented by prophylactic infusion of calcium (164).

The risk of hypokalemia is reduced by ensuring the presence of potassium in the replacement fluid. Metabolic alkalosis can result from the infusion of citrate and its subsequent metabolism to release bicarbonate. In most patients, this is compensated and no rise in serum bicarbonate is seen (165). However, alkalosis may develop following repeated treatments if renal failure is also present (166). These patients are also at particular risk of accumulating aluminum, present in albumin solutions, although bone deposition of aluminum in a patient with normal renal function has been described (167,168).

When albumin is used as the replacement fluid, there is significant depletion of all the coagulation factors to between 20% and 50% of the original levels; however, bleeding episodes are rare (162,169,170). Following a single plasma exchange, the recovery of coagulation-factor levels is biphasic, with an initial rapid increase in the first 4 hours, followed by a more gradual increase over the next 4 to 24 hours. Antithrombin III (AT III) and fibrinogen require 72 hours for complete recovery. The partial thromboplastin time is doubled immediately posttreatment and returns to normal 4 hours later, whereas the prothrombin ratio increases by 30% posttreatment and requires 24 hours to normalise (169). When multiple cycles are performed over a relatively short time such as three times a week, spontaneous recovery of coagulation-factor levels may take several days, and their replacement with FFP is advised (171,172).

Platelet counts may also fall, and this is usually more profound with the centrifugal method when a decrease of 50% may occur (173,174). Paradoxically, episodes of thrombosis (such as pulmonary embolism, cerebral ischemia, or myocardial infarction) suggesting a hypercoagulable state may occur, possibly related to the lowering of AT III levels (175). Hemolysis is a theoretic concern with membrane-based techniques, but does not seem to occur (159).

Infection may develop postplasmapheresis as a result of depletion of immunoglobulin levels; however, the true incidence of this is difficult to estimate as patients will often also be receiving immunosuppressive drugs. Early studies described an increase in opportunistic infections following plasmapheresis, but these patients often had a neutropenia, more likely as a result of immunosuppressive drugs than plasmapheresis per se (176). Neither the Lupus Nephritis Collaborative Study Group (177) nor reports of the treatment of patients with myasthenia gravis showed an increased incidence of infection (121,124). However, should a severe infection develop in the period following plasmapheresis, infusion of immunoglobulin may be prudent, in a dose similar to that recommended for patients with hypogammaglobulinemia (178).

Transmission of infection may occur rarely with FFP. Albumin and immunoglobulin are heat treated, which inactivates hepatitis and the human immunodeficiency virus (179), although these may survive in FFP, as may bacteria and endotoxin (180). There has been recent concern about the theoretic possibility of the transfer of transmissible spongiform encephalopathy by blood products.

Reactions to albumin are unusual (1.4% in the above study) but relatively common when FFP is used (20%). These are anaphylactoid in nature, comprising fever, rigors, urticaria, wheezing, and hypotension (181). The majority of deaths associated with plasmapheresis occur in those patients where FFP is given (182,183). Potential reasons for the anaphylaxis seen with FFP include the presence of a prekallikrein activator and bradykinin (or rarely, bacteria or endotoxin). In patients deficient in immunoglobulin A (IgA), anti-IgA antibodies may develop, giving a reaction when IgA-containing fluids are infused. The rare intolerance to albumin may be caused by the formation of antibody to polymerized albumin created by heat treatment (184). Membrane bioincompatibility, similar to that described during hemodialysis may occur (185), as may sensitivity to ethylene oxide used as a sterilizing agent (186).

Drug removal by plasmapheresis depends on the extent to which protein binding occurs. For example, only low levels of cyclophosphamide are bound, and therefore clearance is not significant, whereas azathioprine is 30% protein bound, and moderate amounts may be removed (187). Prednisolone is only minimally cleared by plasmapheresis (188). To avoid any potential lowering of blood levels, it is usual to administer all drugs following plasmapheresis.

Future Prospects

With increasing understanding of the mechanisms of autoimmunity, it should be possible to develop specific IA in a number of disorders. The feasibility of this approach has already been demonstrated in myasthenia gravis and SLE. Good candidates for future specific IA include anti-GBM disease and the systemic vasculitides, since the autoantigens involved have been identified. The expression of these antigens as recombinant proteins, which has already been achieved, should soon allow development of specific IA for clinical studies.

Another possible application for IA in the future is in the management of patients receiving xenografts. Xenotransplantation is an attractive alternative to allotransplantation because of the general lack of donor organs. Although there are a number of different immune barriers to be overcome, the removal of naturally occurring IgM xenoantibodies is likely to be important. These antibodies have cytotoxic effects and cause the equivalent of hyperacute rejection. Their removal may be achieved by IA, using columns bearing the appropriate synthetic antigen Gal (α1–3) Gal (189).

References

1. Abel JJ, Rowntree LG, Turner BB. Plasma removal with return of corpuscles. J Pharmacol Exp Ther 1914;5:625–641.
2. Skoog WA, Adams WS. Plasmapheresis in a case of Waldenstrom's macroglobulinaemia. Clin Res 1959;7:96–97.
3. Soloman A, Fahey JL. Plasmapheresis therapy in macroglobulinaemia. Ann Intern Med 1963;58:789–800.
4. Lockwood CM, Boulton-Jones JM, Lowenthal RM, et al. Recovery from Goodpasture's syndrome after immunosuppressive treatment and plasmapheresis. Br Med J 1975;2:252–254.
5. Mason PD, Pusey CD. Plasma exchange. 5th ed. Oxford, England: Blackwell Scientific, 1993:885–908.
6. Rock GA, Shumak KH, Buskard NA, et al. Comparison of plasma exchange with plasma infusion in the treatment of thrombotic thrombocytopaenic purpura. N Engl J Med 1991;325:393–397.
7. Malchesky PS, Bambauer R, Horiuchi T, et al. Apheresis technologies: an international perspective. Artif Organs 1995;19:315–324.
8. Derkson RHWM, Schuurman HJ, Gmelig Meyling FHJ, et al. The efficiency of plasma exchange in the removal of plasma components. J Lab Clin Med 1984;104:346–354.
9. Chopek M, McCullogh J. Protein and biochemical changes during plasmapheresis. Washington, DC: American Association of Blood Banks, 1980:13–52.
10. Gjorstrup P, Watt RM. Therapeutic protein A immunoadsorption: a review. Transfus Sci 1990;11:281–302.
11. Schiedu KM. Plasmapheresis and immunoadsorption: different techniques and their current role in medical therapy. Kidney Int 1998;53(S64):S61–S65.
12. Pinching AJ, Peters DK, Newsom-Davis J. Remission of myasthenia gravis following plasma exchange. Lancet 1976;2:1373–1376.
13. Newsom-Davis J, Murray N. Plasma exchange and immunosuppressive drug treatment in the Lambert-Easton syndrome. Neurology 1984;34:480–485.
14. Sturgill BC, Worzniak MJ. Stimulation of proliferation of 19S antibody-forming cells in the spleens of immunised guinea pigs after exchange transfusion. Nature 1970;228:1304–1305.
15. Schroeder JO, Euler HH, Loffler H. Synchronisation of plasmapheresis and pulse cyclophosphamide in severe lupus erythematosus. Ann Intern Med 1987;107:344–346.
16. Lockwood CM, Worlledge S, Nicholas A, et al. Reversal of impaired splenic function in patients with nephritis or vasculitis (or both) by plasma exchange. N Engl J Med 1979;300:524–530.
17. Frank MM, Hamburger MI, Lawley TJ, et al. Defective reticuloendothelial system Fc receptor function in systemic lupus erythematosus. N Engl J Med 1979;300:518–523.
18. Walport MJ, Peters AM, Elkon KB, et al. The splenic extraction ratio of antibody-coated erythrocytes and its response to plasma exchange and pulse methylprednisolone. Clin Exp Immunol 1985;60:465–473.
19. Law A, Hotze A, Krapf F, et al. The non-specific clearance function of the reticuloendothelial system in patients with immune complex–mediated diseases before and after plasmapheresis. Rheumatol Int 1985;5:69–72.
20. Kadar JG, Borberg H. Biocompatability of extracorporeal immunoadsorption systems. Extracorporeal Immunoadsorption Sys 1990;11:223–239.
21. Verrier-Jones J. Staphylococcal protein A as an extracorporeal immunosorben: theoretical and practical considerations. Transfus Sci 1990;11:153–159.
22. Turner N, Mason PJ, Brown R, et al. Molecular cloning of the Goodpasture antigen demonstrates it to be the alpha 3 chain of type IV collagen. J Clin Invest 1992;89:592–601.
23. Benoit FL, Rulon DB, Theil GB, et al. Goodpasture's syndrome: a clinicopathological entity. Am J Med 1964;37:424–444.
24. Proskey AJ, Weatherbee L, Easterling RE, et al. Goodpasture's syndrome: a report of 5 cases and a review of the literature. Am J Med 1970;48:162–173.
25. Lerner RA, Glassock RJ, Dixon FJ. The role of antiglomerular basement membrane antibody in the pathogenesis of human glomerulonephritis. J Exp Med 1967;126:989–1004.
26. Kincaid-Smith P, D'Apice AJF. Plasmapheresis in rapidly progressive glomerulonephritis. Am J Med 1978;65:564–566.
27. Erickson SB, Kurtz SB, Donadio JV, et al. Use of combined plasmapheresis and immunosuppression in the treatment of Goodpasture's syndrome. Mayo Clin Proc 1979;54:714–720.
28. Walker RG, Scheinkestal C, Becker GJ, et al. Clinical and morphological aspects of the management of crescentic anti-glomerular basement membrane antibody (anti-GBM) nephritis/Goodpasture's syndrome. Q J Med 1985;54:75–89.
29. Bygren P, Freiburghaus C, Lindholm T. Goodpasture's syndrome with staphylococcal protein A immunoadsorption. Lancet 1985;2:1295–1296.
30. Savage COS, Pusey CD, Bowman C, et al. Anti-glomerular basement membrane antibody mediated disease in the British Isles 1980–1984. Br Med J 1986;1:301–304.
31. Pusey CD, Lockwood CM, Peters DK. Plasma exchange and immunosuppressive drugs in the treatment of glomerulonephritis due to antibodies to the glomerular basement membrane. Int J Artif Organs 1983;6:15–18.
32. Johnson JP, Moore J, Austin HA, et al. Therapy of anti-glomerular basement membrane antibody disease: analysis of prognostic significance of clinical, pathologic and treatment factors. Medicine 1985;64:219–227.
33. Kelly PT, Haponik EF. Goodpasture syndrome: molecular and clinical advances. Medicine 1994;73:171–185.
34. Briggs WA, Johnson JP, Teichman S, et al. Anti-GBM antibody mediated glomerulonephritis and Goodpasture's syndrome. Medicine 1979;58:348–361.
35. Simpson IJ, Doak PB, Williams LC, et al. Plasma exchange in Goodpasture's syndrome. Am J Nephrol 1982;2:301–311.

36. Hind CRK, Paraskevakou H, Lockwood CM, et al. Prognosis after immunosuppression of patients with crescentic nephritis. Lancet 1983;1:263–265.

37. Flores JC, Taube D, Savage COS. Clinical and immunological evolution of oligoanuric anti-GBM nephritis treated by haemodialysis. Lancet 1986;1:5–8.

38. van der Woude FJ, Lobatto S, Permin H, et al. Autoantibodies against neutrophils and monocytes: a tool for diagnosis and marker of disease activity in Wegener's granulomatosis. Lancet 1985;1:425–429.

39. Savage COS, Winearls CG, Jones S, et al. Prospective study of radioimmunoassay for antibodies against neutrophil cytoplasm in diagnosis of systemic vasculitis. Lancet 1987;1:1389–1393.

40. Johnson RJ. The mystery of the antineutrophil cytoplasmic antibodies. Am J Kidney Dis 1995;26:57–61.

41. Kallenberg CGM, Brouwer E, Weening JJ, et al. Antineutrophil cytoplasm antibodies: current diagnostic and pathophsiological potential. Kidney Int 1994;46:1–15.

42. Glassock RJ. Intensive plasma exchange in crescentic glomerulonephritis: help or no help? Am J Kidney Dis 1992;20:270–275.

43. Becker GJ, D'Apice AJF, Walker RG, et al. Plasmapheresis in the treatment of glomerulonephritis. Med J Aust 1977;2:693–696.

44. D'Apice AJF, Kincaid-Smith P. Plasma exchange in the treatment of glomerulonephritis. In: Kincaid-Smith P, d'Apice AJF, Atkins RC, eds. Progress in glomerulonephritis. New York: Wiley, 1979:371–385.

45. Pusey CD, Lockwood CM. Plasma exchange for glomerular disease. In: Robinson RR, ed. Nephrology. New York: Springer Verlag, 1984:1474–1485.

46. Stevens ME, McConnell M, Bone JM. Aggressive treatment with pulse methylprednisolone or plasma exchange in rapidly progressive glomerulonephritis. Proc Eur Dial Transplant Assoc 1982;19:724–731.

47. Thysell H, Bygren P, Bengtsson U, et al. Immunosuppression and the additive effect of plasma exchange in the treatment of rapidly progressive glomerulonephritis. Acta Med Scand 1982;212:107–114.

48. Stevens ME, Bone JM. Follow-up prednisolone dosage in rapidly progressive crescentic glomerulonephritis treated with pulse methylprednisolone or plasma exchange. Proc Eur Dial Transplant Assoc 1984;21:594–599.

49. Burran WP, Avasthi P, Smith KJ, et al. Efficacy of plasma exchange in severe idiopathic rapidly progressive glomerulonephritis: a report of 10 cases. Transfusion 1986;26:382–387.

50. Glöckner WM, Sieberth HG, Wichmann H, et al. Plasma exchange and immunosuppression in rapidly progressive glomerulonephritis: a controlled, multicentre study. Clin Nephrol 1988;29:1–8.

51. Bruns FJ, Adler S, Fraley RS, et al. Long-term follow-up of aggressively treated idiopathic rapidly progressive glomerulonephritis. Am J Med 1989;86:400–406.

52. Bolton WK, Sturgill BC. Methylprednisolone therapy for acute crescentic rapidly progressive glomerulonephritis. Am J Nephrol 1989;9:368–375.

53. Kunis CL, Kiss B, Williams G, et al. Intravenous pulse cyclophosphamide therapy of crescentic glomerulonephritis. Clin Nephrol 1992;37:1–7.

54. Pusey CD, Rees AJ, Evans DJ, et al. Plasma exchange in focal necrotising glomerulonephritis without anti-GBM antibodies. Kidney Int 1991;40:757–763.

55. Cole E, Cattran D, Magil A, et al. A prospective randomised trial of plasma exchange as additive therapy in idiopathic crescentic glomerulonephritis. Am J Kidney Dis 1992;20:261–269.

56. Palmer A, Cairns T, Dische F, et al. Treatment of rapidly progressive glomerulonephritis by extracorporeal immunosorption, prednisolone and cyclophosphamide. Nephrol Dial Transplant 1991;6:536–542.

57. Esnault VL, Testa A, Jayne DRW, et al. Influence of immunoadsorption of the removal of immunoglobulin G autoantibodies in crescentic glomerulonephritis. Nephron 1993;65:180–184.

58. Jayne DRW, Rasmussen N. Treatment of antineutrophil cytoplasm autoantibody-associated systemic vasculitis: initiatives of the European Community Systemic Vasculitis Clinical Trials Study Group. Mayo Clin Proc 1997;72:737–747.

59. Appel GB, Cohen DJ, Pirani CL, et al. Long-term follow-up of patients with lupus nephritis: a study based on the WHO classification. Am J Med 1987;83:877–885.

60. Verrier-Jones J, Cumming RH, Bucknall RC, et al. Plasmapheresis in the management of acute systemic lupus erythematosus? Lancet 1976;1:709–711.

61. Verrier-Jones J, Cumming RH, Bacon PA, et al. Evidence for a therapeutic effect of plasmapheresis in patients with systemic lupus erythematosus. Q J Med 1979;48:555–576.

62. Lockwood CM, Pusey CD, Rees AJ, et al. Plasma exchange in the treatment of immune complex disease. Clin Immunol Allergy 1981;1:433–455.

63. Lewis EJ. Plasmapheresis for the treatment of severe lupus nephritis: uncontrolled observations. Am J Kidney Dis 1982;2:182–187.

64. Moriconi L, Ferri C, Fanara G, et al. Plasma exchange in the treatment of lupus nephritis. Int J Artif Organs 1983;6:35–38.

65. Leaker BR, Becker GJ, Dowling JP, et al. Rapid improvement in severe lupus glomerular lesions following intensive plasma exchange associated with immunosuppression. Clin Nephrol 1986;25:236–244.

66. Jordan SC, Ho W, Ettenger R, et al. Plasma exchange improves the glomerulonephritis of systemic lupus erythematosus in selected paediatric patients. Pediatr Nephrol 1987;1:276–280.

67. Wei N, Klippel JH, Huston DP, et al. Randomised trial of plasma exchange in mild systemic lupus erythematosus. Lancet 1983;1:17–22.

68. Haworth SJ, Pusey CD, Lockwood CM. Plasma exchange in lupus nephritis. Proc EDTA-ERA 1985;22:699–704.

69. Lewis EJ, Hunsicker LG, Lan S-P, et al. A controlled trial of plasmapheresis therapy in severe lupus nephritis. N Engl J Med 1992;326:1373–1379.

70. Euler HH, Schroeder JO. Lupus Plasmapheresis Study Group. Plasmapheresis for lupus nephritis. N Engl J Med 1992;327:1028.

71. Robinson JA. Plasmapheresis for lupus nephritis. N Engl J Med 1992;327:1028–1029.

72. Fukuda M, Kamiyama Y, Kawahara K, et al. The favourable effect of cyclophosphamide pulse therapy in the treatment

of massive pulmonary haemorrhage in systemic lupus erythematosus. Eur J Paediatr 1994;153:167–170.

73. Kinoshita M, Aotsuka S, Funahashi I, et al. Selective removal of anti–double-stranded DNA antibodies by immunoadsorption with dextran sulphate in a patient with systemic lupus erythematosus. Ann Rheum Dis 1989; 48:856–860.

74. Suzuki K, Hara M, Harigai M, et al. Continuous removal of anti-DNA antibody using a new extracorporeal immunoadsorption system in patients with systemic lupus erythematosus. Arthritis Rheum 1991;34:1546–1552.

75. Traeger J, Laville M, Serres P-F, et al. A new device for specific extracorporeal immunoadsorption of anti-DNA antibodies. Ann Med Interne (Paris) 1992;143:9–12.

76. Hoyer JR, Vernier RL, Najarian JS, et al. Recurrence of idiopathic nephrotic syndrome after renal transplantation. Lancet 1972;2:343–348.

77. Pinto J, Lacerda G, Cameron JS, et al. Recurrence of focal segmental glomerulosclerosis in renal allografts. Transplantation 1981;32:83–89.

78. Munoz J, Sanchez M, Perez-Garcia R, et al. Recurrent focal segmental glomerulosclerosis in renal transplants: proteinuria relapsing following plasma exchange. Clin Nephrol 1985;24:213–214.

79. Laufer J, Ettenger RB, Ho WG, et al. Plasma exchange for recurrent nephrotic syndrome following renal transplantation. Transplantation 1988;46:540–542.

80. Dantal J, Baatard R, Hourmant M, et al. Recurrent nephrotic syndrome following renal transplantation in patients with focal glomerulosclerosis: a one-centre study of plasma exchange effects. Transplantation 1991;52:827–831.

81. Sharma M, Sharma R, McCarthy ET, et al. "The FSGS factor": enrichment and in vivo effect of activity from focal segmental glomerulosclerosis plasma. J Am Soc Nephrol 1999;10:552–561.

82. Artero ML, Biava C, Amend W, et al. Recurrent focal glomerulosclerosis: natural history and response to therapy. Am J Med 1992;92:375–383.

83. Vincenti F, Biava C, Tomlanovitch S, et al. Inability of cyclosporin to completely prevent the recurrence of focal glomerulosclerosis after kidney transplantation. Transplantation 1989;47:595–598.

84. Banfi G, Colturi G, Montagnino G, et al. The recurrence of focal segmental glomerulosclerosis in kidney transplant patients treated with cyclosporin. Transplantation 1990;50: 594–596.

85. Meyrier A, Noel L-H, Auriche P, et al. Long-term renal tolerance of cyclosporin A treatment in adult idiopathic nephrotic syndrome. Kidney Int 1994;45:1446–1456.

86. Artero ML, Sharma R, Savin VJ, et al. Plasmapheresis reduces proteinuria and serum capacity to injure glomeruli in patients with recurrent glomerulosclerosis. Am J Kidney Dis 1994;23:574–581.

87. Dantal J, Bigot E, Bogers W, et al. Effect of plasma protein adsorption on protein excretion in kidney transplant recipients with recurrent nephrotic syndrome. N Engl J Med 1994;330:7–14.

88. Mitwalli AH. Adding plasmapheresis to corticosteroids and alkylating agents: does it benefit patients with focal segmental glomerulosclerosis? Nephrol Dial Transplant 1998;13:1524–1528.

89. Taube DH, Williams DG, Cameron JS, et al. Renal transplantation after removal and prevention of resynthesis of HLA antibodies. Lancet 1984;1:824–826.

90. Fauchald P, Leivestad T, Bratlie A, et al. Plasma exchange and immunosuppressive therapy before renal transplantation in allosensitised patients. Transplant Proc 1987;14: 3748–3749.

91. Fehrman I, Barany P, Bjork S, et al. Measures to decrease HLA antibodies in immunised patients awaiting kidney transplantation. Transplant Proc 1990;22:147–148.

92. Kupin WL, Venkat KK, Hayashi H, et al. Removal of lymphocytotoxic antibodies by pretransplant immunoadsorption therapy in highly sensitised renal transplant recipients. Transplantation 1991;51:324–329.

93. Kriaa F, Rousseau P, Hiesse C, et al. Anti-HLA antibodies depletion on protein A sepharose columns in hyperimmunised patients awaiting renal transplantation. Ann Internal Med 1992;143:39–42.

94. Ross CN, Gaskin G, Gregor-Macgregor S, et al. Renal transplantation following immunoadsorption in highly sensitised recipients. Transplantation 1993;55:785–789.

95. Palmer A, Welch K, Gjorstrup P, et al. Removal of anti-HLA antibodies by extra-corporeal immunoadsorption to enable renal transplantation. Lancet 1989;1:10–12.

96. Higgins RM, Bevan DJ, Carey BS, et al. Prevention of hyperacute rejection by removal of antibodies to HLA immediately before renal transplantation. Lancet 1996;348:1208–1211.

97. Esnault VL, Bignon JD, Testa A, et al. Effect of protein A immunoadsorption on panel lymphocyte reactivity in hyperimmunised patients awaiting a kidney graft. Transplantation 1990;50:449–453.

98. Alrabi AA, Wikstrom B, Backman U, et al. Pretransplantation immunoadsorption therapy in patients immunised with human lymphocyte antigen: effect of treatment and three years follow-up of grafts. Artif Organs 1993;17:702–707.

99. Agishi T, Takahashi K, Yagisawa T, et al. Immunoadsorption of anti-A or anti-B antibody for successful kidney transplantation between ABO incompatible pairs and its limitation. ASAIO Trans 1991;37:496–498.

100. Renard TH, Andrews WH. An approach to ABO-incompatible liver transplantation in children. Transplantation 1992;53:116–121.

101. Paul LC, Carpenter CB. Antibodies against renal endothelial alloantigens. Transplant Proc 1980;12:43–48.

102. Vangelista A, Frasca GM, Nanni Cosa A, et al. Value of plasma exchange in renal transplant rejection induced by anti-HLA antibodies. ASAIO Trans 1982;28:599–603.

103. Franco A, Anaya F, Niembro E, et al. Plasma exchange in the treatment of vascular rejection. Transplant Proc 1987;14: 3661–3663.

104. Allen N, Smith J, Tate D, et al. Intensive plasma exchange in acute renal allograft rejection—a controlled trial. Transplant Proc 1983;15:1060–1062.

105. Soulillou JP, Guyot C, Guimbretiere J, et al. Plasma exchange in early graft rejection associated with anti-donor antibodies. Nephron 1983;35:158–162.

106. Gurland HJ, Blumenstein M, Lysaght MJ, et al. Plasmapheresis in renal transplantation. Kidney Int 1983;23:82–84.

107. Bonomini V, Vangelista A, Frasca GM, et al. Effects of plasmapheresis in renal transplant rejection: a controlled study. Trans Am Soc Intern Organs 1985;31:698–703.
108. Cardella CJ, Sutton DMC, Uldall RR, et al. Factors influencing the effect of intensive plasma exchange on acute transplant rejection. Transplant Proc 1985;17:2777–2778.
109. Bodziak KA, Hammond WS, Molitoris BA. Inherited diseases of the glomerular basement membrane. Am J Kidney Dis 1994;23:605–618.
110. Flinter F. Molecular genetics of Alport's syndrome. Q J Med 1993;86:289–292.
111. Gobel J, Olbicht CJ, Offner G, et al. Kidney transplantation in Alport's syndrome: long-term outcome and allograft anti-GBM nephritis. Clin Nephrol 1992;38:299–304.
112. Cameron JS. Recurrent disease in renal allografts. Kidney Int 1993;43:91–94.
113. Kauffman RH, Houwert DA. Plasmapheresis in rapidly progressive Henoch-Schonlein purpura and the effect on circulating IgA immune complexes. Clin Nephrol 1981;16:155–160.
114. Nicholls K, Walker RG, Kincaid-Smith P, et al. Malignant IgA nephropathy. Am J Kidney Dis 1984;5:42–46.
115. Kincaid-Smith P, Walker RG. The case for plasmapheresis. In: Nairns RG, ed. Controversies in nephrology and hypertension. New York: Churchill Livingstone, 1984:463–469.
116. Roujeau J-C, Quaranta J-F, Guillevin L, et al. Les echanges plasmatique therapeutiques: indications et resultats. Ann Med Interne (Paris) 1984;135:308–327.
117. McGinley E, Watkins R, McLay A, et al. Plasma exchange in the treatment of mesangiocapillary glomerulonephritis. Nephron 1985;40:385–390.
118. Coppo R, Basolo B, Roccatello D, et al. Immunological monitoring of plasma exchange in primary IgA nephropathy. Artif Organs 1985;9:351–360.
119. Lai KN, Lai FM, Leung ACT, et al. Plasma exchange in patients with rapidly progressive idiopathic IgA nephropathy: a report of two cases and review of the literature. Am J Kidney Dis 1987;10:66–70.
120. Espinal E, Valles M, Rodriguez JA, et al. Crescentic mesangiocapillary glomerulonephritis and plasmapheresis. Proceedings of the Ninth International Congress of Nephrology 1984;85A.
121. Dau PC, Lindstrom JM, Cassel CK, et al. Plasmapheresis and immunosuppressive drug therapy in myasthenia gravis. N Engl J Med 1997;297:1134–1140.
122. Nielsen VK, Paulson OB, Rosenkvist, et al. Rapid improvement of myasthenia gravis after plasma exchange. Ann Neurol 1982;11:160–169.
123. Newsom-Davis J, Pinching AJ, Vincent A, et al. Function of circulating antibody to acetylcholine receptor in myasthenia gravis: investigation by plasma exchange. Neurology 1978;28:266–272.
124. Newsom-Davis J, Wilson SG, Vincent A, et al. Long-term effects of repeated plasma exchange in myasthenia gravis. Lancet 1979;1:464–468.
125. Somnier FE, Langvad E. Plasma exchange with selective immunoadsorption of anti-acetylcholine receptor antibodies. J Neuroimmunol 1989;22:123–127.
126. Hosokawa S, Oyamaguchi A. Safety, stability and effectiveness of immunoadsorption under membrane plasmapheresis for myasthenia gravis. ASAIO Trans 1990;36:207–208.
127. Nakaji S, Oka K, Tanihara M, et al. Development of a specific immunoadsorbent containing immobilised synthetic peptide of acetylcholine receptor for treatment of myasthenia gravis. Utrecht: VSP, 1993:573–576.
128. Guillain-Barre Study Group. Plasmapheresis and acute Guillain-Barre syndrome. Neurology 1985;1105–1107.
129. Raphael JC, Chastang C. Cooperative randomised trial of plasma exchange in Guillain-Barre syndrome: preliminary results. Ann Med Interne (Paris) 1984;8:135–138.
130. Rosenow F, Haupt WF, Grieb P, et al. Plasma exchange and selective adsorption in Guillain-Barre syndrome—a comparison of therapies by clinical course and side effects. Transfus Sci 1993;14:13–15.
131. van der Meche FGA, Schmitz PIM, and the Dutch Guillain-Barre Study Group. A randomised trial comparing intravenous immunoglobulin and plasma exchange in Guillain-Barre syndrome. N Engl J Med 1992;326:1123–1129.
132. Dyck PJ, Daube J, O'Brien P, et al. Plasma exchange in chronic demyelinating polyradiculopathy. N Engl J Med 1986;14:461–465.
133. Canadian Cooperative Multiple Sclerosis Study Group. The Canadian cooperative trial of cyclophosphamide and plasma exchange in progressive multiple sclerosis. Lancet 1991;337:441–446.
134. Hosokawa S, Oyamaguchi A, Yoshida O. Successful immunoadsorption with membrane plasmapheresis for multiple sclerosis. ASAIO Trans 1989;35:576–577.
135. Pozzi C, Pasquali S, Donini U, et al. Prognostic factors and effectiveness of treatment in acute renal failure due to multiple myeloma: a review of 50 cases. Clin Nephrol 1987;28:1–9.
136. Zucchelli P, Pasquali S, Cagnoli L, et al. Controlled plasma exchange trial in acute renal failure due to multiple myeloma. Kidney Int 1988;33:1175–1180.
137. Johnston WJ, Kyle RA, Pineda AA, et al. Treatment of renal failure associated with multiple myeloma: plasmapheresis, haemodialysis and chemotherapy. Arch Intern Med 1990;150:863–869.
138. Berkman EM, Orlin JB. Use of plasmapheresis and partial plasma exchange in the management of patients with cryoglobulinaemia. Transfusion 1980;20:171–178.
139. Frankel AH, Singer DRJ, Winearls CG, et al. Type II essential mixed cryoglobulinaemia: presentation, treatment and outcome in 13 patients. Q J Med 1992;82:101–124.
140. Valbonesi M. Plasmapheresis in the management of cryoglobulinaemia. Milano: Wichtig Editore, 1986:89–96.
141. Furlan M, Robles R, Galbusera M, et al. Von Willebrand factor–cleaving protease in thrombotic thrombocytopaenic purpura and the heamolytic uraemic syndrome. N Engl J Med 1998;339:1578–1584.
142. Tsai H-M, Lian EC-Y. Antibodies to von Willebrand factor–cleaving protease in acute thrombotic thrombocytopaenic purpura. N Engl J Med 1998;339:1585–1594.
143. Caggiano V. Apheresis in the treatment of TTP. Milano: Wichtig Editore, 1986:135–142.
144. Bell WR, Braine HG, Ness PM, et al. Improved survival in thrombotic thrombocytopaenic purpura-haemolytic uraemic syndrome—clinical experience in 108 patients. N Engl J Med 1991;325:398–403.

145. Marder VJ, Nusbacher J, Anderson FW. One-year follow-up of plasma exchange therapy in 14 patients with idiopathic thrombocytopaenic purpura. Transfusion 1981;21:291–298.

146. Blanchette VS, Hogan VA, McCombie NE, et al. Intensive plasma exchange in ten patients with idiopathic thrombocytopaenic purpura. Transfusion 1984;24:388–394.

147. Slocombe GW, Newland AC, Colving MP, et al. The role of intensive plasma exchange in the prevention and management of haemorrhage in patients with inhibitors to factor VIII. Br J Haematol 1981;47:577–585.

148. Nilsson IM, Jonsson S, Sundqvist S-B, et al. A procedure for removing high titre antibodies by extracorporeal protein A sepharose adsorption in haemophilia: substitution therapy and surgery in patients with haemophilia B antibodies. Blood 1981;58:38–44.

149. Rock G. Apheresis in the treatment of immune-mediated haematologic disease. Milano: Wichtig Editore, 1986:127–134.

150. Winkelstein A, Starz TW, Agarwal A. Efficacy of combined therapy with plasmapheresis and immunosuppressants in rheumatoid vasculitis. J Rheumatol 1981;11:162–166.

151. Miller FW, Leitman SF, Cronin ME, et al. Controlled trial of plasma exchange and leukopheresis in polymyositis and dermatomyositis. N Engl J Med 1992;326:1380–1384.

152. O'Reilly MJG, Talpos G, Roberts VC, et al. Controlled trial of plasma exchange in Raynaud's syndrome. Br Med J 1979;2:1113–1115.

153. Ruocco V, Rossi A, Argenziano G, et al. Pathogenicity of the intercellular antibodies of pemphigus and their periodic removal from the circulation by plasmapheresis. Br J Dermatol 1978;98:237–241.

154. Ruocco V, Astarita C, Pisani M. Plasmapheresis as an alternative or adjunctive therapy in problem cases of pemphigus. Dermatologica 1984;168:219–233.

155. Guillaume J-C, Ronjeau J-C, Morel P, et al. Controlled study of plasma exchange in pemphigus. Arch Dermatol 1988;124:1659–1663.

156. Roujeau J-C, Guillaume J-C, Morel P, et al. Plasma exchange in bullous pemphigoid. Lancet 1984;2:484–486.

157. Coffe C. Plasma exchange in dermatological disease. Milano: Wichtig Editore, 1986:97–106.

158. Turner AM, Whittaker S, Banks I, et al. Plasma exchange in refractory cutaneous vasculitis. Br J Dermatol 1990;122:411–415.

159. Mokrzycki MH, Kaplan AA. Therapeutic plasma exchange: complications and management. Am J Kidney Dis 1994;23:817–827.

160. Aufeuvre JP, Morin-Hertal F, Cohen-Solal M, et al. Hazards of plasma exchange. Stuttgart: FK Schattauer Verlag, 1980:143–148.

161. Ziselman EM, Bongiovanni MB, Wurzel HA. The complications of therapeutic plasma exchange. Vox Sang 1984;46:270–276.

162. Sutton DMC, Nair RC, Rock G, et al. Complications of plasma exchange. Transfusion 1989;29:124–127.

163. Hester JP, McCullogh J, Mishler JM, et al. Dosage regimes for citrate anticoagulants. J Clin Apheresis 1983;1:149–157.

164. Buskard NA, Varghese Z, Wills MR. Correction of hypocalcaemic symptoms during plasma exchange. Lancet 1976;2:344–345.

165. Orlin JB, Berkman EM. Partial plasma exchange using albumin replacement: removal and recovery of normal plasma constituents. Blood 1980;56:1055–1059.

166. Pearl RG, Rosenthal MH. Metabolic alkalosis due to plasmapheresis. Am J Med 1985;79:391–393.

167. Milliner DS, Shinaberger JH, Shurman P, et al. Inadvertent aluminium administration during plasma exchange due to aluminium contamination of albumin replacement solutions. N Engl J Med 1985;312:165–167.

168. Mousson C, Charhon SA, Ammar M, et al. Aluminium bone deposits in normal renal function patients after long-term treatment by plasma exchange. Int J Artif Organs 1989;12:664–667.

169. Chirnside A, Urbank SJ, Prowse CV, et al. Coagulation abnormalities following intensive plasma exchange on the cell separator. Br J Haematol 1981;48:627–634.

170. Rossi PL, Cecchini L, Minichella G, et al. Comparison of the side effects of therapeutic cytopheresis and those of other types of haemapheresis. Haematologica 1991;76:75–80.

171. Gelabert A, Puig L, Maragall S, et al. Coagulation alterations during massive plasmapheresis. Stuttgart: FK Schattauer Verlag, 1980:71–75.

172. Kaplan AA, Haley SE. Plasma exchange with a rotating filter. Kidney Int 1990;38:160–166.

173. Keller AJ, Chirnside A, Urbaniak SJ. Coagulation abnormalities produced by plasma exchange on the cell separator with special reference to fibrinogen and platelet levels. Br J Haematol 1979;42:593–603.

174. Gurland HJ, Lysaght MJ, Samtleben W, et al. A comparison of centrifugal- and membrane-based apheresis formats. Int J Artif Organs 1984;7:35–38.

175. Sultan Y, Bussel A, Maisonneuve P, et al. Potential dangers of thrombosis after plasma exchange in the treatment of patients with immune disease. Transfusion 1979;19:588–593.

176. Wing EJ, Bruns FJ, Fraley DS, et al. Infectious complications with plasmapheresis in rapidly progressive glomerulonephritis. JAMA 1980;244:2423–2426.

177. Pohl MA, Lan SP, Berl T, et al. Plasmapheresis does not increase the risk for infection in immunosuppressed patients with severe lupus nephritis. Ann Intern Med 1991;114:924–929.

178. Consensus on IVIG. Lancet 1990;1:470–472.

179. Hass A. Use of intravenous immunoglobulin in immunoregulatory disorders. Ann Intern Med 1987;107:367–382.

180. The risk of transfusion transmitted diseases. N Engl J Med 1992;327:419–421. Editorial.

181. Ring J, Messmer K. Incidence and severity of anaphylactoid reactions to colloid volume substitutes. Lancet 1977;2:466–469.

182. Huesis DW. Mortality in therapeutic haemapheresis. Lancet 1983;1:1043.

183. Aufeuvre JP, Morin-Hertel F, Cohen-Solal M, et al. Clinical tolerance and hazards of plasma exchanges: a study of 6200 plasma exchanges in 1033 patients. Basel: Karger, 1982:65–177.

184. Apter AJ, Kaplan AA. An approach to immunologic reactions with plasma exchange. J Clin Immunol 1992;90:119–124.

185. Jorstad S. Biocompatibility of different haemodialysis and plasmapheresis membranes. Blood Purif 1987;5:123–137.
186. Nicholls AJ, Platts MM. Anaphylactoid reactions due to haemodialysis, haemofiltration or membrane plasma separation. Br Med J 1982;258:1607–1609.
187. Jones JV. The effect of plasmapheresis on therapeutic drugs. Dial Transplant 1985;14:225–226.
188. Stigelman WH, Henry DH, Talbert RL, et al. Removal of prednisone and prednisolone by plasma exchange. Clin Pharmacol 1984;3:402–407.
189. Sandrin MS, Vaughan HA, Dabkowski PL, et al. Anti-pig IgM antibodies in human serum react predominantly with Gal(alpha 1–3)Gal epitopes. Proc Natl Acad Sci USA 1993;90:11385–11391.

Chapter 45

Drug Therapy for HIV Infection

John P. Doweiko
Jerome E. Groopman

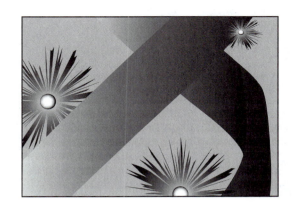

Retroviruses were discovered in the late 1970s. Type 2 human immunodeficiency virus (HIV-2) was first reported and is still predominant in Africa and India; sporadic cases appear in the United States and Europe. Type 1 HIV, previously known as HTLV-III, is a member of the *Retroviridae* family and *Lentivirinae* subfamily (1,2). Other strains of lentivirus are known to infect nonhuman primates and animal species.

Phylogenetic origins suggest that HIV-1 is a result of cross-transmission from simian viruses (3), although the exact ancestral point is still unknown. HIV-1 has now evolved into at least seven different subspecies (clades). Types A through F are considered the major group (group M), all descending from the same point, while group O ("outliers") probably descended from an earlier point. These strains of HIV-1 differ in ease and mode of transmission, virulence, and global distribution (3,4). This is consistent with the hypothesis that most regional epidemics started with the introduction of a variant that locally diversified.

HIV-1 infection may have had its origins in the 1940s and reached epidemic proportions in 1981. By the end of the 20th century, it will be the greatest lethal epidemic in the history of civilization (5). At its peak in the 14th century, the bubonic plague killed 25 million people; influenza A killed 20 million people in the earlier part of this century. Thus far, HIV-1 infection has killed 28 million people (5). Currently, it is estimated that over one million people in the United States, and over 30 million worldwide, have been infected with this virus (4).

To realize potential therapies for HIV infection, it is necessary to understand the structure and life cycle of the virus, as well as the dynamics and pathophysiology of the infection. Only in this way can we come to understand what aspects of the virus are amenable to exploitation as therapeutic strategies.

Structure of HIV-1

Although HIV-1 has a relatively simple structure, it has an elaborate mechanism of replication (6). The genome of HIV-1 is encoded within a single strand of RNA that is enclosed within a cone-shaped "shell" of P-24 protein, the "core antigen" of HIV-1 (7). This is contained within a lipid bilayer envelope, derived largely from the host cell membrane, which is studded with the transmembrane P-41 protein to which is attached the Gp-120

protein (1,2). The latter envelope protein is necessary for binding to the CD-4 protein of target cells (8).

The Gp-120 glycoprotein of HIV-1 attaches to the CD-4 molecule with high affinity (8–11). The latter protein is contained on T lymphocytes and cells of the monocyte/macrophage line, as well as fibroblasts, glial cells, and bone-marrow stromal cells. It is a member of the immunoglobulin superfamily (10). The process of binding of HIV-1 to the CD-4 antigen allows the virus to enter the cell. In addition, it results in inhibition of signal transduction by the T-cell CD-3 receptor and leads to secretion of cytokines by the T cell that include interleukin-1B, IL-6, TNF-alpha, and GM-CSF (9).

HIV-1 is genetically more complex than other members of the *Retroviradae* family (2). It has a genome that is 9.7 Kb in total length and contains three genes that are characteristic of replicative retroviruses (1,2): the *Gag* gene that encodes for the core structural protein of the virus, the *Pol* gene that encodes for the viral enzymes (reverse transcriptase, integrase, and protease), and the *Env* gene encoding for the surface glycoproteins of the virus. In addition, the genome of HIV-1 also includes six other genes that are not present in other retroviruses, but are important to the pathogenesis of HIV-1 infection (1,10).

Life Cycle of HIV-1

HIV-1 uses more than the CD-4 receptor to attack immune cells with high efficiency. It also makes use of chemokine receptors, cell-surface receptors that are part of the immune system (12). These receptors belong to the seven-transmembrane G-protein–coupled super-family and include CXCR4 (formerly called fusin or LESTR) and CCR5 (also known as CC-CKR5). Other chemokine receptors such as CCR2b and CCR3 may also serve as coreceptors for HIV-1 infection.

Cells expressing both the CD-4 and CCR5 (or fusin) molecules bind HIV-1 10,000-fold more avidly than cells that lack these proteins. HIV-1 uses the CD-4 and CKR-5 receptors to invade cells of monocytic lineage. As disease progresses, however, HIV switches trophism and uses the CD-4 molecule and CXCR4 receptor to infect T-helper cells (13).

HIV-1 can bind to cells by means of receptors other than CD-4 and chemokine receptors. The alternative receptors include galactosylceramide on cells of the nervous system and the gastrointestinal tract and Fc receptors when the virus is part of an immune complex. Although these receptors do not promote cellular invasion as efficiently as the CD-4 and chemokine receptors, they do allow HIV-1 to enter cells other than lymphocytes and monocytes.

After the virus enters the target cell, the protein coat is shed and there is activation of the genes contained within the RNA (1). The *Tat* gene (transactivator of transcription) encodes for a protein that is required for viral replication and enhances expression of other viral genes (1). The reverse transcriptase of HIV-1 is the viral DNA polymerase that converts the viral genomic RNA into double-stranded DNA (1,7). Catalysis of a DNA copy of the HIV-1 genome by the reverse transcriptase copy is an essential step in HIV replication that converts the single-stranded RNA of the infecting virus into a circularized copy of double-stranded DNA (14,15).

Some of this DNA enters the nucleus of the cell and is incorporated into the host genome in a reaction catalyzed by the HIV-1–encoded enzyme integrase (14,16). The viral genome that is incorporated into the genome of the host cell is never truly "latent," however, since there is always at least low-level production of new HIV virions (1). Inhibitors of HIV-1 integrase are currently under investigation for their therapeutic potential.

Acceleration of the pace of viral replication is controlled by a complicated interplay between host factors and the viral regulatory proteins and is in part caused by agonists that can bind to specific elements of the proviral DNA, leading to an increase in the rate of transcription of HIV DNA (1,17). These agonists include cytokines such as GM-CSF, IL-3, IL-6, and TNF-alpha (17–20). Manipulation of the complicated interaction between HIV and cytokines to form a therapeutic strategy for this viral infection is being actively explored (21). Recent discoveries include the beta chemokines (MIPIa and RANTES) that are released by CD-8+ T cells and macrophages (22,23). These molecules limit HIV replication in vitro and offer a possible therapeutic strategy (22,23). Another finding is that interleukin-16 down-regulates HIV, offering another avenue of research (24).

The final stages of HIV replication involve the *Rev* protein. This is a regulatory factor, encoded by the HIV-1 genome, that is important to the synthesis of the *Gag* and *Env* proteins (18). Some of the proteins that are required for assembly of new virions require posttranscriptional processing such as cleavage by HIV-specific proteases or the addition of carbohydrates by the enzyme glycosylase (25,26). HIV particles are assembled in the cytoplasm of the host cell, and then, as is typical of enveloped viruses, new virions from the infected cell are released by budding through the cell membrane (14), taking a portion of the host cell membrane as a new viral envelope. During this process, there is incorporation of host molecules within the new viral envelope (27). Since MCH-II is the natural ligand for the CD-4 molecule, having the MHC-II molecule incorporated into its outer envelope allows HIV-1 to attach to new, susceptible cells with stronger affinity (27).

Dynamics of HIV Infection

It was previously thought that, after viremia occurs with the onset of HIV infection, the virus entered a "latent phase" during which replication took place at a very reduced rate. More recent studies have shown that viral replication actively persists throughout the course of the HIV infection (28,29) with billions of viral particles being produced and destroyed each day. HIV-infected persons produce and destroy about 30% of the total body viral burden daily, and the clearance of HIV virions is relatively constant during the course of the HIV infection, regardless of CD-4 lymphocyte counts (30,31).

One life cycle for HIV is about 1.2 days in vivo. About 0.9 of a day of this time is intracellular with the remainder of time representing the half-life of the virion within the tissues and/or blood (30–32); the time that the virus exists as a virion in plasma is estimated to be about 10 minutes. Each infected lymphocyte produces about 4000 new viral particles, and this number seems to be independent of the stage of HIV infection, the treatment status, or the plasma viral load. Therefore, about 99% of the virus that is present at any one time is derived from activated CD-4+ lymphocytes that were infected within the previous 2 weeks; the remaining small fraction is derived from monocytes and resting CD-4+ lymphocytes.

In vivo, HIV-1 undergoes 3000 to 5000 replication cycles per day (30,31,33). This gives rise to over 10^{12} viral particles produced during the patient's lifetime (10^{12} seconds = 317 years!). Given that there is a mutation rate of 10^{-4} per base pair of the genome of HIV-1, there exists the possibility that one of every three viral progeny has at least one mutation. Therefore, HIV-1 has an enormous potential to diversify within a single patient. Infection with HIV-1 occurs with a single genotype that rapidly evolves into multiple viral substrains. With late-stage disease, a patient may harbor up to a *billion* viral substrains. This is important to the development of drug resistance that occurs with time.

During the clinical "latent" phase, in which those infected may be only minimally symptomatic, there is a large reservoir of HIV sequestered in the lymphoid tissues wherein HIV replication is ongoing, and there is ceaseless destruction of the architecture and function of the lymphoid tissue (28,34,35). The destruction of the follicular dendritic cells and the germinal centers of lymph nodes results in the decreasing ability of these cells to carry out their normal functions of nurturing CD-4+ lymphocytes. The loss of the capacity to produce antibody of high specificity thus results from the effect(s) of HIV-1 on the lymph nodes.

There is a brisk cytotoxic CD-8+ lymphocyte response early in the course of the HIV infection. This response is markedly augmented by HIV-specific CD-4 lymphocytes (36–38). This HIV-1–specific T-helper response is lost early in HIV infection in the majority of people and does not recover even with successful antiretroviral therapy. This HIV-specific immune response controls viral replication during the "set point" and may play a major role in disease progression. Quantitative variations in this response in some patients may account, in part, for the longer asymptomatic periods in some patients and may also contribute to the dissimilarities in disease course that occurs among patients (35,36).

Associated with this brisk viral replication rate is a brisk replication response on the part of the CD-4+ lymphocytes. The peripheral blood CD-4+ lymphocyte count represents only about 2% of the total body CD-4+ lymphocyte pool. Productively infected CD-4+ lymphocytes have a life span of only about 2.2 days, so that about 5% of the CD-4+ lymphocyte population turns over each day and the entire CD-4+ lymphocyte pool may turn over each 10 to 14 days (30,31). Unlike the viral production rate that tends to be fairly constant, there is a large variation in the CD-4+ lymphocyte production rate from patient to patient (30,31). As the disease progresses, the ability of the body to replenish CD-4+ lymphocytes is stressed: viral destruction eventually outpaces production. The decline in the CD-4+ lymphocyte count that occurs with progression of HIV infection is the result of the gradual failure of the immune system to match lymphocyte production with destruction by the virus (30,31,33–35). The productive capacity of the cellular system (and eventually of the humoral immune system also) is simply overwhelmed.

Pathogenesis of HIV Infection

The fundamental morbidity of this infection is degradation of the cellular immune system (39). The clinical manifestations are largely caused by opportunistic infections and neoplasms, as well as by the cytokines produced in response to the infection (40,41). The latter result in a prolonged and ultimately detrimental inflammatory response that disrupts metabolism and the integrity of normal physiology and contributes to the suppression of immunity.

The initial infection with HIV-1 is quickly followed by a burst of replication of virions that results in an intense viremia (42). Viremia decreases following the development of humoral immunity that results in immune complexes. These are trapped by the follicular dendritic cell network of the lymph nodes (10,14). The cellular immune system also responds, as noted above. During the clinical "latent phase" of the infection, there is low-grade but continuous replication of virus in the lymphatic tissues (43,44).

The monocyte, as well as the CD-4+ lymphocyte, plays an important role in the pathogenesis of HIV infection. In the early phases of infection, monocytotropic strains of HIV-1 predominate over lymphocytotrophic strains (39,45). Infection of cells of the monocyte/macrophage line is not lethal for these cells, making them important reservoirs of the virus and vectors for spread throughout the body (4,46), particularly the central nervous system. Derivatives of the monocyte/macrophage cell line such as glial cells of the central nervous system may be infected by, and harbor, the virus (18). Within these cells, the virus may replicate more rapidly than in other tissues (18) and is relatively hidden from the immune system.

Infection of T lymphocytes results in both qualitative *and* quantitative aberrations in these cells (47). Altered function of the CD-4+ T cells may occur before, and independently of, T-cell depletion (47). Causes of T-lymphocyte dysfunction include interference with T-cell activation by GP-120, Gp-41–mediated inhibition of protein kinase C–dependent T-cell activation, formation of Gp-41 cross-reactive antibodies that react with MHC class II antigens, transforming growth factor-beta (TGF-beta)–mediated immunosuppression, and decreased functions of antigen-presenting cells such as macrophages and bone marrow–derived dendritic cells (47).

Depletion of CD-4+ lymphocytes results from syncytia formation, antibody-dependent cytolysis, and Gp-120–specific T-cell–mediated cytolysis (47). In addition, an important factor in T-cell depletion is accelerated cell death by apoptosis (10,48,49). Apoptosis occurs by HIV-1 envelope protein–mediated CD-4 cross-linking and also by cytokine-induced up-regulation of proapoptotic genes and down-regulation of genes that normally inhibit apoptosis (48).

The humeral immune system is also altered during the course of HIV-1 infection. B-cell activation depends on the follicular dendritic cell, a nonmotile cell within the lymph node follicles. During infection, antigens and B lymphocytes localize on the surfaces of these cells, and the follicular dendritic cell organizes a process that results in selection of those B cells that produce the most specific antibody for the antigen. With HIV lymphadenopathy, follicular dendritic cells are continuously destroyed within the progressively degenerating germinal centers, and the ability of the host to produce high-affinity antibody is degraded.

"Surrogate" Markers of Prognosis of HIV Infection

The CD-4+ lymphocyte count has been used as a "surrogate marker" of disease activity (49,50). This count correlates with the stage of HIV infection, risk of progression to AIDS, and survival (51–55). The percentage of CD-4+ cells is perhaps a better predictor of disease progression than is the absolute number (51). The risk of opportunistic infection and of progression to AIDS increases substantially as the CD-4 count declines to less than 20% of the total lymphocyte count (56).

The presence of p-24 antigenemia is a poor prognostic sign (54,57–59). It is not clear that the magnitude of the p-24 antigen level has any prognostic relevance (7). The serum beta-2-microglobulin correlates with the presence of p-24 antigenemia and progression of HIV infection (54,57,58). Other markers include endogenous interferon and serum triglyceride levels (59,60).

Until recently, the CD-4 lymphocyte count and percentage were thought to be the best clinically available surrogate markers of disease activity. The CD-4 lymphocyte count is, however, an incomplete marker of the clinical benefit of antiretroviral therapy (51). The CD-4 lymphocyte counts also fail to explain the seemingly benign clinical course of some patients who have persistently low T-helper lymphocyte counts. Moreover, the CD-4

Table 45-1. Overview of Antiretrovirals

| Fusion | Reverse Transcription | | | Integrase | Protease |
	Nucleoside	Nonnucleo	Nucleotide		
Chemokines	AZT	Neviripine	*Adefovir*		Saquinavir
MIPI-a	ddI	Delaverdine	*Tenofovir*		Ritonavir
MIPI-b	ddC	Efavirenz			Indinavir
RANTES	d4T	*Loviridine*		*Zintevir*	Nelfinavir
Anti CD-4	3TC	*HBY-997*			Amprenavir
T-20	Abacavir				*Lopinavir*
	Emticitabine				*[ABT-378]*
	[FTC]				
					PNU-140690
	Lodenosine				*Tipranavir*
	[Fdd-A]				
					MKC-442

Drugs in *italics* are not yet FDA approved.

lymphocyte count tends to be an indicator of *damage already done* to the immune system.

A more useful marker of disease activity is the "viral load" (61). This is a measure of the number of copies of HIV-1 RNA per mL of blood, measured either directly by polymerase chain reaction or indirectly by the branched chain DNA assay. The "viral load" provides information about *pending damage* to the immune system. In an untreated patient, a level of 10,000 RNA copies/mL or lower suggests a good prognosis, and values above this level are associated with progressively greater risk of disease progression. It is recommended that any person with a viral load exceeding 2000 to 5000 copies/mL should begin antiretroviral therapy regardless of clinical status.

The plateau concentration of plasma viral RNA after the initial HIV-1 viremia of seroconversion (the "set point") predicts long-term clinical outcome (62). Following initiation of therapy, the viral load is predictive of the long-term response to therapy and prognosis. The minimum indication of a response to therapy is at least a 2.5-fold ($0.39 \log_{10}$) decrease in the baseline viral load. Anything smaller than this may be normal diurnal variation.

When potent antiretroviral therapy is initiated, there is a two-stage decline in the HIV-1 plasma RNA levels: a rapid and profound drop of usually 100-fold within the first 7 to 14 days, followed by a slower decline over the next 4 to 16 weeks (63). Patients with viral loads of 1000 copies or less at this time after starting an antiretroviral regimen have a 98% chance of a response at week 24, whereas those with more than this number have only a 25% chance of adequate response at week 24 (64). Treatment effects on the CD-4+ lymphocyte counts occur more slowly than the responses seen with the viral load (65). The initial increase in CD-4 counts that occurs with therapy may be redistribution of cells from lymphoid follicles, while the subsequent increase in CD-4 numbers reflects decreased destruction of these cells (36–38).

While the viral load has been shown to reflect the activity of the HIV infection within tonsillar lymphoid tissue, it is not yet

Table 45-2. Recommendations for Initiating Antiretroviral Therapy*

All symptomatic patients
Patients with CD-4 <500
For patients with CD-4 >500, use the plasma viral load as the guideline:
    >2000–5000 copies/mL: Start therapy
    >1000 copies/mL: Many would start therapy
    <1000 copies/mL: Could observe

*Data from Carpenter CC, Fischl MA, Hammer SM, et al. Antiretroviral therapy for HIV infection in 1998: updated recommendations of the International AIDS Society—USA Panel. JAMA 1998;280:78.

known if it reflects the activity of the HIV infection in *all* tissues. There are "sanctuary sites" that include the central nervous system, long-lived lymphocytes, and dendritic cells of the skin and other sites. Evidence is collecting that HIV can be compartmentalized in genital secretions in levels that far exceed the levels in the blood.

The Nucleoside Antiretroviral Agents

Until recently, the major emphasis of antiretroviral therapy has been directed toward inhibition of reverse transcriptase (1,65). It is likely that any step in the replicative process of HIV-1 that is different from that of human cells could be targeted for therapy (65). At this time, inhibitors of this enzyme are the prevailing, clinically available, therapeutic agents against this relentless infection (Tables 45-1, 45-2) (66,67).

In 1985 nucleosides with a 2′,3′-dideoxyribose moiety were identified to have inhibitory effects against HIV-1 in vitro (68). Following phosphorylation to the triphosphate form by the host cell kinases, these dideoxynucleoside-5′-triphosphates compete with physiologic nucleotides for binding with reverse transcriptase of HIV-1 (68–70). Unlike naturally occurring deoxynucleosides, these analogs lack a hydroxyl group in the 3′ position of the sugar ring (71). This prevents formation of the 3′,5′-phosphodiester bond that is necessary for DNA chain elongation, resulting in inhibition of reverse transcriptase, as well as premature termination of the DNA chain (68,69,72).

A major advantage of the nucleoside analogs is that they have a 10-fold to 20-fold greater affinity for retroviral reverse transcriptase (the RNA-directed DNA polymerase of HIV-1) than they do for cellular DNA polymerase alpha (73,74). The latter enzyme is important for DNA synthesis and repair. Mitochondrial DNA polymerase-gamma and DNA polymerase-beta are, however, more susceptible to inhibition by these analogs (74). Inhibition of these latter enzymes may account for some of the toxic effects of these drugs.

The purine and pyrimidine nucleoside analogs act on the preintegrational stages of the HIV-1 life cycle and therefore inhibit the early stages of virus infection (18,69). They have relatively little effect on chronically infected cells containing latent virus (69,73–75). Each nucleoside inhibitor has adverse effects that are noted below. All of them, however, can cause a rare but potentially fatal syndrome of lactic acidosis with hepatic steatosis (Table 45-3) (76).

Zidovudine (AZT)

Zidovudine was synthesized in 1964 as a potential chemotherapeutic agent (77). In 1974 it was found to inhibit retroviruses (78), and in 1985 it was found to inhibit HIV-1 in vitro (79). In 1985 it was taken into phase I clinical trials (80,81).

Zidovudine is the structural analog of thymidine, with an azido (N₃) group in place of the hydroxyl group at the 3′ position of the ribose ring (14). The active form of the drug is the triphosphate form that competes with deoxythymidine triphosphate for binding to the reverse transcriptase of HIV-1, subsequently inhibiting this enzyme and causing premature termination of the growing DNA chain (82). Zidovudine-monophosphate may also inhibit ribonuclease H, which functions in transcriptional processing of HIV-1 (83). In addition, zidovudine may also interfere with assembly and/or packaging of the HIV-1 particles at the cell membrane (84). This drug also hinders replication of other retroviruses, hepatitis B virus, and some bacteria as well (83).

Pharmacology

Although the plasma half-life is only 0.5 to 1.1 hours, like most nucleoside analogs, the intracellular half-life is relatively long (14,72). Passage of the drug into the host cells is by passive (nonfacilitated) diffusion (85). The lipophilic nature of the molecule is important in this regard (86).

On entering the host cells, it is phosphorylated in the cytosol by thymidine kinase (87). As with other anlaogs of thymidine, zidovudine is preferentially phosphorylated in proliferating (active) cells in which thymidine kinase levels are increased (88). This fact is important when considering the use of this drug in combination therapy. Since zidovudine-monophosphate is a substrate inhibitor of cellular thymidine kinase (87), it thus inhibits its own phosphorylation to the triphosphate form (88). It is this property of zidovudine monophosphate to inhibit thymidine kinase that makes it a potentially useful antineoplastic drug (89). However, the inhibition of thymidine kinase by zidovudine results in lower intracellular levels of the active triphosphate form of the drug (69,88) so that administration of higher doses of zidovudine does *not* result in higher intracellular levels of active drug.

Zidovudine enters the cerebrospinal fluid with peak levels of 60% of those of plasma (90). Within the CNS, it inhibits HIV-1 within brain macrophages and perhaps glial cells (91). Because of the ability to cross the blood-brain barrier, administration of

Table 45-3. Nucleoside Analog Inhibitors of Reverse Transcriptase

	Zidovudine (AZT)	Didanosine (ddI)	Zalcitabine (ddC)	Stavudine (d4T)	Lamivudine (3TC)	Abacavir (1589)
Analog of	Thymidine	Inosine → adenosine	Cyosine	Thymidine	Cytosine	Guanosine
CNS levels (% Serum)	60%	25%	30%	50%	~6%	20%
Metabolism (excretion)	Hepatic (85%) renal (15%)	Metabolism to urate; renal (50%)	Renal (75%)	Renal (50%) liver (50%)	Renal (50%)	Hepatic (alcoh dehydrog)
Toxicity	Bone marrow myopathy; headache; GI upset; insomnia	Pancreatitis neuropathy; GI upset	Neuropathy; stomatitis	Neuropathy	Nausea; Hepatitis	

Lactic acidosis and hepatic steatosis may occur with all NRTIs.

zidovudine to those with HIV dementia may result in significant cognitive improvement (91). It has been administered to pregnant patients in whom the pharmacodynamics were similar to those of nongravid adults and with no significant adverse effects on the fetus or neonate (92).

Zidovudine is predominately cleared from the body by hepatic glucuronidation to inactive metabolites that are subsequently eliminated by glomerular filtration and renal tubular secretion (41,83,93,94). About 15% of these metabolites are cleared by the biliary system (83). Preexisting hepatic disease in HIV-infected hemophilia patients does not alter toxicity or efficacy of the drug (41). Severe liver disease, however, with altered synthetic function, is an indication to reduce the drug dose and/or dose frequency (83). With markedly impaired renal function, plasma levels of the drug and metabolites may accumulate, dictating dose reduction or a decrease in dose frequency (83).

Several drugs, when given concurrently, alter the metabolism and/or clearance of zidovudine (83,95). Probenecid inhibits hepatic metabolism of zidovudine and results in higher levels of the active drug in the serum and cerebrospinal fluid (94,96). There is synergistic myelotoxicity, but no pharmacokinetic interactions, with concurrent administration of zidovudine with pyrimethamine, dapsone, sulfonamides, and ganciclovir (95). The contraindication between acetaminophen and zidovudine that came out of earlier studies has not been demonstrated in later studies (83,95).

Doses of Zidovudine

Zidovudine was initially prescribed in maintenance doses as high as 1200 to 1500 mg/day (97), doses that were associated with considerable toxicity (98). Subsequent studies revealed and confirmed that reduced maintenance doses of 600 mg/day were as effective as 1500 mg/day (99–101). Twice daily dosing of 300 mg of zidovudine is as effective as more-frequent dosing with better compliance. Preliminary data have shown that doses as low as 300 mg/day may be as effective (101,102), but doses below 300 mg/day seem to be suboptimal (103). Given these findings, it is recommended that the maintenance doses of zidovudine as first-line therapy of HIV infection should be 500 to 600 mg/day given in divided doses (99,101). Higher doses may be advisable for nervous-system dysfunction manifesting either as cognitive deficits or neuropathy (83).

Toxicity of Zidovudine

The most outstanding toxicity of zidovudine is bone-marrow suppression (81), particularly megaloblastic erythropoiesis (81). Marrow toxicity from zidovudine correlates with the stage of HIV infection and the dose of the drug (97). The ability of zidovudine to interfere with the phosphorylation of thymidine, as well as a hepatically produced metabolite of zidovudine (3′-amino-3′-deoxythymidine) that is toxic to bone-marrow precursor cells, may account for the bone-marrow toxicity (104,105). Zidovudine specifically inhibits globulin gene expression, and this may account for its greater cytotoxicity on erythroid cells

(106). The toxicity of zidovudine on red-blood-cell production can be substantially alleviated by administration of erythropoietin (107).

Administration of zidovudine may be associated with a myopathy that can be difficult to distinguish from HIV-related myopathy; both are associated with muscle wasting, myalgias, and elevations in serum levels of muscle enzymes (108,109). Cardiomyopathy may also occur (110). Myopathy is related to the cumulative dose of the drug (68). In tissues, zidovudine has its highest concentrations in skeletal and cardiac muscle (109). Inhibition of mitochondrial DNA polymerase gamma by zidovudine adversely alters mitochondrial functions, particularly oxidation-phosphorylation coupling, and results in morphophologic changes in the mitochondria that include enlarged, abnormal cristae containing electron-dense deposits in the matrix (109,111).

Nausea is a common adverse effect of zidovudine and is less sensitive to dose or stage of disease than are some of the other side effects of this drug (112). Other adverse effects include fatigue and headache that can be seen in about 50% of people for a period after initiation of therapy (112). Other toxicities include microvesicular steatosis of hepatocytes (113), central-nervous-system side effects such as agitation, confusion, lethargy, headaches (14), and esophageal ulcers (113).

Didanosine: ddI

Pharmacology

Didanosine was the second agent approved for clinical use for therapy of infection with HIV-1 (83). Unlike zidovudine, it is acid labile, so it must be administered along with a buffer (114,115). It is converted within human cells to 2′,3′-dideoxyadenosine, which is then phosphorylated by cellular enzymes to the 5′-triphosphate form (69,116). The latter is the active form of the drug that, like other dideoxynucleosides, competes with natural substrates, causing premature termination of the growing DNA chain, and inhibits the reverse transcriptase of HIV-1 (69,116,117).

The active metabolite of didanosine, dideoxy-adenosine 5′-triphosphate, has an intracellular half-life of 12 to 24 hours (117). Unlike zidovudine, which is more readily phosphorylated in active cells, didanosine may be more easily phosphorylated in resting cells (118,119). The drug is metabolized to uric acid that is excreted by the kidney (117). This accounts for the elevation in serum uric acid levels in those on this medication.

Didanosine is less lipophilic than is zidovudine and thus has reduced levels within the cerebrospinal fluid compared with zidovudine (91,115). Cerebrospinal fluid levels of the drug are 20% to 25% of those of the plasma (14). This may correlate with the clinical observation that cognitive improvements in HIV dementia are seen to a greater extent with zidovudine than with didanosine. Didanosine has at least additive, if not synergistic, antiretroviral activity when used with either zidovudine or stavudine (120–122).

Doses of Didanosine

The recommended doses for an adult are 125 mg PO twice a day for 35 to 49 kg weight, 200 mg PO twice a day for 50 to 74 kg of body weight, and 300 mg twice daily for adults more than 75 kg in weight (120,123). Because of the relatively long intracellular half-life of didanosine (~12 hours), once-daily dosing of the drug is as clinically effective as more-frequent dosing and is associated with less peripheral neuropathy (124,125).

Toxicity

Didanosine has a toxicity profile unlike that of zidovudine. In vitro, it has little effect on hematopoiesis at doses that affect HIV replication (123,126). The dose-limiting toxicities of didanosine were found to be pancreatitis and peripheral neuropathy (121). Other toxicities that have been seen include xerostomia (123), hepatitis (121), and increases in blood uric acid levels (121). Infrequently, higher doses of the drug were associated with hypocalcemia (69); central nervous system abnormalities such as restlessness, insomnia, and seizures (18); abnormalities of cardiac conduction; and elevations in skeletal muscle enzyme levels (121).

The annual risk of pancreatitis associated with didanosine is 4% to 7% in those on 500 mg/day and up to 23% in those on 750 mg/day of didanosine (120,127). Pancreatitis was seen in 3% (120) of those on zidovudine and in only 1.5% of age-matched seropositive controls not on antiviral therapy (128). The onset of pancreatitis varies between 6 to 24 weeks after institution of therapy (128,129), and it may be fatal in up to 10% (129).

Risk factors for pancreatitis associated with didanosine include the use of high doses of the drug; a history of prior pancreatitis; advanced HIV infection; the use of other pancreatotoxic medications such as ganciclovir, rifampin, ethambutol, and ethanol; and a history of increased hepatic transaminases (128,129). The pathophysiology of pancreatitis may be related to the release of reactive oxygen species during the catabolism of the drug by xanthine oxidase (18). Use of didanosine may also be associated with asymptomatic increases in serum amylase levels (129) in up to 39%, and this may be related to salivary-gland toxicity by the drug (128,129).

Neuropathy is another major toxicity associated with didanosine (130,131). In phase I studies using 750 mg twice daily, it was seen in up to 30% of patients within 3 months of entry into the study (69). It often begins with symmetric dyesthesiae of the feet and progresses to an uncomfortable ascending axonal neuropathy (131). Although it typically reverses with discontinuation of the drug (69), it may progress after withdrawal of the medication (131). The pathophysiology may be related to inhibition of DNA polymerase-gamma in nerve-cell mitochondria (14).

Zalcitabine: ddC

Zalcitabine has an oral bioavailability of over 80% (14,132), a plasma half-life of about 1 hour, and an intracellular half-life of about 2.5 hours (14). Like didanosine, phosphorylation of this drug by cellular kinases may occur more readily in resting cells (118). Zalcitabine may also have activity against hepatitis B virus

(96). Penetration of the drug into the cerebrospinal fluid is on the order of about 20% that of plasma concentrations (14), and 75% of the drug is excreted unchanged into the urine (93). Currently, the drug has limited utility in the antiretroviral arsenal, and its role is limited to a component of combination therapy with zidovudine (122). Because of overlapping and synergistic neurotoxicities, it should not be used in conjunction with didanosine. The recommended dose is 0.75 mg orally three times daily (99).

Toxicity of Zalcitabine

Adverse effects associated with zalcitabine include aphthous stomatitis and rash (133–135). Rash typically occurs during the first 6 weeks of study and may subside despite continued therapy with the drug (134). Other reported side effects include transient thrombocytopenia, arthralgias, and low-grade fevers (133,134).

The dose-limiting toxicity of zalcitibine is peripheral neuropathy, a symmetric, distal, primarily sensory neuropathy characterized by aching, burning, or lancinating pain (133–135). It is typically seen after the first 6 weeks of therapy and less commonly occurs after 24 weeks on the drug (133,134). Motor dysfunction, if seen at all, is generally limited to loss of the Achilles reflex (136). The neuropathy associated with zalcitabine may be caused by ddC diphosphate choline, a metabolic by-product of the drug that is a neurotoxin, or by the effect of zalcitabine on mitochondrial DNA polymerase gamma (74).

Stavudine: d4T

Stavudine, 2′,3′-didehydro-3′-deoxythymidine, is a structural analog of thymidine. Similar to the other dideoxynucleoside analogs, stavudine is phosphorylated by cellular enzymes (93,137–141). After metabolism to the triphosphate form, it is incorporated into the growing DNA chain resulting in inhibition of reverse transcriptase, as well as truncation of the growing DNA strand (138). In addition to the inhibitory effects on HIV reverse transcriptase, stavudine inhibits cellular DNA polymerases beta and gamma and thus reduces synthesis of mitochondrial DNA. These latter effects may be responsible for the side effects of this drug. They occur at much higher doses than those needed to inhibit HIV.

Stavudine is metabolized by the same enzymes that phosphorylate thymidine. Unlike zidovudine, however, it does not inhibit these enzymes (142). Therefore, it does not accumulate as the monophosphate form and is readily metabolized to the active triphosphate form. The drug has a relatively long intracellular half-life of about 200 minutes (138–140). Since it does not inhibit the enzymes responsible for phosphorylation of thymidine; however, it has less hematologic toxicity than zidovudine (104,142).

Stavudine has additive antiviral effects when given concurrently with didanosine. Zidovudine, however, inhibits thymidine kinase, so that concurrent administration of stavudine and zidovudine results in decreased activity of the former drug as a result of inhibition of conversion to the active (triphosphate) form (91). Excretion of this drug is divided between renal and non-renal routes (93), with approximately 40% of the drug being excreted unchanged in the urine (93) with active tubular secretion taking place. The drug dose needs to be modified with renal dysfunction.

The major toxicity of stavudine is peripheral neuropathy, that is dose-related, predominately affecting sensory nerves. This is encountered in up to 55% of those on greater than 1 mg/kg/day of the drug (137). It is characterized by paresthesiae, numbness, cramping, and decreased deep-tendon reflexes or abnormal sensory examination (137). Neuropathy occurs in 15% to 21% of those on less than 1 mg/kg/day and usually resolves after discontinuation of the drug. It may, however, temporarily worsen or continue after the drug is stopped. Those patients with a prior history of neuropathy or other predisposing factors for neuropathy are at increased risk of stavudine-induced, peripheral-nerve damage. Increases on liver function tests, predominately transaminases, may be seen in about 11% of patients (136,137). Erythrocytic macrocytosis is seen in about 50% of patients on the drug, and 14% develop anemia (136,137).

Lamivudine (3TC)

The pyrimidine, cytidine, has been modified to form nucleosides with antiretroviral activity. One modification results in 2',3'-dideoxy 3'-thiacytidine (3TC) that has a sulfur atom in place of the 3'-carbon atom in the ribose ring (143). The negative enantiomer of the molecule, which has the ribose ring in a different conformation than the physiologic nucleosides (18), is relatively resistant to exonucleases, making it more active as an antiviral compound (144). This forms a potent inhibitor of reverse transcriptase that is less toxic than zalcitabine (ddC) (18).

Lamivudine is preferentially phosphorylated in resting CD-4+lymphocytes. Penetration of this drug into CSF is less than 10% of serum levels but within the concentrations that suppress HIV replication (145–147). The inhibitory activity of lamivudine on reverse transcriptase is synergistic with that of zidovudine and at least additive with that of zalcitabine and didanosine (146).

The simultaneous presence of the most commonly encountered mutations in the reverse transcriptase gene that confers resistance to both zidovudine (codon 215) and lamivudine paradoxically restores zidovudine sensitivity. Those clones with both of these mutations are more susceptible to zidovudine than are clones with only the codon 215 mutation (which confers zidovudine resistance) (146).

Moreover, while the M184V mutation in reverse transcriptase that occurs with lamivudine may promote resistance to lamivudine (3TC), it has the beneficial effect of increasing the fidelity of the reverse transcriptase with respect to the nucleoside inserted (66). This makes the enzyme more susceptible to inhibition by other nucleoside analogs that are used in combination with lamuvidine (148).

Abacavir

Abacavir is an analog of guanosine. The drug is largely metabolized by hepatic glucuronidation (over 80%), with the remaining 20% metabolized by alcohol dehydrogenase (149). Since these two metabolic pathways are compensatory, the dose of the drug need not be altered in the presence of renal failure.

While resistance to this drug tends to develop slowly, the first mutation that occurs is often M184V, which also gives rise to cross-resistance to lamivudine (3TC) (150). Therefore, although the drug may be an addition to the antiretroviral armamentarium in drug-naïve patients, it offers only limited advantages to patients with resistant viral strains. In those patients with one to two mutations that confer resistance to reverse transcriptase inhibitors, about 75% respond to abacavir; with more than three such mutations, less than 25% will benefit from abacavir. The addition of mycophenolic acid may increase serum levels of abacavir by tenfold, while the addition of hydroxyurea may provide mild synergy.

Major side effects of abacavir include nausea (the intensity of which correlates with serum levels of the drug), headache, diarrhea, and insomnia. A hypersensitivity reaction to the drug may occur in up to 5% of patients. This typically develops within an average of 11 days after initiation of therapy, with over 90% of those who develop the reaction doing so within 6 weeks of starting the drug. The reaction consists of a morbilliform eruption, fever, nausea, and possible respiratory distress. The hypersensitivity symptoms tend to progress if the drug is continued, and they intensify within an hour of drug dosing. Rechallenge with the drug after such a reaction may be fatal (149,150).

Adefovir

Adefovir is a nucleotide and therefore does not require intracellular monophosphorylation. HIV-1 strains that are resistant to nucleoside inhibitors of reverse transcriptase are sensitive to this drug. This drug has the advantage of being active in stimulated and resting lymphocytes, as well as in monocytes and macrophages. Adefovir is also active against HIV-2 and a range of herpes viruses.

The parent formulation of adefovir has poor bioavailability, but the prodrug dipivoxil is 40% bioavailable and is converted by the liver to adefovir. It is transported across the plasma membrane by a protein transporter that is saturable. The drug has an intracellular half-life of approximately 18 hours, so once-daily administration is possible (147). The drug has at least additive activity with other antiretroviral medications, and no other medications seem to be antagonistic.

Adefovir has the potential side effect of nephrotoxicity consisting of a "Fanconi-like syndrome." Hypophosphatemia, proteinuria, glycosuria, lowered serum bicarbonate levels, and elevations in serum creatinine levels may result and require discontinuation of the drug. A rare minority (1% of 1500 patients in one study) experienced renal tubular necrosis associated with the use of this drug. Other potential adverse effects of the drug include an increase in hepatic transaminases in 4% of patients, an increase in bilirubin in 1%, and increased muscle enzymes in 2%. All patients on this medication experience a decrease in serum carnitine levels caused by binding of this molecule with a metabolite of adefovir (pivalic acid) and subsequent renal excretion of the complex by the kidney. Tenofovir (PMPA) is a nucleotide inhibitor of HIV-1 reverse transcriptase that is related to adefovir, but may have less renal toxicity. It is currently entering clinical trials.

The Purine Analogs

The purine 2′,3′-dideoxynucleosides tend to be acid labile (117) and therefore vulnerable to destruction by gastric acid unless administered in a buffered form (69). Dideoxyadenosine is an analog of adenosine that is converted by adenosine deaminase to dideoxyinosine and ultimately to hypoxanthine (69). It is therefore a prodrug of didanosine (69,151). The major disadvantage of dideoxyadenosine is that it has metabolites that cause renal dysfunction (117). Additions to the sugar ring of adenosine (152–154) may result in a molecule that has much less toxicity. This drug, lodenosine (FddA), is active against strains of HIV that have the Q151M mutation, one that promotes cross-resistance to all of the other nucleoside analogs and has little cross-resistance with these other nucleoside-analog inhibitors of reverse transcriptase.

Pyrimidine Analogs

Because of the poor affinity of 2′,3′-dideoxyuridine (ddU) for cellular nucleoside kinases, it cannot be biotransformed to the active 5′-triphosphate form and is therefore not effective at inhibiting HIV-1 in human T cells (69,155,156).

A modification of cytidine that is being studied is the addition of a fluorine atom to the negative stereoisomer of 3′-thia′2′-deoxycytidine (FTC) (emtricitabine) (157). A disadvantage of this compound is that a small amount is converted to the toxic metabolite 4-fluorouracil (157). However, the drug has activity against hepatitis B, as well as HIV, and is up to tenfold more potent than lamivudine (3TC). Its resistance pattern is the same as 3TC.

The compound 3-fluoro-2′,3′-dideoxy-thymidine, a derivative of thymidine, is efficiently converted to the active triphosphate form (69). In this form in vitro it has activity against the reverse transcriptase of HIV-1 (158). Similar to zidovudine, which is also an analog of thymidine, hematologic side effects are seen in the majority (158).

Combination Therapy with Nucleoside Analogs

Infection with HIV-1 is associated with a progressive qualitative, as well as quantitative, decline in CD-4+ lymphocytes (159). Monotherapy with nucleoside analogs in a drug-naïve patient is associated with an increase in CD-4 lymphocyte numbers with a maximum effect in 6 to 12 weeks following initiation of therapy (51,54,58). The persistance and magnitude of the increase in CD-4+ lymphocyte counts varies with the severity of immunodepletion at the start of therapy (51,54,98,160).

Only a small part of the effect of the nucleoside analogs on morbidity and mortality is related to the effects on CD-4 counts (51). In vitro, administration of these drugs is associated with at least a transient increase in CD-4+ lymphocyte functions such as lymphocyte blastogenesis and production of interferon-gamma; in vivo, there is an increase in natural-killer cell-function (161). The durability of the qualitative changes in lymphocyte function varies from 10 weeks to 2 years (159,162). These qualitative improvements in CD-4+ lymphocyte function do not correlate very well with improvements in surrogate markers of HIV infection (48,54,159–161).

The benefits of nucleoside analogs on disease progression are less durable if they are initiated later in the course of the HIV infection when the burden of virus is higher and the host immune response is less able to control viral replication (97,98,162–169). When used with advanced disease, decreases in disease progression and increases in survival still occur (81,98), indicating that therapy is efficacious in advanced disease for at least a limited duration of time (163,169).

Analogs of thymidine (zidovudine and stavudine) inhibit HIV-1 replication in activated CD-4+ lymphocytes, while purine (didanosine) and cytosine (zalcitabine, lamivudine) analogs are more effective in inhibiting viral replication in resting CD-4+ T cells. Combinations of these nucleoside analogs thus provide synergistic inhibition of reverse transcriptase (103,170–173). Combination therapy with nucleoside analog inhibitors of reverse transcriptase (a drug that is more active in stimulated CD-4 lymphocytes along with one that is active in resting CD-4+ lymphocytes and monocytes) is now the standard of care and forms the basis of almost all currently recommended drug regimens.

Effective combinations of nucleoside inhibitors of reverse transcriptase include the following:

> zidovudine + lamivudine
> stavudine + lamivudine
> zidovudine + didanosine
> stavudine + didanosine

The combination of zidovudine + zalcitabine is less effective, and because of pharmacologic antagonism zidovudine + stavudine is not recommended.

A third drug, and sometimes a fourth, is added to the double-nucleoside combination, either a nonnucleoside inhibitor of reverse transcriptase and/or a protease inhibitor. Other combinations, for which data are currently more limited, include the following:

1 protease inhibitor + 1 nucleoside inhibitor + 1 nonnucleoside inhibitor

2 protease inhibitors + 1 nucleoside inhibitor + 1 nonnucleoside inhibitor

Abacavir + 2 nucleoside inhibitors

2 protease inhibitors (in full doses)

The Nonnucleoside Reverse Transcriptase Inhibitors

The nonnucleoside inhibitors of reverse transcriptase are a class of structurally unrelated compounds (15,18) that have in common the ability to directly inhibit the RNA-directed DNA polymerase of HIV-1. Unlike the nucleoside analog inhibitors of reverse transcriptase, these compounds do *not* require phosphorylation to be active and are *not* incorporated into the DNA chain (47,174). These drugs have little, if any, inhibitory activity on human DNA polymerases and therefore lack some of the side effects of the nucleoside analogs. For the most part, this class of compounds is inactive against other retroviruses (175,176).

Unlike the nucleoside analogs of reverse transcriptase discussed above, these substances act on nonsubstrate binding sites, rather than the catalytic site, of the enzyme. They alter the conformation of the enzyme in a manner that inhibits its catalytic action (143). These compounds have the advantage of being non–cross-resistant with nucleoside analog inhibitors of reverse transcriptase (175) and therefore offer the possibility of at least additive inhibition of this enzyme (177–179). These drugs tend to have greatest activity in those with viral loads of less than 50,000 copies/mL and are less effective in those with viral loads exceeding 100,000 copies/mL.

The rapid development of resistance has been a major disadvantage of these compounds (175–177). Mutations that confer resistance to one nonnucleoside reverse transcriptase inhibitor may induce cross-resistance to other nonnucleoside inhibitors. Cross-resistance between first-generation, nonnucleoside inhibitors is likely because they share a key mutation at position 181 of the reverse transcriptase enzyme. Administration of nucleoside analogs does not prevent, or significantly delay, the emergence of resistance.

Specific Drugs

The largest group of nonnucleoside reverse transcriptase inhibitors are derivates of TIBO (4,5,6,7-**T**etrahydro-5-methyl-**I**midazo**B**enzo-[4,5,1] [1,4] benzo-diazepi-2 (1H)-**O**ne) (180,181). This group includes delavirdine, nevirapine, and the pyridinone derivatives L-697,661 (Table 45-4) (175,181).

Nevirapine was the first nonnucleoside inhibitor of reverse transcriptase to be clinically available. It has excellent bioavailability after oral absorption, with over 93% of the drug being absorbed from the gastrointestinal tract (179,182). The drug is very lipophilic and therefore crosses the blood-brain barrier in levels close to 90% of those of serum levels. The dose of the drug is 200 mg PO daily for the first 10 days and then 200 mg PO twice daily thereafter.

A major side effect of this drug is rash; about 30% have a rash that is mild to moderate. About 7% of patients on this drug have to discontinue the drug because of rash that may progress to Stevens-Johnson syndrome. The majority of rashes occur within the first 6 weeks of therapy.

Like all of the nonnucleoside reverse transcriptase inhibitors, however, there is rapid emergence of resistance to nevirapine (181). HIV isolates with 100-fold to 250-fold reduced susceptibility to the drug emerge in vitro by 8 weeks of nevirapine monotherapy. The time to emergence of resistant strains is not altered by combination therapy with other inhibitors of reverse transcriptase.

Delavirdine was the second NNRTI to become clinically available and has a profile similar to that of nevirapine. Both of

Table 45-4. Profile of the Nonnucleoside Inhibitors of Reverse Transcriptase

	Nevirapine (Viramune)	Delavirdine (Rescriptor)	Efavirenz (Sustiva)
Dose	200 mg/d ×14 days; then 200 mg bid	400 mg tid	600 mg hs
	(See dose modifications for use with protease inhibitors.)		
Elimination	All are metabolized by hepatic cytochrome 450		
	80% urinary	50% urinary	30% urinary
	20% biliary	45% biliary	60% biliary
Drug interactions	Induces P-450	Inhibits P-450	Induces P-450

Doses of protease inhibitors need to be adjusted when used with NNRTIs:
- Indinavir levels are decreased 30%, so increase the dose to 1000 mg tid.
- Saquinavir levels are decreased up to 70%, so avoid concurrent use.
- Amprenavir levels are decreased up to 30%, so the doses of amprenavir may have to be increased to 1200 mg tid or ritonavir added 200 mg bid to block the P-450 system.
- Nelfinavir levels are *probably* not significantly altered by NNRTIs.
- Ritonavir levels are not significantly altered by NNRTIs. Ritonavir can be used in low doses to decrease activity of P-450 to enhance the levels of other protease inhibitors in the presence of NNRTIs.

these drugs are extensively biotransformed by the hepatic P-450 cytochrome system, with glucuronide conjugation and urinary excretion of the metabolites being the major excretory route. While nevirapine is an inducer of these enzymes, delavirdine is an inhibitor of the hepatic P-450 enzymes. Therefore, nevirapine may decrease the serum levels of protease inhibitors by increasing their metabolism, while delavirdine may increase the serum levels.

The most recent addition to the class of nonnucleoside inhibitors of reverse transcriptase is efavirenz (DMP-266, Sustiva[R]). Compared with nevirapine and delavirdine, this drug requires a few more mutations within the reverse transcriptase before high-level resistance occurs; however, cross-resistance does still occur. Efavirenz, like nevirapine, induces the hepatic P-450 system, and this must be taken into account when it is used with protease inhibitors. This drug shares the propensity for allergic rash that the former two drugs have, and, in addition, because it has greater penetration into the central nervous system, efavirenz may be associated with side effects not seen with the others such as dizziness, sleep disturbances, and a "dissociative feeling." However, efavirenz, as a hepatic P-450 inducer, increases its own metabolism, so within 10 days a steady state is reached and side effects may abate.

Second-generations, nonnucleoside inhibitors of reverse transcriptase that are currently in clinical trials, including quinoxalone and derivatives of oxanthiin carboxanilide, are active against HIV-1 strains that contain the 181 mutation (182).

Ancillary Agents

Hydroxyurea

Hydroxyurea inhibits the enzyme ribonucleotide reductase, which is present in replicating cells but detectable in only very low amounts in resting cells, and thus inhibits deoxynucleotide synthesis. This results in decreased intracellular deoxynucleotide levels and inhibited DNA synthesis, so that cells are arrested in the G1/S phase of the cell cycle (183,184). This action of hydroxyurea is nonspecific, affecting cells that have been infected with HIV, as well as uninfected cells.

Monotherepay with hydroxyurea is not an effective antiretroviral regimen (184,185). Hydroxyurea may be used in low doses to augment the antiviral activity of nucleoside analog inhibitors of reverse transcriptase (186). This potential is greater with didanosine than it is with zalcitabine (ddC) or zidovudine (AZT) (184). Enhancement of the viral activity of didanosine arises from a specific depletion of dATP by hydroxyurea, resulting in a shift in the ratio of 2′,3′-dideoxyadenosine 5′-triphosphate to dATP (185,187). This shift increases the intracellular metabolism of didanosine to its active form, dideoxyadenosine triphosphate (185,187).

Concomitant administration of hydroxyurea and didanosine has been shown to be well tolerated and effects synergistic inhibitory activity on HIV-1 with significant decreases in viral titers and increases in CD-4 lymphocyte counts after 3 months of therapy (188). Hydroxyurea also has the advantage of crossing the blood-brain barrier (185). There is often little or no change in the CD-4+ lymphocyte count with the use of hydroxyurea because of hydroxyurea-related lymphopenia (189).

Agents Used to Treat Other Viral Infections

The use of acyclovir may decrease morbidity and mortality from HIV-1 infection despite the fact that acyclovir has little if any antiretroviral activity as a single agent (190–193). Herpes viruses result in up-regulation of HIV replication (192,194); by controlling herpesvirus infections, acyclovir is useful in the therapy of HIV-1 infection. Some studies have shown that acyclovir potentiates the anti-HIV effects of zidovudine in vitro, and in vivo there is a transient increase in CD-4 counts and a decrease in p24 antigen levels (193).

Another drug that may have some utility in HIV infection is foscarnet (trisodium phosphono-formate hexahydrate) (195). This drug inhibits the reverse transcriptase of HIV-1 (195). While some studies have shown that concurrent administration of foscarnet and zidovudine may yield a synergistic increase in survival time (195), others have not found this to be true (196).

Agents Directed Toward the CD-4+ Receptor

Recombinant soluble CD-4 is a part of the N-terminal domain of the extracellular portion of the CD-4 molecule (65). In vitro it may be able to bind the Gp-120 glycoprotein of the HIV-1 viral envelope and thus hinder binding of the virus to the target cell (65). Despite successes in vitro (65), recombinant soluble CD-4 has had disappointing results in vivo (65,197). This agent may have a role as prophylaxis against HIV-1 after an acute exposure such as a needle stick (65).

Dextran sulfate is a weak inhibitor of binding of HIV-1 to target cells (198) and may have inhibitory activity against the reverse transcriptase of HIV-1 (190). Despite an in vitro therapeutic index at least equivalent to that of zidovudine (190), nonrandomized studies have shown no significant changes in surrogate markers of disease activity (199). The anti-HIV-1 activity of dextran sulfate is largely the result of the sulfate (190,198).

In vitro, pretreatment of human monocytes with 1-alpha 25-dihydroxyvitamin D3 reduced HIV-1 infection of these cells by decreasing HIV-1 binding by mechanisms that are as yet poorly defined (200). This approach has not proven to be clinically useful (200). Other approaches that alter binding of HIV-1 to the CD-4 receptor such as pyridoxal 5-phosphate, which binds to the CD-4 receptor; modifications of the CD-4 receptor into antibody-like molecules; or recombinant proteins consisting of parts of the HIV envelope glycoproteins that are linked to various toxins have not met with great success (201,202). Inhibition of viral binding to host cells would seem to be a logical therapeutic strategy. Despite intensive research in this area, however, this potential has remained elusive (22).

Inhibitors of Viral Replication

Interferons inhibit HIV-1 in vitro largely by inhibition of viral assembly and budding (7). In vitro, the inhibitory activity of interferon-alpha toward HIV-1 replication is synergistic with that of zidovudine (83). In vivo, coadministration of zidovudine and interferon-alpha results in a transient decrease in surrogate markers of viral infection, but no beneficial long-term results (7).

Replication of HIV-1 depends on the activity of the Tat gene. This encodes for the Tat protein that functions to enhance expression of other viral genes (203). Agents that interfere with the functions of the Tat protein hinder replication and maintain the virus in dormancy (204). While toxicity has been a problem for this line of agents, one candidate, currently known as Ro24-7429, is being investigated (203,204).

Integrase is another unique viral enzyme, the inhibition of which could potentially offer therapy for HIV-1 infection (98). To date, however, inhibitors of viral integrase have had toxicity precluding clinical use (205).

Similar to the Tat protein, tumor necrosis factor-alpha also stimulates HIV-1 replication in acutely and chronically infected CD-4+ lymphocytes, as well as monocytes/macrophages (20). This cytokine activates cellular transcription factors that result in augmentation of replication (20). In vitro, soluble TNF-receptors have been shown to limit HIV-1 transcription (20). Chemical inhibitors of TNF-alpha production such as thalidomide (19), vesnarine (206), and cimetidine also limit HIV-1 replication in vitro (19). Inhibitors of tumor necrosis factor-alpha tend to be more effective against acutely infected cells than chronically infected cells.

Antisense oligonucleotides offer the potential of being able to decrease HIV-1 mRNA transcription (207). For a successful outcome, these agents must be stable in vivo and must be able to enter target cells (208). Obstacles to the use of these agents occur because different viral strains may have different mRNA types, and there may be variable transport of the antisense construction into target cells (207). Ampligen, poly(i)n: poly(C12U)n, is a double-stranded synthetic RNA with immunomodulatory activities that may decrease viral replication (208). Although uncontrolled studies have shown actions that are synergistic with zidovudine (208), there is considerable toxicity and lack of significant benefits in vivo (208).

As noted above, HIV-1 requires the CD-4 antigen and a co-antigen for high-efficiency binding and entry into target cells (12). The coreceptors are the chemokine receptors, CXCR4 (also called fusin) and CCR5; other chemokine receptors such as CCR2b and CCR3 may also serve as coreceptors for HIV-1. About 1% of the population has two copies of a 32-base pair deletion-mutation form of chemokine receptor CCR5, and these people are relatively resistant to HIV infection. About 10% to 15% of the population has one mutant gene, and in these people HIV infection takes two to three times as long to progress as in those with wild-type genes. These people with mutant genes and therefore mutant receptors seem to be healthy. These mutant alleles are tenfold more common in the Caucasian population than in other populations.

It is known that CD-8+ lymphocytes make soluble factors that inhibit HIV infection of other cells. These factors have been identified as the chemokines RANTES, MIP-1-alpha, and MIP-1-beta. These factors block and down-regulate production of chemokine receptors so that they are not as available, and thus HIV-1 is unable to infect target cells with its usual avidity (12,23,209). Given this new data, the concept of chemokine receptor blockers has therefore emerged and is being explored (23).

Interleukin-2 is also being explored for its potential as a therapeutic agent in HIV-1 infection. Infection by HIV-1 is known to be associated with decreased production of IL-2 and with CD-8+ lymphocytes being rendered nonfunctional; these cells are stuck in the G-1 phase of the cell cycle. Interleukin-2, given either intravenously or subcutaneously, has been shown to support CD-8+ lymphocyte maturation by permitting these cells to overcome the G1/2 "hump." IL-2 also enhances the function and number of NK, B, and T cells and promotes the secondary release of cytokines that enhance antigen processing (210–212). The response of patients to IL-2 infusions (4.5 to 9 M units SQ twice daily for 5 days every 4 to 8 weeks) correlates with the initial CD-4 count.

Other Agents Being Investigated

Several compounds are in development for potential use in HIV-1 infection (213). One drug, FP-21399, a bis-azo dye, inhibits the postabsorptive stage of viral replication. Pentafuside is a synthetic peptide HIV-fusion inhibitor. ISIS 5320 is a phosphorothioate oligonucleotide that binds GP120. Resobene is a sulfonated dye that inhibits HIV attachment and fusion.

Therapies directed toward the postattachment phases of viral replication include CNI-HO294 as an inhibitor of the HIV preintegration-complex nuclear translocation. Calanolide A is a reverse transcriptase inhibitor that is active against both zidovudine-resistant and nonnucleoside inhibitor–resistant strains that contain the Y181C genotype. NSC 687025 is a bisimidazo-acridone that inhibits the formation of single and unspliced viral RNA transcripts. MSI-1436 is an aminosterol that inhibits IL-6–induced viral expression.

Disulfide-containing macrolides have antiretroviral activity by forming a complex that has a chemical-binding motif known as a zinc finger. These structures allow HIV-1 to bind zinc. Disulfide-containing macrolides bind zinc and dislodge it from the pocket in which the virus normally holds it (214).

T-20 (pentafuside) is a 36 amino acid peptide that corresponds to the extracellular portion of the transmembrane segment of the HIV envelope glycoprotein (p41). It inhibits viral fusion to the host cell membrane. The durability of its activity, however, seems to be limited.

Protease Inhibitors

The protein products of the HIV-1 genome are initially translated as high-molecular-weight polyproteins that are then cleaved into the various structural proteins and enzymes by a protease that is also encoded for by the viral genome (75). The site of cleavage by HIV-1 protease is a Phe (or Tyr)-Pro dipeptide that is not recognized by eukaryotic proteases. Since mammalian protease enzymes are aspartyl proteases, they are not able to subserve the function(s) of the HIV-1 protease enzyme (2). This gives the HIV-1 protease inhibitors an in vitro therapeutic index of greater than one-thousand when compared with eukaryotic proteases (25,45,215).

Inhibition of reverse transcriptase blocks viral replication in previously uninfected cells, but has little effect on virus in cells in which integration has already occurred. Functional protease is essential for the release of infectious virus. Although protease inhibitors interfere with later stages of infection by HIV-1 (75), these agents also block early steps in HIV-1 replication possibly by interfering with production of viral nucleocapsid protein (75).

The protease inhibitors are transition-state mimetics of the Phe (Tyr)-Pro substrate moiety and were developed using a three-dimensional, computer-generated model of the active site of the protease enzyme of HIV-1. Unlike the nucleoside analog inhibitors of reverse transcriptase, they do not require metabolic activation (215). Analysis of the structure of HIV-1 protease protein has identified many compounds that may inhibit it such as the curious finding that haloperidol has this function (2).

A potential disadvantage of these agents is that their uptake by target cells is by passive diffusion and is therefore both dose and time dependent (216). Consequently, uptake of these substances by target cells is slower than the receptor-mediated entry of the virus, so that infection of target cells and incorporation of the viral genome into that of the host cell may occur before the protease inhibitors can start to act (75). Moreover, the CNS penetration of these drugs is poor. The problem of resistance to protease inhibitors is significant and is discussed below.

The protease inhibitors tend to be highly bound to plasma proteins, particularly albumin. A minor component of the plasma-binding capacity, however, is provided by alpha$_1$-acid glycoprotein (AAG). While albumin is constitutively produced and binds drugs with high capacity but low affinity, AAG is produced in an inducible manner (up-regulated by infection, hormones, and inflammation) and binds drugs with low capacity but high affinity. Thus, a potential problem with protease inhibitors is increased binding by AAG during times of physiologic stress. Since only the free drug is available to inhibit HIV-1 protease, resistance may emerge.

The protease inhibitors have effects on human metabolism that are still poorly defined. Diabetes mellitus occurs in about 2% of patients who are on any of the protease inhibitors, and glucose intolerance may occur more frequently. Hyperlipidemia also occurs in about one out of three patients who are on these drugs. This may reach a magnitude that merits therapy, and this is complicated by the drug interactions of the lipid-lowering drugs and the protease inhibitors. The "statin" drugs are metabolized by the P-450, 3A subset of hepatic enzymes and may result in clinically significant alterations in protease-inhibitor levels. Gemfibrazole

is not metabolized by this system and thus can be used with protease inhibitors. Cholestyramine should be avoided because of its ability to bind medications in the GI tract.

All of the protease inhibitors decrease the activity of the hepatic P-450 cytochromes. This needs to be taken into consideration when other medications are introduced, since toxicity from the latter may become a problem. The rank order of CYP3A4 inhibition is as follows (213,215,216):

Ritonavir ≫ indinavir = nelfinavir = ampenavir > saquinavir

The cytochromes consist of over thirty isoenzymes located in the endoplasmic reticulum of hepatocytes. The 3A subset of the P-450 enzymes make up approximately 60% of the hepatic P-450 enzymes. Although other P-450 enzymes have genetic polymorphism, there is no evidence as yet of polymorphism within the 3A subset. *The P450, 3A4 subset is the major enzymatic route of metabolism of the protease inhibitors.* Coadministration of other drugs that are metabolized by the 3A subsystem is relatively contraindicated. Drugs that interact with protease inhibitors do so by altering the levels of the protease inhibitor (creating the potential for decreased serum levels) and/or the other drug, resulting in alterations in the levels of the second drug with potentially life-threatening reactions. (Table 45-5).

Clinical Use of Combination Regimens Containing Protease Inhibitors

The combination of a protease inhibitor and two nucleoside analog inhibitors of reverse transcriptase has emerged as the current standard of care. However, other combinations may be as active in suppression of HIV-1 replication (217,218). Treatment strategies that include induction, maintenance, and intensification are being studied, but no conclusions have been reached to date.

Neither the initial CD-4+ lymphocyte count nor the initial viral load indicates the nadir in the viral load that can be attained with triple-drug therapy. The viral load response at week 12 of therapy, however, is predictive of the ultimate response that can be expected. Patients with 1000 copies or less at 12 weeks had a 98% chance of response at week 24 (an undetectable viral load). Those patients with more than 1000 copies at 12 weeks had only a 25% chance of attaining this desirable response by week 24 (216).

Resistance to Antiviral Agents

The result of advancing HIV-1 infection is decreased immune surveillance (219), allowing for increasing rates of viral replication and a greater viral burden. Compounding this problem is the tendency for the viral pool within a particular patient to gradually mutate toward a population of closely related genomes ("quasispecies") from which resistant viral strains may develop (118,219–221). The high mutation rate of HIV combined with

Table 45-5. Profiles of the First-Generation Protease Inhibitors

	Saquinavir (Invirase)	Indinavir (Crixivan)	Ritonavir (Norvir)	Nelfinavir (Viracept)	Amprenavir (Agenerase)
Oral bioav	4%	30%	70–80%	20–80%	—
Effect of food	Incr	Decr	Incr	Incr	Unchanged (avoid high fat)
Protein binding	98%	60%	90%	>80%	~90%
Half-life (hours)	1.5–2	1.5–2	3–4	3.5–5	7.1–10.6
Metab	All are cleared by hepatic cytochrome P-450-3A4 with rapid but saturable metabolism. Other drugs that are metabolized by the P-450 system may markedly decrease or increase serum protease levels.				
Fecal %	88	83	86	87	75
Urine %	12	17	14	2	14
CNS pentr	Generally poor, but indinavir may reach concentrations in CSF that inhibit HIV-1 since it is less protein-bound than the other protease inhibitors.				
Dose	600 mg tid	800 mg tid	600 mg bid	750 mg tid 1250 mg bid	1200 mg bid
Adverse effects	Diarrhea, nausea, and increases in liver-function tests. Gilbert's syndrome may occur with all. Hyperlipidemia has been seen with ritonavir and increases in CPK with nelfinavir. Headache and kidney stones in those on indinavir.				

the large daily turnover of virus results in a broad diversity of genomic variants over time.

The reverse transcriptase gene is error-prone (175,221,222), and HIV lacks the corrective 3'–5' exonuclease activity that is encountered in higher forms of life. This inherent genetic instability allows drug-resistant strains to appear de-novo, without prior drug exposure (222). More commonly, drug resistance develops in the presence of one of the antiretroviral drugs (223–225). Horizontal transmission of these resistant strains is possible (222).

Although a single amino-acid change may confer resistance to a particular antiretroviral medication (14), high-level resistance is caused by sequential accumulation of multiple amino-acid mutations in the reverse transcriptase enzyme (226–228). These substitutions typically are not in proximity to the catalytic site of the enzyme (229) and therefore often do not greatly alter the function of the enzyme.

Strains of virus with resistance to various nucleoside analogs have a growth advantage in the presence of the drug compared with the wild-type virus (222). When the selective pressure of the drug is removed, the predominant HIV population tends to revert toward the wild-type strains again (230,231). This reversion tends to occur relatively slowly, indicating that the resistant strains continue to have replicative and pathogenic capacity (39). Some of these resistant strains have been reported to persist for over a year after discontinuation of the medication (219).

Several, specific amino-acid changes in reverse transcriptase may confer cross-resistance to other nucleoside analog inhibitors of reverse transcriptase (224,232–236). Particular codon changes in the gene for reverse transcriptase may promote relative cross-resistance to the other nucleoside inhibitors (Table 45-6) (235–240). It is important to consider these changes when prescribing either initial or subsequent therapy with nucleoside inhibitors of reverse transcriptase.

Resistance to the Nonnucleoside Reverse Transcriptase Inhibitors

Rapid emergence of resistance to the nonnucleoside reverse transcriptase inhibitors occurs after as little as 2 weeks of therapy (Table 45-7) (243). Concurrent administration of other antiretroviral medications does not prevent the emergence of resistant viral strains (80,243). Resistance to one first-generation NNRTI tends to confer cross-resistance to the entire class of drugs, but not to other classes of antiretroviral medications (175–180,243,244).

Resistance to Protease Inhibitors

Selection of viral strains that are resistant to the protease inhibitors is a gradual process during which mutations accumulate at different sites in the protease gene, generating populations with increasing levels of resistance (Table 45-8). Once viral resis-

Table 45-6. Codon Changes in Reverse Transcriptase Associated with Resistance

Zidovudine (AZT)	41 (4×)		67	70	**<u>215</u>** (16×)	219

Combinations of mutations yield synergistic resistance:
215 + 41 = 60-fold resistance
215 + 67 + 70 = 31-fold resistance
215 + 67 + 70 + 41 = 179-fold resistance
215 + 67 + 70 + 219 = 166-fold resistance

Didanosine (DDI)	<u>65</u> (10×)	**<u>74</u>** 10×)	<u>75</u> 10×)	<u>184</u> (5×)
Zalcitabine (ddC)	<u>65</u>	**69**	**74** (10×)	<u>184</u>
Lamivudine (3TC)	<u>65</u>			**184** (1000×)
Stavudine (d4T)	50		**75** (7×)	
Abacavir	65 (3×)	<u>74</u> (4×)	115 (5×)	**184**
Adefovir	65 (15×)	70 (10×)		

Those in **bold** are most significant, and those that are in *italic* are associated with cross-resistance. The number below the codon change refers to the magnitude of decreased sensitivity.
Adapted from references 133, 219, 224, 234–236, 241, and 242.

Table 45-7. Patterns of Codon Changes Associated with Resistance to Nonnucleoside Inhibitors of Reverse Transcriptase

	98	100	101	103	106	108	179	181	188	190	236
Nevirapine (Viramune)	98 (2×)	100 (5×)	101 (12×)	**103** (40×)	**106** (100×)	108		**181** (100×)	**188** (100×)	**190** (100×)	
Delavirdine (Rescriptor)		**100** (35×)	101 (5×)	**103** (25×)	**106** (15×)			**181** (25×)	**188** (20×)	**190** (20×)	236 70×
Loviride				103				**181**			236
Efaverenz (Sustiva)		**100** (20×)	101 (8×)	**103** (20×)		108	179	181 (4×)	**188** (100×)	**190** (100×)	

Codons in **bold** confer high-level resistance. The numbers below the mutation are the magnitude of resistance conferred.

tance emerges, it tends to progress despite increases in drug doses. High plasma HIV-1 RNA levels or low CD-4 counts at the onset of therapy with protease inhibitors do not predict the occurrence of genotypic resistance (245). Unfortunately, many of the amino-acid changes that promote resistance to the protease inhibitors increase the fitness of the virus. To delay the emergence of resistance for as long as possible, protease inhibitors need to be used in combination with other antiretroviral drugs (245,246). Also, the highest possible doses of the protease inhibitor should be used from the onset. Drugs holidays may occur if necessary, but the dose of the drug should *never* be decreased.

The nadir (trough) levels of protease inhibitors in blood tend to be critically near the level at which some strains of HIV-1 can replicate. Because of this, even minor breaks in the adherence to the protease inhibitors can result in breakthrough replication of HIV-1 and, consequently, resistance (247).

Adherence (%)	Complete Viral Suppression (%)
>95	81
90	64
85	50
75	25
<75	6

Table 45-8. Patterns of Amino Acid Substitutions that Promote Resistance to Protease Inhibitors*

	Saquin	Riton	Indin	Nelfin	Ampren
L10I, V, R		*	*		
K20R		*	*		
L24I			*		
D30N				0	
M46I, L	*	*	0		*
G48V, Y	0				
I50V					0
I54V	*	*	*		
L63P	*		*		
I64V			*		
A71V, T	*	*	*	*	
V82A, T, F	*	*	0		
I84V	*	*	*	0	
L90M	0	*	*	0	

* A combination of 3–5 amino acid substitutions are needed for high-level resistance. Those noted 0 promote high-level resistance.

Conclusions

The epidemic of HIV-1 infection continues to grow both in the United States and worldwide. Left untreated, this infection results in a relentless degradation of the cellular immune system (39). The clinical manifestations are largely the result of opportunistic infections and neoplasms, as well as metabolic disturbances caused by the cytokines produced in response to the infection (40,41).

Despite its relatively simple structure, HIV- has a complicated mechanism of replication (6). It is likely that any step in the replicative process of HIV-1 that is different from that of human cells could be targeted for therapy (175). At this time, inhibitors of reverse transcriptase are the prevailing clinically available therapeutic agents against this relentless infection (76). A major issue of the nucleoside reverse transcriptase inhibitors is that the benefits with respect to survival and disease progression tend to dissipate with time. The nonnucleoside inhibitors of reverse transcriptase initially offered promise for effective therapy. Rapid emergence of resistance to these agents, however, has been a major disadvantage of these compounds (175,176).

Resistance to antiretroviral agents is a major therapeutic problem. Recent studies have shown that a significant minority of people with newly diagnosed HIV-1 infection have some degree of resistance to at least one class of antiretroviral agents: 5% are resistant to protease inhibitors, 7% to zidovudine, and 15% to NNRTIs; 3% have multidrug resistance (248–252).

Initial virologic response rates to HAART range from 60% to 90% (251–253). Those with more advanced disease at the time of diagnosis may not fare as well. Age may be a prognostic factor, as the progressive loss of thymic activity after the age of 25 is associated with less immunologic recovery after the institution of antiretroviral therapy (252,253). The strongest predictor of prognosis is the plasma HIV-1 RNA level at week 4 after institution of therapy (ACTG-320). For those who fail an initial, highly active, antiretroviral regimen, salvage therapy offers only a 26% to 40% chance of a good response (251).

Significant improvement in the morbidity associated with HIV infection and a decline in the death rate have occurred with combination antiretroviral therapy (50). It is likely that therapeutic advances in the near future will temper the pace of infection. This would incline HIV-1 infection toward a more chronic illness, allowing for a better quantity and quality of life of afflicted patients.

References
1. Hirsch MS, Kaplan JC. The biomedical impact of the AIDS epidemic. In: Broder S, Merigan TC, Bolognesi D, eds. Textbook of AIDS medicine. Baltimore: Williams & Wilkins, 1994:3–12.
2. Huff JR. HIV protease. A novel chemotherapeutic target for AIDS. J Med Chem 1991;34:2305–2314.
3. Essex ME. Origin of acquired immunodeficiency syndrome. In: DeVita VT, Hellman S, Rosenberg S, et al, eds. AIDS: biology, diagnosis, treatment and prevention. 4th ed. Philadelphia: Lippincott-Raven, 1997.
4. Kessler HA, Bick JA. Pottage JC Jr, Benson CA. AIDS: Part I. Dis Mon 1992;38:633–690.
5. Bartlett JG. Update in infectious diseases. Ann Intern Med 1997;127:217–224.
6. Jeffries DJ. Targets for antiviral therapy of human immunodeficiency virus infection. J Infect 1989;1:5–13.
7. Edlin BR, Weinstein RA, Whaling SM, et al. Zidovudine-interferon-alpha combination therapy in patients with advanced human immunodeficiency virus type 1 infection: biphasic response of p24 antigen and quantitative polymerase chain reaction. J Infect Dis 1992;165:793–798.
8. Capon DJ, Ward RHR. The CD-4-gp 120 interaction and AIDS pathogenesis. Annu Rev Immunol 1991;9:649–678.
9. Oyaizu N, McCloskey TW, Coronesi M, et al. Accelerated apoptosis in peripheral blood mononuclear cells (PBMCs) from human immunodeficiency virus type-1–infected patients and in CD-4 cross-linked PBMCs from normal individuals. Blood 1993;82:3392–3400.
10. Langner KD, Niedrig M, Fultz P, et al. Antiviral effects of different CD4-immunoglobulin constructs against HIV-1 and SIV: immunological characterization, pharmacokinetic data and in vivo experiments. Arch Virol 1993;130:157–170.
11. Haertle T, Carrera CJ, Wasson DB, et al. Metabolism of antihuman immunodeficiency virus-1 activity of 2-halo-2', 3'-dideoxyadenosine derivatives. J Biol Chem 1988;263:5870–5875.
12. Littman DR. Chemokine receptors: keys to AIDS pathogenesis? Cell 1998;93:677–679.
13. Deichmann M, Kronenwett R, Haas R. Expression of the human immunodeficiency virus type-1 coreceptors CXCR-4 (Fusin, LESTR) and CKR-5 in CD-34+ hematopoietic progenitor cells. Blood 1997;89:3522–3528.
14. Volberding PA, Fischl MA, Merigan TC. Strategies for antiretroviral therapy in adult HIV disease. In: Broder S, Merigan TC, Bolognesi D, eds. Textbook of AIDS medicine. Baltimore: Williams & Wilkins, 1994:773–787.

15. Byrnes VW, Sardana VV, Schleif WA, et al. Comprehensive mutant enzyme and viral variant assessment of human immunodeficiency virus type-1 reverse transcriptase resistant to nonnucleoside inhibitors. Antimicrob Agents Chemother 1993;37:1576–1579.

16. Fesen MR, Kohn KW, Leteurtre F, Pommier Y. Inhibitors of HIV integrase. Proc Nat Acad Sci USA 1993;90:2399–2403.

17. McNair A, Main J, Goldin R, Thomas HC. Liver disease and AIDS. In: Broder S, Merigan TC, Bolognesi D, eds. Textbook of AIDS medicine. Baltimore: Williams & Wilkins, 1994: 581–594.

18. Mitsuya, H, Yarchoan R. Development of antiretroviral therapy for AIDS and related disorders. In: Broder S, Merigan TC, Bolognesi D, eds. Textbook of AIDS medicine, 2nd ed. Baltimore: Williams & Wilkins, 1999:721–742.

19. Makonkawkeyoon S, Limson-Pobre RN, Moreira AL, et al. Thalidomide inhibits the replication of human immunodeficiency virus type 1. Proc Nat Acad Sci USA 1993;90:5974–5978.

20. Howard OM, Clouse KA, Smith C, et al. Soluble tumor necrosis factor receptor: inhibition of human immunodeficiency virus activation. Proc Nat Acad Sci USA 1993;90:2335–2339.

21. Mosmann TR. Cytokine patterns during the progression to AIDS. Science 1994;265:193–196.

22. Chan DC, Kim PS. HIV entry and its inhibition. Cell 1998;93:681–685.

23. Cocchi F, DeVico AL, Garzino-Demo A, et al. Identification of RANTES, MIP-1a, and MIP-1b as the major HIV-suppressive factors produced by CD8+ T cells. Science 1995;270:1811–1813.

24. Baier M, Werner A, Bannert N, et al. HIV suppression by interleukin-16. Nature 1995;378:563–566.

25. Meek TD, Lambert DM, Dreyer GB, et al. Inhibition of HIV-1 protease in infected T-lymphocytes by synthetic peptide analogues. Nature 1990;343:90–92.

26. Roberts NA, Martin JA, Kinchington D, et al. Rational design of peptide-based HIV proteinase inhibitors. Science 1990;248:348–361.

27. Cantin R, Fortin J-F, Lamontagne G, Tremblay M. The acquisition of host-derived major histocompatibility complex class II glycoproteins by human immunodeficiency virus type 1 accelerates the process of virus entry and infection in human T-lymphoid cells. Blood 1997;90:1091–1100.

28. Ho DD. Presentation at the Thirty-fifth Interscience Conference on Antimicrobial Agents and Chemotherapy, San Francisco, September 1995.

29. Piatak M Jr, Saag MS, Yang LC, et al. High levels of HIV-1 in plasma during all stages of infection determined by competitive PCR. Science 1993;259:1749–1754.

30. Ho DD, Neumann AU, Perelson AS, et al. Rapid turnover of plasma virions and CD-4 lymphocytes in HIV-1 infection. Nature 1995;373:123–126.

31. Wei X, Ghosh SK, Taylor ME, et al. Viral dynamics in human immunodeficiency virus type 1 infection. Nature 1995;373:117–122.

32. Kim SY, Byrn R, Groopman J, Baltimore D. Temporal aspects of DNA and RNA synthesis during human immunodeficiency virus infection: evidence for differential gene expression. J Virol 1989;63:3708–3713.

33. McLean AR. The balance of power between HIV and the immune system. Trends Microbiol 1993;1:9–13.

34. Pantaleo G, Graziosi C, Demarest JF, et al. HIV infection is active and progressive in lymphoid tissue during the clinically latent stage of disease. Nature 1993;362:355–358.

35. Kalams SA, Walker BD. The cytotoxic T-lymphocyte response in HIV-1 infection. Clin Lab Med 1994;14:271–299.

36. Hellerstein M, Hanndley MB, Cesar D, et al. Directly measured kinetics of circulatory T lymphocytes in normal and HIV-1 infected humans. Nat Med 1999;5:83–89.

37. O'Brien WA, Hartigan PM, Martin D, et al. Changes in plasma HIV-1 RNA and CD4+ lymphocyte count relative to treatment and progression to AIDS. N Engl J Med 1996;334:426–431.

38. Wei X, Ghosh SK, Taylor ME, et al. Viral dynamics in human immunodeficiency virus type 1 infection. Nature 1995;373:117–122.

39. Albert J, Wahlberg J, Lundeberg J, et al. Persistence of azidothymidine-resistant human immuno-deficiency virus type 1 RNA genotypes in posttreatment sera. J Virol 1992;66:5627–5630.

40. Hersh EM, Brewton G, Abrams D, et al. Ditiocarb sodium (diethyldithiocarbamate) therapy in patients with symptomatic HIV infection and AIDS. A randomized, double-blind, placebo-controlled, multicenter study. JAMA 1991;265:1538–1544.

41. Merigan TC, Amato DA, Balsley J, et al. NHF-ACTG 036 Study Group. Placebo-controlled trial to evaluate zidovudine in treatment of human immunodeficiency virus infection in asymptomatic patients with hemophilia. Blood 1991;78:900–906.

42. Clark SJ, Saag MS, Decker WD, et al. High titers of cytopathic virus in plasma of patients with symptomatic primary HIV-1 infection. N Engl J Med 1991;324:954–960.

43. Piatak M Jr, Saag MS, Yang LC, et al. High levels of HIV-1 in plasma during all stages of infection determined by competitive PCR. Science 1993;259:1749–1754.

44. Fauci AS. CD4+ T-lymphocytopenia without HIV infection—no lights, no camera, just facts. N Engl J Med 1993;6:429–431.

45. Perno CF, Bergamini A, Pesce CD, et al. Inhibition of the protease of human immunodeficiency virus blocks replication and infectivity of the virus in chronically infected macrophages. J Infect Dis 1993;168:1148–1156.

46. Crowe SM, McGrath MS, Elbeik T, et al. Comparative assessment of antiretrovirals in human monocyte-macrophages and lymphoid cell lines acutely and chronically infected with the human immunodeficiency virus. J Med Virol 1989;29:176–180.

47. Ruegg CL, Engleman EG. Impaired immunity in AIDS. The mechanisms responsible and their potential reversal by antiviral therapy. Ann N Y Acad Sci 1990;616:307–317.

48. Hashimoto F, Oyaizu N, Kalyanaraman VS, Pahwa S. Modulation of Bcl-2 protein by CD4 cross-linking: a possible mechanism for lymphocyte apoptosis in human immunodeficiency virus infection and for rescue of apoptosis by interleukin-2. Blood 1997;70:745–753.

49. O'Brien WA, Hartigan PM, Martin D, et al. Changes in plasma HIV-1 RNA and CD-4+ lymphocyte counts and the

risk of progression to AIDS. N Engl J Med 1996;334:426–429.

50. Palella FJ Jr. Delaney KM, Moorman AC, et al. Declining morbidity and mortality among patients with advanced human immunodeficiency virus infection. N Engl J Med 1998;338:853–857.

51. Choi S, Lagakos SW, Schooley RT, Volberding PA. CD4+ lymphocytes are an incomplete surrogate marker for clinical progression in persons with asymptomatic HIV infection taking zidovudine. Ann Intern Med 1993;118:674–680.

52. Nightingale SC, Jockusch JD, Haslund I, et al. Logarithmic relationship of the CD4 count to survival in patients with human immunodeficiency virus infection. Arch Intern Med 1993;153:1313–1318.

53. Yarchoan R, Venzon DJ, Pluda JM, et al. CD4 count and the risk for death in patients infected with HIV receiving anti-retroviral therapy. Ann Intern Med 1991;115:184–189.

54. Stein DS, Korvick JA, Vermund SH. CD4+ lymphocyte cell enumeration for prediction of clinical course of human immunodeficiency virus disease: a review. J Infect Dis 1992;166:1198–1199.

55. Jacobson MA, Bacchetti P, Kolokathis A, et al. Surrogate markers for survival in patients with AIDS and AIDS-related complex treated with zidovudine. Br Med J 1991; 302:63–64.

56. Kessler HA, Bick JA, Pottage JC Jr, Benson CA. AIDS: Part II. Dis Mon 1992;38:691–764.

57. Jacobson MA, Abrams DI, Volberding PA, et al. Serum beta 2-microglobulin decreases in patients with AIDS or ARC treated with azidothymidine. J Infect Dis 1989;159:1029–1036.

58. Mildvan D, Machado SG, Wilets I, Grossberg SE. Endogenous interferon and triglyceride concentrations to assess response to zidovudine in AIDS and advanced AIDS-related complex. Lancet 1992;339:453–456.

59. Allain JP, Laurian Y, Paul DA, et al. Long-term evolution of HIV antigen and antibodies to p24 and gp41 in patients with hemophilia. N Engl J Med 1987;317:1114–1121.

60. Mulder JW, Cooper DA, Mathiesen L, et al. Zidovudine twice daily in asymptomatic subjects with HIV infection and a high risk of progression to AIDS: a randomized, double-blind placebo-controlled study. AIDS 1994;8:313–321.

61. Shepp DH, Ashraf A. Effect of didansine on human immunodeficiency virus viremia and antigenemia in patients with advanced disease: correlation with clinical response. J Infect Dis 1993;167:30–35.

62. Ho DD. Time to hit HIV: early and hard. N Engl J Med 1995;333:450–451.

63. Saag MS. Use of HIV viral load in clinical practice: back to the future. Ann Intern Med 1997;126:983–985.

64. Mellors JW, Munoz A, Giorgi JV, et al. Plasma viral load and CD-4 lymphocytes as prognostic markers of HIV-1 infection. Ann Int Med 1997;126:946–954.

65. Hughes MD, Johnson VA, Hirsch MS, et al. Monitoring plasma HIV-1 RNA levels in addition to CD-4+ lymphocyte counts improves assessment of antiretroviral therapeutic response. Ann Intern Med 1997;126:929–938.

66. Carpenter CC, Fischl MA, Hammer SM, et al. Antiretroviral therapy for HIV infection in 1998: updated recommendations of the International AIDS Society—USA Panel. JAMA 1998;280:78–82.

67. Buckheit RW Jr, Hollingshead MG, Germany-Decker J, et al. Thiazolobenzimidasole: biological and biochemical anti-retroviral activity of a new nonnucleoside reverse transcriptase inhibitor. Antiviral Res 1993;21:247–265.

68. Mitsuya H, Broder S. Inhibition of the in vitro infectivity and cytopathic effect of human T-lymphotrophic virus type III/lymphadenopathy virus–associated virus (HTLV-III/LAV) by 2′,3′-dideoxynucleosides. Proc Natl Acad Sci USA 1986;83:1911–1915.

69. Balzarini J, De Clercq E. Biochemical pharmacology of nucleoside analogues. In: Broder S, Merigan TC, Bolognesi D, eds. Textbook of AIDS medicine. Baltimore: Williams & Wilkins, 1994:751–772.

70. Mitsuya H, Jarrett RF, Matsukura M, et al. Long-term inhibition of human T-lymphotrophic virus type III/lymphadenopathy–associated virus (human immunodeficiency virus) DNA synthesis and RNA expression in T cells protected by 2′,3′-didooxynucleosides in vitro. Proc Natl Acad Sci USA 1987;84:2033–2037.

71. Meng T-C, Fischl MA, Richman DD. AIDS clinical trials group: phase I/II study of combination 2′,3′-dideoxycytidine and zidovudine in patients with acquired immunodeficiency syndrome (AIDS) and advanced AIDS-related complex. Am J Med 1990;88(suppl 5B):27S–30S.

72. Fischl MA, Richman DD, Grieco MH, et al. The efficacy of aziodothymidine (AZT) in the treatment of patients with AIDS and AIDS-related complex: a double-blind, placebo-controlled trial. N Engl J Med 1987;317:185–191.

73. Starnes MC, Cheng Y-C. Cellular metabolism of 2′,3′-dideoxycitidine, a compound active against human immunodeficiency virus in vitro. J Biol Chem 1987;262:988–991.

74. Broder S. Pharmacodynamics of 2′,3′-dideoxycytidine: an inhibitor of human immunodeficiency virus. Am J Med 1990;88(suppl 5B):2S–7S.

75. Nagy K, Young M, Baboonian C, et al. Antiviral activity of human immunodeficiency virus type 1 protease inhibitors in a single cycle of infection: evidence for a role of protease in the early phase. J Virol 1994;68:757–765.

76. Drugs for HIV infection. Med Lett 2000;42:1–6.

77. Horwitz JP, Chua J, Noel M. Nucleosides: the monomesylates of 1-(2′-deoxy-beta-D-lyxofuranosyl)thymine. J Organic Chem 1964;29:2076–2078.

78. Ostertag W, Roesler G, Krieg CJ, et al. Induction of endogenous virus and of thymidine kinase by bromo-deoxyuridine in cell cultures transformed by Friend virus. Proc Natl Acad Sci USA 1974;71:4980–4985.

79. Mitsuya H, Weinhold KJ, Furman PA, et al. 3′-Azido-3′deoxythymidine (BW A509U): an antiviral agent that inhibits the infectivity and cytopathic effect of human T-lymphotropic virus type III/lymphadenopathy–associated virus in vitro. Proc Natl Acad Sci USA 1985;82:7096–7100.

80. Yarchoan R, Klecker RW, Weinhold KJ, et al. Administration of 3′-azido-3′-deoxythymidine, an inhibitor of HTLV-III/LAV replication, to patients with AIDS or AIDS- related complex. Lancet 1986;1:575–580.

81. Fischl MA, Richman DD, Grieco MH, et al. The efficacy of 3′-azido 3′-deoxythymidine (azidothymidine) in the treatment of patients with AIDS and AIDS-related complex: a double-blind, placebo-controlled trial. N Engl J Med 1987;317:185–191.

82. Vrang L, Oberg B, Lower J, Jurth R. Reverse transcriptases from human immunodeficiency virus type 1 (HIV-1), HIV-2, and simian immunodeficiency virus (SIM Mac) are susceptible to inhibition by foscarnet and 3'-azido-3'-deoxythymidine triphosphate. Antimicrob Agents Chemother 1988;32:1733–1734.

83. McLeod GX, Hammer SM. Zidovudine: five years later. Ann Intern Med 1992;117:487–501.

84. Rooke R, Tremblay M, Wainberg MA. AZT (zidovudine) may act postintegrationally to inhibit generation of HIV-1 progeny virus in chronically infected cells. Virology 1990; 176:205–215.

85. Zimmerman TP, Mahony WB, Prus KL. 3'-Azido 3'deoxythymidine. An unusual nucleoside analogue that permeates the membrane of human erythrocytes and lymphocytes by nonfacilitated diffusion. J Biol Chem 1987;262:5748–5754.

86. Balzarini J, Cools M, De Clerq E. Estimation of the lipophilicity of anti-HIV nucleoside analogues by determination of the partition coefficient and retention time on a lichrospher 60 RP-8 HPLS column. Biochem Biophys Res Commun 1989;158:413–422.

87. Furman PA, Tyfe JA, St. Clair MH, et al. Phosphorylation of 3'-azido-3'-deoxythymidine and selective interaction of the 5'-triphosphate with human immunodeficiency virus reverse transcriptase. Proc Natl Acad Sci USA 1986;83:8333–8337.

88. Richman D. Viral resistance to antiretroviral therapy. In: Broder S, Merigan TC, Bolognesi D, eds. Textbook of AIDS medicine. Baltimore: Williams & Wilkins, 1994:795–806.

89. Scanlon KJ, Kashani-Sabet M, Sowers LC. Overexpression of DNA replication and repair enzymes in cisplatin-resistant human colon carcinoma HCT8 cells and circumvention by azidothymidine. Cancer Commun 1989;1:269–275.

90. Fischl M, Richman DD, Hansen N, et al. The safety and efficacy of zidovudine (AZT) in the treatment of subjects with mildly symptomatic human immunodeficiency virus type I (HIV) infection. A double-blind, placebo controlled trial. Ann Intern Med 1990;112:272–237.

91. Geleziunas R, Arts EJ, Boulerice F, et al. Effect of 3'-azido-3'-deoxythymidine on human immunodeficiency virus type 1 replication in human fetal brain macrophages. Antimicrob Agents Chemother 1993;37:1305–1312.

92. O'Sullivan MJ, Boyer PJ, Scott GB, et al. The pharmacokinetics and safety of zidovudine in the third trimester of pregnancy for women infected with human immunodeficiency virus and their infants: phase I acquired immunodeficiency syndrome clinical trials group. Am J Obstet Gynecol 1993;168:1510–1516.

93. Dudley MN, Graham KK, Kaul S, et al. Pharmacokinetics of stavudine in patients with AIDS or AIDS-related complex. J Infect Dis 1992;166:480–485.

94. Kornhauser DM, Petty BG, Hendrix CW, et al. Probenecid and zidovudine metabolism. Lancet 1989;2:473–475.

95. Burger DM, Meenhorst PL, Koks CHW, Beijnen JH. Drug interactions with zidovudine. AIDS 1993;7:445–460.

96. Patel PH, Preston BD. Marked infidelity of human immunodeficiency virus type 1 reverse transcriptase at RNA and DNA template ends. Proc Natl Acad Sci USA 1994;91:549–553.

97. Volberding PA, Lagakos SW, Koch MA, et al. The AIDS Clinical Trials Group of the National Institute of Allergy and Infectious Diseases. Zidovudine in asymptomatic human immunodeficiency virus infection. A controlled trial in persons with fewer than 500 CD4-positive cells per cubic millimeter. N Engl J Med 1990;322:941–949.

98. Hamilton JD, Hartigan PM, Simberkoff MS, et al. A controlled trial of early versus late treatment with zidovudine in symptomatic human immunodeficiency virus infections. Results of the Veterans Affairs Cooperative Study. N Engl J Med 1992;326:437–443.

99. Sande MA, Carpenter CCJ, Cobbs G, et al. Antiretroviral therapy for adult HIV-infected patients. Recommendations for a state-of-the-art conference. JAMA 1993;27:2583–2589.

100. Fischl MA, Parker CB, Pettinelli C, et al. The AIDS Clinical Trials Group. A randomized controlled trial of a reduced daily dose of zidovudine in patients with the acquired immunodeficiency syndrome. N Engl J Med 1990;323:1009–1014.

101. Mulder JW, Cooper DA, Mathiesen L, et al. Zidovudine twice daily in asymptomatic subjects with HIV infection and a high risk of progression to AIDS: a randomized, double-blind placebo-controlled study. AIDS 1994;8:313–321.

102. Collier AC, Bozzette S, Coombs RW, et al. A pilot study of low-dose zidovudine in human immunodeficiency virus infection. N Engl J Med 1990;323:1015–1021.

103. Meng T-C, Fischl MA, Boota AM, et al. Combination therapy with zidovudine and dideoxycytidine in patients with advanced human immunodeficiency virus infection. Ann Intern Med 1992;116:13–20.

104. Mansuri MM, Hitchcock MJM, Buroker RA, et al. Comparison of in vitro biological properties and mouse toxicities of three thymidine analogs active against human immunodeficiency virus. Antimicrob Agents Chemother 1990;34:637–641.

105. Cretton EM, Xie M-Y, Bevan RJ, et al. Catabolism of 3'-azido-3'deoxythymidine in hepatocytes and liver microsomes with evidence of formation of 3'amino-3'deoxythymidine, a highly toxic catabolite for human bone marrow cells. Mol Pharmacol 1991;39:258–266.

106. Weidner DA, Sommadossi J-P. 3'-Azido-3'-deoxythymidine (AZT) inhibits globulin gene transcription in human K-562 leukemia cells. Proc Am Assoc Cancer Res 1990;31:422–425.

107. Lutton JD, Jiang S, Abraham NG, et al. Therapeutic usefulness of heme and erythropoietin for AZT hematotoxicity. Abstracts and Proceedings of the Eighth International Conference on AIDS, The Netherlands, June 1992.

108. Fischl MA. Strategies for antiretroviral therapy in adult HIV disease: the Miami perspective. In: Broder S, Merigan TC, Bolognesi D, eds. Textbook of AIDS medicine. Baltimore: Williams & Wilkins, 1994:787–791.

109. Lamperth L, Dalakas MC, Dagani F, et al. Abnormal skeletal and cardiac muscle mitochondria induced by zidovudine (AZT) in human muscle in vitro and in an animal model. Lab Invest 1991;65:742–751.

110. Herskowitz A, Willoughby SB, Baughman KL, et al. Cardiomyopathy associated with antiretroviral therapy in patients with HIV infection: a report of six cases. Ann Intern Med 1992;116:3111–3113.

111. Bessen LH, Greene JB, Louie E, et al. Severe polymyositis-like syndrome associated with zidovudine therapy of AIDS and ARC. N Engl J Med 1988;318:708–712.

112. Gelmon K, Montaner JS, Fanning M, et al. Nature, time course and dose dependence of zidovudine-related side effects: results from the Multicenter Canadian Azidothymidine Trial. AIDS 1989;3:555–561.

113. Freiman JP, Helfert KE, Hamrell MR, Stein DS. Hepatomegaly with severe steatosis in HIV-seropositive patients. AIDS 1993;7:379–385.

114. Lambert JS, Seidlin M, Reichman RC, et al. 2′,3′-dideoxyinosine (ddI) in patients with the acquired immunodeficiency syndrome or AIDS-related complex. N Engl J Med 1990;322:1333–1340.

115. Hartman NR, Yarchoan R, Pluda JM, et al. Pharmacokinetics of 2′,3′-dideoxyadenosine and 2′,3′-dideoxyinosine in patients with severe HIV infection. Clin Pharmacol Ther 1990;47:647–654.

116. Mitsuya H, Broder S. Strategies for antiviral therapy in AIDS. Nature 1987;325:773–778.

117. Yarchoan R, Mitsuya H, Thomas RV, et al. In vivo activity against HIV and favorable toxicity profile of 2′,3′-dideoxyinosine. Science 1989;245:412–415.

118. Gao W-Y, Shirasaka T, Johns DG, et al. Differential phosphorylation of azidothymidine, dideoxycytidine, and dideoxyinosine in resting and activated peripheral blood mononuclear cells. J Clin Invest 1993;91:2326–2333.

119. Spruance SL, Pavia AT, Peterson D, et al. Didanosine compared with continuation of zidovudine in HIV-infected patients with signs of clinical deterioration while receiving zidovudine. Ann Intern Med 1994;120:360–368.

120. Kahn JO, Lagakos SW, Richman DD, et al. The NIAID AIDS Clinical Trials Group. A controlled trial comparing continued zidovudine with didansine in human immunodeficiency virus infection. N Engl J Med 1992;327:581–587.

121. Cooley TP, Kunches LM, Saunders CA, et al. Once-daily administration of 2′,3′-dideoxyinosine (ddI) in patients with acquired immunodeficiency syndrome or AIDS-related complex. N Engl J Med 1990;322:1386–1388.

122. Abrams DI, Goldman AI, Launer C, et al. A comparative trial of didanosine or zalcitabine after treatment with zidovudine in patients with human immunodeficiency virus infection. N Engl J Med 1994;330:657–662.

123. Allan JD, Connolly KJ, Fitch H, et al. Long-term follow-up of didanosine administered orally twice daily to patients with advanced human deficiency virus infection and hematologic intolerance of zidovudine. Clin Infect Dis 1993;16(suppl 1):S46–S51.

124. Reynes J. Once daily administration of didanosine in combination with stavudine in antiretroviral-naive patients. European Zerit Symposium, Cannes, France, March 22, 1997.

125. Drusani GL, Yuen GJ, Morse G, et al. Impact of bioavailability on determination of the maximal tolerated dose of 2′3′-dideoxyinosine in phase I trials. AAC 1992;36(suppl 6):1280–1282.

126. Schacter LP, Rozencweig M, Beltangaday M, et al. Effects of therapy with didanosine on hematologic parameters in patients with advanced human immunodeficiency virus disease. Blood 1992;80:2969–2976.

127. Valentine C, Deenmamode J, Sherwood R. Xerostomia associated with didanosine. Lancet 1992;340:1542. Letter.

128. Maxson CJ, Greenfield SM, Turner JL. Acute pancreatitis as a common complication of 2′-3′-dideoxyinosine therapy in the acquired immunodeficiency syndrome. Am J Gastroenterol 1993;88:459–460.

129. Capell MS. The pancreas in AIDS. In: Broder S, Merigan TC, Bolognesi D, eds. Textbook of AIDS medicine. Baltimore: Williams & Wilkins, 1994:555–566.

130. Yarchoan R, Pluda JM, Thomas RV. Long-term toxicity/activity profile of 2′,3′-dideoxyinosine in AIDS or AIDS-related complex. Lancet 1990;2:526–529.

131. Kieburtz KD, Seidlin M, Lambert JS, et al. Extended follow-up of peripheral neuropathy in patients with AIDS and AIDS-related complex treated with didioxyinosine. J AIDS 1992;5:60–64.

132. Broder S, Yarchoan R. Dideoxycytidine: current clinical experience and future prospects. Am J Med 1990;88(suppl 5B):31S–33S.

133. Fischl MA, Olson RM, Follansbee SE, et al. Zalcitabine compared with zidovudine in patients with advanced HIV-1 infection who received previous zidovudine therapy. Ann Intern Med 1993;118:762–769.

134. Merigan TC, Skowron G. Safety and tolerance of dideoxycytidine as a single agent. Am J Med 1990;88(suppl 5B):11S–15S.

135. McNeely MC, Yarchoan R, Broder S, Lawley TJ. Dermatologic complications associated with administation of 2′,3′-dideoxycytidine in patients with human immunodeficiency virus infection. J Am Acad Dermatol 1989;21:1213–1217.

136. Bozette SA, Richman DD. Salvage therapy for zidovudine-intolerant HIV-infected patients with alternating and intermittent regimens of zidovudine and dideoxycytidine. Am J Med 1990;88(suppl 5B):24S–26S.

137. Browne MJ, Mayer KH, Chafee SB, et al. 2′-3′-didehydro-3′-deoxythymidine (d4T) in patients with AIDS or AIDS-related complex: a phase I trial. J Infect Dis 1993;167:21–29.

138. August EM, Marongui ME, Lin T-S, Prusoff WH. Initial studies on the cellular pharmacology of 3′-deoxythymidine-2′-ene (d4T): a potent and selective inhibitor of human immunodeficiency virus. Biochem Pharmacol 1988;37:4419–4422.

139. Sommadossi JP, Carlisle R. Toxicity of 3′-azido-3′-deoxythymidine and 9-(1,2 dihydroxy-2″ propoxymethyl) guanine for normal human hematopoietic progenitor cells in vitro. Antimicrob Agents Chemother 1987;31:452–454.

140. Zhu Z, Ho HT, Hitchcock MJ, Sommadossi J-P. Cellular pharmacology of 2′,3′-didehydro-2′,3′-dideoxythymidine (d4T) in human peripheral blood mononuclear cells. Biochem Pharmacol 1990;39:R14–R19.

141. Balzarini J, Pauwels R, Baba M, et al. The in-vitro and in-vivo antiretroviral activity and intracellular metabolism of 3′-azido-2′3-dideoxythymidine and 2′-3′-dideoxycytidine are highly dependent on cell species. Biochem Pharmacol 1988;37:897–903.

142. Larfer BA, Darby G, Richman DD. HIV with reduced sensitivity zidovudine (AZT) isolated during prolonged therapy. Science 1989;243:1731–1734.

143. Coates JAV, Cammack N, Jenkinson HJ, et al. The separated enantiomers of 2′-deoxy-3′-thiacytidine (BCH 189) both

inhibit human immunodeficiency virus replication in vitro. Antimicrob Agents Chemother 1992;36:202–205.

144. Skalski V, Chang CN, Dutschman G, Cheng YC. The biochemical basis for the differential anti-human immunodeficiency virus activity of two *cis* enantiomers of 2',3'-dideoxy-3'-thiacytidine. J Biol Chem 1993;268:23234–23238.

145. Foudraine NA, Hoetelmans RM, Lange JM, et al. Cerebrospinal-fluid HIV-1 RNA and drug concentrations after treatment with lamivudine plus zidovidine or stavudine. Lancet 1988;351:154–157.

146. Foudraine N, DeWolf F, Hoetel-Mans P, et al. CSF and serum HIV-RNA levels during AZT/3TC and d4T/3TC treatment. Fourth Conference on Retroviruses and Opportunistic Infections, Washington, DC, 1997.

147. Johnson MA, Moore KH, Yuen GJ, et al. Clinical pharmacokinetics of lamivudine. Clin Pharmacokinet 1999;36:41–60.

148. Wainberg MA, Drosopoulos WC, Salomon H, et al. Enhanced fidelity of ETC-selected mutant HIV-1 reverse transcriptase. Science 1996;271:1282–1286.

149. Daluge SM, Good SS, Faletto MB, et al. 1592 uccinate—a novel carbocyclic nucleoside analog with potent, selective anti-HIV activity. Antimicrob Agents Chemother 1997;41:1099–1103.

150. Tisdale M, Alnadaf T, Cousens D. Combination of mutations in HIV-1 reverse transcriptase required for resistance to carbocyclic nucleoside 1592U89. Antimicrob Agents Chemother 1997;41:1094–1099.

151. Hao Z, Cooney DA, Farqhar D, et al. Potent DNA chain termination activity and selective inhibition of human immunodeficiency virus reverse transcriptase by 2',3'-dideoxyurindine-5'-triphosphate (ddUTP). Mol Pharmacol 1990;37:157–163.

152. Pauwels R, Balzarini J, Schols D, de Clercq E. Phosphonylmethoxyethyl purine derivatives, a new class of anti-human immunodeficiency virus (HIV) in vitro. Antimicrob Agents Chemother 1988;32:1025–1030.

153. De Clercq E. Broad-spectrum anti-DNA virus and anti-retrovirus activity of phosphonylmethoxyalkyl purines and pyrimidines. Biochem Pharmacol 1991;42:963–972.

154. Votruba I, Travnicek M, Rosenberg I, et al. Inhibition of avian myeloblastosis virus reverse transcriptase by diphosphates of acyclic phosphonylmethyl nucleotide analogues. Antiviral Res 1990;13:287–293.

155. Sastry JK, Nehete PN, Khan S, et al. Membrane-permeable dideoxyuridine 5'-monophosphate analogue inhibits human immunodeficiency virus infection. Mol Pharmacol 1992;41:441–445.

156. Zelphati O, Degols G, Loughrey H, et al. Inhibition of HIV-1 replication in cultured cells with phosphorylated dideoxyuridine derivatives encapsulated in immuno-liposomes. Antiviral Res 1993;21:181–195.

157. Frick LW, St John L, Taylor LC, et al. Pharmacokinetics, oral bioavailability, and metabolic disposition in rats of *cis*-5-fluoro-1-[2-(hydroxymethyl)-1,3-oxathiolan-5-yl] cytosine, a nucleoside analog active against human immun- odeficiency virus and hepatitis B virus. Antimicrob Agents Chemother 1993;37:2285–2292.

158. Cox SW, Albert J, Wahlberg J, et al. Loss of synergistic response to combinations containing AZT in AZT-resistant HIV-1. AIDS Res Hum Retroviruses 1992;8:1229–1234.

159. Clerici M, Landay AI, Kessler HA, et al. Reconstitution of long-term T helper cell function after zidovudine therapy in human immunodeficiency virus–infected patients. J Infect Dis 1992;166:723–730.

160. Cooper DA, Gatell JM, Kroon S, et al. Zidovudine in person with asymptomatic HIV infection and CD4+ cell counts greater than 400 per cubic millimeter. N Engl J Med 1993;329:297–303.

161. Rinaldo C, Huang XL, Piazza P, et al. Augmentation of cellular immune function during the early phase of zidovudine treatment of AIDS patients. J Infect Dis 1991;164:638–645.

162. Longini IM Jr, Clark WS, Karon JM. Effect of routine use of therapy in slowing the clinical course of human immunodeficiency virus (HIV) infection in a population-based cohort. Am J Epidemiol 1993;137:1229–1240.

163. Inserm SCIO, Aboulker J-P (MVR HIV Clinical Trials Centre), Swart AM (Concorde Coordinating Committee). Preliminary analysis of the Concorde trial. Lancet 1993;341:889–890.

164. Carpenter CCJ, Fischl MA, Hammer SM, et al. Antiretroviral therapy for HIV in 1998. JAMA 1998;280:78–86.

165. Graham NMH, Zeger SL, Park LP, et al. The effects on survival of early treatment of human immunodeficiency virus infection. N Engl J Med 1992;326:1037–1042.

166. Moore RD, Hidalgo J, Sugland BW, Chaisson RE. Zidovudine and the natural history of the acquired immunodeficiency syndrome. N Engl J Med 1991;325:1311–1313.

167. Cooper DA, Pedersen C, Aiuti F, et al. The efficacy and safety of zidovudine therapy in early asymptomatic HIV infection. AIDS 1991;5:933–943.

168. Kinloch-de Loes S, Hirschel BJ, Hoen B, et al. A controlled trial of zidovudine in primary human immunodeficiency virus infection. N Engl J Med 1995;333:408–413.

169. Iannidis JPA, Cappelleri JC, Lau J, et al. Early or deferred zidovudine therapy in HIV-infected patients without an AIDS-defining illness. A meta-analysis. Ann Intern Med 1995;122:856–866.

170. Eron JJ Jr, Johnson VA, Merrill DP, et al. Synergistic inhibition of replication of human immunodeficiency virus type-1, including that of a zidovudine-resistant isolate by zidovudine and 2',3'-dideoxycytidine in vitro. Antimicrob Agents Chemother 1992;36:1559–1562.

171. Ragni M, Dafni R, Amato DA, et al. Combination zidovudine and dideoxyinosine in asymptomatic HIV (+) patients. The Eighth International Conference on AIDS/III STD World Congress, The Netherlands, June 1992.

172. Collier AC, Coombs RW, Fischl MA, et al. Combination therapy with zidovudine and didanosine with zidovudine alone in HIV-1 infection. Ann Intern Med 1993;119:786–793.

173. Cox SW, Albert J, Ljungdahl-Stahle E, Wahren B. Effect of resistance on combination chemotherapy for human immunodeficiency virus infection. Adv Enzyme Regul 1993;33:27–36.

174. Baba M, Tanaka H, De Clercq E, et al. Highly specific inhibition of human immunodeficiency virus type 1 by a novel 6-substituted acyclouridine derivative. Biochem Biophys Res Commun 1989;165:1375–1381.

175. Saag MS, Emini EA, Laskin OL, et al. A short-term clinical evaluation of L-697, 661, a non-nucleoside inhibitor

of HIV-1 reverse transcriptase. N Engl J Med 1993;329: 1065–1072.

176. Mellors JW, Dutschman GE, IM G-J, et al. In vitro selection and molecular characterization of human immunodeficiency virus-1 resistant to non-nucleoside inhibitors of reverse transcriptase. Mol Pharmacol 1992;41:446–451.

177. Nunberg JH, Schleif WA, Boots EJ, et al. Viral resistance to human immunodeficiency virus type 1–specific pyridinone reverse transcriptase inhibitors. J Virol 1991;65:4887–4892.

178. Balzarini J, Karlsson A, De Clercq E. Human immunodeficiency virus type 1 drug-resistance patterns with different 1-[(2-hydro-oxyethoxy)methyl]-6-(phenylthio)thymine derivatives. Mol Pharmacol 1993;44:694–701.

179. Koup RA, Brewster F, Grob P, Sullivan JL. Nevirapine synergistically inhibits HIV-1 replication in combination with zidovudine, interferon or CD4 immunoadhesion. AIDS 1993;7:1181–1184.

180. Balzarini J, Karlsson A, Perez-Perez MJ, et al. Treatment of human immunodeficiency virus type 1 (HIV-1)–infected cells with combinations of HIV-1–specific inhibitors results in a different resistance pattern than does treatment with single-drug therapy. J Virol 1993;67:5353–5359.

181. Davey RT Jr, Dewar RL, Reed GF, et al. Plasma viremia as a sensitive indicator of the antiretroviral activity of L-697, 661. Proc Natl Acad Sci USA 1993;90:5608–5612.

182. Buckheit RW, Snow MF, Fliakas-Boltz V, et al. Highly potent oxanthiin carboxanilide derivatives with efficacy against nonnucleoside reverse transriptase inhibitor-resistant human immunodeficiency virus isolates. Aintmicrob Agents Chemother 1997;41:831–837.

183. Lori F, Malykh A, Cara A, et al. Hydroxyurea as an inhibitor of human immunodeficiency virus-type 1 replication. Science 1994;266:801–805.

184. Clotet B, Ruiz L, Cabrera C, et al. Short-term anti-HIV activity of the combination of didanosine and hydroxyurea. Antiviral Ther Q 996;1:189–193.

185. Gas WY, Johns DG. Antihuman immunodeficiency virus type 1 activity of hydroxyurea in combination with 2′,3′-dideoxynucleosides. Mol Pharmacol 1994;46:767–772.

186. Gao WY, Mitsuya H, Driscoll JS, Johns DG. Enhancement by hydroxyurea of the anti-human immunodeficiency virus type 1 potency of 2′-beta-fluoro-2′,3′-dideoxyadenosine in peripheral blood mononuclear cells. Biochem Pharmacol 1995;50:274–276.

187. Gao WY, Johns DG, Chokekuchai S, Mitsuya H. Disparate actions of hydroxyurea in potentiation of purine and pyrimidine 2′,3′-di-deoxynucleoside activities against replication of human immunodeficiency virus. Proc Nat Acad Sci USA 1995;92:8333–8337.

188. Biron F, Lucht F, Peyramond D, et al. Anti-HIV activity of the combination of didano-sine and hydroxyurea in HIV-1–infected individuals. J Acquir Immune Def Syndr 1995;10:36–40.

189. Kelleher AD, Roggensack M, Emery S, et al. Effects of IL-2 therapy in asymptomatic HIV-infected individuals on proliferative responses to mitogen recall antigens and HIV-related antigens. Clin Exp Immunol 1998;113:85–91.

190. Chang RS, Tabba HD, He YS, Smith KM. Dextran sulfate as an inhibitor against the human immunodeficiency virus. Proc Soc Exp Biol Med 1988;189:304–309.

191. Cooper DA, Pehrson PO, Pedersen C, et al. The efficacy and safety of zidovudine alone or as cotherapy with acyclovir for the treatment of patients with AIDS and AIDS-related complex: a double-blind, randomized trial. AIDS 1993;7:197–207.

192. Youle MS, Gazzard BD, Johnson MA, et al. Effects of high dose oral acyclovir on herpes virus disease and survival in patients with advanced HIV disease: a double-blind, placebo controlled study. AIDS 1994;8:641–649.

193. Nyuyen BY, Shay LE, Wyvill KM, et al. A pilot study of sequential therapy with zidovudine plus acyclovir, dideoxyinosine, and dideoxycytidine in patients with severe human immunodeficiency virus infection. J Infect Dis 1993;168:810–817.

194. Jault FM, Spector SA, Spector DH. The effects of cytomegalovirus on human immunodeficiency virus replication in brain-derived cells correlate with permissiveness of the cells for each virus. J Virol 1994;68:959–973.

195. Polis MA, deSmet MD, Baird BF, et al. Increased survival of a cohort of patients with acquired immunodeficiency syndrome and cytomegalovirus retinitis who received sodium phosphonoformate (foscarnet). Am J Med 1993;94:175–180.

196. Harb GE, Bacchetti P, Jacobson MA. Survival of patients with AIDS and cytomegalovirus disease treated with ganciclovir or foscarnet. AIDS 1991;5:959–965.

197. Schooley RT, Herigan TC, Gaut P, et al. Recombinant soluble CD4 therapy in patients with the acquired immunodeficiency syndrome (AIDS) and AIDS-related complex. Ann Intern Med 1990;112:247–253.

198. Nakashima H, Yoshida O, Baba M, et al. Anti-HIV activity of dextran sulphate as determined under different experimental conditions. Antiviral Res 1989;11:233–246.

199. Abrams DI, Kuno S, Wong R, et al. Oral dextran sulfate (UA001) in the treatment of the acquired immunodeficiency syndrome (AIDS) and AIDS-related complex. Ann Intern Med 1989;110:183–188.

200. Connor R, Rigby WF. 1-Alpha, 25-dihydroxyvitamin D3 inhibits productive infection of human monocytes by HIV-1. Biochem Biophys Res Commun 1991;176:852–859.

201. Ashorn P, Moss B, Berger EA. Anti-HIV effects of CD4-*Pseudomonas* exotoxin on human lymphocyte and monocyte-macrophage cell lines. Ann N Y Acad Sci 1990;616:149–154.

202. Salhany JM, Schopfer LM. Pyridoxal 5′-phosphate binds specifically to soluble CD4 protein, the HIV-1 receptor. Implications for AIDS therapy. J Biol Chem 1993;268:7643–7645.

203. Rosen CA, Pavlakis GN. Tat and Rev: positive regulations of HIV gene expression. AIDS 1990;4:499–509.

204. Hsu MC, Dhingra U, Earley JV, et al. Inhibition of type 1 human immunodeficiency virus replication by a Tat antagonist to which the virus remains sensitive after prolonged exposure in vitro. Proc Nat Acad Sci USA 1991;90:6395–6399.

205. Cushman M, Sherman P. Inhibition of HIV-1 integration protein by aurintricarboxylic acid monomers, monomer analogs, and polymer fractions. Biochem Biophys Res Commun 1992;185:85–90.

206. Maruyama I, Maruyama Y, Nakajima T, et al. Vesnarinone inhibits production of HIV-1 in cultured cells. Biochem Biophys Res Commun 1993;195:1264–1271.

207. Matsukura M, Zon G, Shinozuka K, et al. Regulation of viral expression of human immunodeficiency virus in vitro by an antisense phosphorothioate oligodeoxynucleotide against Rev in chronically infected cells. Proc Nat Acad Sci USA 1989;86:4244–4248.

208. Stein CA, Cheng YC. Antisense oligonucleotides as therapeutic agents—is the bullet really magical? Science 1993; 261:1004–1012.

209. Margolis LB, Glushakova S, Grivel J-C, Murphy PM. Blockade of CC chemokine receptor 5 (CCR5)–tropic human immunodeficiency virus-1 replication in human lymphoid tissue by CC chemokines. J Clin Invest 1998;101:1876–1881.

210. Lori F, Malykh AG, Foli A, et al. Overcoming drug resistance to HIV-1 by the combination of cell and virus targeting. Abstract 589. Fourth Conference on Retroviruses and Opportunistic Infections, Washington, DC, 1997.

211. Davey RT, Chaitt D, Piscitelli S, et al. Subcutaneous administrtion of interleukin-2 in human immunodeficiency virus type-1–infected persons. J Infect Dis 1997;175:781–789.

212. Carr A, Emery S, Lloyd A, et al. Australian IL-2 Study Group. Outpatient continuous intravenous interleukin-2 or subcutaneous, polyethylene glycol-modified interleukin-2 in human immunodeficiency virus–infected patients: a randomized, controlled, multicenter study. J Infect Dis 1998; 178:992–999.

213. Inouye RT, Hammer SM. Update on developments in antiretroviral therapy. Fourth Conference on Retroviruses and Opportunistic Infections, Washington, DC, 1997.

214. Witvrouw M, Balzarini J, Pannecouque C, et al. SRR-SB3, a disulfide-containing macrolide that inhibits a late stage of the replicative cycle of human immunodeficiency virus. Antimicrob Agents Chemother 1997;41:262–268.

215. Kageyama S, Mimoto T, Murakawa Y, et al. In vitro antihuman immunodeficiency virus (HIV) activities of transition state mimetic HIV protease inhibitors containing allophenylnorstatine. Antimicrob Agents Chemother 1993; 37:810–817.

216. Markowitz M, Saag M, Powderly WG, et al. A preliminary study of ritonavir, an inhibitor of HIV-1 protease, to treat HIV-1 infection. N Engl J Med 1995;333:1534–1539.

217. Montaner JS, Reiss P, Cooper D, et al. The Netherlands, Canada and Australia Study. A randomized, doubleblind trial comparing combinations of neviripine, didanosine, and zidovudine for HIV-infected patients: the INCAS trial, Italy. JAMA 1998;279:930–991.

218. Vella S, Floridia M, Tomino C, et al. Zidovudine plus didanosine plus nevirapine versus zidovudine plus didanosine in antiretroviral-naïve patients with very advanced disease. Abstract 57. Abstracts of the Fifth International Workshop on HIV Drug Resistance, Treatment Streategies and Eradication. St. Petersburg, FL, 1998.

219. Smith MS, Koerber KL, Pagano JS. Long-term persistence of zidovudine resistance mutations in plasma isolates of human immunodeficiency virus type 1 of dideoxyinosine-treated patients removed from zidovudine therapy. J Infect Dis 1994;169:184–188.

220. Wahlbert J, Albert J, Lundeberg J, et al. Dynamic changes in HIV-1 quasispecies from azidothymidine (AZT)–treated patients. Faseb J 1992;6:2843–2847.

221. Husson RN, Shirasaka T, Butler KM, et al. High-level resistance to zidovudine but not to zalcitabine or didanosine in human immunodeficiency virus from children receiving antiretroviral therapy. J Pediatr 1993;123:9–16.

222. Mohri H, Singh MK, Ching WT, Ho DD. Quantitation of zidovudine-resistant human immunodeficiency virus type 1 in the blood of treated and untreated patients. Proc Nat Acad Sci USA 1993;90:25–29.

223. Chow Y-K, Hirsch MS, Merrill DP, et al. Use of evolutionary limitations of HIV-1 multidrug resistance to optimize therapy. Nature 1993;361:650–654.

224. Larder BA, Darby G, Richman DD. HIV with reduced sensitivity to zidovudine (AZT) isolated during prolonged therapy. Science 1989;243:1731–1734.

225. Erice A, Mayers D, Strike L, et al. Primary infection with zidovudine-resistant human immunodeficiency virus type 1. N Engl J Med 1993;328:1163–1193.

226. Richman DD. Susceptibility to nucleoside analogues of zidovudine-resistant isolates of human immunodeficiency virus. Am J Med 1990;88(suppl 5B):8S–10S.

227. Kellam P, Boucher CA, Larder BA. Fifth mutation in human immunodeficiency virus type 1 reverse transcriptase contributes to the development of high-level resistance to zidovudine. Proc Natl Acad Sci USA 1992;89:1934–1938.

228. Richman DD, Guatelli JC, Grimes J, et al. Detection of mutations associated with zidovudine resistance in human immunodeficiency virus utilizing the polymerase chain reaction. J Infect Dis 1991;164:1075–1081.

229. Kohlstaedt LA, Wang J, Friedman JM, et al. Crystal structure at 3.5 *A* resolution of HIV-1 reverse transcriptase complexed with an inhibitor. Science 1992;256:1783–1790.

230. Land S, McGavin K, Birch C, Lucas R. Reversion from zidovudine resistance to sensitivity on cessation of treatment. Lancet 1991;338:830–831.

231. McLeod GX, McGrath JM, Ladd EA, Hammer SM. Didanosine and zidovudine resistance patterns in clinical isolates of human immunodeficiency virus type 1 as determined by a replication endpoint concentration assay. Antimicrob Agents Chemother 1992;36:920–925.

232. Larder BA, Kemp SD. Multiple mutations in HIV-1 reverse transcriptase confer high-level resistance to zidovudine (AZT). Science 1989;246:1155–1158.

233. Smith MS, Koerber KL, Pagano JS. Zidovudine-resistant human immunodeficiency virus type 1 genomes detected in plasma distinct from viral genomes in peripheral blood mononuclear cells. J Infect Dis 1993;167:445–448.

234. Larder BA, Chesebro B, Richman DD. Susceptibilities of zidovudine susceptible and resistant human immunodeficiency virus isolates to antiviral agents determined by using a quantitative plaque reduction assay. Antimicrob Agents Chemother 1990;34:436–441.

235. St Clair MH, Martin JL, Tudor-Williams G, et al. Resistance to ddI and sensitivity to AZT induced by a mutation in HIV-1 reverse transcriptase. Science 1991;253:1557–1559.

236. Shirasaka T, Yorchoan R, O'Brien MC, et al. Changes in drug sensitivity of human immunodeficiency virus type 1 during therapy with halothymidine, dideoxycytidine, and

dideoxyinosine: an in vitro comparative study. Proc Natl Acad Sci USA 1993;90:562–566.

237. Gu Z, Gao Q, Li X, et al. Novel mutation in the human immunodeficiency virus type-1 reverse transcriptase gene that encodes cross-resistance to 2′,3′-dideoxyinosine and 2′,3′-dideoxycytidine. J Virol 1992;66:7128–7135.

238. Fitzgibbon JE, Howell RE, Harberzettl CA, et al. Human immunodeficiency virus type 1 *pol* gene mutations which cause decreased susceptibility to 2′,3′-dideoxycytidine. Antimicrob Agents Chemother 1991;36:153–157.

239. Yarchoan R, Mitsuya H, Myers C, Broder S. Clinical pharmacology of 3′-azido-2′,3′dideoxythymidine (zidovudine) and related dideoxynucleosides. N Engl J Med 1989;321: 726–738.

240. Gao Q, Gu Z, Parniak MA, et al. The same mutation that encodes low-level human immunodeficiency virus type 1 resistance to 2′,3′-dideoxyinosine and 2′,3′-dideoxy-cytidine confers high-level resistance to the (-) enantiomer of 2′,3′-didooxy-3′-thiacytidine. Antimicrob Agents Chemother 1993;37:1390–1392.

241. Mayers D. Rational approaches to resistance: nucleoside analogues. AIDS 1996;10(suppl 1):S9–S13.

242. Tisdale M, Alnadaf T, Cousens D. Combinations of mutations in human immunodeficiency virus-1 reverse transcriptase required for resistance to the carbocyclic nucleoside 1592U89. Antimicrob Agents Chemother 1997; 41:1094–1098.

243. Richman DD. Loss of nevirapine activity associated with the emergence of resistance in clinical trials. [Abstract PoB 3576]. Eighth International Conference on AIDS, The Netherlands, June 1992.

244. Goldman ME, O'Brien JA, Ruffing TL, et al. A nonnucleoside reverse transcriptase inhibitor active on human immunodeficiency virus type 1 isolates resistant to related inhibitors. Antimicrob Agents Chemother 1993;37: 947–949.

245. Patick AK, Duran M, Cao Y, et al. Genotypic analysis of HIV-1 variants isolated from patients treated with protease inhibitor nelfinavir, alone or in combination with d4T or AZT and 3TC. Fourth Conference on Retroviruses and Opportunistic Infections, Washington, DC, 1997.

246. Roberts NA. Drug resistance patterns of saquinavir and other HIV protease inhibitors. AIDS 1995;9(suppl 2): 27–32.

247. Gallavort JE. Strategies for long-term success in the treatment of HIV infection. JAMA 2000;283:1329–1334.

248. Imrie A, Beveridge A, Glenn W, et al. Transmission of HIV type 1 resistance to nevirapine and zidovudine. J Infect Dis 1997:175:1502–1506.

249. Wegner S, Mascola J, Barile A, et al. High frequency of antiretroviral drug resistance in HIV-1 from recently infected therapy-naive individuals. Sixth Conference on Retroviruses and Opportunistic Infections, Chicago, IL, 1999. Abstract #LB9.

250. Erice A, Mayers DL, Strike DG, et al. Brief report: primary infection with zidovudine-resistance HIV type 1. N Engl J Med 1993;328:1163–1165.

251. Hecht FM, Grant RM, Petropoulos CJ, et al. Sexual transmission of an HIV-1 variant resistance to multiple reverse-transcriptase and protease inhibitors. N Engl J Med 1998;339:307–311.

252. Markowitz M, Vesanen M, Tenner-Racz K, et al. The effect of commencing combination antiretroviral therapy soon after HIV type 1 infection on viral replication and antiviral immune responses. J Infect Dis 1999;179:525–537.

253. Schacker T, Ollier AC, Highes J, et al. Clinical and epidemiologic features of primary HIV infection. Ann Intern Med 1996;125:257–264.

Index

MCP-1 (monocyte chemotactic protein-1), 207
M-CSF. *See* Monocyte colony-stimulating factor
Measles-mumps-rubella vaccine (MMR), 415*t*, 417
Measles vaccine, 415*t*, 417
Mediators
in graft-versus-host disease, 505
mast cell-delivered, 150
in specific allergen injection immunotherapy, 353
tumor necrosis factor effects on, 314*t*, 315
Melanoma, malignant
genetically engineered vaccine, 577
human clinical trials, adoptive cellular immunotherapy, 562
interleukin-2 for, 243–244
Membrane cofactor protein (MCP), 289
Memory, DNA-raised, 433
Meningococcus vaccine, 402*t*
Meperidine (Demerol), for acute HAE attacks, 305
6-Mercaptopurine
degradation, 52
mechanism of action, 52
structure, 52
Mesalamine. *See* 5-Aminosalicylic acid
Metchnikoff, Eli, 240
Methotrexate
administration, 71
carcinogenicity, 73
chemical structure, 65, 66
development, 65
discontinuation of, 70–71
dosage, 71
with etanercept, for adult rheumatoid arthritis, 256*f*, 257
hematologic toxicity, 72
mechanisms of action, 65–68
monitoring, 75
pharmacology, 68–69
for rheumatoid arthritis, 66–68
teratogenicity, 72–73
therapeutic indications, 69–71, 75
toxicity, 72–75
vs. etanercept, for psoriatic arthritis, 260
Methotrexate polyglutamates, 66
Methyltestosterone, for hereditary angioedema, 304
MHC. *See* Major histocompatibility complex
Micopolyspora faeni lung inflammation, TNFR:Fc efficacy in, 253, 254
Microemulsion cyclosporine (Neoral), 479

Minor histocompatibility antigens, 559–560
Mixed hematopoietic cell chimerism, 542
MMF. *See* Mycophenolate mofetil
MMR (measles-mumps-rubella vaccine), 415*t*, 417
Molecular chimerism, 542–543
Molecular immunology, historical aspects, 242–243
Moloney murine leukemia virus (MoMLV), as gene-transfer system, 582, 583*f*
Monoclonal antibodies (mAbs), 4. *See also specific monoclonal antibodies*
anti-IgE. *See* Anti-IgE antibody
anti-T-cell, species specificity, 332
CD3. *See* CD3 antibody
chimeric humanized, 327, 328*f*
IL-2 receptor as target for, 327–329
for renal allograft recipients, 328–329
historical aspects, 241–242
with interleukin-2, 247
rodent antihuman
advantages of, 327
therapeutic response, 327
Monocyte chemotactic protein-1 (MCP-1), 207
Monocyte colony-stimulating factor (M-CSF)
biological activity, 180*t*
indications, 180*t*
for neutrophil recovery, after bone marrow transplantation, 184
for osteopetrosis, 189
Monocyte/macrophage, 8
Monomethylfumarate, 206*t*
Mononuclear phagocyte system, 3
Montelukast (Singulair), 133
for chronic persistent asthma, 135
for exercise-induced asthma, 133–134
with inhaled corticosteroids, for asthma, 136
side effects, 136–137
MR1 antibody (anti-CD40L), 442, 445
for human immune disease, 450–451, 450*t*
in vivo effects, 446–450, 446*t*, 447*t*
Mucociliary clearance, theophylline stimulation of, 140
Multiple myeloma
IVIG for, 271
plasma cell CD28 expression, 384–385
plasmapheresis, 603–604
Multiple sclerosis
cyclophosphamide for, 44
interferon therapy for, 234

IVIG for, 278
murine model, 447*t*, 448
plasmapheresis, 603
Mumps vaccine, 415*t*, 417
Mx protein, 227
Myasthenia gravis, treatment, 278, 603
Mycobacterium avium infection susceptibility, 231–233
Mycobacterium chelonei infection susceptibility, 231–233
Mycobacterium fortuitum infection susceptibility, 231–233
Mycobacterium tuberculosis, 407
Mycophenolate mofetil (MMF)
adverse effects, 58–59
history, 57
for immunosuppression, 462*t*, 463, 478–479
indications, 58
asthma, 360, 360*f*
rheumatoid arthritis, 58
transplantation, 58
mechanism of action, 57–58
pharmacology, 57–58
structure, 57
Myelodysplasia
hematopoietic growth factors for, 185
with monosomy 7, 191
Myelodysplastic syndromes, stem cell transplantation for, 502
Myeloid leukemia
acute, 191, 501
interferon therapy for, 233–234
stem cell transplantation for, 501–502
Myoblast transplantation, 521
Myocyte transplantation, 521
Myopathy, glucocorticoid-induced, 111

N

Naproxen, 125
Natural antibodies, preformed, hyperacute rejection of xenotransplant and, 537–539, 539*t*
Natural killer cells (NK)
in cellular immune response, 550, 551
historical aspects, 241
interferon-γ biosynthesis, 221
interleukin-10 and, 209
Negative selection (central tolerance), 7, 8, 9, 10
Neoral (microemulsion cyclosporine), 479
Neupogen, for cyclophosphamide therapy, 39
Neural tissue transplantation, 522